Dictionary of Psychology and Psychiatry
Wörterbuch der Psychologie und Psychiatrie

Dictionary of Psychology and Psychiatry

Volume 1 English–German

2nd, completely revised and expanded edition

Wörterbuch der Psychologie und Psychiatrie

Band 1 Englisch–Deutsch

2., vollständig überarbeitete und erweiterte Auflage

Roland Haas, Dipl. Psych.

HOGREFE

Library of Congress Cataloging-in-Publication Data

is now available via the Library of Congress Marc Database under the

LC Control Number: 2002111975

National Library of Canada Cataloguing in Publication

Haas, Roland
Dictionary of psychology and psychiatry: English–German = Wörterbuch der Psychologie und Psychiatrie : Englisch–Deutsch / Roland Haas. — 2nd completely rev. and expanded ed.

Includes bibliographical references.
Contents: v. 1. English-German / Englisch-Deutsch. — v. 2.
German-English / Deutsch-Englisch.
ISBN 978-0-88937-302-0 (hardcover set).— ISBN 978-0-88937-300-6 (v. 1).—
ISBN 978-0-88937-301-3 (v. 2)

ISBN 978-0-88937-450-8 (softcover set)

1. Psychology–Dictionaries. 2. Psychology–Dictionaries–German.
3. Psychiatry–Dictionaries. 4. Psychiatry–Dictionaries–German.
5. English language–Dictionaries–German. 6. German language–Dictionaries–English.
I. Title. II. Title: Wörterbuch der Psychologie und Psychiatrie.

BF31.H22 2003 150'.3'31 C2003-903285-X

PUBLISHING OFFICES
USA: Hogrefe Publishing, 875 Massachusetts Avenue, 7th Floor, Cambridge, MA 02139
Phone (866) 823-4726, Fax (617) 354-6875, E-mail customerservice@hogrefe-publishing.com
Europe: Hogrefe Publishing, Merkelstr. 3, D-37085 Göttingen, Germany
Phone +49 551 99950-0, Fax +49 551 99950-425, E-mail publishing@hogrefe.com

SALES & DISTRIBUTION
USA: Hogrefe Publishing, Customer Services Department, 30 Amberwood Parkway, Ashland, OH 44805
Phone (800) 228-3749, Fax (419) 281-6883, E-mail customerservice@hogrefe.com
Europe: Hogrefe Publishing, Merkelstr. 3, D-37085 Göttingen, Germany
Phone +49 551 99950-0, Fax +49 551 99950-425, E-mail publishing@hogrefe.com

OTHER OFFICES
Canada: Hogrefe Publishing, 660 Eglinton Ave. East, Suite 119 - 514, Toronto, Ontario M4G 2K2
Switzerland: Hogrefe Publishing, Länggass-Strasse 76, CH-3000 Bern 9

Hogrefe Publishing
Incorporated and registered in the Commonwealth of Massachusetts, USA, and in Göttingen, Lower Saxony, Germany

Printed and bound in Germany
ISBN 978-0-88937-450-8

Contents

Preface vi
Explanatory Notes viii
Bibliography x
English-German Dictionary 1
List of Abbreviations 527

Inhalt

Vorwort vii
Benutzerhinweise ix
Bibliographie x
Englisch-Deutsches Wörterverzeichnis 1
Abkürzungsverzeichnis 527

Preface

In this new edition, the *Dictionary of Psychology and Psychiatry* has been fully revised and updated, and substantially expanded by the addition of new entries. For instance, all the terms and vocabulary from the field of psychiatry have been carefully reviewed and brought up to date by inclusion of the terminology used in DSM–IV and ICD–10, as well as numerous other entries from this evolving subject area. The increasing standardization of scientific terminology in the field of psychiatry has thus been taken account of in the new edition.

Overall, around 4,000 terms from the fields of psychology and psychiatry have been added. In addition to numerous words and terms from psychology and psychiatry in general that have been added, particular importance was also placed on including new terminology from the areas of cognitive neuroscience, biological psychology, personality psychology, methodology, and computer–based assessment, as well, of course, as relevant terms from fields such as computing and the Internet. At the same time, corrections and changes of usage since the previous edition have been included, and some terms that have in the meanwhile become obsolete have been removed. The new German spelling and orthography is used throughout.

The author and publisher trust that, like the first edition, this new revised edition of the Dictionary will meet the expectations and needs of its users and readers from both science and practice.

Finally, I would like to extend my thanks to the numerous helpful readers who have provided valuable ideas and suggestions for the new edition. Particular thanks go to Lisa Bennett, Karen Fries, Kathrin Rothauge, Nadine Schuchart, and Robert Dimbleby of the Hogrefe publishing group, who have supported the work on this 2nd edition of the Dictionary, and whose helpful suggestions and constructive criticism contributed to the successful completion of this work.

Neuhäusel, October 2003 **Roland Haas**

Vorwort

Mit der vorliegenden Neuauflage wurde das Wörterbuch vollständig überarbeitet und durch viele Neueinträge stark erweitert. So wurde vor allem der gesamte Wortschatz der Psychiatrie überarbeitet und durch die Einbeziehung der Nomenklaturen aus ICD–10 und DSM–IV auf den neuesten Stand gebracht. Der fortschreitenden Vereinheitlichung der wissenschaftlichen Terminologie in der Psychiatrie wird damit Rechnung getragen. Darüber hinaus wurde eine Vielzahl neuer Begriffe aus diesem Wissenschaftsgebiet berücksichtigt.

Insgesamt etwa 4.000 Begriffe aus Psychologie und Psychiatrie wurden in die 2. Auflage des Wörterbuches neu aufgenommen. Neben vielen Allgemeinbegriffen der Psychologie wurde dabei insbesondere die neuere Terminologie aus den Bereichen kognitive Neurowissenschaften, biologische Psychologie, Persönlichkeitspsychologie, psychologische Methodenlehre und computerunterstützte Diagnostik sowie die für Psychologen und Psychiater relevanten Begriffe aus dem Internet berücksichtigt. Dagegen wurden einige Korrekturen vorgenommen und obsolet gewordene Begriffe aus dem Wörterbuch entfernt. Auch die neue deutsche Rechtschreibung wurde eingearbeitet.

Damit wird hoffentlich auch die 2. Auflage des Wörterbuches den Anforderungen von Wissenschaft und Praxis in vollem Umfang gerecht werden.

Für wertvolle Anregungen und Beiträge zu dieser Neuauflage möchte sich der Autor bei den vielen fachkundigen Benutzern herzlich bedanken. Ein besonderer Dank geht an Frau Lisa Bennett, Frau Karen Fries, Frau Kathrin Rothauge, Frau Nadine Schuchart und Herrn Robert Dimbleby vom Verlag Hogrefe, die mit unermüdlichem Einsatz die 2. Auflage dieses Wörterbuches kritisch begleitet und durch viele Anregungen zum Gelingen des Werkes beigetragen haben.

Neuhäusel, im Oktober 2003 **Roland Haas**

Explanatory Notes

1. All items are arranged alphabetically. Current abbreviations are recorded in a separate list in the appendix of this dictionary. Compound entries can be found under the first noun of the term.

e.g.	**Abhängigkeit des Ichs**
see	**Abhängigkeit**
but	**psychologisches Profil**
see	**Profil, psychologisches**

2. Besides British, also the American spellings have been recorded in most cases, e. g.

   behaviour, behavior
   colour, color
   centre, center
   etc.

   However, the following word endings have not been recorded separately: **–ise**, **–ize** and **–isation**, **–ization**.

3. The following abbreviations and signs are used in this dictionary:

   m = male
   f = female
   n = neutral
   pl = plural
   ~ = repetition of main entry
   – = hyphen
   - = word break
   ’ = apostrophe
   / = new entry
   ( ) = parentheses
   | = marks part of entry repeated

4. Some words appearing in this dictionary are simultaneously proprietary names or registered trademarks. The lack of designation of this fact does not, however, indicate that a term is not a proprietary name or registered trademark.

Benutzerhinweise

1. Alle Begriffe sind in alphabetischer Reihenfolge geordnet. Gebräuchliche Abkürzungen sind in einem separaten Abkürzungsverzeichnis als Anhang diesem Wörterbuch beigefügt. Zusammengesetzte Begriffe sind grundsätzlich unter dem ersten Substantiv des Begriffes zu suchen, also

z.B.	**Abhängigkeit des Ichs**
siehe unter	**Abhängigkeit**
aber	**psychologisches Profil**
siehe unter	**Profil, psychologisches**

2. Es werden neben den britischen meistens auch amerikanische Varianten der Schreibweise aufgeführt, also z. B.

   behaviour, behavior
   colour, color
   centre, center
   etc.

   Nicht separat aufgeführt wurden Varianten in der Schreibweise von Wortendungen, wie **–ise**, **–ize** and **–isation**, **–ization**.

3. Folgende Abkürzungen und Zeichen werden benutzt:

   m = männlich
   f = weiblich
   n = sächlich
   pl = Plural
   ~ = Wiederholung des Hauptbegriffs
   – = Bindestrich
   - = Worttrennung
   ’ = Apostroph
   / = neuer Begriff
   ( ) = Klammern
   | = bezeichnet den zu wiederholenden Teil des Begriffes

4. Einige der in diesem Wörterbuch aufgenommen Begriffe sind zugleich eingetragene Warenzeichen. Das Fehlen eines entsprechenden Hinweises bedeutet jedoch nicht, dass es sich im Einzelfall um einen freien Warennamen handelt.

Bibliography / Bibliographie

American Psychiatric Association. (2000). *Diagnostic and Statistical Manual of Mental Disorders* (4th ed., Text Revision). Washington, DC: Author.

Batinic, B. (Ed.). (1999). *Internet für Psychologen* (2. Aufl.). Göttingen: Hogrefe.

Beigel, H. G. (1971). *Dictionary of psychology and related fields. German–English.* New York: Ungar.

Berger, A. H. (1977). *Dictionary of psychology. English–German.* New York: Ungar.

Birnbaumer, N., & Schmidt, R. F. (1999). *Biologische Psychologie* (4th ed.). Berlin: Springer–Verlag.

Boer–Hoff, L. E. (1977). *Engels–Nederlands psychologisch woordenboek.* Deventer: Van Loghum Slaterus.

Bunjes, W. E. (1974). *Medical and pharmaceutical dictionary. English–German* (3rd ed.). Stuttgart: Thieme.

Burkhardt, D. (1971). *Wörterbuch der Neurophysiologie* (2. Aufl.). Jena: Fischer.

Castonguay, J. (1973). *Dictionary of psychology and related sciences: English–French. Dictionnaire de la psychologie et des sciences connexes: Français–Anglais.* Quebec: Edisem.

Dilling, H., Mombour, W., & Schmidt, M. H. (Ed.). (1999). *Internationale Klassifikation psychischer Störungen.* Bern: Huber.

Drever, J., & Fröhlich, W. D. (1975). *Wörterbuch zur Psychologie* (9. Aufl.). München: Deutscher Taschenbuch Verlag.

Duijker, H. C. J., & Van Rijswijk, M. J. (1975). *Trilingual psychological dictionary.* Bern: Huber.

Edgerton, J. E., & Campbell III, R. J. (Ed.). 1994. *American psychiatric glossary* (7th ed.). Washington DC: American Psychiatric Press.

English, H. B., & English, A. C. (1974). *A comprehensive dictionary of psychological and psychoanalytical terms* (2nd ed.). London: Longmans.

Frances, A., First, M. B., & Pincus, H. A. (1995). *DSM–IV Guidebook.* Washington DC: American Psychiatric Press.

Gove, P. B. (Ed.). 1971. *Webster's third new international dictionary.* Chicago: Merriam.

Höcker, H., Stapf, K. H., & Kurt, H. (Eds.). (1998). *Dorsch Psychologisches Wörterbuch* (13. überarb. und erw. Aufl). Bern: Verlag Hans Huber.

Kendall, M. G., & Buckland, W. R. (1971). *A dictionary of statistical terms* (3. Aufl.). London: Longman Group.

Laplanche, J., & Pontalis, J. B. (1973). *Das Vokabular der Psychoanalyse.* Frankfurt a. M.: Suhrkamp.

Lejeune, F., & Bunjes, W. E. (1968). *Wörterbuch für Ärzte. Deutsch–Englisch.* Stuttgart: Thieme.

Linnert, P., Müller–Seydlitz, U., & Neske, F. (1972). *Lexikon angloamerikanischer und deutscher Managementbegriffe*. Gernsbach: Deutscher Betriebswirte–Verlag.

Moor, L. (1969). *Lexique Français–Anglais–Allemand des termes usuels en psychiatrie, neuropsychiatrie infantile et psychologie pathologique* (2nd ed.). Paris: Expansion.

Oppermann, A. (1969). *Wörterbuch Kybernetik. Deutsch–Englisch / Englisch–Deutsch*. München–Pullach: Verlag für Dokumentation.

Paetzel, H. W. (1972). *Praktisches Wörterbuch für Presse und Werbung. Deutsch–Englisch–Französisch*. Essen: Stamm–Verlag.

Peters, U. H. (1999). *Wörterbuch der Psychiatrie, Psychotherapie und medizinischen Psychologie* (5. Aufl.). München–Wien: Urban & Schwarzenberg.

Reuter, P., & Reuter, C. (1995). *Thieme Leximed — Medical Dictionary. English–German*. Stuttgart: Thieme.

Reuter, P., & Reuter, C. (1999). *Thieme Leximed — Medizinisches Wörterbuch. Deutsch–Englisch*. Stuttgart: Thieme.

Roche Lexikon Medizin (4. Aufl.). (1998). München: Urban & Schwarzenberg.

Sass, H., Wittchen, H–U., Zaudig, M., & Houben, I. (Ed.). (1998). *Diagnostische Kriterien DSM–IV*. Göttingen: Hogrefe.

Terrell, P., Schnorr, V., Morris, W. V. A., & Breitsprecher, R. (1999). *Pons Collins Großwörterbuch für Experten und Universität. Deutsch–Englisch / Englisch–Deutsch* (4. Aufl.). Stuttgart: Ernst Klett Verlag.

Theodorson, G. A., & Theodorson, A. G. (1969). *A modern dictionary of sociology*. New York: Crowell.

World Health Organization. (1992). *The ICD–10 classification of mental and behavioural disorders*. Geneva: WHO.

Wildhagen, K., & Heraucourt, W. (1973). *Englisch–Deutsches / Deutsch–Englisches Wörterbuch* (12. Aufl.). Wiesbaden: Brandstetter.

Wolman, B. B. (1988). *Dictionary of behavioral science* (2nd ed.). San Diego: Academic Press.

Zeier, H. (1976). *Wörterbuch der Lerntheorien und der Verhaltenstherapie*. München: Kindler.

Zentralstelle für psychologische Information und Dokumentation. (Ed.). (1997). *PSYNDEX Terms* (5th ed.). Trier: ZPID.

Zetkin, M., & Schaldach, H. (Ed.). (1974). *Wörterbuch der Medizin* (5. Aufl.) Stuttgart: Thieme.

A

abac Kurvendiagramm *n*, Kurvenblatt *n*

abaca Manilahanf *m*

abacus Rechenbrett *n*, Rechenmaschine *f* mit Kugeln

abandon Ungezwungenheit *f*, Ausgelassenheit *f*, Hemmungslosigkeit *f*

abandonment Vernachlässigung *f*, Verlassenheit *f*, Hingabe *f*, Überlassen *n* / **~ complex** Verlassenheitskomplex *m*

abarognosis Verlust *m* des Gewichtssinnes

abasement Erniedrigung *f*, Demütigung *f* / **~ need** Selbsterniedrigungstrieb *m* / **repressed ~** verdrängte Demütigung *f*

abasia Gehstörung *f*, Abasie *f* / **ataxic ~** Ataxie *f* / **choreic ~** spastische Gehstörung *f* / **paralytic ~** paralytische Gehstörung *f*

abasic gehgestört

abaxial nicht in der Achse liegend, abaxial

ABBA order Reihenfolge A–B–B–A *f*

abdomen Bauch *m*, Abdomen *m*

abdominal abdominal, Unterleibs–, Bauch–, Abdominal–

abducens Nervus abducens *m*, sechster Gehirnnerv *m* / **~ nerve** Nervus abducens *m*

abduction Abduktion *f*, Wegbewegung *f* von der Mittellinie, Auswärtsbewegung *f*

Abel complex Abel–Komplex *m*

aberrant abweichend, abartig

aberration Aberration *f*, Abweichung *f*, Abirrung *f*, Geistesverwirrung *f*, Brechungsabweichung *f* / **~ of light** Lichtbrechung *f* / **chromatic ~** chromatische Aberration *f* / **chromosomal ~** Chromosomenaberration *f* / **dioptric ~** sphärische Aberration *f* / **mental ~** Geisteskrankheit *f*, Geistesstörung *f*, geistige Umnachtung *f*, Irrsinn *m*, Wahnsinn *m* / **sexual ~** Perversität *f*, geschlechtliche Abartigkeit *f* / **spherical ~** sphärische Aberration *f*

abience, abiency Vermeidung *f*, Rückzug *m*

abient Vermeidungs–

ability Fähigkeit *f*, Eignung *f*, Begabung *f*, Leistungsvermögen *n* / **~ to adapt** Anpassungsfahigkeit *f*, Gewöhnungsfähigkeit *f* / **~ to concentrate** Konzentrationsfähigkeit *f* / **~ to dissociate** Dissoziationsvermögen *n* / **~ grouping** Einstufung *f* nach Fähigkeit, Fähigkeitsgruppierung *f* / **~ level** Leistungsniveau *n*, Eignungsniveau *n* / **~ to repress** Verordnungsfähigkeit *f* / **~ test** Eignungstest *m*, Fähigkeitstest *m* / **~ to think** Denkfähigkeit *f* / **apperceptual ~** Apperzeptionsfähigkeit *f* / **arithmetic ~** Rechenfähigkeit *f* / **artistic ~** künstlerische Begabung *f*, künstlerische Fähigkeit *f* / **basic ~** Grundfähigkeit *f* / **cognitive ~** kognitive Fähigkeit *f*, Denkvermögen *n* / **crystallized ~** kristallisierte Fähigkeit *f*, kristallisierte Begabung *f* / **differential ~ test** differentieller Eignungstest *m* / **discerning ~** Einsichtsfähigkeit *f* / **final ~** Endfähigkeit *f* / **fluid ~** flexible, veränderliche Fähigkeit *f* / **general ~** Allgemeinbegabung *f* / **initial ~** Anfangsfähigkeit *f* / **intellectual ~** geistige Fähigkeit *f*, Begabung *f* / **manual ~** handwerkliche Begabung *f* / **mathematical ~** mathematische Begabung *f* / **mechanical ~** technische Begabung *f*, mathematische Fähigkeit *f* / **mental ~** psychisches Leistungsvermögen *n*, geistige Fähigkeit *f* / **musical ~** musikalische Begabung *f*, musikalische Fähigkeit *f* / **nonverbal ~** nichtsprachliche Fähigkeit *f* / **numerical ~** Rechenfähigkeit *f*, Rechengewandtheit *f* / **occu-**

pational ~ Berufseignung *f* / **prehensil ~** Greiffähigkeit *f* / **primary ~** Primärfähigkeit *f* / **primary mental ~** primäre geistige Fähigkeit *f*, Intelligenzfaktor *m* / **reflective ~** Besinnungsfähigkeit *f* / **spatial ~** räumliches Vorstellungsvermögen *n*, Raumvorstellungsvermögen *n* / **special ~** Sonderbegabung *f*, Spezialbegabung *f*, spezielles Talent *n* / **specific ~** besondere Fähigkeit *f*, Begabung *f* / **verbal ~** sprachliche Fähigkeit *f*, Sprachbeherrschung *f* / **visual ~** Sehvermögen *n* / **visuospatial ~** visuell–räumliche Fähigkeit *f* / **vocational ~** Berufseignung *f*

abiogenesis Urzeugung *f*, Abiogenese *f*

abiotrophy, abiotrophia Vitalitätsverlust *m*, Nachlassen *n* der Lebenskraft, Abiotrophie *f*

abirritant beruhigend, Erregung herabsetzend / Beruhigungsmittel *n*

abirritation Verminderung *f* der Erregung, Herabsetzung *f* der Erregung

abjection Erniedrigung *f*, Verworfenheit *f*

ablation Amputation *f*, Entfernung *f*, Wegnahme *f* / **~ experiments** Versuche *mpl* mit Gehirnabtragung, Ablationsexperiment *n*

ablutomania Ablutomanie *f*, Waschzwang *m*, Waschmanie *f*

abmodality Typabweichung *f*, Abweichung *f* vom Modalwert

abnormal abnorm, abartig, krankhaft, pathologisch, anomal

abnormality, abnormity Anomalie *f*, Abweichung *f* von der Norm, Missbildung *f*, Unregelmäßigkeit *f*, Störung *f* / **~ in behavior** Verhaltensauffälligkeit *f* / **~ of growth** Wachstumsanomalie *f* / **~ of volition** Willensschwäche *f*, Abulie *f* / **sexual ~** sexuelle Abartigkeit *f*, Perversität *f*

aboral vom Mund weg, mundfern

aboriginal eingeboren, einheimisch / Ureinwohner *m*, Eingeborener *m*

abortion Fehlgeburt *f*, Abort *m*, Abtreibung *f*, Schwangerschaftsunterbrechung *f* / **~ law** Gesetz *n* über die Schwangerschaftsunterbrechung, Abtreibungsgesetz *n* / **~ psychosis** Abortpsychose *f* / **elective ~** freiwillige Abtreibung *f* / **induced ~** Schwangerschaftsabbruch *m*, künstlicher Abort *m*, Abtreibung *f* / **spontaneous ~** Fehlgeburt *f* / **therapeutic ~** medizinisch indizierter Abort *m*

aboulia Willenlosigkeit *f*, Willensschwäche *f*, Entschlusslosigkeit *f*, Abulie *f*

abreact abreagieren

abreaction Abreaktion *f*, Abreagieren *n*, Ableitung *f*, Katharsis *f*

abscess Abszess *m*, Eiterung *f*, Geschwür *n* / **cerebellar ~** Kleinhirnabszess *m* / **cerebral ~** Hirnabszess *m*, Gehirnabszess *m*

abscissa Abszisse *f*, X–Achse *f*, X–Koordinate *f*

abscission natürliche Trennung *f* von Interaktionssystemen

absence Abwesenheit *f*, Fehlen *n*, kurzzeitiger Bewusstseinsausfall *m* bei Epilepsie, Absence *f* / **~ of appetite** Appetitmangel *m*, Anorexie *f* / **~ of ejaculation** fehlender Samenerguss *m* / **~ of mind** Geistesabwesenheit *f*, Gedankenlosigkeit *f*, Zerstreutheit *f* / **~ of orgasm** Ausbleiben n des Orgasmus, Anorgasmie *f* / **~ of reaction** Reaktionsausfall *m* / **~ of response** Reaktionsausfall *m* / **~ of sensibility to pain** Schmerzunempfindlichkeit *f* / **~ seizure** Absence *f*, Petit mal *m* / **~ status** Petit–mal–Status *m* / **myoclonic ~** myoklonisches Petit mal *n*, Petit mal impulsif *n* / **parental ~** Fehlen *n* der Eltern

absenteeism Arbeitsversäumnis *n*, Fernbleiben *n* von der Arbeit, Abwesenheit *f*

absentminded geistesabwesend, zerstreut, gedankenlos

absentmindedness Geistesabwesenheit *f*, Zerstreutheit *f*, Gedankenlosigkeit *f*

absinthism Absinthvergiftung *f*, Absinthismus *m*

absolute absolut

absolutism Absolutismus *m*, unumschränkte Herrschaft *f*

absorb absorbieren, resorbieren, aufnehmen

absorbed zerstreut, vertieft, versunken, beschäftigt, absorbiert, resorbiert

absorption Vertieftsein *n*, Beschäftigtsein *n*, Versunkensein *n*, Aufnahme *f*, Absorption *f*, Resorption *f* / ~ **line** Absorptionslinie *f*, Absorptionskurve *f* / ~ **of light** Lichtabsorption *f* / ~ **spectrum** Absorptionsspektrum *n* / **physiological** ~ Resorption *f*

abstinence Enthaltsamkeit *f*, Abstinenz *f* / ~ **delirium** Entzugsdelir *n* / ~ **symptom** Entziehungssymptom *n*, Abstinenzsymptom *n* / **sexual** ~ sexuelle Enthaltsamkeit *f*, freiwillige Keuschheit *f*

abstinent abstinent, enthaltsam

abstract abstrakt, theoretisch / abstrahieren, gesondert betrachten

abstraction Abstraktion *f*, abstraktes Denken *n* / ~ **factor** Abstraktionsfaktor *m*, Faktor *m* des abstrakten Denkens

absurd sinnlos, absurd

absurdity Absurdität *f*, Sinnlosigkeit *f* / ~ **test** Absurditätentest *m*

abulia Willensschwäche *f*, Willenlosigkeit *f*, Entschlusslosigkeit *f*, Abulie *f*

abulic willenlos, willensschwach, entschlusslos

abulomania totaler Willensverlust *m*

abuse Missbrauch *m*, Abusus *m* / ~ **liability** Abhängigkeitspotenzial *n*, Suchtpotenzial *n* / ~ **of alcohol** Alkoholmissbrauch *m* / ~ **of morphia** Morphiumsucht *f* / ~ **of narcotics** Rauschgiftsucht *f* / ~ **of non–dependence–producing substances** Missbrauch *m* von Substanzen, die keine Abhängigkeit erzeugen / ~ **of power** Machtmissbrauch *m* / ~ **of tobacco** Nikotinsucht *f*, Tabakabusus *m* / ~ **reporting** Missbrauchsanzeige *f* / **emotional** ~ psychische Misshandlung *f* / **physical** ~ **of a child (of a adult)** körperliche Misshandlung *f* eines Kindes (eines Erwachsenen) / **sexual** ~ sexueller Missbrauch *m*, sexuelle Gewalt *f* / **sexual** ~ **of a child (of a adult)** sexueller Missbrauch *m* eines Kindes (eines Erwachsenen)

academic akademisch, Hochschul–, schulisch, philosophisch, theoretisch

acalculia Rechenstörung *f*, Akalkulie *f*, Rechenunvermögen *n*

acarophobia Krätzeangst *f*, Akarophobie *f*

acatalepsia, acatalepsy Akatalepsie *f*, Unfähigkeit *f* zu begreifen, Geistesschwäche *f*

acataleptic geistesschwach, begriffsschwach

acatamathesia Unfähigkeit *f* Sprache zu verstehen, Akatamathesie *f*, sensorische Aphasie *f*

acataphasia Akataphasie *f*, Agrammatismus *m*, Verlust *m* der sprachlichen Ausdrucksfähigkeit, sprachliche Entgleisung *f* infolge von Hirnstörungen

acathexis fehlende Kathexis *f*, mangelnde Libidobesetzung *f*

acathisia Akathisie *f*, Unfähigkeit *f* zum ruhigen Sitzenbleiben, hysterischer Bewegungsdrang *m*

accelerate beschleunigen / Hochbegabter *m*, Klassenspringer *m* / **developmental** ~ Schnellentwickler *m*

acceleration Beschleunigung *f*, Akzeleration *f* / ~ **effect** Beschleunigungswirkung *f*, Beschleunigungseffekt *m* / ~ **sensor** Beschleunigungssensor *m* / **angular** ~ Drehbeschleunigung *f* / **bodily** ~ körperliche Akzeleration *f* / **developmental** ~ Entwicklungsbeschleunigung *f* / **educational** ~ Überspringen *n* von Schulklassen / **gravitational** ~ Gravitationsbeschleunigung *f* / **negative** ~ negative Beschleunigung *f*, Verzögerung *f* / **positive** ~ positive Beschleunigung *f* / **retarded** ~ Verzögerung *f*, negative Beschleunigung *f* / **rotational** ~ Drehbeschleunigung *f* / **scholastic** ~ Überspringen *n* von Schulklassen / **translational** ~ Translationsbeschleunigung *f*

accelerometer Beschleunigungsmesser *m*

accent Akzent *m*, Betonung *f* / **subjective** ~ subjektiver Rhythmus *m*

accept annehmen, entgegennehmen, akzeptieren

acceptability Annehmbarkeit *f*

acceptance Annahme *f*, Akzeptierung *f* / ~ **boundary** Akzeptanzgrenze *f* / ~ **of life** Lebensbejahung *f* / ~ **need** Bedürfnis *n* akzeptiert zu werden / ~ **remark** Bestätigung *f* einer Aussage in der Psychotherapie / ~ **therapy** kathartische Psychotherapie *f* / **social** ~ soziale Akzeptanz *f*, soziale Akzeptierung *f*

access, lexical lexikalischer Zugang *m*

accessibility Ansprechbarkeit *f*, Erreichbarkeit *f*, Zugänglichkeit *f*

accessible zugänglich, ansprechbar, erreichbar

accessory zusätzlich, akzessorisch, Neben–, untergeordnet

accident Unfall *m*, Zufall *m* / ~ **neurosis** Unfallneurose *f*, traumatische Neurose *f*, posttraumatische Neurose *f* / ~ **prevention** Unfallverhütung *f* / **~–prone** unfallgeneigt / ~ **proneness** Unfallneigung *f*, Unfalltendenz *f*, Unfallanfälligkeit *f* / **~–prone person** Unfäller *m* / **cerebrovascular** ~ Schlaganfall *m*, Apoplexie *f* / **industrial** ~ Betriebsunfall *m*, Arbeitsunfall *m* / **occupational** ~ Arbeitsunfall *m*, Berufsunfall *m* / **on–duty** ~ Betriebsunfall *m*, Arbeitsunfall *m* / **pedestrian** ~ Fußgängerunfall *m*

accidental zufällig, Zufalls–, Unfall–

acclimate, acclimatize akklimatisieren, eingewöhnen

acclimation, acclimatisation Anpassung *f*, Gewöhnung *f*, Akklimatisation *f* / ~ **to high altitude** Höhenakklimatisation *f* / **thermal** ~ Wärmeanpassung *f*, Wärmeakklimatisierung *f*

accomodate anpassen, akkommodieren

accommodating entgegenkommend, gefällig, behilflich

accommodation Anpassung *f*, Akkommodation *f* / ~ **constant** Akkommodationskonstante *f* / ~ **difficulty** Akkommodationsstörung *f* / ~ **dream** Annehmlichkeitstraum *m* / ~ **to light and darkness** Hell–Dunkel–Adaptation *f* / ~ **mechanism** Akkommodationsmechanismus *m* / ~ **time** Akkommodationszeit *f* / **absolute** ~ getrennte Augenakkommodation *f* / **binocular** ~ beidäugige Akkommodation *f* / **consensual** ~ übereinstimmende Akkommodation *f* beider Augen / **ocular** ~ okulare Akkommodation *f* / **pupillary** ~ Pupillenreflex *m* / **social** ~ soziale Anpassung *f*

accomplishment Leistung *f*, Fertigkeit *f* / ~ **quotient** Leistungsquotient *m* / ~ **test** Leistungstest *m*

account Kunde *m*, Etatkunde *m* einer Werbeagentur, Zugangsberechtigung *f* zu einem Rechner / ~ **executive** Kontakter *m*, Sachbearbeiter *m* eines Werbeetats / ~ **supervisor** Kontakter *m*

accountability Verantwortung *f*, Verantwortlichkeit *f*

accredition berufliche Zulassung *f*

accretion Zunahme *f*, Wachstum *n* / ~ **learning** Lernzuwachs *m* durch Aneignung beziehungsloser Einzelfakten

acculturation Akkulturation *f*, Kulturaneignung *f*, Hineinwachsen *n* in eine Kultur / ~ **problem** kulturelles Anpassungsproblem *n*, Angleichung *f* an eine fremde Kultur

accumulation Anhäufung *f*, Ansammlung *f*, Häufung *f*, Akkumulation *f*, Kumulation *f*

accuracy Genauigkeit *f*, Richtigkeit *f*, Sorgfalt *f* / ~ **compulsion** Pedanterie *f*, Zwang *m* zur Genauigkeit / ~ **score** Zahl *f* der richtigen Antworten, Genauigkeitswert *m* / ~ **test** Genauigkeitstest *m*, Präzisionstest *m* / **clerical** ~ Genauigkeit *f* bei Büroarbeiten, Arbeitssorgfalt *f* bei Büroarbeiten / **predictive** ~ Vorhersagegenauigkeit *f*

accurate genau, sorgfältig, richtig, fehlerfrei

accurateness Fehlerfreiheit *f*, Genauigkeit *f*

accustom gewöhnen, angewöhnen

acedia Apathie *f*, geistige Stumpfheit *f*, Azedie *f*

acenaesthesia, acenesthesia Gefühl *n* der Unwirklichkeit des Körpers

acetaldehyde Azetaldehyd *n*

acetazolamide Azetazolamid *n*

acetylcholine Azetylcholin *n*

acetylcholinesterase Azetylcholinesterase *f*

ache anhaltender Schmerz *m*

acheiria Acheirie *f*, angeborenes Fehlen *n* beider Hände

achieved erreicht, erzielt

achievement Leistung *f*, Fertigkeit *f* / ~ **age** Leistungsalter *n* / ~ **anxiety** Leistungsangst *f* / ~ **battery** Testbatterie *f* mit Leistungstests / ~ **curve** Leistungskurve *f* / ~ **drive** Leistungsmotiv *n* / ~ **measure** Leistungsmaß *n*, Leistungsmessung *f*, Leistungstest *m* / ~ **motivation** Leistungsmotivation *f* / ~ **motive** Leistungsmotiv *n*, Leistungsmotivation *f* / ~ **need** Leistungsbedürfnis *n* / ~ **pleasure** Erfolgslust *f*, Lust *f* an der eigenen Leistung / ~ **potential** Leistungspotential *n* / ~ **quotient** Leistungsquotient *m* / ~ **striving** Streben *n* nach Leistung / ~ **testing** Leistungsmessung *f* / ~ **want** Leistungsmotiv *n* / **academic** ~ Schulleistung *f* / **academic** ~ **motivation** Schulleistungsmotivation *f* / **academic** ~ **prediction** Vorhersage *f* der Schulleistung, Schulleistungsprognose *f* / **scholastic** ~ Schulleistung *f* / **test** ~ Leistungstest *m*

Achilles| jerk Achillessehnenreflex *m* / ~ **tendon reflex** Achillessehnenreflex *m*

aching schmerzhaft, schmerzend

achloropsia, achloroblepsia Grünblindheit *f*, Achloropsie *f*, Deuteranopie *f*, Deuteranopsie *f*

achondroplasia, achondroplasty Störung *f* des Knorpelwachstums, Achondroplasie *f*

achromate gänzlich Farbenblinder *m*

achromatic farblos, achromatisch

achromatism Achromatismus *m*, Fehlen *n* der chromatischen Aberration

achromatopsia totale Farbenblindheit *f*, Achromatopsie *f*, Farbenblindheit *f*

acid Säure *f* / ~ **phosphatase** saure Phosphatase *f* / **acetylsalicylic** ~ Azetylsalizylsäure *f* / **amino** ~ Aminosäure *f* / **aminobutyric** ~ Aminobuttersäure *f* / **ascorbic** ~ Askorbinsäure *f* / **aspartic** ~ Asparaginsäure *f* / **barbituric** ~ Barbitursäure *f* / **cyanic** ~ Blausäure *f* / **deoxyribonucleic** ~ Desoxyribonukleinsäure *f*, DNS *f* / **2,5–dihydroxyphenylacetic** ~ 2,5–Dihydroxyphenylessigsäure *f* / **fatty** ~ Fettsäure *f* / **folic** ~ Folsäure *f* / **glutamic** ~ Glutaminsäure *f* / **glutaminic** ~ Glutaminsäure *f* / **gymnemic** ~ Gymnemasäure *f* / **homogentisic** ~ Homogentisinsäure *f*, 2,5–Dihydroxyphenylessigsäure *f* / **homovanillic** ~ Homovanillinsäure *f* / **hydrochloric** ~ Salzsäure *f* / **hydroxyindoleacetic** ~ Hydroxyindolessigsäure *f* / **ibotenic** ~ Ibotensäure *f* / **kainic** ~ Kainsäure *f* / **lactic** ~ Milchsäure *f* / **lysergic** ~ Lysergsäure *f* / **lysergic** ~ **diethylamide** Lysergsäurediäthylamid *n*, LSD *n*, Lysergid *n* / **nicotinic** ~ Niazin *n*, Nikotinsäure *f* / **nicotinic** ~ **amide** Niazinamid *n*, Nikotinsäureamid *n* / **nucleic** ~ Nukleinsäure *f* / **phosphoric** ~ Phosphorsäure *f* / **ribonucleic** ~ Ribonukleinsaure *f*, RNS *f* / **uric** ~ Harnsäure *f* / **valproic** ~ Valproinsäure *f*

acidity Azidität *f*, Säuregrad *m*

acidosis Azidose *f* / **compensated** ~ kompensierte Azidose *f* / **decompensated** ~ dekompensierte Azidose *f* / **diabetic** ~ diabetische Azidose *f* / **metabolic** ~ metabolische Azidose *f* / **nonrespiratory** ~ metabolische Azidose *f* / **renal tubular** ~ renal–tubuläre Azidose *f* / **respiratory** ~ respiratorische Azidose *f*

acinesia Bewegungsarmut *f*, Unbeweglichkeit *f*, Akinesie *f*

acinetic akinetisch, bewegungsarm, unbeweglich

acknowledgment Anerkennung *f*, Bestätigung *f*

acmaesthesia, acmesthesia schmerzlose, stichartige Hautempfindung *f*, Akrognosie *f*

acme Gipfel *m*, Höhepunkt *m*, Orgasmus *m*

acoasma, acousma Gehörhalluzination *f*, Gehörtäuschung *f*, Akoasma *n*

acoenaesthesia, acoenesthesia Gefühl *n* der Unwirklichkeit des Körpers

aconative willensunabhängig, triebunabhängig

acoria unersättlicher Hunger *m*, dauernder Heißhunger *m*, Akorie *f*

acouaesthesia Überempfindlichkeit *f* des Gehörs

acoumeter, acouometer Hörschärfemesser *m*, Akumeter *n*, Audiometer *n*

acoumetry Hörprüfung *f*, Hörschärfemessung *f*, Akumetrie *f*

acousmatamnesia Unfähigkeit *f* Klänge zu behalten und zu erinnern

acousmatognosis Seelentaubheit *f*, Unfähigkeit *f* Klänge zu erkennen, Akusmatognosie *f*

acoustic akustisch, Hör–

acoustician Akustiker *m*, Akustikfachmann *m*

acousticophobia krankhafte Angst *f* vor Tönen, Akustikophobie *f*

acoustics Akustik *f*, Schallehre *f*

acoutometer Hörschärfemesser *m*, Akumeter *n*, Audiometer *n*

acquaintance Bekanntschaft *f*, Kenntnis *f* / **~ index** Zahl *f* der Bekanntschaften / **~ rape** Vergewaltigung *f* durch Bekannte / **~ volume** Zahl *f* der Bekanntschaften

acquiescence Jasagetendenz *f*, Akquieszenz *f*, Zustimmungstendenz *f* / **~ response set** Jasagetendenz *f* / **~ tendency** Jasagetendenz *f*

acquired erworben, erlernt

acquisition Erwerb *m*, Aneignung *f*, Errungenschaft *f*, Lernen *n* / **~ curve** Lernkurve *f* / **~ need** Lernbedürfnis *n* / **~ of behaviour** Verhaltenslernen *n* / **~ of knowledge** Wissenserwerb *m*

acquisitive gewinnsüchtig, erwerbssüchtig

acquisitiveness Erwerbssinn *m*, Erwerbstrieb *m*, Gewinnsucht *f*

acrasia, acrasy mangelnde Selbstbeherrschung *f*, krankhafte Maßlosigkeit *f*, Akrasie *f*

acratia Kraftlosigkeit *f*, Schwäche *f*

acroaesthesia, acroesthesia Schmerzen *mpl* in den Extremitäten

acroagnosis, acroagnosia Unfähigkeit *f* zu Reizunterscheidungen in den Extremitäten

acroanaesthesia, acroanesthesia Gefühllosigkeit *f* in den Extremitäten, Störung *f* der Sensibilität in den Akren, Akroanästhesie *f*

acroataxia Ataxie *f* der Finger und Zehen

acrocephalia, acrocephaly Spitzköpfigkeit *f*, Akrozephalie *f*

acrocinesis, acrokinesis, acrocinesia, acrokinesia übermäßige Beweglichkeit *f*

acrocinetic übermäßig beweglich

acrognosis Lagesinn *m* bezüglich der Extremitäten

acromania unheilbare, starke Psychose *f*, Akromanie *f*

acromegalia, acromegaly Akromegalie *f*, übermäßiges Wachstum *n* der Akren

acromicria Kleinheit *f* der Akren, Akromikrie *f* / **congenital ~** Down Syndrom *n*

acroneurosis Akroneurose *f*, Angioneurose *f* an den Enden der Körperglieder, Sensibilitätsstörung *f* an den Enden der Gliedmaßen

acroparaesthesia, acroparesthesia Akroparästhesie *f*, Sensibilitätsstörungen *fpl* im Bereich der Hände und Füße, Gefühllosigkeit *f* und Steife *f* der Finger und Zehen

acrophobia Höhenangst *f*, Akrophobie *f*

act Handlung *f*, Akt *m* / handeln / **~ out** abreagieren, agieren, ausleben / **~ psychology** Aktpsychologie *f* / **~ regression** Handlungsregression *f* / **~ of volition** Willensakt *m* / **adaptive ~** Anpassungshandlung *f* / **affective ~** Affekthandlung *f* / **aimed ~** zielgerichtete Handlung *f* / **compulsive ~** Zwangshandlung *f* / **consummatory ~** Endhandlung *f* / **destructive ~** zerstörerische Handlung *f* / **emotional ~** Affekthandlung *f* / **faulty ~** Fehlhandlung *f*, Fehlleistung *f* / **ideomotor ~** psychomotorische Handlung *f* / **imperious ~** unwiderstehliche Triebhandlung *f* / **impulsive ~** Impulshandlung *f*, Kurzschlughandlung *f* / **instinctive ~** Triebhandlung *f*, Instinkthandlung *f* / **obsessional ~** Zwangshandlung *f* / **obsessive ~** Zwangshandlung *f* / **predominantly compulsive ~s (obsessional rituals)** vorwiegend Zwangshandlungen *fpl* (Zwangsrituale) / **purposive ~** zielgerichtete Handlung *f* / **sexual ~** Geschlechtsverkehr *m*, Koitus *m* / **signalizing ~** Signalfunktion *f* / **subconscious ~** unterbewusste Handlung *f*, Automatismus *m* / **successful ~** erfolgreiche Handlung *f* / **symptomatic ~** Symptomhandlung *f* / **unintentional ~** unfreiwillige Handlung *f* / **unsuccessful ~** erfolgloser Versuch *m*

actin Aktin *n* / **~ filament** Aktinfilament *n*

acting out Lösung *f* von Konflikten im Handeln, Abreagieren *n*, Ausagieren *n*, Kurzschlussreaktion *f* / **antisocial ~** asoziales Benehmen *n*

action Handlung *f*, Aktion *f*, Tätigkeit *f* / **~–and–state orientation** Handlungs– und Lageorientierung *f* / **~ current** Aktionsstrom *m* / **~ mechanism** Handlungssystem *n* / **~ orientation** Handlungsausrichtung *f* / **~ pattern** Handlungsstruktur *f*, Verhaltensmuster *n* / **~ planning** Maßnahmenplanung *f*, Aktionsplanung *f* / **~ potential** Aktionspotenzial *n* / **~ probability** Handlungswahrscheinlichkeit *f* / **~ quotient** Aktionsquotient *m* / **~ research** Handlungsforschung *f*, Begleitforschung *f*, Aktionsforschung *f* / **~ reversibility** Handlungsumkehr *f* / **~ sequence** Handlungsfolge *f*, Handlungsabfolge *f* / **~ space** Handlungsraum *m* / **~–specific** handlungsspezifisch / **~ substance** Aktionssubstanz *f* / **~ system** Handlungssystem *n* / **~ theory** Handlungstheorie *f* / **~ time** Empfindungszeit *f* / **~ unit** Handlungseinheit *f* / **abnormal ~** Fehlhandlung *f* / **accidental ~** Zufallshandlung *f* / **affirmative ~** Förderung *f* diskriminierter Gruppen / **aimed ~** beabsichtigte Handlung *f*, gezielte Aktion *f* / **autochthonous ~** autochthone Handlung *f*, Handlung *f* mit Eigenmotivation / **automatic ~** Automatismus *m* / **autorhythmic ~** Autorhythmie *f*, autonome rhythmische Tätigkeit *f* / **biphasic ~ potential** biphasisches Aktionspotenzial *n* / **cholinergic ~** cholinergische Wirkung *f* / **compound ~ potential** Summenaktionspotenzial *n* / **compulsive ~** Zwangshandlung *f* / **consensual ~** Handlung *f* mit beiderseitigem Einverständnis / **consummatory ~** Endhandlung *f* / **cumulative ~** Kumulationswirkung *f* / **defective ~** Defekthandlung *f* / **deferred ~** nachträgliche Handlung *f* / **faulty ~** Fehlhandlung *f*, Fehlleistung *f* / **fixed pattern ~** fixierte Handlungsstruktur *f* / **ideomotor ~** ideomotorische Handlung *f* / **impulsive ~** Triebhandlung *f*, Impulshandlung *f* / **intelligent ~** vernünftiges Handeln *n* / **interrupted ~** unterbrochene Handlung *f* / **involuntary ~** unwillkürliche Handlung *f*, Automatismus *m* / **irrelevant ~s** Komfortverhalten *n* / **least law ~** Gesetz *n* der geringsten Anstrengung / **microphonic ~** Cochlea–Mikrophonpotential *n* / **purposeful ~** zielgerichtete Handlung *f* / **reciprocal ~** Interaktion *f*, Wechselwirkung *f* / **retinal ~ time** Empfindungszeit *f* der Netzhaut / **secretory ~** Drüsentätigkeit *f* / **specific ~** spezifische Aktion *f* / **specific ~ potential** spezifisches Aktionspotential *n* / **social ~** Gemeinschaftsaktion *f*, Sozialreform *f* / **supplemental ~** zusätzliche Handlung *f* / **symptomatic ~** Symptomhandlung *f* / **vital ~** physiologischer Vorgang *m* / **voluntary ~** Willkürhandlung *f*

actionism Aktionismus *m*

activation Aktivierung *f*, Anregung *f*, Aktivation *f* / **~ research** Kaufentschlussanalyse *f* / **~ syndrome** Aktivationssyndrom *n* / **~ theory** Aktivierungstheorie *f* / **behavioural ~ system** Annäherungssystem *n*

activator Aktivator *m*, Aktivierungsmittel *n*, Stimulans *n*

active aktiv, wirksam, Aktiv–

activism Aktivismus *m*

activist movement Aktivistenbewegung *f*

activity Aktivität *f*, Tätigkeit *f* / **~ analysis** Tätigkeitsanalyse *f* / **~ cage** Handlungskäfig *m* / **~ cycle** Aktivitatsperiodik *f* / **~ concept** Aktivitätstheorie *f* / **~ decrease** Aktivitätsabfall *m* / **~ drive** Tätigkeitsdrang *m* / **~ factor** Aktivitätsfaktor *m* / **~ group** Aktivgruppe *f* / **~ inventory** Tätigkeitsanalyse *f* / **~ level** Aktivitätsniveau *n* / **~ motive** Handlungsmotiv *n* / **~ need** Tätigkeitsdrang *m* / **~ of daily life** Alltagsfertigkeit *f* / **~ pleasure** Freude *f* an einer Tätigkeit / **~ questionnaire** Fragebogen *m* zur Erfassung von Tätigkeiten / **~ quotient** Aktionsquotient *m* / **~ rating** Tätigkeitsbewertung *f* / **~ sampling** Multimomentaufnahme *f* / **~ system** Handlungssystem *n* / **~ therapy** Aktivitätstherapie *f* / **~ wheel** Laufrad *n* / **cerebral ~** Gehirntätigkeit *f*, Gehirnfunktion *f* / **cortical ~** kortikale Aktivität *f* / **electrical ~** elektrische Aktivität *f* / **extracurricular ~** außerschulisches Engagement *n*, Freizeitbetätigung *f*, extrakurrikulare Aktivität *f* / **glandular ~** Drüsentätigkeit *f*, Drüsenfunktion *f* / **gross motor ~** Grobmotorik *f* / **higher nervous ~** höhere Nerventätigkeit *f* / **imaginative ~** Phantasietätigkeit *f* / **immanent ~** immanente Aktivität *f* / **intellectual ~** geistige Aktivität *f*, Denktätigkeit *f* / **irrelevant ~** Übersprunghandlung *f* / **maintained ~** Daueraktivität *f* / **mental ~** geistige Aktivität *f* / **minute motor ~** Feinmotorik *f* / **motor ~** motorische Aktivität *f* / **nervous ~** Nerventätigkeit *f* / **partial ~** Teilaktivität *f* / **perceptual ~** Wahrnehmungstätigkeit *f* / **permanent ~** Daueraktivität *f* / **psychomotor ~** Psychomotorik *f* / **purposive ~** zielgerichtete Aktivität *f* / **random ~** zufällige Handlung *f*, Zufallsbewegung *f* / **resting ~** Ruheaktivität *f*, Ruhetätigkeit *f* / **sensorimotor ~** sensomotorische Aktivität *f* / **sexual ~** sexuelle Aktivität *f*, Brunst *f* / **signalizing ~** Signalfunktion *f* / **social ~** Aktivität *f* in einem sozialen Feld / **spontaneous ~** Spontanaktivität *f* / **substitutive ~** Ersatzhandlung *f* / **thalamic ~** Thalamusfunktion *f* / **thyroid ~** Schilddrüsentätigkeit *f* / **vascular ~** Gefäßtätigkeit *f* / **vital ~** lebensnotwendige Tätigkeit *f*, lebenswichtige Funktion *f* / **voluntary ~** Willenshandlung *f*

actor Schauspieler *m*, handelnde Person *f*, Täter *m*

actual wirklich, tatsächlich, gegenwärtig

actualisation Verwirklichung *f*, Aktualisation *f*

actuarial statistisch, versicherungsmathematisch

acuaesthesia, acuesthesia abnorm feines Empfinden *n*

acuity Schärfe *f* / **~ of colour perception** Farbtüchtigkeit *f*, Schärfe *f* der Farbwahrnehmung / **~ grating** Sehschärfegitter *n* / **auditory ~** Hörscharfe *f* / **olfactory ~** Geruchsschärfe *f* / **sensory ~** Sinnesschärfe *f*, sensorisches Differenzierungsvermögen *n* / **tactile ~** taktile Sinnesschärfe *f*, Tastschärfe *f* / **tactual ~** Tastschärfe *f* / **visual ~** Sehschärfe *f*

acumeter Audiometer *n*, Akumeter *n*, Hörschärfemesser *m*

acupuncture Akupunktur *f*

acupuncturist Akupunktur–Fachmann *m*, Akupunkteur

acusticus Hörnerv *m*, Nervus acusticus *m*

acute akut, scharf, fein

acuteness Schärfe *f* / **~ of hearing** Hörschärfe *f* / **~ of sight** Sehschärfe *f*, Sehleistung *f*

acyanoblepsia, acyanopsia Blaublindheit *f*, Azyanoblepsie *f*, Azyanopsie *f*

ad Anzeige *f*, Inserat *n*

adapt anpassen, adaptieren

adaptability Anpassungsfähigkeit *f*, Anpassungsvermögen *n*, Flexibilitit *f* / **social ~** soziales Anpassungsvermögen *n*

adaptable anpassungsfähig, flexibel

adaptation Anpassung *f*, Gewöhnung *f*, Adaptation *f* / **~ board** Adaptionsbrett *n* / **~ disease** Adaptationskrankheit *f* / **~ level** Adaptationsniveau *n*, Anpassungsniveau *n* / **~ to reality** Realitätsanpassung *f*, Anpassung *f* an die Wirklichkeit / **~ of receptor** Rezeptoranpassung *f* / **~ syndrome** Adaptationssyndrom *n* / **~ time** Anpassungszeit *f* / **alloplastic ~** Anpassung *f* durch Veränderung der Umwelt / **autoplastic ~** Anpassung *f* durch Veränderung des Selbst / **chromatic ~** chromatische Adaptation *f* / **dark ~** Dunkelanpassung *f* / **environmental ~** Anpassung *f* an die Umwelt, Umweltanpassung *f* / **general ~ syndrome** allgemeines Adaptationssyndrom *n* / **local ~** Lokaladaptation *f* / **negative ~** negative Adaptation *f*, negative Anpassung *f* / **photopic ~** Anpassung *f* ans Tageslicht, photopische Adaptation *f* / **physical ~** physikalische Adaptation *f* / **retinal ~** Adaptation *f* des Auges / **scotopic ~** Dunkeladaptation *f*, Anpassung *f* an die Dämmerung / **sensory ~** Sinnesanpassung *f*, sensorische Adaptation *f* / **social ~** soziale Anpassung *f* / **visual ~** Adaptation *f* des Auges

adaptational Anpassungs–, adaptiv

adaption Anpassung *f*, Adaptation *f* / **~ time** Adaptionszeit *f*

adaptive anpassungsfähig, adaptiv

adaptometer Adaptometer *n*, Gerät *n* zur Schwellenprüfung des Lichtsinnes

adaptometry Adaptometrie *f*, Schwellenprüfung *f* des Lichtsinnes

addict Süchtiger *m*, Suchtkranker *m*

addiction Sucht *f*, Süchtigkeit *f*, Gewöhnung *f* / **~ to cocaine** Kokainsucht *f* / **~ to hashish** Haschischsucht *f* / **~ to morphine** Morphinismus *m* / **~ to opium** Opiumsucht *f* / **~ reaction** Suchtreaktion *f* / **alcoholic ~ test** Test *m* zur Feststellung der Alkoholsucht / **gambling ~** Spielleidenschaft *f* / **sexual ~** Sexsucht *f*

addictology Wissenschaft *f* von den Süchten, Lehre *f* von den Süchten

addictologist Spezialist *m* für Suchtkrankheiten

Addison's disease Addisonsche Krankheit *f*, Nebenniereninsuffizienz *f*, Bronzekrankheit *f*

addition Addition *f*, Zusammenrechnung *f* / **~ theorem** Additionssatz *m*

additional zusätzlich, nachträglich

additive additiv

additivity Additivität *f* / **countable ~** zählbare Menge *f* / **finite ~** endliche Menge *f*

adduction Adduktion *f*, Bewegung *f* zur Mittellinie des Körpers, Anziehung *f*

adenine Adenin *n*

adenohypophysis Hypophysenvorderlappen *m*, Adenohypophyse *f*

adenoma Adenom *n*, Drüsengeschwulst *f*

adenosine Adenosin *n* / **~ diphosphate** Adenosindiphosphat *n* / **~ triphosphate** Adenosontriphosphat *n* / **cyclic ~ monophosphate** zyklisches Adenosinmonophosphat *n*

adenylate cyclase Adenylatcyclase *f*

adephagia Vielfresserei *f*, Völlerei *f*, Heißhunger *m*

adequate angemessen, adäquat

adherence Festhalten *n*, Hängenbleiben *n* / **subjective ~** subjektives Festhalten *n*

adhesion Adhäsion *f* / **~ principle** Adhäsionsprinzip *n* / **genetic ~** genetische Adhäsion *f*

adhesiveness Klebrigkeit *f*, Fähigkeit *f* zur Fixierung / **~ of the libido** Klebrigkeit *f* der Libido

adhesivity Haften *n*, Kleben *n*

adiadochokinesis Unfähigkeit *f* rasch antagonistische Bewegungen auszuführen, Adiadochokinese *f*

adient Annäherungs–

Adie's syndrome Adie–Syndrom *n*, Pupillotonie *f* mit Reflexausfall an den unteren Extremitäten

adipose adipös, fett

adiposis, adipositas Fettsucht *f*, Fettleibigkeit *f*, Adipositas *f* / **~ dolorosa** Adipositas dolorosa *f*, Dercum–Krankheit *f*

adiposogenital adiposogenital

adipsia fehlendes Durstgefühl *n*, Adipsie *f*

adjudication Urteil *n*, richterliche Entscheidung *f*, Rechtsspruch *m*

adjustment Anpassung *f* / **~ defect** Anpassungsstörung *f* / **~ disorder** Anpassungsstörung *f* / **~ disorder with depressed mood** Anpassungsstörung *f* mit depressiver Stimmung / **~ disorder with mixed anxiety and depressed mood** Anpassungsstörung *f* mit Angst und depressiver Stimmung / **~ disorder with mixed disturbance of emotions and conduct** Anpassungsstörung *f* mit emotionalen Störungen und Störungen des Sozialverhaltens, gemischt / **~ of equivalent stimulus procedure** Herstellungsverfahren *n* / **~ inventory** Liste *f* zur Erfassung der Anpassung / **~ level** Anpassungsniveau *n* / **~ of equivalent stimulus method** Herstellungsverfahren *n* / **~ of measurements** Messwertausgleich *m*, Glättung *f* / **~ mechanism** Anpassungsmechanismus *m* / **~ method** Herstellungsverfahren *n* / **~ of observations** Beobachtungsausgleich *m* / **~ problem** Anpassungsschwierigkeit *f* / **~ procedure** Herstellungsverfahren *n* / **~ scale** Anpassungsskala *f* / **~ therapy** Einstellungstherapie *f* / **emotional ~** emotionale Anpassung *f* / **good ~** Anpassung *f* / **interpersonal ~** interpersonale Anpassung *f*, soziale Anpassung *f* / **marital ~** Anpassung *f* an den Ehepartner / **occupational ~** berufliche Anpassung *f* / **personal ~** persönliche Anpassung *f* / **social ~** soziale Anpassung *f* / **statistical ~** statistischer Ausgleich *m* / Glättung *f* / **visuo–motor ~** visuell–motorische Anpassung *f* / **vocational ~** berufliche Anpassung *f*

Adler's theory Adler'sche Psychologie *f*, Lehre *f* von Adler

ad–lib improvisieren, aus dem Stehgreif reden

administration Verwaltung *f* / **~ of a test** Testdarbietung *f*, Testdurchführung *f* / **educational ~** Schulverwaltung *f*

administrator Verwalter *m*, Administrator *m*, Systemverwalter *m* in einem Netzwerk

admissible zulässig

admission Eingeständnis *n*, Zugeständnis *n*, / Aufnahme *f (ins Krankenhaus)*

adolescence Jugendalter *n*, Adoleszenz *f*, Jugend *f*

adolescent Heranwachsender *m*, jugendlicher *m* / jugendlich, heranwachsend

adopt adoptieren, an Kindes Statt annehmen

adoptee adoptierte Person *f*

adoption Annahme *f* an Kindes Statt, Adoption *f* / **interracial ~** interkulturelle Adoption *f*

adoptive angenommen, Adoptiv–

adrenal Nebennieren–

adrenalectomy Nebennierenentfernung *f*, Nebennierenexzision *f*

adrenalin, adrenaline Adrenalin *n*

adrenalinaemia Adrenalinämie *f*

adrenergic adrenergisch

adrenin Adrenalin *n*

adrenochrome Adrenochrom *n*

adrenocorticotrophin Kortikotropin *n*

adrenocorticotropic adrenokortikotrop

adualistic nicht–dualistisch

adult Erwachsener *m* / erwachsen, reif / **~ antisocial behaviour** antisoziales Verhalten *n* im Erwachsenenalter / **~ attitude** Erwachseneneinstellung *f* / **~ day care** Tagesbetreuung *f* für Erwachsene / **~ development** Entwicklung *f* im Erwachsenenalter, Erwachsenenentwicklung *f* / **~ education** Erwachsenenbildung *f* / **~ intelligence** Erwachsenenintelligenz *f* / **~ learning** Lernen *n* im Erwachsenenalter / **~ offspring** erwachsene Nachkommen *m* / **~ psychology** Erwachsenenpsychologie *f* / **superior ~ test** Intelligenztest *m* für Erwachsene mit höherer Intelligenz / **young ~** junger Erwachsener *m*

adulterous ehebrecherisch

adultery Ehebruch *m*

adulthood Erwachsenenalter *n*, Erwachsensein *n*

adultomorphism Erklärung *f* kindlichen Verhaltens in Analogie zum Erwachsenenverhalten, Zuerkennung *f* von Erwachsenencharakteristika an Kinder, Adultomorphismus *m*

advanced fortgeschritten

advantage Vorteil *m*, Nutzen *m* / **~ by illness** Krankheitsgewinn *m* / **epinosic ~** sekundärer Krankheitsgewinn *m* / **secondary ~ by illness** sekundärer Krankheitsgewinn *m*

advertise werben, inserieren

advertisement Anzeige *f*, Inserat *n* / **~ department** Werbeabteilung *f*

advertising Werbung *f*, Anzeigenwerbung *f* / werblich, Werbe– / **~ activity** Werbeaktion *f* / **~ agency** Werbeagentur *f* / **~ appeal** Werbeappel *m* / **~ approach** Werbeaspekt *m*, Erregung *f* der Aufmerksamkeit / **~ area** Werbebereich *m* / **~ campaign** Werbekampagne *f*, Werbefeldzug *m* / **~ character** Werbefigur *f* / **~ conception** Werbekonzeption *f* / **~ consultant** Werbeberater *m* / **~ control** Werbeerfolgskontrolle *f* / **~ department** Werbeabteilung *f* / **~ design** Werbeentwurf *m* / **~ device** Werbeslogan *m*, Motto *n* / **~ effect** Werbewirkung *f*, Werbeeffekt *m* / **~ effectiveness** Werbewirksamkeit *f* / **~ effectiveness study** Werbeerfolgskontrolle *f* / **~ efficiency** Werbewirksamkeit *f* / **~ figure** Werbefigur *f* / **~ horizons** Werbemöglichkeiten *fpl* / **~ idea** Werbeidee *f* / **~ manager** Werbeleiter *m* / **~ measures** Werbemaßnahmen *fpl* / **~ medium** Werbemittel *n*, Werbeträger *m* / **~ message** Werbeaussage *f*, Werbebotschaft *f* / **~ objectives** Werbeziele *mpl* / **~ point** Werbeargument *n* / **~ practice** Werbebrauch *m* / **~ psychology** Werbepsychologie *f* / **~ purpose** Werbezweck *m* / **~ research** Werbeforschung *f* / **~ result** Werbeerfolg *m* / **~ schedule** Werbeplan *m*, Terminplan *m* eines Werbefeldzuges / **~ slogan** Werbeslogan *m*, Motto *n* / **~ support** Werbeunterstützung *f* / **~ test** Testwerbung *f* / **~ theme** Werbethema *n* / **~ value** Werbewert *m* / **accessory ~** Ergänzungswerbung *f*, zusätzliche Werbung *f* / **acoustic ~** akustische Werbung *f* / **appealing ~** ansprechende Werbung *f* / **attractive ~** zugkräftige Werbung *f* / **audio–visual ~** audiovisuelle Werbung *f* / **comparative ~** vergleichende Werbung *f* / **direct ~** Direktwerbung *f* / **direct mailing ~** Direktwerbung *f* per Post / **educational ~** belehrende Werbung *f* / **subliminal ~** unterschwellige Werbung *f* / **suggestive ~** Suggestivwerbung *f*

advice Rat *m*, Ratschlag *m*, Beratung *f* / **~ therapy** Beratung *f*, psychotherapeutische Beratung *f*

advise raten, ernpfehlen, sich beraten

advocacy Befürwortung *f*, offenes Eintreten *n*, Hilfsinitiative *f*

advocate verfechten, verteidigen

adynamia, adynamy Adynamie *f*, Kraftlosigkeit *f*

aeroasthenia Aeroasthenie *f*

aeroneurosis Aeroneurose *f*, Fliegerneurose *f*

aerophagia Luftschlucken *n*, Aerophagie *f*

aerophobia Luftscheu *f*, Aerophobie *f*, Angst *f* vor Luft (z. B. Durchzug)

aerotaxis Aerotaxis *f*

aerotherapy Aerotherapie *f*, Klimatherapie *f*

aesthesia Empfindung *f*, Empfindlichkeit *f*, Ästhesie *f*, Empfindungsvermögen *n*

aesthesiology Lehre *f* von den Empfindungen und Empfindungsorganen

aesthesiometer Empfindlichkeitsmesser *m*, Tasterzirkel *m*, Ästhesiometer *n*

aesthesiometry Empfindlichkeitsmessung *f*

aesthesiophysiology Sinnesphysiologie *f*

aesthete Ästhet *m*, Ästhetiker *m*

aesthetic ästhetisch

aesthetics Ästhetik *f* / **psychological ~** psychologische Ästhetik *f*, Kunstpsychologie *f*

aesthetism Ästhetizismus *m*, Schöngeisterei *f*

aetiology Lehre *f* von den Ursachen der Krankheiten, Ätiologie *f*, Entstehung *f* einer Krankheit

A factor Abstraktionsfaktor *m*, Faktor *m* des abstrakten Denkens

affect Affekt *m*, Erregung *f*, Gemütsbewegung *f*, Emotion *f* / wirken auf, beeinflussen, affizieren / **~ block** Affektsperre *f* / **~ conversion** Affektumwandlung *f* / **~ displacement** Affektverschiebung *f* / **~ epilepsy** Affektepilepsie *f* / **~ equivalent** affektives Äquivalent *n* / **~ explosion** Affektausbruch *m* / **~ hunger** starkes Bedürfnis *n* nach affektiver Zuneigung, Affekthunger *m* / **~ incontinence** Affektinkontinenz *f* / **~ irradiation** Affektirradiation *f* / **~-produced spasm** Affektkrampf *m* / **associated ~** Begleitaffekt *m* / **asthenic ~** niederdrückender Affekt *m* / **dissociated ~** abgespaltener Affekt *m* / **externally aroused ~** von außen hervorgerufener Affekt *m* / **floating ~** freiflottierender Affekt *m* / **internally aroused ~** organisch bedingter Affekt *m* / **labile ~** labiler Affekt *m* / **shut-in ~** eingeklemmter Affekt *m* / **split-off ~** abgespaltener Affekt *m* / **sthenic ~** erregender Affekt *m* / **strangulated ~** eingeklemmter Affekt *m*

affectation übertriebene Vorliebe *f*, Affektiertheit *f*, Heuchelei *f*

affected unnatürlich, affektiert, gekünstelt, behaftet mit / **mentally ~** geisteskrank

affection Zuneigung *f*, Erkrankung *f*, Affektion *f* / **cerebral ~** Hirnveränderung *f* / **localised cerebral ~** zerebrale Herderkrankung *f* / **masked ~** maskierte Zuneigung *f*, verborgene Zuneigung *f* / **Platonic ~** platonische Liebe *f*

affectional affekthaft, affektbedingt, affektiv

affectionate zärtlich, liebevoll

affective affektiv, affektbehaftet, affektbetont, Affekt–

affectivity Affektivität *f*, Stimmungslage *f* / **labile ~** Affektlabilität *f* / **restrained ~** gebremste Affektivität *f*

afference Afferenz *f*, afferenter Einstrom *m*

afferent zum Zentralnervensystem leitend, afferent / Afferenz *f* / **visceral ~** viszerale Afferenz *f*

afferentiation afferente Reizung *f*

affiliation Angliederung *f*, Anschließung *f* / **~ motivation** Geselligkeitsbedürfnis *n*, Anschlussmotiv *n* / **~ motive** Geselligkeitsbedürfnis *n* / **~ need** Geselligkeitsbedürfnis *n*, Affiliationsbedürfnis *n* / **~ want** Geselligkeitsbedürfnis *n* / **religious ~** religiöse Bindung *f*, Religionszugehörigkeit *f*

affiliative affiliativ, Anschluss–

affinity Verwandtschaft *f*, Affinität *f* / **elective ~** Wahlverwandtschaft *f*

afflicted niedergeschlagen, bedrückt, betrübt, leidend, behaftet mit

affliction Niedergeschlagenheit *f*, Kummer *m*, Leid(en) *n*, Krankheit *f*

afflux Zustrom *m*, Zuflug *m*, Zufuhr *f* / **~ of stimulus** Reizzufuhr *f*

affordance handlungsauffordernde Umweltgegebenheit *f*

after nach, hinter / **~ brain** Nachhirn *n*, Myelenzephalon *n* / **~-care** Nachbehandlung *f*, Nachsorge *f*, Nachbetreuung *f* / **~-**

contraction Nachzuckung *f* / **~–cure** Nachkur *f*, Nachbehandlung *f* / **~ discharge** nachwirkender Reflex *m*, Nachentladung *f* / **~–discharge reflex** reflektorische Nachentladung *f* / **~–effect** Nachwirkung *f*, Spätwirkung *f* / **~–effect of motion** Bewegungsnachbild *n*, Nachbewegung *f* / **~–effect of movement** Bewegungsnachbild *n*, Nachbewegung *f* / **perceptual ~–effect** perzeptiver Nacheffekt *m* / **~–hearing** Nachhören *n* / **~ image** Nachbild *n* / **negative ~ image** negatives Nachbild *n* / **positive ~ image** positives Nachbild *n* / **~–impression** Nacheindruck *m* / **~–movement** Bewegungsnachbild *n*, Nachbewegung *f* / **~–only design** Versuchsplan *m* mit Nachtest / **~–perception** Nachempfindung *f*, Nachempfinden *n* / **~–potential** Nachpotenzial *n* / **depolarizing ~potential** depolarisierendes Nachpotential *n* / **hyperpolarizing ~potential** hyperpolarisierendes Nachpotenzial *n* / **~–sensation** Nachempfinden *n*, Nachempfindung *f* / **~–sound** Nachklang *m*, Nachschall *m* / **~–taste** Nachgeschmack *m*, Beigeschmack *m* / **~–treatment** Nachbehandlung *f* / **~–vision** Nachbildsehen *n*, Wahrnehmen *n* eines Nachbildes / **figural ~–effect** figurale Nachwirkung *f* / **perceptual ~–effect** Nachbild *n* / **spiral ~–effect** Spiral–Nachwirkung *f*

afterexpulsion Sekundärverdrängung *f*

afunctional funktionslos, nicht arbeitend

agamic geschlechtslos, ungeschlechtlich

agapism Agapetheorie *f*, Erotismus *m*

age Alter *n* / **~ of achievement** Leistungsalter *n* / **~ calibration** Altersnormung *f* / **~ difference** Altersunterschied *m* / **~ discrimination** Altersdiskriminierung *f* / **~ equivalent** Altersäquivalent *n*/ **~ group** Altersgruppe *f*, Altersschicht *f* / **~ limit** Altersgrenze *f* / **~–mates** Gleichaltrige *pl* / **~ norm** Altersnorm *f* / **~–progress curve** altersabhängige Entwicklungskurve *f* / **~ of puberty** Pubertätsalter *n* / **~ ratio** Altersquotient *m* / **hypnotic ~ regression** hypnotische Altersregression *f* / **~–related cognitive decline** altersbedingter kognitiver Abbau / **~ scale** Altersskala *f* / **~ score** Alterswert *m*, Altersäquivalent *n* / **anal ~** anale Stufe *f*, anales Alter *n* / **anatomical ~** anatomisches Alter *n* / **basal ~** Grundalter *n* / **calendar ~** tatsächliches Alter *n*, Lebensalter *n* / **carpal ~** Handwurzelknochenalter *n* / **chronological ~** Lebensalter *n*, chronologisches Alter *n* / **crawling ~** Krabbelalter *n*, Kriechalter *n* / **dental ~** Zahnalter *n* / **developmental ~** Entwicklungsalter *n* / **educational ~** Lernalter *n*, Schulleistungsalter *n* / **emotional ~** emotionales Alter *n* / **full ~** Volljährigkeit *f* / **involutional ~** Involutionsalter *n*, Rückbildungsalter *n* / **lunar ~** Alter *n* ausgedrückt in Mondmonaten / **maximal ~** Höchstalter *n* / **mental ~** Intelligenzalter *n*, geistiges Alter *n* / **normal ~** normales Alter *n* / **old ~** hohes Alter *n*, Greisenalter *n* / **ontogenetic ~** Lebensalter *n* / **organismic ~** organismisches Alter *n* / **physiological ~** physiologisches Alter *n* / **preschool ~** Vorschulalter *n*, frühe Kindheit *f* / **reading ~** Lesealter *n* / **reproductive ~** gebärfähiges Alter *n* / **skeletal ~** Knochenbildungsalter *n* / **social ~** Sozialalter *n* / **talking ~** Sprechalter *n* / **true ~** tatsächliches Alter *n* (inkl. Zeit vor der Geburt) / **ungrateful ~** undankbares Alter *n* / **walking ~** Lauflernalter *n*

aged betagt, alt, im Alter von / Senior *m*, alter Mensch *m* / **middle ~** im mittleren Alter / **middle ~** Person *f* mittleren Alters, Erwachsener *m* mittleren Alters

agency Instanz *f*, Agentur *f* / **selective ~** Auswahlbüro *n*

agenesia, agenesis fehlende Organentwicklung *f*, Agenesie *f*, Fehlen *n* eines Körperteils, Aplasie *f*

agenetic agenetisch, aplastisch

agenitalism Fehlen *n* der Geschlechtsorgane, Agenitalismus *m*

agent Mittel *n*, Medium *n* / **~ of intellect** Mittel *n* des Verstandes / **anti–anxiety ~** Ataraktikum *n* / **anti–fertility ~** Empfängnisverhütungsmittel *n* / **ataractic ~** Ataraktikum *n* / **excitatory ~** Reizmittel *n* / **fermenting ~** Biokatalysator *m* / **ganglionic blocking ~** Ganglienblocker *m* / **hypoglycaemic ~** blutzuckersenkendes Mittel *n* / **parasympathetic blocking ~** vagusdämpfendes Mittel *n* / **psychopharmacological ~** Psychopharmakon *n* / **psychotherapeutic ~** psychotherapeutisches Mittel *n* / **soothing ~** Beruhigungsmittel *n* / **sympathicolytic ~** Sympathikolytikum *n*

agerasia jugendliches Aussehen *n* trotz hohem Alter

ageusia, ageustia Geschmacksverlust *m*, Geschmacksblindheit *f*, Geschmackslähmung *f*, Ageusie *f*

aging process Alterungsprozess *m*, Altersprozess *m*

agglutinate agglutinieren

agglutination Zusammenballung *f*, Agglutination *f*

agglutinin Agglutinin *n* / **immune ~** Agglutinin *n*

agglutinogen Agglutinogen *n*

aggravate verschlechtern, verschlimmern, erschweren, aggravieren

aggravation Verschlechterung *f*, Verschlimmerung *f*, Aggravation *f*

aggregate Aggregat *n*, Anhäufung *f*, Ansammlung *f* / **social ~** soziales Aggregat *n*

aggregation Ansammlung *f*, soziales Aggregat *n* / **~ theory** Aggregationstheorie *f*

aggregative zusammengestellt, Sammel–

aggression Aggression *f*, Angriff *m* / **~–frustration hypothesis** Aggressions–Frustrations–Hypothese *f* / **~ need** Aggressionstrieb *m* / **direct ~** direkte Aggression *f* / **displaced ~** verschobene Aggression *f* / **normal sexual ~** normale sexuelle Aggression *f* / **repressed ~** verdrängte Aggression *f*

aggressive aggressiv, angriffslustig

aggressiveness, aggressivity Aggressivität *f*, aggressive Haltung *f*, Angriffslust *f* / **competitive ~** wettbewerbsbedingte Aggressivität *f*

aggrith heterogene Stichprobe *f*, nicht–spezifizierte Gruppe *f*

agility Beweglichkeit *f*, Agilität *f* / **physical ~** körperliche Beweglichkeit *f*, Bewegungsdrang *m*

aging Altwerden *n*, Altern *n* / alternd / **physiological ~** physiologisches Altern *n*, natürliches Altern *n*

agitated erregt, unruhig, aufgeregt, nervös, agitiert

agitation Erregung *f*, Unruhe *f*, Aufregung *f*, Agitiertheit *f*, Agitation *f* / **~ and anxiety** ängstliche Erregtheit *f*

agitographia Agitographie *f*, abnorm schnelles, undeutliches Schreiben *n*

agitolalia, agitophasia Agitophasie *f*, hastige Sprache *f*, anomal schnelles Sprechen *n*

aglossia Aglossie *f*, organischer Mutismus *m*, angebotenes Fehlen *n* der Zunge

agnoea, agnea Nichterkennen *n* von Gegenständen oder Personen

agnosia Agnosie *f*, agnostische Störung *f*, Unfähigkeit *f* trotz Funktionstüchtigkeit Wahrnehmbares zu erkennen / **auditory ~** Seelentaubheit *f*, akustische Agnosie *f* / **ideational ~** pragmatische Agnosie *f*, fehlendes Wiedererkennen *n*, Objektagnosie *f* / **optic ~** Seelenblindheit *f*, optische Agnosie *f* / **tactile ~** Tastblindheit *f*, taktile Agnosie *f* / **visual ~** Seelenblindheit *f*, optische Agnosie *f*

agnosticism Agnostizismus *m*

agogigs Agogik *f*

agonist Synergist *m*, Primärmuskel *m*, Agonist *m*

agony, agonia Todeskampf *m*, Agonie *f*, Qual *f* / **~ of mind** Seelenqual *f* / **mental ~** Seelenqual *f*

agoraphobia Agoraphobie *f*, Platzangst *f* / **~ without panic attacks** Agoraphobie *f* ohne Panikattacke / **~ without history of panic disorder** Agoraphobie *f* ohne Panikstörung in der Vorgeschichte

agrammatism, agrammaphasia Agrammatismus *m*, ungrammatische Sprechweise *f*

agranulocytosis Agranulozytose *f*

agraphia Agraphie *f*, Verlust *m* der Schreibfähigkeit / **absolute ~** völlige Agraphie *f*, totale Agraphie *f* / **acoustic ~** akustische Agraphie *f* / **aphasic ~** aphasische Agraphie *f* / **apraxic ~** apraktische Agraphie *f* / **atactic ~** ataktische Agraphie *f*, völlige Agraphie *f* / **cerebral ~** zerebrale Agraphie *f* / **congenital ~** angeborene Agraphie *f* / **literal ~** völlige Agraphie *f* / **mental ~** zerebrale Agraphie *f* / **motor ~** motorische Agraphie *f* / **optic ~** optische Agraphie *f* / **verbal ~** Unfähigkeit *f* Worte zu schreiben

agraphic agraphisch, unfähig zu schreiben

agreeableness Verträglichkeit *f*

agreement Übereinstimmung *f*, Übereinkunft *f* / **~ coefficient** Koeffizient *m* der Übereinstimmung / **~ tendency** Zustimmungstendenz *f*, Jasagetendenz *f* / **interjudge ~** Übereinstimmung *f* zwischen Beurteilern

agriothymia psychotischer Wutanfall *m*

agromania pathologischer Trieb *m* zur Einsamkeit, intensiver Drang *m* abgesondert zu leben

agrypnia Schlaflosigkeit *f*, Agrypnie *f*, Asomnie *f*, Insomnie *f*

agrypnotic schlaflindernd, Schlaflosigkeit verursachend / Wachhaltemittel *n*

agyiphobia Straßenangst *f*, krankhafte Furcht *f* auf der Straße zu gehen

aha experience Aha–Erlebnis *n*

ahedonia Unlust *f*

ahistorical unhistorisch, aktuell

Ahlfeld| breathing movements Ahlfeld'sche Atembewegungen *fpl* des Fötus / **~'s sign** Ahlfeld'sches Schwangerschaftszeichen *n*

ahypnia, ahypnosis krankhafte Schlaflosigkeit *f*, Ahypnie *f*

aichmophobia krankhafte Furcht *f* vor spitzen Gegenständen, Aichmophobie *f*

aid Hilfe *f*, Unterstützung *f*, Hilfsmittel *n* / **audio–visual ~** audiovisuelles Hilfsmitteln *n* / **educational audio–visual ~s** audiovisuelle Lehrmittel *npl*, audiovisuelle Unterrichtsmedien *npl* / **instructional ~s** Lehrmittel *npl*, Unterrichtshilfen *fpl* / **mnemonic ~** Gedächtnisstütze *f* / **optical ~** Sehhilfe *f* / **visual ~s** Anschauungsmaterial *n*

aide Helfer *m*, Helferin *f*, Hilfspfleger *m* / **psychiatric ~** psychiatrischer Hilfspfleger *m*, psychiatrische Hilfspflegerin *f*

aidoiomania Aidoiomanie *f*, krankhaft gesteigerter Geschlechtstrieb *m*

AIDS| dementia AIDS–Demenz *f* / **~ prevention** AIDS–Prävention *f*

ailurophobia krankhafte Furcht *f* vor Katzen, Ailurophobie *f*

aim Ziel *n*, Absicht *f*, Intention *f*, Vorsatz *m*, Zweck *m*, Streben *n* / **~–cathected** zielbesetzt / **~–cathexis** Zielbesetzung *f* / **~–inhibited** zielgehemmt / **~ inhibition** Zielhemmung *f* / **~ of instinct** Triebziel *n* / **~ transference** Zieländerung *f* / **external ~** äußeres Ziel *n* / **instinctual ~** Triebziel *n* / **internal ~** innerer Zweck *m* / **partial ~** Teilziel *n*, Partialziel *n*

aiming Zielbewegung *f*, Zielbewegungskoordination *f* / **~ test** Zielbewegungstest *m*

air Luft *f* / **~ conduction** Luftleitung *f* / **~ encephalogram** Pneumenzephalogramm *n* / **~ encephalography** Pneumenzephalographie *f*, Luftenzephalographie *f* / **~ hunger** Lufthunger *m* / **~ sickness** Luftkrankheit *f* / ~ **traffic accident** Luftverkehrsunfall *m* / ~ **traffic control** Flugsicherung *f* / ~**–way resistance** Atemwegswiderstand *m* / **alveolar** ~ Alveolarluft *f*

akataphasia Akataphasie *f*, Agrammatismus *m*, Verlust *m* der sprachlichen Ausdrucksfähigkeit

akathisia Akathisie *f*, Unfähigkeit *f* zum ruhigen Sitzenbleiben, hysterischer Bewegungsdrang *m*

akinaesthesia, akinesthesia Verlust *m* des Muskelsinnes, Akinästhesie *f*

akinesia, akinesis Bewegungslosigkeit *f*, Unbeweglichkeit *f*, Akinesie *f*, Akinese *f*, Bewegungssperre *f*

akinesic, akinetic akinetisch, bewegungsarm, unbeweglich

akoasm Akoasma *n*, Gehörhalluzination *f*, Gehörtäuschung *f*

akoria unersättlicher Hunger *m*, beständiger Hunger *m*, Akorie *f*

alalia Alalie *f*, Sprachlosigkeit *f*, Nichtsprechenkönnen *n* / **idiopathic** ~ idiopathische Alalie *f* / **logographic** ~ Agraphie *f* / **mental** ~ mentale Alalie *f* / **relative** ~ mentale Alalie *f*, relative Alalie *f*

alalic sprachlos, stumm aufgrund einer Alalie

alanine Alanin *n*

alarm Alarm *m* / ~ **call** Alarmschrei *m*, Alarmruf *m* / ~ **function** Alarmfunktion *f* / ~ **reaction** Alarmreaktion *f* / ~ **response** Alarmreaktion *f*

alarming beunruhigend, unheimlich, alarmierend

albedo Albedo *f*, Reflexionsgrad *m* des Lichtes / ~ **perception** Albedowahrnehmung *f*

albinic, albinotic albinoartig, albinotisch

albinism Albinismus *m*

albino Albino *m* / ~ **rat** Albinoratte *f*

albumin Albumin *n*

alcadd test Test *m* zur Feststellung der Alkoholsucht

alcohol Alkohol *m* / ~ **abuse** Alkoholmissbrauch *m* / ~ **addict** Alkoholiker *m*, Alkoholabhängige *m,f* / ~ **addiction** Alkoholabhängigkeit *f*, Alkoholismus *m*, Trunksucht *f*, Äthylismus *m* / ~**–antabuse–reaction** Disulfiram–Alkohol–Reaktion *f* / ~ **deconditioning** Alkoholentziehungskur *f* / ~ **dehydrogenase** Alkoholdehydrogenase *f* / ~ **detoxication treatment** Alkoholentziehungskur *f* / ~ **drinking attitude** Einstellung *f* zum Alkoholtrinken / ~ **drinking pattern** Trinkgewohnheit *f*, Alkoholkonsumgewohnheit *f* / ~ **idiosyncratic intoxication** idiosynkratische Alkoholintoxikation *f* / ~**–induced anxiety disorder** alkoholinduzierte Angststörung *f* / ~**–induced mood disorder** alkoholinduzierte affektive Störung *f* / ~**–induced persisting amnestic disorder** persistierende alkoholinduzierte amnestische Störung *f* / ~**–induced persisting dementia** persistierende alkoholinduzierte Demenz *f* / ~**–induced psychotic disorder** alkoholinduzierte psychotische Störung *f* / ~**–induced sexual dysfunction** alkoholinduzierte sexuelle Funktionsstörung *f* / ~**–induced sleep disorder** alkoholinduzierte Schlafstörung *f* / ~ **intolerance** Alkoholintoleranz *f* / ~ **intoxication** Alkoholisierung *f*, Alkoholintoxikation *f*, Alkoholvergiftung *f*, Alkoholrausch *m* / **pathological** ~ **intoxication** pathologischer Rausch *m* / ~ **intoxication delirium** Alkoholintoxikationsdelir *n* / ~ **rehabilitation** Alkoholrehabilitaion *f* / ~**–resistant** alkoholfest / **fetal** ~ **syndrome** Alkoholembryopathie *f* / ~ **withdrawal** Alkoholentzug *m* / ~ **withdrawal delirium** Alkoholentzugsdelir *n* / **denatured** ~ denaturierter Alkohol *m*, vergällter Alkohol *m* / **ethyl** ~ Äthylalkohol *m* / **methyl** ~ Methylalkohol *m*, Methanol *n*

alcoholaemia, alkoholemia Alkohol *m* im Blut

alcoholic Trinker *m*, Alkoholiker *m*, Säufer *m* / alkoholisch / **~s Anonymous** Anonyme Alkoholiker *mpl* / **epileptoid ~** epileptoider Trinker *m* / **excessive ~** exzessiver Trinker *m*

alcoholism Alkoholismus *m*, Alkoholabhängigkeit *f*, Äthylismus

alcoholomania Trunksucht *f*, Alkoholismus *m*

alcoholophilia Neigung *f* zum Trinken

aldehyde dehydrogenase Aldehyddehydrogenase *f*

aldolase Aldolase *f*

aldosterone Aldosteron *n*

alert wachsam, wach, munter, rege

alertness Wachheit *f*, Vigilanz *f*, Munterkeit *f* / **~ test** Aufmerksamkeitstest *m* / **cortical ~** kortikale Wachheit *f*

alexia Alexie *f*, Wortblindheit *f*, Buchstabenblindheit *f*, Schriftblindheit *f*, visuelle Aphasie *f* / **congenital ~** Legasthenie *f* / **motor ~** motorische Alexie *f* / **musical ~** musikalische Alexie *f* / **sensory ~** sensorische Alexie *f*

alexithymia Unfähigkeit *f* Gefühle zu äußern, Alexithymie *f*

algaesthesis, algaesthesia Schmerzempfindung *f*, Schmerzsinn *m*

algebra, Boolean Boole'sche Algebra *f*

algebraic algebraisch

algedonia Schmerzlustempfindung *f*

algedonic Schmerzlust empfindend, alghedonisch

algesia, algesis Algesie *f*, Schmerzempfindlichkeit *f*

algesimeter, algesiometer Algesimeter *n*, Schmerzprüfer *m*, Schmerzmesser *m*

algesimetry, algesiometry Algesimetrie *f*, Messung *f* der Schmerzintensität

algesiogenic schmerzauslösend

algesiology Algesiologie *f*, Lehre *f* von der Schmerzempfindung

algesthesia, algesthesis Schmerzempfindung *f*, Schmerzsinn *m*

algetic schmerzerzeugend, Schmerz betreffend

algochronometer Algochronometer *n*, Gerät *n* zur Messung der Reaktionszeit auf Schmerzreize, Algesimeter *n*

algogenesia, algogenesis Schmerzquelle *f*, Schmerzursache *f*, Schmerzauslösung *f*

algolagnia Schmerzwollust *f*, Algolagnie *f* / **active ~** Sadismus *m* / **passive ~** Masochismus *m*

algolagnic algolagnisch

algolagnist Sado–Masochist *m* / **active ~** Sadist *m* / **passive ~** Masochist *m*

algometer Schmerzprüfer *m*, Algometer *n*, Algesimeter *n*

algopareunia Schmerz *m* beim Koitus, Dyspareunie *f*

algophilia, algophily Masochismus *m*, Algophilie *f*

algophobia Angst *f* vor Schmerzen, Überempfindlichkeit *f* gegen Schmerz, Algophobie *f*

algorithm Algorithmus *m*

algorithmic algorithmisch

"alibi" remark Alibibemerkung *f*, Rechtfertigungsbemerkung *f*

Alice–in–Wonderland syndrome Alice–im–Wunderland–Syndrom *n*, Depersonalisationssyndrom *n*

alien fremd, andersartig, artfremd / **~ to the ego** ichfremd

alienate entfremden

alienation Entfremdung *f* / **~ of affection** Entzug *m* der Zuneigung / **~ coefficient** Alienationskoeffizient *m* / **~ of mind** Geistesgestörtheit *f*, Geisteskrankheit *f*, Psychopathie *f* / **mental ~** Geistesgestörtheit *f*, Geisteskrankheit *f* Psychopathie *f*

alienism Lehre *f* von den Geisteskrankheiten

alienist Psychiater *m*, Gerichtspsychiater *m*

alignment Richtung *f*, Anordnung *f*, Ausrichtung *f* / **graphic ~** Schreibrichtung *f*

alimentary Ernährungs–, Nahrungs–, Verdauungs–

alimentation Ernährung *f*, Nutrition *f*

alkaline alkalisch, basisch

alkaloid Alkaloid *n*

allachaesthesia, allaesthesia Allachästhesie *f*, Reizlokalisation *f* an einer anderen als der gereizten Stelle

allegorization Allegorisation *f*

allele, allel Allel *n*, Allegon *n*, Genpaar *n*

allelomimetic allelomimetisch, handlungsangleichend

allelomorph Allelomorph *n*, Allel *n* bei Diploidie, allelomorphes Gen *n*

allelomorphic allelomorph

allelomorphism Allelomorphie *f*

allergen Allergen *n*, allergieerzeugender Stoff *m*

allergology Lehre *f* von den allergischen Erkrankungen

allergy Allergie *f*, allergische Reaktion *f*, Überempfindlichkeitsreaktion *f*

allesthesia Allachästhesie *f*, Reizlokalisation *f* an einer anderen als der gereizten Stelle

alleviate erleichtern, mildern, lindern

alleviation Erleichterung *f*, Milderung *f*

alley Allee *f*, Durchgang *m* / **~ problem** Parallelitätstäuschung *f* / **blind ~ of a maze** Sackgasse *f* in einem Labyrinth

alliaceous knoblauchartig

alliance Allianz *f* / **therapeutic ~** therapeutische Allianz *f*

allness Gesamtheit *f*, Totalität *f*, Ganzes *n*, Vollständigkeit *f*

allocation Zuteilung *f*, Zuweisung *f*, Allokation *f*, Aufteilung *f*

allocentric allozentrisch, nach außen verlagert

allocentrism Allozentrismus *m*

allochaesthesia Allachästhesie *f*, Reizlokalisation *f* an einer anderen als der gereizten Stelle

allocheiria, allochiria Allocheirie *f*, Reizlokalisation *f* auf der anderen Körperseite

allochthonous allochthon, an anderer Stelle entstanden

allodynia Allodynie *f*

alloerotic alloerotisch

alloeroticism, alloerotism Alloerotismus *m*, Objekterotik *f*

allogamic, allogamous allogamisch

allogamy Allogamie *f*

allokinesis, allocinesia passive Bewegung *f* Allokinese *f*

allolalia Allolalie *f*, Fehlsprechen *n* bei Geisteskranken

allomnesia Allomnesie *f*, fehlerhafte Erinnerung *f*

allopath Vertreter *m* der gegenwärtigen Schulmedizin, Allopath *m*

allophasia, allophasis unzusammenhängendes Sprechen *n*, Sprechverwirrung *f*, Allophasie *f*

allophemy Versprechen *n*, Heterophasie *f*, Lapsus linguae *m*

allophone Allophon *n*

allophthalmia Heterochromie *f* Heterophthalmus *m*, Verschiedenheit *f* beider Augen

alloplastic alloplastisch

alloplasty Alloplastie *f*

allopsychic allopsychisch, psychisch auf die Außenwelt gerichtet

allopsychosis Geisteskrankheit *f* mit gestörter Außenweltorientierung, Allopsychose *f*

all–or–none alles oder nichts / **~ law** Alles–oder–Nichts–Gesetz *n*

all–or–nothing alles oder nichts

allosome Allosom *n*, Geschlechtschromosom *n*, Gonosom *n*, Heterochromosom *n*

allotriogeusia, allotriogeustia Geschmackstäuschung *f*, Allotriogeusie *f*, Halluzination *f* des Geschmackssinnes

allotriophagia, allotriophagy Allotriophagie *f*, Hunger *m* auf absonderliche Dinge, Genuss *m* ungewöhnlicher Dinge

allotriosmia Geruchstäuschung *f*, Geruchshalluzination *f*, Allotriosmie *f*

allotropic auf andere eingestellt

alloxan Alloxan *n*, Mesoxalylharnstoff *m*

alogia Alogie *f*, motorische Aphasie *f*, Sprechunvermögen *n*

aloof zurückhaltend, distanziert, unnahbar

alopecia Alopezie *f*, Haarausfall *m*, Kahlheit *f*

alpha alpha / **~ angle** Alpha–Winkel *m* / **~–blocker** Alphablocker *m*, Alpha–Adrenorezeptorenblocker *m* / **~ blocking agent (drug)** Alphablocker *m* / **~ blockade** Alpha–Blockierung *f* / **~ coefficient** Alpha–Koeffizient *m*, Interitem–Konsistenzkoeffizient *m* / **~ examination** Alpha–Test *m* / **~ feedback** Alphatraining *n* / **~ hypothesis** Alpha–Hypothese *f* / **~ methylparatyrosine** Alpha–Methylparatyrosin *n* / **~ motion** Alpha–Bewegung *f*, Scheinbewegung *f* / **~ movement** Alpha–Bewegung *f*, Scheinbewegung *f* / **~ response** Alpha–Reaktion *f* / **~ rhythm** Alpha–Rhythmus *m* / **~ test** Alpha–Test *m* / **~ variant rhythm** Alpha–Variante *f* / **~ wave** Alpha–Welle *f* / **~ wave training** Alphatraining *n*

alphabet Alphabet *n* / **~ content** Buchstabendeutung *f* / **deaf–and–dumb ~** Taubstummenalphabet *n* / **manual ~** Fingeralphabet *n* / **phonetic ~** phonetisches Alphabet *n*

alprazolam Alprazolam *n*

alter ego alter ego *n*, zweites Ich *n*, anderes Ich *n*, Doppelgänger *m*

alterable veränderlich, wandelbar, veränderbar

alteration Änderung *f* Veränderung *f*, Umwandlung *f*, Umformung *f*, Umgestaltung *f*, Verwandlung *f* / **~ of consciousness** Bewusstseinsveränderung *f* / **~ of the ego** Ich–Veränderung *f* / **~s in function** Funktionsveränderungen *fpl* / **~s in structure** Strukturveränderungen *fpl*

alternate wechselseitig, abwechselnd

alternating alternierend, abwechselnd

alternation Wechsel *m*, Abwechslung *f*, Alternieren *n* / **~ cycle** Permutationsreihe *f*, Wechselzyklus *m* / **~ of generations** Generationswechsel *m* / **~ phase** alternierende Reihe *f*, Wechselzyklus *m* / **delayed ~** verzögerter Wechsel *m*, verzögerte Alternierung *f* / **spontaneous ~** spontaner Wechsel *m*, spontane Alternation *f*

alternative alternativ, abwechselnd / Alternative *f* / **fixed–~** Mehrfachwahl–, mit gebundener Aufgabenbeantwortung

altitude Höhe *f* / **~ effect** Höhenwirkung *f* / **~ of intelligence** Intelligenzhöhe *f* / **high–~ intoxication** Höhenrausch *m* / **high–~ sickness** Höhenkrankheit *f* / **~ test** Höhentest *m*

altrigenderism zwischengeschlechtliche Kameradschaft *f*, Freundschaft *f* mit Partnern des anderen Geschlechts

altruism Altruismus *m*, Selbstlosigkeit *f*

altruistic altruistisch, selbstlos

alveolus Alveole *f*

Alzheimer|'s disease Alzheimer Krankheit *f* / **~'s psychosis** Alzheimer–Demenz *f*

amacrine amakrine Zelle *f*, Amakrine *f*

amalgamation Amalgamierung *f*, Amalgamation *f*, Vermengung *f*

amantadine, amatadine Amantadin *n*

amathophobia Staubangst *f*, krankhafte Furcht *f* vor Staub

amaurosis Amaurose *f*, Blindheit *f*, vollständige Erblindung *f*

amaurotic amaurotisch, blind

amaxophobia Furcht *f* in einem Fahrzeug zu fahren, Amaxophobie *f*

ambidexter mit beiden Händen gleich geschickter Mensch *m*, Ambidexter *m*

ambidexterity, ambidextrousness gleiche Geschicklichkeit *f* beider Hände, Ambidextrie *f*

ambidextrous, ambidextral beidhändig, mit beiden Händen gleich geschickt, ambidexter

ambidextrality Doppelhändigkeit *f*

ambient umgebend, Umgebungs–

ambiequal ambiäqual

ambiguity, ambiguousness Mehrdeutigkeit *f*, Zweideutigkeit *f*, Doppelsinn *m* / **~ tolerance** Fähigkeit *f* mit mehrdeutigen Situationen zu leben

ambiguous mehrdeutig, zweideutig, doppelsinnig

ambilateral beidseitig, ambilateral

ambilevous gleich ungeschickt mit beiden Händen, ambisinister

ambisexual doppelgeschlechtlich, mit Eigenschaften beider Geschlechter, bisexuell

ambisexuality Bisexualität *f*, Zwittertum *n*, auf beide Geschlechter gerichteter Sexualtrieb *m*

ambisinister, ambisinistrous gleich ungeschickt mit beiden Händen, ambisinister

ambitendency Ambitendenz *f*, Ambivalenz *f*, gleichzeitiges Bestehen *n* entgegengesetzter Antriebe

ambitendent ambitendent, ambivalent, entschlusslos, hin– und hergerissen

ambition Ehrgeiz *m*, Ambition *f*

ambitious ehrgeizig

ambivalence, ambivalency Ambivalenz *f*, gleichzeitiges Bestehen *n* entgegensetzter Gefühle oder Motive, Bipolarität *f* der Gefühle

ambivalent ambivalent

ambiversion Ambiversion *f*, Zustand *m* zwischen Introversion und Extraversion

ambiversive ambivertiert

ambivert Ambivertierter *m,f*

amblyopia Amblyopie *f*, Schwachsichtigkeit *f*, Sehschwäche *f* / **hysterical ~** hysterische Amblyopie *f* / **nocturnal ~** schwache Nachtsichtigkeit *f*

amblyopic sehschwach, schwachsichtig, amblyop

amblyoscope, amblyscope Amblyoskop *n*

amboceptor Immunkörper *m*, Ambozeptor *m*

ambrosiac, ambrosial ambrosisch

ambulatory ambulant

ameba Amöbe *f*

ameboidism, amebism amöbenartige Bewegung *f*

ameliorate verbessern, besser werden, sich bessern

amenomania krankhafter Fröhlichkeitswahn *m*, manische Phase *f* einer Zyklothymie

amenorrhoea, amenorrhea Ausbleiben *n* der Regel, Amenorrhoe *f*

ament Schwachsinnige *m,f*, Idiot *m*

amential amentiell, schwachsinnig

amentia Amentia *f*, Amenz *f*, amentielles Syndrom *n*, Verwirrtheit *f*, Schwachsinn *m* / **agitated ~** Amentia agitata *f* / **paranoid ~** Amentia paranoides *f* / **phenylpyruvic~** Phenylbrenztraubensäureschwachsinn *m* / **subcultural ~** unterdurchschnittliche Intelligenz *f*

Ames demonstration Ames–Vorführung *f*, Honi–Phänomen *n*

ametropia Ametropie *f*, Fehlsichtigkeit *f*

ametropic ametrop, fehlsichtig

amianthinopsy Violettblindheit *f*

amimia Mimikverlust *m*, Amimie *f*, Verlust *m* des Minenspiels, fehlende mimische Ausdrucksfähigkeit *f* / **amnesic ~** amnestischer Mimikverlust *m*

amine Aminverbindung *f*, Aminkörper *m* / **~ oxidase** Aminooxidase *f* / **~ oxidase inhibitor** Aminooxidase–Hemmer *m* / **biogenic ~** biogene Aminverbindung *f* /

sympathomimetic ~ sympathikomimetische Aminverbindung *f*, Weckamin *n*, sympathomimetisches Amin *n*

aminotransferase Aminotransferase *f*, Transaminase *f*

amitosis Amitose *f*, direkte Zellteilung *f*

amitotic amitotisch, Zellteilung betreffend

amitriptyline Amitriptylin *n*

ammeter Amperemeter *n*, Strommesser *m*

ammonium| base, quaternary quartäre Ammoniumbase *f* / **~ bromide** Ammoniumbromid *n*

Ammon's horn Ammonshorn *n*, Hippocampus *m*

amnesia Amnesie *f*, Erinnerungslücke *f*, Gedächtnislücke *f*, Erinnerungsverlust *m*, Gedächtnisstörung *f* / **anterograde ~** anterograde Amnesie *f* / **auditory ~** auditorische Amnesie *f*, Tontaubheit *f*, akustische Agnosie *f* / **autohypnotic ~** autohypnotische Amnesie *f*, Vergessen *n* durch Verdrängen / **circumscribed ~** lakunäre Amnesie *f*, auf umgrenzte Ereignisse beschränkter Gedächtnisverlust *m* / **continuous ~** dauernde Amnesie *f* / **dissociative ~** dissoziative Amnesie *f* / **dynamic ~** dynamische Amnesie *f* / **episodic ~** episodische Amnesie *f* / **epochal ~** epochale Amnesie *f* / **global ~** totale Amnesie *f*, globale Amnesie *f* / **hypnotic ~** hypnotische Amnesie *f* / **hysteric ~** hysterische Amnesie *f* / **infantile ~** infantile Amnesie *f*, Kindheitsamnesie *f* / **lacunar ~** lakunäre Amnesie *f* / **localised ~** Gedächtnislücke *f* / **organic ~** organische Amnesie *f* / **posthypnotic ~** posthypnotische Amnesie *f* / **posttraumatic ~** posttraumatische Amnesie *f* / **psychogenic ~** psychogene Amnesie *f* / **retroactive ~** retroaktive Amnesie *f*, retrograde Amnesie *f* / **retrograde ~** retrograde Amnesie *f* / **temporary ~** vorübergehende Amnesie *f* / **transitory ~** vorübergehende Amnesie *f* / **transient global ~** transitorische globale Amnesie *f* / **verbal ~** verbale Amnesie *f*, amnestische Aphasie *f* / **visual ~** visuelle Amnesie *f*, Wortblindheit *f*, optische Agnosie *f*

amnesiac amnestischer Patient *m*

amnesic, amnestic amnesisch, amnestisch, Amnesie verursachend

amniotic Amnion–, innere Eihülle betreffend

amobarbital Amobarbital *n* / **~ sodium** Amobarbital–Natrium *n*

amodal amodal, ohne Sinnesreizung wahrnehmend

amoeba Amöbe *f*

amoeboidism, amoebism amöbenartige Bewegung *f*

amoenomania leichte Manie *f*, krankhaft heitere Stimmungslage *f*, Amönomanie *f*

amok Amok *m* / **to run ~** Amok laufen

amor Liebe *f*, Erotik *f* / **~ lesbicus** lesbische Liebe *f*, weibliche Homosexualität *f*

amoral unmoralisch

amoralism Amoralität *f*, moralischer Defekt *m*

amorous verliebt, Liebes–

amorphia, amorphism Amorphismus *m*, Formlosigkeit *f*

amorphosynthesis amorphe Synthese *f*

amorphous amorph, formlos, missgestaltet

amount Betrag *m*, Summe *f*, Menge *f* / **~ of information** Informationsmenge *f*

ampere Ampere *n*

amphetamine Amphetamin *n* / **~ abuse** Amphetaminmissbrauch *m* / **~ addiction** Weckaminsucht *f* / **~ dependence** Amphetaminabhängigkeit *f* / **~ derivative** Amphetaminabkömmling *m* / **~–induced** amphetamininduziert / **~ intoxication** Amphetaminintoxikation *f*, Amphetaminvergiftung *f* / **~ intoxication delirium** Amphetaminintoxikationsdelir *n* / **~ sulphate** Amphetaminsulfat *n* / **~ withdrawal** Amphetaminentzug *m*

amphierotic amphierotisch, bisexuell

amphierotism Amphierotik *f*, Bisexualität *f*

amphigenic, amphigenous, amphigenetic, amphogenic geschlechtlich gezeugt, amphigen

amphigony geschlechtliche Fortpflanzung *f*, geschlechtliche Zeugung *f*, Amphigonie *f*

amphimixis Amphimixis *f*, Vereinigung *f* väterlicher und mütterlicher Erbanlagen, Vereinigung *f* von prägenitaler, urethraler und analer Erotik

amphioxus Lanzettfischchen *n*, Amphioxus *m*

amplification Amplifikation *f*, Erweiterung *f* (eines Trauminhaltes)

amplifier Verstärker *m* / **differential ~** Differenzialverstärker *m*, Gegentaktverstärker *m*

amplitude Amplitude *f*, Schwingungsbreite *f*, Weite *f* / **~ of accommodation** Akkommodationsbreite *f* / **~ of light wave** Amplitude *f* einer Lichtwelle / **effective ~** durchschnittliche Amplitude *f* / **maximum ~** maximale Amplitude *f*

amputation Amputation *f*

amputee Amputierter *m*

amuck Amok *m* / **to run ~** Amok laufen

amulet Talisman *m*, Amulett *n*

amusia Amusie *f*, Unfähigkeit *f* zu musizieren oder Musik zu erfassen / **motor ~** motorische Amusie *f*, vokale Amusie *f*, instrumentelle Amusie *f* / **sensory ~** sensorische Amusie *f*, Tontaubheit *f*, Melodientaubheit *f*

amusic amusisch

amychophobia Amychophobie *f*, krankhafte Furcht *f* gekratzt zu werden

amygdala Mandelkern *m*, Mandelkörper *m*

amygdaloid mandelförmig, mandelartig

amylase Amylase *f*

amylobarbitone Amobarbital *n*

amyloid Amyloid *n*

amyostasia amyostatischer Symptomenkomplex *m*, Störungen *fpl* im statischen Zusammenwirken von Muskelgruppen

amyostatic amyostatisch

amyosthenia Myasthenie *f*, Muskelschwäche *f*

amytal Amobarbital *n* / **~ interview** Exploration *f* unter Amobarbitalgaben

anabasis Anabasis *f*, mystisches Gefühl *n* des Emporschreitens

anabolic anabolisch, aufbauend

anabolism Aufbaustoffwechsel *m*, Anabolismus *m*

anacamptometer Gerät *n* zur Messung der Reflexstärke

anachoresis Anachorese *f*

anaclisis Anlehnung *f*, emotionale Abhängigkeit *f*

anaclitic anaklitisch, Anlehnungs–, emotionell abhängig

anacoluthia Anakoluthie *f*, krankhafte Wort– und Silbenauslassungen *fpl*

anacoluthic anakoluth

anacousia, anacusia, anacusis völlige Taubheit *f*, Anakusis *f*

anadipsia unstillbarer Durst *m*

anaemia Anämie *f*

anaesthesia Anästhesie *f*, Empfindungslosigkeit *f*, Gefühllosigkeit *f* / **dissociative ~ and sensory loss** dissoziative Sensibilitäts– und Empfindungsstörungen *fpl* / **hysterical ~** hysterische Schmerz– und Empfindungslosigkeit *f* / **local ~** Lokalanästhesie *f*, örtliche Betäubung *f* / **moral ~** moralische Gefühllosigkeit *f* / **regional ~** örtliche Betäubung *f*, Lokalanästhesie *f* / **sexual ~** Frigidität *f*, sexuelle Gefühllosigkeit *f* / **spinal ~** Spinalanästhesie *f*, Leitungsanästhesie *f* der Spinalnerven / **tactile ~** Aufhebung *f* der Berührungsempfindlichkeit, taktile Anästhesie *f*

anaesthesiology Anästhesiologie *f*, Lehre *f* von der Schmerzausschaltung

anaesthetic unempfindlich, anästhetisch / Anästhetikum *n*, Betäubungsmitteln, Narkotikum *n* / **general ~** Allgemeinanästhetikum *n*, Narkosemittel *n* / **local ~** Lokalanästhetikum *n*

anaesthetisation Narkose *f*, Betäubung *f*, Anästhesie *f*

anaesthetise anästhesieren, betäuben, narkotisieren

anaesthetist Narkosefacharzt *m*, Anästhesist *m*

anaglyph Anaglyphe *f*, stereoskopes Bild *n*

anaglyphoscope, anaglyptoscope Gerät *n* zur Darstellung des perspektivischen Schlagschattens, Anaglyptoskop *n*

anagogic anagogisch, anagog, zum Geistigen hinaufführend

anagram Anagramm *n*, Buchstabenversetzrätsel *n* / **~ problem solving** Lösen *n* von Anagrammen

anal anal / **~-erotic** analerotisch / **~-expulsive** analexpulsiv / **~-retentive** analretentiv / **~-sadistic** analsadistisch

analeptic analeptisch, stärkend, belebend / Stärkungsmittel *n*, Anregungsmittel *n*, Analeptikum *n*

analgesia Gefühllosigkeit *f*, Schmerzunempfindlichkeit *f*, Analgesie *f*

analgesic, analgetic schmerzunempfindlich, schmerzstillend, analgetisch / Schmerzmittel *n*, Analgetikum *n* / **~**/ **~ addiction** Analgetikasucht *f*

analgesimeter Analgesimeter *n*, Gerät *n* zur Messung der Schmerzempfindlichkeit

analgia Schmerzlosigkeit *f*, Analgie *f*

analgize schmerzunempfindlich machen, Schmerzen aufheben

anality Analität *f*

analog, analogue Analogon *n*, Vergleichbares *n*, Ähnliches *n* / analog / **~ computer** Analogrechner *m* / **~ data** analoge Daten *npl* / **~ digital converter** Analog-Digital-Wandler *m*, Analog-Digital-Umsetzer *m* / **~ process** analoges Verfahren *n*, Analogieverfahren *n*

analogous analog, entsprechend

analogy Analogie *f* / **~ test** Analogietest *m*

analphabetism Analphabetentum *n*

analysand Analysand *m*, Person *f* die psychoanalytisch untersucht wird

analyse analysieren, genau untersuchen, bestimmen

analyser, analyzer Analytiker *m*, Analysator *m*, Zerstreuungsprisma *n* / **neural ~** Analysator *m* von Sinnesreizen, Nervenimpulsanlysator *m*

analysis Analyse *f*, Untersuchung *f* / **~ of consistency** Konsistenzanalyse *f* / **~ of covariance** Kovarianzanalyse *f* / **~ of data** Datenanalyse *f* / **~ of discrimination** Diskriminanzanalyse *f* / **~ of life history** Lebenslaufanalyse *f* / **~ of the ego** Ich-Analyse *f* / **~ of variance** Varianzanalyse *f* / **active ~** aktive Analyse *f* / **aspective ~** Aspektanalyse *f*, psychokulturelle Eigenschaftsanalyse *f* / **Bayesian ~** Bayes-Statistik *f* / **bi-factorial ~** Bifaktorenanalyse *f* / **blind ~** Blindanalyse *f*, Blindversuch *m* / **causal ~** Kausalanalyse *f* / **clinical ~** klinische Untersuchung *f* / **comparative ~** vergleichende Analyse *f*, Vergleichsanalyse *f* / **componential ~** Komponentenanalyse *f* / **controlled ~** kontrollierte Analyse *f* / **didactic ~** Lehranalyse *f* / **direct ~** direkte Analyse *f* / **discriminant ~** Diskriminanzanalyse *f* / **discriminatory ~** Diskriminanzanalyse *f* / **existential ~** Daseinsanalyse *f* / **figural ~** figurale Analyse *f* / **focused ~** gezielte Analyse *f* / **focal ~** Fokalanalyse *f* / **functional ~** Funktionsanalyse *f* / **graphic ~** graphische Auswertung *f* / **harmonic ~** Fourrier'sche Analyse *f* / **interactional ~** Interaktionsanalyse *f* / **lay ~** Laienanalyse *f* / **linguistic ~** sprachwissenschaftliche Analyse *f* / **meta ~** Metaanalyse *f* / **Mendelian ~** Erbanalyse *f* / **mental ~** Geistesanalyse *f* / **molar ~** molare Analyse *f* / **multivariate ~** multivariate Analyse *f* / **occupational ~** Arbeitsplatzanalyse *f*, Tätigkeitsanalyse *f* / **orthodox ~** orthodoxe Analyse *f* / **parametric ~** parametrischer Test *m* / **passive ~** passive Analyse *f* / **phonetic ~** Lautanalyse *f*, phonetische Analyse *f* / **qualitative ~** qualitative Analyse *f* / **quantitative ~** quantitative Analyse *f* / **reductive ~** Analyse *f*, Reduktionsanalyse *f* / **relational ~** Strukturanalyse *f*, Beziehungsanalyse *f* / **sequential ~** Sequenzanalyse *f*, sequentielle Analyse *f*, schrittweises Vorgehen *n* / **situational ~** Situationsanalyse *f* / **statistical ~** statistische Analyse *f* / **structural ~** Strukturanalyse *f* / **supervised ~** kontrollierte Analyse *f* / **supervisory ~** Kontrollanalyse *f* / **transactional ~** Transaktionsanalyse *f* / **urinary ~** Harnuntersuchung *f*, Urinanalyse *f* / **vectorial ~** Vektorenanalyse *f* / **wild ~** wilde Psychoanalyse *f*

analyst Analytiker *m*, Psychoanalytiker *m* / **lay ~** Laienanalytiker *m*

analytic, analytical analytisch

analytics Analytik *f*

analyzability Analysierbarkeit *f*

anamnesis Anamnese *f*, Vorgeschichte *f* eines Falles, Krankengeschichte *f* / **associative ~** Assoziationsanamnese *f*

anamnestic anamnestisch

anancasm, anancastia, anankastia Anankasmus *m*, Zwangsneurose *f*

anancastic anankastisch, zwangsneurotisch

anancotropic anankotrop, zu Zwangsneurosen neigend

ananda Ananda *f*, Glückseligkeit *f*, höchste Wonne *f*

anandria Unmännlichkeit *f*, männliche Impotenz *f*, Anandrie *f*

anaphia Tastsinnverlust *m*, Anaphie *f*

anaphrodisia Anaphrodisie *f*, Störung *f* der Geschlechtslust, Fehlen *n* des sexuellen Wollustgefühles

anaphrodisiac Anaphrodisiakum *n*, Geschlechtslust hemmendes Mittel *n*, Anaphrodisie hervorrufendes Mittel *n* / Geschlechtslust hemmend

anaphrodite geschlechtlichen Dingen abgeneigter Mensch *m*

anaphylaxis Überempfindlichkeit *f*, Anaphylaxie *f* / **psychic ~** psychische Überempfindlichkeit *f*

anarchy Anarchie *f*, Gesetzlosigkeit *f* / **political ~** politische Anarchie *f*

anarithmia Zählunvermögen *n*, Unfähigkeit *f* zu zählen

anarthria gestörte Sprachartikulation *f*, Anarthrie *f*

anarthric sprachgestört, unartikuliert, anarthrisch

anastigmatic ohne Astigmatismus, anastigmatisch

anatomical anatomisch

anatomy Anatomie *f* / **~ response** Anatomiedeutung *f*, Anatomieantwort *f* / **regional ~** topographische Anatomie *f* / **topographic ~** topographische Anatomie *f*

anaudia Artikulationsunvermögen *n*, Sprachverlust *m*

ancestor Vorfahr *m*, Ahn *m* / **~ worship** Ahnenkult *m*

anchor ankern, verankern / Anker *m*, Bezugspunkt *m* / **~ age** Bezugsalter *n* / **internal ~** innerer Bezugspunkt *m*

anchorage Bezugssystem *n*, Bezugspunkt *m*, Bezug *m* / **~ effect** Auswirkung *f* des Bezugssystems / **interdisciplinary ~** interdisziplinäres Bezugssystem *n* / **social ~** soziales Bezugssystem *n*

anchoring Bezug *m*, Verankerung *f* / **~ of ego** Ich–Verankerung *f*, Identifikation *f* / **~ point** Bezugspunkt *m* / **perceptual ~** Wahrnehmung *f* innerhalb eines Bezugssystems / **social ~** sozialer Bezug *m*

ancillary Hilfs–, untergeordnet

andragogic andragogisch, Erwachsenenbildung betreffend

andragogics Erwachsenenbildung *f*, Andragogik *f*

androgen männliches Geschlechtshormon *n*, Androgen *n*

androgenic, androgenous androgen, männliches Hormon betreffend

androgyne Hermaphrodit *m*, Zwitter *m*

androgyneity, androgynism, androgyny Hermaphroditismus *m*, Androgynie *f*, Zwittertum *n*

androgynous androgyn

andromania Nymphomanie *f*, Andromanie *f*, Mannstollheit *f*

andropause Andropause *f*, Aufhören *n* der sexuellen Funktion beim Manne

androphany männlicher Habitus *m* einer Frau

androphobia Androphobie *f*, Männerscheu *f*, Angst *f* vor Männern

androphonomania Androphonomanie *f*, Mordsucht *f*

androsterone Androsteron *n*

anecdotal anekdotisch

anechoic echofrei

anelectrotonus Anelektrotonus *m*

anemia Anämie *f*

anemometer Windmesser *m*

anemophobia Angst *f* vor Wind, Anemophobie *f*

anemotropism, anemotaxis Anemotropismus *m*, Anemotaxis *f*, Orientierung *f* zur Windrichtung

anencephalia, anencephaly Anenzephalie *f*, Fehlen *n* des Hirns

anencephalic hirnlos, anenzephal

aneneia Taubstummheit *f*, Hörstummheit *f*

anepia Unfähigkeit *f* zu sprechen

anergasia Anergasie *f*, herabgesetzte oder fehlende Funktion *f*, Herabsetzung *f* der funktionalen Aktivität, Intelligenzdefekt *m*

anergastic anergastisch, fehlende Funktion betreffend

anergia, anergy Anenergie *f*, Anergie *f*, Energiemangel *m*, Mangel *m* an Aktivitat, Asthenie *f* / **producing ~~** schlafmachend, passiv machend

anergic energielos, anergisch, anergetisch

anerotism Anerosie *f*, Anerotismus *m*, Fehlen *n* erotischer Gefühle, mangelnde Geschlechtslust *f*

anerythroblepsia, anerythropsia Rotblindheit *f*, Anerythropsie *f*

anesthesia, anesthesis Anästhesie *f*, Empfindungslosigkeit *f*, Gefühllosigkeit *f* / **general ~~** Allgemeinnarkose *f* / **hysterical ~~** hysterische Schmerz– und Empfindungslosigkeit *f* / **sexual ~~** Frigidität *f*, sexuelle Gefühllosigkeit *f*

anesthesiology Anästhesiologie *f*, Lehre *f* von der Schmerzausschaltung

anesthetic unempfindlich, anästhetisch / Anästhetikum *n*, Betäubungsmitteln, Narkotikum *n*

anesthetist Narkosefacharzt *m*, Anästhesist *m*

anesthetization Narkose *f*, Betäubung *f*, Anästhesierung *f*

anesthetize anästhesieren, betäuben, narkotisieren

aneuria mangelnde Nervenkraft *f*

aneuric nervenschwach

aneurin, aneurine Aneurin *n*, Vitamin B_1 *n*

aneurysm Aneurysma *n*

anger Wut *f*, Zorn *m*, Ärger *m*, Unwille *m* / **~ call** Wutschrei *m* / **~ control** Ärgerkontrolle *f* / **sudden ~** Jähzorn *m*

angiasthenia Gefäßschwäche *f*, Labilität *f* der Gefäßnerven, Angiasthenie *f*

anginophobia Anginophobie *f*, Angst *f* vor Angina pectoris, Angst *f* vor einem Angina pectoris Anfall

angiography Röntgenaufnahme *f* der Gefäße, Angiographie *f*, Vasographie *f*, Gefäßdarstellung *f*

angioneurosis Gefäßneurose *f*, Vasoneurose *f*, Angioneurose *f* neurotische Störung *f* des Vasomotorensystems

angiospasm Gefäßkrampf *m*, Angiospasmus *m*

angiostenosis Gefäßverengung *f*, Angiostenose *f*

angiotensin Angiotensin *n* / **~ase** Angiotensinase *f* / **~ogen** Angiotensinogen *n*

angiotonase Angiotensinase *f*

angle Winkel *m* / **~ of aberration** Aberrationswinkel *m* / **~ of convergence** Konvergenzwinkel *m* / **~ of emission** Austrittswinkel *m* / ~ **illusion** Winkeltäuschung *f* / ~ **of incidence** Einfallswinkel *m* / ~ **of inclination** Neigungswinkel *m* / ~ **of refraction** Brechungswinkel *m* / **facial** ~ Gesichtswinkel *m*, Sehwinkel *m* / **optic** ~ Sehwinkel *m*, Gesichtswinkel *m* / **visual** ~ Sehwinkel *m*, Gesichtswinkel *m*

angophrasia Angophrasie *f*, stoßweises Sprechen *n* und Einschieben *n* unartikulierter Laute, Embolophrasie *f*, Gaxen *n*

angry zornig, böse, aufgebracht

angström unit Angströmeinheit *f*

anguish Pein *f*, Qual *f*, qualvolle Angst *f* / ~ **of mind** Seelenqual *f*

angular winklig, eckig, ungelenk, steif

angularity Ungelenkigkeit *f*, steifes Benehmen *n*, Unumgänglichkeit *f*, Steifheit *f*

anhedonia Anhedonie *f*, affektive Verödung *f*, Fehlen *n* des sexuellen Wollustgefühls

anhidrosis, anidrosis verminderte Schweißabsonderung *f*, Anhidrosis *f*

anhormia Antriebsstörung *f*, Antriebsmangel *m*, Anhormie *f*

anhydrase Anhydrase *f* / **carbonic** ~ Carboanhydrase *f*, Kohlensäureanhydratase *f*

anianthinopsy Violettblindheit *f*

aniconia Fehlen *n* der bildlichen Vorstellung

aniconic das Fehlen der bildlichen Vorstellung betreffend

anideation fehlende Ideenbildung *f*, mangelnde Vorstellung *f*

anile altweiberlich

anilinction, anilinctus Anilingus *m*

anima Anima *f*, Seele *f*

animal Tier *n*, Lebewesen *n* / animalisch, tierisch, sinnlich / ~ **aggressive behaviour** Aggressionsverhalten *n* bei Tieren / ~**-assisted therapy** tierunterstützte Therapie *f* / ~ **behaviour** Tierverhalten *n* / ~ **biological rhythm** biologischer Rhythmus *m* bei Tieren / ~ **breeding** Tierzucht *f*, Aufzuchtverhalten *n* bei Tieren / ~ **captivity** gefangenlebendes Tier *n* / ~ **circadian rhythm** tierischer Schlaf–Wach–Rhythmus *m*, Tagesrhythmus *m* bei Tieren / ~ **coloration** Körperfärbung *f* bei Tieren / ~ **communication** Tiersprache *f*, Kommunikation *f* bei Tieren / ~ **content** Tierdeutung *f*, Tierantwort *f* / ~ **courtship behaviour** Werbeverhalten *n* bei Tieren / ~ **courtship display** Werberitual *n* bei Tieren / ~ **defensive behaviour** Verteidigungsverhalten *n* bei Tieren / ~ **development** Entwicklung *f* bei Tieren / ~ **distress call** Klageschrei *m* bei Tieren / ~ **division of labour** Arbeitsteilung *f* bei Tieren / ~ **domestication** Domestikation *f* von Tieren / ~ **dominance** Dominanzverhalten *n* bei Tieren / ~ **drinking behaviour** Trinkverhalten *n* bei Tieren / ~ **emotionality** Emotionalität *f* bei Tieren / ~ **environment** Tierumwelt *f* / ~ **escape behaviour** Fluchtverhalten *n* bei Tieren / ~ **ethology** Tierethologie *f*, Wissenschaft *f* vom tierischen Verhalten / ~ **experiment** Tierversuch *m* / ~ **exploratory behaviour** Explorationsverhalten *n* bei Tieren / ~ **feeding behaviour** Fütterungsverhalten *n* bei Tieren / ~ **figure** Tierfigur *f*, Tierform *f* / ~ **grooming behaviour** Putzverhalten *n* bei Tieren / ~ **hoarding behaviour** tierisches Hamsterverhalten *n*, Vorratssammeln *n* bei Tieren / ~ **homing** Heimkehrverhalten *n* bei Tieren / ~ **locomotion** Fortbewegungsverhalten *n* bei Tieren / ~ **mate selection** Partnerwahl *f* bei Tieren / ~ **maternal behaviour** Mutterverhalten *n* bei Tieren / ~ **maternal deprivation** Mutterdeprivation *f* bei Tieren / ~ **mating behaviour** Paarungsverhalten *n* bei Tieren / ~ **migratory behaviour** Wanderverhalten *n* bei Tieren / ~ **model** Tiermodell *n* / ~ **motivation** Motivation *f* bei Tieren / ~ **navigation** tierische Orientierung *f* / ~ **nocturnal behaviour** Nachtverhalten *n* von Tieren / ~ **open field behaviour** tierisches Verhalten *n* in Freiheit / ~ **parental behaviour** Elternverhalten *n* bei Tieren / ~ **paternal behaviour** Vaterverhalten *n* bei Tieren / ~ **play** Spielverhalten *n* bei Tieren / ~ **predatory behaviour** tierisches Raubverhalten *n* / ~ **rearing** Aufzucht *f* von Tieren / ~ **psychology** Tierpsychologie *f* / ~ **scent marking** Reviermarkierung *f* / ~ **sex difference** Geschlechtsunterschied *m* bei Tieren / ~ **sexual behaviour** Sexualverhalten *n* bei Tieren / ~ **sexual receptivity** Empfängnisfähigkeit *f* bei Tieren / ~ **social behaviour** tierisches Sozialverhalten *n* / ~ **sociology** Tiersoziologie *f* / ~ **strain differences** Rassemerkmale *npl* bei Tieren / ~ **totemism** Tiertotemismus *m* / ~ **type** Tier–Typus *m* / ~ **vocalisation** Lautbildung *f* bei Tieren, Vokalisation *f* bei Tieren / ~ **welfare** Tierschutz *m* / **experimental** ~ Versuchstier *n* / **macrosmatic** ~ Lebewesen *n* mit besonders gutem Riechvermögen / **microsmatic** ~ Lebewesen *n* mit schwach entwickeltem Riechvermögen / **sociable** ~**s** Gesellschaftstiere *npl* / **spinal** ~ Rückenmarkstier *n*

animalism Animalismus *m*, Lebenstrieb *m*, Sinnlichkeit *f*

animality Tierheit *f*, Tiernatur *f*

animate beleben, anregen, stimulieren, motivieren / belebt, beseelt, angeregt

animation Belebtsein *n*, Anregung *f*, Stimulierung *f*, Motivation *f*

animism, animatism Animismus *m*, Naturbeseelung *f*

animistic animistisch

animosity Animosität *f*, Hass *m*, Feindseligkeit *f*

animus Animus *m*, Seele *f*

anion Anion *n*

aniseikonia, aniseiconia Größendisparität *f* der Netzhautbilder, Aniseikonie *f*

anisocoria ungleiche Pupillenweite *f*, Pupillendifferenz *f*

anisodominance ungleiche Dominanz *f*

anisometrope Anisometroper *m*, Mensch *m* mit verschieden brechenden Augen

anisometropia Anisometropie *f*, ungleiche Brechkraft *f* beider Augen

anisometropic anisometrop, mit verschiedener Brechkraft beider Augen

anisophoria latentes Höhenschielen *n*, Anisophorie *f*

anisopia Anisopie *f*, ungleiche Sehqualität *f* beider Augen

anisotropy Anisotropie *f*, Verschiedenartigkeit *f* der Raumwahrnehmung

anisotropic, anisotropous anisotrop, heterotrop

ankle Fußknöchel *m* / ~ **clonus** Fußklonus *m* / ~ **reflex** Achillessehnenreflex *m*

annihilate vernichten, zerstören

annihilation Vernichtung *f*, völlige Zerstörung *f*

anniversary reaction Jahrestagsreaktion *f*

annoyance Störung *f*, Beunruhigung *f*

annoyer unangenehmer Reiz *m*

annoying störend, lästig

annulment Ungeschehenmachen *n* / ~ **of marriage** Aufhebung *f* der Ehe

anodal Anoden–

anode Anode *f* / ~ **break excitation** Anodenöffnungserregung *f*

anodyne schmerzstillendes Mittel *n*, Schmerzlinderungsmittel *n* / schmerzstillend

anoegenetic anoogen, keine neuen Erkenntnisse erzielend

anoesia Unverstand *m*, Stumpfsinn *m*, Stupor *m*, Blödsinn *m*, Anoia *f*, Idiotie *f*

anoesis Anoese *f*

anoestrous paarungsungünstig

anoestrum, anoestrus paarungsungünstige Zeit *f*, Anöstrus *m*

anoetic ohne Verstandesbeteiligung, anoetisch, stumpfsinnig, idiotisch

anoia Idiotie *f*, Schwachsinn *m*, Stupor *m*

anomaloscope Anomaloskop *n*, Apparat *m* zur Erkennung von Farbenblindheit

anomalous anomal, abnorm, abweichend, abartig, ungewöhnlich

anomaly Anomalie *f*, Abnormität *f*, Abartigkeit *f*, Abweichung *f* vom Normalen, Fehlanlage *f* / **sexual ~** sexuelle Abartigkeit *f*

anomia Anomie *f*

anomic orientierungslos, vereinsamt, sozial disintegriert

anomie, anomy, anomia Anomie *f*, Gesetzlosigkeit *f*, innere Orientierungslosigkeit *f*, Zustand *m* der Vereinsamung, soziale Disintegration *f*

anonymity Anonymität *f*

anonymous anonym, namenlos

anoopsia, anopsia Aufwärtsschielen *n*, Anopsie *f*

anoretic appetitlos, appetitzügelnd, anorektisch

anorexia Anorexie *f*, Appetitlosigkeit *f*, Inappetenz *f* / **~ nervosa** Anorexia nervosa *f*, Pubertätsmagersucht *f* / **atypical ~ nervosa** atypische Anorexia nervosa *f*

anorexiant Appetitzügler *m*, Appetithemmer *m*, Anorektikum *n*

anorexic appetitlos, appetitzügelnd, anorektisch

anorgasmy Ausbleiben *n* des Orgasmus beim Koitus, Anorgasmie *f*

anorthography motorische Agraphie *f*, Anorthographie *f*

anorthopia Schielen *n*, Strabismus *m*, verzerrtes Sehen *n*

anorthoscope Stroboskop *n*

anosmia Anosmie *f*, Geruchsblindheit *f*, Fehlen *n* des Geruchssinnes / **partial ~** partielle Anosmie *f*

anosmic, anosmatic anosmisch, ohne Geruchssinn

anosognosia Anosognosie *f*, Uneinsichtigkeit *f*

anosphrasia, anosphresia Geruchsverlust *m*

anoxia, anoxaemia, anoxemia Sauerstoffmangel *m*, Anoxie *f* / **cerebral ~** Sauerstoffmangel *m* des Gehirns

answer Antwort *f*, Reaktion *f* / reagieren, antworten, beantworten / **~ key** Antwortschlüssel *m* / **selective-~ test** Test *m* mit Wahlantworten / **short-~ test** Test *m* mit gebundener Aufgabenbeantwortung

ant Ameise *f*

Antabuse Antabus *n*, Disulfiram *n*

antagonism Antagonismus *m*, Gegenwirkung *f*, Gegensatz *m* / **~ of muscles** Muskelgegenwirkung *f*

antagonist Antagonist *m*, Gegenmuskel *m*, antagonistischer Muskel *m* / **narcotic ~** Gegenmittel *n* zu Narkotika, Betäubungsmittelantagonist *m*, Opiatantagonist *m*

antagonistic antagonistisch, entgegenwirkend, entgegengesetzt wirksam

antalgic schmerzlinderndes Mittel *n*, Analgetikum *n*

antaphrodisiac Antiaphrodisiakum *n*, den Geschlechtstrieb reduzierendes Mittel *n*

antecedent vorhergehend, vorausgegangen, früher / **~s** vorausgegangene Ereignisse *npl*, Vorleben *n*, frühere Erlebnisse *npl*

antedating antizipatorisch, vorhergehend, vorempfindend

antenatal pränatal, vorgeburtlich

antenna Fühler *m*, Fühlhorn *n*, Antenne *f*

antergia, antergy Widerstand *m*, Gegenwirkung *f*, Antagonismus *m*

antergic antagonistisch, entgegenwirkend

anterior Vorder–, vorne liegend

anterograde anterograd, vorangehend

anthophobia krankhafte Angst *f* vor Blumen

anthropobiology Anthropobiologie *f*, Biologie *f* des Menschen und der Menschenaffen

anthropocentric anthropozentrisch, den Menschen in den Mittelpunkt stellend

anthropocentrism Anthropozentrismus *m*

anthropogenesis, anthropogeny Entwicklungsgeschichte *f* des Menschen, Anthropogenese *f*, Anthropogenie *f*

anthropogenetic anthropogenetisch, anthropogon

anthropognomics Anthropognomik *f*, menschliche Wesens– und Erkenntnislehre *f*

anthropoid anthropoid, menschenähnlich / Anthropoid *m*, Menschenaffe *m*

anthropoidea pl Menschenaffen *mpl*, Anthropoide *mpl*, Menschen *mpl* und Menschenaffen *mpl*

anthropological anthropologisch

anthropologist Anthropologe *m*

anthropology Anthropologie *f*, Lehre *f* vom Menschen / **applied ~** angewandte Anthropologie *f* / **criminal ~** Kriminalanthropologie *f* / **cultural ~** Kulturanthropologie *f* / **physical ~** Somatologie *f*, Körperlehre *f* / **social ~** Sozialanthropologie *f*, Kulturanthropologie *f*

anthropometric anthropometrisch

anthropometry Anthropometrie *f*, Körpermessung *f*

anthropomorphic, anthropomorphous anthropomorph, menschenähnlich

anthropomorphism Anthropomorphismus *m*

anthroponomy Verhaltenslehre *f*, Lehre *f* vom menschlichen Verhalten, Behaviorismus *m*, Anthroponomie *f*

anthropopathy Anthropomorphismus *m*

anthropophagy Menschenfresserei *f*, Kannibalismus *m*, Anthropophagie *f*

anthropophobia Menschenscheu *f*, Anthropophobie *f*

anthropophobic menschenscheu

anthroposcopy Typeneinteilung *f* nach dem Erscheinungsbild

anthroposophy Anthroposophie *f*

anthypnotic schlafverhindernd / schlafverhinderndes Mittel *n*

antialcoholic Antialkoholiker *m*

antiandrogen Antiandrogen *n*

antibiotic Antibiotikum *n* / antibiotisch

antibody Antikörper *m*

anticathexis Gegenbesetzung *f*

anticholinesterase Anticholinesterase *f* / **~ drug** Azetylcholinesterase–Hemmer *m*

anticipate vorwegnehmen, erwarten, antizipieren, ahnen

anticipation Vorwegnahme *f*, Erwartung *f*, Antizipation *f* / **~ anxiety** Erwartungsangst *f* / **~ error** Erwartungsfehler *m* / **~ image** Erwartungsvorstellung *f*, Zielvorstellung *f* / **~ response** Erwartungsfehler *m*, Erwartungsreaktion *f* / **serial ~** serielle Antizipation *f* / **serial ~ method** Souffliermethode *f*, Methode *f* der Lernhilfen

anticipative, anticipatory vorwegnehmend, erwartend, vorgreifend, antizipatorisch

anticonceptive empfängnisverhütend

anticoncipiens Empfängnisverhütungsmittel *n*, antikonzeptionelles Mittel *n*

anticonvulsant krampflösend, krampfhemmend, antikonvulsiv / Krampfmittel *n*, Antikonvulsivum *n*

anticonvulsive krampflösend, krampfhemmend, antikonvulsiv / Krampfmittel *n*, Antikonvulsivum *n*

anti–democratic antidemokratisch

antidepressant antidepressiv / Antidepressivum *n* / **tricyclic ~s** trizyklische Antidepressiva *npl*, Trizyklika *npl*

antidepressive antidepressiv

antidiuresis Antidiurese *f*

antidromic gegenläufig, antidrom

antiemetic antiemetisch, gegen Erbrechen wirkend / Antiemetikum *n*, Mittel *n* gegen Erbrechen

antieroticum die Geschlechtslust herabsetzendes Mittel *n*, Antiaphrodisiakum *n*

antiestrogen Antiöstrogen *n*, Östrogenhemmer *m*

antifetishism Antifetischismus *m*

antigen Antigen *n* / **~–antibody complex** Antigen–Antikörperkomplex *m* / **~–antibody–reaction** Antigen–Antikörperreaktion *f*

antihistamine Antihistaminikum *n*, Antihistamin *n*

antihistaminic antihistaminisch

antihormone Gegenhormon *n*, Antihormon *n*

antihygienic unhygienisch, unsauber

anti–intellectualism Anti–Intellektualismus *m*

anti–intraception Ablehnung *f* von individuellen Gefühlsäußerungen und Nachgiebigkeit

antikinesis Antikinese *f*

antimetropia Brechungsgegenläufigkeit *f* der Augen, Brechungsdisparität *f* der Augen

antinarcotic gegen Rauschgifte wirksam / Antinarkotikum *n*

antineuralgic antineuralgisch, Neuralgie behebend

antineurotic antineurotisch

antinomy Antinomie *f*, Widerspruch *m* in sich selbst

antinormative antinormativ, gegen die Norm gerichtet

antiovulant Ovulationshemmer *m*

antipathetic, antipathetical antipathisch, Antipathie hervorrufend

antipathy Antipathie *f*, Abneigung *f*, Widerwille *m*

antiphone Lärmschutzmittel *n*

antipsychotic antipsychotisch

anti–Semitism Antisemitismus *m*

antisocial asozial, unsozial, antisozial, gesellschaftsfeindlich

antisocialism gesellschaftsfeindliche Haltung *f*

antithesis Antithese *f*, Gegensatz *m* / **~ of primal words** Gegensinn *m* der Urworte / **neurotic ~** neurotische Antithese *f*

antithetical antithetisch, gegensätzlich

antitoxin Antitoxin *n*, Gegengift *n*, Abwehrstoff *m*

antonym Antonym *n*, entgegengesetzter Begriff *m* / **~ test** Antonymentest *m*

antuitary den Hypophysenvorderlappen betreffend

anuresis, anuria Harnverhaltung *f*

anus Anus *m*, After *m*

anvil Amboss *m* des Ohres

anxiety Angst *f*, Angstzustand *m* / **~ affect** Angstaffekt *m* / **~ attack** Angstanfall *m* / **~ battery** Angsttest *m* / **~–cathected** angstbesetzt / **~ complex** Angstkomplex *m* / **~ component** Angstkomponente *f* / **~ condition** Angstzustand *m* / **~ conservation** Angsterhaltung *f* / **~ depression** Angstdepression *f*, ängstliche Depression *f* / **~ discharge** Angstabfuhr *f* / **~ disorder** Angststörung *f* / **~ disorder due to a general medical condition** Angststörung *f* aufgrund eines medizinischen Krankheitsfaktors / **amphetamine–induced ~ disorder** amphetamininduzierte Angststörung *f* / **atypical ~ disorder** atypisches Angstsyndrom *n* / **generalized ~ disorder** generalisierte Angststörung *f*, generalisiertes Angstsyndrom *n* / **hallucinogen–induced ~ disorder** halluzinogeninduzierte Angststörung *f* / **mixed ~ disorder** gemischte Angststörung *f* / **mixed ~ and depressive disorder** Angst *f* und depressive Störung *f*, gemischt / **organic ~ disorder** organische Angststörung *f* / **~ dream** Angsttraum *m* / **~ equivalent** Angstäquivalent *n* / **~ fit** anfallsweiser Angstzustand *m* / **~ fixation** Angstfixierung *f* / **~ hierarchy** Angsthierarchie *f* / **~ hysteria** Angsthysterie *f* / **~ indicator** Angstindikator *m* / **~ management** Angstverarbeitung *f* / **~ management training** Angstbewältigungstraining *n* / **~ neurosis** Angstneurose *f*, Angstzustand *m* / **~ object** Angstobjekt *n* / **~–phobic behaviour** durch eine Angstphobie bestimmtes Verhalten *n* / **~ pleasure** Angstlust *f* / **~ preparedness** Angstbereitschaft *f* / **~ reaction** Angstreaktion *f* / **~ readiness** Angstbereitschaft *f* / **~–reducing drug** Anxiolytikum *n*, Mittel *n* gegen Angst / **~ regression** Angstregression *f* / **~ relief response** Angstunterbrechungsreaktion *f* / **~ response** Angstreaktion *f* / ~ **scale** Angsttest *m* / ~ **situation** Angstsituation *f* / ~ **state** Angstzustand *m* / ~ **symptom** Angstsymptom *n* / ~ **tolerance** Angsttoleranz *f* / **actual** ~ Aktualangst *f* / **anticipatory** ~ Erwartungsangst *f* / **automatic** ~ automatische Angst *f* / **basal** ~ grundsätzliche Angst *f* / **basic** ~ Urangst *f* / **depressive** ~ Depressionsangst *f* / **episodic paroxysmal** ~ episodisch paroxysmale Angst *f* / **erotized** ~ Angstliebe *f* / **expectant** ~ Erwartungsangst *f* / **free** ~ latente Angst *f* / **free floating** ~ freiflottierende Angst *f* / **high unbound** ~ hohe ungebundene Angst *f* / **instinctual** ~ Triebangst *f*, instinktive Angst *f* / **manifest** ~ manifeste Angst *f* / **manifest** ~ **scale** Test *m* der manifesten Angst / **moral** ~ Gewissensangst *f* / **neurotic** ~ neurotische Angst *f* / **objective** ~ objektive Angst *f* / **oral** ~ orale Angst *f* / **organic** ~ organisch bedingte Angst *f* / **organic** ~ **syndrome** organisch bedingtes Angstsyndrom *n* / **other** ~ **disorders** sonstige Angststörungen *fpl* / **over–**~ übertriebene Ängstlichkeit *f* / **pervasive** ~ durchdringende Angst *f* / **phobic** ~ **disorder** phobische Störung *f* / **phobic** ~ **disorder of childhood** phobische Störung *f* des Kindesalters / **phobic** ~ **disorder, unspecified** nicht näher bezeichnete phobische Störung *f* / **precordial** ~ Herzangst *f* / **prepared for** ~ angstbereit / **primal** ~ Urangst *f* / **ready for** ~ angstbereit / **real** ~ objektive Angst *f*, Realangst *f* / **realistic** ~ Realangst *f* / **situational** ~ Situationsangst *f* / **social** ~ soziale Angst *f* / **social** ~ **disorder of childhood** Störung *f* mit sozialer Ängstlichkeit des Kindesalters / **unattached** ~ freiflottierende Angst *f*

anxiolysis Anxiolyse *f*

anxiolytic angstlösend / Anxiolytikum *n*

anxious ängstlich, bange, besorgt, unruhig

anxiousness Ängstlichkeit *f*, Angst *f*, Besorgtheit *f*

apareunia Unfähigkeit *f* den Koitus zu vollziehen, Unfähigkeit *f* Geschlechtsverkehr zu haben

apartheid Rassentrennung *f*, getrennte Rassenentwicklung *f*, Apartheid *f*

apathetic apathisch, teilnahmslos, stumpf, gefühllos, gleichgültig, ohne Antrieb

apathy Apathie *f*, Teilnahmslosigkeit *f*, Gleichgültigkeit *f*, Indifferenz *f*, Desinteresse *n*, Affektlosigkeit *f*, geistige Stumpfheit *f* / ~ **syndrome** Apathie–Syndrom *n* / **mental** ~ Denkfaulheit *f* / **sceptical** ~ skeptische Zurückhaltung *f*

ape Menschenaffe *m* / nachäffen, nachmachen / **anthropoid** ~ Menschenaffe *m*

aperiodic unregelmäßig

aperture Öffnung *f*, Blende *f* / ~ **colour** Flächenfarbe *f*

apex beat Herzspitzenstoß *m*

aphacic, aphakic, aphakial ohne Linse, aphakisch

aphagia Unfähigkeit *f* zu schlucken, Aphagie *f* / **algesic** ~ Aphagia algera *f*

aphakia, aphacia Fehlen *n* der Augenlinse, Aphakie *f*

aphanisis Aphanisis *f*, Verschwinden *n* des sexuellen Bedürfnisses

aphasia Aphasie *f*, Sprachstörung *f* / ~ **area** Aphasieareal *n*, Aphasiezone *f* / ~ **universalis** verbale Aphasie *f* / ~ **zone** Aphasiezone *f*, Aphasieareal *n*/ ~ Worttaubheit *f*, Sprachtaubheit *f*, Aphasie *f* / **acquired** ~ **with epilepsy (Landau–Kleffner syndrome)** erworbene Aphasie *f* mit Epilepsie (Landau–Kleffner Syndrom) / **amnesic** ~ amnestische Aphasie *f* / **anomic** ~ anomische Aphasie *f* / **ataxic** ~ motorische Aphasie *f*, Wortstummheit *f* / **auditory** ~ Worttaubheit *f*, Sprachtaubheit *f*, Aphasie *f* / **commissural** ~ Leitungsaphasie *f* / **complete** ~ vollständige Aphasie *f* / **cortical** ~ kortikale Aphasie *f* / **cortical motor** ~ kortikale motorische Aphasie *f*, Broca–Aphasie *f* / **cortical sensory** ~ kortikale sensorische Aphasie *f*, Wernicke–Aphasie *f* / **de-**

velopmental ~ Entwicklungsaphasie *f* / **emotional** ~ Affektaphasie *f*, Schreckaphasie *f* / **expressive** ~ motorische Aphasie *f* / **global** ~ globale Aphasie *f* / **grapho–motor** ~ Verlust *m* der Schreibfähigkeit, Schriftverlust *m*, Aphasie *f* / **manual** ~ Agraphie *f* / **motor** ~ motorische Aphasie *f*, Aphemie *f* / **musical** ~ musikalische Aphasie *f*, Notenblindheit *f* / **nominal** ~ Namensaphasie *f* / **optic** ~ optische Aphasie *f* / **parieto–occipital** ~ kombinierte Aphasie *f* und Apraxie *f* / **partial** ~ Paraphasie *f* / **perceptive** ~ Wortblindheit *f* / **receptive** ~ sensorische Aphasie *f* / **semantic** ~ semantische Aphasie *f* / **sensory** ~ sensorische Aphasie *f*, Sprachtaubheit *f*, Worttaubheit *f* / **subcortical** ~ subkortikale Aphasie *f* / **subcortical motor** ~ subkortikale motorische Aphasie *f* / **subcortical sensory** ~ subkortikale sensorische Aphasie *f* / **syntactical** ~ Agrammatismus *m*, syntaktische Aphasie *f* / **temporoparietal** ~ kortikale sensorische Aphasie *f*, Wernicke–Aphasie *f* / **total** ~ totale Aphasie *f* / **transcortical** ~ transkortikale Aphasie *f* / **transcortical motor** ~ transkortikale motorische Aphasie *f* / **transcortical sensory** ~ transkortikale sensorische Aphasie *f* / **verbal** ~ verbale Aphasie *f* / **visual** ~ Alexie *f*, Buchstabenblindheit *f*, Schriftblindheit *f*, Wortblindheit *f*

aphasiac, aphasic aphasisch, aphatisch / Aphasiekranker *m*

aphemaesthesia Wortblindheit *f* und Worttaubheit *f*

aphemia Aphemie *f*, motorische Aphasie *f*, Wortstummheit *f*

aphemic aphatisch, aphasisch / Aphasiekranke *m*

aphonia, aphony Aphonie *f*, Stimmlosigkeit *f*, Sprachverlust *m*, Stimmverlust *m* / **functional** ~ funktionelle Aphonie *f* / **hysterical** ~ hysterische Stimmlosigkeit *f*

aphonic, aphonous aphonisch, stimmlos, ohne Stimme, klanglos

aphrasia Aphrasie *f*, Satztaubheit *f*, Unvermögen *n* ganze Sätze zu sprechen / **amnesic** ~ amnestische Aphrasie *f*

aphrenia Aphrenie *f*, Demenz *f*, Blödsinn *m*

aphrodisia Aphrodisie *f*, gesteigerte Geschlechtslust *f*, gesteigerter Sexualtrieb *m*

aphrodisiac aphroditisch, den Geschlechtstrieb anregend, den Geschlechtstrieb reizend / Aphrodisiakum *n*, den Geschlechtstrieb anregendes Mittel *n*

aphrodisiomania Aphrodisiomanie *f*, Liebeszwang *m*, krankhaft gesteigerter Geschlechtstrieb *m*

aphronesia Verwirrtheit *f*, Blödsinn *m*, Orientierungsverlust *m*

aphtongia Reflexaphasie *f*, Aphthongie *f*, Sprechkrampf *m*

apiphobia Apiphobie *f*, krankhafte Angst *f* vor Bienen

apish affenartig, nachäffend, nachmachend, albern

aplasia mangelnde Entwicklung *f* eines Organes, Fehlen *n* eines Organes, Aplasie *f*

aplastic aplastisch, unterentwickelt

apnoea, apnea Apnoe *f*, Atemstillstand *m*, Atemlähmung *f*

apochromatic aberrationsfrei, apochromatisch

apodemialgia Wandertrieb *m*, Heimatflucht *f*, Wandersucht *f*

apoenzyme Apoenzym *n*, Apoferment *n*, Zwischenferment *n*

apollonian apollinisch, harmonisch, ausgeglichen, maßvoll

apomorphine Apomorphin *n* / ~ **hydrochloride** Apomorphinhydrochlorid *n*

apopathetic apopathetisch, sich aufspielend, angeberisch

apoplectic apoplektisch, Schlaganfall–

apoplexia, apoplexy Apoplexie *f*, Gehirnschlag *m*, Schlaganfall *m*, Schlag *m*, apoplektischer Anfall *m* / ~ **hysterica** Apoplexia hysterica *f* / **cerebellar** ~ Kleinhirnapoplexie *f* / **cerebral** ~ Gehirnschlag *m*, Gehirnapoplexie *f* / **fulminating** ~

plötzliche, blitzartige Apoplexie *f* / **functional ~** funktionelle Apoplexie *f*, hysterische Apoplexie *f* / **meningeal ~** durch Hirnhautblutung verursachte Apoplexie *f* / **nervous ~** funktionelle Apoplexie *f*, hysterische Apoplexie *f*

apopnixis hysterisches Erstickungsgefühl *n*, Apopnixis *f*, Globus hystericus *m*

apoptosis Apoptose *f*

a posteriori empirisch, induktiv, von der Wirkung auf die Ursache schließend, a posteriori

apostilb Apostilb *n*

apotropaic apotropaisch, das Böse abwendend

apotropaism Vornahme *f* magischer Handlungen zur Abwendung des Bösen

apparatus Apparat *m*, Gerät *n*, Instrument *n*, Vorrichtung *f* / **~ of the mind** psychischer Apparat *m*, seelischer Apparat *m* / **genital ~** Geschlechtsapparat *m* / **jumping ~** Sprungapparat *m* / **measuring–~** Messgerät *n*, Messapparat *m* / **mental ~** psychischer Apparat *m* / **olfactory ~** Geruchsapparat *m* / **psychic ~** psychischer Apparat *m* / **vestibular ~** Vestibularapparat *m* / **visual ~** Sehapparat *m* / **vocal ~** Stimmapparat *m* / **transistorized ~** Transistorgerät *n*

apparent offenbar, augenscheinlich, sichtbar, anscheinend, scheinbar, Schein–

apparition Erscheinung *f*, Halluzination *f*, Geist *m*, Phantom *n*

appeal Aufforderungscharakter *m*, Anziehungskraft *f* / **~ erg** Appellationsmotiv *n* / **long–circuit ~** lang dauernder Aufforderungscharakter *m* / **short–circuit ~** kurz dauernder Aufforderungscharakter *m*

appearance Erscheinen *n*, äußeres Erscheinungsbild *n*, Auftreten *n* / **general ~** Allgemeinbild *n*, Aussehen *n*, Allgemeinerscheinung *f* / **outward ~** Äußeres *n* / **physical ~** äußere Erscheinung *n*, Habitus *m* / **visual ~** sichtbares Erscheinungsbild *n*

appeasement, appeasing Beruhigung *f*, Beschwichtigung *f* / **~ behaviour** Beschwichtigungsverhalten *n*, Befriedungsverhalten *n* / **~ gesture** beruhigende Geste *f*

appeaser Beruhigungsmittel *n*

appendix Anhang *m*, Appendix *m*, Blinddarm *m* / **~ cerebri** Hirnanhang *m*, Hypophyse *f*

apperceive apperzipieren, aneignen

apperception Apperzeption *f*, Erfassen *n*, Auffassen *n*, Aneignung *f* / **~ category** Apperzeptionskategorie *f*, Apperzeptionsstadium *n* / **~ phase** Apperzeptionsstadium *n* / **~ test** Apperzeptionstest *m*, Auffassungstest *m* / **~ type** Auffassungstypus *m* / **active ~** aktive Apperzeption *f* / **dynamic ~ test** Test *m* der dynamischen Apperzeption / **passive ~** passive Apperzeption *f* / **tendentious ~** autistische Apperzeption *f*, tendenziöse Apperzeption *f* / **thematic ~ test** thematischer Apperzeptionstest *m*, TAT *m*

apperceptionism Apperzeptionspsychologie *f*

apperceptive apperzeptiv, Apperzeptions–

appetence, appetency Appetenz *f* Verlangen *n*, Begierde *f*, Streben *n*

appetent appetent, begierig, verlangend

appetite Appetit *m*, Hunger *m*, Trieb *m*, Gier *f*, Verlangen *n*, Gelüste *npl* / **~ depressing drug** Appetitzügler *m*, Appetithemmer *m* / **~ disorder** Essstörung *f* / **excessive ~** Heißhunger *m*, Fressgier *f* / **failing ~** Appetitlosigkeit *f*, fehlender Appetit *m* / **impaired ~** gestörter Appetit *m*, schlechter Appetit *m* / **morbid ~** Heißhunger *m*, Unersättlichkeit *f* / **perverted ~** Trieb *m* zum Genuss absonderlicher Dinge / **ravenous ~** Heißhunger *m* / **sexual ~** Geschlechtslust *f* / **voracious ~** Heißhunger *m*

appetition Verlangen *n*, Triebrichtung *f*

appetitive Appetenz–

applicability Anwendbarkeit *f*

applicable anwendbar

application Anwendung *f*, Applikation *f*, Bewerbung *f* / **~ blank** Bewerbungsbogen *m*

applicator Instrument *n*, Applikator *m*, Hilfsmittel *n*

applied angewandt

apply anwenden, verwenden, applizieren

appointed ernannt, offiziell

appointment Ernennung *f*, Termin *m* / **permanent ~** feste Ernennung *f*, Bestallung *f*

apport Apport *m*

appraisal Beurteilung *f*, Bewertung *f* / **~ of behaviour** Verhaltensbeurteilung *f* / **~ interview** Beurteilungsgespräch *n* / **comparative ~** vergleichende Bewertung *f*

appraise abschätzen, beurteilen

appreciable abschätzbar, merklich, wahrnehmbar

appreciate würdigen, schätzen, einsehen

appreciation Würdigung *f*, Schätzung *f*, Verständnis *n* / **~ of space** Raumbegriff *m* / **aesthetic ~ test** Kunstverständnistest *m* / **artistic ~** Kunstgenuss *m*

apprehend begreifen, erfassen, verstehen

apprehensible begreiflich, wahrnehmbar

apprehension Auffassung *f*, Wahrnehmung *f*, Auffassungsvermögen *n*, Vorstellung *f*, Begriff *m*, Begreifen *n* / **~ span** Aufmerksamkeitsumfang *m*, Auffassungsumfang *m*, Auffassungsbereich *m* / **~ span test** Test *m* des Auffassungsumfanges / **collective ~** kollektive Auffassung *m* / **implicit ~** unbemerkte Wahrnehmung *f* / **ocular ~** visuelles Erfassen *n* / **synthetic ~** synthetische Auffassung *f*

apprehensive empfindlich, furchtsam, angstbereit, besorgt

apprehensiveness Besorgnis *f*, Befürchtung *f*, Angstbereitschaft *f*

apprentice Auszubildender *m*, Lehrling *m*, Anfänger *m* / **~–training** Lehrlingsausbildung *f*, Lehrzeit *f*

apprenticeship Lehrzeit *f*, Ausbildungszeit *f*, Lehre *f*

approach Annäherung *f*, Hinwendung *f*, Ansatz *m* / sich nähern, herantreten / **~–approach conflict** Konflikt *m* zwischen Annäherungstendenzen, Appetenz–Appetenz–Konflikt *m*, Konflikt *m* zwischen Appetenztendenzen / **~–avoidance conflict** Annäherungs–Vermeidungs–Konflikt *m*, Appetenz–Aversions–Konflikt *m*, Ambivalenzkonflikt *m* / **~–avoidance gradient** Annäherungs–Vermeidungs–Gradient *m* / **~ gradient** Annäherungsgradient *m*, Appetenzgradient *m* / **~ response** Annäherungsreaktion *f* / **actuarial ~** versicherungsmathematischer Ansatz *m* / **behavioural ~ system** Annäherungssystem *n* / **biopsychosocial ~** biopsychosozialer Ansatz *m* / **clinical ~** klinischer Ansatz *m* / **conceptual ~** konzeptionelle Vorgehensweise *f* / **cross–cultural ~** Methode *f* des Kulturvergleichs / **dispositional ~** Dispositionsansatz *m* / **empirical ~** empirische Methode *f* / **functional ~** funktionale Vorgehensweise *f* / **historical ~** historische Vorgehensweise *f* / **idiographic ~** idiographischer Ansatz *m* / **indirect ~ method** indirekte Interviewmethode *f* / **logic ~** rationale Vorgehensweise *f* / **mental ~** Anstrengungsbereitschaft *f*, Arbeitsbereitschaft *f* / **nomothetic ~** nomothetischer Ansatz *m* / **psychotherapeutic ~** psychotherapeutische Methode *f*, psychotherapeutisches Verfahren *n* / **stereotactic ~** stereotaktische Vorgehensweise *f*

approachable zugänglich, kontaktfähig

approbation Billigung *f*, Genehmigung *f*, Zustimmung *f*

appropriate angemessen, entsprechend, geeignet

approval Billigung *f*, Genehmigung *f* / **social ~** soziale Billigung *f*

approximate, approximative annähernd, approximativ

approximation Näherung *f*, Annäherung *f*, Näherungswert *m* / **~ conditioning** approximatives Bedingen *n* / **~ and correction** Versuch– und Irrtumslernen *n* / **~ er-**

ror Schätzfehler *m*, Aufrundungsfehler *m* / **~ method** Näherungsverfahren *n* / **~ procedure** Näherungsverfahren *n* / **linear ~** lineare Approximation *f* / **successive ~** sukzessive Näherung *f*

appurtenance Zugehörigkeit *f*, Zubehör *n*

apractognosia Apraktagnosie *f*, Agnosie *f* verbunden mit Apraxie

apragmatism Apragmatismus *m*

apraxia Apraxie *f*, Unfähigkeit *f* zu zweckmäßigem Handeln / **~ with agnosia** Agnosie *f* verbunden mit Apraxie / **alimentary ~** Unfähigkeit *f* zu essen / **amnestic ~** amnestische Apraxie *f* / **constructional ~** konstruktive Apraxie *f* / **cortical ~** kortikale Apraxie *f* / **dressing ~** Ankleide–Apraxie *f* / **ideational ~** ideatorische Apraxie *f* / **ideokinetic ~** ideokinetische Apraxie *f* / **ideomotor ~** ideomotorische Apraxie *f* / **limb–kinetic ~** gliedkinetische Apraxie *f*, kortikale Apraxie *f* / **motor ~** motorische Apraxie *f* / **oculomotor ~** okulomotorische Apraxie *f* / **optic ~** optische Apraxie *f* / **unilateral ~** einseitige Apraxie *f*

apraxic, apractic apraxisch, Apraxie betreffend

a priori deduktiv, von der Ursache auf die Wirkung schließend

aprioristic apriorisch

aprosexia Aprosexie *f*, Denkunfähigkeit *f*, Unfähigkeit *f* zu geistiger Anstrengung, Teilnahmslosigkeit *f*

aprosopia angeborener Gesichtsdefekt *m*, Gesichtsverkümmerung *f*, Aprosopie *f*

apselaphesia Störung *f* des Tastsinnes, Tastlähmung *f*

apsychia Bewusstlosigkeit *f*, Ohnmacht *f*

apsithyria Apsithyrie *f*

apt geeignet, tauglich, geschickt, fähig, geneigt

aptitude Eignung *f*, Begabung *f*, Fähigkeit *f*, Befähigung *f*, Veranlagung *f* / **~ measure** Eignungsmessung *f*, Eignungstest *m* / **~ test** Eignungstest *m*, Begabungstest *m*, Fähigkeitstest *m* / **academic ~** Schuleignung *f* / **basic ~** Grundfähigkeit *f* / **clerical ~** Eignung *f* für Büroberufe / **differential ~ test** differentieller Begabungstest *m*, differentieller Eignungstest *m* / **general ~** Allgemeinbegabung *f* / **general ~ test battery** allgemeine Berufseignungstestbatterie *f* / **manual ~** manuelle Geschicklichkeit Handgeschicklichkeit *f*, manuelle Fähigkeit *f* / **mechanical ~** mechanisch–technische Eignung *f*, technische Begabung, mechanisch–technische Fähigkeit *f*, mechanisch–technische Veranlagung *f* / **mechanical ~ test** Test *m* der technischen Begabung / **motor ~** Geschicklichkeit *f*, motorische Veranlagung *f* / **multiple ~ test** Eignungstestbatterie *f* / **musical ~ test** Musik–Begabungstest *m* / **numerical ~** rechnerische Begabung *f* / **perceptual ~** Wahrnehmungsfähigkeit *f* / **professional ~** Berufseignung *f* / **psychomotor~** psychomotorische Veranlagung *f* / **scholastic ~** Schuleignung *f* / **scholastic ~ test** Schuleignungstest *m* / **special ~** Begabung *f*, Sonderbegabung *f* / **special ~ test** spezieller Eignungstest *m*, Test *m* für Sonderbegabung / **vocational ~** Berufseignung *f* / **vocational ~ test** Berufseignungstest *m*, Berufseignungsprüfung *f*

aquaphobia Wasserscheu *f*, Angst *f* vor Wasser

aqueduct Aquaeductus *m*, Kanal *m* / **~ of midbrain** Aquaeductus cerebri *m*, Aquaeductus mesencephali *m* / **~ of Sylvius** Aquaeductus Sylvii *m* / **cerebral ~** Aquaeductus cerebri *m*

aqueous wässrig

arachnephobia, arachnophobia Furcht *f* vor Spinnen, Arachnophobie *f*

arachnoid(al) arachnoid

arachnid Spinnentier *n*

arachnoid spinnwebartig / Arachnoidea *f* Spinnwebenhaut *f*

arachnoiditis, arachnitis Arachnoiditis *f*, Entzündung *f* der Arachnoidea, Entzündung *f* der Spinnwebenhaut

arbitrary willkürlich, eigenmächtig

arbitration Schlichtung *f*, Schiedsgerichtsbarkeit *f*

arborisation Verzweigung *f* einer Nervenzelle, Arborisation *f* / **terminal ~** Endverzweigung *f*

arbor vitae Arbor vitae *m*, Zeichnung *f* des Kleinhirns im Mittelschnitt

arc Bogen *m*, Kreis *m* / **~ de cercle** Arc de cercle *m*, hysterischer Körperbogen *m* / **nervous ~** Nervenbogen *m*, Reflexbogen *m* / **neural ~** Nervenbogen *m*, Reflexbogen *m*

arch of Corti Corti–Bogen *m*, Corti–Kanal *m*

archaic archaisch, veraltet

archaism Archaismus *m*, veralteter Ausdruck *m*

archencephalon Urhirn *n*, Archencephalon *n*

archetype Archetyp *m*, Archetypus *m*, Urbild *n*, Urtyp *m*

archetypical archetypisch, urbildlich

archicortex Archicortex *m*, stammesgeschichtlich alter Hirnrindenabschnitt *m*

archipallium Archipallium *n*, Rhinenzephalon *n*, Riechhirn *n*

architectural architektonisch, Architektur–

arcuate bogenförmig

area Gebiet *n*, Fläche *f*, Zone *f*, Bereich *m*, Areal *n* / **~ and block sampling** Flächenstichprobenverfahren *n*, Klumpenstichprobenverfahren *n* / **~ of the body** Körpergegend *f*, Körperbezirk *m* / **~s of constancy** Konstanzbereiche *mpl* / **~ of examination** Untersuchungsfeld *n* / **~ of freedom** Freiheitsbereich *m* / **~ of intelligence** Intelligenzbereich *m* / **~ of interest** Interessengebiet *n* / **~ of propagation** Ausbreitungsgebiet *n* / **~ sampling** Gebietsstichprobentechnik *f*, Area–Technik *f* / **~ striata** Area striata *f* / **~ study** Untersuchung *f* eines geographischen Gebietes / **~ thinking** Technik *f* des kreativen Denkens / **auditopsychic ~** Hörassoziationszentrum *n* / **auditory ~** Hörzentrum *n*, Gehörzentrum *n*, Hörsphäre *f* / **cognitive ~** Erkenntnisbereich *m* / **cortical ~** Rindensphäre *f*, Rindenfeld *n* / **motor ~** motorisches Feld *n*, Bewegungsfeld *n*, motorische Region *f* / **olfactory ~** Riechfläche *f* der Nase, Riechzentrum *n* / **postcentral ~** postzentrale Region *f* / **precentral ~** präzentrale Region *f* / **prefrontal ~** präfrontale Region *f* / **preoptic ~** Area prae–optica *f* / **primary sensory ~** primäres sensorisches; Rindenfeld *n* / **psycho–algesic ~** Körperfühlsphäre *f* / **pyramidal ~** motorisches Feld *n* / **segmental ~** Segmentbereich *m* / **sensory ~** sensorisches Rindenfeld *n* / **septal ~** Scheidewandbereich *m* / **social analysis ~** Analyse *f* von Wohnbezirken nach soziologischen Merkmalen / **striate ~** Area striata *f* / **suppressive ~** Suppressorfeld *n* / **visual ~** Sehrinde *f*, Sehzentrum *n*, Sehsphäre *f*

arecoline Arecolin *n* / **~ hydrobromide** Arecolinhydrobromid *n*

areflexia Areflexie *f*, Fehlen *n* der normalen Reflexe

argument Argument *n*, Beweis *m* / **~s** Streit *m* / **~–completion** freie Fortführung *f* einer Argumentation / **strong ~** starkes Argument *n*

argumentative streitsüchtig

argumentativeness Streitsucht *f*

Argyll–Robertson pupil Argyll–Robertson'sches Phänomen *n*, reflektorische Pupillenstarre *f*

aridity Reizlosigkeit *f*, Schalheit *f*, Trockenheit *f*

aristogenic mit hervorragendem genetischen Potential ausgestattet

Aristotelian aristotelisch, von Aristoteles stammend

Aristotle Aristoteles / **~'s experiment** Aristotelischer Versuch *m* / **~'s illusion** Aristotelischer Versuch *m*, Aristotelische Täuschung *f*

arithmetic arithmetisch, rechnerisch

arithmomania Zählzwang *m*, Arithmomanie *f*

armchair psychology Schreibtischpsychologie *f*

armor–plating Panzerung *f*

aromatic würzig, aromatisch

aromatisation Aromatisierung *f*

arousal Erregung *f*, Aktivation *f*, Wachbeit *f*, Arousal *f* / **~ function** Erregungsfunktion *f* / **~ index** Erregbarkeitsindex *m* / **~ level** Aktivationsniveau *n* / **~ reaction** Weckreaktion *f* / **~ system** thalamoretikuläres Projektionssystem *n*, Erregungssystem *n* / **~ threshold** Erregungsschwelle *f* / **~ of wants** Erweckung *f* von Bedürfnissen / **affective ~ theory** Theorie *f* der Gefühlsaktivation / **ascending reticular ~ system** aufsteigendes retikuläres Erregungssystem *n* / **emotional ~** Gefühlserregung *f*, Gefühlsaktivation *f* / **female sexual ~ disorder** Störung *f* der sexuellen Erregung bei der Frau / **physiological ~** physiologische Aktivierung *f* / **preparatory ~** vorbereitende Aktivierung *f* / **sexual ~** sexuelle Erregung *f*, sexuelle Aktivierung *f*

arpeggio paradox Humphrey–Paradox *n*, Humphrey–Prinzip *n*

arrangement Anordnung *f*, Gliederung *f*, Arrangement *n* / **~ of chromosomes** Chromosomenanordnung *f* / **~ of the neurosis** Arrangement *f* der Neurose / **experimental ~** Versuchsanordnung *f* / **neurotic ~** neurotisches Arrangement *n* / **segmental ~ of the nervous system** Neuromere *f*, segmentale Gliederung *f* des Nervensystems / **topographical ~** topographische Gliederung *f*

array Reihe *f*, Rangreihe *f*, Rangordnung *f*

arrest Stillstand *m*, Hemmung *f*, Stockung *f*, Festnahme *f*, Haft *f* / **~ of development** Entwicklungshemmung *f*, Entwicklungsstillstand *m* / **~ of growth** Wachstumshemmung *f* / **legal ~** Festnahme *f*

arrhythmia Arrhythmie *f*, Rhythmusstörung *f*

arrhythmic, arrhythmous arrhythmisch, unrhythmisch

arrow–head and feather illusion Müller–Lyer'sche Täuschung *f*

arson Brandstiftung *f*

arsonvalisation Arsonvalisation *f*, Behandlung *f* mit hochfrequenten und hochgespannten Strömen

arsphenamine Salvarsan *n*, Arsphenamin *n*

art Kunst *f* / **~ director** künstlerischer Leiter *m* einer Werbeagentur / **~ education** Kunsterziehung *f* / **~ judgment test** Kunstverständnistest *m* / **~ therapy** Kunsttherapie *f* / **creative ~s therapy** kreative Therapie *f* / **black ~** Magie *f*, Schwarze Kunst *f* / **healing ~** Heilkunst *f* / **martial ~** Kampfsport *m* / **performing ~s** darstellende Künste *fpl* / **photographic ~** Photographie *f* / **plastic ~** bildende Kunst *f*

artefact, artifact Kunsterzeugnis *n*, Kunstprodukt *n*, Artefakt *n*

artefactitious, artifactitious artefaktisch, künstlich erzeugt

arterenol Noradrenalin *n*

arteriography Arteriographie *f*, Arteriendarstellung *f*

arteriole Arteriole *f*, kleinste Arterie *f*

arteriosclerosis Arteriosklerose *f*, Aderverkalkung *f* / **cerebral ~** Zerebralsklerose *f* / **coronary ~** Koronarsklerose *f*

arteriosclerotic arteriosklerotisch, verkalkt

artery Arterie *f*, Schlagader *f*, Pulsader *f* / **carotid ~** Halsschlagader *f* / **coronary ~** Herzkranzgefäß *n*, Koronaraterie *f*

arthralgia Gelenkschmerz *m*

arthropod Gliederfüßler *m*

articular artikulär, Gelenk–

articulate artikulieren, deutlich sprechen, verbinden, gliedern / deutlich, artikuliert, klar erkenntlich

articulation Artikulation *f*, deutliche Aussprache *f*, Gelenkverbindung *f* / **developmental ~ disorder** entwicklungsbezogene Artikulationsstörung *f* / **~ intelligibility** verständliche Aussprache *f*, deutliches Artikulieren *n* / **~ test** Aussprachetest *m*

articulatory Artikulations–

artifact Kunsterzeugnis *n*, Kunstprodukt *n*, Artefakt *n*

artificial künstlich, artifiziell

artificialism Betonung *f* des Gekünstelten

artistic Kunst–, künstlerisch

asapholalia Gemurmel *n*, Gemummel *n*, undeutliche Aussprache *f*

A scale A–Skala *f*

ascend aufsteigen

ascendance, ascendancy, ascendence, ascendency Überlegenheit *f*, Übergewicht *n*, Dominanz *f*, Aszendenz *f* / **~–submission relation** Überlegenheits–Unterlegenheits–Beziehung *f* / **social ~** sozialer Aufstieg *m*, soziale Dominanz *f*

ascendant, ascendent, ascending aufsteigend, ansteigend, aszendierend

ascetic asketisch / Asket *m*

asceticism Askese *f*, Aszese *f*, einfachste Lebensweise *f*

aschematia Körperschemastörung *f*, Aschematie *f*

asemia, asemasia Asemie *f*, Verständigungsunfähigkeit *f*, Asymbolie *f*

asexual asexuell, agamisch, geschlechtslos, ungeschlechtlich

asexualisation Kastrierung *f*, Sterilisation *f*

asexuality Asexualität *f*, Mangel *m* an Geschlechtslust, geschlechtlich indifferentes Verhalten *n*

asitia Abscheu *f* beim Anblick von Speisen, Verlust *m* des Appetits, Asitie *f*

asocial asozial, unsozial

asociality Asozialität *f*, Unfähigkeit *f* sich gesellschaftlich einzuordnen

asomatous asomatisch, immateriell, körperlos

asomnia Schlaflosigkeit *f*, Asomnie *f*

asonia Tontaubheit *f*, Tonempfindlichkeit *f*

aspartate Aspartat *n*

aspect Anblick *m*, Erscheinung *f*, Aussehen *n*, Aspekt *m* / **~ of behaviour** Verhaltensaspekt *m* / **anthropological ~** anthropologischer Aspekt *m* / **clinical ~** klinisches Bild *n* / **double ~ theory** Zwei–Aspekten–Lehre *f* / **facial ~** Gesichtsausdruck *m* / **general ~** allgemeiner Eindruck *m*, Gesamteindruck *m* / **objective ~** objektiver Aspekt *m* / **sociopsychological ~** sozialpsychologischer Aspekt *m* / **topographic ~** topographischer Aspekt *m*

Asperger's disorder Asperger–Störung *f* / **~ syndrome** Asperger–Syndrom *n*

aspermia Fehlen *n* der Ejakulation, Fehlen *n* des Samenergusses, Aspermie *f*

asphyxia Asphyxie *f*, Ersticken *n*, Sauerstoffmangel *m*

asphyxial asphyktisch, Erstickungs–

asphyxiant Erstickung hervorrufendes Mittel *n*

asphyxiate ersticken, an Sauerstoffmangel zugrunde gehen

asphyxiation Ersticken *n*, Asphyxie *f*

aspiration Aspiration *f*, Anspruch *m*, Hoffnung *f* / **~ level** Anspruchsniveau *n* / **educational ~** Erziehungsziel *n*, Bildungsanspruch *m* / **occupational ~** berufliche Zielvorstellung *f*, berufliches Ziel *n* / **vocational ~** berufliche Zielvorstellung *f*, beruflicher Anspruch *m*

AS ratio Assoziations–Empfindungs–Quotient *m*

assassination Ermordung *f* / **political ~** politischer Mord *m*

assault Angriff *m*, Anschlag *m*, Übergriff *m* / **criminal ~** Körperverletzung *f* / **indecent ~** Sittlichkeitsverbrechen *n* / **sexual ~** sexuelle Nötigung *f*

assay Prüfung *f*, Erprobung *f*, Analyse *f*, Versuch *m*

A–S scale Antisemitismus–Skala *f*

assemblage Versammlung *f*, Vereinigung *f*, Haufen *m*

assembly Versammlung *f*, Zusammenbau *m* / **~ line** Fließband *n* / **~ line work** Fließbandarbeit *f* / **~ test** Mosaiktest *m*

assert behaupten, beteuern, bestehen auf, verfechten, verteidigen

assertion Behauptung *f*, Aussage *f*, Feststellung *f*, Versicherung *f*

assertive bejahend, positiv, ausdrücklich, bestimmt

assertiveness selbstbewusstes Verhalten *n*, selbstbewusstes Vorgehen *n*, Durchsetzungsfähigkeit *f*, Selbstsicherheit *f* / **~ of movement** Beständigkeit *f* der Bewegung / **~ of posture** Beständigkeit *f* der Körperhaltung / **~ training** Selbstbehauptungstraining *n*, Selbstsicherheitstraining *n*

assess beurteilen, schätzen, bewerten, werten, veranschlagen

assessment Beurteilung *f*, Einschätzung *f*, Bewertung *f*, Wertung *f* / **~ centre** Beurteilungszentrum *n*, Assessment–Center *n* / **~ of the course of a disease** Verlaufsbeurteilung *f* einer Krankheit / **~ programme** Beurteilungsprogramm *n* / **affective ~** affektive Messung *f* / **behavioural ~** Verhaltensdiagnostik *f* / **cognitive ~** kognitive Messung *f* / **geriatric ~** geriatrische Diagnostik *f* / **neuropsychological ~** neuropsychologische Messung *f* / **psychological ~** psychologische Messung *f*

assets Anlagen *fpl* / **~–liabilities technique** Soll–Haben–Technik *f*

assiduity Beharrlichkeit *f*, Fleiß *m*, Ausdauer *f*

assiduous beharrlich, fleißig, ausdauernd

assign bestimmen, zuweisen, zuteilen

assignment Auftrag *m*, Aufgabe *f*, Zuweisung *f*, Position *f* / **~ therapy** Sozialtherapie *f*, Soziotherapie *f*

assimilability Assimilierbarkeit *f*

assimilable assimilierbar

assimilate assimilieren, angleichen, aneignen, aufnehmen, umwandeln

assimilation Assimilation *f*, Assimilierung *f*, Angleichung *f* Umwandlung *f* / **~ illusion** Assimilationstäuschung *f* / **cultural ~** kulturelle Assimilation *f* / **social ~** soziale Assimilation *f*, soziale Anpassung *f*

assimilative assimilierend, assimilatorisch

assist unterstützen, beistehen, helfen

assistance Hilfe *f*, Beistand *m*, Unterstützung *f* / **~–seeking** hilfesuchend / **educational financial ~** Ausbildungsbeihilfe *f*, Studienbeihilfe *f*

assistant Assistent *m*, Assistentin *f*, Helfer *m*, Helferin *f*, Beistand *m*, Gehilfe *m*, Gehilfin *f* / **psychological ~** psychologischer Assistent *m*, psychologische Assistentin *f*

associability Vereinbarkeit *f*, Fähigkeit *f* der Mitempfingung

associate eng zusammengehörig, begleitend, nicht vollamtlich angestellt / Kollege *m*, Mitarbeiter *m*, außerordentliches Mitglied *n* / assoziieren, verbinden, in Zusammenhang bringen / **paired ~s** zusammengehörige Paare *npl*, Paarassoziationen *fpl* / **paired ~ learning** paarweises Assoziieren *n*, Paarassoziationslernen *n* / **paired ~s test** Paarvergleichsverfahren *n* / **remote ~s test** sekundärer Assoziationsversuch *m* / **right ~s procedure** Treffermethode *f*, Paarwortmethode *f*

association Assoziation *f*, Gedankenverbindung *f*, Vereinigung *f*, Verband *m* / **~ area** Assoziationsareal *n*, Assoziationsfeld *n* / **~ centre** Assoziationszentrum *n* / **~ coefficient** Assoziationsquotient *m* / **~ by contiguity** Berührungsassoziation *f* / **~ by contrast** heterosensorielle Assoziation *f* / **~ cortex** Assoziationszentrum *n* / **~ experiment** Assoziationsversuch *m*, Assoziationsexperiment *n* / **~ fibres** Assoziationsfasern *fpl* / **~ field** Assoziationsfeld *n* / **~–frequency table** Liste *f* der häufigsten Assoziationen / **~ of a generic concept** totalisierende Assoziation *f* / **~ group** Vereinigung *f* / **~ of ideas** Ideenassoziation *f*, Gedankenassoziation *f*, Gedankenverknüpfung *f*, Ideenverbindung *f* / **~ mass** Apperzeptionsmasse *f* / **~ method** Assoziationsmethode *f* / **~ neuron** Assoziationsneuron *n* / **~ nucleus** Assoziationskern *m* / **~ path** Assoziationsbahn *f*, assoziative Verbindung *f*, Assoziationsweg *m* / **~ of a part to a whole** partialisierende Assoziation *f* / **~ psychology** Assoziationspsychologie *f* / **~ reaction time** Reaktionszeit *f* bei Assoziationen / **~ reflex** bedingte Reaktion *f*, bedingter Reflex *m* / **~ region** Assoziationszentrum *n* / **~–sensation ratio** Assoziations–Empfindungs–Quotient *m* / **~ by similarity** homosensorielle Assoziation *f* / **~ test** Assoziationsversuch *m*, Assoziationstest *m* / **~ time** Reaktionszeit *f* bei Assoziationen / **~ tract** Assoziationsbahn *f*, Assoziationsweg *m*, assoziative Verbindung *f* / **~ word** Assoziationswort *n* / **affective ~** gefühlsmäßige Assoziation *f* / **auditory ~** Gehörassoziation *f* / **backward ~** retrograde Assoziation *f*, rückwärtsgerichtete Assoziation *f* / **constrained ~** festgelegte Assoziation *f* / **contextual ~** Kontextassoziation *f*, kontextgebundene Assoziation *f* / **controlled ~** kontrollierte Assoziation *f*, gerichtete Assoziation *f*, gebundene Assoziation *f* / **direct ~** gerichtete Assoziation *f* / **evidential ~** bedeutsame Assoziation *f* / **false ~** Assoziationstäuschung *f* / **forward ~** vorwärtsgerichtete Assoziation *f* / **free ~** freie Assoziation *f*, freier Einfall *m* / **frontal ~ area** frontales Assoziationsfeld *n* / **immediate ~** direkte Assoziation *f* unmittelbare Assoziation *f* / **induced ~** gerichtete Assoziation *f* / **mediate ~** mittelbare Assoziation *f*, überspringende Assoziation *f* / **negative ~** negative Assoziation *f* / **paired ~s** paarweise Assoziationen *fpl* / **positive ~** positive Assoziation *f* / **remote ~** mittelbare Assoziation *f*, seltene Assoziation *f*, überspringende Assoziation *f* / **retroactive ~** retroaktive Assoziation *f*, rückwirkende Assoziation *f* / **serial ~** Reihenassoziation *f*, Reihenlernen *n* / **social ~** soziale Gruppierung *f* / **verbal ~** Wortassoziation *f*

associationism Assoziationslehre *f*, Assoziationismus *m*, Assoziationspsychologie *f*, assoziative Psychologie *f*

associative assoziativ, Assoziations–

associativity Assoziativität *f*

assonance Gleichklang *m*, Assonanz *f*, Klangähnlichkeit *f*

assonant assonierend, gleichklingend, anklingend

assumed angenommen

assumption Annahme *f*, Postulat *n*, Voraussetzung *f*

assurance Zuversicht *f*, Vertrauen *n*, Sicherheit *f* / **self–~** Selbstsicherheit *f*

astasia Astasie *f*, motorische Koordinationsstörung *f* beim Stehen / **~–abasia** Unvermögen *n* zu gehen und zu stehen, Astasie–Abasie *f*

astereognosis, astereognosy Tastlähmung *f*, Tastblindheit *f*, Verlust *m* des feinen Tastsinnes, Astereognosie *f*, Stereoagnosie *f*, taktile Agnosie *f*

asthenia Asthenie *f*, Schwäche *f*, Körperschwäche *f*, asthenischer Zustand *m*, Anergie *f* / **congenital universal ~** Asthenia *f* universalis congenita / **irritable ~** reizbare Schwäche *f* / **mental ~** Asthenia *f* mentalis / **neurocirculatory ~** neurozirkulatorische Asthenie *f*, Herzangstsyndrom *n*

asthenic asthenisch, kraftlos

asthenope Schwachsichtiger *m*, im Nahsehen Gestörter *m*

asthenopia Schwachsichtigkeit *f*, Asthenopie *f*, Störung *f* des Nahsehens / **accomodative ~** akkomodative Asthenopie *f* / **nervous ~** nervöse Asthenopie *f*

asthenopic asthenopisch, im Nahsehen gestört

asthma Asthma *n* / **bronchial ~** Asthma bronchiale *n*, Bronchialasthma *n* / **nervous ~** Asthma nervosum *n*, nervöses Asthma *n*, stressbedingtes Asthma *n* / **sexual ~** Asthma sexuale *n*

asthmatic asthmatisch, kurzatmig

astigmatic, astigmic astigmatisch, stabsichtig / Astigmatiker *m*

astigmatism, astigmia Astigmatismus *m*, Stabsichtigkeit *f*

astigmatometry, astigmoscopy, astigmatoscopy Astigmatismusmessung *f* Astigmatismusbestimmung *f*

astigmograph, astigmometer, astigmatometer Astigmatoskop *n*, Astigmometer *n*

astraphobia, astrophobia, astrapophobia Gewitterangst *f*, Astraphobie *f*

astrocyte Sternzelle *f*, Astrozyt *m*, Makroglia *f*

astroglia Astroglia *f*

astrology Astrologie *f*, Sterndeutung *f*

asyllabia Unvermögen *n* Silben zu bilden, Asyllabie *f*

asylum Asyl *n*, Heim *n*, Anstalt *f* / **~ for alcoholics** Trinkerheilstätte *f*, Entwöhnungsanstalt *f* / **~ for the insane** Irrenanstalt *f*, psychiatrische Klinik *f* / **lunatic ~** Irrenanstalt *f*, Nervenklinik *f*

asymbolia Asymbolie *f*, Asemie *f*, Unverständnis *n* von Zeichen und Symbolen / **~ to pain** Schmerzasymbolie *f*

asymmetric, asymmetrical asymmetrisch, symmetrielos, schräg, schief, ungleichförmig

asymmetry Asymmetrie *f*, Schiefe *f*, Ungleichförmigkeit *f*, Symmetrielosigkeit *f*, Schräge *f* / **facial ~** Gesichtsschiefe *f*, ungleichförmiges Gesicht *n*

asymptomatic asymptomatisch, symptomlos, ohne Symptome

asymptote Asymptote *f*, Näherungslinie *f*

asymptotic asymptotisch

asynapsis Asynapsis *f*, fehlende Paarung *f* homologer Chromosomen in der Meiose

asynchronism Koordinationsstörung *f*, Fehlen *n* des Zusammenspiels

asynchronous asynchron, unkoordiniert

asyndesis fehlende Paarung *f* homologer Chromosomen in der Meiose

asynergia, asynergy Koordinationsstörung *f*, Asynergie *f* / **verbal ~** Koordinationsstörung *f* beim Sprechen / **vocal ~** Sprachstörung *f*

asystematic unsystematisch, diffus

ataractic, ataraxic ataraktisch / Ataraktikum *n*, Psychosedativum *n*

ataraxia, ataraxy Ataraxie *f*, Seelenruhe *f*, Unerschütterlichkeit *f*, Gelassenheit *f*

atavism Atavismus *m*, Entwicklungsrückschlag *m*, Auftreten *n* von Eigenschaften der Ahnen, Rückschlag *m*

atavistic atavistisch

ataxaphasia, ataxiaphasia Unfähigkeit *f* Wörter zu Sätzen zu ordnen

ataxia, ataxy Ataxie *f*, Koordinationsstörung *f* / **acute ~** akute Ataxie *f* / **alcoholic ~** Alkoholataxie *f* / **articulative ~** Silbenstolpern *n* / **bulbar ~** bulbäre Ataxie *f* / **cerebellar ~** zerebelläre Ataxie *f*, Kleinhirnataxie *f* / **cerebral ~** zerebrale Ataxie *f* / **cortical ~** Rindenataxie *f* / **frontal ~** Stirnhirnataxie *f*, frontale Ataxie *f* / **hereditary ~** hereditäre Ataxie *f*, Friedreich–Ataxie *f* / **intrapsychic ~** intrapsychische Ataxie *f* / **labyrinthic ~** Labyrinth–Ataxie *f* / **locomotor ~** lokomotorische Ataxie *f*, Bewegungsataxie *f*, Tabes dorsalis *f* / **mental ~** geistige Ataxie *f* / **motor ~** Ataxie *f*, Koordinationsstörung *f* / **ocular ~** Nystagmus *m* / **optic ~** optische Ataxie *f* / **psychic ~** psychische Ataxie *f* / **sensory ~** sensorische Ataxie *f* / **spinal ~** Hinterstrangataxie *f*, spinale Ataxie *f* / **static ~** statische Ataxie *f* / **vasomotor ~** vasomotorische Ataxie *f*, Gefäßataxie *f* / **vestibular ~** vestibuläre Ataxie *f*

ataxiameter, ataxiagraph Ataxiameter *n*, Gerät *n* zur Registrierung unwillkürlicher Bewegungen

ataxiaphasia Unfähigkeit *f* Sätze zu bilden

ataxic ataktisch

ataxiophemia, ataxophemia Koordinationsschwäche *f* der Sprechmuskeln

ateleiosis, ateliosis Zwergwuchs *m*, Ateleiosis *f*

atelia Unvollkommenheit *f*, Unvollendetsein *n*, Mangelhaftigkeit *f*

atheism Atheismus *m*, Gottesleugnung *f*

atherosclerosis Atherosklerose *f*

atherosclerotic atherosklerotisch

athetoid, athetosic, athetotic athetotisch, Athetose betreffend

athetosis Athetose *f*, ungeordnete Bewegung *f* besonders der Hände und Finger, bizarre unwillkürliche Bewegungen *fpl* der Gliedmaßen

athletic athletisch

athletosome athletischer Typ *m*, athletischer Typus *m*, Athletiker *m*

athymia Athymie *f*, Antriebslosigkeit *f*, Schwermut *f*, mutlose Lebensstimmung *f*, Melancholie *f*

athyreosis mangelnde Funktion *f* der Schilddrüse, Zustand *m* bei fehlender Schilddrüse

atmosphere Atmosphäre *f* / **~ of anxiety** Atmosphäre *f* der Angst / **~ effect** Atmosphäreneffekt *m* / **~ of tension** Atmosphäre *f* der Spannung / **authoritarian ~** autoritäre Atmosphäre *f* / **democratic ~** demokratische Atmosphäre *f* / **psychic ~** seelische Atmosphäre *f*

atom Atom *n* / **social ~** soziale Einheit *f*, soziometrische Einheit *f*

atomism Atomismus *m* / **mental ~** geistiger Atomismus *m* / **psychological ~** atomistische Psychologie *f*

atomistic atomistisch

atonement Wiedergutmachung *f*, Sühne *f*

atonia, atony, atonicity Atonie *f*, Erschlaffung *f*, Tonusmangel *m*, atonischer Zustand *m*

atonic atonisch, kraftlos, schlaff, tonuslos

atopognosia, atopognosis Unvermögen *n* Berührungsreize zu lokalisieren, Atopognosie *f*

atopy Veranlagung *f* zu allergischen Erkrankungen, Atopie *f*

atoxic ungiftig, atoxisch

atrabiliar, atrabilious melancholisch, schwermütig, deprimiert

atrabilarian schwermütiger Mensch *m*, Depressiver *m*

atrabilariousness Schwermut *m*, Melancholie *f*

atriopeptin, atriopeptide Atripeptin *n*, Atriopeptid *n*

atrium Vorkammer *f* des Herzens, Vorhof *m*

atrophia, atrophy Atrophie *f*, Schwund *m*, Schrumpfung *f* / **~ of the brain** Gehirnschwund *m*, Hirnatrophie *f* / **~ of the tissues** Atrophie *f* der Gewebe / **cerebral ~** Hirnatrophie *f*, Gehirnschwund *m*, zerebrale Atrophie *f* / **diffuse progressive cerebrocortical ~** diffuse progressive Großhirnrindendegeneration *f* / **gray ~** Sehnervenatrophie *f* / **muscular ~** Muskelatrophie *f*, Muskelschwund *m* / **neural ~** neuropathische Atrophie *f* / **neuropathic ~** neuropathische Atrophie *f* / **neurotrophic ~** neurotrophe Atrophie *f* / **normal ~ of the thymus gland** normale Atrophie *f* der Thymusdrüse / **olivopontocerebellar ~** Brückenatrophie *f* / **optic ~** Sehnervenatrophie *f*, Optikusatrophie *f* / **progressive nervous ~** progressive Nervenatrophie *f* / **senile ~** Altersatrophie *f*, Altersschwund *m* / **spinal ~** Rückenmarkschwund *m*, spinale Atrophie *f* / **spinoneural ~** spinoneurale Atrophie *f* / **trophoneurotic ~** trophoneurotische Atrophie *f*

atropin Atropin *n*

atropinism, atropism Atropinsucht *f*, Belladonnaabusus *m*

attach binden, fixieren

attachment Fixierung *f*, Bindung *f*, Besetzung *f*, angehängte Datei *f* an einem E–Mail / **~ behaviour** Bindungsverhalten *n* / **~ disorder** Beziehungsstörung *f* / **disinhibited ~ disorder of childhood** Bindungsstörung *f* im Kindesalter mit Enthemmung / **reactive ~ disorder of childhood** reaktive Bindungsstörung *f* im Kindesalter / **reactive ~ disorder of infancy or early childhood** reaktive Bindungsstörung *f* im Säuglingsalter oder in der frühen Kindheit / **~ to the father** Vaterbindung *f*, Fixierung *f* an den Vater / **~ to the mother** Mutterbindung *f*, Fixierung *f* an die Mutter / **anaclitic ~** anaklitische Bindung *f* / **emotional ~** emotionale Bindung *f* / **libidinal ~** Libidobindung *f*, Libidofixierung *f*, libidinöse Fixierung *f* / **social ~** soziale Bindung *f*

attack Angriff *m*, Anfall *m*, Schub *m* / **~ of acute mania** Tobsuchtsanfall *m* / **~ behaviour** Angriffsverhalten *n* / **~ of catatonia** Katatonieanfall *m* / **acute ~** akuter Anfall *m* / **akinetic ~** akinetischer Anfall *m*, Anfall *m* von Bewegungslosigkeit / **apoplectiform ~** apoplektiformer Anfall *m* / **epileptic ~** epileptischer Anfall *m* / **hysterical ~** hysterischer Anfall *m*, psychogener Anfall *m* / **negative ~** Gegenargumentation *f*, Technik *f* des „advocatus diaboli" / **nervous ~** Nervenanfall *m* / **psychogenetic ~** psychogener Anfall *m*, hysterischer Anfall *m* / **psycholeptic ~** psycholeptischer Anfall *m* / **psychomotor ~** psychomotorische Attacke *f*, psychomotorrischer Anfall *m* / **psychosensory ~** psychosensorischer Anfall *m* / **syncopal ~** Ohnmachtsanfall *m*, Kollaps *m*

attainment Errungenschaft *f*, Fertigkeit *f*, Leistung *f* / **~ discrepancy** Leistungsdiskrepanz *f* / **educational ~ level** Bildungsabschluss *m* / **~ test** Leistungstest *m* / **initial ~** Anfangsfertigkeit *f*

attempt Versuch *m*

attempted versucht

attend achten, beachten, merken

attendant Wärter *m*, Pfleger *m* / anwesend

attensity sensorische Klarheit *f*

attention Aufmerksamkeit *f*, Beachtung *f* / **~ deficit disorder** Störung *f* mit Aufmerksamkeitsdefizit, Aufmerksamkeitsstörung *f* / **~ deficit disorder with hyperactivity** Störung *f* mit Aufmerksamkeitsdefizit bei Hyperaktivität / **~ deficit disorder without hyperactivity** Störung *f* mit Aufmerksamkeitsdefizit ohne Hyperaktivität / **~ deficit disorder, residual type** Störung *f* mit Aufmerksamkeitsdefizit, Residualtyp / **~–deficit / hyperactivity disorder** Aufmerksamkeitsdefizit– / Hyperaktivitätsstörung *f* / **~–deficit syndrome** Aufmerksamkeitsdefizit–Syndrom *n* / **~ disorder** Aufmerksamkeitsstörung *f* / **~ factor** Aufmerksamkeitsfaktor *m* / **~ getter** Aufmerksamkeitserreger *m* / **~–getting** Aufmerksamkeit erzeugend / **~ level** Aufmerksamkeitsniveau *n* / **~ reflex** Aufmerksamkeitsreflex *m* / **~ span** Aufmerksamkeitsumfang *m*, Aufmerksamkeitsspanne *f* / **~ test** Aufmerksamkeitstest *m* / **~ value** Aufmerksamkeitswert *m*, Zugkraft *f* / **arrest ~** Aufmerksamkeit *f* fesseln / **attract ~** Aufmerksamkeit *f* erregen / **call ~** Aufmerksamkeit *f* lenken (auf) / **concentrated ~** konzentrierte Aufmerksamkeit *f* / **derived primary ~** unwillkürliche Aufmerksamkeit *f* / **distributive ~** distributive Aufmerksamkeit *f* / **divert ~** Aufmerksamkeit *f* ablenken / **divided ~** geteilte Aufmerksamkeit *f* / **draw ~** Aufmerksamkeit *f* lenken (auf) / **evenly hovering ~** gleichschwebende Aufmerksamkeit *f* / **evenly poised ~** gleichschwebende Aufmerksamkeit *f* / **evenly suspended ~** gleichschwebende Aufmerksamkeit *f* / **exaggerated ~** übertriebene Aufmerksamkeit *f* / **fixed ~** konzentrierte Aufmerksamkeit *f* / **fluctuating ~** schwankende Aufmerksamkeit *f* / **divided ~** gespaltene Aufmerksamkeit *f* / **focused ~** gerichtete Aufmerksamkeit *f* / **forced ~** unwillkürliche Aufmerksamkeit *f* / **give ~** achtgeben / **involuntary ~** unwillkürliche Aufmerksamkeit *f* / **one–level ~** engzentrierte Aufmerksamkeit *f* / **poised ~** gleichschwebende Aufmerksamkeit *f*/ **primary ~** primäre Aufmerksamkeit *f* / **punctual ~** punktuelle Aufmerksamkeit *f* / **secondary ~** sekundäre Aufmerksamkeit *f* / **selective ~** selektive Aufmerksamkeit *f*, Filterung *f* / **spontaneous ~** spontane Aufmerksamkeit *f* / **suspended ~** gleichschwebende Aufmerksamkeit *f* / **sustained ~** Daueraufmerksamkeit *f* / **unremitting ~ test** Test *m* der Daueraufmerksamkeit

attentive aufmerksam, bedacht, wachsam, achtsam

attentiveness Aufmerksamkeit *f*, Wachsamkeit *f*

attenuation Abnahme *f*, Dämpfung *f*, Schwächerwerden *n*, Reduktion *f*

attitude Einstellung *f*, Attitüde *f*, Haltung *f*, Gesinnung *f* / **~ change** Einstellungsänderung *f*, Wandel *m* der Einstellung / **~ cluster** Einstellungskonstellation *f* / **~ constellation** Einstellungskomplex *m* / **~ development** Einstellungsbildung / **~ formation** Einstellungsbildung *f*, Entwicklung *f* einer Einstellung / **~ generality** Einstellungsbreite *f* / **~ interconnectedness** Interdependenz *f* von Einstellungen / **~ inventory** Einstellungstest *m*, Einstellungsfragebogen *m* / **~ measurement** Einstellungsmessung *f* / **~ measures** Einstellungstests *mpl*, Einstellungsskalen *fpl* / **~ of mind** Geisteshaltung *f* / **~ questionnaire** Einstellungsfragebogen *m* / **~ scale** Einstellungsskala *f*, Attitüdenskala *f*, Einstellungstest *m* / **~ similarity** Ählichkeit *f* der Einstellung / **~ survey** Einstellungsbefragung *f*, Meinungsbefragung *f* / **~ test** Einstellungstest *m* / **~ therapy** Einstellungstherapie *f* / **~ toward disabled** Einstellung *f* zu Behinderten / **~ toward handicapped** Einstellung *f* gegenüber Behinderten / **~ toward homosexuality** Einstellung *f* zur Homosexualität / **~ toward mental illness** Einstellung *f* zu Geisteskrankheiten / **~ type** Einstellungstyp *m* / **~ universe** Gesamtheit *f* der Einstellungen / **abstract ~** abstrakte Einstellung *f*, semantisches Klassifikationsvermögen *n* / **acquired ~** erlernte Einstellung *f* / **adolescent ~** Jugendlicheneinstellung *f* / **authoritarian ~** autoritäre Einstellung *f* / **blocking ~** Sperrung *f* / **cognitive ~** kognitive Einstellung *f* / **collective ~** Gruppenhaltung *f* / **conceptual ~** abstrakte Einstellung *f* / **concrete ~** konkrete Haltung *f* / **conscious ~** Bewusstseinslage *f* / **cramped ~** Krampfhaltung *f* / **cultural ~** gesellschaftliche Einstellung *f*, kulturelle Einstellung *f* / **cumulative ~ scale** additive Einstellungsskala *f* / **drinking ~** Einstellung *f* zum Alkoholgenuss / **environmental ~** Einstellung *f* zur Umwelt / **ergic ~** Einstellungserg *n* / **exhibitionistic ~** exhibitionistische Gesinnung *f* / **faulty ~** Fehlhaltung *f* der Persönlichkeit / **giving–up ~** Resignationshaltung *f* / **integrative ~** integrierende Einstellung *f* / **intersibling ~s** Einstellungen *fpl* zwischen Geschwistern / **intrafamilial ~s** Einstellungen *fpl* innerhalb der Familie / **moralistic ~** Tugendwächtertum *n*, moralistische Einstellung *f* / **negative ~ change** negative Einstellungsänderung *f* / **objectifying ~** Bemühen *n* um Objektivität / **occupational ~** berufliche Einstellung *f*, Einstellung *f* zum Beruf / **parental ~** Einstellung *f* der Eltern, elterliche Einstellung *f* / **political ~** politische Einstellung *f* / **private ~** private Einstellung *f* / **public ~** öffentlich bekundete Einstellung *f* / **racial and ethnic ~** rassische und nationale Einstellung *f* / **receptive ~** aufgeschlossene Haltung *f* / **religious ~** religiöse Einstellung *f* / **scientific ~** wissenschaftliche Einstellung *f* / **sexual ~** sexuelle Einstellung *f*, Einstellung *f* zur Sexualität / **social ~** soziale Einstellung *f* / **stereotyped ~** stereotype Einstellung *f*, Stereotypie *f* / **verbalized ~** mitteilbare Einstellung *f*

attitudinal Einstellungs–, Haltungs–

attitudinize posieren, eine gezierte Haltung einnehmen

attraction Anziehung *f*, Attraktion *f*, Attraktivität *f* / **~–aversion** Anziehung *f* — Abneigung *f* / **~ to the group** Gruppenanziehung *f* / **interpersonal ~** zwischenmenschliche Anziehung *f*, Attraktion *f* zwischen Personen, interpersonale Anziehung *f*

attractive attraktiv, anziehend

attractiveness Attraktivität *f*, Anziehungskraft *f* / **physical ~** körperliche Anziehungskraft *f*, physische Attraktivität *f*

attribute Attribut *n* / **~ of being conscious** Bewusstheit *f* / **subjective ~** subjektives Merkmal *n* / **tonal ~** Klangattribut *n*

attribution Attribuierung *f*, Attribution *f*, ursächliche Zuschreibung *f* / **~ error** Attribuierungsfehler *m*

attrition Schwund *m*, Verlust *m*, Abnutzung *f* / **experimental ~** Stichprobenschwund *m*

attune anpassen, einspielen, abstimmen

atypia Atypie *f*

atypical atypisch, heterolog

Aubert| diaphragm Aubert–Blende *f* / **~–Förster phenomenon** Aubert–Förster'sches Phänomen *n*, Aubert–Förster'scher Satz *m* / **~ phenomenon** Aubert'sches Phänomen *n*

audibility Hörbarkeit *f*, Vernehmbarkeit *f* / **~ curve** Hörkurve *f* / **~ limit** Hörgrenze *f* / **~ range** Hörbereich *m*, Hörfeld *n* / **~ threshold** Hörschwelle *f*

audible hörbar, vernehmlich

audience Zuhörerschaft *f*, Publikum *n*, Auditorium *n* / **~ analysis** Höreranalyse *f*, Leseranalyse *f* / **~ effect** Zuhörereffekt *m* / **~ measurement** Höreranalyse *f*

audile auditiv, akustisch ausgerichtet / auditiver Typus *m*

audimutism motorische Hörstummheit *f*, Audimutitas *f*

audio–frequency Tonfrequenz *f*, Tonbreite *f*

audiogenic durch Töne verursacht, audiogen

audiogram Audiogramm *n*, Hörkurve *f*

audiology Audiologie *f*, Wissenschaft *f* vom Hören

audiometer Audiometer *n*, Instrument *n* zur Hörprüfung, Hörmessgerät *n*

audiometric audiometrisch

audiometry Audiometrie *f*, Gehörmessung *f*, Hörprüfung *f*

audio–oscillator Summer *m*, akustischer Schwingungserzeuger *m*, Audiooszillator *m*

audiotape Tonband *n*

audiovisual audiovisuell

audition Hören *n*, Hörvermögen *n*, Hörkraft *f*, Hörfähigkeit *f* / **~ of thoughts** Gedankenhören *n*, Gedankenlautwerden *n* / **chromatic ~** Farbwahrnehmung *f* beim Hören, Audition colorée *f* / **gustatory ~** Geschmackswahrnehmung *f* beim Hören

auditive auditiv, Hör–

auditooculogyric akustisch bedingte Sehbewegungs–

auditopsychic Hörassoziationszentrums–

auditory auditiv, Hör–

auditosensory Hörzentrums–

Auersperg effect Auersperg–Effekt *m*, Auersperg–Phänomen *n*

aura Aura *f*, Vorzeichen *n* eines Anfalls / **~ cursoria** Aura cursativa *f* / **~ hysterica** hysterische Aura *f* / **auditory ~** akustische Aura *f* / **epigastric ~** epigastrische Aura *f*, viszerale Aura *f* / **epileptic ~** epileptische Aura *f* / **gustatory ~** Geschmacksaura *f* / **intellectual ~** traumhafte Bewusstseinsstörung *f* bei einem psychomotorischen Anfall / **motor ~** motorische Aura *f* / **olfactory ~** olfaktorische Aura *f*, Geruchsaura *f* / **sensible ~** sensible Aura *f* / **visceral ~** viszerale Aura *f* / **visual ~** optische Aura *f*, Skotom *n*, Funkensehen *n*

aural aural, Ohren–, Ohr–

auralize akustisch vorstellen, als Hörbild vorstellen

aureola, aureole Aureole *f*, Hof *m*

auride Ohrmuschel *f*, äußeres Ohr *n*

auriscope Ohrenspiegel *m*, Otoskop *n*

aurist Ohrenarzt *m*, Otologe *m*

aurometer Gehörmesser *m*, Hörschärfemesser *m*

autacoid Autacoid *n*, autopharmakologische Substanz *f*

autarchy Autarkie *f*, unumschränkte Herrschaft *f*

autemesia Erbrechen *n* (der Hysterischen)

authentic authentisch, echt, glaubwürdig

authenticity Authentizität *f*, Echtheit *f*, Glaubwürdigkeit *f*

authoritarian autoritär, autoritativ / autoritäre Person *f*, Autoritärer *m*

authoritarianism autoritäre Einstellung *f*, autoritäre Gesinnung *f*, Autoritarismus *m* / **parental ~** autoritäre Einstellung *f* der Eltern

authoritative gebieterisch, herrisch, autoritativ

authoritativeness herrisches Verhalten *n*, diktatorisches Verhalten *n*

authority Autorität *f*, Einfluss *m*, Macht *f*, Glaubwürdigkeit *f* / **~ complex** Autoritätskomplex *m* / **~ conflict** Autoritätskonflikt *m* / **~ figure** Autoritätsperson *f* / **medical ~ therapy** Autoritätstherapie *f* / **parental ~** elterliche Autorität *f* / **paternal ~** väterliche Autorität *f* / **political ~** politische Macht *f* / **social ~** soziale Autorität *f*, Status *m*

autia exzentrisches Verhalten *n*, Überspanntheit *f*, autistische Unbekümmertheit *f*

autism Autismus *m* / **akinetic ~** akinetischer Mutismus *m* / **atypical ~** atypischer Autismus *m* / **early infantile ~** frühkindlicher Autismus *m* / **infantile ~** infantiler Autismus *m* / **normal ~** normaler Autismus *m* / **primary ~** angeborener Autismus *m*

autistic autistisch

autoactivation Selbstaktivierung *f*

autoanalysis Selbstanalyse *f*, Autoanalyse *f*

autoanamnesis, automnesia Autoanamnese *f*, Eigenanamnese *f*

autocastration Selbstkastration *f*

autocentric egozentrisch

autochthon Eingeborener *m*, Ureinwohner *m*

autochthonal, autochthonous autochthon, systemimmanent, von selbst entstehend, eingeboren

autocompetition Wettbewerb *m* mit sich selbst, Wettbewerb *m* durch Höherstecken der eigenen Ziele

autocorrelation Autokorrelation *f*, Korrelation *f*, aufeinanderfolgender Meßwerte in Zeitreihen / **~ coefficient** Autokorrelationskoeffizient *m* / **~ function** Autokorrelationsfunktion *f*

autocratic autokratisch, selbstherrlich

autocriticism Selbstkritik *f*

autodiagnosis Selbstdiagnose *f*

autodiagnostic selbstdiagnostisch

autodivinization Selbstvergötterung *f* / **~ complex** Selbstvergötterungskomplex *m*

autoecholalia stereotype Wiederholung *f* einzelner Wörter, Autoecholalie *f*

autoechopraxia unaufhörliches Wiederholen *n* stereotyper Handlungen

autoerotic autoerotisch, sich selbst liebend

autoerotism, autoeroticism Autoerotismus *m*, Autoerotik *f*, Insichselbstverliebtsein *n*

autofetishism Autofetischismus *m*

autoflagellation Selbstgeißelung

autogenetic, autogenic, autogenous autogen, selbstentstanden

autogenital die eigenen Genitalien betreffend

autognosis Selbsterkenntnis *f*, Autognosis *f*

autohypnosis, autohypnotism Selbsthypnose *f*, Autohypnose *f*

autohypnotic autohypnotisch

autoimmune autoimmun

autointoxication Selbstvergiftung *f*, Autointoxikation *f*

autokinesis willkürliche Bewegung *f*

autokinetic autokinetisch

autolesion Selbstverstümmelung *f*

automata theory Automatentheorie *f*

automatic automatisch, selbsttätig, willensunabhängig

automation Automation *f*, Verwendung *f* von Maschinen, Automatisierung *f*

automatisation Automatisierung *f*, Verfestigung *f* von Handlungsabläufen

automatism Automatismus *m*, Automatie *f*, willensunabhängige Handlung *f* / **acquired ~** erworbener Automatismus *m* / **ambulatory ~** Wandertrieb *m*, Poriomanie *f*, Automatismus ambulatorius *m*, Davonlaufen *n* / **compulsive ~** Befehlsautomatie *f* / **epileptic ~** postparoxysmaler Dämmerzustand *m* / **mental ~** geistiger Automatismus *m*, Automatismus mentalis *m*, Assoziationismus *m* / **partial ~** partieller Automatismus *m* / **psychological ~** psychischer Automatismus *m* / **sensory ~** sensorischer Automatismus *m* / **total ~** totaler Automatismus *m*

automatograph Automatograph *m*, Gerät *n* zur Aufzeichnung unwillkürlicher Handlungen

automaton Automat *m*, abstrakter Automat *m*, mechanisch handelnder Mensch *m*

automorphic automorph, am eigenen Maßstab gemessen

automorphism Automorphismus *m*, Beurteilung *f* des Verhaltens anderer nach eigenem Maßstab

automysophobia krankhafte Furcht *f* vor körperlicher Beschmutzung, Automysophobie *f*

autonomasia Autonomasie *f*, Unfähigkeit *f* sich an Namen zu erinnern

autonomic, autonomous autonom, selbstgesteuert

autonomy Autonomie *f*, Selbständigkeit *f*, Eigengesetzlichkeit *f* / **~ drive** Autonomiestreben *n*, Streben *n* nach Unabhängigkeit / **~ need** Autonomiestreben *n*, Streben *n* nach Unabhängigkeit / **functional ~** funktionelle Autonomie *f* / **functional ~ of motives** funktionelle Autonomie *f* der Motive / **functional ~ principle** Prinzip *n* der funktionellen Autonomie / **moral ~** moralische Autonomie *f* / **organismic ~** organismische Autonomie *f* / **relative ~ of certain organs** relative Autonomie *f* einzelner Organe

autopathy Krankheit *f* ohne feststellbare Ursache

autophagy Autophagie *f*, krankhafte Neigung *f* sich selbst zu beißen

autophilia Selbstliebe *f*, Narzissmus *m*

autophobia krankhafte Furcht *f* vor der Einsamkeit, krankhafte Furcht *f* vor dem Alleinsein, Autophobie *f*

autophonomania Selbstmordtrieb *m*

autophony, autophonia Autophonie *f*, verstärktes Hören *n* der eigenen Stimme

autoplastic autoplastisch

autoplasticity, autoplasty Autoplastie *f*

autopsy Obduktion *f*, Autopsie *f*, Leichenöffnung *f*, Sektion *f* / **psychological ~** psychische Autopsie *f*

autopsychic autopsychisch

autopsychoanalysis Autopsychoanalyse *f*, Selbstanalyse *f*, Autoanalyse *f*

autopsychorhythmia Autopsychorhythmie *f*

autopsychosis Autopsychose *f*, Störung *f* des Ichgefühls

autopsychotherapy Selbstpsychotherapie *f*

autopsychotic autopsychotisch

autopunition Selbstbestrafung *f*

autoradiography Autoradiographie *f*

autoregulation Selbststeuerung *f*, Autoregulation *f*

autorivalry Wettbewerb *m* mit sich selbst, Wettbewerb *m* durch Höherstecken der eigenen Ziele

autosadism Autosadismus *m*

autoscope Autoskop *n*, Gerät *n* zur Aufzeichnung unwillkürlicher Körperbewegungen

autoscopy optische Halluzination *f* des eigenen Körperschemas

autoshaping Selbstformung *f*

autosomal autosom, autosomal

autosomatognosis Phantomgefühl *n*, Gefühl *n* des Nochvorhandenseins amputierter Glieder, Autosomatognosie *f*

autosome Autosom *n*, Euchromosom *n* / **~ disorder** Autosomenstörung *f*

auto–stereotype Autostereotyp *n*

autostimulation Selbsterregung *f*

autosuggestibility Fähigkeit *f* zur Selbstsuggestion

autosuggestion Autosuggestion *f*, Selbstsuggestion *f*

autosuggestive autosuggestiv

autotelic autotelisch, den Zweck in sich selbst habend

autotomy Selbstverstümmelung *f*, Autotomie *f*, spontanes Abwerfen *n* von Körperteilen bei niederen Tieren

autotopagnosia Verlust *m* der Orientierung über die eigenen Körperteile, Autotopagnosie *f*

autotopoamnesia Verlust *m* der Erinnerung über die eigenen Körperteile, Autotopoamnesie *f*

auxiliary helfend, mitwirkend, Hilfs– / Helfer *m*, Assistent *m*

availability Verfügbarkeit *f*, Bereitschaft *f*, Disponibilität *f* / **~ principle** Bereitschaftsprinzip *n*

avalanche conduction Auxomerie *f*, Lawinenreaktion *f*

avarice Habsucht *f*, Gier *f*

avaricious gierig, habgierig, geizig

a–v block Atrioventrikularblock *m*

average Durchschnitt *m*, Mittel *n*, Durchschnittswert *m*, Mittelwert *m* / durchschnittlich, Durchschnitts–, mittler(r, –s), Mittel– / **~ deviation** mittlere Abweichung *f* / **~ error** mittlerer Fehler *m* / **~ error procedure** Herstellungsverfahren *n* / **~ inaccuracy** mittlerer Schätzfehler *m* / **~ increase** durchschnittliche Zunahme *f* / **~ individual** Durchschnittsmensch *m* / **~ variation** mittlere Abweichung *f* / **above ~** über dem Durchschnitt / **abstract ~** abstrakter Mittelwert *m* / **calculated ~** berechneter Durchschnittswert *m* / **concrete ~** tatsächlicher Mittelwert *m* / **descriptive ~** beschreibender Mittelwert *m* / **geometric ~** geometrisches Mittel *n* / **guessed ~** geschätzter Mittelwert *m*, angenommenes Mittel *n* / **harmonic ~** harmonisches Mittel *n* / **moving ~ method** Methode *f* des gleitenden Durchschnitts / **typical ~** tatsächlicher Mittelwert *m*, typischer Durchschnittswert *m* / **weighted ~** gewogenes Mittel *n*

aversion Abneigung *f*, Widerwille *m*, Ekel *m*, Aversion *f* / **~ centre** Aversionszentrum *n* / **~ to colours** Farbenscheu *f*, Abneigung *f* gegen Farben / **~ conditioning** Aversionskonditionierung *f* / **~ conditioning treatment** Aversionskur *f* / **~ therapy** Aversionstherapie *f* / **~ to work** Arbeitsunlust *f*, Arbeitsscheu *f* / **sexual ~ and lack of sexual enjoyment** sexuelle Aversion *f* und mangelnde sexuelle Befriedigung *f* / **sexual ~ disorder** Störung *f* mit sexueller Aversion

aversive aversiv, abgeneigt, feindlich, widerwillig

aversiveness Abgeneigtheit *f*, Widerwille *m*

aviation| psychology Luftfahrtpsychologie *f*, Fliegerpsychologie *f* / **~ safety** Flugsicherheit *f*

avitaminosis Avitaminose *f*, Vitaminmangelkrankheit *f*

avocation Nebenbeschäftigung *f*, Nebentätigkeit *f*, Hobby *n*

avoid vermeiden, meiden

avoidance Vermeidung *f*, Meidung *f* / **~–avoidance conflict** Konflikt *m* zwischen Vermeidungstendenzen, Konflikt *m* zwischen Aversionstendenzen, Aversions–Aversions–Konflikt *m* / **~ behaviour** Vermeidungsreaktion *f*, Vermeidungsverhalten *n* / **~ conditioning** Vermeidungskonditionieren *n*, Vermeidungslernen *n* / **~ gradient** Vermeidungsgradient *m* / **~ learning** Vermeidungslernen *n* / **~ motive** Vermeidungstrieb *m*, Fluchtmotiv *n* / **~ reaction** Vermeidungsreaktion *f* / **~**

response Vermeidungsreaktion *f* / **~ training** Vermeidungslernen *n*, Fluchttraining *n* / **active ~** aktive Vermeidungsreaktion *f* / **conditioned ~** konditionierte Vermeidungsreaktion *f* / **free operant ~** kontinuierliche Vermeidung *f* / **passive ~** passive Vermeidungsreaktion *f*

avolition Willenssperrung *f*

avow eingestehen, gestehen, bekennen

avowal Bekenntnis *n*, Geständnis *n*, Erklärung *f*

awake wach, munter, bewusst / erwecken, aufwachen, bewusst werden, gewahr werden

awakening Erwachen *n* / **dissociated ~** dissoziiertes Erwachen *n*

aware bewusst, wissend

awareness Bewusstsein *n*, Bewusstwerden *n*, Auffassen *n*, Bewusstheit *f* / **perceptual ~** Wahrnehmungsbewusstsein *n* / **unconscious ~** unbewusstes Bewusstsein *n*

awe Ehrfurcht *f*, Scheu *f*

aweless furchtlos, unehrerbietig

awkward ungeschickt, linkisch, unbeholfen, verlegen, peinlich

awkwardness Ungeschicklichkeit *f*, unbeholfenes Wesen *n*, Unbeholfenheit *f*

axanthopsia Gelbblindheit *f*, Axanthopsie *f*

axes *siehe* **axis**

axial, axile axial, achsenförmig

axillary axillar, Achsel–

axiological wertend, interpretierend, deutend, axiologisch

axiology Wertlehre *f*, Axiologie *f*

axiom Axiom *n*, Grundsatz *m*

axiomatic axiomatisch, grundsätzlich, durch sich selbst erwiesen, ohne Beweis vorausgesetzt

axis Achse *f*, Ordinate *f*, Koordinate *f* / **~ cylinder** Achsenzylinder *m*, Axon *n*, Neurit *m* / **~ I disorder** Achse–I–Störung *f* / **~ of the eye** Augenachse *f* / **~ of reference** Bezugsachse *f* / **~ of rotation** Drehachse *f*, Rotationsachse *f* / **anatomical ~ of reference** anatomische Bezugsachse *f* / **cerebrospinal ~** Zerebrospinalachse *f* / **longitudinal ~** Längsachse *f* / **mathematical ~** mathematische Achse *f* / **neural ~** Rückgrat *n*, Rückenmark *n* / **oblique ~** schiefwinklige Achsen *fpl* / **optical ~** Sehachse *f* / **orthogonal ~** rechtwinklige Achsen *fpl*, orthogonale Achsen *fpl* / **principal ~** Hauptachse *f* / **proximodistal ~** Proximodistalachse *f* / **sagittal ~** Sagittalebene *f*, Dorsoventralachse *f* / **vertical ~** Körperlängsachse *f* / **visual ~** Sehachse *f*, Sehlinie *f*

axite Axon *n*, Neuron *n*, Nervenendast *m*

axoaxonal axo–axonal, zwischen zwei Axonen verbindend

axodendrite Achsenzylinder *m* mit Dendrit

axodendritic axo–dendritisch, zwischen einem Axon und einem Dendriten verbindend

axofugal zentrifugal

axon, axone Axon *n*, Achsenzylinder *m*, Neurit *m*, Körperachse *f*, Rückgrat *n* / **~ hillock** Axonhügel *m* / **~ reflex** Axonreflex *m*

axoneuron, axoneurone Neurit *m*, Zerebrospinalzelle *f*

axopetal zentripetal

axoplasm Axoplasma *n*, Zytoplasma *n* des Achsenzylinders

axosomatic axo–somatisch, zwischen einem Axon und einem Zellkörper verbindend

Ayres| Handwriting Scale Ayres–Handschriftenskala *f* / **~ Spelling Scale** Ayres–Buchstabierskala *f*

azidothymidine Azidothymidin *n*, AZT *n*

B

babble plappern, stammeln, schwatzen, nachschwatzen / Plappern *n*, Nachplappern *n* / **~ stage** Babbelstadium *n*, Plapperstadium *n*

babblement, babbling Geplapper *n*, Geschwätz *n* / **~ stage** Babbelstadium *n*, Plapperstadium *n*, Lallphase *f*, Lallperiode *f* / **vocal ~** Lallen *n*

Babinski| phenomenon Babinski–Reflex *m* / **~ reflex** Babinski–Reflex *m* / **~ sign** Babinski–Reflex *m*, Großzehenreflex *m* / **~–Weil test** Babinski–Weil–Blindgang–Versuch *m*

baboon Pavian *m*

baby Säugling *m*, Kleinkind *n*, Baby *n* / **~ farm** Säuglingsheim *n* / **~ sitter** Babysitter *m*, Kinderbetreuer(in) *m,f* / **~ sitting** Kinderbetreuung *f* / **~ talk** Babysprache *f*, Ammensprache *f* / **~–test** Entwicklungstest *m* für Kleinkinder / **premature ~** Frühgeburt *f*, zu früh geborenes Kind *n*

babyhood Säuglingsalter *n*, Kleinkindalter *n*

bacillophobia Bazillenangst *f*, Bazillophobie *f*

back Rücken *m* / **~ bone** Rückgrat *n*, Wirbelsäule *f*, Hauptverkehrsadern *fpl* des Internets / **~ pain** Rückenschmerzen *mpl*

backcross Rückkreuzung *f*

background Grund *m*, Hintergrund *m*, Umgebung *f* / **~ depression** Hintergrundverstimmung *f* / **~ noise** Hintergrundgeräusch *n*, Geräuschkulisse *f*, Störgeräusch *n* / **cultural ~** kultureller Hintergrund *m*, Lebensmilieu *n* / **educational ~** Ausbildungsgang *m*, Ausbildungsweg *m* / **personal ~** persönlicher Werdegang *m*

backing Unterstützung *f*, Hilfe *f*

backlash Umkehrreaktion *f*, Rückstoß *m*, Spielraum *m*, Rückwärts–Schrägstrich *m*

backward zurückgeblieben, retardiert, retroaktiv, retrograd

backwardness Zurückgebliebenheit *f*, Retardation *f* / **affective ~** affektive Zurückgebliebenheit *f* / **mental ~** geistig–seelische Zurückgebliebenheit *f* / **psychic ~** psychische Retardierung *f*

baclofen Baclofen *n*

bacteriophobia Bakterienangst *f*, Bakteriophobie *f*

bad–me böses Ich *n*

balance Gleichgewicht *n*, Ausgleich *m*, Gleichgewichtsorientierung *f* / **~ of mind** geistiges Gleichgewicht *n* / **~ of minus judgments** Differenz *f* zwischen der Anzahl positiver und negativer Urteile bei zwei objektiv gleichen Reizen / **~ test** Gleichgewichtsprüfung *f* / **~ theory** Theorie *f* des Gleichgewichts kognitiver Systeme / **autonomic ~** autonomes Gleichgewicht *n* / **biological ~** biologisches Gleichgewicht *n* / **cognitive ~** kognitives Gleichgewicht *n* / **emotional ~** seelisches Gleichgewicht *n* / **genic ~** Gengleichgewicht *n* / **mental ~** geistiges Gleichgewicht *n* / **oculomotor ~** okulomotorisches Gleichgewicht *n* / **psychic ~** seelisches Gleichgewicht *n* / **structural ~** strukturelles Gleichgewicht *n* / **unstable ~** labiles Gleichgewicht *n*

balanced ausgeglichen, ausgewogen, im Gleichgewicht befindlich / **well–~** gut ausgeglichen

balbuties Stottern *n*, Stammeln *n*, Dysarthrie *f*, Balbuties *f*

Bales category system Kategoriensystem *n* von Bales

Balint| group Balint–Gruppe *f* / **~'s syndrome** Balint–Syndrom *n*, Seelenlähmung *f* des Schauens

Ballard's phenomenon Ballard–Williams–Phänomen *n*

ballism Ballismus *m*, ballistisches Syndrom *n*

ballistic ballistisch, schleudernd, Schleuder–

ballistophobia Ballistophobie *f*, krankhafte Angst *f* vor Geschossen

balsamic balsamisch

Bamberger's disease Bamberger'sche Krankheit *f*

band Band *n* / **~ chart** Banddiagramm *n* / **~ pass filter** Bandpass *m* / **spectral ~** Band *n* des Spektrums

bandwagon effect Mitläufereffekt *m*

bandwidth Bandbreite *f*

bar Balken *m*, Stange *f*, Stab *m* / **~ chart** Balkendiagramm *n*, Stabdiagramm *n* / **~ diagram** Balkendiagramm *n*, Stabdiagramm *n*, Säulendiagramm *n* / **~ graph** Balkendiagramm *n*, Stabdiagramm *n* / **horizontal ~** Querstrich *m* / **parallel ~** Parallelstrich *m*

baraesthesia, baresthesia, baresthesis Drucksinn *m*, Barästhesie *f*

baraesthesiometer, baresthesiometer Drucksinnmesser *m*, Barästhesiometer *n*

baragnosis Verlust *m* des Gewichtssinnes, Baragnosie *f*

Barany| noise box Barany–Lärmtrommel *f*, Barany–Lärmapparat *m* / **~'s chair** Barany–Stuhl *m*, Drehstuhl *m* / **~'s chair test** Drehstuhlversuch *m* / **~'s pointing test** Barany–Zeigeversuch *m* / **~'s syndrome** Barany–Symptomenkomplex *m*

barbaralalia Barbaralalie *f*, schwer verständliche Sprache *f*

barbital Barbital *n*, Diäthylbarbitursäure *f* / **~ ism** Barbituratvergiftung *f*

barbiturate Barbitursäurepräparat *n*, Barbiturat *n* / **~ poisoning** Barbituratvergiftung *f*, Barbitursäurevergiftung *f*

barbiturism Barbituratabusus *m*, Barbituratvergiftung *f*, Barbitursäurevergiftung *f*

bargaining Verhandeln *n*

Barnum effect Barnum–Efekt *m*

baroceptor, baroreceptor Barorezeptor *m*, Druckrezeptor *m*

barognosis Gewichtssinn *m*, Drucksinn *m*, Barognose *f*

barotropism Barotropismus *m*, Barotaxis *f*

barrenness Unfruchtbarkeit *f*, Sterilität *f* / **~ of intellect** Geistesarmut *f* / **~ of mind** Geistesarmut *f*

barrier Barriere *f*, Schranke *f*, Grenze *f* / **~ against incest** Inzestschranke *f* / **schizophrenic ~** schizophrene Barriere *f*

baryecoia partieller Hörverlust *m*

baryencephalia Stupidität *f*, Stumpfsinn *m*, Dummheit *f*

baryglossia schwerfälliges, unartikuliertes Sprechen *n*, Baryglossie *f*

barylalia organisch bedingtes, schwerfälliges Sprechen *n*, Barylalie *f*

baryphonia, baryphony tiefe, schwere Stimme *f*, Dysphasie *f*, Sprechschwierigkeit *f*

barythyinia, barythymy Schwermut *m*, Melancholie *f*

basal basal, an der Basis liegend, basilar, Basal–

base Basis *f*, Grundlinie *f*, Grundfläche *f* / basieren, gründen (auf) / **~ age** Grundalter *n* / **~ frequency** Basisfrequenz *f* / **~ line** Grundlinie *f*, Nullinie *f*, Ausgangswert *m*, Ausgangsniveau *n* / **~ line data** Ausgangsdaten *pl* / **~ of stapes** Steigbügelplatte *f* / **~ of the brain** Hirnbasis *f*, Gehirnfuss *m* / **~ period** Bezugszeitraum *m* / **~ rate** Ausgangsniveau *n* / **~ year** Grundalter *n* / **fractured ~** Schädelbasisbruch *m*

basedowoid basedowoid

Basedow|'s disease Basedow–Krankheit *f*, Hyperthyreose *f* / **~ psychosis** Basedow–Psychose *f* / **~'s triad** Basedow–Trias *f*

basedowian Basedowkranker *m*, an Basedow Leidender *m*

basement layer Basalmembran *f*

bashful scheu, schüchtern, verschämt

bashfulness Schüchternheit *f*, Scheu *f*, Verschämtheit *f*

basic grundlegend, Grund–

basilar basilar, Basal–, Schädelbasis betreffend

basis Basis *f*, Grundlage *f* / **anterior ~ bundle** Vorderstranggrundbündel *n* / **empiric ~** empirische Basis *f* / **endothymic ~** endothymer Grund *m* / **lateral ~ bundle** Seitenstranggrundbündel *n* / **operational ~** operationale Basis *f*

basket nerve ending Korbzelle *f*

basophobia Basophobie *f*, Gehfurcht *f*

basophobic basophob

bastard unehelich, unecht / Bastard *m*

bastardy uneheliche Geburt *f*, Bastardschaft *f*

batch Menge *f*, Partie *f* / **~ production** Serienproduktion *f* / **~ storage** Datenspeicher *m*

bathophobia Höhenangst *f*, Tiefenangst *f*, Bathophobie *f*

bathyaesthesia, bathyesthesis Tiefensensibilität *f*, Tiefenempfindlichkeit *f*, Bathyästhesie *f*

bathyanaesthesia Verlust *m* der Tiefensensibilität, Verlust *m* der Tiefenempfindlichkeit, Tiefenanästhesie *f*

bathyphobia Höhenangst *f*, Tiefenangst *f*, Bathophobie *f*

bathypsychology Tiefenpsychologie *f*

batrachophobia Batrachophobie *f*, krankhafte Furcht *f* vor Fröschen

battarism Battarismus *m*, Stottern *n* durch überstürzte Sprechweise

battery Batterie *f* / **~ procedure** Testen *n* mittels Testbatterien

battle Kampf *m* / **~ exhaustion** Kampfneurose *f*, Frontkoller *m* / **~ fatigue** Kampfneurose *f*, Frontkoller *m*, Kriegsneurose *f*

baud Baud *n*

Bayes|' estimation Bayes–Schätzung *f* / **~' postulate** Bayes–Postulat *n* / **~' principle** Bayes–Gesetz *n*, Bayes–Theorem *n* / **~ian risk** Bayes–Risiko *n* / **~ian solution** Bayes–Lösung *f* / **~ ian statistics** Bayes–Statistik *f*, Bayes–Theorem *n* / **~ian strategy** Bayes–Strategie *f* / **~' theorem** Bayes–Theorem *n*, Bayes–Gesetz *n*, Bayes–Statistik *f*

Bayle's disease Bayle–Krankheit *f*, progressive Paralyse *f*, Dementia paralytica *f*

B coefficient B–Koeffizient *m*, Zugehörigkeitskoeffizient *m*

beaker cell Becherzelle *f*

Beale|'s ganglion cell Beale–Ganglionzelle *f* / **~ fibre** Beale–Faser *f*, Spiralnervenfaser *f*

Beard's disease Neurasthenie *f*, Nervenschwäche *f*, Beard–Syndrom *n*

beat Schwebung *f* / **~ effect** Schwebungseffekt *m* / **~ frequency** Schwebungsfrequenz *f* / **~ tone** Differenzton *m* / **binaural ~** Differenzschwebung *f* links–rechts

beatitude Seligkeit *f*, Glückseligkeit *f*, passive Euphorie *f*

Bechterew|–Mendel reflex Bechterew–Mendel–Reflex *m* / **~ technique** Bechterew–Technik *f*

bed Bett *n* / **~ craving** Bettsucht *f* / **~ restraint** Fixierung *f*, Fesselung *f* ans Bett / **~–wetter** Bettnässer *m*, Enuretiker *m* / **~–wetting** Bettnässen *n*, Enuresis nocturna *f* / **capillary ~** Kapillarnetz *n*

bee Biene *f*

beetle Käfer *m*

beg bitten, erbitten, betteln

begetter Erzeuger *m*, Vater *m*, Kindesvater *m*

behave sich verhalten, sich benehmen, sich betragen

behavioral, behavioural Verhaltens–, verhaltensbestimmt

behaviorism Behaviorismus *m*, Verhaltensforschung *f*, Verhaltenspsychologie *f* / **descriptive ~** deskriptiver Behaviorismus *m* / **operational ~** Operationalismus *m* / **purposive ~** zielgerichteter Behaviorismus *m*

behaviorology Ethologie *f*, Verhaltenslehre *f* / **comparative ~** vergleichende Verhaltensforschung *f*

behaviour, behavior Verhalten *n*, Benehmen *n* / **~ adjustment** Verhaltensanpassung *f* / **~ analysis** Verhaltensanalyse *f* / **~ cards** Karten *fpl* mit aufgelisteten Verhaltensweisen / **~ change** Verhaltensänderung *f* / **~ check list** Verhaltensprüfliste *f* / **~ clinic** Klinik *f* fürVerhaltenstherapie / **~ component** Verhaltenskomponente *f* / **~ contagion** ansteckendes Verhalten *n* / **~ contracting** Verhaltensverträge *mpl* / **~ criterion** Verhaltenskriterium *n* / **~ deficit** Verhaltensdefizit *n* / **~-description record** Aufzeichnung *f* einer Verhaltensbeschreibung / **~ determinant** Verhaltensdeterminante *f* / **~ disorder** Verhaltensstörung *f* / **~ disturbance** Verhaltensstörung *f* / **~ dynamics** Verhaltensdynamik *f* / **~ environment** Verhaltensfeld *n*, Verhaltensumfeld *n*, Milieu *n* / **~ field** Verhaltensfeld *n* / **~ formation** Verhaltensformung *f* / **~ function** geistige Funktion *f*, Verhaltensfunktion *f* / **~ generalisation** Verhaltensgeneralisation *f* / **~ integration** Verhaltensintegration *f* / **~ method** behavioristische Methode *f* / **~ modification** Verhaltensänderung *f*, Modifikation *f* des Verhaltens / **~ object** Verhaltensobjekt *n*, Zielobjekt *n* / **~ pattern** Verhaltensmuster *n*, Verhaltensgefüge *n*, Verhaltensweise *f*, Art *f* und Weise *f* des Verhaltens / **~ potential** Reaktionspotential *n* / **~ problem** Verhaltensproblem *n* / **~ psychology** Verhaltenspsychologie *f*, Behaviorismus *m* / **~ rating** Verhaltensbeurteilung *f* / **~ ratio** Verhaltensquotient *m* / **~ record** Verhaltensaufzeichnung *f* / **~ rehearsal** Verhaltensübung *f* / **~ repertoire** Verhaltensrepertoire *n* / **~ sampling** Erhebung *f* einer Verhaltensstichprobe / **~ segment** Verhaltenssegment *n*, Verhalteneinheit *f* / **~ set** Verhaltenskonstellation *f* / **~ setting** Verhaltensanordnung *f*, institutionalisierte Verhaltenssituation *f* / **~ shaping** Verhaltensformung *f* / **~ space** Lebensraum *m*, Verhaltensbereich *m* / **~ support** Verhaltensunterstützung *f* / **~ system** Verhaltenssystem *n* / **~ theory** Verhaltenstheorie *f*, Neobehaviorismus *m* / **~ therapy** Verhaltenstherapie *f* / **cognitive ~ therapy** kognitive Verhaltenstherapie *f*, Erkenntnistherapie *f* / **~ trait** Verhaltenseigenschaft *f*, Verhaltenszug *m*, Wesenszug *m* des Verhaltens / **~ unit** Verhalteneinheit *f* / **aberrant ~** abweichendes Verhalten *n* / **abient ~** Vermeidungsverhalten *n* / **abnormal ~** Verhaltensstörung *f* / **abstract ~** abstraktes Verhalten *n* / **acquired ~** erworbenes Verhalten *n*, angeeignetes Verhalten *n* / **adaptive ~** Adaptationsverhalten *n*, adaptives Verhalten *n* / **addictive ~** Suchtverhalten *n* / **adient ~** Annäherungsverhalten *n* / **adjunctive ~** kontingenzunabhängiges Verhalten / **affiliate ~** Gesellungsverhalten *n* / **aggressive ~** aggressives Verhalten *n*, Aggressionsverhalten *n* / **agonistic ~** Kampfverhalten *n* / **aimed ~** zielgerichtetes Verhalten *n* / **allelomimetic ~** allelomimetisches Verhalten *n*, Handlungsangleichung *f* / **allochthonous ~** allochthones Verhalten *n* / **ambivalent ~** ambivalentes Verhalten *n* / **antisocial ~** antisoziales Verhalten *n*, pathologisches Verhalten *n* / **apopathetic ~** apopathetisches Verhalten *n* / **appetitive ~** Appetenzverhalten *n* / **asocial ~** asoziales Verhalten *n*, asiziale Gesinnung *f* / **autochthonous ~** autochthones Verhalten *n* / **aversive ~** Vermeidungsverhalten *n*, Vermeidungsreaktion *f* / **charitable ~** karitatives Verhalten *n*, Wohltätigkeitsverhalten *n* / **cognitive ~** kognitives Verhalten *n* / **collective ~** Gruppenverhalten *n*, Kollektivverhalten *n* / **compulsive ~** Zwangsverhalten *n* / **concrete ~** konkretes Verhalten *n* / **conflicting ~** widersprüchliches Verhalten *n* / **conformist ~**

konformistisches Verhalten *n*, Konformismus *m* / **constructive ~** konstruktives Verhalten *n* / **coping ~** Aktionsverhalten *n*, Bewältigungsverhalten *n* / **coronary prone ~** koronargefährdendes Verhalten *n* / **corporate ~** Gruppenverhalten *n* / **covert ~** nach außen nicht erkennbares Verhalten *n* / **demonstrative ~** demonstratives Verhalten *n* / **deviant ~** abweichendes Verhalten *n*, Dissozialität *f* / **disorganized ~** desorganisiertes Verhalten *n*, unorganisiertes Verhalten *n* / **disruptive ~ disorder** expansive Verhaltensstörung *f* / **drinking ~** Trinkverhalten *n* / **ego–dystonic ~** ich–fremdes Verhalten *n* / **elicited ~** ausgelöstes Verhalten *n* / **emitted ~** nicht–reizbedingtes Verhalten *n*, Wirkverhalten *n* / **emotional ~** emotionales Verhalten *n*, affektives Verhalten *n* / **epistemic ~** epistemisches Verhalten *n*, intellektuell–suchendes Verhalten *n* / **ergic ~** zielstrebiges Verhalten *n* / **exaggerated ~** übersteigertes Verhalten *n*, demonstratives Verhalten *n* / **explicit ~** explizites Verhalten *n*, offenkundiges Verhalten *n*, manifestes Verhalten *n* / **exploratory ~** Explorationsverhalten *n*, Suchverhalten *n*, forschendes Verhalten *n* / **expressive ~** Ausdrucksverhalten *n* / **extrinsic ~** von außen verursachtes Verhalten *n* / **food–getting ~** Fütterungsverhalten *n* / **frozen ~** beschriebenes Verhalten *n* / **genotypic ~** genotypisches Verhalten *n* / **haphazard ~** Zufallsverhalten *n* / **help–seeking ~** hilfesuchendes Verhalten *n* / **hostile paranoid ~** aggressiv–paranoides Verhalten *n* / **human ~** menschliches Verhalten *n* / **ideational ~** Einsicht *f* / **imitative ~** Nachahmungsverhalten *n*, Imitation *f* / **implicit ~** implizites Verhalten *n* / **impulsive ~** Drang *m*, impulsive Handlung *f* / **inborn ~** angeborenes Verhalten *n* / **individual ~** individuelles Verhalten *n* / **innate ~** angeborenes Verhalten *n* / **innate ~ repertoire** angebotene Verhaltensweisen *fpl* / **instinctive ~** Instinktverhalten *n*, triebbedingtes Verhalten *n* / **intentional ~** Willenshandlung *f* beabsichtigtes Verhalten *n* / **interpersonal ~** zwischenmenschliches Verhalten *n* / **intrinsic ~** von innen verursachtes Verhalten *n* / **learned ~** erlerntes Verhalten *n* / **locomotor ~** Lokomotion *f*, Bewegung *f* / **maladaptive ~** fehlangepasstes Verhalten *n* / **maladjusted ~** unangepasstes Verhalten *n* / **manipulative ~** manipulierendes Verhalten *n* / **matched–dependent ~** Imitation *f* / **matching ~** Nachahmung *f*, Imitation *f* / **maternal ~** mütterliches Verhalten *n* / **mediating ~** Überbrückungsverhalten *n* / **metanergic ~** metanergisches Verhalten *n* / **migratory ~** Wanderungsverhalten *n*, Zugverhalten *n* / **mimetic ~** Nachahmungsverhalten *n* / **molar ~** molares Verhalten *n* / **molecular ~** molekulares Verhalten *n* / **motor ~** motorisches Verhalten *n*, Motorik *f* / **neurotic pattern ~** neurotische Verhaltensweise *f* / **non–adjustive ~** unangepasstes Verhalten *n* / **nonverbal ~** sprachfreies Verhalten *n* / **operant ~** operantes Verhalten *n*, nichtreizbedingtes Verhalten *n*, Aktionsverhalten *n* / **organizational ~** Organisationsverhalten *n* / **orienting ~** Orientierungsverhalten *n* / **ostentatious ~** demonstratives Verhalten *n* / **overt ~** manifestes Verhalten *n* / **parental ~** Elternverhalten *n*, elterliches Verhalten *n* / **planned ~** geplantes Verhalten *n* / **pluralistic ~** pluralistisches Verhalten *n* / **prenatal ~** vorgeburtliches Verhalten *n*, pränatales Verhalten *n* / **primitive ~** Primitivverhalten *n*, primitives Verhalten *n* / **problematic ~** Problemverhalten *n* / **prosocial ~** prosoziales Verhalten *n* / **protean ~** veränderliches Verhalten *n*, unbeständiges Verhalten *n*, proteanisches Verhalten *n* / **psychosexual ~** Sexualverhalten *n*, psychosexuelles Verhalten *n* / **puerilistic ~** läppisches Verhalten *n* / **purposive ~** zielstrebiges Verhalten *n*, zielgerichtetes Verhalten *n*, zweckgerichtetes Verhalten *n*, zielorientiertes Verhalten *n* / **rational ~** rationales Verhalten *n*, vernünftiges Verhalten *n* / **regressive ~** regressives Verhalten *n*, Regression *f* / **regulatory ~** regelndes Verhalten *n* / **required ~** vorgeschriebenes Verhalten *n*, gefordertes Verhalten *n* / **respondent ~** Reaktionsverhalten *n*, reaktives Verhalten *n* / **ritualistic ~** rituelles Verhalten *n*, Ritualverhalten *n* / **rotational ~** Rotationsverhalten *n* / **serial ~** ständig gleichbleibender Verhaltensablauf *m* / **sexual ~** Sexualverhalten *n* / **skipping ~** Sprungverhalten *n* / **social ~** Sozialverhalten *n*, soziales Verhalten *n* / **species-specific ~** artspezifisches Verhalten *n* / **spontaneous ~** Spontanverhalten *n* / **stereotyped ~** stereotypes Verhalten *n* / **superstitious ~** abergläubisches Verhalten *n* / **symbolic ~** symbolisches Verhalten *n* / **thymergastic ~** pathologisch-affektives Verhalten *n* / **unlearned ~** angeborenes Verhalten *n*, Triebverhalten *n*, Instinktverhalten *n* / **unselfish ~** altruistisches Verhalten *n* / **verbal ~** Sprachverhalten *n*, Verbalverhalten *n*, verbales Verhalten *n* / **voting ~** Wählerverhalten *n*

behaviourist, behaviorist Behaviorist *m*, Verhaltensforscher *m*, Verhaltenspsychologe *m*

behaviouristic, behavioristic behavioristisch, verhaltenspsychologisch, Verhaltens–

behaviouristics, behavioristics Verhaltenswissenschaft *f*

being Sein *n*, Existenz *f*, Leben *n*, Wesen *n*, Lebewesen *n* / **human ~** Mensch *m*

bel Bel *n* (10 Dezibel)

belief Glaube *m*, Meinung *f*, Überzeugung *f* / **~ system** Überzeugungssystem *n* / **~–value matrix** Wertsystem *n*, Wertorientierung *f*, Wertematrix *f*, Überzeugungswertmatrix *f* / **cultural ~** überlieferter Glaube *m* / **irrational ~** irrationale Überzeugung *f* / **religious ~** religiöser Glaube *m*, religiöse Überzeugung *f*

bell Glocke *f* / **~–shaped** glockenförmig, normalverteilt / **tonal ~** Klangglocke *f*

Bell|'s disease Bell'sche Krankheit *f*, Bell–Delirium *n* / **~'s law** Bell'sches Gesetz *n*, Bell–Magendie'sches Gesetz *n* / **~–Magendie law** Bell–Magendie–Regel *f* / **~'s mania** Bell–Delirium *n*, Bell'sche Krankheit *f* / **~ palsy** Bell–Lähmung *f*, Fazialislähmung *f* / **~ paralysis** Bell–Lähmung *f*, Fazialislähmung *f* / **~'s phenomenon** Bell–Phänomen *n*, Bell–Zeichen *n* / **~'s spasm** Fazialis–Tic *m*

belladonna alkaloid Belladonna–Alkaloid *n*

belonephobia krankhafte Angst *f* vor Nadeln, Belonephobie *f*

belonging, belongingness Zugehörigkeit *f* / **~ coefficient** Zugehörigkeitskoeffizient *m*, B–Koeffizient *m*

bemigride Bemigrid *n*

benactyzine Benactyzin *n* / **~ hydrochloride** Benactyzin–Hydrochlorid *n*

benadryl Benadryl *n*

bench–mark Festpunkt *m*, Bezugspunkt *m*, Orientierungspunkt *m*

beneceptive Wohlbefinden vermittelnd

beneceptor Wohlbefinden vermittelndes Nervenendorgan *n*, Benerezeptor *m*

beneficial vorteilhaft, nützlich, heilsam

benefit Nutzen *m*, Vorteil *m*, Gewinn *m* / nützen, begünstigen, fördern, Nutzen ziehen

benevolence Wohlwollen *n*, Güte *f*, Wohltätigkeit *f*

benevolent wohlwollend, gütig, Wohltätigkeits–, Unterstützungs–

benign, benignant gutartig, günstig, gütig, mild

benignity Gutartigkeit *f*, Güte *f*, Milde *f*

bent Hang *m*, Neigung *f*, Tendenz *f*, Disposition *f*

Benussi|'s experiment Benussi–Versuch *m* / **~ illusion** Benussi–Täuschung *f*

benzedrine Benzedrin *n*, Amphetamin *n*

benzodiazepine Benzodiazepin *n* / **~ agonist** Benzodiazepinagonist *m* / **~ antagonist** Benzodiazepinantagonist *m*

berdache Transvestit *m*

bereavement schmerzlicher Verlust *m*, einfache Trauer *f*

Berger rhythm Berger–Rhythmus *m*, Alphawellen *fpl*

Bernouilli| curve Bernouilli–Kurve *f*, Bernouilli–Verteilung *f* / **~ distribution** Bernouilli–Verteilung *f*, Binomialverteilung *f* / **~ theorem** Bernouilli–Theorem *n*

berserk amok, wütend, rasend, fanatisch

bestial bestialisch, tierisch, gemein

bestiality Bestialität *f*, Bestialismus *m*, Geschlechtsverkehr *m* mit Tieren, Sodomie *f*, Unzucht *f* mit Tieren

bet Wette *f*

beta Beta / **~–adrenergic** beta–adrenerg / **~–adrenergic receptor blocking agent** Beta–Rezeptorenblocker *m*, Beta–Blocker *m* / **~ amyloid** Beta–Amyloid *n* / **~–blocker** Betablocker *m*, Beta–Rezeptorenblocker *m* / **~–blocking drug** Betablocker *m*, Beta–Rezeptorenblocker *m* / **~–carboline** Beta–Carbolin *n* / **~–endorphin** Beta–Endorphin *n* / **~ coefficient** Beta–Koeffizient *m*, Beta–Gewicht *n* / **~ distribution** Beta–Verteilung *f* / **~ hypothesis** Beta–Hypothese *f* / **~ movement** Scheinbewegung *f*, Beta–Bewegung *f* / **~ regression coefficient** Beta–Koeffizient *m*, Standard–Partial–Regressionskoeffizient *m* / **~ response** Beta–Reaktion *f* / **~ rhythm** Beta–Rhythmus *m* / **~ test** Beta–Test *m* / **~ wave** Beta–Welle *f* / **~ weight** Beta–Gewicht *n*, Beta–Koeffizient *m*

between–brain Zwischenhirn *n*, Dienzephalon *n*

Betz cell Betz–Pyramidenzelle *f*

bewildered verwirrt

bewilderment Verwirrung *f*

Bezold–Brücke phenomenon Bezold–Brücke–Phänomen *n*

bhang Marihuanagetränk *n*

bias Vorurteil *n*, konstanter Fehler *m*, systematischer Verzerrungseffekt *m*, Bias *m* / **~ in responding** systematische Antworttendenz *f* / **emotional ~** emotionelles Vorurteil *n* / **experimental ~** Versuchsleiterfehler *m*

biased, biassed voreingenommen, in eine Richtung neigend, mit einem konstanten Fehler behaftet, subjektiv

biblio|clasty Biblioklasie *f* / **~kleptomania** Bibliokleptomanie *f* / **~kleptomaniac** Kleptomaner *m* der nur Bücher stiehlt, krankhafter Bücherdieb *m* / **~later** Bibelverehrer *m*, Büchernarr *m* / **~latry** übertriebene Bibelgläubigkeit *f*, übertriebene Bücherverehrung *f*, krankhafte Büchersammelwut *f* / **~mania** krankhafte Bücherliebhaberei *f*, Büchersucht *f*, Bücherleidenschaft *f*, Bibliomanie *f* / **~maniac** Büchernarr *m*, Bibliomaner *m*, an krankhafter Büchersammelwut Leidender *m* / biblioman, in Bücher vernarrt / **~phile** Bücherfreund *m*, Bibliophiler *m* / **~philia** Bibliophilie *f* / **~phobia** Bibliophobie *f* / **~therapy** Bibliotherapie *f*, Einsatz *m* von Lesestoff in der Therapie

bicoloured zweifarbig

bicycle ergometer Fahrradergometer *n*

bidactyly Bidaktylie *f*, Zweifingerigkeit *f*

bidigital mit zwei Fingern

bidirectional bidirektional, doppeltgerichtet

Bidwell's ghost zweites Nachbild *n*

Bielschowsky–Jansky disease Bielschowsky–Jansky–Schob Syndrom *n*

bifactor Zweifaktoren–

bifactorial bifaktoriell, Bifaktoren–, Zweifaktoren–

bifurcate spalten, teilen, zweiteilen

bifurcation Gabelung *f* Teilung *f*, Zweiteilung *f*

bigamist in Doppelehe Lebender *m*, Bigamist *m*

bigamous bigamisch, in Doppelehe lebend

bigamy Bigamie *f*, Doppelehe *f*

bigeminal doppelt, Zwillings–, zweikeimig, zweifach

biglottal zweisprachig

biglottism Zweisprachigkeit *f*

bilateral zweiseitig, doppelseitig, beiderseitig

bilaterality Zweiseitigkeit *f*, Doppelseitigkeit *f*

bile Galle *f*, Gallenflüssigkeit *f*

bilingual zweisprachig, bilingual

bilingualism Zweisprachigkeit *f*, Bilingualismus *m* / **combined ~** koordinierter Bilingualismus *m* / **compound ~** zusammengesetzter Bilingualismus *m*

bilious Gallen–, biliös, reizbar, cholerisch *n*

bimanual zweihändig, mit beiden Händen ausgeführt

bimodal bimodal, zweigipfelig

binary binär, aus zwei Teilen bestehend

binaural, binauricular beidohrig, binaural

bind binden, festbinden, festmachen / **~–web** Neuroglia *f*, Glia *f*, Nervenkitt *m*

binding bindend, verbindend / Bindung *f* / **~ of libido** Bindung *f* der Libido / **capable of ~** bindungsfähig

binge eating Heißhungerattacke *f*

binocular binokular, für beide Augen bestimmt

binomial binomial

binotic beidohrig, binaural

Binswanger dementia Binswanger–Demenz *f* / **~'s disease** Binswanger–Enzephalopathie *f* / **~'s encephalopathy** Binswanger–Enzephalopathie *f* / **~ treatment** Binswanger–Behandlung *f*

bio|–analysis Bioanalyse *f* / **~–assay** biologische Prüfung *f*, Bioassay *m*, Drogenerprobung *f* am lebenden Tier / **~ availability** Bioverfügbarkeit *f*

biocatalyst Biokatalysator *m*

biocentric biozentrisch

biochemical biochemisch

biochemistry Biochemie *f*

bioclimatology Bioklimatologie *f*, Lehre *f* vom Einfluss des Klimas auf Lebensvorgänge, Bioklimatik *f*

biocoenosis, biocenosis Biozönose *f*, Lebensgemeinschaft *f* zwischen Pflanzen und Tieren

biocoenotic, biocenotic biozönotisch

biocycle Biozyklus *m*, Lebenszyklus *m*

biodynamic biodynamisch

biodynamics Biodynamik *f*, Lehre *f* von den Lebenskräften, Biodynamismus *m*

bioelectric bioelektrisch

bioenergetics Bioenergetik *f*

bioengineering Biotechnologie *f*

bioequivalence Bioäquivalenz *f*

biofeedback Biofeedback *m*, physiologische Rückkopplung *f*, biologische Rückmeldung *f* / **~ training** Biofeedbacktraining *n*, Training *n* physiologischer Regelmechanismen

biogenesis, biogeny Biogenese *f*, Entwicklungsgeschichte *f* / **~ law** biogenetisches Grundgesetz *n*, Rekapitulationstheorie *f*

biogenetics Genmanipulation *f*, genetische Manipulation *f*

biogenic, biogenous biogen, biogenetisch

biogerontology biologische Altersforschung *f*

biogram standardisierte Lebensaufzeichnung *f*

biographical biographisch

biography Biographie *f*, Lebensbeschreibung *f*, Lebensgeschichte *f*

biological biologisch, Lebens–

biologism Biologismus *m*, Überbetonung *f* des biologischen Prinzips, Erklärung *f* allen Seins vom biologischen Standpunkt

biologist Biologe *m*

biology Biologie *f*, Lehre *f* von den Lebensvorgängen, Lehre *f* vom Leben

biomagnetism tierischer Magnetismus *m*, Mesmerismus *m*

biomechanics Biomechanik *f*, Ergonomie *f*, human engineering *n*, Ingenieurpsychologie *f*

biometrics, biometry Biometrie *f*, Biometrik *f*

biomorphosis Biomorphose *f*, Biometamorphose *f*

bionegativity organische Fehlorganisation *f*

bionergy Lebenskraft *f*

bionics Bionik *f*, vergleichende Wissenschaft *f* von Biologie und Technik

bionomics, bionomy Bionomie *f*, Lehre *f* von den Lebensgesetzen, bionome Ordnung *f*

biophobia Lebensangst *f*

biophore Biophore *f*, kleinstes Lebenselement *n*

biophysical biophysikalisch

biophysics Biophysik *f*

biopolymer Biopolymer *n*

biopsy Biopsie *f*, Probeexzision *f* und Untersuchung *f* lebenden Gewebes

biopsychic biopsychisch

biopsychism Biopsychismus *m*, Biopsychik *f*

biopsychology Psychobiologie *f*

biorhythm Biorhythmus *m*, endogene Rhythmik *f*, Lebensrhythmus *m*

biosocial biosozial

biosphere Biosphäre *f*

biospheric biosphärisch

biostatics Biostatik *f*

biostatistics Biostatistik *f*, Lebensstatistik *f*

biosynthesis Biosynthese *f*

biotechnology Biotechnologie *f*

biotherapy Behandlung *f* mit biologischen Substanzen

biotic biotisch, Leben betreffend, Umweltleben betreffend

biotics Lehre *f* vom Leben und seinen Funktionen

biotin Biotin *n*, Vitamin H *n*

biotonus Biotonus *m*

biotropic biotrop

biotropism Biotropismus *m*, Biotropie *f*

biotype Biotypus *m*, Biotyp *m*, reiner Typus *m*, Erbstamm *m*

biotypic biotypisch

biotypology Biotypologie *f*

biparental von beiden Eltern stammend

biped zweifüßig / Zweifüßler *m*

biphasic biphasisch, Zweiphasen–

bipolar bipolar, zweipolig, gegensätzlich

bipolarity Bipolarität *f* / **~ of traits** Bipolarität *f* von Eigenschaften

birth Geburt *f*, Abstammung *f* / **~ control** Geburtenkontrolle *f*, Geburtenbeschränkung *f* / **~ control methods** empfängnisverhütende Methoden *fpl* / **~ cry** Geburtsschrei *m*, erster Schrei *m* / **~ haemorrhage** Geburtsblutung *f* / **~ injury** Geburtsschaden *m*, Geburtstrauma *n* / **~ order** Geburtenfolge *f* / **~ palsy** Entbindungslähmung *f* / **~ rate** Geburtenrate *f* / **~ rite** Geburtsritus *m* / **~ symbolism** Geburtssymbolik *f* / **~ trauma** Geburtstrauma *n* / **~ weight** Geburtsgewicht *n* / **dead ~** Totgeburt *f* / **difficult ~** schwere Geburt *f* / **early ~** Frühgeburt *f* / **falling ~ rate** Geburtenrückgang *m* / **immature ~** Frühgeburt *f* / **infantile ~ theories** kindliche Geburtstheorien *fpl* / **monstrous ~** Missgeburt *f* / **multiple ~** Mehrlingsgeburt *f* / **premature ~** Frühgeburt *f* / **retarded ~** Spätgeburt *f*, Übertragen *n* des Kindes / **rising ~ rate** Geburtenanstieg *m* / **viable ~** Lebendgeburt *f*

birthmark Muttermal *n*, Geburtsfleck *m*

bisect halbieren, in zwei gleiche Teile teilen, sich teilen

bisection Halbierung *f* Zweiteilung *f* / **~ scaling method** Halbierungsmethode *f*, Halbierungsverfahren *n*

bisector Mittellinie *f*, Halbierungslinie *f*

bisensory bisensorisch, zwei Sinne gleichzeitig betreffend

biserial biserial

bisexual bisexuell, zweigeschlechtig, zwitterig

bisexuality Bisexualität *f*, Zweigeschlechtlichkeit *f*, Hermaphroditismus *m*

bit Bit *n*, Binärziffer *f*

bitter bitter

bitterness Bitterkeit *f*

bivalence Bivalenz *f*, Doppelwertigkeit *f*

bivariate bivariat, zwei Variablen enthaltend, in zwei Dimensionen variierend

bizarre bizarr

bizarreness Bizarrheit *f*, Bizarrerie *f*

black schwarz, Neger–

blackbox schwarzer Kasten *m*, black–box *f*

blackmail Erpressung *f* / **emotional ~** emotionelle Erpressung *f*, emotioneller Druck *m*

blackout Bewusstseinslücke *f*, Bewusstseinspause *f*, Blackout *n*, Fliegeramaurose *f* / **~ of consciousness** Bewusstseinslükke *f*, temporärer Bewusstseinsverlust *m* / **~ threshold** Schwelle *f* zum Bewusstseinsverlust / **inteffectual ~** geistiger Block *m*, mentale Blockierung *f*

bladder Blase *f*, Harnblase *f* / **~ control** Beherrschung *f* der Blase, Blasenkontrolle *f* / **~ evacuation reflex** Blasenentleerungsreflex *m* / **automatic ~** Reflexblase *f*

blamavoidance need Bedürfnis *n* Tadel zu vermeiden durch Kontrolle unsozialer Triebimpulse

blame Beschuldigung *f*, Tadel *m*

blamescape need Bedürfnis *n* Tadel zu vermeiden durch Flucht oder Verheimlichung tadelnswerter Situationen

blame–shifting Schuldverschiebung *f*

blaming others andern die Schuld geben

blanch erbleichen, blass werden

bland bland, mild, sanft, erträglich

blank weiße Stelle *f*, kurzzeitige Bewusstseinsstörung *f*, Formular *n*

blanket group Gruppe „Sonstige" *f*

blankness flüchtige Bewusstseinsstörung *f*

blast–injection technique Verfahren *n* der Zufuhr von Druckwellen

blastocoele Blastozöl *n*, Blastulahöhle *f*

blastocyte Blastozyt *m*, undifferenzierte Embryonalzelle *f*

blastoderm Keimhaut *f*, Blastoderm *n*

blastodermic blastodermal

blastogenesis, blastogeny Blastogenese *f*, Keimentwicklung *f*

blastogenic blastogen, aus der Keimanlage stammend

blastomere Blastomere *f*, Furchungszelle *f* des Eies

blastophthoria Keimschädigung *f*, Blastophthorie *f*

blastosphere, blastosphore Blastula *f*, Keimblase *f*

blastula Blastula *f*, Keimblase *f*

blastular blastulär, Keimblasen–

blastulation Blastulabildung *f*, Keimblasenbildung *f*

bleeding Bluten *n*, Blutung *f* / **~ into the dura** Durahämatom *n* / **cerebral ~** Gehirnblutung *f* / **menstrual ~** Periodenblutung *f*, Regelblutung *f* / **subdural ~** Subduralblutung *f*

blend Mischung *f*

blepharospasm Blepharospasmus *m*, Lidkrampf *m*

Bleuler's syndrome Bleuler–Psychosyndrom *n*

blind blind, nicht sehend / blenden, blind machen / **~ from birth** blindgeboren, blind seit Geburt / **the ~** die Blinden *mpl*

blinding Erblindung *f* / **~ headache** Augenmigräne *f*, Migraine ophtalmique *f*

blindism Verhaltensweisen *fpl* eines Blinden

blindness Blindheit *f*, Nichtsehenkönnen *n*, Einsichtslosigkeit *f* / **blue ~** Blaublindheit *f*, Azyanopsie *f*, Tritanopie *f* / **blue–yellow ~** Blaugelbblindheit *f*, Erythrochloropie *f* / **cerebral ~** zerebrale Blindheit *f* / **congenital ~** angeborene Blindheit *f* / **cortical ~** Rindenblindheit *f* / **deaf–and–dumb ~** Taubstummblindheit *f* / **emotional ~** hysterische Blindheit *f* / **functional ~** funktionelle Blindheit *f* / **green ~** Grünblindheit *f*, Achloropie *f*, Deuteranopie *f* / **hereditary ~** angeborene Blindheit *f*, vererbte Blindheit *f* / **hysterical ~** hysterische Blindheit *f* / **mental ~** geistige Blindheit *f* / **psychic ~** zerebrale Blindheit *f*, optische Agnosie *f* / **psychogenic ~** psychogene Blindheit *f* /

red–green ~ Rotgrünblindheit *f*, Xanthozyanopie *f* / **selective** ~ selektive Blindheit *f* / **spatial** ~ Raumblindheit *f* / **yellow** ~ Gelbblindheit *f*, Axanthopsie *f*

blink blinzeln, zwinkern / **~–eyed** (neurotisch) blinzelnd

blinking unwillkürliches Zwinkern *n*, Blinzeln *n* / ~ **reflex** Blinzelreflex *m*

bliss Glückseligkeit *f*, höchste Wonne *f*, Ananda *f*

Blix's temperature experiment Blix's Temperaturversuch *m*

block Block *m*, Leitungsunterbrechung *f*, Blockade *f* / blockieren, hemmen, sperren / ~ **counting test** Würfelanalyse *f*, Steinhaufentest *m* / ~ **design test** Würfeltest *m*, Mosaikspiel *n* / ~ **diagram** Blockdiagramm *n*, Blockschaltbild *n* / ~ **frequency** Blockdarstellung *f* der Häufigkeit / ~ **of the ganglia** Ganglienblockade *f* / ~ **of impulse** Antriebshemmung *f* / ~ **sampling** Erhebung *f* einer Gebietsstichprobe / ~ **situation test** Würfeltest *m* / **anaesthetic** ~ Leitungsanästhesie *f* / **anodic** ~ anodischer Block *m* / **atrioventricular (heart)** ~ Atrioventrikularblock *m* / **mental** ~ mentaler Block *m*, Unterbrechung *f* des Gedankenzuflusses / **spinal** ~ Lumbalanästhesie *f*

blockage Blockade *f*, Widerstand *m*, Sperrung *f*, Blockierung *f* / **emotional** ~ emotionelle Sperrung *f*, Affektsperre *f*

blocked gesperrt, unpassierbar, blockiert

blocker Blocker *m* / **adrenergic** ~ Ganglienblocker *m* / **ganglionic** ~ Ganglienblocker *m*

blocking Blockieren *n*, Blockierung *f*, plötzlicher Stopp *m* in einer Assoziationsbildung bei Durchbruch eines Komplexes, Sperrung *f* / ~ **of affect** Affektsperre *f* / ~ **of impulse** Frustration *f*, Impulssperre *f* / ~ **of thought** Denkhemmung *f*, Gedankensperre *f* / ~ **of thought processes** Denkstörung *f*

blood Blut *n* / ~ **alcohol** Blutalkohol *m* / ~ **alcohol concentration** Blutalkoholkonzentration *f* / ~ **and lymphatic disorder** Blut– und Lymphsystemerkrankung *f* / **~–brain barrier** Blut–Hirn–Schranke *f* / ~ **cell** Blutzelle *f*, Blutkörperchen *n* / ~ **circulation** Blutkreislauf *m*, Blutzirkulation *f* / ~ **clot** Blutgerinnsel *n* / ~ **coagulation** Blutgerinnung *f* / ~ **concentration** Blutkonzentration *f* / ~ **constituents** Blutbestandteile *mpl* / ~ **corpuscle** Blutkörperchen *n* / ~ **count** Blutbild *n*, Blutkörperchenzählung *f* / ~ **disorder** Bluterkrankung *f* / ~ **flow** Blutstrom *m*, Blutfluss *m*, Durchblutung *f*, Perfusion *f* / **coronary** ~ **flow** Koronardurchblutung *f* / ~ **glucose** Blutzucker *m* / ~ **group** Blutgruppe *f* / ~ **group incompatibility** Blutgruppenunverträglichkeit *f* / ~ **grouping** Blutgruppenbestimmung *f*, Feststellen *n* der Blutgruppe / **~–injection–injury type** Blut–Spritzen–Verletzungs–Typus *m* / ~ **level** Blutkonzentration *f* / ~ **macrophage** Monozyt *m* / ~ **picture** Blutbild *n* / ~ **plasma** Blutplasma *n* / ~ **platelet** Blutplättchen *n*, Thrombozyt *m* / ~ **poisoning** Blutvergiftung *f* / ~ **pressure** Blutdruck *m* / ~ **pressure disorder** Blutdruckkrankheit *f* / ~ **pressure measurement** Blutdruckmessung *f* / ~ **protein** Bluteiweiß *n* / ~ **serum** Blutserum *n* / ~ **specimen** Blutprobe *f* / ~ **stain** Blutfleck *m*, Blutspur *f* / **~–stained** blutbefleckt, blutig / ~ **sugar** Blutzucker *m* / ~ **test** Blutprobe *f*, Bluntuntersuchung *f* / ~ **transfusion** Blutübertragung *f*, Bluttransfusion *f* / ~ **type** Blutgruppe *f* / **~–typing** Blutgruppenbestimmung *f* / ~ **vessel** Blutgefäß *n* / ~ **volume** Blutmenge *f*, Blutvolumen *n* / **cerebral** ~ **flow** zerebrale Durchblutung *f* / **diastolic** ~ **pressure** diastolischer Blutdruck *m* / **differential** ~ **count** Differentialblutbild *n* / **differential** ~ **picture** Differentialblutbild *n* / **high** ~ **pressure** hoher Blutdruck *m*, Hypertonie *f* / **imcompatible** ~ Blut *n* einer inkompatiblen Blutgruppe / **menstrual** ~ Menstruationsblut *n* / **systolic** ~ **pressure** systolischer Blutdruck *m* / **white** ~ **cell**

weißes Blutkörperchen *n*, Leukozyt *m* / **white ~ count** Leukozytenzahl *f*

bloodthirst Blutdurst *m*

bloom Überstrahlung *f*, Aureole *f*

blue blau / **~-eyed** blauäugig / **~-sighted** blausichtig, blauüberempfindlich

blunt dumm, geistig schwerfällig / **~-witted** schwer von Begriff

blur Verschwommenheit *f*, Verschwommensein *n* / **hyperopic ~** durch Weitsichtigkeit bedingte Verschwommenheit *f*

blurred undeutlich, verschwommen

blush rot werden, erröten / Erröten *n*, Röte *f* / **emotional ~** Erröten *n* durch seelische Erregung, Affekterythem *n*

blushing errötend

board Ausschuss *m*, Behörde *f* / **~ of education** Schulbehörde *f* / **~ school** Volksschule *f*

boarding| house Pensionat *n*, Schülerheim *n*, Schülerinnenheim *n* / **~ school** Internat *n*

Boas' algesimeter Boas–Algesimeter *n*

boast prahlen, angeben / Prahlerei *f*, Angeberei *f*

boasting Prahlerei *f*, Angeberei *f*

body Körper *m*, Leib *m* / **~ awareness** Körperbewusstsein *n* / **~ balance** Körpergleichgewicht *n* / **~-build** Körperbau *m* / **~-build index** Körperbauindex *m* / **~ cell** Körperzelle *f* / **~ concept** Körpervorstellungsbild *n* / **~ control** Körperbeherrschung *f* / **~ dysmorphic disorder** körperdysmorphe Störung *f* / **~ ego** Körper–Ich *n*, körperliches Ich *n* / **~-ego technique** Körper–Ich–Technik *f* / **~ fluid** Körperflüssigkeit *f* / **~ hallucination** Körperhalluzination *f* / **~ height** Körpergröße *f* / **~ image** Körperbild *n*, Körperschema *n* / **~ image agnosia** Verlust *m* des Körpergefühls, Somatoagnosie *f* / **~ image disturbance** Körperbildstörung *f* / **~ jerk** Körperreflex *m* / **~ language** Körpersprache *f* / **~ length** Körperlänge *f* / **~ of the lens** Linsenkörper *m* / **~ mass index** Körpermasseindex *m* / **~ measurement** Körpermessung *f*, Körpermaß *n* / **~ mechanics** Körpermechanik *f* / **~ memory** Körpererinnerung *f* / **~-mind problem** Leib–Seele–Problem *n* / **~ odour** Körpergeruch *m* / **~ protest** Protest *m* des Körpers / **~ rocking** Körperschaukeln *n*, Körperschwanken *n* / **~ schema** Körperschema *n* / **~ size** Körpergröße *f* / **~-soul problem** Leib–Seele–Problem *n* / **~ structure** Körperbau *m* / **~ sway** Körperschwingung *f* / **~ temperature** Körpertemperatur *f* / **~ therapy** Körpertherapie *f* / **~ type** Körperbautyp *m*, Körperbautypus *m* / **~ type index** Körperbauindex *m* / **~ weight** Körpergewicht *n* / **~ zone** Körperzone *f*, Körpergegend *f* / **~ zone fixation** Fixierung *f* auf eine Körperzone / **adrenal ~** Nebenniere *f* / **amygdaloid ~** Mandelkörper *m* / **anal ~ zone** anale Körperzone *f* / **asthenic ~ type** asthenischer Typus *m*, Astheniker *m* / **astral ~** Astralleib *m* / **black ~ radiation** Wärmestrahlung *f* eines schwarzen Körpers, Planck'sche Strahlung *f* / **carotid ~** Karotisknötchen *n*, Glomus caroticum *n* / **chromatin ~** Chromatinkörper *m*, Chromosom *n* / **ciliary ~** Ziliarfortsatz *m*, Ziliarkörper *m*, Ziliarmuskel *m* / **conoid ~** Epiphyse *f*, Zirbeldrüse *f* / **elementary ~** Elementarkörperchen *n* / **epithelial ~** Epithelkörperchen *n*, Nebenschilddrüse *f* / **foreign ~** Fremdkörper *m* / **geniculate ~** Corpus geniculatum *n*, Kniehöcker *m* / **human ~** menschlicher Körper *m* / **infundibular ~** Hypophysenhinterlappen *m* / **mammillary ~** Mammilarkörper *m* / **medial geniculate ~** medialer Kniehöcker *m* / **microsomatic ~ build** Zwergwuchs *m* / **olivary ~** Olivenkörper *m*, Olive *f* / **oral ~ zone** orale Körperzone *f*, Oralraum *m* / **out-of-~ experience** außerkörperliche Erfahrung *f* / **pineal ~** Epiphyse *f*, Zirbeldrüse *f* / **pituitary ~** Hypophyse *f*, Hirnanhang *m* / **polar ~** Polkörperchen *n* / **quadrigeminal ~s** Vierhügel *mpl* / **simple ~** Grundstoff *m*, Element *n* / **striate ~** Corpus striatum *n*, Streifenhügel *m* / **subthalamic ~** Hypothalamus *m* / **suprarenal ~** Nebenniere *f*

/ **thyroid** ~ Schilddrusenkörper *m*, Schilddrüse *f*, Thyreoidea *f* / **trapezoid** ~ trapezförmiger Körper *m* / **vertebral** ~ Wirbelkörper *m* / **yellow** ~ Gelbkörper *m*, Corpus luteum *n*

Bogardus scale Bogardus–Skala *f* / ~ **of social distance** Bogardus–Skala *f* zur Bestimmung der sozialen Distanz

Bogen cage Käfig–Test *m* von Bogen

bogey system Quotensystem *n*, Akkordsystem *n*

bogus| erudition Scheingelehrsamkeit *f*, vorgetäuschte Bildung *f* / ~ **pipeline** Scheindirektleitung *f*

bolometer Bolometer *n*, Messapparat *m* für schwache Wärmestrahlen

bombesin Bombesin *n*

bond Verbindung *f*, Verknüpfung *f*, Verkettung *f*, Assoziation *f* / ~ **of friendship** Freundschaftsbündnis *n* / ~ **hypothesis** Verknüpfungshypothese *f*, Assoziationshypothese *f* / **emotional** ~ seelische Verbindung *f*, seelischer Kontakt *m* / **neural** ~ Nervenverbindung *f*

bone Knochen *m*, Bein *n* / ~ **cell** Knochenzelle *f* / **~–conduction** Knochenleitung *f*, Kopfknochenleitung *f*, Osteoakusis *f* / **~–conduction test** Knochenleitungstest *m* / **~–conduction audiometry** Knochenleitungsaudiometrie *f* / **~s of the cranium** Gesichtsschädel *m* / ~ **disorder** Knochenerkrankung *f* / ~ **marrow** Knochenmark *n* / ~ **sensibility** Vibrationsempfindung *f*, Vibrationsgefühl *n*, Pallästhesie *f* / **back** ~ Rückgrat *n*, Wirbelsäule *f* / **brittle** ~ **syndrome** Osteoporose *f* / **cortical** ~ Knochenrinde *f*, Knochenschale *f* / **cranial** ~ Schädelbein *n*, Schädelknochen *m* / **ethmoid** ~ Siebbein *n* / **frontal** ~ Stirnbein *n*, Os frontale *n* / **medullary** ~ Markknochen *m* / **occipital** ~ Hinterhauptbein *n*, Os occipitale *n* / **otic** ~ Ohrknöchelchen *n* / **palate** **~s** Gaumenknochen *mpl* / **palatine** ~ Gaumenbein *n*, Gaumendach *n* / **parietal** ~ Scheitelbein *n* / **pectineal** ~ Schambeinkamm *m* / **pubic** ~ Schambein *n*, Os pubis *n* / **pyramidal** ~ Dreiecksbein *n* / **sacred** ~ Kreuzbein *n* / **temporal** ~ Schläfenbein *n*, Os temporale *n* / **tympanic** ~ Paukenbein *n*

bonelet Knöchelchen *n*

Bonhoeffer|'s symptom Bonhoeffer–Zeichen *n*

bonus Zulage *f*, Gratifikation *f*, Prämie *f*

book Buch *n* / ~ **mark** Lesezeichen *n* / **scrambled** ~ Lehrprogrammbuch *n* mit verzweigtem Programm

boomerang effect Bumerang–Effekt *m*

boopia Boopie *f*, Kuhauge *n*, schmachtender Augenausdruck *m*

boorishness unkultiviertes Wesen *n*, Ungeschliffenheit *f*

booster session Unterstützungssitzung *f*, Auffrischungssitzung *f*

bootstrap method Münchhausen–Methode *f*, Methode *f* sich an den Haaren selbst aus dem Wasser zu ziehen

borderline Borderline *n* / ~ **case** Grenzfall *m*, Borderline–Fall *m* / ~ **contrast** Grenzkontrast *m*, Randkontrast *m* / ~ **defect** Borderline–Defekt *m*, Grenzfall *m* eines Defektes / ~ **disorder** Borderline–Störung *f* / ~ **intellectual functioning** Grenzbereich *m* der intellektuellen Leistungsfähigkeit / ~ **intelligence** Grenzfall *m* der Intelligenz / ~ **mental retardation** Grenzfall *m* der geistigen Retardierung, Geistigbehinderte *m,f* im Grenzbereich / ~ **personality** Borderline–Persönlichkeit *f* / ~ **personality disorder** Borderline–Persönlichkeitsstörung *f*, Borderline–Persönlichkeit *f*, Grenzpsychose *f* / ~ **personality organization** Borderline–Persönlichkeitsstruktur *f* / ~ **psychosis** Borderline–Psychose *f*, Borderline–Schizophrenie *f*, Grenzfall *m* einer Psychose / ~ **state** Grenzzustand *m*, Borderline–Zustand *m* / ~ **syndrome** Borderline–Syndrom *n*

bore langweilen, belästigen / langweilige, lästige Sache *f*, langweiliger Mensch *m*

boredom Langeweile *f*, Lästigkeit *f*

boring langweilig

born geboren / **~ before term** zu früh geboren / **first–~** erstgeboren / **prematurely ~** vorzeitig geboren

borstal Jugendstrafanstalt *f*, Jugendgefängnis *n* / **~ institution** Jugendstrafanstalt *f* mit Resozialisierungscharakter / **~ system** Resozialisierungssystem *n* in Jugendstrafanstalten

bosom Busen *m*, weibliche Brust *f*

bossiness herrisches Wesen *n*

botanical botanisch, zum Pflanzenreich gehörig

botanist Botaniker *m*, Pflanzenkundler *m*

botany Botanik *f*, Pflanzenkunde *f*

bottle Flasche *f* / **~–fed** mit der Flasche großgezogen / **~–fed child** Flaschenkind *n* / **~–feeding** Flaschenfütterung *f* / **~–neck** Engpass *m*, Stagnation *f*

botulism Botulismus *m*, spezifische Nahrungsmittelvergiftung *f*

boulimia Heißhunger *m*, Bulimie *f*

bound gebunden / **constitutionally ~** konstitutionell bedingt, konstitutionell verankert / **upward ~** nach oben tendierend

boundary Grenze *f*, Schranke *f*, Barriere *f* / **boundaries of the ego** Ich–Grenzen *fpl*, interpersonelle Abgrenzung *f* / **sexual ~ violation** Überschreiten *n* sexueller Grenzen

bounder unfeiner Mensch *m*, Plebejer *m*, Außenseiter *m*

bourgeois bürgerlich

Bourneville's disease Bourneville–Syndrom *n*, tuberöse Sklerose *f*

bout Anfall *m*

boutons terminaux Endknöpfe *mpl*, Boutons terminaux *mpl*

bovarism, bovarysm unrealistisches Selbstkonzept *n*, unrealistisches Selbstbild *n*, Selbsttäuschung *f*

bow movement Scheinbewegung *f* in Bogenform

bowel Darm *m*, Eingeweide *npl* / **~ control** Darmbeherrschung *f* / **~ disorder** Darmstörung *f* / **~ motility** Darmmotilität *f* / **~ training** Sauberkeitsgewöhnung *f* / **irritable ~** Reizkolon *n*, Colon irritabile *n*, Reizdarm *m*, irritables Kolon *n* / **regular ~s** normaler Stuhlgang *m* / **small ~** Dünndarm *m*

box Kasten *m* / **black ~** black–box *f*, schwarzer Kasten *m* / **jumping ~** Sprungkasten *m*

boxer's| dementia Boxerdemenz *f* / **~ encephalopathy** Boxerenzephalopathie *f*

brachybasia Trippelgang *m*, Brachybasie *f*

brachycephalia, brachycephaly, brachycephalism Brachyzephalie *f*, Kurzköpfigkeit *f*, Breitköpfigkeit *f*

brachycephalic, brachycephalous kurzköpfig, breitköpfig, brachyzephal

brachycephalus Brachyzephalus *m*, Kurzkopf *m*, Breitkopf *m*

brachydactylia, brachydactyly Kurzfingerigkeit *f*, Kurzzehigkeit *f*, Brachydaktylie *f*

brachydactylic, brachydactylous kurzfingerig, mit kurzen Fingern

brachymetropia Kurzsichtigkeit *f*

brachymetropic kurzsichtig

brachymorphic untersetzt, von kleiner Gestalt

brachymorphy Kleinheit *f* der Gestalt

brachytype breitwüchsiger Typ *m*

bradyacousia, bradyacusia Taubheit *f*, Schwerhörigkeit *f*

bradyaesthesia, bradyesthesia verlangsamte Empfindung *f*

bradyarthria langsame Sprache *f*, Bradyarthrie *f*

bradycardia verlangsamter Puls *m*, langsamer Herzschlag *m*, Bradykardie *f*

bradycinesia, bradycinesis verlangsamte Bewegungen *fpl*, Bradykinesie *f*

bradycinetic bradykinetisch

bradyecoia partielle Taubheit *f*

bradyglossia verlangsamte Sprache *f*, zögernde Sprache *f*, Bradyglossie *f*

bradykinesia, bradykinesis verlangsamte Bewegungen *fpl*, Bradykinesie *f*

bradykinetic bradykinetisch

bradykinin Bradykinin *n*

bradylalia verlangsamte Sprache *f*, zögernde Sprache *f*, Bradylalie *f*

bradylexia langsames Lesen *n*, Bradylexie *f*

bradylogia, bradylogy gehemmte Sprache *f*, Bradylogie *f*

bradyphagia Bradyphagie *f*, langsames Essen *n*, Bradyphagie *f*

bradyphasia verlangsamtes Sprechen *n*, Bradyphasie *f*

bradyphrasia langsames Sprechen *n*, langsame Sprache *f*, Bradyphrasie *f*

bradyphrenia Verlangsamung *f* aller psychischen Abläufe, verlangsamte Denkweise *f*, Bradyphrenie *f*

bradypnea Bradypnoe *f*

bradypragia verlangsamter Bewegungsablauf *m*, langsames Handeln *n*, Bradypragie *f*, Bradypraxie *f*

bradypsychia verlangsamte psychische Abläufe *mpl*, Bradypsychie *f*

bradypsychic bradypsychisch, psychisch verlangsamt

bradyscope Bradyskop *n*, Gerät *n* zur verlangsamten Projektion von Bilderserien

bradyspermatism verzögerte Ejakulation *f*, Bradyspermie *f*

bradyteleokinesis Bradyteleokinese *f*, krankhaftes Abbremsen *n* begonnener Bewegungen, Bremsungsphänomen *n*

Braidism, braidism Braidismus *m*, Hypnotismus *m*

Braille Blindenschrift *f*, Schrift *f* und Druck *m* für Blinde, Brailleschrift *f* / **~ instruction** Braille–Unterricht *m*, Unterricht *m* in Blindenschrift

brain Gehirn *n*, Hirn *n*, Enzephalon *n* / **~s** Verstand *m*, Intelligenz *f*, Köpfchen *n* / **~ ablation** Dezerebrierung *f* / **~ activity** Hirntätigkeit *f* / **~ aneurysm** Gehirnaneurysma *n* / **~ area** Gehirnregion *f*, Gehirnzentrum *n* / **~ axis** Gehirnstamm *m* / **~ basement** Basalhirn *n* / **~ cell** Gehirnzelle *f* / **~ centre** Hirnzentrum *n*, Gehirnzentrum *n* / **~ compression** Hirndruck *m* / **~ concussion** Gehirnerschütterung *f* / **~ contusion** Hirnkontusion *f*, Hirnquetschung *f*, Hirnprellung *f* / **~ cortex** Hirnrinde *f*, Großhirnrinde *f* / **~ damage** Hirnschädigung *f* / **infantile ~ damage** frühkindlicher Hirnschaden *m* / **minimal ~ damage** minimaler Hirnschaden *m* / **~ damaged** hirngeschädigt / Hirngeschädigte *m,f* / **~ death** Hirntod *m* / **~ defect** Hirnschaden *m* / **~ disease** Gehirnkrankheit *f*, Gehirnleiden *n*, Gehirnerkrankung *f* / **~ disorder** Hirnfunktionsstörung *f* / **~ dominance** zerebrale Dominanz *f*, Hemisphärendominanz *f* / **~ dynamism** Gehirndynamismus *m* / **~ dysfunction** Hirnfunktionsstörung *f* / **minimal ~ dysfunction** minimale Hirnleistungsstörung *f* / **~–fag** geistige Überanstrengung *f*, Gehirnermüdung *f* / **~–fever** Gehirnfieber *n*, Hirnhautentzündung *f* / **~–field dominance** Gehirnfelddominanz *f* / **~ function** Gehirnfunktion *f* / **~ injury** Hirnverletzung *f*, Gehirnschädigung *f* / **~ lesion** Hirnläsion *f*, Hirnverletzung *f* / **traumatic ~ injury** traumatische Hirnverletzung *f* / **~ localisation** Gehirnlokalisation *f* / **~–localised psychosyndrome** hirnlokales Psychosyndrom *n* / **~ mantle** Gehirnmantel *m*, Gehirnrinde *f* / **~ map** Gehirnatlas *m*, Hirnkarte *f* / **dynamic ~ mapping** EEG–Brain–Mapping *n* / **~ metabolism** Gehirnstoffwechsel *m* / **~ murmur** Gehirngeräusch *n* / **~ neoplasm** Hirntumor *m*, Gehirngeschwulst *f* / **~ nerve** Hirnnerv *m* / **~ operation** Gehirnoperation *f* / **~–pan** Hirnschädel *m* / **~ potential** Gehirnpotenzial *n* / **~ pressure** Gehirndruck *m*, Hirndruck *m* / **~ removal** Enthirnung *f*, Dezerebrierung *f* / **~ sand** Gehirnsand *m*, Hirnsand *m* / **~ size** Gehirnumfang *m*, Gehirngröße *f* / **~ spot hypothesis** Lokalisationstheorie *f* / **~ stem** Hirnstamm *m*, Gehirnstamm *m*, Hirnachse *f* / **~ stem**

evoked response audiometry Messung *f* akustisch evozierter Hirnstammpotentiale, BERA / **~ stem reflex** Hirnstammreflex *m* / **~ stimulation** Hirnreizung *f*, Hirnstimulation *f* / **chemical ~ stimulation** chemische Gehirnstimulation *f* / **electrical ~ stimulation** elektrische Gehirnstimulation *f* / **~ storm** plötzliche geistige Umnachtung *f* / **~ storming** „Brainstorming" *n*, schöpferische Ideenassoziation *f*, kreative Ideenfindungstechnik *f* / **~ subdivision** Hirnabschnitt *m* / **~ substance** Gehirnmasse *f* / **~ sugar** Gehirnzucker *m* / **~ surgery** Gehirnchirurgie *f* / **~ syndrome** Zerebralsyndrom *n* / **chronic ~ syndrome** chronisches psychoorganisches Syndrom *n* / **organic ~ syndrome** organisches Hirnsyndrom *n* / **~ trauma** Hirntrauma *n*, Hirnverletzung *f* / **~ tumour** Gehirntumor *m*, Gehirngeschwulst *f*, Hirngeschwulst *f*, Hirntumor *m* / **~ volume** Hirnvolumen *n* / **~–wash** Gehirnwäsche vornehmen / **~–washing** Gehirnwäsche *f*, geistige Umerziehung *f* / **~ wave** Gehirnwelle *f*, telepathische Schwingung *f*, Eingebung *f*, Geistesblitz *m* / **~ weight** Gehirngewicht *n* / **~ work** geistige Arbeit *f* / **acute ~ disorder** akute Gehirnerkrankung *f* / **acute organic ~ syndrome** akutes hirnorganisches Psychosyndrom *n* / **chemical ~ stimulation** chemische Hirnreizung *f* / **chronic ~ syndrome** chronisches Gehirnleiden *n* / **congenital ~ defect** angeborener Hirnschaden *m* / **developmental ~ defect** erworbener Hirnschaden *m* / **electrical ~ stimulation** elektrische Hirnreizung *f* / **expanding ~ lesion** raumbeengender Hirnprozess *m* / **focal ~ damage** Herdschaden *m* des Gehirns / **left ~** linke Hirnhemisphäre *f* / **little ~** Kleinhirn *n* / **minimal ~ disorder** minimale zerebrale Dysfunktion *f* / **minimal ~ dysfunction in children** frühkindliches exogenes Psychosyndrom *n* / **minimally ~–damaged** minimal Hirngeschädigter *m* / **olfactory ~** Riechhirn *n*, Rhinenzephalon *n* / **open ~ injury** offene Hirnverletzung *f* / **organic ~ damage** organischer Hirnschaden *m* / **organic ~ syndrome** organisches Psychosyndrom *n*, hirnorganisches Syndrom *n* / **primitive ~** Urhirn *n* / **right ~** rechte Hirnhemisphäre *f* / **split–~** split–brain, gespaltenes Gehirn *n* / **upper ~** Großhirn *n* / **wet ~** Hirnödem *n*

brained mit Gehirn versehen / **crack–~** verrückt / **shallow–~** hohlköpfig, dumm, einfältig

brainless dumm, blöde, einfältig, hirnlos

branch Zweig *m*, Ast *m*, Abzweigung *f* / **~ of the nerve** Nervenast *m* / **communicating ~** Verbindungsast *m* / **lateral ~** Nebenzweig *m* / **main ~** Hauptast *m* / **side ~** Seitenast *m*, Nebenast *m* / **terminal ~** Endast *m*

branched verzweigt, gegabelt

branching Verzweigung *f*, Verzweigen *n* von Programmen, Verästelung *f* / verzweigt, sich verzweigend / **backward ~** zurückverweisende Verzweigung *f* von Programmen / **forward ~** weiterführende Verzweigung *f* von Programmen

brand Marke *f* / **~ image** Markenbild *n* / **~ leader** Marktführer *m* / **~ manager** Product–Manager *m* / **~ name** Markenname *m* / **~ preference** Markenpräferenz *f*

brandy addiction Branntweinsucht *f*

bravery Tapferkeit *f* Unerschrockenheit *f*, Mut *m*, Courage *f*

b reaction b–Reaktion *f*

breadth Breite *f*, Ausdehnung *f* in der Breite, Weite *f*, Ausmaß *n*

break Erholungspause *f*, Unterbrechung *f*

breaking of taboo Tabuverletzung *f*

breakdown Zusammenbruch *m*, Aufgliederung *f*, Auffächerung *f* / **~ of marriage** Zerrüttung *f* der Ehe / **mental ~** Seelenkrise *f* / **nervous ~** Nervenzusammenbruch *m*, nervöse Erschöpfung *f*

break phenomenon Brechungsphänomen *n*

breakthrough Durchbruch *m* / **~ of drive** Triebdurchbruch *m* / **~ of instinct** Triebdurchbruch *m* / **~ of the repressed** Wiederkehr *f* des Verdrängten, Rückkehr *f* des Verdrängten / **psychotherapeutic ~** psychotherapeutischer Durchbruch *m*

breakup of a relationship Beendigung *f* einer Beziehung

breast Brust *f* / **~ cancer** Brustkrebs *m*, Mammakarzinom *n* / **~ examination** Brustuntersuchung *f* / **~ feeding** Stillen *n*, Brusternährung *f* / **~–fed** brustgenährt / **~–fed child** Brustkind *n* / **~–feeding** Säugen *n*, Nähren *n* mit Muttermilch, Brusternährung *f* / **~ neoplasm** Brustgeschwulst *f*, Brustkrebs *m*

breathing Atmen *n*, Respiration *f* / **~–exercises** Atemübungen *fpl* / **~–related sleep disorder** atmungsgebundene Schlafstörung *f* / **abdominal ~** Bauchatmung *f*, Zwerchfellatmung *f* / **difficult ~** Atemnot *f*, Dyspnoe *f* / **heavy~** Atembeschwerden *fpl* / **nasal ~** Nasenatmung *f* / **oppressed ~** erschwerte Atmung *f*, Atemnot *f* / **regular ~** regelmäßige Atmung *f* / **short ~** Kurzatmigkeit *f* / **thoracic ~** Brustatmung *f*, Rippenatmung *f*

breathless außer Atem, atemlos

bred gezüchtet / **cross–~** gekreuzt / **pure–~** reinrassig

breed züchten, aufziehen, erziehen / Brut *f*, Rasse *f*, Art *f*, Stamm *m*, Züchtung *f* / **cross–~** kreuzen

breeding Züchten *n*, Zucht *f*, Aufzucht *f*, Züchtung *f* / **~–ground** Brutplatz *m* / **cross–~** Kreuzung *f* / **selective ~** Zuchtselektion *f*

brevi|lineal kurzwüchsig / **~ type** kurzwüchsiger Typ *m*, kurzwüchsiger Typus *m*, Bréviligne *f*

bridge Brücke *f* / **~ circuit** Brückenschaltung *f* / **~ insulator** Brückenisolator *m*

briefing spezifizierter Arbeitsauftrag *m*, Arbeitsanweisung *f*, genaue Instruktion *f* / **~ conference** Auftragsbesprechung *f* einer Agentur

bright klar, glänzend, klug, aufgeweckt, begabt

brighten aufmuntern, günstiger werden

brightness Helligkeit *f*, Klarheit *f*, Scharfsinn *m* / **~ adaptation** Helligkeitsanpassung *f* / **~ of colour** Farbintensität *f*, Farbhelligkeit *f* / **~ constancy** Helligkeitskonstanz *f* / **~ contrast** Helligkeitskontrast *m* / **~ discrimination** Helligkeitsunterschied *m*, Helligkeitsunterscheidung *f* / **~ invariance** gleichbleibende Helligkeit *f* / **~ perception** Helligkeitswahrnehmung *f* / **~ threshold** Helligkeitsschwelle *f* / **absolute ~ threshold** absolute Helligkeitsschwelle *f* / **tonal ~** Klanghelligkeit *f*, Tonhelligkeit *f*

bril Bril *n*, 0,01 Millilambert *n*

brilliance Helligkeit *f* Klarheit *f*, Scharfsinn *m* / **~ contrast** Helligkeitskontrast *m* / **~ limen** Lichtschwelle *f* / **~ threshold** Lichtschwelle *f*

brilliant hochbegabt, ausgezeichnet, genial

bring up erziehen, aufziehen

Briquet syndrome Briquet–Syndrom *n*

Brissaud|–Marie syndrome Brissaud–Syndrom *n* / **~ syndrome** Brissaud–Syndrom *n*

broad breit, weit / **~–minded** tolerant, großzügig, vorurteilslos, weitherzig / **~–mindedness** Toleranz *f*, Großzügigkeit *f*, Vorurteilslosigkeit *f*, Weitherzigkeit *f* / **~–set** untersetzt

broadcast Rundfunksendung *f* / **~ advertising** Funkwerbung *f* / **~ research** Hörerforschung *f*

broadcasting of thought Gedankenausbreiten *n*

Broca|'s aphasia motorische Aphasie *f*, Broca–Aphasie *f* / **~'s area** Broca'sches Zentrum *n* / **~'s centre** Brocasches Zentrum *n* / **~'s centre of speech** Broca'sches Sprachzentrum *n* / **~'s convolution** Broca'sche Windung *f*

Brodmann areas, Brodmann's areas Brodmann–Felder *npl*, Brodmann–Areale *npl*

bromide Bromid *n*, Bromsalz *n* / **~ intoxication** chronische Bromvergiftung *f*, Bromismus *m*

bromidrosiphobia Bromidrosiphobie *f*

bromine cachexia Bromkachexie *f*

bromism, brominism chronische Bromvergiftung *f*, Bromismus *m*

bromocriptine Bromocriptin *n*

bronchi Luftröhren *fpl*, Bronchien *pl*

bronchial bronchial, Bronchial–

bronchiole Bronchiole *f*

bronchoconstriction Bronchokonstriktion *f*

brontophobia krankbafte Angst *f* vor Gewittern, Astraphobie *f*

brooding Grübeln *n* / **~ person** Grübler *m* / **compulsive ~** Grübelzwang *m* / **obsessive ~** Grübelzwang *m*

broody brütend, nachdenklich

brother Bruder *m* / **~s and sisters** Geschwister *pl* / **~ complex** Bruderkomplex *m* / **~–sister incest** Bruder–Schwester–Inzest *m*

Brown|–Séquard syndrome Brown–Séquard–Syndrom *n*, Halbseitenlähmung *f* des Rückenmarks / **~–Spearman formula** Spearman–Brown–Formel *f*

browser Browser *m*, Programm *n* zum Durchblättern des Internets

Bruch's membrane Bruch–Membran *f*

bruise Quetschung *f*

Brunswik ratio Brunswik–Beziehung *f*, Brunswik–Quotient *m*

brutal brutal, roh, grausam, unmenschlich

brutality Brutalität *f*, Grausamkeit *f*, Roheit *f*

brute gefühflos, brutal

bruxism Zähneknirschen *n* im Schlaf, Bruxismus *m*

bruxomania nervöses Zähneknirschen *n*, Bruxomanie *f*

B score B–Wert *m*

B type B–Typ *m*

buccal buccal, Backen–, Wangen–

bud Knospe *f*, Keim *m* / **gustatory ~** Geschmacksknospe *f* / **olfactory ~** Geruchsknospe *f*

budding Aufkeimen *n*, Aufblühen *n*, Knospen *n*

Buddhism Buddhismus *m*

buffer Puffer *m* / **~ item** Pufferfrage *f*, Pufferaufgabe *f*

bufotenin Bufotenin *n*

bugger Unzucht treiben / Sodomit *m*

buggery Unzucht *f*, Sodomie *f*

build bauen, aufbauen / Körperbau *m*, Figur *f* / **general ~** Allgemeinerscheinung *f* / **macrosplanchnic ~** viszeraler Körperbau *m* / **structural ~** Körperbau *m*, Körperbeschaffenheit *f*

bulb, bulbus Zwiebel *f*, Knolle *f*, Bulbus *m* / **~ of the eye** Augapfel *m* / **gustatory ~** Geschmacksknospe *f* / **olfactory ~** Riechkolben *m*, Bulbus olfactorius *m* / **sensory ~** Sinnesknospe *f* / **spinal ~** verlängertes Mark *n*, Medulla oblongata *f*, Nachhirn *n*, Myelanzephalon *n* / **terminal ~** Nervenendknospe *f*, Nervenendkolben *m*

bulbar bulbär, Bulbo–

bulbonuclear Medulla oblongata und deren Nervenzentren betreffend

bulimarexia Bulimarexie *f*

bulimia Bulimie *f*, Heißhunger *m*, Essgier *f*, krankhafter Hunger *m*, Hyperorexie *f* / **~ nervosa** Bulimia nervosa *f* / **atypical ~ nervosa** atypische Bulimia nervosa *f*

bulimic heißhungrig

bulimy Bulimie *f*, Heißhunger *m*

Bumke's| pupil Bumke–Zeichen *n* / **~ symptom** Bumke–Zeichen *n*

bump of locality Ortssinn *m*, Orientierungssinn *m*

bundle Bündel *n* / **~ of fibers** Faserbündel *n* / **~ of His** His–Bündel *n*, Atrioventrikularbündel *n* / **~ hypothesis** Mosaikauffassung *f* / **atrioventricular ~** His–Bündel *n*, Atrioventrikularbündel *n* / **main ~** Hauptbündel *n* / **medial longitudinal ~** hinteres Längsbündel *n* / **medullary ~** Markbündel *n* / **olfactory ~** Riechbündel *n* / **sinu–atrial ~** Sinusknoten *m*, Keith–Flack–Knoten *m*

Bunsen–Roscoe law Bunsen–Roscoe–Gesetz *n*, Reizmengengesetz *n*

Burdach|'s column Burdach–Strang *m* / **~'s nucleus** Burdach–Kern *m*, keilförmiger Kern *m*

bureaucracy Bürokratie *f*, Amtsschimmel *m*

bureaucratic bürokratisch

bureaucratisation Bürokratisierung *f*, Ausdehnung *f* bürokratischen Verhaltens

burn–out Ausgebranntsein *n*

burnt gebrannt, verbrannt

burst bersten, zerplatzen, zerspringen / Aufplatzen *n*, Bersten *n*, Durchbruch *m*, Ausbruch *m* / **~ with rage** vor Wut platzen / **~ into tears** in Tränen ausbrechen

business Geschäftsleben *n*, Geschäft *n*, Betrieb *m*, Industrie *f* und Handel *m* / **~ education** kaufmännische Ausbildung *f*, betriebswirtschaftliche Ausbildung *f* / **~ and industrial personnel** Beschäftigte *mpl* in Wirtschaft und Industrie / **~ judgement test** Test *m* zur Erfassung der kaufmännischen Urteilsfähigkeit / **~ management** Unternehmensleitung *f*, Betriebsführung *f* / **~ organization** Firma *f*, Unternehmen *n* / **~ student** Betriebswirtschaftsstudent *m* / **coordinated ~ neurosis** Berufsneurose *f*

businessman Geschäftsmann *m*, Kaufmann *m*

button Knopf *m* / **gustatory ~** Geschmacksknospe *f*

butyrylpiperazine Butyrylpiperazin *n*

buyer Käufer *m*/ **~'s market** Käufermarkt *m* / **~'s resistance** Kaufhemmung *f*

buying Einkauf *m* / **~ decision** Kaufentschluss *m*, Kaufentscheidung *f* / **~ habits** Kaufgewohnheiten *fpl* / **~ motive** Kaufmotiv *n* / **~ power** Kaufkraft *f*

buzz–session Diskussionsmethode „Diskussion 66" *f*

buzzer Summer *m*, Lärmtrommel *f*

buzzing Ohrensausen *n*, Brummen *n*, Sausen *n*

by–product Nebenprodukt *n*

bystander–behaviour Zuschauerverhalten *n*

byte Byte *n*

byword Sprichwort *n*, Schlagwort *n*

C

cacaesthesia, cacesthesia schlechtes Gefühl *n*, Unlustempfinden *n*, Kakästhesie *f*

cacergasia mangelhafte Funktion *f*, geistiger Defekt *m*

cachectic kachektisch, Kachexie–

cache memory Cache–Speicher *m*

cachexia, cachexy Kachexie *f*, schlechter Körperzustand *m*, Kräfteverfall *m* / ~ **hypophysea** Simmonds–Krankheit *f*, Hypophysenvorderlappeninsuffizienz *f*

cachinnate übermäßig laut lachen, hysterisch lachen

cachinnation übermäßig lautes Lachen *n*, hysterisches Lachen *n*

cacodaemonomania Besessenheit *f*, Dämonomanie *f*

cacogenic den Gesetzen der Eugenik zuwiderlaufend

cacogeusia übler Geschmack *m*, Empfindung *f* schlechten Geschmacks, Kakogeusie *f*

cacolalia Kakolalie *f*

cacology schlechte Aussprache *f*, fehlerhafte Ausdrucksweise *f*

cacopathia schwere Geistesstörung *f*

cacophonia, cacophony Misston *m*, Missklang *m*, Kakophonie *f*

cacosmia schlechter Geruch *m*, Kakosmie *f*

cacothymia Geistesstörung *f*

cadence Rhythmus *m*, Ton *m*, Tonfall *m*

cadre Kerngruppe *f*, Führungsgruppe *f*, Stamm *m* / ~ **formation** Kaderschulung *f*

caecitas völlige Erblindung *f*

caenogenesis Zänogenese *f*, Entwicklung *f* durch Anpassung

caesaromania Cäsarenwahn *m*, Größenwahn *m*

caesarotomy Kaiserschnitt *m*

cafard Depression *f*, schwere Apathie *f*

cafeteria feeding Fütterung *f* mit selbst ausgewähltem Essen, Selbstbedienungsfütterung *f*

caffeine Koffein *n* / ~ **intoxication** Koffeinvergiftung *f*, Koffeinintoxikation *f*, Koffeinismus *m*

caffeine–induced koffeininduziert

caffeinism chronische Koffeinvergiftung *f*, Koffeinismus *m*

cage Käfig *m*, Gefängniszelle *f* / ~ **apparatus** Käfig *m* / ~ **consciousness** Haftbewusstsein *n*

cainophobia Neophobie *f*, Furcht *f* vor Neuerungen, krankhafte Abneigung *f* gegen Neuerungen, Misoneismus *m*

caisson disease Caisson–Krankheit *f*

calamity Unglück *n*, Unheil *n*, Elend *n* / **social** ~ soziales Elend *n*

calamus scriptorius Calamus scriptorius *m*, unterster Abschnitt *m* des 4. Ventrikels

calcarine spornförmig

calcification Verkalkung *f*, Kalkablagerung *f* / ~ **of the wall of a vessel** Gefäßwandverkalkung *f* / **arterial** ~ Arterienverkalkung *f*

calcify verkalken

calcitonin Calcitonin *n*, Kalzitonin *n*

calcium Kalzium *n* / ~ **antagonist** Kalziumantagonist *m* / ~ **blocking agent** Kalziumantagonist *m* / ~ **bromide** Kalziumbromid *n* / ~ **channel blocker** Kalziumantagonist *m* / ~ **ion** Kalziumion *n* / ~ **metabolism disorder** Kalzium–Stoffwechsel–Störung *f* / ~ **pump** Kalziumpumpe *f*

calculation Berechnung *f*, Rechnung *f*

calculator Rechenmaschine *f* / **rotary ~** Rechenscheibe *f*

calculus Rechnung *f* / **~ of interpolation** Interpolationsrechnung *f* / **infinitesimal ~** Infinitesimalrechnung *f* / **integral ~** Integralrechnung *f*

calibrate eichen, kalibrieren

calibration Eichung *f*, Kalibrierung *f*, Standardisierung *f*

call Ruf *m*, Lockruf *m* / **maternal ~** Lockruf *m* der Mutter

callback Kontrollinterview *n*, Besuchswiederholung *f*

calfigraphy Kalligraphie *f*, Kunst *f* des Schönschreibens

calling Berufung *f*, Vokation *f*

callosity Gefühllosigkeit *f*, Abstumpfung *f*, Gefühlskälte *f*, Gemütsarmut *f*

callosum Corpus callosum *n*

callous gefühllos, abgestumpft, gefühlskalt, gemütsarm

callousness Gefühllosigkeit *f*, Abstumpfung *f*, Gefühlskälte *f*

calm ruhig, still, beruhigen, besänftigen / Ruhe *f*, Stille *f*

calmative beruhigend, mildernd / Beruhigungsmittel *n*, Sedativum *n*

calming Beruhigung *f*, Dämpfung *f* / beruhigend

calmness Gemütsruhe *f* / **~ of mind** Ataraxie *f*, Seelenruhe *f*

caloric kalorisch, thermisch

calorific Wärme–, Wärme erzeugend

calorimeter Wärmemesser *m*, Kalorimeter *n*

calvarium Schädeldecke *f*

camouflage Tarnung *f* / tarnen

camp Lager *n*, Ferienlager *n* / **therapeutic ~** therapeutisches Ferienlager *n*

campaign Kampagne *f*, Feldzug *m* / **~ plan** Werbeplan *m* / **national ~** nationale Werbekampagne *f*, überregionaler Werbefeldzug *m* / **political ~** politische Kampagne *f*

campimeter Gesichtsfeldmesser *m*

campimetry Gesichtsfeldmessung *f*

camptocormia Haltungshysterie *f*

campus Hochschulgelände *n*

can Können *n* / können

canal Gang *m*, Kanal *m* / **~ of Cloquet** Cloquet'scher Kanal *m* / **~ of Schlemm** Schlemm'scher Kanal *m* / **alimentary ~** Verdauungstrakt *m*, Magen–Darm–Kanal *m*, Verdauungskanal *m*, Digestionstrakt *m* / **auditory ~** Gehörgang *m* / **auricular ~** Ohrgang *m*, innerer Gehörgang *m* / **central ~ of the spinal cord** Zentralkanal *m* / **cerebrospinal ~** Hirn–Rückenmarkskanal *m* / **cochlear ~** Schneckenkanal *m*, Schneckengang *m* / **digestive ~** Verdauungskanal *m*, Verdauungstrakt *m*, Digestionstrakt *m* / **endocervical ~** Zervikalkanal *m* / **gastro–intestinal ~** Magen–Darm–Kanal *m*, Verdauungstrakt *m*, Verdauungswege *mpl*, Gastrointestinaltrakt *m* / **genital ~** Geschlechtswege *mpl*, Genitalkanal *m* / **medullary ~** Markkanal *m* / **neural ~** Vertebralkanal *m*, Neuralrohr *n* / **semicircular ~** Bogengang *m* / **spinal ~** Wirbelkanal *m* / **tympanic ~** Paukengang *m* / **vertebral ~** Wirbelkanal *m* / **vestibular ~** Vorhoftreppe *f*

canalboat children Kanalboot–Kinder *npl*

canalis centralis Zentralkanal *m* im Rückenmark, Canalis centralis *m*

canalisation Kanalisierung *f*, Kanalisation *f* / **~ formation** Kanalbildung *f*, Bahnung *f* / **~ strength** Stärke *f* der Kanalisierung / **neural ~** Balmung *f*

canalise kanalisieren

cancellation Durchstreichung *f*, Streichung *f* / **~ test** Durchstreichtest *m*

cancer Krebs *m*, Karzinom *n* / **~ cell** Tumorzelle *f*, Krebszelle *f* / **~ screening** Krebsvorsorgeuntersuchung *f* / **terminal ~** letaler Krebs *m*, unheilbarer Krebs *m*

cancerophobia Karzinophobie *f*, Furcht *f* vor Krebserkrankung

candle Kerze *f* / **~ power** Kerzenstärke *f*

cannabinoid Cannabinoid *n*

cannabinomania Haschischsucht *f*, Cannabismus *f*

cannabis Cannabis *f*, Hanf *m* / **~ abuse** Cannabismissbrauch *m* / **~ delusional disorder** cannabisinduziertes Syndrom *n* / **~ dependence** Haschischsucht *f* / **~ indica** indischer Hanf *m* / **~ intoxication** Cannabisintoxikation *f*, Haschischsucht *f* / **~ intoxication delirium** Cannabisintoxikationsdelir *n* / **~ organic mental disorders** cannabisinduzierte organisch bedingte psychische Störungen *fpl*

cannabis|–induced cannabisinduziert / **~–related** im Zusammenhang mit Cannabis

cannabism Cannabismus *m*, Haschischsucht *f*, Haschischvergiftung *f*, chronische Intoxikation *f* der Haschischraucher

cannibal Kannibale *m*, Menschenfresser *m*

cannibalism Kannibalismus *m*, Menschenfresserei *f*, Anthropophagie *f*

cannibalistic kannibalisch

Cannon's theory Cannon–Syndrom *n*, Notfallsfunktion *f*, Notfallsreflex *m*

canon Kanon *m*, Regel *f* / **~ of agreement** Regel *f* der Übereinstimmung / **~ of differences** Unterschiedsregel *f* / **~ of residues** Residualregel *f*

capability Fähigkeit *f*, Eignung *f*

capacitance Kapazitanz *f*, kapazitive Reaktanz *f*

capacitor Kondensator *m*

capacity Kapazität *f*, Fähigkeit *f*, Leistungsvermögen *n*, Leistungsfahigkeit *f* / **~ for criminal responsibility** Zurechnungsfähigkeit *f* / **~ for getting into rapport** Rapportfähigkeit *f* / **~ model** Leistungsmodell *n* / **~ test** Fähigkeitstest *m*, Eignungstest *m* / **~ variable** Leistungsvariable *f* / **abstractive ~** Abstraktionsfähigkeit *f* / **accommodative ~** Akkommodationsfähigkeit *f* / **cranial ~** Schädelvolumen *n* / **eidetic ~** eidetische Fähigkeit *f*, eidetische Anlage *f* / **electrical ~** Kapazitanz *f* / **functional ~** Leistungsvermögen *n*, Leistungsfähigkeit *f* / **functional residual ~** funktionelle Residualkapazität *f* / **inherent ~** Fähigkeit *f*, Leistungsvermögen *n* / **integrative ~** Integrationsfähigkeit *f* / **intracranial ~** Schädelkapazität *f* / **legal ~** Geschäftsfähigkeit *f* / **limited ~** begrenzte Kapazität *f* / **maximum ~** Höchstleistung *f* / **mental ~** geistige Fähigkeit *f*, geistig–seelisches Leistungsvermögen *n* / **procreative ~** Zeugungsfähigkeit *f*, Potenz *f* / **vital ~** Vitalkapazität *f*

Capgras syndrome Capgras–Syndrom *n*, Doppelgänger–Illusion *f*

capillary haarfein, kapillar / Haargefäß *n*, Kapillargefäß *n*, Kapillare *f*

caprice Laune *f*

capricious launenhaft, unberechenbar, launisch, unbeständig

caprylic kaprylisch, nach Ziegenbock stinkend

capsaicin Capsaicin *n*

capsula, capsule Kapsel *f*, Hülle *f* / **adrenal ~** Nebenniere *f* / **external ~** Capsula externa *f* / **internal ~** Capsula interna *f* / **reducing ~** Reduktionskapsel *f* / **suprarenal ~** Nebenniere *f*

captation Hingerissensein *n*, Gebanntsein *n*, Kaptation *f*, Zustand *m* des Gebundenseins an den Hypnotiseur

captivation schlafähnlicher Zustand *m*, Pseudohypnose *f*, Kaptivation *f*

captivity Gefangenschaft *f*, Gebanntsein *n*

captopril Captopril *n*

car accident Autounfall *m*

carbachol Karbachol *n*, Carbachol *n*

carbamazepine Carbamazepin *n*

carbidopa Carbidopa *n*

carbohydrate metabolism Kohlenhydratstoffwechsel *m*

carbon Kohle *f*, Kohlenstoff *m* / **~ dioxide** Kohlensäure *f*, Kohlendioxyd *n* / **~ dioxide partial pressure** CO_2–Partialdruck *m* / **~ dioxide therapy** Kohlensäurebehandlung *f* / **~ monoxide** Kohlenoxydgas *n*,

Kohlenmonoxyd *n* / ~ **monoxide poisoning** Kohlenmonoxydvergiftung *f* / ~ **tetrachloride** Tetrachlorkohlenstoff *m*

carboxyhaemoglobinaemia Carboxyhämoglobinämie *f*

carcinogen krebserzeugender Stoff *m*, Karzinogen *n*

carcinoma Krebs *m*, Karzinom *n*, bösartiger Tumor *m*

carcinomatophobia, carcinophobia Krebsangst *f*, Karzinophobie *f*

card Karte *f* / ~ **index** Kartei *f*, Kartothek *f* / ~ **sorting** Bilderordnen *n* / ~**–sorting test** Karteitest *m*, Katalogtest *m*, Bilderordnen *n* / **medical** ~ Krankenblatt *n*

cardiac Herz–

cardialgia Herzschmerz *m*, Kardialgie *f*, Magenschmerz *m*, Magenkrampf *m*

cardiazol, cardiazole Cardiazol *n* / ~ **convulsive shock therapy** Cardiazolschockbehandlung *f* / ~ **spasm** Cardiazolkrampf *m* / ~ **shock** Cardiazolschock *m*

cardinal Kardinal–, Haupt–

cardiochronograph Gerät *n* zur Aufzeichnung der Herzschlagdauer, Kardiochronograph *m*

cardiodynia Herzschmerz *m*, Schmerz *n* in der Herzgegend, Kardialgie *f*

cardiogram Kardiogramm *n*

cardiograph Kardiograph *m*, Herzkurvenschreiber *m*

cardiographic kardiographisch

cardiography Kardiographie *f*, Kurvendarstellung *f* der Herztätigkeit

cardiology Lehre *f* vom Herzen, Kardiologie *f*

cardioneurosis Herzneurose *f*

cardiophobia Kardiophobie *f*, Angst *f* vor Herzkrankheit

cardiosphygmograph Herzkurvenschreiber *m*, Kardiosphygmograph *m*

cardiotachometer Kardiotachometer *n*, Herzimpulsmesser *m*

cardiovascular kardiovaskulär, Kreislauf–

care Sorge *f*, Pflege *f*, Betreuung *f* / **intensive** ~ Intensivbehandlung *f* / **long–term** ~ Langzeitpflege *f*, Langzeitbetreuung *f* / **palliative** ~ palliative Versorgung *f* / **prenatal** ~ Schwangerschaftsvorsorge *f*, pränatale Versorgung *f* / **preventive** ~ Vorsorge *f* / **residential** ~ **institution** Wohn– und Pflegeeinrichtung *f* / **respite** ~ Kurzzeitpflege *f*

career Laufbahn *f*, Karriere *f* / ~ **aspiration** berufliche Zielvorstellung *f* / ~ **change** Berufswechsel *m* / ~ **choice** Berufswahl *f* / ~ **counselling** Berufsberatung *f*, Laufbahnberatung *f* / ~ **development** berufliche Entwicklung *f* / ~ **education** Berufsausbildung *f*, Berufsvorbereitung *f* / ~ **goal** Karriereziel *m* / ~ **guidance** Berufsberatung *f* / ~ **ladder** Karriereleiter *f* / ~**s master** Studienberater *m*, Ausbildungsberater *m* / ~ **maturity** Berufsreife *f* / ~ **preference** berufliche Bevorzugung *f*, Berufsinteresse *n* / ~ **woman** berufstätige Frau *f* / **dual** ~ Berufstätigkeit *f* beider Partner / **nontraditional** ~ untypische Berufswahl *f*

careful vorsichtig, achtsam

carefulness Achtsamkeit *f*, Sorgfalt *f*, Vorsicht *f*, Gründlichkeit *f*

caregiver Pflegeperson *f*, pflegender Angehöriger *m* / ~ **burden** Belastung *f* pflegender Angehöriger

careless sorglos, unbekümmert, unachtsam, nachlässig

carelessness Sorglosigkeit *f*, Unachtsamkeit *f*, Nachlässigkeit *f*, Fahrlässigkeit *f*, Leichtsinn *m*

caress liebkosen, streicheln / Liebkosung *f*

carotid Karotis *f*, Halsschlagader *f* / ~ **sinus** Karotissinus *m* / ~ **sinus reflex** Karotissinusreflex *m*

carpal Handwurzel–, karpal

Carpenter effect Carpenter–Effekt *m*, ideomotorisches Gesetz *n*, Ideo–Realgesetz *n*

carphenazine Carphenazin *n*

carphology Karphologie *f*, Flockenlesen *n*, Krozidismus *m*

carrier molecule Carriermolekül *n*, Trägermolekül *n*

carry–over Übertragung *f*, Übertrag *m*, Transfer *m* / **~ effect** Transferwirkung *f*, Bedingungsreihenfolge *f*

car–sickness Reisekrankheit *f* beim Autofahren

cartilage Knorpel *m* / **thyroid ~** Schildknorpel *m*, Adamsapfel *m*

cartoon Karikatur *f*, Cartoon *n*

case Fall *m* / **~ control** Verlaufsüberwachung *f*, Fallkontrolle *f* / **~ history** Anamnese *f*, Vorgeschichte *f* / **~ load** Zahl *f* der betreuten Fälle / **~ in point** typisches, charakteristisches Beispiel *n* / **~ management** Fallbetreuung *f* / **~ report** Krankenbericht *m*, Fallbericht *m* / **~ study** Fallstudie *f* / **~ study method** Fallstudienmethode *f*, Fallmethode *f* / **~work** Betreuung *f* einzelner Sozialfälle, individuelle Fürsorgearbeit *f* / **~ worker** Sozialarbeiter *m* / **custodial ~** Anstaltsfall *m* / **equal–and–unequal ~s method** Methode *f* der gleichen und ungleichen Intervalle / **fatal ~** Fall *m* mit tödlichem Ausgang / **mental ~** psychiatrischer Fall *m* / **mild ~** leichter Fall *m* / **obstinate ~** hartnäckiger Fall *m* / **poisoning ~** Vergiftungsfall *m* / **psychiatric ~** Geisteskranker *m* / **right–and–wrong ~s method** Methode *f* der richtigen und falschen Fälle / **severe ~** schwerer Fall *m* / **single–~ analysis** Einzelfallanalyse *f* / **social ~work** soziale Einzelfallarbeit *f* / **special ~** Sonderfall *m* / **trivial ~** Bagatellfall *m* / **urgent ~** Dringlichkeitsfall *m*

casework Fallarbeit *f* / **social ~** soziale Fallarbeit *f*, Sozialarbeit *f*, soziale Einzelbetreuung *f*

caste Kaste *f* / **~ system** Kastenwesen *n*, Kastensystem *n*

castrate kastrieren, entmannen

castration Kastration *f*, Kastrierung *f*, Entmannung *f* / **~ anxiety** Kastrationsangst *f* / **~ complex** Kastrationskomplex *m* / **~ fear** Kastrationsfurcht *f*, Kastrationsangst *f* / **~ phantasy** Kastrationsphantasie *f* / **~ threat** Kastrationsdrohung *f* / **anal ~ anxiety** anale Kastrationsfurcht *f* / **male ~** Kastration *f* bei Männern, Entmannung *f* / **symbolic ~** symbolische Kastration *f*

casuistry Kasuistik *f*, Fallsammlung *f*

catabolic katabolisch, abbauend

catabolism Katabolismus *m*, Abbaustoffwechsel *m*

catabolite Katabolit *m*

catagelphobia Furcht *f* sich lächerlich zu machen

catalepsy Katalepsie *f*, Starrkrampf *m*, Starrsein *n* / **hypnotic ~** hypnotische Starre *f* / **rigid ~** kataleptische Starre *f* / **spontaneous ~** spontane Katalepsie *f*

cataleptic kataleptisch, starr, in Starrkrampf verfallend

cataleptoid starrkrampfähnlich, katalepsieähnlich, kataleptoid

catalexia Dyslexie *f*, Katalexie *f*, Tendenz *f* Worte und Sätze zu wiederholen

catalogia Kataphasie *f*, krankhafte Wiederholung *f* von Antworten, Verbigeration *f*

catalytic katalytisch

catalysis Katalyse *f*

catalyst Katalysator *m*

catamenia Katamenien *npl*, Menstruation *f*

catamenial menstrual

catamnesis Katamnese *f*, Krankenbericht *m*

cataphasia Kataphasie *f*, Verbigeration *f*, krankhafte Wiederholung *f* von Antworten

cataphora Cataphora *f*

cataplexia, cataplexy Kataplexie *f*, Schrecklähmung *f*, Schreckstarre *f*, Geloplegie *f*, affektiver Tonusverlust *m* / **matutinal ~** Wachanfall *m*

cataract Katarakt *m*, grauer Star *m*, Linsentrübung *f*

catathymia Katathymie *f*, katathymer Wahn *m*

catathymic katathym

catatonia, catatony Katatonie *f*, katatone Schizophrenie *f* / **degenerative ~** Defektkatatonie *f*

catatonic kataton

catch Fang *m*, Sperrung *f* / **~ experiment** Fangexperiment *n* / **~ muscle** Schließmuskel *m* / **~ phrase** Werbespruch *m* / **~ trial** Fangdurchgang *m* / **~ word** Slogan *m*, Schlagwort *n*

catecholamine Katecholamin *n* / **~ hypothesis** Katecholamin–Hypothese *f*

catecholaminergic katecholaminerg

categorical kategorisch, unbedingt

categorisation, categorizing Kategorisierung *f*, Klassifikation *f*

category Kategorie *f*, Klasse *f*, Ordnung *f* / **~ of apperception** Apperzeptionskategorie *f* / **~ of persons** Personenkreis *m* / **lower ~** untere Kategorie *f* / **occupational ~** Berufsschicht *f* / **social ~** soziale Kategorie *f*, soziale Schicht *f*

catharsis Katharsis *f*, seelische Entspannung *f*, Abreagieren *n*, Läuterung *f*

cathartic kathartisch

cathect besetzen

cathected besetzt / **~ as to aim** zielbesetzt / **affectively ~** affektbesetzt / **highly ~** hochbesetzt / **purposively ~** zielbesetzt / **regressively ~** regressiv besetzt

cathectibility Besetzbarkeit *f*

cathectible besetzbar

cathection Vorgang *m* der Besetzung, Besetzung *f*

catheterization Katheterisierung *f*

cathexis Kathexis *f*, Besetzung *f* / **~ as to aim** Zielbesetzung *f* / **~ of the ego** Ich–Besetzung *f* / **~ of an image** Vorstellungsbesetzung *f* / **~ by instinct** Triebbesetzung *f* / **~ of an instinct** Triebbesetzung *f* / **~ by libido** Libidobesetzung *f* / **~ of an object** Objektbesetzung *f* / **~ of a symbol** Symbolbesetzung *f* / **~ of thought** Denkbesetzung *f* / **affective ~** affektive Besetzung *f* / **aimed ~** Zielbesetzung *f* / **with a high ~** hochbesetzt / **instinctual ~** Triebbesetzung *f* / **purposive ~** Zielbesetzung *f* / **regressive ~** regressive Besetzung *f* / **retroactive ~** Rückbesetzung *f* / **susceptible to ~** besetzbar

cathisophobia Kathisophobie *f*

cathode Kathode *f* / **~–ray** Kathodenstrahl *m* / **~–ray oscillograph** Kathodenstrahloszillograph *m* / **~–ray oscilloscope** Elektronenstrahloszillograph *m*

cation Kation *n*

catoptrics Reflexionslehre *f*, Katoptrik *f*

catoptromancy Wahrsagen *n* mit einer Kristallkugel

Cattell's factorial theory of personality Cattells Faktorentheorie *f* der Persönlichkeit, Cattells faktorielle Persönlichkeitstheorie *f*

cauda equina Cauda equina *f*, Pferdeschweif *m*

caudal caudal, schwanzwärts, steißwärts

causal kausal, ursächlich

causalgia Kausalgie *f*, brennender Schmerz *m*

causality Kausalität *f*, Kausalzusammenhang *m* / **~ by generation** Kausalität *f* durch eigenes Erzeugen / **animistic ~** animistische Kausalität *f* / **dynamic ~** dynamische Kausalität *f* / **final ~** finale Kausalität *f* / **intentional ~** Veranlassungskausalität *f* / **magical ~** magische Kausalität *f* / **mechanical ~** technische Kausalität *f* / **moral ~** moralische Kausalität *f* / **phenomenistic ~** phänomenale Kausalität *f* / **psychological ~** psychische Kausalität *f*

causation Entstehung *f*, Verursachung *f*, Ursache *f* / **historical ~** historische Verursachung *f*, frühere Ursachen *fpl* / **multiple ~** multiple Verursachung *f* / **systematical ~** systematische Entstehung *f*

causative kausal, verursachend, ursächlich

cause Ursache *f*, Grund *m* / hervorrufen, verursachen, auslösen / **to ~ anxiety** Angst hervorrufen / **~ of dream** Traumanlass *m* / **~ and effect** Ursache *f* und

Wirkung *f* / **to ~ pain** Schmerz erzeugen / **concomitant ~** Mitursache *f* / **efficient ~** tatsächliche Ursache *f* / **exciting ~** Erregungsgrund *m* / **formal ~** formeller Grund *m* / **material ~** materieller Grund *m* / **occasional ~** zufällige Ursache *f*, Gelegenheitsursache *f* / **original ~** Entstehungsursache *f* / **partial ~** Teilgrund *m* / **predisposing ~** prädisponierende Ursache *f* / **prime ~** Hauptgrund *m* / **secondary ~** Nebenursache *f* / **structural ~** strukturelle Ursache *f* / **superimposed psychic ~** Überlagerung *f*

caused verursacht, hervorgerufen, bedingt

cautiousness Vorsicht *f*

cavernous kavernös, Hohlräume betreffend

cavity Höhle *f*, Hohlraum *m* / **cerebral ~** Hirnventrikel *n* / **cranial ~** Schadelhöhle *f* / **medullary ~** Markhöhle *f* / **nasal ~** Nasenhöhle *f* / **oral ~** Mundraum *m* / **pleural ~** Pleuralspalt *m* / **thoracic ~** Brusthöhle *f*, Brustraum *m* / **tympanic ~** Paukenhöhle *f*, Gehörtrommel *f* / **ventricular ~** Ventrikelhöhle *f*

cebocephalia Affenköpfigkeit *f*, Kebozephalie *f*, Zebozephalie *f*

ceiling Höchstgrenze *f*, Höchstwert *m* / **~ effect** Begrenzungseffekt *m*, Nivellierungseffekt *m*, ceiling–Effekt *m*, Deckeneffekt *m* / **~ of a test** Grenze *f* der Testdifferenzierung

celerity Schnelligkeit *f*, Geschwindigkeit *f*

celibacy Zölibat *n,m*, Ehelosigkeit *f*, Keuschheit *f*

cell Zelle *f* / **~ activity** Zelltätigkeit *f* / **~ of the anterior gray** Vorderhornzelle *f* / **~ assembly** Zellverbund *m*, funktionelle Zellorganisation *f* / **~ atrophy** Zellenschwund *m* / **~ body** Zellkörper *m* / **~ death** Zelltod *m* / **~ division** Zellteilung *f* / **~ frequency** Zellenhäufigkeit *f* / **~ fusion** Zellverschmelzung *f* / **~ layer** Zellschicht *f* / **~ membrane** Zellmembran *f*, Zellhaut *f* / **~ metabolism** Zellstoffwechsel *m*, Zellmetabolismus *m* / **~ nest** Zellanhäufung *f* / **~ nucleus** Zellkern *m* / **~ respiration** Zellatmung *f*, Gewebebeatmung *f* / **~ structure** Zellstruktur *f* / **~ substance** Zellsubstanz *f* / **acid ~** Belegzelle *f* / **acoustic ~** Hörzelle *f* / **amacrine ~** amakrine Zelle *f* / **basal ~** Basalzelle *f* / **binary ~** binäres Speicherelement *n* / **bipolar ~** bipolare Zelle *f* / **elementary ~** Urzelle *f*, Elementarzelle *f* / **embryonal ~** Embryonalzelle *f*, Stammzelle *f* / **embryonic ~** Embryonalzelle *f*, Stammzelle *f* / **epithelial ~** Epithelzelle *f*, Oberflächenzelle *f* / **excitable ~** erregbare Zelle *f* / **flagellate ~** Geißelzelle *f*, Flimmerzelle *f* / **ganglionic ~** Ganglienzelle *f* / **glial ~** Gliazelle *f* / **gustatory ~** Geschmackszelle *f* / **horizontal ~** Horizontalzelle *f* / **initial ~** Urzelle *f*, Keimzelle *f* / **interstitial ~–stimulating hormone** Gelbkörperreifungshormon *n* / **male generative ~** männliche Samenzelle *f* / **marrow ~** Markzelle *f* / **medullary ~** Markzelle *f* / **mesenchymal ~** Mesenchymzelle *f* / **motor ~** motorische Nervenzelle *f*, Motoneuron *n* / **multipolar ~** multipolare Zelle *f* / **myocardial ~** Herzmuskelzelle *f* / **neuromuscular ~** Neuromuskelzelle *f* / **non–nucleated ~** kernlose Zelle *f* / **olfactory ~** Riechzelle *f* / **osseous ~** Knochenzelle *f* / **padded ~** Gummizelle *f* / **parietal ~** Belegzelle *f* / **photoelectric ~** Photozelle *f*, photoelektrische Zelle *f* / **polar ~** Polkörperchen *n* / **primary ~** Urzelle *f*, Embryonalzelle *f* / **primordial ~** Stammzelle *f* / **pyramidal ~** Pyramidenzelle *f* / **retinal ~** Netzhautzelle *f* / **sensory ~** Sinneszelle *f* / **sexual ~** Geschlechtszelle *f*, Keimzelle *f* / **spermatic ~** Samenzelle *f* / **spermatogenic ~** Samenbildungszelle *f* / **supporting ~** Stützzelle *f* / **tactile ~** Tastzelle *f*, Tastkörperchen *n* / **undifferentiated ~** Embryonalzelle *f* undifferenzierte Zelle *f* / **visual ~** Sehzelle *f*

cellular zellulär, aus Zellen bestehend, zellig

cellularity Zellenförmigkeit *f*, zellartiger Aufbau *m*

cellule, cellula kleine Zelle *f*, Zellchen *n*

cenesthesia, cenesthesis Existenzbewusstsein *n*, Gefühl *n* physischer Existenz, Gemeingefühl *n*, Leibgefühl *n*

cenesthesiopathy gestörtes Existenzbewusstsein *n*

cenesthetic, cenesthesic das Gefühl körperlicher Existenz habend, das Gemeingefühl betreffend

cenesthopathia, cenesthopathy allgemeines Krankheitsgefühl *n*

cenophobia Raumangst *f*, Angst *f* vor hohen Gebäuden

cenotrope Trieb *m*, Instinkt *m*, allgemeine Hinwendung *f*, Triebausrichtung *f*

censor of dreams Traumsensor *m*

censorship Zensur *f* / **~ in dreams** Traumzensur *f* / **social ~** Zensur *f* durch die Gesellschaft, gesellschaftliche Zensur *f*

census Volkszählung *f*, Erhebung *f* / **~ data** Erhebungsdaten *npl* einer Volkszählung

cent Maß *n* der Tonhöhe, Cent *n*

center *siehe* **centre**

centering Zentrierung *f*, Aufmerksamkeitszentrierung *f* / **~ effect** Zentrierungseffekt *m* / **~ experiment** Zentrierungsexperiment *n*

centesimal hundertste(r, s), zentesimal

centigrade Grad *n* Celsius

centile Perzentil *n*, Zentil *n*, Hundertstel *n*, Hundertstelwert *m* / **~ curve** Perzentilkurve *f*, Zentilkurve *f* / **~ rank** Perzentilrang *m*, Zentilrang *m* / **~ scale** Prozentrangskala *f* / **~ score** Zentilwert *m* / **fiftieth ~** Median *m*

central zentral, im Zentrum liegend

centralism Zentralismus *m*, auf Vorgänge im Zentralnervensystem orientierte Psychologie *f*

centralist psychology auf Vorgänge im Zentralnervensystem orientierte Psychologie *f*

centrality Zentralität *f*, Ausgerichtetsein *n* auf einen Mittelpunkt / **individual ~** individuelle Ausrichtung *f* auf den Gruppenmittelpunkt

centre, center Zentrum *n*, Mittelpunkt *m* / **~ of accommodation** Akkommodationszentrum *n* / **~ of association** Assoziationszentrum *n* / **~ of attraction** Anziehungspunkt *m* / **~ clipping** Auslassen *n* der Sprachteile im mittleren Amplitudenbereich / **~ of gravity** Schwerpunkt *m* / **~ of gravity method** Zentroidmethode *f* / **~ of interest** Hauptinteresse *n* / **~ of perception** Wahrnehmungszentrum *n* / **~ of rotation** Drehpunkt *m* / **acoustic ~** Hörzentrum *n* / **advisory ~** Beratungsstelle *f* / **afferent ~** Sinneszentrum *n* / **associative ~** Assoziationszentrum *n* / **audito–psychic ~** Wahrnehmungsfeld *n* / **auditory ~** Hörzentrum *n* / **autonomic ~** vegetatives Zentrum *n* / **cardiovascular ~** Kreislaufzentrum *n* / **cerebral ~** Gehirnzentrum *n* / **cheirokinaesthetic ~** Schreibzentrum *n* / **cortical ~** Rindenzentrum *n* / **functional ~** Funktionszentrum *n* / **gustatory ~** Geschmackszentrum *n* / **higher ~** höheres Gehirnzentrum *n* / **ideomotor ~** Zentrum *n* der Ideomotorik / **inhibitory ~** Hemmzentrum *n* / **locomotor ~** Bewegungszentrum *n* / **lower ~** niederes Gehirnzentrum *n* / **mnestic ~** Erinnerungszentrum *n* / **motor ~** motorisches Zentrum *n* / **neural ~** Nervenzentrum *n* / **oculomotor ~** Okulomotoriuzentrum *n* / **olfactory ~** Riechzentrum *n* / **optic ~** Sehzentrum *n* / **psychomotor ~** psychomotorisches Zentrum *n* / **receptive ~** Rezeptionszentrum *n* / **reflex ~** Reflexzentrum *n* / **respiratory ~** Atemzentrum *n* / **sensory ~** sensorisches Zentrum *n*, Sinneszentrum *n* / **spinal ~** Rückenmarkszentrum *n* / **subcortical ~** subkortikales Zentrum *n* / **sympathetic ~** sympathisches Zentrum *n* / **tactile ~** Tastzentrum *n* / **vasomotor ~** Gefäßzentrum *n* / **visual ~** Sehzentrum *n*

centrifugal zentrifugal, vom Zentrum zur Peripherie verlaufend, efferent

centrifugality Efferenz *f*, Zentrifugalität *f*

centripetal zentripetal, afferent, zum Zentrum verlaufend

centripetality Afferenz *f*, Zentripetalität *f*

centroid Zentroid *n*, Kern *m*, Schwerpunkt *m* / ~ **factors** Zentroidfaktoren *mpl* / ~ **method** Zentroidmethode *f*, Centroidmethode *f*

centrosphere Zentrosphäre *f*

centrotonic zentrotonisch

centroversion Zentroversion *f*, Selbsterhaltung *f* / **considered** ~ besonnene Zentroversion *f*, Individuation *f*

cephalalgia Kopfschmerz *m*

cephalea schwerer chronischer Kopfschmerz *m* mit Lichtempfindlichkeit

cephalic cephal, Kopf–, Haupt–, Schädel–

cephalisation Enzephalisation *f*, Zerebration *f*

cephalocaudal kephalokaudal, in Längsrichtung des Körpers liegend, vom Kopf bis zum Rumpfende

cephalogram Röntgenaufnahme *f* des Kopfinnern, Kephalogramm *n*

cephalographic kephalografisch

cephalography Kephalographie *f*, Hirnaufnahme *f*

cephalogyric Schädelwindung betreffend, kephalogyrisch

cephalometer Schädelmessgerät *n*, Schädelmessinstrument *n*

cephalometric kephalometrisch, Schädelmessung betreffend

cephalometry Kephalometrie *f*, Schädelmessung *f*

cephalopathy Kopfleiden *n*

cephalopod Kopffüßler *m*, Kephalopod *m* / ~ **brain** Kephalopodenhirn *n*

cerea flexibilitas wachsartige Biegsamkeit *f*, Flexibilitas cerea *f*, Katalepsie *f*

cerebellar zerebellar, Kleinhirn–

cerebellum Cerebellum *n*, Zerebellum *n*, Kleinhirn *n*

cerebral zerebral, Hirn–, Gehirn–, zum Gehirn gehörig

cerebration Gehirntätigkeit *f*, Geistestätigkeit *f*, Denkprozess *m*, Zerebration *f*

cerebrifugal hirnabgewandt

cerebripetal hirnzugewandt

cerebroatrophia Hirnatrophie *f*

cerebroid hirnartig, zerebroid

cerebrology Hirnkunde *f*, Lehre *f* vom Zentralnervensystem

cerebromalacia Hirnerweichung *f*, Enzephalomalazie *f*

cerebromedullary zerebrospinal

cerebro–organic hirnorganisch

cerebropathy Hirnleiden *n*, Gehirnleiden *n*, Gehirnerkrankung *f*

cerebropenia Gehirnmangel *m*, Zerebropenie *f*

cerebropsychosis somatisch bedingte Psychose *f*

cerebrosclerosis Hirnsklerose *f*

cerebroscopy Augenhintergrundspiegelung *f*, Hirnsektion *f*

cerebrosis Gehirnerkrankung *f*

cerebrospinal zerebrospinal

cerebrostimulant Hirnstimulans *n*

cerebrotomy Gehirnsektion *f*, Schädelobduktion *f*

cerebrotonia Zerebrotonie *f*, zurückhaltendes und gehemmtes Temperament *n*

cerebrotonic zerebrotonisch

cerebrovascular zerebrovaskulär, Gehirngefäß—

cerebrum Gehirn *n*, Hirn *n*, Zerebrum *n*, Encephalon *n* / ~ **affecting drug** gehirnwirksames Medikament *n*

ceremonial zeremoniell / Zeremoniell *n* / **compulsory** ~ Zwangsritus *m* / **defensive** ~ Beschwörungshandlung *f*

ceremony Zeremonie *f*, Feierlichkeit *f*, Förmlichkeit *f*

certainty Gewissheit *f*, feste Überzeugung *f*, Sicherheit *f*, Bestimmtheit *f*

certifiable meldepflichtig (z.B. Geisteskranke)

certification Bescheinigung *f*, Beglaubigung *f*, Zulassung *f* / **compulsory** ~ obligatorische Zulassungsprüfung *f* / **legal** ~ gesetzliche oder staatliche Zulassungsprüfung *f* / **professional ~** Berufszulassung *f*, beruflicher Qualifikationserwerb *m*

certitude innere Gewissheit *f*, Überzeugung *f*

cervical zervikal, Hals–

cervix Hals *m*, Gebärmutterhals *m*

cessation Aufhören *n*, Beendigung *f*, Stillstand *m* / **~ of male sexual activity** Andropause *f*, Aufhören *n* der sexuellen Funktion beim Manne

C factor C–Faktor *m*, Faktor *m* der geistigen Wendigkeit und Originalität

C group Kontrollgruppe *f*

chaeromania, chairomania krankhafte Heiterkeit *f*, Chaeromanie *f*

chaerophobia krankhafte Angst *f* vor dem Frohsein

chain Kette *f* / **~ of association** Assoziationskette *f* / **~ break** Werbeeinblendung *f* / **~ of behaviour** Verhaltenskette *f* / **~ of neuron(e)s** Neuronenkette *f* / **~ reaction** Kettenreaktion *f* / **~ reflex** Kettenreflex *m* / **~ smoker** Kettenraucher *m* / **associative ~ theory** assoziative Kettentheorie *f* / **ossicular ~** Gehörknöchelchen *npl*, Gehörknöchelchenkette *f* / **sympathetic ~** Grenzstrang *m*

chained verbunden, verknüpft, Ketten–, Verkettung–

chaining Reaktionsverkettung *f*, Erlernen *n* einer Verhaltensfolge, Verkettung *f* / **conversational ~** Barlow–Kette *f* / **verbal ~** verbale Kettenbildung *f*

chalice cell Becherzelle *f*

challenge Herausforderung *f*, Aufforderung *f* / herausfordern, auffordern, in Frage stellen

chalone hernmendes Hormon *n*

chamber Zimmer *n*, Raum *m* / **~ of eye** Augenkammer *f* / **~ of the middle ear** Paukenhöhle *f* / **anterior ~ of eye** vordere Augenkammer *f* / **posterior ~ of eye** hintere Augenkammer *f*

chamecephalic, chamecephalous flachköpfig, platyzephal, chamazephal

chamecephaly Flachköpfigkeit *f*, Platyzephalus *m*

chance Zufall *m*, Chance *f* / **~ difference** zufälliger Unterschied *m* / **~ error** Zufallsfehler *m* / **~ expectancy** Zufallserwartung *f* / **~ forms** Zufallsformen *fpl*, Zufallsbilder *npl* / **~ halves correlation** Korrelation *f* zweier nach Zufall ausgewählter Hälften, Split–half–Korrelation *f* / **~ hit** Zufallstreffer *m* / **~ meeting** Zufallsbegegnung *f*, zufälliges Treffen *n* / **~ occurence** Zufallsereignis *n* / **~ test** freie Assoziationen *fpl* / **~ variation** Zufallschwankung *f*, Zufallsabweichung *f*

change Änderung *f*, Veränderung *f*, Wechsel *m*, Umgestaltung *f*, Umwandlung *f* / ändern, verändern, wechseln, umwandeln, umgestalten / **~ of attitude** Einstellungsänderung *f* / **~ for the better** Besserung *f* / **~ of character** Charakterveränderung *f* / **~ of dominance** Dominanzwechsel *m* / **~ in excitability** Erregbarkeitsänderung *f* / **~ of life** Wechseljahre *npl*, Klimakterium *n*, Menopause *f* / **~ in mood** Stimmungsschwankung *f* / **~ of mood** Gemütsveränderung *f*, Stimmungswechsel *m* / **~–over** Übergang *m*, Umstellung *f* / **~ of paradigms** Paradigmenwechsel *m* / **~ of personality** Persönlichkeitsveränderung *f*, Charakterveränderung *f*, Wesensänderung *f* / **~ of polarity** Umpolarisierung *f* / **~ in state of consciousness** Bewusstseinsstörung *f* / **~ for the worse** Verschlechterung *f*, Verschlimmerung *f* / **autonomous ~** autonomer Wechsel *m* / **cognitive ~** kognitive Änderung *f* / **cryptic genetic ~** latente genotypische Veränderung *f* / **dramatic ~** durchgreifende Veränderung *f* / **environmental ~** Umweltveränderung *f* / **mental ~** psychische Veränderung *f* / **minimal ~s method** Annäherungsmethode *f* / **morbid ~** krankhafte Veränderung *f* / **organizational ~** Organisationsänderung *f*, Änderung *f* der Organisationsform / **pathological ~** krankhafte Veränderung *f* / **social ~** sozialer Wandel *m*, gesellschaftliche Veränderungen *fpl* / **structural ~** Strukturänderung *f* / **substantial ~** wesentliche Änderung *f* / **technological ~** technologischer Wandel *m*

changeable veränderlich, unbeständig, wandelbar

changeless unveränderlich

changelessness Unveränderlichkeit *f*

channel Kanal *m* / kanalisieren / **~ capacity** Kanalkapazität *f* / **~ of communication** Kommunikationsweg *m* / **~ programme** Kanalprogramm *n* / **~ protein** Kanalprotein *n* / **multi–~ recorder** Mehrkanalschreiber *m*

chaos theory Chaostheorie *f*

character Charakter *m*, Merkmal *n* / **~ analysis** Charakteranalyse *f* / **~ armor** Charakterpanzerung *f*, triebgehemmter Charakter *m* / **~ defect** Charaktermangel *m*, Charakteranomalie *f* / **~ defence** Charakterabwehr *f* / **~ development** Charakterentwicklung *f* / **~ disorder** Charakterstörung *f*, Charakterveränderung *f* / **~–education–inquiry** Untersuchung *f* zur charakterlichen Erziehung / **~ formation** Charakterbildung *f* / **~ forming** Charaktererziehung *f* / **~ neurosis** Charakterneurose *f*, Charakterose *f* / **~ quality** Charaktereigenschaft *f* / **~ research** Persönlichkeitsforschung *f* / **~ set** Zeichenvorrat *m* / **~ structure** Charakterstruktur *f*, Charakteraufbau *m*, Charaktergefüge *n* / **~ test** Charaktertest *m*, Persönlichkeitstest *m* / **~ training** Charakterbildung *f*, Charakterschulung *f*, Charaktererziehung *f* / **~ trait** Charakterzug *m*, Charaktermerkmal *n*, Charaktereigenschaft *f* / **~ types** Charaktertypen *mpl* / **acquired ~** erworbene Eigenschaft *f* / **affective ~** Grundstimmung *f*, Charakterstimmung *f* / **anal ~** Analcharakter *m*, analer Charakter *m* / **anal–erotic ~** analerotischer Charakter *m* / **anomalous ~** Charakteranomalie *f* / **antinomic ~** antinomischer Charakter *m* / **authoritarian ~** autoritäre Persönlichkeit *f* / **compliant ~** neurotisch unterwürfiger Charakter *m* / **degenerative ~** degenerativer Charakter *m* / **demonic ~** dämonischer Charakter *m* / **dependent ~** abhängiger Charakter *m* / **depressive ~** depressiver Charakter *m*, Charakterdepression *f* / **dominant ~** dominanter Charakter *m* / **genital ~** genitaler Charakter *m* / **histrionic ~** theatralischer Charakter *m* / **hysterical ~** hysterischer Charakter *m* / **impulsive ~** impulsiver Charakter *m* / **inadequate ~** unangepasste Persönlichkeit *f* / **linked ~s** gleiche Charaktere *mpl* / **moral ~** Charakter *m*, Moral *f* / **national ~** Nationalcharakter *m* / **neurotic ~** neurotischer Charakter *m* / **obsessional neurotic ~** Zwangsneurotiker *m* / **optical ~ recognition** optisches Beleglesen *n*, maschinell lesbare Schreibmaschinenschrift *f* / **oral ~** oraler Charakter *m* / **paranoid ~** paranoide Persöhnlichkeit *f*, paranoischer Charakter *m* / **phallic ~** phallischer Charakter *m* / **positive ~** gefestigte Persönlichkeit *f* / **receptive ~** aufnehmender Charakter *m* / **recessive ~** rezessive Merkmale *npl* / **strong ~** starker Charakter in / **tonal ~** Klangfarbe *f* / **urethral ~** urethraler Charakter *m* / **without ~** charakterlos

characterisation Charakterisierung *f*, Kennzeichnung *f* / **lean ~** enge Deutung *f*

characteristic Merkmal *n*, Eigenschaft *f*, Charakteristikum *n* / charakteristisch, kennzeichnend, bezeichnend / **acquired ~** erworbene Eigenschaft *f* / **demographic ~** demographisches Merkmal *n*, Merkmal *n* einer Population / **dominant inherited ~** dominante Erbeigenschaft *f* / **elementary cognitive ~s** Bedeutungselemente *npl* / **emotional ~s** Erlebnischarakter *m* / **external ~** äußeres Kennzeichen *n* / **facial ~** Gesichtsmerkmal *n* / **formal ~** formale Eigenschaft *f* / **functional ~** funktionale Eigenschaft *f* / **inherited ~** Erbeigenschaft *f* / **national ~** Nationaleigenschaft *f* / **operating ~** Leistungsfunktion *f* / **organisational ~** Organisationsmerkmal *n* / **parental ~** Elternmerkmal *n* / **physical ~** körperliches

Kennzeichen *n* / **primary sexual ~s** primäre Geschlechtsmerkmale *npl* / **qualitative ~** qualitatives Merkmal *n* / **racial ~** Rassenmerkmal *n* / **recessive ~s** rezessive Merkmale *npl* / **regressive inherited ~** rezessive Erbeigenschaft *f* / **secondary sexual ~s** sekundäre Geschlechtsmerkmale *npl* / **sexual ~** Geschlechtsmerkmal *n*

characterize charakterisieren, beschreiben, kennzeichnen

characterless charakterlos, ohne Charakter

characterollogy Charakterkunde *f*, Charakterologie *f* / **~ pathy** Charakteropathie *f*

Charcot|'s disease Charcot–Krankheit *f* / **~'s syndrome** Charcot–Syndrom *n*, intermittierendes Hinken *n* / **~'s sign** Charcot–Zeichen *n* / **~ zones** hysterogene Zonen *fpl*

charge Besetzung *f*, Kathexis *f* / **~ of affect** affektive Besetzung *f*, Kathexis *f*

charisma Charisma *n*, Begnadung *f*

charitable wohltätig, Wohltätigkeits–

charlatan Scharlatan *m*, Schwindler *m*

Charlier's checks Charlier–Kontrollen *fpl*

charm Charme *f*, Zauber *m*, Amulett *n*, Talisman *m* / bezaubern

Charpentier|'s bands Charpentier–Streifen *mpl* / **~'s law** Charpentier'sches Gesetz *n*

chart Tafel *f*, Tabelle *f*, Kurve *f*, Diagramm *n* / **optical ~** Sehtafel *f* / **pseudoisochromatic ~s** pseudoisochromatische Tafeln *fpl*, Ishihara–Tafeln *fpl*

chasmus hystericus hysterischer Gähnkrampf *m*

chaste keusch, rein

chastisement Bestrafung *f*, Strafe *f*, Züchtigung *f*

chastity Keuschheit *f*, Reinheit *f*

chatterbox effect Cocktailparty–Syndrom *n*

cheat Betrug *m*, Betrüger *m* / betrügen

cheating Betrügen *n*, Vortäuschen *n*

check Kontrolle *f*, Überprüfung *f*, Prüfung *f* / kontrollieren, prüfen, nachprüfen, überprüfen, untersuchen / **~ coding** Kontrollkodierung *f* / **~ experiment** Kontrollexperiment *n* / **~ list** Prüfliste *f*, Kontrollliste *f* / **~ point** Anhaltspunkt *m*, Bezugspunkt *m* / **~ reading** Vergleichskontrolle *f* / **~ test** Gegenprobe *f*

checking Kontrolle *f*, Überprüfung *f*

cheek Wange *f*, Backe *f* / **painless ~–area** schmerzfreier Wangenbereich *m*

cheerful heiter, froh, munter

cheerfulness, cheeriness Heiterkeit *f*, Munterkeit *f*, Frohsinn *m*, Fröhlichkeit *f*

cheirognomy Handlesekunst *f*, Chirognomik *f*, Chirologie *f*

cheirology Taubstummensprache *f*, Fingersprache *f*, Chirologie *f*, Handlesekunst *f*

cheiromancy Handlesekunst *f*, Chiromantik *f*, Chirologie *f*

cheirospasm Schreibkrampf *m*, Handkrampf *m*

chemical chemisch / Chemikalie *f*

chemistry Chemie *f* / **biological ~** Biochemie *f* / **mental ~ viewpoint** Standpunkt *m* dass geistige Elemente durch Assoziation miteinander verschmelzen / **physiological ~** physiologische Chemie *f*, Biochemie *f*

chemophysiology physiologische Chemie *f*

chemoreceptor, chemoceptor Chemorezeptor *m*

chemoreflex Chemoreflex *m*

chemosensor Chemosensor *m*

chemotactic chemotaktisch

chemotaxis, chemotaxy, chemotaxis Chemotaxis *f*

chemotherapeutical chemotherapeutisch

chemotherapy, chemotherapeutics Chemotherapie *f*, Behandlung *f* mit chemischen Mitteln

chemotropism Chemotropismus *m*, Chemotaxis *f*

cheromania krankhafte Heiterkeit *f*, Chaeromanie *f*

chess–board–illusion Schachbrettillusion *f*

chest Brust *f*, Thorax *m*

chewing Kauakt *m*, Kauvorgang *m* / ~ **tobacco** Kautabak *m*

Cheyne–Stokes| breathing Cheyne–Stokes–Atmung *f* / ~ **respiration** Cheyne– Stokes–Atmung *f*

chiaroscuro Chiaroscuro *n*, Helldunkel *n*, Licht– und Schattenwirkung *f*

chiasm, chiasma Sehnervenkreuzung *f*, Chiasma *n*, Kreuzung *f*, Überkreuzung *f* / **optic** ~ Sehnervenkreuzung *f*, Chiasma opticum *n*

chiasmal gekreuzt, Chiasma–

child Kind *n* / ~ **abuse** Kindesmisshandlung *f* / ~ **abuse reporting** Kindesmissbrauchsanzeige *f* / ~ **advocacy** Eintreten *n* für die Kinder / ~ **analysis** Kinderanalyse *f* / ~ **attitude** kindliche Einstellung *f* / **~–battering** körperliche Kindesmisshandlung *f* / **~–bearing** Geburt *f*, Niederkunft *f* / **~–bearing age** gebärfähiges Alter *n* / ~ **behaviour diagnostic inventory** Verfahren *n* zur Kinder–Verhaltensdiagnostik / ~ **care** Kinderbetreuung *f* / ~ **care worker** Jugendsozialarbeiter *m* / **~–centered** auf das Kind ausgerichtet, kinderfreundlich / ~ **custody** Sorgerecht *n*, elterliche Sorge *f* / ~ **day care** Kinderganztagsversorgung *f*, Kindertagesstätte *f* / ~ **delivered by forceps** Zangengeburt *f* / ~ **development** Entwicklung *f* des Kindes / ~ **discipline** kindliche Disziplin *f*, kindlicher Gehorsam *m* / ~ **education** Kindererziehung *f* / ~ **guidance** Erziehungsberatung *f* / ~ **guidance clinic** Erziehungsberatungsstelle *f* / ~ **marriage** Kinderehe *f* / ~ **neglect** Kinderverwahrlosung *f*, Kindervernachlässigung *f* / **~–parent fixation** Kind–Eltern–Bindung *f*, Fixierung *f* an die Eltern / ~ **prodigy** Wunderkind *n* / ~ **psychiatric clinic** Klinik *f* für Kinderpsychiatrie / ~ **psychiatrist** Kinderpsychiater *m* / ~ **psychiatry** Kinderpsychiatrie *f* / ~ **psychology** Kinderpsychologie *f*, Psychologie *f* des Kindes / ~ **psychotherapy** Kinderpsychotherapie *f* / ~ **rearing** Kindererziehung *f* / ~ **of school age** Schulkind *n* / ~ **self–care** kindliche Selbstversorgung / ~ **study** Erforschung *f* der kindlichen Entwicklung / ~ **support** Kindesunterhalt *m*, Unterhaltspflicht *f* / ~ **visitation** Besuchsrecht *n* / ~ **welfare** Kinderfürsorge *f*, Jugendwohlfahrtspflege *f* / **abandoned** ~ vernachlässigtes Kind *n* / **abnormal** ~ gestörtes Kind *n* / **adopted** ~ Adoptivkind *n* / **asocial** ~ schwererziehbares Kind *n* / **autistic** ~ autistisches Kind *n* / **backward** ~ zurückgebliebenes Kind *n* / **battered** ~ misshandeltes Kind *n* / **battered ~ syndrome** Misshandlungssyndrom *n* bei Kindern / **defective** ~ anomales Kind *n* / **difficult** ~ schwieriges Kind *n*, schwererziehbares Kind *n* / **disadvantaged** ~ (sozial) benachteiligtes Kind *n* / **exceptional** ~ hochbegabtes Kind *n* / **female** ~ Mädchen *n* / **feral** ~ wildes Kind *n* / **gifted** ~ begabtes Kind *n*, talentiertes Kind *n* / **growing** ~ heranwachsendes Kind *n*, größeres Kind *n* / **handicapped** ~ behindertes Kind *n* / **hyperactive ~ syndrome** kindliches Hyperkinesesyndrom *n* / **illegitimate** ~ uneheliches Kind *n*, außereheliches Kind *n* / **incorrigible** ~ unverbesserliches Kind *n* / **institutionalized** ~ Heimkind *n*, Anstaltskind *n* / **later–born** ~ Nachkömmling *m* / **maladjusted** ~ unangepasstes Kind *n* / **new–born** ~ Neugeborenes *n*, neugeborenes Kind *n* / **obstreperous** ~ eigenwilliges Kind *n*, lautes Kind *n* / **only** ~ Einzelkind *n* / **pre–school** ~ Vorschulkind *n* / **retarded** ~ zurückgebliebenes Kind *n*, retardiertes Kind *n*, Spätentwickler *m* / **sharp** ~ aufgewecktes Kind *n* / **spoiled** ~ verwöhntes Kind *n*, verzogenes Kind *n* / **superior** ~ begabtes Kind *n*, überlegenes Kind *n* / **wanted** ~ Wunschkind *n* / **wayward** ~ widerspenstiges Kind *n*, eigenwilliges Kind *n*

childbirth Geburt *f*, Niederkunft *f*, Entbindung *f* / **~ training** Geburtsvorbereitungskurs *m*, Schwangerengymnastik *f* / **natural ~** natürliche Geburt *f*, schmerzlose Entbindung *f*

childhood Kindheit *f*, Kindesalter *n*, frühe Jugend *f* / **~ autism** frühkindlicher Autismus *m* / **~ development** Entwicklung *f* in der Kindheit / **~ disease** Kinderkrankheit *f* / **~ disintegrative disorder** desintegrative Störung *f* im Kindesalter / **~ disorder of social functioning** Störung *f* sozialer Funktionen mit Beginn in der Kindheit / **~ emotional disorder** emotionale Störung *f* des Kindesalters / **~ experience** Kindheitserlebnis *n* / **~ history** Kindheitsgeschichte *f* / **~ memory** Kindheitserinnerung *f* / **~ neurosis** Kindheitsneurose *f* / **~ phobia** Phobie *f* in der Kindheit / **~ play behaviour** Spielverhalten *n* bei Kindern / **~ play development** Entwicklung *f* des kindlichen Spielens / **~ psychosis** infantile Psychose *f*, Kindheitspsychose *f* / **~ schizophrenia** kindliche Schizophrenie *f*, Kindheitsschizophrenie *f* / **~ suicide** Kinderselbstmord *m* / **early ~** frühe Kindheit *f* / **early ~ development** frühkindliche Entwicklung *f*, Entwicklung *f* in der frühen Kindheit / **late ~** spätes Kindesalter *n* / **mid ~** mittleres Kindesalter *n*

childish kindisch, kindlich, infantil

childlessness Kinderlosigkeit *f*

childlike kindlich, wie ein Kind, unschuldig

childrearing Kindererziehung *f* / **~ attitudes** Erziehungsnormen *fpl*, Einstellungen *fpl* zur Kindererziehung / **~ practices** Erziehungspraktiken *fpl*, Erziehungsstile *mpl*

children Kinder *npl* / **~'s apperception test** Kinder–Apperzeptionstest *m* / **~'s manifest anxiety scale** Test *m* zur Erfassung der manifesten kindlichen Angst / **~'s personality questionnaire** Kinder–Persönlichkeitsfragebogen *m* / **~'s psychologist** Kinderpsychologe *m* / **~'s recreational games** Kinder–Freizeitspiele *npl* / **~ village** Kinderdorf *n*

chill Kältegefühl *n*, Frostgefühl *n* / **~s** Schüttelfrost *m*

chimaera, chimera Schimaref, Hirngespinst *n*

chimpanzee Schimpanse *m*

chionophobia Angst *f* vor Schnee, Schneeangst *f*, Chionophobie *f*

chirography Handschrift *f*, Schönschrift *f*

chiromancy, chirognomy, chirosophy Chiromantik *f*, Chiromantie *f*, Handlesekunst *f*, Handdeutung *f*

chiromancer Handliniendeuter *m*, Handleser *m*, Chiromant *m*

chirospasm Schreibkrampf *m*, Chirospasmus *m*

chi–square Chi–Quadrat *n* / **~ distribution** Chi–Quadrat–Verteilung *f* / **~ method** Chi–Quadrat–Methode *f* / **~ test** Chi–Quadrat–Test *m* / **~ test of goodness of fit** Chi–Quadrat–Test *m* zur Prüfung der Güte der Anpassung

chlor gelbgrün

chloral hydrate Chloralhydrat *n*

chloralism Chloralismus *m*, Sucht *f* sich mit Chloralpräparaten zu betäuben, chronische Chloralvergiftung *f*, Chloralomanie *f*

chloralose Chloralose *f*

chlordiazepoxide Chlordiazepoxid *n*, Methamindiazepoxid *n*

chloride ions Chloridionen *npl*

chlorimipramine Chlorimipramin *n*

chlorisondamine Chlorisondamin *n*

chloroform Chloroform *n* / **~ ism** Chloroformismus *m*, Chloroformomanie *f*, Chloroformsucht *f*, Chloroformvergiftung *f*

chlorophane grün schimmernd, grün erscheinend

chloropia, chloropsia Grünsehen *n*, Chloropsie *f*

chlorpheniramine Chlorpheniramin *n*

chlorpromazine Chlorpromazin *n*

chlorprothixene Chlorprothixen *n*

choice Wahl *f* / **~ behaviour** Wahlverhalten *n* / **~ experiment** Wahlreaktionsexperiment *n* / **~ of neurosis** Neurosenwahl *f* / **~ point** Entscheidungspunkt *m* / **~ reaction** Wahlreaktion *f*, Wahlhandlung *f* / **~ shift** Entscheidungsumschwung *m* / **forced ~** Zwangswahl *f*, gebundene Wahlantwort *f* / **forced–~ item** Aufgabe *f* mit gebundener Wahlantwort / **~ method** Methode *f* der gebundenen Wahlantwort / **forced–~ technique** Methode *f* der gebundenen Wahlantwort / **free ~ method** Freiwahlmethode *f* / **multiple ~** Mehrfachwahl *f*, Multiple–Choice *f* / **multiple–~ box** Mehrfachwahlbox *f* / **multiple–~ experiment** Mehrfachwahlversuch *m* / **multiple–~ method** Mehrfachwahlmethode *f*, Multiple–Choice–Methode *f* / **multiple–~ programme** Mehrfachwahlprogramm *n* / **multiple–~ question** Auswahlfrage *f* / **multiple–~ response** Auswahlantwort *f* / **multiple–~ test** Alternativantworten–Test *m* / **occupational ~** Berufswahl *f* / **simple ~ situation** Einfachwahlsituation *f* / **sociometric ~** soziometrische Wahl *f* / **vocational ~** Berufswahl *f*

cholecystokinin Cholezystokinin *n*

cholelith Gallenstein *m*

choler Zorn *m*

choleric cholerisch, jähzornig

cholesterin, cholesterol Cholesterin *n*

choline Cholin *n*, Bilineurin *n* / **~ acetylase** Cholinacetylase *f*, Cholinacetyltransferase *f* / **~ acetyltransferase** Cholinacetyltransferase *f* / **~ chloride** Cholin *n*

cholinergic cholinergisch / Cholinergikum *n*

cholinesterase Cholinesterase *f* / **~ inhibitors** Cholinesterase–Hemmer *mpl*

cholinomimetic cholinomimetisch, parasympathikomimetisch

chord Akkord *m*, Band *n*, Strang *m* / **spinal ~** Rückenmark *n* / **vocal ~** Stimmband *n*

chorda Strang *m*, Band *n*, Chorda *f* / **~ dorsalis** Chorda dorsalis *f*, primitives Achsenskelett *n* / **~ tympani** Paukensaite *f*, Chorda tympani *f*

chordata Chordaten *mpl*, Wirbeltiere *npl*

chordotomy Durchtrennung *f* der Vorderseitenstränge, Chordotomie *f*

chorea Chorea *f*, Veitstanz *m* / **~ minor** Chorea minor *f*, Sydenham–Chorea *f* / **chronic progressive heriditary ~** Huntington–Chorea *f* / **epidemic ~** Chorea major *f*, Chorea saltatoria *f* / **Parkinsonian ~** Parkinsonismus *m*

choreal, choreatic, choreic choreatisch

choreiform, choreoid choreiform, veitstanzartig

choreoathetosis Choreoathetose *f*

choreomania Choreomanie *f*, Chorea major *f*, schwerer hysterischer Anfall *m*

choreomaniac Choreomane *m* / choreomanisch

chorioidea Aderhaut *f* des Auges, Chorioidea *f*

choroid Aderhaut *f* des Auges, Chorioidea *f* / **~ coat** Aderhaut *f* / **~ layer** Aderhaut *f* / **~ membrane** Aderhaut *f* / **~ plexus** Plexus choroideus *m*

chrematophobia Furcht *f* vor Geld

chroma Farbsättigung *f* / **~–brilliance coefficient** Koeffizient *m* der Farbsättigung und Helligkeit / **spectral ~ scale** Skala *f* der Spektralfarben / **tonal ~** Farbton *m*

chromaesthesia, chromesthesia Farbenhören *n*, Chromatismus *m*, Chromästhesie *f*, Synästhesie *f*

chromascale Farbenband *n* / **spectral ~** Spektralfarbenband *n*

chromatelopsia, chromatelopsis partielle Farbenblindheit *f*

chromatic chromatisch

chromaticity Farbeigenschaft *f* / **~ coordinates** dreidimensionale Farbenkoordinaten *fpl* / **~ diagram** Farbtondiagramm *n*, Farbendreieck *n*

chromaticness subjektiv empfundene Farbigkeit *f*, Farbqualität *f*

chromatics Farbenlehre *f*, Farbentheorie *f*

chromatid Chromatide *f*, Tochterchromosom *n*

chromatin Chromatin *n*, Kernsubstanz *f*

chromatism Chromatismus *m*, Synästhesie *f*

chromatodysopia, chromatodysopsia fast totale Farbenblindheit *f*

chromatology Farbenlehre *f*, Farbtheorie *f*

chromatolysis Chromatolyse *f*, Auflösen *n* der Nissl–Schollen

chromatometer Farbenmesser *m*, Chromatometer *n*, Kolorimeter *n*

chromatometric chromatometrisch

chromatometry Messung *f* des Farbsehvermögens, Kolorimetrie *f*

chromatophobia, chromophobia Angst *f* vor Farben, Chromatophobie *f*

chromatophore Pigmentzelle *f*, Farbträger *m*, Chromatophore *f*

chromatopseudopsis, chromatopseudopsia Farbenblindheit *f*

chromatopsia Farbensehen *n*, Chromopsie *f*

chromatoptometer Instrument *n* zur Bestimmung der Farbentüchtigkeit, Chromatoptometer *n*

chromatoptometry Farbtüchtigkeitsmessung *f*

chromesthesia Farbenhören *n*, Chromatismus *m*, Chromästhesie *f*, Synästhesie *f*

chromogen Chromogen *n*, Farbbildner *m*

chromogenesis Farbbildung *f*, Pigmentbildung *f*

chromogenic farbbildend, chromogen

chromometry Farbmessung *f*, Messung *f* des Farbsehvermögens, Kolorimetrie *f*

chromophoric farbtragend

chromophototherapy Chromophototherapie *f*, Buntlichttherapie *f*

chromopsia Farbensehen *n*, Chromatopsie *f*, Chromopsie *f*

chromoptometer Instrument *n* zur Messung der Farbtüchtigkeit

chromoptometry Bestimmung *f* der Farbtüchtigkeit, Messung *f* der Farbtüchtigkeit

chromosomal chromosomal, Chromosomen–

chromosome Chromosom *n* / **~ aberration** Chromosomenaberration *f* / **~ abnormality** Chromosomenaberration *f* / **~ count** Chromosomenzahl *f* / **~ deletion** Chromosomendeletion *f* / **~ disorder** Chromosomenstörung *f* / **~ pattern** Chromosomenmuster *n* / **~ theory** Chromosomentheorie *f* / **~ translocation** Translokation *f*, Chromosomenstückaustausch *m* / **X ~** X–Chromosom *n* / **Y~** Y–Chromosom *n*

chromotherapy Chromotherapie *f*, Farbentherapie *f*

chromotropism Farbtropismus *m*

chronaxia, chronaxie, chronaxy Chronaxie *f*, Kennzeit *f*

chronaximeter Chronaximeter *n*

chronaximetry Chronaximetrie *f*

chronic chronisch

chronicity chronischer Zustand *m*, chronischer Verlauf *m* von Krankheiten

chrono|biology Chronobiologie *f* / **~gnosis** Chronognosie *f* / **~graph** Chronograph *m* / **~meter** Chronometer *n*, Präzisionsuhr *f* / **~metry** Zeitmessung *f* / **~phobia** krankhafte Angst *f* vor der Zeit, Chronophobie *f* / **~scope** Chronoskop *n* / **simple ~scope** einfaches Chronoskop *n* / **~taraxis** zeitliche Desorientierung *f*, Verwirrtheit *f* in der zeitlichen Orientierung / **~tropism** chronotrope Wirkung *f*

chrono|logical chronologisch

chrysotherapy Goldtherapie *f*, Behandlung *f* mit Goldpräparaten

chthonophagia Erdessen *n*, Geophagie *f*

Chvostek|'s reflex Chvostek–Zeichen *n*, Fazialisphänomen *n* / **~'s sign** Chvostek–Zeichen *n*, Fazialisphänomen *n*

chymotrypsin Chymotrypsin *n*

cibophobia krankhafte Angst *f* vor Nahrung, Cibophobie *f*

cigarette smoking Zigarettenrauchen *n* / **~ habit** Rauchergewohnheit *f*

cilia Augenwimpern *fpl*, Zilien *fpl*

ciliary Wimpern–, ziliär

cilium Wimper *f*, Flimmerhaar *n*

cimetidine Cimetidin *n*

cinaesthesia Kinästhesie *f*, Muskelsinn *m*, Kraftsinn *m*, kinetischer Sinn *m*

cinaesthesiometer Kinästhesiometer *n*, Instrument *n* zum Messen des Muskelsinnes

cinaesthetic kinästhetisch, Kinästhesie

cinematograph Kinematograph *m*

cinematography Kinematographie *f*

cinesia Kinetose *f*, Bewegungskrankheit *f*

cinesitherapy, cinesiatrics Bewegungstherapie *f*

cingulectomy, cingulectomia operative Entfernung *f* des Gyrus cinguli, Zingulektomie *f*

cingulotomy Durchtrennung *f* des Gyrus cinguli, Zingulotomie *f*

circadian zirkadian, tageszyklisch, tagesperiodisch

circle Kreis *m*, Ring *m*, Zyklus *m* / **functional ~** Funktionskreis *m* / **tactile ~** Raumschwelle *f* / **vicious ~** Circulus vitiosus *m*, Teufelskreis *m*

circuit Kreis *m*, Kreislauf *m* / **closed ~** geschlossener Kreislauf *m* / **closed–~ television** innerbetriebliches Fernsehen *n* / **local ~ theory** Strömchentheorie *f* / **multineuronal ~ of Papez** Neuronenkreis *m* von Papez / **regulatory ~** Regelkreis *m* / **reverberatory ~** Erregungskreis *m*, reverberatorischer Kreislauf *m* / **short ~** Kurzschluss *m*

circular kreisförmig, zirkulär, ringförmig

circularity Kreisform *f*, Zirkularität *f*

circulation Kreislauf *m*, Blutkreislauf *m*, Durchblutung *f* / **major ~** Körperkreislauf *m* / **minor ~** Lungenkreislauf *m* / **pulmonary ~** Lungenkreislauf *m* / **systemic ~** Körperkreislauf *m*

circulatory Kreislauf–

circumcision Beschneidung *f*

circumference Umfang *m* / **~ of the head** Kopfumfang *m* / **~ of the skull** Schädelumfang *m*

circumscribed eng umschrieben, begrenzt

circumstances Verhältnisse *npl*, Umstände *mpl*, Situation *f*

circumstantial umständlich, eingehend, detailliert

circumstantiality Umständlichkeit *f*, Detailliertheit *f*, Einzelheit *f*

circumventricular zirkumventrikulär

citizen Bürger *m*, Bürgerin *f* / **senior ~s** ältere Mitbürger *mpl*, Senioren *mpl*

civic, civil bürgerlich, staatsbürgerlich, Bürger–

civilization Zivilisation *f*, Kultur *f*

civism Staatsbürgersinn *m*, Bürgertugend *f*

claim Anspruch *m*, Anrecht *n*, Forderung *f* / **neurotic ~** neurotischer Anspruch *m*

clairaudience Hellhören *n*, Hellhörigsein *n*

clairvoyance Hellsehen *n*

clairvoyant hellsehend / Hellseher *m*, Hellseherin *f*

clan Clan *m*, Stamm *m*, Sippe *f*, Clique *f* / **~–spirit** Stammesbewusstsein *n*

clang Klang *m* / **~ association** Klangassoziation *f* / **~ colour** Klangfarbe *f*, Timbre *n* / **~ quality** Klangqualität *f*, Klangfarbe *f* / **~ tint** Timbre *n*, Klangfarbe *f*

clarification Verdeutlichung *f*, Klärung *f*, Läuterung *f* / **~ remark** verdeutlichende Wiederholung *f* einer Aussage / **sudden ~** plötzliche Erleuchtung *f*

Clarke's column Clarke–Säule *f*, Clarke–Kern *m*, Columna thoracica *f*

clasping reflex Umklammerungsreflex *m*

class Klasse *f* / klassifizieren / **~ affiliation** Klassenzugehörigkeit *f* / **~ analysis chart** Analysediagramm *n* einer Klasse / **~ attitudes** Einstellungen *fpl* einer Klasse / **~ boundary** Klassengrenze *f* / **~ conflict** Klassenkampf *m* / **~ conscious** klassenbewusst / **~ consciousness** Klassenbewusstsein *n* / **~ of consumers** Verbraucherschicht *f* / **~ difference** Standesunterschied *m* / **~-free test** kulturunabhängiger Test *m* / **~ frequency** Klassenhäufigkeit *f* / **~ identification** Klassenidentifikation *f* / **~ index** Klassenindex *m*, Klassenbezeichnung *f* / **~ interval** Klassenbreite *f*, Klassengröße *f*, Klassenintervall *n*, Stufenintervall *n* / **~ limits** Klassengrenzen *fpl* / **~ mark** Klassenmittelpunkt *m* / **~mate** Klassenkamerad *m* / **~ mobility** Klassenmobilität *f* / **~ of population** Bevölkerungsschicht *f* / **~ range** Klassenbereich *m*, Klassenbreite *f* / **~ structure** Klassenstruktur *f* / **~ struggle** Klassenkampf *m* / **~ system** Klassensystem *n* / **~-theoretical** klassentheoretisch / **~ theory** Klassentheorie *f* / **~ war** Klassenkampf *m* / **conjunctive ~** Verbundkategorie *f*, konjunktive Klasse *f* / **disjunctive ~** Trennkategorie *f* / **extracurricular ~** freiwillige Schülerarbeitsgemeinschaft *f* außerhalb des regulären Stundenplans / **lower ~** Unterschicht *f*, untere Klasse *f* / **lower-lower ~** unterste Gesellschaftsschicht *f* / **lower-middle ~** untere Mittelschicht *f* / **lower-upper ~** untere Oberschicht *f* / **median ~** Klasse *f* um den Median / **middle ~** Mittelschicht *f*, Mittelstand *m*, Mittelklasse *f* / **relational ~es** Beziehungsklassen *fpl* / **social ~** soziale Klasse *f* / **socio-economic ~** sozioökonomische Schicht *f* / **socio-economic ~ attitude** schichtspezifische Einstellung *f* / **special ~** Sonderklasse *f* / **ungraded ~** Schulklasse *f* ohne Aufteilung nach Leistungsstufen oder Schuljahren / **upper ~** Oberschicht / **upper-lower ~** obere Unterschicht *f* / **upper-middle ~** obere Mittelschicht *f* / **upper-upper ~** obere Oberschicht *f* / **white-collar ~** Angestelltenschicht *f*, Gruppe *f* der Angestellten / **working ~** Arbeiterklasse *f*

classic klassisch, traditionell

classification Klassifikation *f*, Eingruppierung *f*, Aufgliederung *f* / **~ method** Klassifikationsmethode *f* / **~ systems** Klassifikationssysteme *npl* / **~ table** Klassifikationstafel *f* / **~ test** Einstufungstest *m*, Ordnungstest *m* / **Aristotelian ~** aristotelische Klassifikation *f* / **logical-abstract ~** logisch-begriffliche Klassifikation *f* / **psychiatric ~** psychiatrische Klassifikation *f* / **psychodiagnostic ~** psychodiagnostische Klassifikation *f* / **selective ~** selektive Klassifikation *f*

classificatory klassifizierend, Klassifikations-

classifier Klassifikationstafel *f*

classify klassifizieren

classroom Klassenzimmer *n*, Schulraum *m* / **~ behaviour** Verhalten *n* in der Klasse, schulisches Verhalten *n* / **~ behaviour modification** Änderung *f* des schulischen Verhaltens / **~ discipline** Klassendisziplin *f*, Unterrichtsdisziplin *f* / **~ environment** Umfeld *n* der Klasse, Schulklassenumwelt *f* / **~ instruction** Klassenunterricht *m* / **~ teacher** Klassenlehrer *m* / **~ test** Klassenprüfung *f*, unstandardisierter Klassentest *m* / **open ~ method** offener Unterricht *m*

clastomania Zerstörungsdrang *m*, Zerstörungswut *f*, Klastomanie *f*

claudication intermittierendes Hinken *n*

Claudius' cells Claudius-Zellen *fpl*

clause Satzteil *m*, kurzer Satz *m* / **phonemic ~** segmentierbare Phonemkette *f*

claustral eingeschlossen

claustrophilia Klaustrophilie *f*, Neigung *f* sich einzuschließen

claustrophobia Klaustrophobie *f*, Angst *f* in geschlossenen Räumen

claustrum Claustrum *n*

clavus hystericus schwerer Kopfschmerz *m*

clean sauber, rein / reinigen, säubern

cleanliness Reinlichkeit *f*, Sauberkeit *f* / **~ compulsion** Waschzwang *m* / **~ training** Reinlichkeitserziehung *f*, Sauberkeitsgewöhnung *f*

clear hell, klar, rein / klären, reinigen, säubern, hell werden

clearness Klarheit *f*, Deutlichkeit *f*

cleavage Furchungsteilung *f* / **~ of the ovum** Eiteilung *f* / **discoid ~** Keimscheibenteilung *f*

cleft Spalte *f* / **~ lip** Hasenscharte *f* / **~ palate** Gaumenspalte *f*

cleptomania Kleptomanie *f*, Stehlsucht *f*

cleptomaniac Kleptomane *m* / kleptoman

cleptophobia Kleptophobie *f*, krankhafte Angst *f* vor Dieben, Angst *f* kleptoman zu werden

Clérambault–Kadinsky's complex Clérambault–Syndrom *n*, psychischer Automatismus *m*, schizophrene Ichstörung *f*

clergy Klerus *m*, Geistlichkeit *f*, Geistliche *mpl*

clerical Büro–, Schreib–

clerk Bürokraft *f*, Sachbearbeiter(in) *m,f*, Kontoristin *f*

cleverness geistige Wendigkeit *f*, Schlauheit *f*, Pfiffigkeit *f*, Einfallsreichtum *m*

cliché Klischee *n*, Gemeinplatz *m*, stereotype Wendung *f*

click Schnalzen *n* / klicken

client Patient *m*, Klient *m* / **~ attitude** Klienteneinstellung *f* / **~–centered** nicht–direktiv, klientbezogen, klientenzentriert / **~ characteristics** Klientenmerkmale *npl*, Klientencharakteristika *npl* / **~–counselor interaction** Interaktion *f* zwischen Patient und Therapeut / **~ education** Patientenaufklärung *f* / **~ participation** Klientenbeteiligung *f* / **~ records** Klientendaten *npl*, Patientenunterlagen *fpl* / **~ rights** Patientenrechte *npl* / **~ satisfaction** Klientenzufriedenheit *f* / **~–server principle** Client–Server–Prinzip *n* / **~ transfer** Überweisung *f* von Patienten / **~–treatment matching** Abstimmung *f* der Klientenbehandlung / **professional–~ sexual relations** sexuelle Bezeihungen *fpl* zu Klienten

cliff Klippe *f* / **visual ~** visuelle Klippe *f*, Bodenabsatz *m*

climacteric klimakterisch / Klimakterium *n*, Menopause *f*, Wechseljahre *npl* / **male ~** Wechseljahre *npl* des Mannes

climacterium Klimakterium *n*, Wechseljahre *npl*, Menopause *f* / **~ virile** Wechseljahre *npl* des Mannes / **male ~** Klimakterium *n* des Mannes

climate Klima *n* / **~ of work** Arbeitsatmosphäre *f* / **affective ~** affektives Klima *n* / **cultural ~** kulturelles Klima *n* / **emotional ~** emotionales Klima *n* / **intellectual ~** intellektuelles Klima *n* / **organizational ~** Organisationsklima *n* / **psychological ~** psychologisches Klima *n* / **social ~** gesellschaftliches Klima *n*, Sozialklima *n*

climax Orgasmus *m*, Klimax *m*, Höhepunkt *m*

climbing Aufstieg *m* / **social ~** sozialer Aufstieg *m*

clinic Klinik *f* / **educational ~** Erziehungsberatungsstelle *f* / **psychoeducational ~** schulpsychologische Beratungsstelle *f* / **psychological ~** psychologische Beratungsstelle *f* / **psychiatric ~** Nervenklinik *f* / **walk–in ~** ambulante psychiatrische Klinik *f*

clinical klinisch

clinician Kliniker *m*

clinocephalic, clinocephaloas sattelköpfig, klinozephal

clinocephalism, clinocephaly Sattelkopf *m*, Klinozephalie *f*

clinomania Klinomanie *f*, Sucht *f* in einer Klinik zu liegen

clinometer Neigungsmesser *m*, Klinometer *n*

clipping Verschlucken *n* von Silben

clique Clique *f*

cliquish, cliquy, cliquey cliquenhaft, Cliquen–

clitoral Klitoris–, klitoridal

clitoris Klitoris *f*, Kitzler *m*

clitoromania Nymphomanie *f*, Klitoromanie *f*, Mannstollheit *f*, krankhaft gesteigerter weiblicher Sexualtrieb *m*

clitrophobia Angst *f* eingeschlossen zu werden

cloaca Kloake *f* / **~ phantasia** Kloakenphantasie *f*, Geburtsphantasie *f* / **~ theory** Kloakentheorie *f*, Kloakenphantasie *f*

clock Uhr *f* / **~wise** im Uhrzeigersinn / **counter ~wise** gegen den Uhrzeigersinn / **biological ~** biologische Uhr *f*, physiologische Uhr *f* / **chemical ~** biologische Uhr *f*, zirkadiane Uhr *f* / **internal ~** innere Uhr *f* / **mental ~** Kopfuhr *f*

clonazepam Clonazepam *n*

clonic klonisch, krampfhaft

clonidine Clonidin *n*

cloning Klonen *n*, Klonung *f*, Klonierung *f*

clonism länger dauernder klonischer Krampf *m*, wiederholt auftretender klonischer Krampf *m*

clonus klonischer Krampf *m*, Klonus *m*, rhythmischer Zuckkrampf *m*

close schließen / **~–mouthed** einsilbig, wenig mitteilsam, schweigsam / **~–tongued** einsilbig, wenig mitteilsam, schweigsam

closed–minded voreingenommen, befangen, starrsinnig, eigenwillig

closed–mindedness Voreingenommenheit *f*, Starrsinn *m*, Dogmatismus *m*

closeness Verschlossenheit *f*, Reserviertheit *f*, verschlossenes Wesen *n*, Annäherung *f*, Vertrautheit *f*

closure Geschlossenheit *f*

clothing fashion Mode *f*, Kleidermode *f*

cloud experiment Wolkenexperiment *n*, Wolkenversuch *m*

cloudiness Umnachtung *f*

clouding Trübung *f* / **~ of consciousness** Bewusstseinstrübung *f*

clownism Clownismus *m*, hysterische Körperverdrehungen *fpl*

clozapine Clozapin *n*

cloze testing „cloze"–Technik *f*

club Club *m*, Verein *m*, gesellschaftlicher Treffpunkt *m* / **preventive ~** im Bereich Vorbeugung tätiger Verein *m*, Präventiv–Verein *m* / **therapeutic social ~** therapeutischer Verein *m*, therapeutische Sozialstation *f*, therapeutischer Patientenclub *m*

clue Schlüssel *m*, Leitfaden *m*, Anhaltspunkt *m*

clumsiness Ungeschicklichkeit *f*, Unbeholfenheit *f*, Dyspraxie *f* / **developmental ~** Dyspraxie *f*

clumsy ungeschickt, unbeholfen, schwerfällig

cluster Menge *f*, Haufen *m*, Gruppe *f*, Bündel *n* / **~ analysis** Faktorenanalyse *f*, Clusteranalyse *f* / **~ correlation** Korrelations–Cluster *n* / **~ headache** Horton–Syndrom *n*, Cluster–Kopfschmerz *m*, Histaminkopfschmerz *m* / **~ sampling** Stichprobenerhebung *f* von geschlossenen Erfassungsgruppen, Klumpenauswahl *f*

clustering Tendenz *f* zur Gruppierung, Tendenz *f* zur Gruppenbildung

clutter stottern / Wirrwarr *m*, Störzeichen *n*

cluttering Silbenverschlucken *n*, Buchstabenschlucken *n*, Wortsalat *m*, Poltern *n*

coach Tutor *m*, Lehrer *m*, Trainer *m* / **~–and–pupil method** Lehrer–Schüler–Methode *f*

coaching Unterricht *m*, private Unterweisung *f*, Lernen *n* mit direkter Überwachung, Einpauken *n*

coacting zusammenarbeitend

coaction compass Interaktionsrahmen *m*

coadaptation gegenseitige Anpassung *f*, gegenseitige Adaptation *f*

coagulation Gerinnung *f* / ~ **disorder** Gerinnungsstörung *f*

coagulum Blutgerinnsel *n*

coalescence Zusammenwachsen *n*, Verschmelzen *n*, Vereinigung *f*

coalition formation Koalitionsbildung *f*, Bildung *f* von Vereinigungen

coarctated, coartated eingeengt, begrenzt, beengt, koartiert

coarctation Begrenzung *f*, Einengung *f*

coarse roh, rauh, grob

coartative koartativ

coat Gefäßwandschicht *f*, Oberzug *m* / **sclerotic** ~ Lederhaut *f* des Auges

cocaine Kokain *n* / ~ **abuse** Kokainmissbrauch *m* / ~ **delirium** Kokaindelirium *n* / ~ **dependence** Kokainabhängigkeit *f* / ~ **intoxication** Kokainintoxikation *f* / ~ **intoxication delirium** Kokainintoxikationsdelir *n* / ~ **withdrawal** Kokainentzug *m* / ~ **use disorders** Störungen *fpl* durch Kokainkonsum

cocaine|-induced kokaininduziert / **~-related** im Zusammenhang mit Kokain

cocainism, cocainomania Kokainsucht *f*, Kokainismus *m*, Kokainomanie *f*

cocainist Kokainsüchtiger *m*, Kokainist *m*

cocainmaniac Kokainsüchtiger *m* / kokainsüchtig

cocculin Pikrotoxin *n*

coccygeal Steißbein–, kokzygeal

coccyx Steißbein *n*

cochlea Cochlea *f*, Kochlea *f*, Schnecke *f*, Ohrschnecke *f* / ~ **microphonic** Cochleapotenzial *n*, Mikrofonpotenzial *m* des Corti–Organs

cochlear kochlear, zur Schnecke gehörig

cochleovestibular Schnecke und Vestibulum betreffend, kochleovestibulär

coconscious mitbewusst

coconsciousness Mitbewusstsein *n*, Mitbewusstes *n*

cocktail|-party conversationalism Cocktailparty–Syndrom *n* / **lytic** ~ lytischer Cocktail *m*

codability Kodierbarkeit *f*, Umsetzbarkeit *f* in Zeichen, Kodabilität *f*

code Kode *m*, Code *m*, Kodex *m* / kodieren / ~ **capacity** Code–Übertragungskapazität *f* / ~ **channel** Code–Übertragungskanal *m* / ~ **character** Codewort *n*, Codezeichen *n* / ~ **conversion** Kode–Umwandlung *f* / ~ **converter** Kode–Umsetzer *m*, Kode–Umformer *m* / ~ **element** Befehlselement *n*, Kode–Element *n* / ~ **group** Kodegruppe *f*, Gruppe *f* von Kode–Elementen / ~ **holes** gestanzte Lochkartenlöcher *npl* / ~ **problem** Kodeproblem *n*, Codeproblem *n* / ~ **set** Codesystem *n* / ~ **structure** Befehlsstruktur *f*, Aufbau *m* eines Kodes, Kodestruktur *f*, Code–Struktur *f* / ~ **switching** Sprachkodewechsel *m* / ~ **test** Code–Test *m* / ~ **translation** Code–Übersetzung *f*, Code–Umwandlung *f* / **binary** ~ Binär–Code *m*, Binärschlüssel *m* / **highway** ~ Straßenverkehrsordnung *f* / **moral** ~ Sittenkodex *m*, Sittengesetz *n* / **professional** ~ Berufskodex *m*, beruflicher Ehrenkodex *m* / **social** ~ gesellschaftliche Norm *f*, soziale Norm *f*

codeine Kodein *n*, Codein *n* / ~ **sulfate** Kodeinsulfat *n*

codeinomania Kodeinsucht *f*, Kodeinismus *m*

codependency Ko–Abhängigkeit *f*

codetermination Mitbestimmung *f*

codetermine mitbestimmen

codification Kodifikation *f*

coding Codierung *f*, Kodieren *n*, Kodifizierung *f* / ~ **key** Kode–Schlüssel *m*, Kodierungsschlüssel *m*

coed Schülerin *f* in einer gemischten Klasse / Koedukations–

coeducation Koedukation *f*, gemeinsame Erziehung *f* beider Geschlechter in der Schule

coefficient Koeffizient *m* / **~ of agreement** Koeffizient *m* der Übereinstimmung / **~ of alienation** Alienationskoeffizient *m* / **~ of association** Assoziationskoeffizient *m* / **~ of belongingness** Zugehörigkeitskoeffizient *m* / **~ of colligation** Verbindungskoeffizient *m* / **~ of concordance** Konkordanzkoeffizient *m* / **~ of consistency** Konsistenzkoeffizient *m* / **~ of contingency** Kontingenzkoeffizient *m* / **~ of correlation** Korrelationskoeffizient *m* / **~ of determination** Determinationskoeffizient *m*, Bestimmtheitsmaß *n* / **~ of dispersion** Zerstreuungskoeffizient *m* / **~ of egocentrism** Egozentrismusindex *m* / **~ of equivalence** Äquivalenzkoeffizient *m*, Stabilitätskoeffizient *m* / **~ of homogeneity** Homogenitätskoeffizient *m* / **~ of internal consistency** Koeffizient *m* der inneren Konsistenz / **~ of multiple correlation** multipler Korrelationskoeffizient *m* / **~ of multiple determination** multipler Determinationskoeffizient *m* / **~ of nondetermination** Unbestimmtheitsmaß *n* / **~ of partial correlation** partieller Korrelationskoeffizient *m* / **~ of partial determination** partieller Determinationskoeffizient *m* / **~ of partial regression** partieller Regressionskoeffizient *m* / **~ of pattern similarity** Koeffizient *m* der Strukturähnlichkeit / **~ of precision** Genauigkeitsindex *m* / **~ of rank correlation** Rangkorrelationskoeffizient *m* / **~ of reality** Realitätsindex *m* / **~ of regression** Regressionskoeffizient *m* / **~ of reliability** Reliabilitätskoeffizient *m* / **~ of reproducibility** Koeffizient *m* der Reproduktionsfähigkeit / **~ of stability** Stabilitätskoeffizient *m* / **~ of stability and equivalence** Stabilitäts– und Äquivalenzkoeffizient *m* / **~ of validity** Validitätskoeffizient *m* / **~ of variability** Variabilitätskoeffizient *m* / **~ of variation** Variationskoeffizient *m* / **binomial ~** Binomialkoeffizient *m* / **inter–item ~** Konsistenzkoeffizient *m*

coenaesthesia, coenaesthesis, coenesthesia, coenesthesis Gefühl *n* physischer Existenz, Existenzbewusstsein *n*, allgemeines Körpergefühl *n*, Gemeingefühl *n*, Koinästhesie *f*

coenaesthesiopathy gestörtes Existenzbewusstsein *n*, Störung *f* des Körpergefühls

coenaesthetic, coenesthetic das Körpergefühl betreffend

coenotrope Trieb *m*, Instinkt *m*, allgemeine Hinwendung *f*, Triebausrichtung *f*

coenzyme Koenzym *n*, Koferment *n*

coercion Zwang *m*, Nötigung *f* / **sexual ~** sexuelle Nötigung *f*

coexist nebeneinander bestehen, koexistieren

coexistence Koexistenz *f*, Nebeneinanderbestehen *n*

cogitative denkend, nachdenklich

cognate verwandt / Verwandter *m*, verwandtes Wort *n*

cognition Erkenntnis *f*, Wahrnehmung *f*, Erkennungsvermögen *n*, Kognition *f* / **paranormal ~** paranormale Wahrnehmung *f*, außersinnliche Wahrnehmung *f* / **social ~** soziale Kognition *f*

cognitive kognitiv

cognizance need Erkundungstrieb *m*, Erkundungsstreben *n* / **repressed ~** Voyeurtum *n*

cognize erkennen, erkunden

cogwheel phenomenon Zahnradphänomen *n*

cohabit Geschlechtsverkehr haben, Beischlaf ausüben, zusammenleben, in nichtehelicher Lebensgemeinschaft leben

cohabitation Beischlaf *m*, Geschlechtsverkehr *m*, nichteheliche Lebensgemeinschaft *f*

coherence Kohärenz *f*, Zusammenhang *m*, logischer Zusammenhang *m*, Folgerichtigkeit *f* / ~ **criterion** Kohärenzkriterium *n* / ~ **factor** Kohärenzfaktor *m* / ~ **of ideas** gedanklicher Zusammenhang *m*

coherent kohärent, logisch zusammenhängend, einheitlich, verständlich

cohesion Kohäsion *f*, Zusammenhang *m* / **figural** ~ Figurenkohäsion *f* / **social** ~ soziale Kohäsion *f*

cohesive kohäsiv, bindend

cohesiveness Zusammenhalt *m*, Kohäsion *f*, Festigkeit *f*, Kohäsivität *f*

cohort analysis Kohortenanalyse *f*

coincidence zufälliges Zusammentreffen *n*, gleichzeitiges Ereignis *n*, Übereinstimmung *f*, Koinzidenz *f*

coincident übereinstimmend, koinzident, korrespondierend

coincidental gleichzeitig, zufällig

coital Koitus–

coition Koitus *m*, Coitus *m*, Geschlechtsverkehr *m*, Beischlaf *m*, Geschlechtsakt *m*

coitophobia krankhafte Angst *f* vor dem Beischlaf, Koitophobie *f*

coitus Koitus *m*, Coitus *m*, Beischlaf *m*, Geschlechtsverkehr *m*, Geschlechtsakt *m* / ~ **interruptus** Coitus interruptus *m* / ~ **reservatus** Vorspiel *n*, Liebesspiel *n*, noch nicht vollzogener Koitus *m*

cold kalt, gemütskalt, gemütsarm / Kälte *f* / ~ **effect** Kältewirkung *f* / **~–hearted** kaltherzig, gefühllos / **~–heartedness** Gefühllosigkeit *f*, Kaltherzigkeit *f* / ~ **point** Kältepunkt *m* / ~ **receptor** Kälterezeptor *m* / ~ **sensation** Kälteempfindung *f* / ~ **sensor** Kältesensor *m* / ~ **spot** Kältepunkt *m* / ~ **stress** Kältebelastung *f* / **common** ~ Erkältung *f* / **paradoxical** ~ paradoxe Kälte *f*

coldavoidance need Bedürfnis *n* Kälte zu vermeiden

coldness Kälte *f* / **sexual** ~ Frigidität *f*

co–learning gemeinsames Lernen *n*

colic, renal Nierenkolik *f*

colitis Colitis *f*, Dickdarmkatarrh *m*, Dickdarmentzündung *f* / **ulcerative** ~ ulzeröse Kolitis *f*, Dickdarmentzündung *f* mit Geschwürsbildung, Colitis ulcerosa *f*

collaborate zusammenarbeiten

collaboration Zusammenarbeit *f*, Mitarbeit *f*

collaborator Mitarbeiter *m*

collapse zusammenbrechen, kollabieren / Kollaps *m*, Zusammenbruch *m* / ~ **delirium** Kollapsdelirium *n* / **nervous** ~ Nervenzusammenbruch *m*

collapsotherapy Kollapsbehandlung *f*

collateral Seitenlinie *f*, Verwandter *m* in der Seitenlinie / begleitend, Seiten–

collecting Sammel–

collective kollektiv, Gruppen–, Kollektiv– / Kollektiv *n*, Masse *f*, Gruppe *f*

collectivity Menge *f*, Kollektivität *f*

college höhere Schule *f*, Hochschule *f*, Fachhochschule *f*, Universität *f* / ~ **ability tests** Hochschulaufnahmetests *mpl* / ~ **academic achievement** Hochschulleistung *f* / ~ **degree** Universitätsgrad *m* / ~ **dropout** Studienabbrecher *m* / ~ **environment** Studienbedingungen *fpl*, Hochschulumgebung *f* / ~ **graduate** Hochschulabgänger *m* / ~ **major** Spezialisierung *f*, Hochschulfachausbildung *f* / ~ **student** Student *m*, Studentin *f* / ~ **teacher** Hochschullehrer *m*, Professor *m* / **junior** ~ Schule *f* welche die zwei letzten Oberstufenklassen des Gymnasiums und die beiden ersten Hochschuljahre umfasst

colliculi Vierhügel *mpl* / **inferior** ~ untere Hügel *mpl* der Vierhügelplatte, Colliculi inferiores *mpl* / **superior** ~ obere Hügel *mpl* der Vierhügelplatte, Colliculi superiores *mpl*

colligation Verbindung *f*

colloid Kolloid *n*

colloquium Kolloquium *n*, Diskussion *f*

collusion geheimes betrügerisches Einverständnis *n*, verabredete rechtswidrige Täuschung *f*, Kollusion *f*

colon Kolon *m*, Dickdarm *m* / ~ **disorder** Darmstörung *f*, Kolonerkrankung *f*, Dickdarmerkrankung *f* / **irritable** ~ Reizdarm *m*, Colon irritabile *n*, Reizkolon *n* / **spastic** ~ Reizkolon *n*, Colon spasticum *n*, Colon irritabile *n*

colonist Siedler *m*, Kolonisator *m*, Kolonist *m*

colorant Farbe *f*, Pigment *n*

coloration Färbung *f*, Farbgebung *f* / **emotional** ~ Affektrötung *f*

colorimeter Farbenmesser *m*, Kolorimeter *n*

colorimetric kolorimetrisch

colorimetry Kolorimetrie *f*, Farbenmessung *f*, Farbenmetrik *f*

colorless farblos, ungefärbt

colostomy Anlegen *n* eines künstlichen Afters, Kolostomie *f*

colour, color Farbe *f* / ~ **adaptation** Farbadaptation *f* / ~ **after–effect** Farbnachbild *n* / ~ **amblyopia** Farbenschwäche *f* / ~ **anomia** Farbenanomie *f* / ~ **antagonism** Farbantagonismus *m* / ~ **antagonists** Gegenfarben *fpl* / ~ **appreciation** Farbenwahrnehmung *f*, Farbempfinden *n* / ~ **attribute** Farbcharakteristik *f*, Farbmerkmal *n* / ~ **blind** farbenblind / ~ **blindness** Farbenblindheit *f*, Farbenfehlsichtigkeit *f* / ~ **blindness test** Farbtüchtigkeitstest *m* / ~ **brightness** Farbhelligkeit *f* / ~ **caste** Kaste *f* der Farbigen / ~ **centre** Zentrum *n* des Farbensinns / ~ **chart** Farbskala *f* / ~ **circle** Farbenkreis *m* / ~ **complementaries** Gegenfarben *fpl*, Komplementärfarben *fpl* / ~ **complementarism** Farbantagonismus *m* / ~ **complements** Gegenfarben *fpl*, Komplementärfarben *fpl* / ~ **composition** Farbkomposition *f* / ~ **constancy** Farbkonstanz *f* / ~ **contrast** Farbkontrast *m*, Farbenkontrast *m* / ~ **conversion** Farbumwandlung *f* / ~ **cycle** Farbenkreis *m* / ~ **deficiency** Farbenfehlsichtigkeit *f* / ~ **description** Farbenbeschreibung *f* / ~ **determinant** Farbdeterminante *f* / ~ **disk** Farbenscheibe *f*, Farbenkreisel *m*, Farbenmischapparat *m* / ~ **dynamics** Farbendynamik *f* / ~ **equation** Farbengleichung *f* / ~**–form test** Farbe–Form–Test *m* / ~ **fundamental** Grundfarbe *f* / ~ **harmony** Farbenharmonie *f* / ~**–hearing** Farbenhören *n*, Synästhesie *f* / ~ **hue** Farbton *m* / ~ **induction** induzierte Farbe *f* / ~ **insistance** Anziehungskraft *f* der Farbe / ~ **invariables** unveränderliche Farben *fpl* / ~ **mixer** Farbenmischapparat *m*, Farbvariator *m* / ~ **mixture** Farbenmischung *f* / ~ **naming** Farbnennung *f* / ~ **notation** Farbbezeichnung *f* / ~ **octaeder** Farbenoktaeder *n*, Farbendoppelkegel *m* / ~ **perception** Farbwahrnehmung *f* Farbentüchtigkeit *f*, Farbensehen *n* / ~ **preference** Farbbevorzugung *f* / ~ **primal** Grundfarbe *f*, Hauptfarbe *f* / ~ **primary** Primärfarbe *f*, Grundfarbe *f* / ~ **purity** Farbreinheit *f* / ~ **pyramid** Farbenpyramide *f* / ~ **pyramid test** Farbpyramidentest *m* / ~ **range** Farbskala *f* / ~ **refraction** Farbenbrechung *f* / ~ **response** Farbantwort *f*, Farbdeutung *f* / ~ **saturation** Farbsättigung *f* / ~ **scale** Farbskala *f* / ~ **scheme** Farbenzusammenstellung *f* / ~ **seer** Farbenseher *m* / ~ **sensation** Farbempfindung *f* / ~ **sense** Farbensinn *m* / ~ **sensibility** Farbenempfindlichkeit *f* / ~ **sensitive** farbenempfindlich / ~ **sensitiveness** Farbenempfindlichkeit *f* / ~ **shade** Farbnuance *f* / ~ **shock** Farbschock *m* / ~ **solid** Farbenkugel *f*, Farbenoktaeder *n* / ~ **sorting test** Farbensortiertest *m*, Wollfadenprobe *f* / ~ **sphere** Farbenkugel *f* / ~ **spindle** Farbenpyramide *f* / ~ **square** Farbenquadrat *n*, Farbenviereck *n* / ~ **substance** Farbsubstanz *f* / ~ **surface** Farbenfläche *f* / ~ **symbolism** Farbensymbolik *f* / ~ **taste** Pseudogeuästhesie *f* / ~ **temperature** Farbtemperatur *f* / ~ **test** Farbentest *m*, Farbenprobe *f* / ~ **theory** Farbtheorie *f*, Farbenlehre *f* / ~ **tint** Farbton *m*, Farbnuance *f* / ~ **tone** Farbton *m* / ~ **top** Farbkreisel *m*, Farbenkreisel *m* / ~ **triad** Farbendreiklang *m* / ~ **triangle** Farbdreieck *n*, Farbendreieck *m* / ~ **value** Farbwert *m*, Helligkeit *f* / ~ **vision** Farbensehen *n* / ~**–vision deficit** Farbsinnesstörung *f* / ~ **vision test chart** Farbprüftafel *f* / ~ **weak** farbenschwach / ~ **weakness** Farbenschwäche *f* / ~ **wheel** Farbenkreisel *m*, Farbenscheibe *f*, Farbenmischapparat *m* / ~ **zone** Farbzone *f* / **achromatic** ~ achromatische Farbe *f*, nicht–bunte Farbe *f* / **achromatic** ~ **response** Farbdeutung *f* zu schwarz und weiß / **antagonistic** ~**s** Komplementärfarben *fpl*, Gegenfarben *fpl* / **bulky** ~ Raumfarbe *f* / **chromatic** ~ bunte Farbe *f* / **cold** ~ kalte Farbe *f* / **complementary** ~**s** Komplementärfarben *fpl* / **double** ~ **pyramid** Farbenoktaeder *n* / **fundamental** ~ Grundfarbe *f* / **glowing** ~ Leuchtfarbe *f* / **hard** ~ harte Farbe *f* / **hysterical** ~ **blindness** hysterische Farbenblindheit *f* / **illuminant** ~ Leuchtfarbe *f* / **induced** ~ Kontrastfarbe *f* / **invariable** ~ unveränderliche Farbe *f* / **metameric** ~**s** metamerische Farben *fpl* / **mirrored** ~ Spiegelfarbe *f* / **mixed** ~ Mischfarbe *f* / **neutral** ~ neutrale Farbe *f* / **normal** ~ **vision** Farbensichtigkeit *f*, normales Farbensehen *n* / **partial** ~ **blindness** partielle Farbenblindheit *f* / **primal** ~ Urfarbe *f* / **primary** ~ Primärfarbe *f* / **principal** ~ Hauptfarbe *f* / **psychological primary** ~ psychologische Grundfarbe *f* / **pure** ~ reine Farbe *f* / **reduced** ~ Flächenfarbe *f* / **reflected** ~ reflektierte Farbe *f*, Reflexionsfarbe *f* / **saturated** ~ satte Farbe *f*, gesättigte Farbe *f* / **soft** ~ weiche Farbe *f* / **spectral** ~ Spektralfarbe *f* / **strong** ~ starke Farbe *f*, kräftige Farbe *f* / **subjective** ~ subjektive Farbe *f* / **symbolic** ~ **response** symbolische Farbdeutung *f* / **total** ~ **blindness** totale Farbenblindheit *f*, Achromatopsie *f*, Daltonismus *m* / **unique** ~ reine Farbe *f* / **warm** ~ warme Farbe *f* / **weak** ~ schwache Farbe *f* / **well differentiated** ~ **vision** Farbentüchtigkeit *f*

coloured farbig, gefärbt, bunt, getönt

colouring Färbung *f* / **emotional** ~ Affektrötung *f* / **protective** ~ Schutzfärbung *f*

columella Säule *f*, kleine Säule *f*

column Säule *f* / ~ **diagram** Säulendiagramm *n*, Balkendiagramm *n* / **cervical vertebral** ~ Halswirbelsäule *f* / **dorsal** ~ Hinterstrang *m* / **lateral** ~ Seitenstrang *m* / **lumbar vertebral** ~ Lendenwirbelsäule *f* / **spinal** ~ Wirbelsäule *f* / **ventral** ~ Vorderstrang *m* / **vertebral** ~ Wirbelsäule *f*

columnar säulenförmig, säulenartig

coma Koma *n*, Coma *n*, Zustand *m* tiefer Bewusstlosigkeit / ~ **vigil** Zustand *m* der Bewusstlosigkeit bei gleichzeitig geöffneten Augen / **agrypnodal** ~ Coma agrypnum *n*, Coma vigile *n* / **alcoholic** ~ Coma alcoholicum *n* / **diabetic** ~ diabetisches Koma *n* / **vigil** ~ vigiles Koma *n*, akinetischer Mutismus *m*

coma–like komaähnlich

comatogenotis Koma hervorrufend, Koma verursachend, komatogen

comatose komatös, im Koma befindlich

combat Kampf *m* / ~ **exhaustion** Kampfneurose *f* / ~ **experience** Gefechtserfahrung *f* / ~ **fatigue** Kriegsneurose *f*, Kampfneurose *f* / ~ **neurosis** Kriegsneurose *f*, Kampfneurose *f*

combative kampfsüchtig, streitlustig

combination Kombination *f* / ~ **principle** Kombinationsprinzip *n* / ~ **test** Kombinationstest *m*, Lückentest *m*, Ergänzungstest *m* / ~ **tone** Kombinationston *m*

combinativity Kombinationsfähigkeit *f*

combined vereinigt, vereint, kombiniert

combustible Brennstoff *m*

comention Konformismus *m*, kulturelle Konformität *f*

cometophobia krankhafte Angst *f* vor einem Kometen

comfort| movement Komfortverhalten *n* / **physical** ~ körperliche Befindlichkeit *f*

comforting tröstlich

comic komisch / Komiker *m*

command Befehl *m*, Herrschaft *f*, Beherrschung *f* / **~ automatism** Befehlsautomatie *f* / **~ negativism** Befehlsnegativismus *m* / **low self–~** geringe Selbstbeherrschung *f*

commensalism Kommensalismus *m*, tierische Symbiose *f*

commensurable vergleichbar, mit gleichem Maße messbar

commensurate angemessen, entsprechend

commerce Handel *m*, Verkehr *m*

commercial Werbesendung *f*, Werbespot *m*, Werbedurchsage *f* / kommerziell, Werbe– / **~ television** Werbefernsehen *n* / **tv–~** Fernsehwerbespot *m*

commissural Kommissur–

commissure Kommissur *f*, Verbindung *f* / **~s of the brain** Commissura *fpl* des Gehirns / **great ~** Gehirnbalken *m*

commissurotomy Split–Brain–Verfahren *m*, Kommissurenschnitt *m*, Kommissurotomie *f*

commitment Engagement *n*, innere Verpflichtung *f*, Verbundenheitsgefühl *n*, Einweisung *f* / **organizational ~** Organisationsverbundenheit *f* / **outpatient ~** ambulante Zwangsbehandlung *f* / **psychiatric ~** psychiatrische Zwangseinweisung *f*

committable anstaltsreif, von Gesetzes wegen in einer geschlossenen Anstalt unterzubringen

committee Komitee *n*, Ausschuss *m*

common gemeinsam, allgemein, Gemein–

commotio Erschütterung *f*, Commotio *f*

cerebri Gehirnerschütterung *f*

commotion Verwirrung *f*, innere Erregung *f*, psychische Erregung *f* / **cerebral ~** Gehirnerschütterung *f*

commotional Kommotions–

communality Kommunalität *f*

commune Gemeinde *f*, Kommune *f*

communicability Mitteilbarkeit *f*, Übertragbarkeit *f*, Kommunizierbarkeit *f*

communicant Kommunikant *m*, Informant *m*

communicate mitteilen, kommunizieren

communication Kommunikation *f* / **~s** Informationen *fpl* / **~ channel** Kommunikationskanal *m* / **~ content** Kommunikationsinhalt *m* / **~ disorder** Kommunikationsstörung *f* / **~ engineering** Nachrichtentechnik *f* / **~ media** Medien *npl*, Kommunikationsmittel *npl* / **~ model** Kommunikationsmodell *n*, Kommunikationsmuster *n* / **~ network** Kommunikationsnetz *n* / **~ skills** Kommunikationsfähigkeiten *fpl*, Geschick *n* zum Kommunizieren / **~ skills training** Kommunikationstraining *n* / **~ system** Kommunikationssystem *n* / **~ theory** Kommunikationstheorie *f* / **~ unit** Kommunikationseinheit *f* / **audiovisual ~ media** audiovisuelle Kommunikationsmedien *npl* / **augmentative ~** Kommunikationshilfe *f* für Behinderte / **consummatory ~** konsummatorische Kommunikation *f* / **cross cultural ~** interkulturelle Kommunikation / **digital ~s** digitale Kommunikation *f*, Digitalkommunikation *f* / **horizontal ~** Kommunikation *f* auf gleicher Ebene / **human ~** menschliche Kommunikation *f* / **instrumental ~** zweckgerichtete Kommunikation *f*, instrumentelle Kommunikation *f* / **interpersonal ~** zwischenmenschliche Kommunikation *f*, interpersonale Kommunikation *f* / **manual ~** manuelle Kommunikation *f*, Kommunikation *f* durch Fingersprache / **nonverbal ~** nichtverbale Kommunikation *f* / **oral ~** mündliche Kommunikation *f*, verbale Kommunikation *f* / **persuasive ~** Überredung *f*, persuasive Kommunikation *f* / **printed ~ media** gedruckte Kommunikationsmittel *npl*, Druckerzeugnisse *npl*, Printmedien *npl* / **privileged ~** Kommunikation *f* unter Schweigepflicht, vertrauliche Mitteilung *f* / **professional ~** wissenschaftliche Mitteilung *f* / **scientific ~** wissenschaftliche Mitteilung *f*, wissenschaftliche Kommunikation *f* / **verbal ~** mündliche Kommunikation *f*, verbale Kommunikation *f* / **written ~** schriftliche Kommunikation *f*

communicative mitteilsam, redselig

communicator Kommunikator *m*

communion Verbindung *f*, enge Gemeinschaft *f*

community Gemeinschaft *f*, Gemeinde *f* / **~ attitude** Einstellung *f* der Öffentlichkeit / **~ care** Gemeindefürsorge *f* / **~ centre** Gemeindezentrum *n*, Gemeindehaus *n*, Bürgerhaus *n* / **~-centrism** Überbewertung *f* der eigenen Gemeinschaft / **~ college** städtische höhere Schule *f* / **~ development** Gemeindeentwicklung *f* / **~ efforts** gemeinschaftliche Bemühungen *fpl* / **~ facilities** öffentliche Einrichtungen *fpl* / **~ feeling** Gruppengeist *m*, Gemeinschaftsgefühl *n* / **~ mental health centers** öffentliche Zentren *npl* für Psychohygiene, gemeindenahe psychosoziale Einrichtungen *fpl* / **~ mental health services** gemeindenahe psychosoziale Dienste *mpl* / **~ of content theory** Theorie *f* der identischen Elemente, Theorie *f* des gemeinsamen Inhalts / **~ of ideas** Ideengleichheit *f*, Gesinnungsgleichheit *f* / **~ psychiatry** gemeindenahe Psychiatrie *f*, Gemeindepsychiatrie *f* / **~ psychology** Gemeindepsychologie *f* / **~ services** öffentliche Dienste *mpl* / **~ therapy** Behandlung *f* in therapeutischen Gemeinschaften / **~ welfare services** öffentliche Wohlfahrtseinrichtungen *fpl* / **conjugal ~** eheliche Gemeinschaft *f* / **therapeutic ~** therapeutische Gemeinschaft *f*

commuter Pendler *m*

commuting Pendelverkehr *m*

comorbidity Komorbidität *f*

companion Kamerad *m*, Gefährte *m* / **imaginary ~** imaginärer Spielgefährte *m*

comparability Vergleichbarkeit *f*

comparable vergleichbar

comparative vergleichend

comparator Komparator *m*, Vergleichsmessinstrument *n*

comparison Vergleich *m* / **~ group** Vergleichsgruppe *f* / **~ level** Vergleichsniveau *n* / **~ by pairs** paarweiser Vergleich *m*, Paarvergleich *m* / **~ stimulus** Vergleichsreiz *m* / **paired ~** Paarvergleich *m* / **paired ~ method** Methode *f* des Paarvergleichs / **social ~** sozialer Vergleich *m* / **successive ~** sukzessiver Vergleich *m*, Sukzessivvergleich *m*

compartment Abteilung *f*, Fach *n*, Feld *n*

compartmentalisation Unterteilung *f*, Untergliederung *f*, psychische Segmentation *f*, psychische Bereichsbildung *f*

compassion Mitleid *n*

compatibility Vereinbarkeit *f*, Verträglichkeit *f*, Kompatibilität *f* / **interpersonal ~** interpersonale Verträglichkeit *f*

compatible vereinbar, verträglich, kompatibel

compeer Gleichgestellter *m*, Kollege *m*, Gefährte *m*, Kamerad *m*

compensate ausgleichen, kompensieren

compensating, compensational, compensatory kompensatorisch, ausgleichend, Kornpensations–

compensation Kompensation *f*, Ausgleich *m* / **~ idea** Kompensationshypothese *f* / **~ neurosis** Rentenneurose *f*, Assekurose *f* / **~ programme** Kompensationsprogramm *n*, Vergütungsprogramm *n* / **~ schedule** Belohnungsplan *m*, Entlohnungsprogramm *n*

compete wetteifern, konkurrieren, in Wettstreit treten

competence, competency Fähigkeit *f*, Fertigkeit *f*, Tüchtigkeit *f*, Leistungsvermögen *n*, Kompetenz *f* / **~ motive** Motiv *n* eine gute Leistung zu erbringen / **~ to stand trial** Verhandlungsfähigkeit *f* vor Gericht / **legal ~** Geschäftsfähigkeit *f* / **minimum ~ test** Grundfähigkeitstest *m* / **professional ~** berufliche Kompetenz *f* / **social ~** Sozialkompetenz *f*

competent fähig, tüchtig, leistungsfähig

competition Wettstreit *m*, Wettbewerb *m*, Konkurrenz *f*, Konkurrenzkampf *m* / **economic ~** wirtschaftlicher Wettbewerb *m*

competitive Konkurrenz–, auf Wettbewerb eingestellt, wetteifernd

competitiveness Konkurrenzfähigkeit *f*, Wettbewerbsfähigkeit *f*

competitor Mitbewerber *m*, Konkurrent *m*, Wettbewerbsteilnehmer *m*

compiler Compiler *m*, Übersetzer–Programm *n*, Compiler–Programm *n*

complacence, complacency Selbstgefälligkeit *f*, Überheblichkeit *f* / **defensive ~** Willensschwäche *f*

complacent selbstgefällig, überheblich

complain klagen, sich beklagen, reklamieren

complaint Klage *f*, Beanstandung *f*, Beschwerde *f* / **~ habit** notorisches Wehklagen *n* / **functional ~s** funktionelle Beschwerden *fpl* / **geriatric ~s** Altersbeschwerden *fpl* / **nervous ~** nervöse Beschwerden *fpl*

complement Ergänzung *f*, Vervollständigung *f*

complemental, complementary komplementär, ergänzend, Komplementär–

complementarism Farbantagonismus *m*, Komplementarismus *m*

completeness Vollständigkeit *f*

completion test Ergänzungstest *m*, Lückentest *m*, Kombinationstest *m*

complex Komplex *m* / komplex / **~ associations** komplexe Assoziationen *fpl* / **~ of Cain** Kainkomplex *m* / **~ indicators** Komplexanzeichen *npl* / **~ of inferiority** Minderwertigkeitskomplex *m* / **~ number** komplexe Zahl *f* / **~ personality** komplexe Persönlichkeit *f* / **~ psychology** komplexe Psychologie *f* / **~ quality** Komplexqualität *f* / **~ reaction** Komplexreaktion *f* / **~ of symptoms** Symptomkomplex *m*, Syndrom *n* / **~ theory** Komplextheorie *f* / **anti–Oedipus ~** Anti–Ödipuskomplex *m* / **autonomous ~** autonomer Komplex *m* / **creative ~** schöpferischer Komplex *m* / **cynical ~** Zynismus–Komplex *m* / **marginal ~** Randkomplex *m* / **nuclear ~** Kernkomplex *m* / **Oedipal ~** Ödipuskomplex *m* / **particular ~** Sonderkomplex *m* / **psychosomatic ~** psychosomatischer Komplex *m* / **repressed ~** verdrängter Komplex *m* / **universal ~** Universalkomplex *m*

complexion Komplexion *f*, fundierter Inhalt *m*

complexity Vielgestaltigkeit *f*, Kompliziertheit *f*, Verflechtung *f*, Komplexität *f* / **cognitive ~** kognitive Komplexität *f*

compliance Compliance *f*, Bereitwilligkeit *f*, Befolgung *f*, Nachgiebigkeit *f*, Unterwürfigkeit *f*, Willfährigkeit *f* / **forced ~** erzwungene Zustimmung *f* / **neurotic ~** neurotische Unterwürfigkeit *f* / **somatic ~** somatisches Entgegenkommen *n*

complication Komplikation *f* / **~ experiment** Komplikationsversuch *m* / **obstetrical ~** Geburtskomplikation *f* / **perinatal ~** Geburtskomplikation *f* / **postsurgical ~** postoperative Komplikation *f* / **surgical ~** Operationskomplikation *f*

component Komponente *f*, Bestandteil *m*, Teil *m* / **~ analysis** Komponentenanalyse *f* / **~ of a drive** Triebkomponente *f* / **~–instinct** Triebkomponente *f*, Partialtrieb *m* / **~ of intelligence** Intelligenzkomponente *f* / **~ of variation** Streuungskomponente *f* / **affective ~** affektive Komponente *f* / **cognitive ~** kognitives Element *n* / **instinctual ~** Triebkomponente *f* / **tactic ~** taktische Komponente *f*

compos mentis geistig normal, zurechnungsfähig

composite zusammengesetzt, gemischt

composition Zusammensetzung *f* / **~ scale** Aufsatzbewertungsskala *f* / **~ theory** geistiger Atomismus *m* / **atomistic ~** atomistische Zusammensetzung *f*

composure Gemütsruhe *f*, Fassung *f*, Gelassenheit *f*

compound Zusammensetzung *f*, Verbindung *f*, Mischung *f*, Kompositum *n* / **~ eye** Facettenauge *n* / **~ reaction** komplexe Reaktion *f* / **~ tone** Mischton *m*, Summationston *m*, zusammengesetzter Ton *m*

comprehend verstehen, begreifen, umfassen

comprehensible begreiflich, verständlich, fassbar

comprehensibility Verständlichkeit *f*, Fassbarkeit *f*

comprehension Verständnis *n*, Einsicht *f*, Auffassung *f*, Inhaltserfassung *f* / **~ test** Verständnistest *m* / **listening ~** akustisches Verständnis *n* / **mechanical ~** mechanisches Verständnis *n* / **mechanical ~ test** mechanisch–technischer Verständnistest *m* / **verbal ~** Sprachverständnis *n*, verbales Verständnis *n*

comprehensive umfassend, komplett, Gesamt–

compressed gepresst, komprimiert

compression Druck *m*, Verdichtung *f* / **cerebral ~** Hirndruck *m*

compromise–formation Kompromissbildung *f*

compulsion Zwang *m*, innerer Zwang *m*, Zwangsantrieb *m*, Zwang *m* zur Vollständigkeit / **~ for cleanliness** Reinlichkeitszwang *m* / **~ of response theory** Theorie *f* der vollständigen Reaktion / **~ to masturbate** Onaniezwang *m*, Masturbationszwang *m* / **~ neurosis** Zwangsneurose *f* / **~ to repeat** Wiederholungszwang *m* / **~ to touch objects** Berührungszwang *m* / **conscientious ~** Gewissenszwang *m* / **hysterical ~** hysterischer Zwang *m* / **inner ~** innerer Zwang *m* / **internal ~** innerer Zwang *m* / **obsessive–~ neurosis** Zwangsneurose *f* / **repetitive ~** Wiederholungszwang *m*

compulsive Zwangs–, zwanghaft, zwangsmäßig, zwingend / **~–neurotic** zwangsneurotisch

compulsiveness, compulsivity Zwanghaftigkeit *f*, Zwangstendenz *f*, zwanghaftes Handeln *n* / **sexual ~** innerer sexueller Zwang *m*

compulsory zwanghaft, zwangsweise, Zwangs–

compunction Gewissensbisse *mpl*, Reue *f*

computable berechenbar, zu berechnend

computation Berechnung *f*, Schätzung *f*

computer Computer *m*, Rechner *m*, Datenverarbeitungsanlage *f* / **~ application** Computeranwendung *f* / **~–assisted design** computerunterstützte Gestaltung *f* / **~–assisted diagnosis** Computerdiagnose *f*, computerunterstützte Diagnostik *f* / **~–assisted instruction** computerunterstützte Unterweisung *f*, computerunterstützter Unterricht *m* / **~–assisted testing** computerunterstütztes Testen *n* / **~ attitude** Einstellung *f* zu Computern / **~–based** rechnergestützt / **~ code** Rechencode *m*, Maschinenkode *m* / **~ game** Computerspiel *n* / **~ instruction** Maschinenbefehl *m* / **human–~ interaction** Mensch–Computer–Interaktion *f* / **~ language** Maschinensprache *f* / **~ literacy** Computerkenntnisse *fpl* / **~ network** Computernetzwerk *n* / **~ peripheral devices** Computerperipherie *f* / **~ programme** Computerprogramm *n* / **~ programming language** Computersprache *f*, Programmiersprache *f*, Maschinensprache *f* / **~ searching** Online–Suche *f* / **~ science** Informatik *f* / **~ simulation** Computersimulation *f* / **~ software** Software *f* / **~ system** EDV–System *n*, Datenverarbeitungssystem *n* / **~ tomography** Computertomografie *f* / **~ training** Computerausbildung *f* / **~ word** Maschinenwort *n* / **analog ~** Analogrechner *m* / **digital ~** Digitalrechner *m*, Digitalcomputer *m*

comradeship Kameradschaft *f*

conation zielgerichtetes Streben *n*, Willenstrieb *m*, Antrieb *m*, Konation *f*

conative konativ, strebend, antriebsgesteuert

conatus zielgerichtetes Streben *n*, Streben *n* nach Selbsterhaltung und Selbstbestätigung

concave konkav, hohlgeschliffen

concavity Konkavseite *f*, Höhlung *f*

conceit Idee *f*, Einfall *m* / Eitelkeit *f*, Stolz *m*

conceivable begreiflich, denkbar

conceive begreifen, ausdenken, ersinnen, denken / schwanger werden

concentrate sich konzentrieren

concentration Konzentration *f* / **~ camp** Konzentrationslager *n* / **~ camp syndrome** Überlebendensyndrom *n* / **~ of mind** Gedankenkonzentration *f* / **~ power** Konzentrationsvermögen *n*, Konzentrationsfähigkeit *f* / **~ test** Konzentrationstest *m* / **bad ~** schlechte Konzentration *f*, Konzentrationsschwäche *f* / **mental ~** Gedankenkonzentration *f* / **weak ~** Konzentrationsschwäche *f*

concept Begriff *m*, Konzept *n*, Begriffsvorstellung *f* / **~ attainment** Begriffsbildung *f*, Konzepterwerb *m* / **~ of character** Charakterbegriff *m* / **~ development** Begriffsentwicklung *f* / **~ differentiation** Begriffsunterscheidung *f* / **~ extension** Begriffserweiterung *f* / **~ formation** Begriffsbildung *f* / **~ generalisation** Konzeptgeneralisierung *f* / **~ learning** Begriffelernen *n*, Konzepterwerb *m* / **~ mastery test** Test *m* zur Prüfung des abstrakten Denkens / **abstract ~** abstrakter Begriff *m*, Konzept *n* / **associative ~** Assoziationskonzept *n* / **chemical ~ of nervous excitation** chemische Theorie *f* der Nervenerregung / **conditional–genetic ~** konditionalgenetischer Begriff *m* / **conjunctive ~** verbindender Begriff *m* / **disjunctive ~** trennender Begriff *m* / **dynamic ~** dynamischer Begriff *m* / **egocentric ~** egozentrisches Konzept *n* / **empirical ~** empirisches Konzept *n* / **general ~** Allgemeinbegriff *m* / **hypothetical ~** hypothetisches Konstrukt *n* / **iconic ~** ikonischer Begriff *m*, anschaulicher Begriff *m* / **mathematical ~** mathematischer Begriff *m* / **relational ~** Strukturkonzept *n* / **representative ~** repräsentativer Begriff *m* / **theoretical ~** theoretisches Konstrukt *n* / **topological ~** topologischer Begriff *m*

conception Auffassung *f*, Begriffsbildung *f*, Begriff *m*, Konzeption *f*, Empfängnis *f* / **structuronomic ~** strukturgesetzliche Auffassung *f*

conceptual begrifflich, Begriffs–, konzeptionell

conceptualisation Begriffsbildung *f*, Strukturierung *f* nach übergeordneten Begriffen

conceptualize Begriffe bilden, nach Begriffen ordnen, begrifflich denken

concert pitch Kammerton *m*

concha Ohrmuschel *f*, Muschel *f*, Concha *f* / **nasal ~** Nasenmuschel *f*

conciliation Versöhnung *f*, Aussöhnung *f*

conclusion Folgerung *f*, Schluss *m* / **~ by analogy** Analogieschluss *m*

concomitant begleitend, Begleit–

concord Einmütigkeit *f*, Eintracht *f*, Harmonie *f*

concordance Übereinstimmung *f*, Konkordanz *f* / **~ coefficient** Konkordanzkoeffizient *m* / **~ reliability** Konkordanzreliabilität *f*

concrete konkret

concreteness Konkretisierung *f*, Veranschaulichung *f*

concretism Konkretismus *m*, Ausgerichtetsein *n* auf die Realität

concretizing Veranschaulichung *f*, Konkretisierung *f*

concubinage Konkubinat *n*, wilde Ehe *f*

concubine Konkubine *f*

concupiscence sinnliche Begierde *f*

concurrence, concurrency Übereinstimmung *f*, Konkurrenz *f*

concurrent gleichzeitig, simultan

concussion Erschütterung *f*, Commotio *f* / **~ of the brain** Gehirnerschütterung *f* / **~ psychosis** Kontusionspsychose *f* / **cerebral ~** Gehirnerschütterung *f*, Commotio cerebri *f*

condemnation Verurteilung *f*

condensation Verdichtung *f*

condense verdichten

condition Bedingung *f*, Zustand *m*, Befinden *n* / bedingen, konditionieren, dressieren / **~ of drive** Bedingung *f* für den Antrieb, Triebzustand *m* / **affective ~** Affektzustand *m* / **atmospheric ~** atmosphärische Bedingung *f* / **depressive ~** Depressionszustand *m* / **emotional ~** Gemütszustand *m* / **environmental ~s** Umweltbedingungen *fpl* / **experimental ~s** Versuchsbedingungen *fpl* / **extraspacial ~s** außerörtliche Bedingungen *fpl* / **general ~** Allgemeinbefinden *n*, Allgemeinzustand *m* / **general medical ~s** medizinische Krankheitsfaktoren *mpl* / **initial psychological ~** psychische Ausgangslage *f* / **mental ~** Geisteszustand *m*, geistige Verfassung *f* / **normal ~** Normalzustand *m* / **optimum ~s** optimale Bedingungen *fpl* / **other ~s that may be a focus of clinical attention** andere klinisch relevante Probleme *npl* / **parathymic ~** Verstimmtheit *f*, Zustand *m* der Verstimmung / **residual ~** Residualzustand *m*, Residualsyndrom *n* / **real–life ~** lebensnahe Bedingung *f* / **schizophrenic ~** Bewusstseinsspaltung *f*, Zustand *m* der Schizophrenie / **social ~s** soziale Verhältnisse *npl* / **working ~s** Arbeitsbedingungen *fpl*

conditionability Konditionierbarkeit *f*

conditional bedingt, konditional

conditionalism Vorherbestimmung *f*, Determinismus *m*

conditionality Bedingtheit *f*, Konditionalität *f*

conditioned bedingt, konditioniert

conditioning Konditionieren *n*, Konditionierung *f*, Bedingen *n*, Dressur *f* / **~ experiments** Konditionierungsexperimente *npl* / **~ shock** Konditionierungsschock *m* / **~ stimulus** konditionierender Reiz *m* / **aversive ~** Abneigungskonditionieren *n*, Aversionstherapie *f* / **avoiding ~** Vermeidungskonditionieren *n* / **backward ~** rückwirkendes Konditionieren *n*, retrograde Konditionierung *f* / **classical ~** klassisches Konditionieren *n*, klassische Konditionierung *f* / **configural ~** Gestaltkonditionieren *n* / **decorticate ~** Konditionieren *n* eines Tieres ohne Großhirn, subkortikales Konditionieren *n* / **delayed ~** verzögertes Konditionieren *n* / **differential ~** differentielles Konditionieren *n* / **emotional ~ test** Prüfung *f* der affektiven Konditionierung / **inhibitory ~** bedingte Hemmung *f* / **instrumental ~** instrumentelles Bedingen *n*, instrumentelle Konditionierung *f* / **interoceptive ~** interozeptive Konditionierung *f* / **negative ~** bedingte Hemmung *f* / **operant ~** operantes Konditionieren *n* / **Pavlovian ~** klassisches Konditionieren *n*, Pawlow'sche Konditionierung *f* / **remote ~** zeitlich verteiltes Konditionieren *n* / **respondent ~** reaktives Konditionieren *n*, reaktives Bedingen *n* / **secondary ~** sekundäres Konditionieren *n*, Konditionierung *f* zweiter Ordnung / **semantic ~** semantische Konditionierung *f* / **sensory ~** Doppelreizkonditionierung *f* / **simultaneous ~** gleichzeitige Konditionierung *f*, Simultankonditionierung *f* / **subconscious ~** unbewusstes Konditionieren *n* / **subcortical ~** subkortikales Konditionieren *n* / **verbal ~** verbale Konditionierung *f* / **vicarious ~** stellvertretendes Konditionieren *n*, Konditionieren *n* durch Beobachten

condom Kondom *n*

conduct Verhalten *n*, Betragen *n*, Benehmen *n* / sich verhalten, sich benehmen, durchführen, leiten / **~ disorder** Störung *f* des Sozialverhaltens / **~ disorder confined to the family context** auf den familiären Rahmen beschränkte Störung *f* des

Sozialverhaltens / **depressive ~ disorder** Störung *f* des Sozialverhaltens mit depressiver Störung / **hyperkinetic ~ disorder** hyperkinetische Störung *f* des Sozialverhaltens / **rational ~** rationales Verhalten *n* / **socialized ~ disorder** Störung *f* des Sozialverhaltens bei vorhandenen sozialen Bindungen / **unsocialized ~ disorder** Störung *f* des Sozialverhaltens bei fehlenden sozialen Bindungen

conductance, conductibility Leitfähigkeit *f*, Leitwert *m*

conduction Leitung *f*, Reizleitung *f* / **~ aphasia** Leitungsaphasie *f* / **~ bundle** Reizleitungsbündel *n* / **~ deafness** Leitungsschwerhörigkeit *f* / **~ with decrement** Dekrementleitung *f* / **~ defect** Reizleitungsstörung *f* / **~ of excitation** Erregungsleitung *f* / **~ path** Leitungsbahn *f*, Bahn *f* / **~ of stimulus** Reizleitung *f* / **~ time** Leitungszeit *f* / **~ unit** Leitungseinheit *f* / **~ velocity** Fortpflanzungsgeschwindigkeit *f*, Leitungsgeschwindigkeit *f* / **active ~** aktive Leitung *f* / **antidromic nervous ~** gegenläufige Nervenleitung *f* / **electrotonic ~** elektrotonische Leitung *f* / **irreciprocal ~** irreversible Leitung *f* / **nervous ~** Nervenleitung *f* / **neural ~** Nervenleitung *f* / **saltatory ~** saltatorische Leitung *f*, saltatorische Erregungsleitung *f* / **synaptic ~** Synapsenleitung *f*

conductive leitend, leitfähig, Leitungs–

conductivity Leitfähigkeit *f*, Leitungsvermögen *n* / **~ disorder** Reizleitungsstörung *f*

cone Zapfen *m*, Konus *m* / **~ adaptation** Zapfenadaptation *f* / **~ cell** Zapfenzelle *f* / **~ curve** kegelförmige Kurve *f* / **retinal ~** Netzhautzapfen *m*

confabulate konfabulieren, phantasieren

confabulation Konfabulation *f*, Phantasieren *n*, sinnlos–phantastische Ausdeutung *f* / **opportune ~** blühende Konfabulation *f*

confact Confact *n*, Übertragung *f* einer gelernten Verhaltensweise

confederate Verbündeter *m*, Komplize *m*, Vertrauter *m* des Versuchsleiters

conference proceedings Kongressberichte *mpl*

confession Beichte *f*, Bekenntnis *n*, Geständnis *n*, Konfession *f*

confidence Vertrauen *n*, Zuversicht *f* / **~ belt** Vertrauensbereich *m* / **~ coefficient** Konfidenzkoeffizient *m* / **~ interval** Vertrauensintervall *n* / **~ level** Konfidenzkoeffizient *m*, Konfidenzbereich *m* / **~ limits** Konfidenzgrenzen *fpl*, Vertrauensgrenzen *fpl* / **~ region** Konfidenzbereich *m*

confidentiality of information Vertraulichkeit *f* der Information

configuration Struktur *f*, Gestalt *f*, Konfiguration *f*, Form *f*, Muster *n*, Gebilde *n* / **~ principle** Gestaltprinzip *n*

configurationism Gestaltpsychologie *f*

confinement Haft *f*, Gefangenschaft *f*, Eingesperrtsein *n*

confirm bestatigen

confirmation Bestätigung *f*, Bekräftigung *f*

conflict Konflikt *m* / im Widerspruch stehen / **~ of ambivalence** Ambivalenzkonflikt *m* / **~ with authority** Autoritätskonflikt *m* / **~ between drives** Triebkonflikt *m* / **~ between instincts** Triebkonflikt *m* / **~–free** konfliktfrei / **~ of motives** Motivkonflikt *m* / **~ regression** Konfliktverminderung *f* / **~ research** Konfliktforschung *f* / **~ resolution** Konfliktlösung *f* / **~ of roles** Rollenkonflikt *m* / **~ situation** Konfliktsituation *f* / **~ of values** Wertekonflikt *m* / **actual ~** aktueller Konflikt *m* / **basic ~** Grundkonflikt *m* / **central ~** zentraler Konflikt *m* / **cultural ~** Kulturkonflikt *m* / **endopsychic ~** innerer Konflikt *m* / **external ~** äußerer Konflikt *m* / **externally cued ~** durch ein äußeres Signal ausgelöster Konflikt *m* / **extrapsychic ~** extrapsychischer Konflikt *m* / **inner ~** innerer Konflikt *m*, seelischer Konflikt *m* / **instinctual ~** Triebkonflikt *m* / **internally cued ~** durch ein inneres Signal ausgelöster Konflikt *m* / **interpersonal ~** interpersonaler Konflikt *m*, zwischenmenschlicher Konflikt *m* / **intrapersonal ~** innerer Konflikt *m*, intrapsychischer Konflikt *m* / **intrapsychic ~** intrapsychischer Konflikt *m*, innerer Konflikt *m* / **marital ~** Ehestreit *m*, Partnerschaftskonflikt *m* / **mental ~** psychischer Konflikt *m* / **motivational ~** Motivationskonflikt *m* / **plus–minus ~** Konflikt *m* zwischen Tendenzen des Annäherns und Meidens / **plus–plus ~** Konflikt *m* zwischen Annäherungstendenzen / **positive–negative ~** Konflikt *m* zwischen Tendenzen des Annäherns und Meidens / **positive–positive ~** Konflikt *m* zwischen Annäherungstendenzen, Konflikt *m* zwischen Appetenztendenzen / **psychical ~** psychischer Konflikt *m* / **social ~** sozialer Konflikt *m* / **triangular ~** Dreieckskonflikt *m* / **unresolved ~** ungelöster Konflikt *m*

conflicting widerstreitend, widersprüchlich, entgegengesetzt

confluence Vereinigung *f*, Zusammenfluss *m* / **~ of aims** Zielverschmelzung *f*

confluent zusammenfließend

conform übereinstimmen, entsprechen, sich anpassen

conformability Gleichförmigkeit *f*, Übereinstimmung *f*, Konformität *f*

conformance Konformität *f*, Übereinstimmung *f* / **social ~** soziale Konformität *f*, konformes Sozialverhalten *n*

conforming konformistisch, konform

conformity Konformität *f*, Konformismus *m*, Gleichförmigkeit *f*, Anpassungsbereitschaft *f* / **~ behaviour** konformes Verhalten *n* / **~ index** Konformitätsindex *m* / **~ need** Konformitätsbedürfnis *n* / **~ pressure** Druck *m* zur Konformität / **~–proneness** Neigung *f* zur Konformität / **enforced ~** Gewissenszwang *m* / **social ~** soziale Konformität *f*

confound vermengen, vereiteln, verwechseln

confused verwirrt, verworren, zerfahren

confusedness Verwirrung *f*, Verwirrtheit *f*

confusion Verwirrung *f*, Verworrenheit *f*, Verwirrtheit *f*, Zerfahrenheit *f* / **~ control** Kontrolle *f* irrelevanter Variablen / **acoustic ~** akustische Verwirrung *f* / **acute hallucinatory ~** Amentia *f*, amentielles Syndrom *n* / **arteriosclerotic ~** arteriosklerotisches Delir *n* / **mental ~** geistige Verwirrung *f*, Verwirrtheit *f* / **psychogenic ~** psychogener Dämmerzustand *m*

confusional Verwirrungs–, Verwirrtheits–, verworren

congenial geistesverwandt, gleichartig

congeniality Geistesverwandschaft *f*

congenic, congenous verwandt, stammverwandt

congenital angeboren, ererbt

congeries Ansammlung *f*, Anhäufung *f*, Masse *f*

congregation Ansammlung *f*, Versammlung *f*

congress Tagung *f*, Kongress *m*, Zusammenkunft *f* / **sexual ~** Geschlechtsverkehr *m*, Beischlaf *m*, Koitus *m*

congruence, congruency, congruity Übereinstimmung *f*, Kongruenz *f* / **~ theory** Kongruenztheorie *f* / **cognitive ~** kognitive Kongruenz *f*

congruent kongruent, übereinstimmend

congruous innerlich zusammenhängend, folgerichtig

conjoint gemeinsam, verbunden

conjugal ehelich

conjugate paarweise, gepaart

conjugation Vereinigung *f*, Konjugation *f*

conjunction Verbindung *f*, Vereinigung *f*

conjunctiva Bindehaut *f*, Konjunktiva *f*

conjunctive verbindend, harmonisierend, konjunktiv

conjunctivity Konjunktivität *f*, Koordination *f* von Handeln und Denken

connate, connatal angeboren, konnatal

connect verbinden

connectedness logischer Zusammenhang *m*, Folgerichtigkeit *f*

connection Verbindung *f*, Verkettung *f*, Verknüpfung *f*, Zusammenhang *m* / ~ **reflex** Verbindungsreflex *m* / ~ **theory** Konnektionismus *m* / **corticothalamic** ~ kortikothalamische Bahn *f* / **cross** ~ Querverbindung *f* / **functional** ~ funktioneller Zusammenhang *m* / **social** ~ soziale Bindung *f* / **suprasegmental** ~**s** Binnenapparat *m*, Binnensystem *n*, Eigenapparat *m* / **temporal** ~ zeitweilige Verbindung *f*, bedingter Reflex *m*

connectionism Konnektionismus *m*

connective Verbindungs–, verbindend

connector, connecter Konnektor *m*, Verbindungselement *n*, Kontaktverbindung *f*

connexon Connexon *n*

conniption Erregung *f*, Wut *f* / ~ **fit** hysterischer Anfall *m*

connotation Bedeutung *f*, Konnotation *f*, Begriffsinhalt *m*

connotative konnotativ, mitbedeutend

connubial ehelich

consanguine, consanguineous blutsverwandt

consanguinity Blutsverwandtschaft *f*

conscience Gewissen *n* / **clear** ~ reines Gewissen *n* / **guilty** ~ schlechtes Gewissen *n*

conscientious gewissenhaft

conscientiousness Gewissenhaftigkeit *f*

conscious bewusst / Bewusstes *n* / **being** ~ Bewusstsein *n*

consciousness Bewusstsein *n*, Bewusstseinszustand *m* / ~ **disorder** Bewusstseinsstörung *f* / ~ **disturbance** Bewusstseinsstörung *f*, Bewusstseinstrübung *f* / ~ **of guilt** Schuldgefühl *n*, Schuldbewusstsein *n* / ~ **of kind** Gattungsbewusstsein *n* / ~ **raising group** bewusstseinserweiternde Gruppe *f*, Selbsterfahrungsgruppe *f* / ~ **of self** Selbstbewusstsein *n*, Ichbewusstsein *n* / ~ **state** Bewusstseinszustand *m* / ~ **of time** Zeitbewusstsein *n* / **approximative** ~ approximatives Bewusstsein *n* / **clouded** ~ getrübtes Bewusstsein *n* / **collective** ~ Kollektivbewusstsein *n*, Wir–Bewusstsein *n* / **cosmic** ~ kosmisches Bewusstsein *n* / **double** ~ doppeltes Bewusstsein *n* / **general** ~ Kollektivbewusstsein *n*, Gruppenbewusstsein *n* / **marginal** ~ Randbewusstsein *n* / **narrowed** ~ Bewusstseinseinengung *f*, eingeengtes Bewusstsein *n* / **objective** ~ Wirklichkeitsbewusstsein *n* / **restricted** ~ eingeengtes Bewusstsein *n* / **social** ~ Sozialbewusstsein *n* / **splitt–off** ~ abgespaltenes Bewusstsein *n* / **subliminal** ~ unterschwelliges Bewusstsein *n*

conselection Mitauslese *f*

consensual übereinstimmend, unwillkürlich, konsensuell

consensus Übereinstimmung *f* / ~ **of opinion** übereinstimmende Meinung *f*

consent zustimmen, einwilligen / Zustimmung *f*, Einwilligung *f* / **informed** ~ Einwilligung *f* (von Patienten oder Versuchspersonen)

consentience intuitive Übereinstimmung *f*, Einmütigkeit *f*

consequence Folge *f*, Folgerung *f*, Schluss *m*, Konsequenz *f*

conservation Erhaltung *f*, Behalten *n*, Beibehaltung *f*, Konservation *f*

conservatism Konservatismus *m*, Konservativismus *m* / **political–economic** ~ politisch–ökonomischer Konservatismus *m*

conservative konservativ / Konservativer *m*

consideration Berücksichtigung *f*, Rücksicht *f*, Beachtung *f* / ~**s of representability** Rücksicht *f* auf Darstellbarkeit

consistency Konsistenz *f*, Folgerichtigkeit *f*, innere Übereinstimmung *f*, Stimmigkeit *f*, Widerspruchsfreiheit *f* / ~ **coefficient** Konsistenzkoeffizient *m* / ~ **index** Konsistenzindex *m* / ~ **reaction** konsistente Reaktion *f* / **interitem** ~ Konsistenz *f*, innere Konsistenz *f* / **interitem** ~ **coefficient** Alpha–Koeffizient *m* / **internal** ~

innere Konsistenz *f* / **internal coefficient ~** Konsistenzkoeffizient *m*, Koeffizient *m* der inneren Konsistenz

consistent konsistent, folgerichtig

consolidation Konsolidierung *f*, Festigung *f* / **~ theory** Perseverationstheorie *f*

consonance Konsonanz *f*, Einklang *m*, Übereinstimmung *f* / **cognitive ~** kognitive Konsonanz *f*, kognitive Ubereinstimmung *f* / **ideational ~** Übereinstimmung *f* der Ideen

consonant Konsonant *m* / konsonant, zustimmend

consonantism Konsonantensystem *n*, Konsonantenabfolge *f*

constancy Konstanz *f*, Unveränderlichkeit *f*, Invarianz *f*, Beständigkeit *f* / **~ attitude** Konstanztheorie *f* / **~ of colour** Farbenkonstanz *f* / **~ of form** Formkonstanz *f* / **~ of Gestalt** Gestaltkonstanz *f*, Formkonstanz *f* / **~ hypothesis** Konstanzannahme *f* / **~ of the IQ** IQ–Konstanz *f* / **~ method** Konstanzverfahren *n* / **~ of movement** Bewegungskonstanz *f* / **~ of organism** Konstanz *f* des Organismus, Konstanz *f* des inneren Milieus, Homöostase *f* / **~ phenomenon** Konstanzphänomen *n* / **~ principle** Konstanzprinzip *n* / **~ of shape** Formkonstanz *f*, Gestaltkonstanz *f* / **~ of size** Größenkonstanz *f* / **~ of the species** Konstanz *f* der Arten / **~ of speed** Geschwindigkeitskonstanz *f* / **perceptual ~** Wahrnehmungskonstanz *f*

constant Konstante *f*, unveränderliche Größe *f* / konstant, unveränderlich, invariabel / **absolute ~** absolute Konstante *f* / **arbitrary ~** willkürlich gewählte Konstante *f* / **numerical ~** numerische Konstante *f*, absolute Konstante *f* / **statistical ~** statistische Konstante *f*

constellation Konstellation *f* / **~ theory** Konstellationstheorie *f*

constipation Verstopfung *f*, Obstipation *f*, Darmverstopfung *f*

constituent Bestandteil *m* / **immediate ~ analysis** Analyse *f* der unmittelbaren Konstituenten

constitution Konstitution *f*, Körperbau *m*, Habitus *m* / **~ of the body** Körperbau *m*, Körperkonstitution *f* / **~ of the ego** Ich–Struktur *f* / **~–specific** körperbauspezifisch, konstitutionsspezifisch / **athletic ~** athletischer Körperbau *m* / **emotional ~** emotionale Konstitution *f* / **hereditary ~** Erbkonstitution *f* / **lymphatic ~** lymphatische Konstitution *f*, Lymphatismus *m* / **physical ~** Körperbau *m*, Körperkonstitution *f* / **psychosexual ~** psychosexuelle Konstitution *f* / **strong ~** robuste Konstitution *f*

constitutional konstitutionell, in der Konstitution begründet, anlagebedingt, Konstitutions–

constrain zwingen, erzwingen

constraint Zwang *m*, Beschränkung *f*, Einschränkung *f*, Zurückhaltung *f* / **~ of movement** Zwangsbewegung *f*, motorischer Automatismus *m* / **material ~** materielle Beschränkung *f*, materielle Einschränkung *f* / **social ~s** soziale Zwänge *mpl*

constrict unterbinden, einengen

constriction Verengung *f*, Einengung *f*, Kontraktion *f*, Konstriktion *f*, eingeengte Spontaneität *f* / **bronchial ~** Bronchokonstriktion *f* / **whole ~** Gesamteinengung *f*

constrictor Schließmuskel *m*, Konstriktor *m*

construct Konstrukt *n*, Konstruktum *n*, hypothetische Vorstellung *f*, Begriff *m* / **~ validity** Konstruktvalidität *f*, theoretisch–logische Validität *f* / **constellatory ~** konstellatorisches Konstrukt *n* / **empirical ~** empirisches Konstrukt *n* / **hypothetical ~** hypothetisches Konstrukt *n* / **personal ~** persönliches Konstrukt *n* / **personal ~ theory** Theorie *f* der personellen Konstrukte, Persönlichkeitstheorie *f* / **pre–emptive ~** Ausschließlichkeitskonstrukt *n* / **preverbal ~** vorsprachliches Konstrukt *n* / **regnant ~** dominantes Konstrukt *n* / **symbolic ~** symbolisches Konstrukt *n*

construction Bau *m*, Aufbau *m*, Struktur *f*, Konstruktion *f* / **~ of the body** Körperbau *m* / **~ erg** Konstruktionsdrang *m* / **~ need** Konstruktionsdrang *m*, Organisationsbedürfnis *n* / **auxiliary ~** Hilfskonstruktion *f*, Hilfskonstrukt *n*

constructive konstruktiv, aufbauend, Konstruktions–

constructivism Konstruktivismus *m*

construe erklären, auslegen, deuten, konstruieren

consuetude Gewohnheit *f*, Brauch *m*

consuetudinary gewohnheitsmäßig, Gewohnheits–

consultant Berater *m* / **~ psychologist** beratender Psychologe *m* / **psychological ~** psychologischer Berater *m*

consultation Beratung *f*, Konsultation *f*, Konsilium *n* / **~ psychiatry** Konsiliarpsychiatrie *f* / **epistemic ~** intellektuelle Diskussion *f* / **professional ~** Fachberatung *f*, Beratung *f* durch Fachleute

consulting, consultative beratend, Beratungs–

consumer Verbraucher *m*, Konsument *m* / **~ acceptance** Kaufbereitschaft *f*, Aufnahmebereitschaft *f* / **~ advertising** Verbraucherwerbung *f*/ **~ attitude** Verbrauchereinstellung *f* / **~ behaviour** Verbraucherverhalten *n* / **~ demand** Verbrauchernachfrage *f* / **~ desire** Verbraucherwunsch *m* / **~ goods** Konsumgüter *npl*, Verbrauchsgüter *npl* / **~ goods advertising** Konsumwerbung *f* / **~ habits** Verbrauchergewohnheiten *fpl* / **~ inquiry** Verbraucherbefragung *f* / **~ interest** Verbraucherinteresse *n* / **~ market** Verbrauchermarkt *m* / **~ panel** Testgruppe *f* von Verbrauchern / **~ protection** Verbraucherschutz *m* / **~ psychology** Verbraucherpsychologie *f* / **~ research** Verbraucherforschung *f*, Erforschung *f* der Verbrauchergewohnheiten / **~ resistance** Kaufunlust *f* / **~ satisfaction** Verbraucherzufriedenheit *f* / **~ survey** Verbraucherbefragung *f*, Verbraucherumfrage *f*

consummate vollziehen, den Eheakt vollziehen

consummation Vollzug *m* / **~ of the sexual act** Vollzug *m* des Beischlafs

consummatory konsummatorisch, End–, Vollzugs–

consumption Verbrauch *m*, Konsum *m* / **~ pattern** Verbrauchsgewohnheiten *fpl*

contact Kontakt *m*, Beziehungsaufnahme *f*, Verbindung *f* / Kontakt aufnehmen, in Verbindung treten / **~ barrier** Kontaktsperre *f* / **~ behaviour** Kontaktverhalten *n* / **~ lenses** Kontaktlinsen *fpl* / **~ sensation** Berührungsempfindung *f* / **favouring social ~** kontaktfördernd / **making ~** Kontaktaufnahme *f*, Kontaktnahme *f* / **physical ~** Körperkontakt *m* / **primary ~** Primärkontakt *m*, persönlicher Kontakt *m* / **secondary ~** oberflächlicher Kontakt *m* / **social ~** sozialer Kontakt *m* / **visual ~** Schaukontakt *m*, Sichtkontakt *m*

contagion Ansteckung *f*, übertragbare Krankheit *f*, krankhafte Übertragung *f* durch Kontakt / **behavioural ~** Verhaltensansteckung *f*, Verhaltensübertragung *f* / **mental ~** psychische Ansteckung *f* / **psychic ~** psychische Ansteckung *f* / **social ~** Ausbreitung *f* einer Mode, Nachahmung *f*, Imitation *f*

contaminate kontaminieren, verunreinigen

contamination Kontamination *f*, Verschmelzung *f* von Wörtern und Sätzen, Verdichtung *f* / **~ of speech** Sprachkontamination *f*

contemplation Kontemplation *f*, beschauliche Betrachtung *f*

contemplative kontemplativ, beschaulich, tiefsinnig, nachdenklich

contemporaneity principle Gleichzeitigkeitspostulat *n*, Gleichzeitigkeitsprinzip *n*

content Inhalt *m* / **~ analysis** Inhaltsanalyse *f* / **~ of anxiety** Angstinhalt *m* / **~ of consciousness** Bewusstseinsinhalt *m* /

~ **factor** intrinsischer Faktor *m*, Faktor *m* der Bedürfnisbefriedigung / ~ **of an idea** Vorstellungsinhalt *m* / ~ **of perception** Wahrnehmungsinhalt *m* / ~ **psychology** Inhaltspsychologie *f* / ~ **response** inhaltliche Deutung *f* / ~ **subject** Lernfach *n* / ~ **validity** inhaltliche Gültigkeit *f* / ~ **word** Inhaltswort *n*, Begriffswort *n* / **conscious** ~ bewusster Inhalt *m*, Bewusstseinsinhalt *m* / **emotional** ~ emotionaler Inhalt *m* / **founded** ~ fundierter Inhalt *m* / **human** ~ menschliche Antwort *f* / **ideational** ~ Vorstellungsinhalt *m* / **intellectual** ~ geistiger Inhalt *m* / **latent** ~ latenter Inhalt *m* / **manifest** ~ manifester Inhalt *m*, erinnerter Trauminhalt *m* / **mental** ~ geistiger Inhalt *m*, Bewusstseinsinhalt *m* / **perceptual** ~ Wahrnehmungsinhalt *m* / **presentational** ~ Vorstellungsinhalt *m* / **representational** ~ Vorstellungsinhalt *m*

contest Wettstreit *m*, Wettkampf *m*, Kampf *m* / wetteifern, streiten, kandidieren

context Kontext *m*, Zusammenhang *m*, Umfeld *n* / ~ **of a construct** Konstruktelement *n*, Konstruktkontext *m* / ~ **factor** extrinsischer Faktor *m*, Hygienefaktor *m* / ~ **free** kontextfrei / ~ **theory** Kontexttheorie *f* / ~ **theory of meaning** Kontexttheorie *f* der Bedeutung

contextual aus dem Zusammenhang ersichtlich, dem Zusammenhang entsprechend, Kontext–

contiguity Kontiguität *f*, enge Aufeinanderfolge *f* / ~ **doctrine** Kontiguitätstheorie *f*, Kontakttheorie *f*, Neuronentheorie *f* / ~ **theory of learning** Kontiguitätsgesetz *n*, Kontiguitätstheorie *f* / **cognitive** ~ kognitive Kontiguität *f*

contiguous angrenzend, benachbart

continence geschlechtliche Enthaltsamkeit *f*, Keuschheit *f*, Mäßigung *f*

continent enthaltsam, mäßig, keusch

contingency Kontingenz *f* / ~ **coefficient** Kontingenzkoeffizient *m* / ~ **management** Kontingenzmanagement *n* / ~ **method** Kontingenzmethode *f*, Kontingenzmaß *n* / ~ **table** Kontingenztafel *f* / ~ **compound table** multivariate Kontingenztafel *f*

contingent abhängig von, bedingt

continuation Fortdauer *f*, Weiterführung *f*, Kontinuität *f* / ~ **school** Fortbildungsschule *f* / ~ **training** berufliche Fortbildung *f* / **good** ~ gute Aufeinanderfolge *f*

continuity Kontinuität *f*, Fortdauer *f* / ~ **doctrine** Kontinuitätstheorie *f*, Fibrillentheorie *f* / ~ **of care** Dauerpflege *f* / ~ **of germ plasm** Kontinuität *f* des Keimplasmas / ~ **theory of learning** Kontinuitätstheorie *f* des Lernens

continuous ununterbrochen, fortdauernd, kontinuierlich, Dauer–

continuum Kontinuum *n* / **polar** ~ bipolares Kontinuum *n*

contour Kontur *f*, Umriss *m*, Linie *f* / **isophonic** ~ Kurve *f* subjektiv gleicher Lautstärken

contraception Empfängnisverhütung *f*, Schwangerschaftsverhütung *f*, Kontrazeption *f*

contraceptive empfängnisverhütend, schwangerschaftsverhütend / empfangnisverhütendes Mittel *n*, Verhütungsmittel *n*, Kontrazeptivum / **oral** ~ orales Kontrazeptivum *n*, orales Empfängnisverhütungsmittel *n*, „Pille" *f*

contract Vertrag *m*, Kontrakt *m* / Vertrag abschließen, kontrahieren, zusammenziehen / ~ **of employment** Arbeitsvertrag *m* / ~ **for services** Dienstvertrag *m* / **social** ~ Gesellschaftsvertrag *m*

contractile, contractible kontraktil

contractility, contractibility Zusammenziehungsvermögen *n*, Kontraktibilität *f*

contraction Kontraktion *f*, Zusammenziehung *f* / ~ **of the field of vision** Gesichtsfeldeinschränkung *f*, Gesichtsfeldeinengung *f* / **afterloaded** ~ Unterstützungskontraktion *f* / **atrial** ~ Vorhofkontraktion *f* / **isometric** ~ isometrische Kontraktion *f* / **isotonic** ~ isotonische Kontraktion *f* / **muscular** ~ Muskelkontraktion *f* / **pha-**

sic ~ Kontraktion *f* in Phasen / **spastic** ~ Verkrampfung *f* / **tetanic** ~ Starrkrampf *m* / **tonic** ~ tonische Kontraktion *f*

contracture Kontraktur *f* / **hysterical** ~ hysterische Kontraktur *f*

contradiction Widerspruch *m*, Unvereinbarkeit *f*

contradictious widerspruchsvoll, widerstreitend

contralateral auf der gegenüberliegenden Seite, gegenüberliegend, kontralateral, gekreuzt

contrast Kontrast *m* / ~ **enhancement** Kontrastverschärfung *f* / ~ **error** Kontrastfehler *m* / ~ **flicker** Kontrastflimmern *n* / ~ **illusion** Kontrastillusion *f* / ~ **imitation** Kontrastimitation *f* / ~ **phenomenon** Kontrasterscheinung *f* / ~ **shadow** Kontrastschatten *m* / ~ **threshold** Kontrastschwelle *f* / **behavioural** ~ Verhaltenskontrast *m* / **chromatic** ~ Farbkontrast *m* / **double** ~ Doppelkontrast *m* / **marginal** ~ Randkontrast *m* / **simultaneous** ~ Simultankontrast *m*, gleichzeitiger Kontrast *m* / **spatial** ~ Raumkontrast *m* / **successive** ~ sukzessiver Kontrast *m* / **visual** ~ visueller Kontrast *m*

contrastimulant reizentgegengesetzt wirkend, reizbeseitigend, beruhigend / Beruhigungsmittel *n*

contrastimulism Behandlung *f* mit Gegenreizen, Reiztherapie *f*

contrastimulus Gegenreiz *m*

contrasuggestibility aktiver Negativismus *m*

contravention Übertretung *f*, Zuwiderhandlung *f*

contravolitional unfreiwillig, gegen den cigenen Willen

contrectation Berühren *n* [des Geschlechtspartners], Kontrektation *f*

contribution Beitrag *m*, Mitwirkung *f* / **professional** ~ Fachbeitrag *m*

control Kontrolle *f*, Regelung *f*, Beherrschung *f*, Prüfung *f*, Regler *m* / ~ **analysis** Kontrollanalyse *f* / ~ **animal** Kontrolltier *n* / ~ **centre** Reglationszentrum *n* / ~ **circuit** Regelkreis *m* / ~ **device** Regeleinrichtung *f*, Steuerglied *n* / ~ **of drive** Triebbeherrschung *f* / ~ **of excitation** Erregungskontrolle *f* / ~ **experiment** Kontrollversuch *m* / ~ **group** Kontrollgruppe *f* / ~ **input** Führungsgröße *f*, Kontrollgröße *f* / ~ **limits** Kontrollgrenzen *fpl* / ~ **pattern** Funktionsstruktur *f* / ~ **of respiration** Atmungskontrolle *f* / ~ **series** Kontrollreihe *f* / ~ **of stimulus** Reizkontrolle *f* / ~ **of substrata** Kontrolle *f* der Stichprobenquoten / ~ **test** Kontrollversuch *m*, Kontrolluntersuchung *f* / **aversive** ~ Verhaltenssteuerung *f* durch Vermeiden / **behavioural** ~ Verhaltenskontrolle *f* / **cognitive** ~ kognitive Kontrolle *f* / **cortical** ~ kortikale Kontrolle *f* / **coverant** ~ verdeckte operante Kontrolle *f* / **efferent** ~ efferente Kontrolle *f* / **emotional** ~ emotionale Kontrolle, Affektbeherrschung *f* / **experimental** ~ Versuchskontrolle *f* / **extrinsic** ~ Fremdkontrolle *f* / **humoral** ~ humorale Steuerung *f* / **hypnotic** ~ Hypnose–Kontrolle *f* / **motor** ~ Bewegungskontrolle *f* / **postural** ~ Haltungskontrolle *f* / **nervous** ~ nervöse Kontrolle *f*, Affektbeherrschung *f* / **neural** ~ Nervenregulation *f* / **oculo–motive** ~ Kontrolle *f* der Augenbewegung / **rigid** ~ strenge Kontrolle *f* / **scientific** ~ wissenschaftliche Kontrolle *f*, Versuchskontrolle *f* / **social** ~ soziale Kontrolle *f*, soziale Regulation *f* / **statistical** ~ statistische Kontrolle *f* / **voluntary** ~ freiwillige Kontrolle *f* / **yoked** ~ verbundene Kontrolle *f*

controlled kontrolliert, überwacht, beaufsichtigt

controller Regler *m*

contusion Prellung *f*, Kontusion *f* / ~ **of the brain** Hirnkontusion *f*, Hirnprellung *f* / **cerebral** ~ Hirnprellung *f*, Hirnkontusion *f*

convenience Bequemlichkeit *f*, Annehmlichkeit *f*, Angemessenheit *f* / **~ dream** Bequemlichkeitstraum *m*

convention Konvention *f*, Übereinkunft *f* / **social ~** gesellschaftliche Konvention *f*

conventionalism Konventionalismus *m*, Schablonenhaftigkeit *f*

conventionality Konventionalität *f*, Gewohnheit *f*, Schablonenhaftigkeit *f*

converge konvergieren, zusammenlaufen

convergence Konvergenz *f*, Zusammenlaufen *n*, Annäherung *f* / **~ theory** Konvergenztheorie *f*

convergent konvergent, konvergierend, zusammenlaufend

conversation Unterhaltung *f*, Gespräch *n*, Konversation *f*, Umgang *m*, Verkehr *m*, Geschlechtsverkehr *m* / **criminal ~** Ehebruch *m*, außerehelicher Geschlechtsverkehr

converse Umkehrung *f*

conversion Konversion *f*, Umwandlung *f*, Somatisierung *f* / **~ of affect** Affektumwandlung *f* / **~ disorder** Konversionsstörung *f* / **~ factor** Umrechnungsfaktor *m* / **~ hysteria** Konversionshysterie *f*, hysterische Reaktion *f* / **~ neurosis** Konversionsneurose *f* / **~ reaction** Konversionsreaktion *f* / **~ of scores** Umwandlung *f* von Rohwerten / **~ symptoms** Konversionssymptome *npl* / **~ table** Umrechnungstabelle *f*

converter Wandler *m*, Umformer *m*

convex konvex, auswärts gewölbt

conviction Überzeugung *f*, innere Gewissheit *f* / **criminal ~** Verurteilung *f* wegen einer Straftat, gerichtliche Verurteilung *f* / **strong ~** feste Überzeugung *f*

convince überzeugen

convolute, convoluted gewunden

convolution Windung *f*, Gyrus *m* / **central ~** Zentralwindung *f* / **cerebellar ~** Kleinhirnwindung *f* / **cerebral ~** Gehirnwindung *f* / **frontal ~** Stirnhirnwindung *f* / **inferior frontal ~** Broca–Windung *f* / **proximal ~** proximales Konvolut *n* / **temporal ~** Schläfenwindung *f*

convulsant krampfauslösendes Mittel *n*, krampferzeugend

convulsibility Krampfbereitschaft *f*

convulsion Krampf *m*, Zuckung *f*, Konvulsion *f* / **~ therapy** Schocktherapie *f*, Konvulsionstherapie *f* / **clonic ~** klonischer Krampf *m*, Klonus *m* / **continuous ~** Dauerkrampf *m* / **dissociative ~** dissoziativer Krampfanfall *m* / **epileptiform ~s** epileptiformer Krampfanfall *m* / **febrile ~** Fieberkrampf *m* / **infantile ~** Kinderkrampf *m* / **Jacksonian ~** Jackson–Epilepsie *f* / **lightening ~s** Blitzkrämpfe *mpl* / **terminal ~** Terminalkrampf *m* / **tetanic ~** Starrkrampf *m*

convulsive konvulsiv, krampfartig, krampfhaft

cookie Cookie *n*

cool Kälte *f*, Kühle *f* / **paradoxical ~** paradoxe Kälte *f*

cooperate zusammenarbeiten, mitarbeiten

cooperation Zusammenarbeit *f*, Zusammenwirken *n*, Mitarbeit *f*, Kooperation *f* / **antagonistic ~** feindselige Kooperation *f* / **intergroup ~** Zusammenarbeit *f* zwischen Gruppen / **social ~** soziale Kooperation *f*

cooperative zusammenarbeitend, mitwirkend, kooperativ

cooptation Kooptation *f*, Zuwahl *f* durch die Gruppe

coordinate koordiniert, beigeordnet / Koordinate *f*, Ordinate *f*/ koordinieren, in Ordnung bringen / **oblique ~s** schiefes Achsensystem *n* / **rectangular ~** rechtwinkliges Achsensystem *n*

coordination Koordination *f*, Übereinstimmung *f* / **~ of movements** Bewegungskoordination *f* / **developmental ~ disorder** entwicklungsbezogene Koordinationsstörung *f* / **hereditary ~** erbliche Übereinstimmung *f* / **impaired ~** Koordinationsstörung *f* / **innate hereditary ~**

angeborene Erbkoordination *f* / **motor ~** motorische Koordination *f*, Bewegungskoordination *f*, Bewegungssteuerung *f* / **normal muscular ~** normale Koordination *f* der Muskeln / **perceptual motor ~** sensumotorische Koordination *f* / **reciprocal ~** Koordination *f* entgegenwirkender Muskeln

coordinator Koordinator *m*

coorientation gemeinsame Ausrichtung *f*, gemeinsame Orientierung *f*

coping Bewältigung *f* / **~ behaviour** Copingverhalten *n* / **~ style** Bewältigungsstil *m* / **active ~** aktive Bewältigung *f* / **passive ~** passive Bewältigung *f*

coprolagnia Koprolagnie *f*, geschlechtliche Erregung *f* durch ekelerregende Vorgänge

coprolalia Koprolalie *f*, Reden *n* in obszönen Worten

coprophagia, coprophagy Koprophagie *f*, Kotessen *n*

coprophagous kotessend

coprophemia obszönes Reden *n*

coprophilia Koprophilie *f*, Interesse *n* an Fäkalien, Freude *f* an Fäkalien

coprophobia Koprophobie *f*, Kotangst *f*

coprophrasia Koprophrasie *f*, Sucht *f* beim Reden obszöne Ausdrücke zu gebrauchen

copula Bindeglied *n*, Ambozeptor *m*

copulate sich begatten, sich paaren, kopulieren

copulation Begattung *f*, Paarung *f*, Kopulation *f*

copulative, copulatory Begattungs–, kopulativ, Paarungs–

copy Nachahmung *f*, Imitation *f* / nachahmen, imitieren / **~ test** Wirkungsprüfung *f* einer Anzeige / **~ testing** Testen *n* von Werbung zur Vorausschätzung des Werbeerfolges / **~ theory** Doppelungstheorie *f*, Widerspiegelungstheorie *f*

cord Strang *m* / **~ block** Lumbalanästhesie *f* / **cranial spinal ~** Hirn–Rückenmark *n* / **lumbar spinal ~** Lendenmark *n* / **sacral spinal ~** Sakralmark *n* / **spinal ~** Rückenmark *n* / **thoracic spinal ~** Brust–Rückenmark–Strang *m* / **umbilical ~** Nabelschnur *f* / **ventral ~** Bauchmark *n*, Strickleiternervensystem *n* / **vocal ~s** Stimmbänder *npl*

core Kern *m* / **~ attributes** Kernmerkmale *npl* / **~ characteristics** Kerneigenschaften *fpl* / **~ course** Kernfach *n* / **~ culture** Kernkultur *f* / **~ curriculum** Hauptausbildung *f*, zentrale Studienfächer *npl* / **~ temperature** Körperkerntemperatur *f* / **~ tendency** zentrale Tendenz *f* / **magnetic–~ storage** Magnetkernspeicher *m*

corium Lederhaut *f*, Korium *n*

cornea Hornhaut *f*, Kornea *f*

corneal Hornhaut–

Cornell method Cornell–Methode *f*, Guttmans Methode *f* zur Feststellung der Skalierbarkeit

corneoretinal Korneoretinal–

cornu Horn *n*, Cornu *n* / **anterior ~** Vorderhorn *n* / **dorsal ~** Hinterhorn *n* / **lateral ~** Seitenhorn *n* / **occipital ~** Hinterhorn *n* / **posterior ~** Hinterhorn *n* / **ventral ~** Vorderhorn *n*

cornual hornförmig, Horn–

corollary Zusatz. *m*, Folgesatz *m*, natürliche Folge *f*

coronal Scheitel–, Stirn–

coronary Koronar–, Herzkranzgefäß—

corpora quadrigemina Corpora quadrigemina *npl*, Vierhügel *mpl*

corporal körperlich, leiblich, somatisch

corporeal körperlich, materiell

corpulence Korpulenz *f*, Fettleibigkeit *f*, Adipositas *f*

corpus Körper *m*, Corpus *n* / **~ callosum** Balken *m*, Corpus callosum *n* / **~ geniculatum** Kniehöcker *m* / **~ luteum** Gelbkörper *m*, Corpus luteum *n* / **~ luteum hormone** Gelbkörperhormon *n* / **~ striatum** Streifenhügel *m*, Corpus striatum *n*

corpuscle, corpuscule Körperchen *n*, Korpuskel *n* / **genital ~** Genitalkörperchen *n*, Wollustkörperchen *n* / **lamellated ~** Pacini–Körperchen *n*, Lamellenkörperchen *n* / **nuclear ~** Kernkörperchen *n* / **Pacinian ~s** Pacini–Körperchen *npl*, Vater–Pacini–Körperchen *npl*, Corpuscula lamellosa *npl* / **tactile ~** Tastkörperchen *n*, Meissner–Körperchen *n*

corpuscular korpuskulär, Korpuskel–

correct korrigieren, ausgleichen / richtig, korrekt, genau

correction Korrektur *f*, Verbesserung *f* / **~ for attenuation** Minderungskorrektur *f* / **~ for chance** Zufallskorrektur *f* / **~ for continuity** Kontinuitätskorrektur *f* / **~ for grouping** Eingruppierungskorrektur *f* / **~ for guessing** Schätzkorrektur *f* / **~ of imbalance** Wiederherstellen *n* des Gleichgewichts

correctional Besserungs–, Straf–

correctness Richtigkeit *f*, Korrektheit *f*

correlate korrelieren, in Wechselwirkung bringen, in Wechselbeziehung stehen / Korrelat *n* / **physical ~** körperliches Korrelat *n* / **physiological ~** physiologisches Korrelat *n* / **psychological ~** psychologische Entsprechung *f*, psychologisches Korrelat *n*

correlation Korrelation *f*, Wechselbeziehung *f*, Zusammenhang *m* / **~ centre** Korrelationszentrum *n* / **~ chart** Korrelationstabelle *f* / **~ cluster** Korrelationshäufung *f* / **~ coefficient** Korrelationskoeffizient *m* / **~ diagram** Korrelationsdiagramm *n*, Streudiagramm *n* / **~ graph** Korrelationsdiagramm *n*, Streudiagramm *n* / **~ hierarchy** Korrelationshierarchie *f* / **~ index** Korrelationsindex *m* / **~ matrix** Korrelationsmatrix *f* / **~ by ranks** Rangkorrelation *f* / **~ ratio** Korrelationsverhältnis *n*, Eta–Verhältnis *n* / **~ surface** Kovariationsdiagramm *n*, Streudiagramm *n* / **~ table** Korrelationstabelle *f* / **biserial ~** biseriale Korrelation *f*, Zweizeilenkorrelation *f* / **bivariate ~** bivariate Korrelation *f*, einfache Korrelation *f* / **curvilinear ~** kurvilineare Korrelation *f* / **direct ~** positive Korrelation *f*, direkte Korrelation *f* / **footrule ~** Spearmans R–Korrelation *f* / **illusory ~** Scheinkorrelation *f* / **indirect ~** negative Korrelation *f* / **interclass ~** Zwischenklassenkorrelation *f* / **interitem ~** Korrelation *f* zwischen Items / **intertrial ~** Korrelation *f* zwischen zwei Versuchsdurchgängen / **intraclass ~** Korrelation *f* innerhalb einer Klasse / **inverse ~** umgekehrte Korrelation *f*, negative Korrelation *f* / **inverted ~** umgekehrte Korrelation *f*, negative Korrelation *f* / **linear ~** lineare Korrelation *f* / **multiple ~** multiple Korrelation *f* / **negative ~** negative Korrelation *f* / **net ~** partielle Korrelation *f* / **neurological ~** neurologische Entsprechung *f* / **nonlinear ~** nicht–lineare Korrelation *f* / **partial ~** partielle Korrelation *f*, Teilkorrelation *f* / **Pearsonian ~** Pearson–Korrelation *f* / **perfect ~** perfekte Korrelation *f* / **phenotypic ~** phänotypische Korrelation *f* / **polychoric ~** polychorische Korrelation *f* / **positive ~** positive Korrelation *f* / **primary ~** primäre Korrelation *f* / **rectilinear ~** lineare Korrelation *f* / **secondary ~** sekundäre Korrelation *f* / **simple ~** einfache Korrelation *f*, bivariate Korrelation *f* / **spurious ~** Scheinkorrelation *f* / **statistical ~** statistische Korrelation *f* / **tetrachoric ~** tetrachorische Korrelation *f* / **total ~** Gesamtkorrelation *f* / **zero ~** Nullkorrelation *f*

correlative korrelativ, voneinander abhängig, in Wechselbeziehung stehend

correspondence Entsprechung *f*, Übereinstimmung *f*, Korrespondenz *f* / **~ course** Fernkurs *m*, Fernstudium *n* / **~ hypothesis** Korrespondenzhypothese *f* / **~ of outcomes** Übereinstimmung *f* der Ergebnisse / **~ theory** Korrespondenztheorie *f*

corresponding korrespondierend, entsprechend

corroboration Bekräftigung *f*, Bestätigung *f*

corrupt verführen, verleiten, bestechen

cortectomy Entfernung *f* der Hirnrinde

cortertia kortikale Wachheit *f*

cortex Cortex *m*, Kortex *m*, Rinde *f* / **~ of the brain** Großhirnrinde *f* / **~ cerebelli** Kleinhirnrinde *f* / **~ cerebri** Großhirnrinde *f* / **adrenal ~** Nebennierenrinde *f* / **adrenal ~ hormone** Nebennierenrindenhormon *n* / **auditory ~** Hörrinde *f*, akustischer Cortex *m* / **calcarine ~** Sehrinde *f* / **cerebellar ~** Kleinhirnrinde *f* / **cerebral ~** Großhirnrinde *f* / **contralateral ~** gegenüberliegende Rinde *f* / **extrinsic ~** extrinsischer Cortex *m* / **intrinsic ~** intrinsischer Cortex *m* / **motor ~** motorisches Rindenzentrum *n*, motorische Rindenregion *f*, motorisches Zentrum *n*, motorischer Kortex *m* / **olfactory ~** Riechhirn *n* / **orbitofrontal ~** orbitofrontaler Kortex *m* / **precentral ~** präzentraler Cortex *m* / **prefrontal ~** präfrontaler Kortex *m*, präfrontale Rinde *f* / **primary visual ~** primäre Sehrinde *f* / **renal ~** Nierenrinde *f* / **sensory ~** sensorisches Rindenfeld *n*, sensibles Rindenzentrum *n* / **sensory–motor ~** sensomotorisches Zentrum *n* / **somatosensory ~** Körperfühlsphäre *f*, sensible Rindenfelder *npl*, somatosensorischer Kortex *m* / **striate ~** primäre Sehrinde *f* / **suprarenal ~** Nebennierenrinde *f* / **visual ~** Sehrinde *f*, visueller Kortex *m*

Corti|'s arch Corti–Kanal *m* / **~'s fibers** Corti–Zellen *fpl* / **~'s ganglion** Hörsinneszelle *f*, Corti–Ganglion *n* / **~'s membrane** Corti–Membran *f* / **organ of ~** Corti–Organ *n* / **~'s rods** Corti–Pfeilerzellen *fpl* / **~'s tunnel** Corti–Kanal *m*

cortical kortikal, Rinden–, zur Rinde gehörig

corticalisation Kortikalisierung *f*, Rindentatigkeit *f*

corticoafferent kortikopetal, zur Hirnrinde hinführend

corticocerebral Hirnrinden–

corticofugal kortikofugal, von der Hirnrinde wegführend

corticoid Kortikoid *n*

corticopetal kortikopetal, zur Hirnrinde hinführend

corticospinal kortikospinal, Hirnrinde und Rückenmark betreffend

corticosteroid Kortikosteroid *n*

corticosterone Kortikosteron *n*, Kortikoid *n*

corticotrophic cortikotrop

corticotrophin, corticotropin Corticotropin *n*, ACTH *n* / **~ releasing factor** Corticoliberin *n* / **~ releasing hormone** Corticoliberin *n*

cortin Kortin *n*, Cortin *n*, Extrakt *m* der Nebennierenrinde

cortisol Cortisol *n*, Hydrocortison *n*

cortisone Cortison *n*, Kortison *n*

coruscation Funkensehen *n*, Lichtfleckensehen *n*, Flimmererscheinung *f*

corybantic tobend, rasend, wahnsinnig

corybantism Raserei *f*, Toben *n*, halluzinatorisches Delirium *n*

cosatiation doppelte Triebbefriedigung *f*

cosine Kosinus *m* / **~ law** Kosinusgesetz *n*

cosmogonic kosmogonisch, Weltentstehungs–

cosmogony Weltentstehung *f*, Kosmogonie *f*

cosmology Kosmologie *f*

cosmos Kosmos *m*, Weltordnung *f*

cost containment Kostendämpfung *f*

Cotard's syndrome Cotard–Syndrom *n*, Verneinungswahn *m*

cotherapy Mitbehandlung *f*, Kotherapie *f*

cotransmitter Kotransmitter *m*

cotwin eineiiger Zwilling *m* / **~ control method** Zwillingsforschung *f* / **~ method** Forschung *f* an eineiigen Zwillingen

coueism Couéismus *m*, Autosuggestion *f* nach Coué

Coué's treatment Coué–Heilweise *f*, Couéismus *m*

cough Husten *m* / **~ reflex** Hustenreflex *m* / **psychogenic ~** psychogener Husten *m*

counsel Beratung *f*, Ratschlag *m* / Rat geben, raten

counselee Klient *m*, Patient *m*, Ratsuchender *m*

counseling Beratung *f*, Beratungstherapie *f* / **~ interview** Beratungsgespräch *n* / **~ ladder** Beratungsstufen *fpl* / **~ psychologist** psychologischer Berater *m*, Beratungspsychologe *m*, Psychagoge *m* / **~ psychology** Beratungspsychologie *f* / **directive ~** direkte Beratung *f*, lenkende Beratung *f* / **educational ~** Erziehungsberatung *f*, Bildungsberatung *f* / **genetic ~** genetische Beratung *f* / **individual ~** Einzelberatung *f* / **nondirective ~** indirekte Beratung *f*, nicht–lenkende Beratung *f* / **pastoral ~** seelsorgerische Beratung *f* / **premarital ~** Beratung *f* vor der Ehe / **psychological ~** psychologische Beratung *f* / **psychotherapeutic ~** psychotherapeutische Beratung *f* / **semantic ~** semantische Erläuterung *f* / **therapeutic ~** Beratungstherapie *f* / **vocational ~** Berufsberatung *f*

counsellor, counselor Berater *m*, psychologischer Berater *m* / **~ attitude** Beratereinstellung *f* / **~ characteristics** Beratermerkmale *npl* / **~ client interaction** Interaktion *f* zwischen Berater und Ratsuchendem / **~ education** Beraterausbildung *f* / **~ effectiveness** Effizienz *f* des Beraters / **~ personality** Beraterpersönlichkeit *f* / **~ role** Beraterrolle *f* / **~ trainee** Berater *m* in Ausbildung / **educational ~** Erziehungsberater *m* / **psychological ~** beratender Psychologe *m*, Psychagoge *m* / **vocational ~** Berufsberater *m*

count Zählung *f*, Zahl *f*

counter Zähler *m*, Zählapparat *m* / entgegen, gegen / **~ ego** Gegenich *n* / **manual controlled ~** Handzähler *m*

counteract entgegenwirken, gegenwirken, neutralisieren

counteraction Gegenwirkung *f*, Widerstand *m* / **~ need** Oppositionsbedürfnis *n*

counteractive entgegenwirkend

counteragent Gegenmittel *n*

counterbalance Gegengewicht *n*, Ausgleich *m* / ausgleichen

counterbalancing Ausgleichen *n*, Kompensieren *n*, Neutralisation *f*

countercathexis Gegenbesetzung *f* / **external ~** äußere Gegenbesetzung *f*

countercharge Gegenbesetzung *f*

countercheck nochmalige Überprüfung *f*, Nachkontrolle *f*, Gegenprobe *f* / nochmals überprüfen, nachkontrollieren

countercompulsion Gegenzwang *m*

counterconditioning Gegenkonditionierung *f*

counterconformity Antikonformität *f*, Opposition *f* zur Gruppenmeinung

counterenquiry Gegenuntersuchung *f*

counterexperiment Gegenversuch *m*, Gegenexperiment *n*

counterfeit falsch, verstellt, erheuchelt / vorgeben, heucheln

counterformity ständige Negierung *f* der Gruppenmeinung, Antikonformität *f*, Kontraformität *f*

counteridentification Gegenidentifikation *f*

counterinvestment Gegenbesetzung *f*

counterirritation Ableitung *f*, Gegenreizung *f*

countermeasure Gegenmaßnahme *f*

counterpart Gegenstück *n*, Gegenwert *m*, Gegenleistung *f*

counterpoise Gegengewicht *n*, Gleichgewicht *n* / entgegenwirken, im Gleichgewicht halten, aufwiegen

counterposition Gegenposition *f*, Partnerposition *f*

counterpower Gegenmacht *f*

counterpressure Gegendruck *m*

counterprobability Gegenwahrscheinlichkeit *f*

counterpropaganda Gegenpropaganda *f*

counterregulation Gegenregulation *f*

countersuggestibility Negativismus *m*, Oppositionsverhalten *n*

countersuggestion Gegensuggestion *f*

countertransference Gegenübertragung *f*

countervaluation Gegenschätzung *f*, Gegenbewertung *f*, Gegengutachten *n*

counterweight Gegengewicht *n*

counterwill Gegenwille *m* / **hysterical ~** hysterischer Gegenwille *m*

counterwish dream Gegenwunschtraum *m*

couple Paar *n* / **~s therapy** Paartherapie *f*, Therapie *f* der Partnerbeziehung / **married ~** Ehepaar *n* / **unmarried ~** unverheiratetes Paar *n*

coupling Kopplung *f*, Paarung *f*, Begattung *f*

courage Mut *m*, Kühnheit *f*, Courage *f*

course Verlauf *m*, Ablauf *m*, Kursus *m* / **~ of action** Handlungsweise *f* / **~ evaluation** Unterrichtsevaluation *f*, Evaluation *f* von Lehrveranstaltungen / **~ of nature** natürlicher Verlauf *m* der Dinge / **~ objectives** Unterrichtsziele *npl* / **~ of reaction** Reaktionsverlauf *m* / **~ of thought** Gedankengang *m* / **dynamic ~** Verlaufsdynamik *f* / **longitudinal ~ specifiers (with and without full interepisode recovery)** Zusatzcodierung *f* des Langzeitverlaufs (mit und ohne Vollremission im Intervall)

court Gericht *n* / **~ referral** gerichtliche Behandlungsanordnung *f* / **juvenile ~** Jugendgericht *n*

courtship Freien *n*, Hofmachen *n*, Werben *n*, Balz *f* / **animal ~ behaviour** tierisches Balzverhalten *n* / **animal ~ display** tierisches Balzverhalten *n* / **human ~** Partnerwerbung *f*, Partnersuche *f*, Freien *n*

cousin Cousin *m*, Vetter *m*, Cousine *f*, Base *f*

couvade Couvade *f*, Männerkindbett *n*

covariance Kovarianz *f* / **~ analysis** Kovarianzanalyse *f* / **~ function** Kovarianzfunktion *f* / **~ matrix** Kovarianzmatrix *f* / **~ technique** Kovarianztechnik *f*

covariation Kovariation *f*, Korrelation *f*, Wechselbeziehung *f* / **~ chart** Kovariationstabelle *f* / **~ table** Kovariationstabelle *f*

coverant nicht beobachtbarer Operant *m*

cover memory Deckerinnerung *f*

covert verdeckt, verborgen, versteckt

covetousness Begierde *f*, heftiges Verlangen *n*, Habsucht *f*

coworker Mitarbeiter *m* / **least preferred ~** am wenigsten beliebter Mitarbeiter *m*

coy scheu, zurückhaltend, spröde

coyness Scheu *f*, Sprödigkeit *f*, Reserviertheit *f*, Koketterie *f*

crack Crack *n*

craft Fertigkeit *f*, Geschicklichkeit *f*, Beruf *m*, Handwerk *n* / **~ neurosis** Berufsneurose *f*, Berufskrämpfe *mpl*

cram einpauken, büffeln, mit Wissen vollstopfen

cramp Krampf *m*, Krampfanfall *m* / krampfen, sich verkrampfen / **clonic ~** klonischer Krampf *m* / **muscular ~** Muskelkrampf *m* / **occupational ~** Berufskrampf *m* / **professional ~** Berufskrampf *m* / **rotatory ~** Drehkrampf *m*

cramping Verkrampfung *f*, krampfhafte Zusammenziehung *f*

cramplike krampfartig

cranial Schädel–, kranial

craniograph Schädelmessinstrument *n*

craniography Schädelmessung *f*, Kraniographie *f*

craniology Schädellehre *f*, Kraniologie *f*

ceraniometer Schädelmessinstrument *n*, Schädelmesser *m*, Kraniometer *n*

craniometry Schädelmessung *f*, Kraniometrie *f*

craniopathy Schädelleiden *n*, Kopfleiden *n*

cranioscopy Untersuchung *f* des Schädels

craniotomy Trepanation *f*, Schädeloperation *f*

craniotopography Schädeltopographie *f*

cranium Schädel *m*, Schädeldecke *f*, Cranium *n*

crave dringend verlangen, begehren

craving heftiges Verlangen *n*, heiße Begierde *f*, Sucht *f*, Gier *f* / **segmental ~** organische Begierde *f*

crawling Kriechen *n*, Krabbeln *n*

craze Verrücktheit *f*, Manie *f*, Fimmel *m* / **~ for objectivity** Objektivitätsdrang *m*

crazy verrückt, geistesgestört, durcheinander

creatine phosphate Kreatinphosphat *n*

creatinine Kreatinin *n* / **~ coefficient** Kreatininkoeffizient *m*

creationism Theorie *f* vom Schöpfungsakt Gottes

creative kreativ, schöpferisch / Kreativer *m*, schöpferischer Mensch *m*

creativeness, creativity Kreativität *f*, schöpferisches Denken *n*, produktives Denken *n*, Originalität *f* / **~ measurement** Kreativitätsmessung *f* / **operational ~** Little–Technik *f*, Gordon–Technik *f*, angewandte Kreativität *f*

crèche Kinderkrippe *f*, Kleinkinderhort *m*

credibility Glaubwürdigkeit *f*

credible glaubwürdig

credit hour Stundengutschrift *f*

credulity, credulousness Leichtgläubigkeit *f*

credulous leichtgläubig

cremnophobia Kremnophobie *f*

creep, creeping Kriechen *n*

crepuscular Dämmerungs–, dämmrig

cresomania eingebildeter Reichtum *m* bei Größenwahn

Crespi effect Crespi–Effekt *m*, Kontrasteffekt *m*

crest Knochenleiste *f*, Kamm *m* / **neural ~** Neuralplatte *f*, Nervenplatte *f*

cretin Kretin *m*, Schwachsinniger *m*

cretinism Kretinismus *m*, Schwachsinn *m*, Idiotie *f*

cretinoid kretinoid

Creutzfeldt–Jacob disease Creutzfeldt–Jakob–Krankheit *f*

crib Kinderkrippe *f*, Kindertagesstätte *f* / **clinical ~** klinische Kindertagesstätte *f*

cri du chat syndrome Cri–du–chat–Syndrom *n*, Katzenschrei–Syndrom *n*

crime Verbrechen *n*, Straftat *f* / **~ passionel** kriminelle Affekthandlung *f* / **~ of violence** Gewaltverbrechen *n* / **~ prevention** Verbrechensverhütung *f* / **~ victim** Kriminalitätsopfer *n*, Verbrechensopfer *n* / **inciting to ~** zu Verbrechen aufhetzend

criminal kriminell, verbrecherisch / Verbrecher *m* / **female ~** Delinquentin *f*, Verbrecherin *f*, weibliche Kriminelle *f* / **habitual ~** Gewohnheitsverbrecher *m* / **male ~** Verbrecher *m*, Delinquent *m*, männlicher Krimineller *m* / **violent ~** Gewaltverbrecher *m*

criminality Kriminalität *f*

criminogenesis Verbrechensentstehung *f*

criminology Kriminologie *f*, Wissenschaft *f* von der Kriminalität / **psychiatric ~** Kriminalpsychopathologie *f*

cripple Krüppel *m*, Behinderter *m* / **mental ~** Geistesbehinderter *m*, geistig Behinderter *m*

crippled verkrüppelt, körperbehindert

crisis Krise *f* / **~ intervention** Krisenintervention *f* / **~ intervention service** Telefonseelsorge *f*, Erste–Hilfe–Station *f* für psychisch Kranke, Kriseninterventionsdienst *m* / **~ team** Krisenteam *n* / **adolescent ~** Reifungskrise *f*, Pubertätskrise *f* / **affective ~** affektive Krise *f* / **developmental ~** Entwicklungskrise *f* / **emotional ~** emotionale Krise *f* / **existential ~** Existenzkrise *f* / **organizational ~** Organisationskrise *f* / **puberal ~** Reifungskrise *f* / **therapeutic ~** therapeutische Krise *f*

crispation krampfhaftes Zusammenziehen *n*, Gänsehaut *f*

crista Crista *f*, Leiste *f*, Kamm *m*

criteriology Kriteriologie *f*

criterion, criterium Kriterium *n*, Merkmal *n*, Kennzeichen *n* / ~ **analysis** Kriterienanalyse *f* / ~ **behaviour** Standardverhalten *n* / ~ **contamination** Verschmelzung *f* von Kriterium und Messvariablen / ~ **of exclusion** Ausschlusskriterium *n* / ~**–frame** Kriteriumtest *m* / ~ **group** Kriteriengruppe *f* / ~ **of inclusion** Einschlusskriterium *n* / ~ **measure** Standardmaß *n*, Standardwert *m* / ~**–oriented validity** empirische Validität *f*, kriteriumsbezogene Validität *f* / ~ **overlap** Kriterienüberlappung *f* / ~**–related validity** empirische Validität *f*, kriteriumsbezogene Validität *f* / ~ **programming** Standardprogrammierung *f* / ~**–referenced test** kriteriumsorientierter Test *m* / ~ **score** Standardwert *m* / ~ **variable** Kriteriumsvariable *f*, abhängige Variable *f*

critical kritisch, entscheidend

criticism kritisches Beurteilen *n*, Kritik *f* / **constructive** ~ konstruktive Kritik *f* / **professional** ~ berufliche Kritik *f* / **professional** ~ **reply** Replik *f* zu einer Fachkritik

critique Kritik *f*

Crohn's disease Crohn–Krankheit *f*, Morbus Crohn *m*

cross quer, kreuzweise, diagonal / kreuzen / ~**–adaptation** Anpassungsgeneralisierung *f* / ~**–breed** Mischrasse *f*, Mischling *m* / ~**–checking** Gegenprobe *f*, Kontrollüberprüfung *f* / ~**–check questioning** Kontrollbefragung *f* / ~**–classification** sich überschneidende Klassifikation *f* / ~**–classification table** Kontingenztafel *f* / ~**–comparison** Kreuzvergleich *m* / ~**–conditioning** Zufallskonditionierung *f* / ~**–correlation** Kreuzkorrelation *f* / ~**–correspondence** sich ergänzende mediale Mitteilungen *fpl* / ~**–cultural** interkulturell / ~**–culture test** kulturfreier Test *m* / ~**–education** Lernübertragung *f* / ~**–out test** Durchstreichtest *m* / ~**–over** Faktorenaustausch *m* / ~**–parent identification** Identifikation *f* mit dem gegengeschlechtlichen Elternteil / ~ **posting** gleichzeitiges Verschicken *n* von Artikeln in mehrere Newsgroups, Crossposten *n* / ~**–section** Querschnitt *m* / ~**–section study** Querschnittuntersuchung *f* / ~**–stroke** Querstrich *m* / ~**–training** Lernübertragung *f*, Doppelausbildung *f* / ~**–transfer** Lernübertragung *f* auf die ungeübte Körperhälfte / ~**–validation** Kreuzvalidierung *f* / ~**–way** Kreuzung *f*, Nervenkreuzung *f*

crossing Kreuzung *f*, Bahnkreuzung *f* / ~ **over** Faktorenaustausch *m*, Überkreuzung *f*

Crouzon's| disease Crouzon–Krankheit *f* / ~ **craniofacial dysostosis** Dystonia craniofacialis *f*, komplexer Turmschädel *m* / ~ **syndrome** Crouzon–Syndrom *n*

crowd Menge *f*, Masse *f*, Ansammlung *f* / ~ **behaviour** Massenverhalten *n* / ~ **mind** Kollektivseele *f*, Massengeist *m* / ~ **psychology** Massenpsychologie *f*, Kollektivpsychologie *f* / **acting** ~ Aktionsgruppe *f* / **casual** ~ zufällige Ansammlung *f*

crowding Überbevölkerung *f*

crucial entscheidend, kritisch

crude roh, unfertig

cruel grausam, hart, gemein

cruelty Grausamkeit *f* / ~ **to children** Kindesmisshandlung *f* / **mental** ~ seelische Grausamkeit *f*

crura Schenkel *mpl*, Stiele *mpl* / ~ **cerebelli** Kleinhirnstiele *mpl* / ~ **cerebri** Großhirnstiele *mpl* / ~ **of the cerebrum** Großhirnstiele *mpl*

crush plötzliche intensive Zuneigung *f*, Verliebtheit *f*, Flirt *m*

crushing Quetschen *n*, Quetschung *f* / ~ **of a nerve** Nervenquetschung *f* / ~ **of the skull** Schädelzertrümmerung *f*

crustacea Krustentiere *npl*, Krustazeen *fpl*

crux Schwierigkeit *f*, kritischer Punkt *m*

cry schreien / Schrei *m* / **epileptic** ~ epileptischer Schrei *m*

cryaesthesia, cryesthesia Kälteüberempfindlichkeit *f*, übermäßige Empfindlichkeit *f* gegenüber Kälte, Kryästhesie *f*

cryanaesthesia, cryanesthesia Unempfindlichkeit *f* gegenüber Kälte, Verlust *m* des Kältegefühls, Kryanästhesie *f*

crying Weinen *n* / **~ cat syndrome** Katzenschrei–Syndrom *n*, Cri du chat–Syndrom *n*

crymotherapy, cryotherapy Kältetherapie *f*, Frigotherapie *f*, Kryotherapie *f*

cryptaesthesia, cryptesthesia Kryptästhesie *f*, Wahrnehmen *n* kaum wahrnehmbarer Eindrücke, Fähigkeit *f* außersinnlicher Wahrnehmung

cryptic verborgen, okkult, kryptisch

cryptogenetic, cryptogenic unbekannten Ursprungs, aus unbekannter Ursache, kryptogenetisch

cryptography Kryptographie *f*, Geheimschrift *f*

cryptomnesia Kryptomnesie *f*, subliminale Erinnerungen *fpl*, unter der Bewusstseinsschwelle liegende Erinnerungen *fpl*

cryptorchidism, cryptorchism Kryptorchismus *m*, Hodenretention *f*

crystal Kristall *n* / **~–gazing** Kristallsehen *n*, Zukunftsdeuten *n* / **~ lens** Kristalllinse *f* / **~ vision** Kristallsehen *n*, Kristallvision *f*

crystallophobia Glasangst *f*, Kristallophobie *f*

C scale C–Skala *f*

cube test Würfeltest *m*

cubital Ellbogen–, kubital

cue Signal *n*, Zeichen *n*, Hinweis *m*, Auslösereiz *m*, Hinweisreiz *m*, Anzeichen *n*, Anhaltspunkt *m* / **~ function** Signalfunktion *f* / **~ pattern** Anregungsmuster *n*, Hinweisreiz *m* / **~–producing response** reizerzeugende Reaktion *f* / **~ recognition** Signalerkennung *f* / **~ reduction** Reduktion *f* des Auslösereizes / **~ reversal** Signalumkehr *f* / **~ utilization** Gebrauch *m* von Signalreizen / **incidental ~** zufälliger Hinweis *m*, zufälliges Signal *n* / **minimal ~** Minimalreiz *m* / **probabilistic ~ learning** Lernen *n* von Hinweisreizen mit unterschiedlichen Reaktionswahrscheinlichkeiten / **sensory ~** sensorisches Signal *n*, sensorischer Bezugspunkt *m*

Cuignet's method Cuignet–Methode *f*, Cuignet–Verfahren *n*, Skiaskopie *f*, Keratoskopie *f*, Schattenprobe *f*

cul–de–sac Sackgasse *f*

Culler's phi process Phi–Funktion *f* von Gamma

culmination Höhepunkt *m*, Kulmination *f* / **~ time** Gipfelzeit *f*

culpability Schuld *f*, Strafbarkeit *f*, Straffälligkeit *f*

cult Kult *m*, Verehrung *f*

cultic, cultual kultisch, Kult–

cultism kultische Verehrung *f*, Kultbegeisterung *f*, Götterverehrung *f*

cultivated gebildet, kultiviert

cultural kulturell, Kultur–

culture Kultur *f*, Zivilisation *f* / **~ area** Kulturkreis *m* / **~ change** Kulturwandel *m*, Kulturveränderung *f* / **~ complex** Kultur *f*, Kultureinheit *f*, kulturelles Wertsystem *n* / **~ conflict** Kulturkonflikt *m* / **~–epoch theory** Kulturzyklentheorie *f* / **~–fair** kulturneutral, sprachfrei, kulturunabhängig / **~–free** kulturunabhängig, sprachfrei / **~–free test** kulturunabhängiger Test *m* / **~ hero** Volksheld *m*, Nationalheiliger *m* / **~ lag** partielle Kulturrückständigkeit *f* / **~ pattern** Kulturnorm *f*, kulturelles Wertsystem *n*, Kulturgefüge *n* / **~ shock** Kulturschock *m* / **~ trait** Kulturmerkmal *n*, Kultureigenschaft *f*, Kulturelement *n* / **adolescent ~** Kultur *f* der Jugendlichen / **explicit ~** sichtbare Kulturgewohnheiten *npl* / **formal ~** formelle Disziplin *f* / **implicit ~** implizite Kulturgewohnheiten *fpl*, kulturelle Selbstverständlichkeiten *fpl* / **personal ~** persönlicher Stil *m*, persönliche Kultur *f*

culturology Kulturwissenschaft *f*

cultus Kult *m*

cumulation Kumulation *f*, Summierung *f*, Anhäufung *f*, Häufung *f* / **~ effect** Kumulationseffekt *m*, kumulative Wirkung *f*, verstärkteWirkung *f*, Summierung *f* der Wirkung

cumulative kumulativ, Kumulations–

cuneus Cuneus *m*, Keil *m* an der Großhirnhemisphäre

cunnilinctus, cunnilinction, cunnilingus Cunnilingus *m*

cunnilinguist den Cunnilingus Ausübender *m*

cunnus Cunnus *m*, weibliche Scheide *f*

cupula Cupula *f*, Kuppel *f*

curare Kurare *n*, Pfeilgift *n*

curarization Kurarisierung *f*

curative, curable heilbar, Heil–

cure Kur *f*, Behandlung *f* / heilen / **sleeping ~** Schlafkur *f* / **spontaneous ~** Spontanheilung *f* / **talking ~** Redekur *f*

curiosity Neugierde *f*, Neugier *f* / **~ drive** Neugiertrieb *m*, Erkundungstrieb *m* / **~ motive** Neugiertrieb *m* / **~ need** Wissbegierde *f* / **infantile ~** kindliche Neugier *f*

current Strom *m* / gegenwärtig, laufend, augenblicklich / **~ of injury** Verletzungsstrom *m* / **~ of rest** Ruhestrom *m* / **alternating ~** Wechselstrom *m* / **anodal ~** Anodenstrom *m* / **direct ~** Gleichstrom *m* / **exciting ~** Erregerstrom *m* / **galvanic ~** galvanischer Strom *m* / **gating ~** Torstrom *m* / **inward ~** Einwärtsstrom *m* / **neural ~** Nervenstrom *m*, Nervenimpuls *m* / **outward ~** Auswärtsstrom *m*

curricular Lehrplan–, kurrikular

curriculum Lehrplan *m*, Ausbildungsgang *m*, Studienweg *m*, Curriculum *n* / **~–based asessment** lehrzielorientierte Diagnostik *f* / **~ development** Lehrplanentwicklung *f*, Curriculumentwicklung *f*

cursive Kursiv–

cursory hastig, flüchtig, oberflächlich

curvature illusion Krümmungstäuschung

curve Kurve *f* / **~ of error** Fehlerkurve *f*, Normalverteilungskurve *f* / **~ fitting** Kurvenglättung *f* / **~ of forgetting** Vergessenskurve *f* / **~ of learning** Lernkurve *f* / **~ of means** Regressionskurve *f* / **~ of normal error** Normalverteilungskurve *f* / **~ of rest** Ruhekurve *f* / **~ smoothing** Kurvenglättung *f* / **abnormal ~** anomale Verteilung *f* / **accelerated ~** beschleunigte Kurve *f* / **ascending ~** ansteigende Kurve *f* / **bell–shaped ~** Glockenkurve *f*, Normalkurve *f* / **bimodal ~** zweigipflige Häufigkeitskurve *f*, zweigipflige Verteilungskurve *f* / **binomial ~** Binomialverteilung *f* / **characteristic ~** Kennlinie *f* / **composite ~** zusammengesetzte Kurve *f* / **corrected ~** ausgeglichene Kurve *f* / **descending ~** abfallende Kurve *f* / **dextrorse ~** rechtsschiefe Kurve *f* / **exponential ~** Exponentialkurve *f* / **Gaussian ~** Gauß'sche Kurve *f* / **Laplacian ~** Laplace–Kurve *f*, Kurve *f* der Normalverteilung / **logarithmic ~** logarithmische Kurve *f* / **logistic ~** logistische Kurve *f* / **normal ~** Normalkurve *f* / **normal ~ of distribution** Normalverteilungskurve *f* / **ogival ~** Ogive *f*, kumulative Häufigkeitskurve *f* / **percentile ~** Prozentrangkurve *f*, Prozentkurve *f* / **polar ~** Kurve *f* im Koordinationssystem / **reversed J shaped ~** umgekehrte J–Kurve *f* / **sigmoid ~** S–förmige Kurve *f* / **sinistrorse ~** linksschiefe Kurve *f* / **smooth ~** glatte Kurve *f* / **smoothed ~** geglättete Kurve *f* / **symmetrical ~** symmetrische Kurve *f* / **U–shaped ~** U–Kurve *f*

curved kurvig, gekrümmt, gebogen

curvilinear kurvilinear

Cushing's syndrome Cushing–Krankheit *f*, Cushing–Syndrom *n*

custodial den Schutz betreffend, Bewachungs–

custody Sorgerecht *n*, Bewachung *f*, Haft *f* / **joint ~** gemeinsames Sorgerecht *n*

custom Brauch *m*, Gewohnheit *f*, Sitte *f* / **social ~** sozialer Brauch *m*, soziale Norm *f*

cut schneiden, abschneiden / Schnitt *m* / **~–off whole response** technische G–Antwort *f* / **~–tail error** Fehler *m* durch Weglassen der Extremfälle

cutaneous kutan, Haut–

cutis Haut *f*, Cutis *f* / **~ anserina** Gänsehaut *f*

cyan blaugrün

cyanic blau

cyanopia, cyanopsia Blausichtigkeit *f*, Blausehen *n*, Zyanopsie *f*

cyanosis Zyanose *f*, Blausucht *f*

cybernetic kybernetisch

cyberneticist Kybernetiker *m*

cybernetics Kybernetik *f*, Lehre *f* von den Steuerungs– und Regelungsmechanismen

cyberspace Cyberspace *m*, künstliche dreidimensionale Computerwelt *f*

cycle Zyklus *m*, Periode *f*, Schwingung *f* / **~s per second** Schwingungen *fpl* pro Sekunde / **lunar synodic ~** Mondmonat *m*, Mondzyklus *m* / **manic–depressive ~** manisch–depressiver Zyklus *m* / **menstrual ~** Menstruationszyklus *m* / **oestrous ~** Brunstzeit *f*, Brunstperiode *f* / **visual ~** sichtbare Schwingung *f*

cycler, rapid Rapidzykler *m*

cyclofusional die Verschmelzung binokularer Netzhautbilder betreffend

cyclogram Sehfeldkurve *f*, Zyklogramm *n*

cycloheximide Cycloheximid *n*

cycloid zykloid / Zykloider *m*

cyclonopathy Wetterfühligkeit *f* bei anrückendem Tiefdruckgebiet

cyclopathia zirkuläre Neuropathie *f*

cyclopean einäugig, Zyklopen–

cyclophrenia Zyklophrenie *f*, manisch–depressive Psychose *f*

cycloplegia Zykloplegie *f*, Akkommodationslähmung *f*

cyclopropane Zyklopropan *n*

cyclorama Rund–Panorama *n*

cycloscope Sehfeldmesser *m*

cyclothyme, cyclothymiac Zyklothyme *m,f*

cyclothymia Zyklothymie *f*, zyklothyme Störung *f*

cyclothymic zyklothym

cylinder Zylinder *m*, Zylinderglas *n*

cylindric, cylindrical zylindrisch, zylinderförmig

cylindriform zylinderförmig

cymbocephalic, cymbocephalous kahnschädelig, mit kahnförmigem Schädel

cymbocephaly Kahnschädel *m*

cynanthropy Kynanthropie *f*, Vorstellung *f* ein Hund zu sein

cynic zynisch / Zyniker *m*

cynical zynisch

cynicism Zynismus *m*

cynophobia Angst *f* vor Hunden, Kynophobie *f*

cynorexia Heißhunger *m*, Wolfshunger *m*, Kynorexie *f*

cypridophobia Angst *f* vor Geschlechtskrankheiten, Kypridophobie *f*

cyproterone Cyproteron *n*

cysteine Cystein *n*

cytoarchitecture Zellaufbau *m*, Zellarchitektur *f*

cytobiology Zellbiologie *f*

cytochrome oxidase Zytochrom–Oxydase, Warburg–Atmungsferment *n*

cytode Zytode *f*, kernlose Protoplasmamasse *f*

cytogenesis, cytogeny Zellbildungf, Zellentwicklung *f*, Zytogenese *f*

cytogenetic, cytogenic zellbildend, zytogenetisch

cytokine Zytokin *n*

cytologic, cytological zytologisch

cytology Zytologie *f*, Lehre *f* von den Zellen, Zellkunde *f*

cyton, cytone Zelle *f*, Nervenzelle *f*

cytophysiological zellphysiologisch

cytophysiology Zellphysiologie *f*

cytoplasm Zellplasma *n*, Protoplasma *n*, Zytoplasma *n*

cytosine Cytosin *n*, Zytosin *n*

cytoskeleton Zytoskelett *n*

cytosol Zytosol *n*

cytotropism Zytotropismus *m*, Anziehungskraft *f* der Zelle

D

Da Costa's syndrome Da Costa Syndrom *n*, Effortsyndrom *n*, Herzangstsyndrom *n*, Hyperventilationssyndrom *n*

dacrygelosis Dakryogelosis *f*

dacryogenic tränenerzeugend, den Tränenfluß anregend

dactylogram Fingerabdruck *m*, Daktylogramm *n*

dactylography Fingerabdruckverfahren *n*, Daktyloskopie *f*

dactylology Fingersprache *f*, Zeichensprache *f*

dactylomegaly abnorm große Finger *mpl*, Daktylomegalie *f*

dactylonomy Daktylonomie *f*, Rechnen *n* durch Abzählen der Finger

dactylophasia Taubstummensprache *f*, Zeichensprache *f*, Daktylophasie *f*

dactyloscopy Fingerabdruckverfahren *n*, Daktyloskopie *f*

dactylotremometer Daktylotremometer *n*, Apparat *m* zur Messung von Zitterbewegungen der Finger

daedaleum Daedaleum *n*, Wundertrommel *f*, einfache, stroboskopische Vorrichtung *f*

Dalton's law Dalton–Gesetz *n*

daltonism Daltonismus *m*, Farbenblindheit *f*, Rot–Grünblindheit *f*

damage Schaden *m*, Schädigung *f* / **genetic ~** Erbschaden *m* / **irreversible ~** irreversible Schädigung *f*

damming up of the libido Libidostauung *f*

damping Abklingen *n*, Dämpfung *f* / **acoustical ~** Schalldämpfung *f*

dance Tanz *m* / **~ therapy** Tanztherapie *f*

danger Gefahr *f* / **~ of addiction** Gewöhnungsgefahr *f* / **~ to the public** Gemeingefährlichkeit *f*

dangerous gefährlich, gefahrvoll

dangerousness Gefährlichkeit *f*

dark–adapted ans Dunkel angepasst, adaptiert

dark–adaptation Dunkeladaptation *f*

darkfield illumination Dunkelfeldbeleuchtung *f*

darkness Dunkelheit *f* / **~ adaptation** Dunkeladaptation *f* / **~ response** Helldunkel–Antwort *f*

darwinian darwinisch

Darwinism, Darwinianism Darwinismus *m*, Darwin'sche Lehre *f* / **social ~** Sozialdarwinismus *m*

darwinist Darwinist *m*, Anhänger *m* der Darwin'schen Lehre

data Daten *npl*, Ergebnisse *npl*, Zahlenmaterial *n* / **~ bank** Datenbank *f* / **~ carrier** Datenträger *m* / **~ collection** Datensammlung *f* / **~ field** Datenfeld *n* / **~ language** Datensprache *f* / **~ matrix** Datenmatrix *f* / **~ processing** Datenverarbeitung *f*, Informationsverarbeitung *f* / **~ processor** Datenverarbeitungsmaschine *f* / **~ set** Datensammlung *f* / **~ theory** Datentheorie *f* / **~ transmission interface** Datenübertragungsschnittstelle *f*, Schnittstelle *f* / **basic ~** Rohergebnisse *npl* / **biographical ~** biographische Angaben *fpl* / **clinical ~** klinische Daten *npl*, Krankheitsbild *n* / **continuous ~** kontinuierliche Daten *npl* / **digital ~** digitale Daten *npl* / **discrete ~** diskrete Daten *npl*, diskontinuierliche Daten *npl* / **electronic ~ processing** elektronische Datenverarbeitung *f* / **experimental ~** Versuchsergebnisse *npl* / **given ~** Gegebenheiten *fpl* / **mechanical ~ processing equipment** mechanische Datenverarbeitungsanlage *f* / **personal ~** persönliche Daten *npl*, biographische Daten *npl* / **personal ~ sheet** Personalbogen *m* / **primary ~** Rohdaten *npl*, Rohwerte *mpl*, ursprüngliche Daten *npl* / **qualitative ~** qualitative Daten *npl* / **quantitative ~** quantitative Daten *npl* / **raw ~** Rohdaten *npl*, Rohwerte *mpl*, Rohergebnisse *npl* / **sensory ~** Sinnesdaten *npl*, Sinnesempfindung *f* / **statistical ~** statistische Daten *pl* / **subjective ~** subjektive Daten *npl*

database Datenbank *f* / **~ language** Datenbanksprache *f*

date Verabredung *f*

dating Verabredung *f*, Rendezvous *n*, Dating *n* / **social ~** geselliges Treffen *n*, gesellschaftliche Kontakte *mpl*

dawdler Trödler *m*, Bummelant *m*

dawdling Trödeln *n*, Bummeln *n*

day Tag *m* / **~ care centre** Tagespflegestätte *f*, Tagesstätte *f* / **~-blindness** Tagblindheit *f*, Nachtsichtigkeit *f* / **~ hospital** Tagesklinik *f* / **~-nursery** Kindertagesstätte *f* / **~ residues** Tagesreste *mpl* / **~ school** Tagesschule *f*, Ganztagsschule *f* / **~ terrors** Pavor diurnus *m*, Tagangst *f* / **~ unit** Tagesklinik *f*

daydream Tagtraum *m*, Wachtraum *m*

daydreamer Tagträumer *m*, Phantast *m*

daydreaming Tagträumerei *f*, Tagträumen *n*

daylight vision Tagessehen *n*, photopisches Sehen *n*

daymare innere Qual *f*, intensive Beklemmung *f*

dazzle blenden / Blendung *f*

deactivation Aktivitätsverlust *m*, Inaktivierung *f*

deaf taub / Taube *m,f* / **~ and dumb** taubstumm / **~-and-dumbness** Taubstummheit *f* / **~ blind** taubblind / Taubblinde *m,f* / **~-mute** taubstumm / Taubstummer *m* / **~-muteness** Taubstummheit *f* / **~-mutism** Taubstummheit *f*, Hörstummheit *f*

deafferentation Deafferentierung *f*, Ausschalten *n* afferenter Nerven

deafness Taubheit *f*, Schwerhörigkeit *f* / **adventitious ~** erworbene Schwerhörigkeit *f* / **cerebral ~** zentral bedingte Taubheit *f* / **conductive ~** Mittelohrschwerhörigkeit *f* / **congenital ~** angeborene Taubheit *f* / **cortical ~** Rindentaubheit *f* / **functional ~** funktionelle Taubheit *f* / **hysterical ~** hysterische Taubheit *f* / **mental ~** Seelentaubheit *f* / **middle ear ~** Mittelohrschwerhörigkeit *f* / **nervous ~** nervöse Schwerhörigkeit *f* / **organic ~** organische Schwerhörigkeit *f* / **progressive ~** fortschreitende Schwerhörigkeit *f* / **psychic ~** Seelentaubheit *f* / **psychogenic ~** psychogene Taubheit *f* / **sensory ~** Seelentaubheit *f* / **total ~** völlige Taubheit *f*

deal Geschäft *n*, Rauschgiftgeschäft *n* / **~er** Rauschgifthändler *m*, Dealer *m*

death Tod *m* / **~ and dying** Tod *m* und Sterben *n* / **~ anxiety** Todesangst *f* / **~ attitude** Einstellung *f* zum Tod / **~ education** Sterbevorbereitung *f* / **~ feigning** Totstellen *n*, Vortauschen *n* des Todes / **~ feint** simulierter Tod *m* / **~ instinct** Todestrieb *m*, Thanatostrieb *m* / **~ penalty** Todesstrafe *f* / **~ rate** Sterberate *f*, Sterblichkeitsziffer *f* / **~ rites** Todesriten *mpl* / **~ trance** Scheintod *m* / **apparent ~** Scheintod *m* / **near ~ experience** todesnahe Erfahrung *f* / **somatic ~** biologischer Tod *m* / **violent ~** gewaltsamer Tod *m* / **voluntary ~** Freitod *m*

debate Diskussion *f*, Debatte *f* / **internal ~** interne Diskussion *f*

debauch Wollust *f*, Ausschweifung *f*

debility Debilität *f*, Schwachsinn *m* / **~ of mobility** motorische Schwäche *f*, motorische Debilität *f* / **emotional ~** emotionale Debilität *f* / **moral ~** moralischer Schwachsinn *m*, moralische Unzurechnungsfähigkeit *f* / **neurotic regressive ~** Regression *f*

debriefing, experimental nachexperimentelle Aufklärung *f*

decadence Dekadenz *f*, geistiger Verfall *m*, geistiger Niedergang *m*

decadent dekadent, entartet

decamethonium Decamethonium *n*

decapitation Dekapitation *f*, Abtrennen *n* des Kopfes, Enthauptung *f*

decarboxylase Decarboxylase *f* / **~ inhibitor** Decarboxylase–Blocker *m*

decay Niedergang *m*, Zerfall *m*, Zersetzung *f*, Auflösung *f* / zerfallen, auflösen / **~ constant** Abfallszeitkonstante *f* / **~ of sensation** Empfindungsrückgang *m* / **~ of stimulus** Reizminderung *f* / **mental ~** Intelligenzverfall *m* / **moral ~** moralischer Niedergang *m*, Dekadenz *f* / **senile ~** Altersdegeneration *f*

decease sterben / Tod *m*, Ableben *n*

deceased verstorben

deceit test Lügentest *m*

deceleration Verzögerung *f*, Verlangsamung *f*, Geschwindigkeitsverminderung *f*

decency Anstand *m*, Sittsamkeit *f*

decentralisation Dezentralisierung *f*

decentration Dezentrierung *f*

deception Sinnenstäuschung *f*, Täuschung *f*, Betrug *m*

decerebrate enthirnt, ohne Gehirn / enthirnen, das Hirn entfernen

decerebration Enthirnung *f*, Entfernung *f* des Hirns, Dezerebration *f*

decibel Dezibel *n*

decide entscheiden, sich entschließen

decile Dezil *n* / **~ rank** Dezilrang *m*, Dezilwert *m*

decision Entscheidung *f*, Entschluss *m* / **~ and choice behaviour** Entscheidungs– und Wahlverhalten *n* / **~ making** Entscheidungsfindung *f* / **~–making process** Entscheidungsprozess *m* / **~ models** Entscheidungsmodelle *npl* / **~ structure** Entscheidungsstruktur *f* / **~ support system** computerunterstützte Entscheidungshilfe *f* / **~ theory** Entscheidungstheorie *f* / **legal ~** Rechtsprechung *f*, juristische Entscheidung *f* / **lexical ~** lexikalische Entscheidung *f*

decline Niedergang *m*, Verfall *m*, Abnahme *f* / abnehmen, verfallen / **~ of life** Lebensabend *m* / **~ in strength** Kräfteverfall *m*

decode entschlüsseln, entziffern, dechiffrieren

decoding Entschlüsselung *f*, Dekodierung *f*

decollation Dekapitation *f*, Trennung *f* von Kopf und Rumpf

decompensated dekompensiert, nicht ausgeglichen

decompensation Kompensationsstörung *f*, Kompensationsmangel *m*, Dekompensation *f*

decomposability Zerlegbarkeit *f*

decompression Druckverminderung *f*, Druckabfall *m*, Dekompression *f* / **~ effect** Dekompressionswirkung *f*, Auswirkung *f* einer Druckverminderung

deconditioning Wegkonditionieren *n*, Dekonditionierung *f*, Entziehungskur *f*

decorticate großhirnlos / entrinden, Rinde entfernen

decortication Dekortikation *f*, Entrindung *f*

decrease Abnahme *f*, Verminderung *f*, Rückgang *m* / **~ in mental tension** geistige Entspannung *f* / **~ in physical ability** körperliche Leistungsminderung *f* / **~ in sensitivity** Empfindlichkeitsminderung *f* / **~ of vital impulse in schizophrenia** Athymhormie *f* / **~ in vitality** Leistungsminderung *f*, Leistungsabfall *m*

decreasing abnehmend

decrement Abnahme *f*, Verminderung *f*, Verringerung *f* / **~ conduction** Dekrementleitung *f* / **social ~** sozial bedingte Leistungsabnahme *f*

decrepitude Gebrechlichkeit *f*, Hinfälligkeit *f*

deculturation Verlust *m* der eigenen Kultur, Dekulturation *f*

decussation Nervenkreuzung *f*, Bahnkreuzung *f*, Decussatio *f* / ~ **of the optic nerve** Chiasma opticum *n* / ~ **of the pyramids** Pyramidenkreuzung *f* / **pyramidal** ~ Pyramidenkreuzung *f*

dedication Hingabe *f*

dedifferentiated entdifferenziert

dedifferentiation Entdifferenzierung *f*

deduction Deduktion *f*, Schlussfolgerung *f*, Schluss *m* / **logical** ~ logische Schlussfolgerung *f*

deductive deduktiv, folgernd

de–efferentation Deefferentierung *f*, Ausschaltung *f* der efferenten Innervation eines Organs

de–escalate deeskalieren

de–escalation Deeskalation *f*

defaecate, defecate den Darm entleeren, Stuhlgang haben, defäzieren

defaecation, defecation Darmentleerung *f*, Defäkation *f*, Stuhlgang *m* / ~ **reflex** Darmentleerungsreflex *m*

defatigation Übermüdung *f*, Überarbeitung *f*, Überanstrengung *f*

defeatism Defätismus *m*

defect Mangel *m*, Fehler *m*, Defekt *m* / ~ **delinquency** Defektkriminalität *f* / ~ **formation** Defektbildung *f* / ~ **in vision** Sehfehler *m* / **acquired** ~ **of intelligence** erworbener Intelligenzdefekt *m* / **auditory** ~ Hörfehler *m* / **cerebral** ~ Gehirnstörung *f* / **congenital** ~ **of intelligence** angeborener Intelligenzdefekt *m* / **developmental** ~ Entwicklungsstörung *f* / **functional** ~ funktionelle Störung *f* / **intellectual** ~ Intelligenzdefekt *m* / **mental** ~ Geistesstörung *f*, geistiger Defekt *m* / **optical** ~ Sehfehler *m* / **perceptual** ~ Wahrnehmungsstörung *f* / **schizophrenic** ~ schizophrener Defekt *m*, Defektschizophrenie *f* / **visual** ~ Sehstörung *f*

defective fehlerhaft, mangelhaft, anomal / Person *f* mit geistigem Defekt / **mental** ~ Schwachsinniger *m* / **mentally** ~ schwachsinnig / **moral** ~ moralisch Kranker *m*, moralisch Gestörter *m*

defectiveness Mangelhaftigkeit *f*, Fehlerhaftigkeit *f* / **mental** ~ Schwachsinn *m*, Oligophrenie *f*, Minderbegabung *f*, geistige Zurückgebliebenheit *f*

defemination, defeminisation Entweiblichung *f*, Defeminisierung *f*

defence, defense Abwehr *f*, Abwehrsystem *n* / ~ **activity** Abwehrmechanismus *m*, Abwehrtätigkeit *f* / ~ **against anxiety** Angstabwehr *f* / ~ **function** Abwehrfunktion *f* / ~ **hysteria** Abwehrhysterie *f* / ~ **mechanism** Abwehrmechanismus *m* / ~ **neuropsychosis** Abwehrpsychoneurose *f* / ~ **neurosis** Abwehrneurose *f* / ~ **reaction** Abwehrreaktion *f* / ~ **reflex** Abwehrreflex *m*, Schutzreflex *m* / ~ **system** Abwehrsystem *n* / **humoral** ~ humorale Abwehr *f* / **manic** ~ manische Abwehr *f* / **muscular** ~ Muskelabwehrreaktion *f* / **personal** ~ Selbstverteidigung *f* / **perceptual** ~ Wahrnehmungsabwehr *f* / **psychical** ~ psychische Abwehr *f* / **social** ~ soziale Abwehr *f* / **unspecific** ~ unspezifische Abwehr *f*

defenceless schutzlos, wehrlos, hilflos

defencelessness Schutzlosigkeit *f*, Wehrlosigkeit *f*

defendance Rechtfertigungsbedürfnis *n*, Verteidigungsbedürfnis *n*

defensive Abwehr–

defensiveness Abwehrhaltung *f*, Verteidigungshaltung *f*, Defensivität *f*

deference Unterwerfung *f*, Unterwürfigkeit *f* / ~ **behaviour** unterwürfiges Verhalten *n* / ~ **need** Bedürfnis *n* sich zu unterwerfen

deferred verzögert, verspätet, nachträglich

defiance Herausforderung *f*, Trotz *m*

defibrillator Defibrillator *m*

deficiency Mangel *m* / ~ **in ability and vitality** Leistungsschwäche *f*, Leistungsdefizit *n* / ~ **disorder** Mangelzustand *m* / ~ **motivation** Mangelmotivation *f*, Defizitmotivation *f* / ~ **of memory** Gedächtnisschwäche *f* / ~ **of will power** Abulie *f*, Willensschwache *f* / **acquired immune** ~

syndrome erworbene Immunschwächekrankheit *f*, AIDS / **affective ~** Affektmattigkeit *f*, Affektlahmheit *f* / **mental ~** Schwachsinn *m*, Oligophrenie *f*, geistige Zurückgebliebenheit *m* / **moral ~** moralischer Defekt *m* / **nutritional ~** Mangelernährung *f*, Ernährungsmangelerscheinung *f* / **parathyroid ~** Hypoparathyreoidismus *m* / **primary mental ~** Geistesschwäche *f*, Oligophrenie *f* / **secondary mental ~** erworbener Schwachsinn *m*

deficient fehlend, mangelnd / **mentally ~** schwachsinnig

defined definiert / **operationally ~** operational definiert

definition Definition *f* / **~ of the situation** Situationsbeurteilung *f* / **circular ~** Zirkeldefinition *f*, zyklische Definition *f* / **formal ~** Nominaldefinition *f* / **operational ~** operationale Definition *f* / **ostensive ~** anschaulische Definition *f* / **recursive ~** rekursive Definition *f*

deflation Deflation *f*

deflection, deflexion Abweichung *f*, Ablenkung *f*

defloration Defloration *f*, Entjungferung *f*

deflower entjungfern, entehren, schanden

deformation Missbildung *f*, Entstellung *f*, Fehlbildung *f*, Verunstaltung *f* / **cranial ~** Schädelmissbildung *f* / **professional ~** berufliche Verunstaltung *f*

deformity Missgestalt *f*, körperliche Missgestaltung *f*, Missbildung *f* / **congenital ~** angeborene Missbildung *f* / **heriditary ~** erbliche Missbildung *f*

defusion Entmischung *f* / **~ of instincts** Triebentmischung *f* / **instinctual ~** Triebentmischung *f*

degeneracy Degeneration *f*, Entartung *f*

degenerate entartet, degeneriert / entarten, degenerieren

degeneration Degeneration *f*, Entartung *f* / **~ psychosis** Degenerationspsychose *f* / **cerebral ~** Gehirnentartung *f* / **cerebromacular ~** amaurotische Idiotie *f*, Tay–Sachs–Krankheit *f* / **mental ~** geistige Degeneration *f*, geistiger Verfall *m*, geistiger Abbau *m* / **myelinic ~** Markscheidendegeneration *f* / **senile ~** Altersdegeneration *f* / **spinal ~** Rückenmarksdegeneration *f* / **social ~** soziale Degeneration *f* / **Wallerian ~** Waller'sche Degeneration *f*

degenerative degenerativ, entartet

deglutition Schlucken *n*, Schluckvorgang *m*

degradation Verfall *m*, Degeneration *f*, Verminderung *f*, Degradierung *f*, Entartung *f* / **~ law** Zerfallgesetz *n*, Degradationsgesetz *n* / **oxidative ~** oxidativer Abbau *m*

degrading entwürdigend, erniedrigend

degree Grad *m* / **~ of accuracy** Genauigkeitsgrad *m* / **~ of brightness** Helligkeitsgrad *m* / **~ of consciousness** Bewusstseinsgrad *m* / **~ of disability** Invaliditätsgrad *m* / **~ of efficacy** Wirkungsgrad *m* / **~ of emotionality** Grad *m* der Emotionalität / **~ of freedom** Freiheitsgrad *m* / **~ of sensitivity** Empfindlichkeitsgrad *m* / **educational ~** Bildungsgrad *m*, Schulabschluss *m*

degustation Schmecken *n*, Geschmackssinn *m*

dehumanisation Entmenschlichung *f*, Verlust *m* des Menschseins

dehumanize entmenschlichen, entseelen, unmenschlich machen

dehydration Dehydration *f*, Wassermangel *m*

dehydroepiandrosterone Dehydroepiandrosteron *n*

dehydrogenase Dehydrogenase *f*, Dehydrase *f* / **lactate ~** Laktatdehydrogenase *f*

dehypnotisation Erwecken *n* aus der Hypnose, Enthypnotisieren *n*

dehypnotize aus der Hypnose erwecken, enthypnotisieren

deification Vergötterung *f*

deintoxicate entgiften, entziehen

deintoxication Entgiftung *f*, Entzug *m*

Deiter's| cell Deiters–Zelle *f* / **~ nucleus** Deiters–Kern *m*

déjà entendu Hörtäuschung *f*, Bekanntheitstäuschung *f*

déjà–entendu phenomenon Déjà–entendu–Erlebnis *n*

déjà–eprouvé phenomenon Déjà—éprouvé–Erlebnis *n*

déjà–fait phenomenon Déjà–fait–Erlebnis *n*

déjà–pensé phenomenon Déjà–pensé–Erlebnis *n*

déjà–raconté phenomenon Déjà–raconté–Erlebnis *n*

déjà–vécu phenomenon Déjà–vécu–Erlebnis *n*

déjà–voulu phenomenon Déjà–voulu–Erlebnis *n*

déjà vu Déjà–vu–Erlebnis *n*

dejected niedergeschlagen, mutlos

dejection, dejectedness Niedergeschlagenheit *f*, Mutlosigkeit *f*

delactation Abstillen *n*, Entwöhnung *f*, Ablaktation *f*

delay verzögern, verschieben / Verzögerung *f*, Aufschub *m*, Retardierung *f*, Latenz *f* / **~ conditioning** Konditionieren *n* mit zeitlicher Verzögerung / **~ of gratification** Verzögerung *f* bei der Befriedigung, Belohnungsaufschub *m* / **~ inhibition** Verzögerungshemmung *f* / **~–path** Sprungweg *m*, Hindernisweg *m* / **~ of reflex** Reflexverzögerung *f*, Reflexlatenz *f* / **~ of reinforcement** Verstärkungsverzögerung *f* / **initial ~** Anfangsverzögerung *f*

delayed verzögert, aufgeschoben, retardiert

Delboeuf| disc Delboeuf–Scheibe *f*, Delboeuf–Kreisel *m* / **~'s illusion** Delboeuf–Täuschung *f*

delegation Delegation *f*, Bevollmächtigung *f*, Übertragung *f* / **~ of responsibility** Delegation *f* von Verantwortung / **~ of power** Bevollmächtigung *f*

deletion Auslöschung *f*

deliberation Überlegung *f* / **regressive ~** Umkehrdenken *n*

delicacy Feingefühl *n*, Takt *m*, Zierlichkeit *f* / **~ of mind** Zartgefühl *n*, Empfindlichkeit

delicate empfindlich, feinfühlend, zierlich

delinquency Kriminalität *f*, Delinquenz *f* / **~ proneness** Neigung *f* zur Kriminalität / **habitual ~** Gewohnheitskriminalität *f* / **juvenile ~** Jugendkriminalität *f* / **potential ~** kriminelle Veranlagung *f* / **sexual ~** Sexualverbrechen *n*, Sittlichkeitsvergehen *n*

delinquent Verbrecher *m*, Delinquent *m*, verbrecherisch / **defective ~** geistig zurückgebliebener Delinquent *m* / **female ~** Verbrecherin *f*, Delinquentin *f* / **juvenile ~** jugendlicher Straftäter *m*, jugendlicher Delinquent *m* / **male ~** Verbrecher *m*, Delinquent *m*

deliramentum Delirament *n*, Deliramentum *n*

délire Wahn *m*, Delirium *n*, Manie *f*, Paranoia *f* / **~ d'emblée** Délire d'emblée *m* / **~ de negation** Verneinungswahn *m* / **~ d'énormité** Délire d'énormité *m* / **~ du toucher** Délire du toucher *m*, Berührungszwang *m*

deliriant Delirium verursachend, delirös machend

delirious delirant, delirös, irre redend, an Delirium leidend

delirium Delirium *n*, Delir *n* / **~ alcoholicum** Alkoholdelir *n*, Delirium tremens *n* / **~ due to a general medical condition** Delirium *n* aufgrund eines medizinischen Krankheitsfaktors / **~ due to multiple etiologies** Delirium *n* aufgrund multipler Ätiologien / **~ ebriosorum** Delirium ebriosorum *n*, Delirium tremens *n* / **~ grandiosum** Größenwahn *m* / **~ mussitans** Delirium mussitans *n*, mussitierendes Delirium *n* / **~, not induced by alcohol and other psychoactive substances** Delir *n*, nicht durch Alkohol oder sonstige psychotrope Substanzen bedingt / **~, not superimposed on dementia, so described** Delir *n* ohne Demenz / **~ of interpretation** Beziehungswahn *m* / **~,**

superimposed on dementia Delir *n* bei Demenz / ~ **tremefaciens** Delirium tremens *n* / ~ **tremens** Delirium tremens *n*, Delirium alcoholicum *n*, Alkoholdelir *n*, Säuferwahn *m* / ~, **unspecified** nicht näher bezeichnetes Delir *n* / **acute** ~ akutes Delirium *n* / **alcoholic** ~ Alkoholdelir *n* / **chronic alcoholic** ~ Korsakow–Psychose *f* / **compulsive** ~ zwangsneurotisches Delirium *n* / **epileptic** ~ Delirium epilepticum *n* / **expansive** ~ Verzückungsdelir *n*, krankhafte Überspanntheit *f* / **febrile** ~ Fieberdelirium *n* / **incipient** ~ Prädelirium tremens *n* / **initial** ~ Initialdelirium *n* / **maniacal** ~ Delirium manicum *n* / **melancholic** ~ délire de ruine / **muttering** ~ Delirium mussitans *n*, mussitierendes Delirium *n* / **occupational** ~ Beschäftigungswahn *m*, Beschäftigungsdelir *n* / **oneiric** ~ oneiroides Delirium *n* / **other** ~ sonstige Formen *fpl* des Delirs / **professional** ~ Beschäftigungswahn *m* / **saturnine** ~ Bleidelirium *n* / **secondary** ~ Folgedelir *n* / **toxic** ~ toxisches Delir *n*, Vergiftungsdelir *n* / **traumatic** ~ Unfalldelirium *n*

delivery Entbindung *f*, Niederkunft *f* / **complicated** ~ Geburtskomplikation *f* / **early** ~ Frühgeburt *f* / **premature** ~ Frühgeburt *f*

delta|activity Delta–Aktivität *f*, Delta–Rhythmus *m* / ~ **alcoholism** Deltaalkoholismus *m* / ~ **movement** Delta–Bewegung *f*, Scheinbebewegung *f* / ~ **rhythm** Delta–Rhythmus *m* / ~ **wave** Delta–Welle *f*

delude täuschen

delusion Wahn *m*, Wahnvorstellung *f*, Wahnidee *f* / ~ **of being harmed** Beeinträchtigungswahn *m* / ~ **of being influenced** Beeinflussungswahn *m* / ~ **of being a prophet** Prophetenwahn *m* / ~ **of culpability** Versündigungswahn *m* / ~ **of dermatozoonosis** Dermatozoenwahn *m* / ~ **of destruction** Zerstörungswahn *m* / ~ **of erotic reference** erotischer Beziehungswahn *m* / ~ **of grandeur** Größenwahn *m* / ~ **of guilt** Schuldwahn *m* / ~ **of immortality** Unsterblichkeitswahn *m* / ~ **of infidelity** Untreuewahn *m* / ~ **of influence** Beeinflussungswahn *m* / ~ **of innocence** Unschuldswahn *m* / ~ **of interpretation** Bedeutungserlebnis *n*, Bedeutungswahn *m* / ~ **of jealousy** Eifersuchtswahn *m* / ~ **of metamorphosis** Verwandlungsdelirium *n* / ~ **of negation** Verneinungswahn *m*, Negationsdelirium *n*, nihilistischer Wahn *m* / ~ **of observation** Beobachtungswahn *m* / ~ **of omnipotence** Allmachtswahn *m* / ~ **of pardon** Begnadigungswahn *m* / ~ **of perception** Einbildungstäuschung *f* / ~ **of persecution** Verfolgungswahn *m* / ~ **of physical influence** körperlicher Beeinflussungswahn *m* / ~ **of poisoning** Vergiftungswahn *m* / ~ **of prejudice** Benachteiligungswahn *m* / ~ **of reference** Beziehungswahn *m*, Bedeutungswahn *m* / ~ **of remembrance** Erinnerungstäuschung *f* / ~ **of revelation** Offenbarungswahn *m* / ~ **of saving the world** Messiaswahn *m* / ~ **of self–accusation** Selbstbeschuldigungswahn *m* / **autochthonous** ~ Primärwahn *m* / **catathymic** ~ katathymer Wahn *m* / **dermatozoic** ~ Dermatozoenwahn *m* / **depressive** ~ depressiver Wahn *m*, depressive Wahnidee *f* / **expansive** ~ Größenwahn *m* / **grandiose** ~ Größenwahn *m* / **hypochondriac** ~ hypochondrischer Wahn *m* / **induced** ~ induzierter Wahn *m* / **jealous** ~ Eifersuchtswahn *m* / **kinaesthetic** ~ kinästhetische Täuschung *f* / **mental** ~ Sinnestäuschung *f* / **Messianic** ~ Erlöseridee *f*, Berufungswahn *m* / **mnemic** ~ Erinnerungstäuschung *f* / **nihilistic** ~ nihilistischer Wahn *m* / **primary** ~ Primärwahn *m* / **primordial** ~ primäre Wahnidee *f* / **religious** ~ religiöser Wahn *m*, Offenbarungswahn *m* / **residual** ~ Residualwahn *m* / **systematised** ~ Wahnsystem *n* / **unsystematised** ~ inkohärenter Wahn *m*

delusional wahnhaft, Wahn– / **~–hallucinatory** wahnhaft–halluzinatorisch

delusive trügerisch, täuschend

demand Nachfrage *f*, Verlangen *n*, Beanspruchung *f*

demarcation Demarkation *f*, Quetschung *f* der Markscheide / ~ **of a nerve fibre** Demarkation *f* einer Nervenfaser / ~ **potential** Demarkationspotential *n*

demasculinization Demaskulinisierung *f*

dematerialize dematerialisieren

dematerialisation Dematerialisation *f*

dement Demente *m,f*, / wahnsinnig machen

demented wahnsinnig, dement

dementia Demenz *f*, Dementia *f* / ~ **apoplectica** Dementia apoplectica *f* / ~ **arising in the senium and presenium** Demenz *f* mit Beginn im Senium und Präsenium / ~ **due to Creutzfeldt–Jacob disease** Demenz *f* aufgrund einer Creutzfeldt–Jacob'schen Erkrankung / ~ **due to head trauma** Demenz *f* aufgrund eines Schädel–Hirn–Traumas / ~ **due to HIV disease** Demenz *f* aufgrund einer HIV–Erkrankung / ~ **due to Huntington's disease** Demenz *f* aufgrund einer Huntington'schen Chorea / ~ **due to multiple etiologies** Demenz *f* aufgrund multipler Ätiologien / ~ **due to other general medical conditions** Demenz *f* aufgrund anderer medizinischer Krankheitsfaktoren / ~ **due to Parkinson's disease** Demenz *f* aufgrund einer Parkinson'schen Erkrankung / ~ **due to Pick's disease** Demenz *f* aufgrund einer Pick'schen Erkrankung / ~ **in Alzheimer's disease** Demenz *f* bei Alzheimer–Krankheit / ~ **in Alzheimer's disease, atypical or mixed type** Demenz *f* bei Alzheimer–Krankheit, atypische oder gemischte Form / ~ **in Alzheimer's disease, unspecified** nicht näher bezeichnete Demenz *f* bei Alzheimer–Krankheit / ~ **in Alzheimer's disease with early (late) onset** Demenz *f* bei Alzheimer–Krankheit mit frühem (spätem) Beginn / ~ **in Creutzfeldt–Jakob disease** Demenz *f* bei Creutzfeldt–Jakob–Krankheit / ~ **infantilis** Dementia infantilis *f* / ~ **in human immunodeficiency virus (HIV) disease** Demenz *f* bei Krankheit durch das humane Immundefizienz–Virus (HIV) / ~ **in Huntington's disease** Demenz *f* bei Huntington–Krankheit / ~ **in other diseases classified elsewhere** Demenz *f* bei sonstigen andernorts klassifizierten Krankheiten / ~ **in Parkinson's disease** Demenz *f* bei Parkinson–Krankheit / ~ **in Pick's disease** Demenz *f* bei Pick–Krankheit / ~ **of the Alzheimer's type** Demenz *f* vom Alzheimer Typ / ~ **paralytica** paralytische Demenz *f* / ~ **paranoides** Dementia paranoides *f* / ~ **praecocissima** Dementia praecocissima *f* / ~ **praecox** Dementia praecox *f*, Jugendirresein *n* / ~ **praesenilis** präsenile Demenz *f* / ~ **pugilista** Boxerenzephalopathie *f*, Boxerdemenz *f* / ~ **senilis** senile Demenz / ~ **simplex** Dementia simplex *f*, einfache Schizophrenie *f* / ~ **without additional symptoms** Demenz *f* ohne zusätzliche Symptome / **acute** ~ Dementia acuta *f* / **alcoholic** ~ Alkoholdemenz *f* / **arteriosclerotic** ~ Demenz *f* bei Zerebralarteriosklerose / **endogenous** ~ endogene Demenz *f* / **epileptic** ~ epileptische Demenz *f*, Dementia epileptica / **infantile** ~ Dementia infantilis *f* / **mixed cortical and subcortical vascular** ~ gemischte (kortikale und subkortikale) vaskuläre Demenz *f*/ **multi–infarct** ~ Multiinfarkt–Demenz *f* / **other vascular** ~ sonstige vaskuläre Demenz *f* / **paralytic** ~ paralytische Demenz *f* / **paranoid** ~ paranoide Schizophrenie *f* / **postapoplectic** ~ postapoplektische Demenz / **posttraumatic** ~ posttraumatische Demenz *f*, Dementia traumatica *f* / **precocious** ~ Jugendirrsein *n* / **presenile** ~ präsenile Demenz *f*, Alzheimer Krankheit *f* / **primary** ~ einfache Schizophrenie *f*, Dementia simplex *f* / **schizophrenic** ~ schizophrene Demenz *f* / **semantic** ~ semantische Demenz *f* / **senile** ~ Altersdemenz *f*, senile Demenz *f*, Altersschwachsinn *m* / **subcortical vascular** ~ subkortikale vaskuläre Demenz *f* / **toxic** ~ toxische Demenz *f* / **traumatic** ~ Dementia posttraumatica *f* / **unspecified** ~ nicht näher bezeichnete Demenz *f* / **vascular** ~ vaskuläre Demenz *f* / **vascular ~, unspecified** nicht näher bezeichnete vaskuläre Demenz *f*

democracy Demokratie *f*

demodulation Demodulation *f*, Gleichrichten *n*

demographic demographisch, Bevölkerungs–

demography Demographie *f*, Bevölkerungswissenschaft *f*, Bevölkerungsstatistik *f*

demoniac Verrückter *m* / rasend, tobend

demonism Dämonismus *m*, Dämonenwahn *m*

demono|logy Lehre *f* von den Dämonen, Lehre *f* vom Dämonenglaube / **~ mania** Dämonenwahn *m*, Besessenheitswahn *m* / **~ maniac** Besessener *m* / **~ melancholia** Dämonomelancholie *f* / **~ pathy** Besessenheit *f* / **~ phobia** Dämonenfurcht *f*, Dämonophobie *f*, Angst *f* vor Teufeln und Geistern

demonstrative demonstrativ, deutlich zeigend, auffällig, anschaulich, ausdrucksvoll

demonstration Darstellung *f*, Demonstration *f*, Vorführung *f* / **social ~** Demonstration *f*, Protestdemonstration *f*

demophobia Demophobie *f*, krankhafte Furcht *f* vor Menschenmengen

demoralisation Demoralisierung *f*, Entmutigung *f*

demoralized demoralisiert, entmutigt

demorphinisation Morphiumentziehung *f*, Morphiumentwöhnung *f*

demutisation Sprechunterricht *m* für Stumme, Verständigungsunterricht *m* für Stumme

demythologisation Entmythologisierung *f*

denatality Geburtenrückgang *m*, Abnahme *f* der Geburtenzahlen

dendrite, dendron Dendrit *m*

denervate denervieren

denervation Denervierung *f*

denial Verweigerung *f*, Verneinung *f*, Negation *f*, Verleugnung *f* / **~ of reality** Realitätsleugnung *f*, Realitätsverleugnung *f*, Skotomisation *f*

denigration Verunglimpfung *f*, Anschwärzung *f*

denotation Bezeichnung *f*, Bedeutung *f*

denotative denotativ, bezeichnend, andeutend

density Dichte *f*, Dichtigkeit *f* / **~ function** Dichtefunktion *f* / **~ mean** Dichtemittel *n* / **~ of population** Bevölkerungsdichte *f* / **social ~** soziale Dichte *f* / **tonal ~** Klanghelligkeit *f*, Tonhelligkeit *f* / **uniform ~** gleichförmige Dichte *f*

dental Zahn–, zahnärztlich

dentition Zahnung *f*, Zahnen *n*, Dentition *f*

denunciation Denunziation *f*, Anzeige *f*, Verrat *m*

deny verneinen, leugnen, ableugnen

deontology Pflichtenlehre *f*, Deontologie *f*

deoxycorticosterone Desoxycorticosteron *n*

deoxyglucose Desoxyglukose *f*

department Abteilung *f* / **~ of psychology** Abteilung *f* für Psychologie, psychologische Abteilung *f*

departmentalized abteilungsgegliedert, in Abteilungen aufgeteilt

dependable zuverlässig

dependant Abhängiger *m*

dependence, dependance Abhängigkeit *f*, Sucht *f* / **~ of the ego** Abhängigkeit *f* des Ichs, Ich–Abhängigkeit *f* / **~ syndrome** Abhängigkeitssyndrom *n* / **oral ~** orale Abhängigkeit *f* / **physical ~** körperliche Abhängigkeit *f* / **physiological ~** körperliche Abhängigkeit *f* / **psychological ~** psychische Abhängigkeit *f* / **stochastic ~** stochastische Abhängigkeit *f*

dependency Abhängigkeit *f*, Unselbstständigkeit *f* / **~ diagram** Abhängigkeitsdiagramm *n* / **~ need** Abhängigkeitsbedürfnis *n* / **linear ~** lineare Abhängigkeit *f*

dependent abhängig, unselbstständig / Abhängige *m,f* / **mutually ~** voneinander abhängig

depersonalization Depersonalisation *f*, Entpersönlichung *f*, Verlust *m* des Persönlichkeitsbewusstseins, Beeinträchtigung *f* des Persönlichkeitsgefühls, Entfremdungsgefühl *n* / **~ depression** Entfremdungsdepression *f* / **~ syndrome** Depersonalisationssyndrom *n*, Derealisationssyndrom *n* / **~ disorder** Depersonalisationsstörung *f* / **~ experience** Entfremdungserlebnis *n* / **~ neurosis** neurotische Depersonalisation *f* / **~ syndrome** Depersonalisationssyndrom *n*

depolarisation Depolarisieren *n*, Depolarisation *f* / **critical ~** Schwellendepolarisation *f*, kritische Depolarisation *f*

depravation moralische Entartung *f*, sittliche Entgleisung *f*

deprave moralisch verderben, verführen

depraved entartet, verdorben

depreciation Herabsetzung *f*, Geringschätzung *f* / **parental ~** Geringschätzung *f* durch die Eltern

depress seelisch bedrücken

depressed niedergedrückt, niedergeschlagen, deprimiert, schwermütig

depressing niederdrückend, deprimierend

depression Depression *f*, Niedergeschlagenheit *f* / **~–pain syndrome** Depressions–Schmerz–Syndrom *n* / **acute ~** akute Depression *f* / **agitated ~** erregte Depression *f*, agitierte Depression *f* / **ambivalent ~** ambivalente Depression *f* / **anaclitic ~** Affektentzugssyndrom *n*, Anlehnungsdepression *f*, anaklitische Depression *f* / **anancastic ~** anankastische Depression *f* / **anodic ~** anodische Depression *f* / **anxious agitated ~** ängstlich agitierte Depression *f* / **arteriosclerotic ~** arteriosklerotische Depression *f* / **autonomous ~** autonome Depression *f* / **averse ~** irreversible Depression *f* / **aversive ~** Involutionsdepression *f* / **circular ~** zirkuläre Depression *f* / **climacteric ~** Depression *f* im Klimakterium / **constitutional ~** konstitutionelle Depression *f* / **cyclothymic ~** zyklothyme Depression *f* / **endogenous ~** endogene Depression *f* / **existential ~** existentielle Depression *f* / **exogenous ~** exogene Depression *f*, reaktive Depression *f* / **gestational ~** Schwangerschaftsdepression *f* / **hypochondriacal ~** hypochondrische Depression *f* / **hysterical ~** hysterische Depression *f* / **infantile ~** infantile Depression *f* / **inhibited ~** gehemmte Depression *f* / **initial ~** beginnende Depression *f* / **involutional ~** Involutionsdepression *f* / **manic ~** manische Depression *f* / **major ~** Major Depression *f* / **menopausal ~** klimakterische Depression *f* / **mild ~** leichte Depression *f* / **neurotic ~** neurotische Depression *f*, depressive Neurose *f* / **nostalgic ~** Heimwehdepression *f* / **periodic ~** periodische Depression / **obsessional ~** Zwangsdepression *f*, anankastische Depression *f* / **permanent ~** Dauerverstimmung *f* / **postinfective ~** postinfektiöse Depression *f* / **post–partum ~** Wochenbettdepression *f* / **post–schizophrenic ~** postschizophrene Depression *f* / **primary ~** primäre Depression *f* / **psychogenic ~** psychogene Depression *f* / **psychotic ~** psychotische Depression *f* / **reactive ~** reaktive Depression *f*, depressive Reaktion *f* / **recurrent ~** periodische Depression *f* / **recurrent major ~ of seasonal pattern** Major Depression *f* mit saisonal abhängiger Verlaufsform / **respiratory ~** Atemdepression *f* / **retarded ~** gehemmte Depression *f* / **secondary ~** sekundäre Depression *f* / **senile ~** senile Depression *f*, Altersdepression *f* / **situational ~** depressive Reaktion *f* / **stuporous ~** schwere Depression *f*, stuporöse Depression *f* / **symptomatic ~** symptomatische Depression *f* / **vernal ~** Frühjahrsdepression *f* / **vital ~** vitale Depression *f*

depressive depressiv, niederdrückend, Depression verursachend / **manic–~** manisch–depressiv

depressor depressorischer Nerv *m*, Musculus depressor *m*, Depressorsubstanz *f*

deprivation, deprival Entzug *m*, Wegnahme *f*, Verlust *m* / **~ of affection** Affektentzug *m* / **~ of freedom** Freiheitsberaubung *f*,

Freiheitsentziehung *f*, Freiheitsentzug *m* / **~ of parental rights** Entzug *m* des elterlichen Sorgerechts / **~ symptom** Entzugssymptom *n* / **cultural ~** kulturelle Benachteiligung *f*, kulturelle Deprivation *f* / **emotional ~ syndrome** Deprivationssyndrom *n* / **maternal ~** Mangel *m* an mütterlicher Zuwendung und Pflege / **perceptual ~** sensorische Deprivation *f* / **relative ~** teilweiser Entzug *m* / **sensory ~** Reizentzug *m*, sensorische Deprivation *f* / **social ~** soziale Isolierung *f*, soziale Deprivation *f*

deprive entziehen, berauben, wegnehmen

deprived beraubt, entzogen, aberkannt / **~ of legal capacity** entmündigt

depth Tiefe *f* / **~ analysis** Tiefenanalyse *f* / **~ of emotions** Tiefe *f* der Gefühle / **~ illusion** Tiefentäuschung *f* / **~ interview** Tiefeninterview *n* / **~ perception** Tiefenwahrnehmung *f* / **~ psychology** Tiefenpsychologie *f* / **~ sensibility** Tiefensensibilität *f*, Tiefenempfindlichkeit *f* / **~ of sleep** Schlaftiefe und –dauer *f* / **~ and time of sleep** Schlafmenge *f* nach Tiefe und Dauer / **binocular ~ perception** binokulare Tiefenwahrnehmung *f* / **monocular ~ perception** monokulare Tiefenwahrnehmung *f* / **visual ~ perception** visuelle Tiefenwahrnehmung *f*

deranged gestört, verwirrt / **mentally ~** geistesgestört, geisteskrank

derangement Störung *f*, Verwirrung *f* / **~ of mind** Geistesstörung *f* / **~ of senses** Bewusstseinsstörung *f* / **mental ~** Geistesstörung *f*, Geisteskrankheit *f*, Irresein *n*, Irrsinn *m*, Wahnsinn *m* / **organic ~** Organstörung *f*

derealization Wirklichkeitsverlust *m*, Derealisation *f*

dereism dereistisches Denken *n*, unlogisches, autistisches Denken *n*

dereistic dereistisch, dereierend, wirklichkeitsfremd, unlogisch–autistisch

derelict Obdachloser *m*, menschliches Wrack *n* / verlassen, aufgegeben, verfallen

dereliction Vernachlässigung *f*, Verlassen *n*

derivate Derivat *n*, Abkömmling *m* / **~ of an instinct** Triebabkömmling *m* / **instinctual ~** Triebabkömmling *m*

derivation Abstammung *f*, Herkunft *f*, Ursprung *m*, Ableitung *f*

derivative abgeleitet, sekundär / Nebenprodukt *n*, Abkömmling *m* / **~ of the unconsciousness** Abkömmling *m* des Unbewussten

derived abgeleitet, sekundär

derma Haut *f* / **~ sense** Hautsinn *m*

dermal dermal, Haut–

dermalgia, dermatalgia, dermatodynia neuralgischer Hautschmerz *m*, Dermatodynie *f*

dermatitis Dermatitis *f*, Hautentzündung *f*

dermato|glyphics Hautstruktur *f* / **~graphia,** Dermographismus *m* / **~graphy** Dermographismus *m* / **~logy** Dermatologie *f*, Lehre *f* von den Hauterkrankungen / **~ mania** Dermatomanie *f* / **~ neurosis** Dermatoneurose *f*, Dermoneurose *f* / **~ phobia** Angst *f* vor Hautkrankheiten, Ekzemangst *f*, Dermatophobie *f* / **~ pathophobia** Angst *f* vor Hautkrankheiten, Ekzemangst *f*, Dermatophobie *f* / **~ siophobia** Dermatosiophobie *f* / **~ thlasia** Dermatothlasia *f*

dermatome Dermatom *n*

dermis Haut *f*

dermographia, dermography, dermographism Dermographismus *m*, Dermographie *f*

dermoneurosis Hautneurose *f*

describable beschreibbar, verbalisierbar

description Beschreibung *f*, Deskription *f*

descriptive beschreibend, deskriptiv

desegregation Aufhebung *f* der Rassentrennung

desensitisation Desensibilisierung *f*, Verlust *m* der Sensibilität, Desensitivierung *f* / **~ therapy** Desensibilisierungstherapie *f* / **systematic ~** systematische Desensibilisierung *f*

desensitise desensibilisieren, die Empfindlichkeit herabsetzen

desexualisation Kastrierung *f*

desexualise kastrieren

design Versuch *m*, Versuchsplan *m*, Gestaltung *f*, Entwurf *m* entwerfen, ausdenken, planen / **double–blind ~** Doppelblindversuch *m* / **experimental ~** Versuchsplan *m*, experimenteller Plan *m* / **factorial ~** faktorieller Versuchsplan *m* / **interior ~** Innenraumgestaltung *f*, Raumdesign *n* / **pictorial ~** Zeichnung *f* / **purposive ~** Versuchsplan *m* / **quasi–experimental ~** quasi–experimenteller Versuchsplan *m* / **randomized ~** auf Zufallsauswahl basierender Versuchsplan *m* / **replicative ~** wiederholbarer Versuchsaufbau *m*

designate bezeichnen, benennen

designation Bezeichnung *f*, Benennung *f*

desinhibition Enthemmung *f*

desintegration Zersetzung *f*, Auflösung *f*, Desintegration *f*

desipramine Desipramin *n*

desirability Erwünschtheit *f* / **personal ~** persönliche Erwünschtheit *f* / **social ~** soziale Erwünschtheit *f*, sozial erwünschte Einstellung *f*

desire Wunsch *m*, Drang *m*, Begierde *f*, Lust *f* / **~ concentration** Wunschkonzentration *f* / **~ for treatment** Behandlungswunsch *m* / **hypoactive sexual ~ disorder** Störung *f* mit verminderter sexueller Appetenz / **inhibited sexual ~** sexueller Triebmangel *m* / **sexual ~** sexuelle Appetenz *f*, sexuelle Lust *f*, Sexualdrang *m*

desk research Marktforschung *f* mittels Sekundärquellen, indirektes Erhebungsverfahren *n*

desmosome Desmosom *n* / **half ~** Halbdesmosom *n*

desocialisation Entsozialisierung *f*

desolate betrübt, bekümmert

desolation Trostlosigkeit *f*, Einsamkeit *f*

despair Verzweiflung *f* / verzweifeln

desperation Verzweiflung *f*

despicable verachtenswert, verabscheuungswürdig, widerwärtig

despise verachten, verschmähen

despondency Mutlosigkeit *f*, Niedergeschlagenheit *f*, Verzagtsein *n* / **subdepressive dysphoric ~** subdepressiv–dysphorische Mutlosigkeit *f*

despondent mutlos, niedergeschlagen, verzagt

destination Bestimmung *f*, Ziel *n* / **~ of message** Bestimmungsort *m* einer Nachricht

destiny Schicksal *n* / **~ of drives** Triebschicksale *npl*

destruction Zerstörung *f*, Destruktion *f*

destructive destruktiv, zerstörend

destructiveness Zerstörungswut *f*, Destruktionstrieb *m*

destrudo Destrudo *f*, Todeswunsch *m*, Todestrieb *m*

desublimation Entsublimierung *f*

desurgency nüchternes, kluges, schweigsames Verhalten *n*

desynchronisation Desynchronisation *f*, Desynchronisierung *f*

detachment Ablösung *f*, Abtrennung *f* / **~ of libido** Libidoablösung *f* / **libidinal ~** Libidoablösung *f* / **retinal ~** Netzhautablösung *f*

detail Einzelheit *f*, Detail *n* / **~ response** Detailantwort *f* / **inside ~** Zwischenfigurdeutung *f* / **large ~ response** Detailantwort *f* / **oligophrenic ~** oligophrenes Kleindetail *n* / **rare ~** Kleindetailantwort *f*, außergewöhnliches Detail *n* / **small ~ response** Kleindetailantwort *f*

detection Entdecken *n*, Wahrnehmung *f* / **~ theory** Theorie *f* von der Signalwahrnehmung / **audio–visual ~** Wahrnehmung *f* audiovisueller Signale / **early ~** Frühwahrnehmung *f*

detector Detektor *m* / **cortical ~** Hirnrindendetektor *m*

detention Zurückbehaltung *f*, Internierung *f*, Arrest *m*, Nachsitzen *n* / **legal ~** Haft *f*, Untersuchungshaft *f*

deter abschrecken, hindern, abhalten

deterioration Verschlechterung *f*, Entartung *f*, Degeneration *f*, Verfall *m*, Abbau *m* / **~ index** Abbauindex *m* / **~ quotient** Abbauquotient *m* / **mental ~** geistige Degeneration *f*, geistiger Verfall *m* / **psychic ~** psychischer Verfall *m*

determinant determinierend, bestimmend Determinante *f* / **~ of anxiety** Angstbedingung *f* / **cultural ~** kulturelle Determinante *f*

determination Bestimmung *f*, Determination *f* / **~ of the absolute threshold** Reizschwellenbestimmung *f* / **multiple ~** Überdeterminierung *f*, mehrfache Determinierung *f*

determinative bestimmend, determinativ

determined entschlossen, zielsicher

determiner Determinante *f*, Bestimmungsfaktor *m*

determining bestimmend, determinierend

determinism Determinismus *m* / **cultural ~** Kulturdeterminismus *m* / **moral ~** moralischer Determinismus *m* / **psychic ~** psychischer Determinismus *m* / **psychological ~** psychologischer Determinismus *m*

deterministic deterministisch

deterrence Abschreckung *f*

deterrent abschreckend / Abschreckungsmittel *n*

detest verabscheuen

detestable verabscheuungswürdig, abscheulich

detour Umweg *m* / **~ action** Umweghandlung *f* / **~ learning** Umweglernen *n* / **~ problem** Umwegproblem *n* / **~ test** Umwegtest *m*

detoxicate, detoxify entgiften

detoxication, detoxification Entgiftung *f* / **~ cure** Entziehungskur *f*, Entwöhnung *f*

detraction Herabsetzung *f*, Beeinträchtigung *f*

detrimental schädlich, nachteilig

detumescence Detumeszenz *f*, Abschwellen *n*

deuteranoid grünschwachsichtig

deuteranomaly Grünschwäche *f*, Deuteranomalie *f*

deuteranope Grünblinder *m*

deuteranopia, deuteranopsia Grünblindheit *f*, Deuteranopie *f*, Deuteranopsie *f*

deuteroscopy Deuteroskopie *f*, Zweites–Gesicht–Sehen *n*, Hellsehen *n*

develop entwickeln, sich entwickeln, entstehen

developed entwickelt, ausgebildet / **badly ~** unterentwickelt, retardiert / **fully ~** vollentwickelt, ausgewachsen / **highly ~** hochentwickelt

development Entwicklung *f* / **~ of affect** Affektentwicklung *f* / **~ age** Entwicklungsalter *n* / **~ anomaly** Entwicklungsanomalie *f*, Entwicklungsfehler *m* / **~ level** Entwicklungsstufe *f* / **~ of the libido** Libidoentwicklung *f* / **~ sequence** Entwicklungsreihe *f*, Entwicklungsfolge *f* / **~ stage** Entwicklungsstufe *f* / **~ of thoughts** Gedankenablauf *m* / **abnormal ~** Fehlentwicklung *f* / **abnormal mental ~** abnorme seelische Entwicklung *f*, erlebnisreaktive Entwicklung *f* / **accelerated ~** Entwicklungsbeschleunigung *f*, beschleunigte Entwicklung *f* / **adolescent ~** Entwicklung *f* im Jugendalter / **animal ~** tierische Entwicklung *f* / **arrested ~** Entwicklungsstillstand *m*, Entwicklungshemmung *f* / **bodily ~** körperliche Entwicklung *f* / **cephalocaudal ~** kephalokaudale Entwicklung *f* / **cognitive ~** kognitive Entwicklung *f* / **defective ~** Fehlbildung *f* / **delayed ~** Entwicklungsverzögerung *f*, verzögerte Entwicklung *f* / **dysharmonic ~** Entwicklungsdysharmonie *f* / **early ~** Frühentwicklung *f*, Frühreife *f* / **emotional ~** Gefühlsentwicklung *f*, emotionale Entwicklung *f* / **faulty ~** Fehlentwicklung *f* / **faulty ~ of character** Charakterfehlentwicklung *f* / **human ~** menschliche Entwicklung *f*, Humanentwicklung *f* / **impaired ~** Entwicklungsstörung *f* / **intellectual ~** geistige Entwicklung *f*, intellektuelle Entwicklung *f* / **late ~** Spätentwicklung *f* / **libidinal ~** Libidoentwicklung *f* / **libidinous ~** Libidoentwicklung *f* / **long–term ~** Längsschnitt *m* / **mental ~** geistige Entwicklung *f*, seelische Entwicklung *f* / **moral ~** moralische Entwicklung *f* / **motor ~** motorische Entwicklung *f* / **neonatal ~** Neugeborenenentwicklung *f* / **neural ~** neurale Entwicklung *f* / **neurotic ~** neurotische Entwicklung *f* / **organizational ~** Organisationsentwicklung *f* / **paranoic ~** paranoische Entwicklung *f* / **perceptual ~** Wahrnehmungsentwicklung *f* / **perceptual–motor ~** sensumotorische Entwicklung *f* / **physical ~** körperliche Entwicklung *f*, physische Entwicklung *f* / **precocious ~** Frühreife *f*, frühreife Entwicklung *f* / **prenatal ~** vorgeburtliche Entwicklung *f*, pränatale Entwicklung *f* / **professional ~** berufliche Entwicklung *f* / **psychomotor ~** psychomotorische Entwicklung *f* / **psychosexual ~** psychosexuelle Entwicklung *f* / **psychosexual ~ disorder** psychosexuelle Entwicklungsstörung *f* / **psychosocial ~** psychosoziale Entwicklung *f* / **psychosomatic ~** psychosomatische Entwicklung *f*, Gesamtentfaltung *f* / **sensorimotor ~** sensumotorische Entwicklung *f* / **sexual ~** sexuelle Entwicklung *f* / **social ~** soziale Entwicklung *f* / **stopped ~** Entwicklungsstillstand *m* / **undesirable ~ of character** charakterliche Fehlentwicklung *f*

developmental Entwicklungs–

deviance, deviancy Devianz *f*, Deviation *f*, Abweichung *f* / **genetic ~** genetische Abweichung *f*

deviant abweichend

deviate abweichen / Perverser *m*, sexuell pervers veranlagte Person *f* / **normal ~** Standardabweichung *f* der Normalverteilung / **psychopathic ~** Psychopath *m*

deviation Abweichung *f* / **~ from normal** Abweichung *f* vom Normalen / **~ of the retinal medians** Abweichung *f* der Augachsen / **~ from trend** Trendabweichung *f* / **~ score** individuelle Abweichung *f* / **average ~** durchschnittliche Abweichung *f*, mittlere Abweichung *f* / **interquartile ~** Quartilabweichung *f*, mittlere Quartilabweichung *f* / **manifest ~** offenkundige Abweichung *f* / **mean ~** mittlere Abweichung *f*, durchschnittliche Abweichung *f* / **mean square ~** mittlere quadratische Abweichung *f* / **median ~** Abweichung *f* des Medians / **probable ~** wahrscheinliche Abweichung *f* / **quartile ~** Quartilabweichung *f*, mittlere Quartilabweichung *f* / **sexual ~** abweichendes Sexualverhalten *n*, Perversion *f*, sexuelle Abnormität *f* / **square ~** quadratische Abweichung *f*

device Apparat *m*, Gerät *n*, Vorrichtung *f* / **contraceptive ~s** empfängnisverhütende Mittel *npl* / **experimental ~** Versuchsvorrichtung *f*, Experimentiergerät *n* / **intra–uterine ~** Intrauterinpessar *n*, intrauterines Empfängnisverhütungsmittel *n* / **medical therapeutic ~** medizinisches Heilgerät *n*, medizinisch–therapeutisches Hilfsmittel *n*

devolution Rückbildung *f*, Abbau *m*, Degeneration *f*, Involution *f*

dexamethasone suppression test Dexamethason–Suppressionstest *m*

dexamphetamine, dexedrine Dexamphetamin *n*, Dextroamphetamin *n*

dexterity Geschicklichkeit *f*, Gewandtheit *f* / **~ apparatus** Geschicklichkeitsprüfer *m* / **~ test** Geschicklichkeitstest *m* / **manual ~** handwerkliche Geschicklichkeit *f* / **physical ~** körperliche Geschicklichkeit *f*

dexterous geschickt, gewandt

dextrad nach rechts, rechtsgerichtet

dextral rechtshändig

dextrality Rechtshändigkeit *f*

dextrasinistral rechts–linkshändig

dextroamphetamine Dextroamphetamin *n*

dextromanual rechtshändig

dextromanuality Rechtshändigkeit *f*

dextrosinistral von rechts nach links, Rechts–links–

dextroversion Rechtsverlagerung *f*, Rechtsdrehung *f*

diabetes Diabetes *m*, Zuckerkrankheit *f* / **~ insipidus** Durstkrankheit *f*, Diabetes insipidus *m* / **~ mellitus** Zuckerkrankheit *f*, Diabetes mellitus *m*

diabolepsy Überzeugung *f* mit übernatürlichen Mächten in Verbindung zu stehen

diabolic diabolisch, teuflisch

diabolism Teufelsverehrung *f*, Teufelei *f*

diacetylmorphine Heroin *n*, Diazetylmorphin *n*

diachronic diachronisch

diacrisis Diakrise *f*, Diakrisis *f*, Unterscheidung *f*

diacritic diakritisch, unterscheidend, scharfsinnig

diad Diade *f*, Dyade *f*, Zweier–Verbindung *f* / **social ~** Zweiergruppe *f*

diadochokinesia, diadochokinesis Diadochokinese *f*, Fähigkeit *f* rasch aufeinanderfolgende antagonistische Bewegungen geordnet auszuführen

diadochokinetic diadochokinetisch

diagnose, diagnosticate diagnostizieren

diagnosis Diagnose *f* / **~ of character** Charakterdiagnose *f* / **~ or condition deferred on axis I** Diagnose *f* oder Zustand auf Achse I zurückgestellt / **~ by exclusion** Ausschlussdiagnose *f* / **blind ~** Blinddiagnose *f*, Blindverfahren *n* / **clinical ~** klinische Diagnose *f* / **differential ~** Differentialdiagnose *f* / **dual ~** Doppeldiagnose *f* / **educational ~** Schulleistungsdiagnose *f* / **false ~** Fehldiagnose *f* / **medical ~** ärztliche Diagnose *f*, medizinische Diagnose *f* / **multidimensional ~** multidimensionale Diagnostik *f* / **neurological ~** neurologische Diagnose *f* / **no ~ on axis II** keine Diagnose *f* auf Achse II / **prenatal ~** pränatale Diagnose *f* / **tentative ~** vorläufige Diagnose *f* / **undetermined ~** unbestimmte Diagnose *f*

diagnostic diagnostisch

diagnostics Diagnostik *f*, Lehre *f* von der Krankheitserkenntnis

diagonal diagonal, querlaufend / Diagonale *f*

diagram Diagramm *n*, Schaubild *n*, Schema *n*

diagrammatic schematisch

diagraph Diagraph *m*

diagraphy perspektivische Zeichnung *f*, Diagraphie *f*

dial Zifferblatt *n*, Skala *f*, Skalenscheibe *f*

dialect Dialekt *m*, Mundart *f*

dialectic dialektisch, logisch, Dialekt–, mundartlich

dialectics Dialektik *f*

dialogue Dialog *m*, Zwiegespräch *n*

dialysis Dialyse *f*

diameter Durchmesser *m* / **frontooccipital ~** frontookzipitaler Durchmesser *m* / **occipitofrontal ~** okzipitofrontaler Durchmesser *m*

Diana complex Dianakomplex *m*

diaphanometer Diaphanometer *n*, Transparenzmesser *m*

diaphanometry Diaphanometrie *f*, Transparenzmessung *f*

diaphanous transparent, durchsichtig

diaphoroscope Gerät *n* zur Untersuchung der Schweißabsonderung

diaphragm Zwerchfell *n*, Diaphragma *n*, Blende *f*, Scheidewand *f*

diaphragmatic phrenisch, Zwerchfell–

diarrhoea, diarrhea Durchfall *m*, Diarrhoe *f*

diary Tagebuch *n*

diaschisis Diaschisis *f*, Assoziationsverlust *m*

diastole Diastole *f*

diastolic diastolisch

diathermia, diathermy Diathermie *f*, Wärmedurchdringung *f*, Thermopenetration *f*

diathesis Krankheitsneigung *f*, Diathese *f* / **neuropathic ~** neuropathische Diathese *f* / **paroxysmal ~** iktaffine Diathese *f* / **psychopathic ~** neuropathische Diathese *f* / **spasmophilic ~** Spasmophilie *f*, Krampfbereitschaft *f*

diatonic diatonisch

diazepam Diazepam *n*

dicaine Dicain *n*, Tetracain *n*

dicephalous dizephal, mit zwei Köpfen

dichloroisoproterenol Dichlorisoproterenol *n*

dichotomisation Zweiteilung *f*, Aufteilung *f* in zwei Gruppen, Dichotomisierung *f*

dichotomous zweigeteilt

dichotomy Zweiteilung *f*, Dichotomie *f* / **graded ~** abgestufte Zweiteilung *f*

dichroic zweifarbig

dichroism Zweifarbigkeit *f*, Dichroismus *m*

dichromasia, dichromasy, dichromatism, dichromatopsia Dichromasie *f*, Dichromatopsie *f*, Zweifarbensehen *n*, dichromatisches Sehen *n*, Fähigkeit *f* nur zwei Grundfarben zu unterscheiden / **anomalous ~** dichromatische Anomalie *f*

dichromat Dichromat *m*, nur dichromatisch sehender Mensch *m*

dichromatic, dichromic zweifarbig

diction Diktion *f*, Sprechweise *f*, Ausdrucksweise *f*, Sprache *f*

dictionary Wörterbuch *n*

didactic didaktisch

didactics Didaktik *f*, Unterrichtslehre *f*

diencephalic dienzephal, zum Zwischenhirn gehörig

diencephalon Zwischenhirn *n*, Dienzephalon *n*

diet Diät *f*, Ernährung *f* / **ketogenic ~** ketogene Diät *f*

dietetics Diätlehre *f*, Ernährungskunde *f*

difference Unterschied *m*, Differenz *f* / **~ canon** Unterschiedsregel *f* / **~ judgment** Unterschiedsurteil *m* / **~ limen** Differenzlimen *n*, Unterschiedsschwelle *f* / **~s of sensation** merkliche Unterschiede *mpl* / **~ threshold** Unterschiedsschwelle *f*, Grenzreiz *m* / **~ tone** Differenzton *m* / **cross–cultural ~s** interkulturelle Unterschiede *mpl* / **cultural ~s** kulturelle Unterschiede *mpl* / **developmental ~** Entwicklungsunterschied *m* / **disappearing ~s method** Methode *f* der verschwindenden Unterschiede / **equally noticeable ~s** gleich wahrnehmbare Unterschiede *mpl* / **ethnic ~s** Volksunterschiede *mpl* / **imperceptible ~** unmerklicher Unterschied *m* / **individual ~s** individuelle Unterschiede *mpl* / **just noticeable ~** eben merklicher Unterschied *m* / **just not noticeable ~** eben nicht merklicher Unterschied *m* / **least–noticeable ~** geringster wahrnehmbarer Unterschied *m* / **least–perceptible ~** eben wahrnehmbarer Unterschied *m* / **liminal ~** eben wahrnehmbarer Unterschied *m*, eben merklicher Unterschied *m* / **marked ~** merklicher Unterschied *m* / **perceptual ~s** Wahrnehmungsunterschiede *mpl* / **potential ~** Potentialdifferenz *f* / **racial ~** Rassenunterschied *m* / **racial and ethnic ~s** ethnische und Rassenunterschiede *mpl* / **regional ~s** regionale Unterschiede *mpl* / **relative ~ threshold** relative Unterschiedsschwelle *f* / **sensed ~** merklicher Unterschied *m* / **significant ~** signifikanter Unterschied *m* / **supraliminal ~** deutlich wahrnehmbarer Unterschied *m*

differential verschieden, differentiell / Differential *n* / **~ diagnostic** differentialdiagnostisch / **semantic ~** semantisches Differential *n*, Polaritätsprofil *n*

differentiate differenzieren

differentiation Differenzierung *f*, Unterscheidung *f* / ~ **of life space** Differenzierung *f* des Lebensraums / ~ **process** Differenzierungsvorgang *m*

difficulty Schwierigkeit *f* / ~ **in education** Erziehungsschwierigkeit *f* / ~ **level** Schwierigkeitsniveau *n* / ~ **scale** Schwierigkeitsabstufung *f* / **adaptive** ~ Anpassungsschwierigkeit *f* / **educational** ~ Erziehungsschwierigkeit *f*

diffidence mangelndes Selbstvertrauen *n*, Schüchternheit *f*, übermäßige Bescheidenheit *f*

diffluent zerfließend

diffraction Brechung *f* / ~ **grating** Reflexionsgitter *n*, Gitterspektrum *n*

diffuse diffus, zerstreut / sich vermischen, verbreiten

diffusion Diffusion *f*, Ausstrahlung *f*, Irradiation *f* / ~ **barrier** Diffusionsbarriere *f* / ~ **circle** Irradiationskreis *m* / ~ **constant** Diffusionskoeffizient *m*, Diffusionskonstante *f* / ~ **potential** Diffusionspotential *n* / **motor** ~ unkoordinierte Bewegungen *fpl*

diffusive Diffusions–, weitläufig

diffusionism Diffusionstheorie *f*

digestion Verdauung *f*

digestive digestiv, Verdauungs–

digit Ziffer *f*, einstellige Zahl *f* / **~–span** kurzzeitiges Zahlengedächtnis *n* / **~–span test** Zahlengedächtnistest *m* / ~ **symbol test** Zahlensymboltest *m* / ~ **transformation** Zahlenumwandlung *f* / **binary** ~ Binärziffer *f*, Bit *n*

digital digital / **~–to–analog converter** Digital–Analog–Wandler *m*

digraph Digraph *m*

digram Digramm *n*

digression Abschweifung *f*, Abweichung *f* vom Normalbereich

dihydro|codeine Dihydrocodein *n* / ~ **ergotamine** Dihydroergotamin *n*, hydriertes Mutterkornalkaloid *n* / ~ **ergotoxine** Dihydroergotoxin *n* / ~ **testosterone** Dihydrotestosteron *n*

3,4–dihydroxyphenylalanine 3,4–Dihydroxyphenylalanin *n*, Dopa *n*

dihydroxytryptamine Dihydroxytryptamin *n*

dilapidation Verfall *m*, Niedergang *m*, Zerstörung *f*

dilatant dilatiert

dilatation Erweiterung *f*, Ausdehnung *f*, Dilatation *f* / ~ **of consciousness** Bewusstseinserweiterung *f*

dilate erweitern, weitermachen, dilatieren

dilemma Dilemma *n*, ausweglos erscheinende Konfliktsituation *f*

dimension Dimension *f* / **~s of personality** Persönlichkeitsdimensionen *fpl* / **psychological** ~ psychologische Dimension *f* / **third** ~ dritte Dimension *f*

dimensionality Dimensionalität *f*

dimethyltryptamine Dimethyltryptamin *n*

2,5–dimethoxy–4–methylamphetamine 2,5–Dimethoxy–4–methylamphetamin *n*

diminishing vermindernd, abklingend / Abschwächung *f*, Verminderung *f*

diminution Verminderung *f*, Verkleinerung *f*, Nachlassen *n*

diminutive klein, verkleinernd

dimming Abblendung *f* / ~ **effect** Abblendeffekt *m* / **chromatic** ~ Farbabschwächung *f*

dimness Sehschwäche *f*

dimorphic, dimorphous dimorph, in zwei Formen vorkommend

dimorphism Dimorphismus *m*, Zweigestaltigkeit *f*

dinomania Tanzwut *f*

dinophobia Angst *f* vor Schwindel, Höhenangst *f*

Diogenes syndrome Diogenes–Syndrom *n*

dionysian, dionysiac dionysisch

diopter, dioptre Dioptrie *f*, Brechkrafteinheit *f*

dioptrics Refraktionslehre *f*, Dioptrik *f*

dioptry Brechkraft *f*

diotic binaural, beide Ohren betreffend

diphasic zweiphasig, biphasisch, diphasisch

diphenhydramine Diphenhydramin *n*, Benadryl *n*

diphenylhydantoin Diphenylhydantoin *n*, Phenytoin *n* / **~ sodium** Diphenylhydantoin *n*, Phenytoin *n*

diphonia Doppelstimme *f*, Diplophonie *f*

diphtong Diphthong *m*, Doppelvokal *m*

diphthongia Doppelstimme *f*, Diplophonie *f*

diplacusis Diplakusis *f*, Doppelhören *n*

diplegia Diplegie *f*, doppelseitige Lähmung *f* / **spastic ~** Littlesche Krankheit *f*

diplegic Diplegie–

diploid diploid, mit zwei Chromosomensätzen versehen

diploidy Diploidie *f*

diplophonia Diplophonie *f*, Doppelstimme *f*

diplopia Diplopie *f*, Doppelsehen *n*, Doppeltsehen *n*, Doppelsichtigkeit *f*

diplopic doppelsichtig

dipolar bipolar, zweipolig

dipole Dipol *m*

dippoldism Dippoldismus *m*, Prügeln *n* von Kindern

diprosopus Fötus *m* mit zwei Gesichtern, Januskopf *m*

dipso|mania Trunksucht *f*, periodischer Alkoholismus *m*, Quartalsäufertum *n*, Dipsomanie *f* / **~maniac** Alkoholiker *m*, Quartalsäufer *m*, Trinker *m*, / trunksüchtig / **~phobia** krankhafte Angst *f* vor alkoholischen Getränken / **~rexia** Dipsorexis *f*

dire schrecklich, schlimm

direct direkt, unmittelbar / lenken, leiten

directed gelenkt, gerichtet, geführt

directedness Gerichtetheit *f*, Einstellung *f* auf ein Ziel

direction Richtung *f*, Leitung *f*, Anweisung *f* / **~ of conduction** Leitungsrichtung *f* / **~ of motion** Bewegungsrichtung *f* / **~ of sound** Schallrichtung *f* / **~ perception** Richtungswahrnehmung *f* / **~ of vision** Sehrichtung *f* / **psychodynamic ~** psychodynamische Gerichtetheit *f*

director Leiter *m*, Direktor *m*, Aufsichtsratsmitglied *n*

dirt Dreck *m*, Schmutz *m*, Kot *m* / **~ eating** Geophagie *f*, Erdessen *n*

dirty schmutzig, gemein, niederträchtig

disability Unfähigkeit *f*, Untauglichkeit *f*, Arbeitsunfähigkeit *f* / **~ assessment** Renteneinstufung *f* / **~ discrimination** Behindertendiskriminierung *f* / **~ evaluation** Invaliditätsbegutachtung *f* / **~ laws** Behindertenrecht *n* / **~ management** betriebliche Maßnahmen *fpl* für Behinderte / **developmental ~** Entwicklungsstörung *f* / **physical ~** körperliche Behinderung *f* / **sensory ~** sensorische Behinderung *f*

disabled Behinderte *m,f* / arbeitsunfähig, versehrt / **adventitiously ~** Behinderte *m,f* mit erworbener Behinderung / **aurally ~** Hörbehinderte *m,f* / **congenitally ~** Behinderte *m,f* mit angeborener Behinderung / **multiply ~** mehrfachbehindert / Mehrfachbehinderte *m,f* / **physically ~** körperbehindert / Körperbehinderte *m,f* / **sensorially ~** sensorisch behindert / sensorisch Behinderte *m,f* / **visually ~** sehbehindert / Sehbehinderte *m,f*

disablement Arbeitsunfähigkeit *f*, Dienstunfähigkeit *f*

disabuse befreien, erleichtern

disadvantaged benachteiligt / Benachteiligte *m,f* / **culturally ~** kulturell benachteiligt / **economically ~** wirtschaftlich benachteiligt / **socially ~** sozial benachteiligt

disaffection Abgeneigtheit *f*, Abneigung *f*

disaggregation Zerfall *m*, Auflösung *f*

disagree nicht übereinstimmen, nicht zustimmen

disagreeable unangenehm, unannehmlich, unliebsam, störend

disagreeableness Unannehmlichkeit *f*

disagreement Unstimmigkeit *f*, Diskrepanz *f*, Uneinigkeit *f*

disappointment Enttäuschung *f*

disapprobation Missbilligung *f*, Tadel *m*, Verurteilung *f*

disapproval Missbilligung *f*, Missfallen *n* / **social ~** soziale Missbilligung *f*

disassociated abgespalten

disassociation Dissoziation *f*, Trennung *f*, Abspaltung *f* / **~ of the ego** Ich–Spaltung *f* / **~ of the personality** Persönlichkeitsspaltung *f*

disaster Katastrophe *f* / **natural ~** Naturkatastrophe *f*

disavowal Verleugnung *f*, Nichtanerkennung *f*

disbelief Unglaube *m*, Zweifel *m*

disc Scheibe *f* / **optic ~** Papille *f*, Sehnerveneintritt *m* / **stroboscopic ~** Stroboskop *n*, Stroboskop–Scheibe *f*

discarnate fleischlos, körperlos

discernible, discernable merklich, unterscheidbar, erkennbar

discernment Unterscheidungsfähigkeit *f*, Urteilskraft *f*, Einsicht *f*

discharge Entladung *f*, Abfuhr *f* / entladen / **~ after reflex** reflektorische Nachentladung *f* / **~ frequency** Entladungsfrequenz *f* / **~ of affect** Affektentladung *f* / **~ of anxiety** Angstabfuhr *f* / **~ of excitation** Reizentladung *f*, Reizabfuhr *f* / **~ of stimulus** Reizentladung *f*, Reizabfuhr *f* / **~ planning** Entlassungsvorbereitung *f* / **~ psychosis** Freiheitspsychose *f* / **catamenial ~** Monatsblutung *f*, Menstruation *f* / **cerebral ~** hirnelektrische Entladung *f* / **epileptic ~** Krampfentladung *f* / **motor ~** motorische Entladung *f* / **nervous ~** Nervenentladung *f* / **neural ~** Nervenentladung *f* / **primary ~** Primärentladung *f* / **seminal ~** Samenerguß *m* / **spontaneous ~** Spontanentladung *f*

discharger Erregerreiz *m*

disciplinary, disciplinarian disziplinarisch, erzieherisch

discipline Disziplin *f*, Unterrichtsfach *n* / **basic ~** Grundlagenfach *n*, Grundfach *n* / **formal ~** formales Bildungsfach *n* / **formal theory ~** Theorie *f* der formalen Bildung

disclosure Enthüllung *f*, Preisgabe *f*

discomfit verwirren / Verwirrung *f*, Enttäuschung *f*

discomfort Unbehagen *n* / Unbehagen verursachen / **~ glare** unangenehme Blendung *f* / **~–relief quotient** Unzufriedenheits–Zufriedenheitsquotient *m* / **diffuse ~** allgemeines Unbehagen *n*

disconnect trennen, abschalten

disconnection Trennung *f*

discontent Unzufriedenheit *f*, Unzufriedener *m* / unzufrieden / unzufrieden machen

discontinuation Unterbrechung *f*, Abbrechen *n*

discontinue unterbrechen, aufgeben, aufhören

discontinuity Diskontinuität *f*, Unterbrechung *f* / **~ theory of learning** Theorie *f* des diskontinuierlichen Lernens

discontinuous unterbrochen, diskontinuierlich

discord Zwietracht *f*, Dissonanz *f*

discordance, discordancy Diskordanz *f*, Missklang *m*

discourage entmutigen, abraten

discourse analysis Diskursanalyse *f*

discover entdecken, einsehen

discovery teaching method nicht–direktive Lehrmethode *f*, entdeckendes Lernen *n*

discrepancy Diskrepanz *f*, Unstimmigkeit *f* / **affective ~** affektive Diskrepanz *f*

discrete einzeln, getrennt, diskret

discretion Besonnenheit *f*, Klugheit *f*, Diskretion *f*, Ermessen *n*

discrimen, discriminandum Unterscheidungsmerkmal *n*

discrimeter, serial Psychergograph *m*

discriminability Unterscheidbarkeit *f*, Unterscheidungsfähigkeit *f*

discriminal Diskriminations–, Unterscheidungs–

discriminate unterscheiden, diskriminieren, benachteiligen

discrimination Unterscheidung *f*, Diskrimination *f*, Unterscheidungsfähigkeit *f*, Unterscheidungsvermögen *n*, Diskriminierung *f* / **~ experiment** Unterscheidungsversuch *m* / **~ learning** Unterscheidungslernen *n*, Diskriminationslernen *n* / **~–reaction time** Reaktionszeit *f* bis zur Unterscheidung / **~ response** Unterscheidungsreaktion *f* / **~ time** Diskriminationszeit *f*, Zeit *f* bis zur Unterscheidung (dargebotener Reize) / **~ training** Unterscheidungsübung *f*, Diskriminationstraining *n* / **auditory ~** akustische Differenzierung *f*, auditive Diskriminierung *f* / **cognitive ~** kognitive Diskrimination *f* / **differential ~** verschiedenartige Diskrimination *f*, multiple Unterscheidung *f* / **errorless ~ learning** fehlerloses Unterscheidungslernen *n* / **kinaesthetic ~** kinästhetische Unterscheidung *f* / **operant ~** nichtreizgebundene Unterscheidung *f*, operantes Diskriminieren *n* / **perceptual ~** Wahrnehmungsunterscheidung *f*, perzeptive Diskrimination *f* / **racial ~** Rassendiskriminierung *f* / **respondent ~** unterscheidende Reaktion *f* / **sensory ~** sensorische Unterscheidung *f* / **simultaneous ~ learning** gleichzeitiges Unterscheidungslernen *n* / **social ~** soziale Diskriminierung *f* / **spatial ~** räumliche Unterscheidungsfähigkeit *f* / **spontaneous ~** spontane Unterscheidung *f* / **successive ~ learning** sukzessives Unterscheidungslernen *n* / **tactile ~** Tastunterscheidung *f* / **tactual ~** Tastunterscheidung *f* / **visual ~** visuelle Diskrimination *f*

discriminative, discriminatory unterscheidend, diskriminierend, Unterscheidungs–

discursive diskursiv

discussion Diskussion *f*, Besprechung *f*, Erörterung *f* / **~ group** Gesprächsgruppe *f* / **~ leader** Diskussionsleiter/in *m,f* / **directed ~ method** Methode *f* der gelenkten Diskussion, gelenkte Gruppendiskussion *f* / **nondirected ~ method** Methode *f* der freien Diskussion, nichtdirektiver Diskussionsstil *m*

disease Krankheit *f*, Erkrankung *f*, Leiden *n* / **~s of the nervous system** Nervenkrankheiten *fpl* / **autoaggressive ~** Autoimmunerkrankung *f* / **autoimmune ~** Autoimmunerkrankung *f*, Autoimmunkrankheit *f* / **catatonic ~** Katatonie *f*, Spannungsirresein *n* / **cerebral ~** Hirnleiden *n*, Enzephalopathie *f* / **constitutional ~** Konstitutionskrankheit *f* / **degenerative ~** degenerative Erkrankung *f* / **demyelinating ~s** Entmarkungskrankheiten *fpl* / **developmental ~** Entwicklungsstörung *f* / **dynamic ~** funktionelle Krankheit *f* / **familial ~** Familienkrankheit *f* / **genetic ~** genetische Erkrankung *f* / **hereditary ~** Erbleiden *n*, Erbkrankheit *f* / **iatrogenic ~** vom Arzt verursachte Krankheit *f* / **idiopathic ~** Grundkrankheit *f* / **local ~** örtliches Leiden *n*, Lokalerkrankung *f* / **masked ~** versteckte Krankheit *f* / **mental ~** Geisteskrankheit *f*, Störung *f* der Geistesfunktion / **nervous ~** Nervenleiden *n* / **occupational ~** Berufskrankheit *f* / **parasitic ~** Parasitenbefall *m*, parasitäre Erkrankung *f* / **psychosomatic ~** psychosomatische Erkrankung *f* / **psychotic ~** Psychose *f*, Geisteskrankheit *f* / **sexual ~** Geschlechtskrankheit *f* / **sexually transmitted ~** sexuell übertragene Krankheit *f* / **somatic ~** körperliches Leiden *n* / **venereal ~** Geschlechtskrankheit *f*

diseased krank, erkrankt

disequilibrium Gleichgewichtsstörung *f* / **mental ~** geistige Unausgeglichenheit *f*

disfiguration, disfigurement Entstellung *f*, Verunstaltung *f* / **physical ~** körperliche Entstellung *f*

disguise maskieren, tarnen, überlagern / Maskierung *f*, Larvierung *f*, Überlagerung *f* / **symbolic ~ of symptom** Maskierungssymptom *n*

disguised maskiert, larviert

disgust Ekel *m*, Widerwille *m*

dishabituation Dishabituation *f*

disharmonious unharmonisch

disharmony Disharmonie *f* / **affective ~** emotionales Ungleichgewicht *n*

dishonesty Unredlichkeit *f*, Unehrlichkeit *f*

disillusion Ernüchterung *f*, Desillusionierung *f*

disinhibition Enthemmung *f*

disintegration Desintegration *f*, Zerfall *m*, Auflösung *f* / **mental ~** psychischer Zerfall *m*, geistige Desintegration *f* / **psychic ~** psychischer Abbau *m*, psychischer Zerfall *m* / **social ~** Gruppenzerfall *m*

disintoxication Entgiftung *f*, Entziehung *f*

disjection Streuung *f*, Zerstreuung *f*

disjunctive trennend, divergent, disjunktiv

disk Datenträger *m*, Platte *f* / **floppy ~** Diskette *f* / **intercalated ~** Glanzstreifen *m* / **magnetic–~ storage** Magnetplattenspeicher *m* / **stroboscopic ~** Stroboskop *n*, Stroboskop–Scheibe *f*

dislike Abneigung *f*, Aversion *f*, Widerwille *m* / ablehnen, nicht mögen / **~ of working** Arbeitsunlust *f*

dismay Bestürzung *f*, Schreck *m* / **reactive ~** Bestürztheit *f*, Bestürzung *f*

disobedience Ungehorsam *m* / **civil ~** ziviler Ungehorsam *m*

disorder Störung *f*, Leiden *n* / **~ of adult personality and behaviour** Persönlichkeits– und Verhaltensstörung *f* / **~ of articulation** artikulatorische Sprachstörung *f* / **~s of balance** Gleichgewichtsstörung *f* / **~ of behaviour** Verhaltensstörung *f* / **~ of the brain** Gehirnerkrankung *f* / **~ of the disposition of emotions** Bereitstellungskrankheit *f* / **~s of excessive somnolence** Störungen *fpl* mit exzessiver Schläfrigkeit / **~s of initiating and maintaining sleep** Einschlaf– und Durchschlafstörungen *fpl* / **~s of sexual preference** Störungen *fpl* der Sexualpräferenz / **~s of social functioning with onset specific to childhood and adolescence** Störungen *fpl* sozialer Funktionen mit Beginn in der Kindheit und Jugend / **~ of sound conduction** Schallleitungsstörung *f* / **~ of speech development** Sprachentwicklungsstörung *f* / **~ of thought process** formale Denkstörung *f* / **~s usually first diagnosed in infancy, childhood, or adolescence** Störungen *fpl*, die gewöhnlich zuerst im Kleinkindesalter, in der Kindheit oder Adoleszenz diagnostiziert werden / **~ of written expression** Störung *f* des schriftlichen Ausdrucks / **acute and transient psychotic ~ (unspecified)** (nicht näher bezeichnete) akute vorübergehende psychotische Störung *f* / **acute paranoid ~** akute paranoide Störung *f* / **acute polymorphic psychotic ~ without symptoms of schizophrenia** akute polymorphe psychotische Störung *f* ohne Symptome einer Schizophrenie / **acute schizophrenia–like psychotic ~** akute schizophreniforme psychotische Störung *f* / **affective ~** affektive Störung *f*, Affektstörung *f*, affektive Psychose *f*, Affektpsychose *f* / **allergic ~** Allergie *f*, allergische Erkrankung *f* / **amnestic ~ due to a general medical condition** amnestische Störung *f* aufgrund eines medizinischen Krankheitsfaktors / **amnestic ~ not otherwise specified** nicht näher bezeichnete amnestische Störung *f* / **amphetamine–induced psychotic ~** amphetamininduzierte psychotische Störung *f* / **atypical dissociative ~** atypische dissoziative Störung *f* / **atypical factitious ~ with physical symptoms** atypische vorgetäuschte Störung *f* mit körperlichen

Symptomen / **atypical paranoid ~** atypische paranoide Störung *f* / **atypical somatoform ~** atypische somatoforme Störung *f* / **autistic ~** autistische Störung *f* / **avoidant ~ of childhood or adolescence** vermeidende Störung *f* in der Kindheit und Jugend / **bacterial ~** bakterielle Erkrankung *f* / **behavioural and emotional ~s with onset usually occurring in childhood and adolescence** Verhaltens– und emotionale Störungen *fpl* mit Beginn in der Kindheit und Jugend / **bipolar ~** bipolare Störung *f*, bipolare Depression *f* / **bipolar I ~** bipolar I Störung *f* / **bipolar II ~** bipolar II Störung *f* / **bipolar affective ~** bipolare affektive Störung *f* / **bipolar affective ~, current episode manic with psychotic symptoms** bipolare affektive Störung *f*, gegenwärtig manische Episode mit psychotischen Symptomen / **bipolar affective ~, current episode severe depression with psychotic symptoms** bipolare affektive Störung *f*, gegenwärtig schwere depressive Episode mit psychotischen Symptomen / **bipolar affective ~, currently in remission** bipolare affektive Störung *f*, gegenwärtig remittiert / **brief psychotic ~** kurze psychotische Störung *f* / **bronchial ~** Bronchialkrankheit *f* / **caffeine–induced ~** koffeininduzierte Störung *f* / **cardiac ~** Herzstörung *f* / **cardiovascular ~** Herz–Kreislauf–Störung *f*, kardiovaskuläre Störung *f* / **catatonic ~** katatone Störung *f* / **cerebral ~** zerebrale Störung *f* / **cerebrovascular ~** Gehirngefäßerkrankung *f*, Hirngefäßstörung *f* / **chronic neuropsychologic ~** chronisches psychoorganisches Syndrom *n* / **circulatory ~** Kreislaufstörung *f* / **clinical ~** klinische Störung *f* / **cognitive ~ not otherwise specified** nicht näher bezeichnete kognitive Störung *f* / **congenital ~** angeborenes Gebrechen *n*, angeborene Krankheit *f* / **convulsive ~** Krampfleiden *n* / **coronary ~** Herzleiden *n*, Koronarerkrankung *f* / **cyclic ~** zirkuläres Irrsein *n* / **cyclothymic ~** zyklothyme Störung *f* / **delusional ~** wahnhafte Störung *f* / **delusional ~, erotomanic type** wahnhafte Störung *f*, Typus mit Liebeswahn / **delusional ~, grandiose type** wahnhafte Störung *f*, Typus mit Größenwahn / **delusional ~, jealous type** wahnhafte Störung *f*, Typus mit Eifersuchtswahn / **delusional ~, persecutory type** wahnhafte Störung *f*, Typus mit Verfolgungswahn / **delusional ~, somatic type** wahnhafte Störung *f*, Typus mit körperbezogenem Wahn / **depressive ~** depressive Störung *f*, Depression *f* / **developmental ~ of motor function** Entwicklungsstörung *f* der motorischen Funktionen / **developmental ~ of scholastic skills** Entwicklungsstörung *f* schulischer Fertigkeiten / **developmental ~ of speech and language** Entwicklungsstörung *f* des Sprechens und der Sprache / **developmental arithmetic ~** entwicklungsbezogene Rechenstörung *f* / **dissociative ~** dissoziative Störung *f* / **dissociative ~s of movement and sensation** dissoziative Störungen *fpl* der Bewegung und der Sinnesempfindung / **dissociative motor ~s** dissoziative Bewegungsstörungen *fpl* / **dysthymic ~** dysthyme Störung *f*, Dysthymie *f* / **emotional ~** Affektstörung *f*, emotionale Störung *f* / **emotional ~ with onset specific to childhood** emotionale Störung des Kindesalters / **endocrine ~** Hormonstörung *f*, endokrine Störung *f* / **endocrine sexual ~** endokrin bedingte Sexualstörung *f* / **ethnic ~** Volkskrankheit *f* / **ethnospecific ~** spezifische Volkskrankheit *f*, ethnospezifische Störung *f* / **factitious ~** vorgetäuschte Störung *f*, simulierte Krankheit *f* / **factitious ~ with combined psychological and physical signs and symptoms** vorgetäuschte Störung *f* mit sowohl psychischen wie körperlichen Zeichen und Symptomen / **factitious ~ with predominantly psychological (physical) signs and symptoms** vorgetäuschte Störung *f* mit vorwiegend psychischen (körperlichen) Zeichen und Symptomen / **female orgasmic ~** weibliche Orgasmusstörung *f* / **focal neurological ~** fokale neurologische Störung *f* / **functional ~** Funktionsstörung *f*, Dysfunktion *f* / **functional nervous ~** nervös bedingte funktionelle Störung *f* / **gastrointestinal ~** Magen–Darm–Störung *f*, gastrointestinale Störung *f* / **genetic ~** genetische Störung *f*, Erbfehler *m* / **genital ~** Sexualstörung *f*, genitale Störung *f*, Erkrankung *f* des Genitalapparats / **gynaecological ~** gynäkologische Störung *f*, Frauenleiden *n* / **hallucinogen–induced psychotic ~** halluzinogeninduzierte psychotische Störung *f* / **hallucinogen–induced organic mental ~** halluzinogeninduzierte organisch bedingte psychische Störung *f* / **hepatic ~** Leberleiden *n* / **hereditary ~** Erbfehler *m*, genetische Störung *f* / **holergastic ~** psychobiologische Funktionsstörung *f* / **hyperkinetic ~** hyperkinetische Störung *f* / **hypochondriacal ~** hypochondrische Störung *f* / **idiopathic ~** idiopathisches Leiden *n* / **immunologic ~** Störung *f* der Krankheitsabwehr, immunologische Störung *f* / **induced delusional ~** induzierte wahnhafte Störung *f* / **induced paranoid ~** induzierte paranoide Störung *f*, Folie à deux *f* / **induced psychotic ~** induzierte psychotische Störung *f*, Folie à deux *f* / **infectious ~** Infektionskrankheit *f* / **intermittent explosive (behavior) ~** Störung *f* mit intermittierend auftretender Reizbarkeit, intermittierende explosible Störung *f* / **isolated explosive ~** isolierte explosive Störung / **laryngeal ~** Kehlkopfleiden *n*, Kehlkopfkrankheit *f* / **lymphatic ~** Erkrankung *f* des lymphatischen Systems / **major depressive ~** Major Depression *f* / **male erectile ~** Erektionsstörung *f* beim Mann / **male genital ~** Erkrankung *f* der männlichen Geschlechtsorgane, genitale Störung *f* bei Männern / **male orgasmic ~** männliche Orgasmusstörung *f* / **material ~ of the mental process** inhaltliche Denkstörung *f* / **menstrual ~** Menstruationsstörung *f* / **mental ~** Geistesstörung *f*, psychische Störung *f*, Geistesgestörtheit *f* / **mental and behavioural ~s associated with the puerperium, not elsewhere classified** psychische oder Verhaltensstörungen *fpl* im Wochenbett, nicht andernorts klassifizierbar / **mental and behavioural ~s due to psychoactive substance use** psychische und Verhaltensstörungen *fpl* durch psychotrope Substanzen / **mental and behavioural ~s due to use of alcohol** psychische und Verhaltensstörungen *fpl* durch Alkohol / **mild cognitive ~** leichte kognitive Störung *f* / **mixed ~ of conduct and emotions** kombinierte Störung *f* des Sozialverhaltens und der Emotionen / **mixed ~ of scholastic skills** kombinierte Störung *f* schulischer Fertigkeiten / **mnestic ~** Gedächtnisstörung *f* / **motor ~** Bewegungsstörung *f*, Bewegungsablaufstörung *f* / **muscular ~** Muskelerkrankung *f* / **musculoskeletal ~** Skelettmuskelerkrankung *f* / **neonatal ~** Neugeborenenerkrankung *f* / **neonatal genetic ~** Neugeborenen–Erbkrankheit *f* / **neurological ~** neurologische Störung *f*, Nervenleiden *n* / **neuromuscular ~** neuromuskuläre Störung *f* / **neurotic ~** neurotische Störung *f*, Neurose *f* / **neurotic, stress–related and somatoform ~s** neurotische, Belastungs– und somatoforme Störungen *fpl* / **nonmood psychotic ~** nicht–affektive psychotische Störung *f* / **nonorganic ~ of the sleep–wake schedule** nichtorganische Störung *f* des Schlaf–Wach–Rhythmus / **obsessional ~** Zwang *m* / **obsessive–compulsive ~** Zwangsstörung *f*, Zwangssyndrom *n* / **oppositional ~** Trotzverhalten *n* / **oppositional defiant ~** Störung *f* mit oppositionellem Trotzverhalten, Störung *f* des Sozialverhaltens mit oppositionellem aufsässigem Verhalten / **organic ~** organische Störung *f* / **organic affective ~s** organische affektive Störungen *fpl* / **organic bipolar affective ~** organische bipolare Störung *f* / **organic catatonic ~** organische katatone Störung *f* / **organic delusional (schizophrenia–like) ~** organische wahnhafte (schizophreniforme) Störung *f* / **organic depressive ~** organische depressive Störung *f* / **organic dissociative ~** organische dissoziative Störung *f* / **organic emotionally labile (asthenic) ~** organische emotional labile (asthenische) Störung *f* / **organic manic ~** organische manische Störung *f* / **organic mental ~** organisch bedingte psychische Störung *f* / **organic mixed affective ~** organische gemischte affektive Störung *f* / **other acute and transient psychotic ~s** sonstige akute vorübergehende psychotische Störungen *fpl* / **other acute predominantly delusional psychotic ~s** sonstige akute vorwiegend wahnhafte psychotische Störungen *fpl* / **other bipolar affective ~s** sonstige bipolare affektive Störungen *fpl* / **other mental ~s due to brain damage or dysfunction or to physical disease** sonstige psychische Störungen *fpl* aufgrund einer Schädigung oder Funktionsstörung des Gehirns oder einer körperlichen Krankheit / **other nonorganic psychotic ~** sonstige nichtorganische psychotische Störung *f* / **other recurrent depressive ~s** sonstige rezidivierende depressive Störungen *fpl* / **other schizoaffective ~s** sonstige schizoaffektive Störungen *fpl* / **other specific affective ~s** sonstige spezifische affektive Störungen *fpl* / **other specified organic mental ~s due to brain damage or dysfunction or to physical disease** sonstige näher bezeichnete organische psychische Störungen *fpl* aufgrund einer Schädigung oder Funktionsstörung des Gehirns oder einer körperlichen Krankheit / **overactive ~ associated with mental retardation and stereotyped movements** überaktive Störung *f* mit Intelligenzminderung und Bewegungsstereotypien / **overanxious ~** Angstsyndrom *n* mit Überängstlichkeit / **overanxious ~ of childhood** Störung *f* mit Überängstlichkeit in der Kindheit / **parasitic ~** parasitäre Krankheit *f* / **parathyroid ~** Erkrankung *f* der Nebenschilddrüse / **paroxysmal ~** anfallsartig auftretende Störung *f* / **persistent affective ~s** anhaltende affektive Störungen *fpl* / **persistent delusional ~** anhaltende wahnhafte Störung *f* / **pervasive developmental ~s** tiefgreifende Entwicklungsstörungen *fpl* / **pharyngeal ~** Rachenerkrankung *f*, Erkrankung *f* des Rachenraums / **phobic ~** phobische Störung *f* / **phonological ~** phonologische Störung *f* / **physical ~** körperliche Krankheit *f* / **pituitary ~** Hypophysenstörung *f* / **primary mental ~** primäre psychische Störung *f* / **psychiatric ~** psychiatrische Erkrankung *f* / **psychic ~** psychische Störung *f* / **psychogenic ~** psychogene Störung *f* / **psychological and behavioural ~s associated with sexual development and orientation** psychische und Verhaltensstörungen *fpl* in Verbindung mit der sexuellen Entwicklung und Orientierung / **psychoneurotic ~** psychoneurotische Störung *f* / **psychophysiologic ~** psychosomatische Erkrankung *f* / **psychosomatic ~** psychosomatische Erkrankung *f*, psychosomatische Störung *f* / **psychotic ~** psychotische Störung *f* / **psychotic ~ due to a general medical condition** psychotische Störung *f* aufgrund eines medizinischen Krankheitsfaktors / **puerperal mental ~, unspecified** nicht näher bezeichnete psychische Störung *f* im Wochenbett / **recurrent depressive ~** rezidivierende depressive Störung *f* / **recurrent depressive ~, current episode severe with psychotic symptoms** rezidivierende depressive Störung *f*, gegenwärtig schwere Episode mit psychotischen Symptomen / **recurrent depressive ~, currently in remission** rezidivierende depressive Störung *f*, gegenwärtig remittiert / **residual affective ~** affektives (Rest–) Zustandsbild *n* / **residual and late–onset psychotic ~** Restzustand *m* und verzögert auftretende psychotische Störung *f* / **schizoaffective ~** schizoaffektive Störung *f* / **schizoaffective ~, depressive type** schizoaffektive Störung *f*, gegenwärtig depressiv / **schizoaffective ~, manic type** schizoaffektive Störung *f*, gegenwärtig manisch / **schizoaffective ~, mixed type** gemischte schizoaffektive Störung *f* / **schizoaffective ~, unspecified** nicht näher bezeichnete schizoaffektive Störung *f* / **schizoid ~ of childhood** schizoide Störung *f* im Kindesalter / **schizophrenic ~**

schizophrene Störung *f* / **schizophreniform ~** schizophreniforme Störung *f* / **schizotypal ~** schizotype Störung *f* / **sensory ~** Störung *f* der Sinnesempfindung / **seasonal affective ~** saisonal bedingte affektive Störung *f* / **sexual ~** Sexualstörung *f*, sexuelle Funktionsstörung *f* / **shared psychotic ~** gemeinsame psychotische Störung *f*, Folie à Deux *f* / **skeletomuscular ~** Skelettmuskelerkrankung *f* / **somatoform ~** somatoforme Störung *f* / **somatogenic ~** somatogene Störung *f* / **specific ~ of arithmetical skills** Rechenstörung *f* / **specific developmental ~s** umschriebene Entwicklungsstörungen *fpl* / **specific developmental ~ of motor function** umschriebene Entwicklungsstörung *f* der motorischen Funktionen / **specific developmental ~s of scholastic skills** umschriebene Entwicklungsstörungen *fpl* schulischer Fertigkeiten / **specific developmental ~s of speech and language** umschriebene Entwicklungsstörungen *fpl* des Sprechens und der Sprache / **thyroid ~** Schilddrüsenerkrankung *f* / **toxic ~** toxische Erkrankung *f*, Vergiftung *f* / **tracheal ~** Luftröhrenerkrankung *f* / **undifferentiated somatoform ~** undifferenzierte somatoforme Störung *f*, undifferenzierte Somatisierungsstörung *f* / **unspecified mental ~ (non–psychotic)** unspezifische psychische Störung *f* (nicht–psychotisch) / **unspecified organic mental ~ due to brain damage or dysfunction or to physical disease** nicht näher bezeichnete organische psychische Störung *f* aufgrund einer Schädigung oder Funktionsstörung des Gehirns oder einer körperlichen Krankheit / **unspecified mental and behavioural ~** nicht näher bezeichnete psychische und Verhaltensstörung *f* / **unspecified organic or symptomatic mental ~** nicht näher bezeichnete organische oder symptomatische psychische Störung *f* / **urogenital ~** Erkrankung *f* des Urogenitalsystems, urogenitale Störung *f* / **vascular ~** Gefäßleiden *n*, Kreislaufstörung *f* / **vegetative ~** vegetative Störung *f* / **viral ~** Viruserkrankung *f* / **visual ~** Sehstörung *f* / **schizoaffective ~** schizoaffektive Störung *f*

disorganization Zerfall *m*, Auflösung *f*, Desorganisation *f* / **~ of personality** Persönlichkeitsabbau *m* / **mental ~** geistiger Zerfall *m* / **schizophrenic ~** Persönlichkeitszerfall *m*

disorganized desorganisiert

disorientate verwirren

disorientated verwirrt, desorientiert

disorientation Desorientiertheit *f*, Bewusstseinstrübung *f*

disparate ungleich, disparat, verschiedenartig

disparity Disparation *f*, Verschiedenheit *f* / **binocular ~** Querdisparation *f* / **retinal ~** disparate Netzhautpunkte *mpl* / **visual ~** Querdisparation *f*

dispersal Verbreitung *f*

dispersion Streuung *f*, Dispersion *f* / **~ area** Streubereich *m* / **~ coefficient** Streuungskoeffizient *m* / **~ law** Dispersionsgesetz *n* / **chromatic ~** Farbenzerstreuung *f*, Farbendispersion *f* / **ergic ~** Reaktionszerfall *m* / **normal ~** normale Streuung *f*

dispersonalisation Persönlichkeitsverlust *m*, Depersonalisation *f*

displaced verschoben

displacement Verschiebung *f* / **~ activity** Ersatzhandlung *f*, Übersprunghandlung *f* / **~ of affects** Affektverschiebung *f* / **visual ~** visuelle Verschiebung *f*, prismatische Verschiebung *f*

display Vorführung *f*, Schaustellung *f*, Imponiergehabe *n*, Werbeauslage *f*, Warenausstellung *f*, Display *n* / **~ behaviour** Imponiergehabe *n* / **auditory ~** Werbedurchsage *f*, Ansage *f*, akustisches Display *n* / **graphical ~** graphische Darstellung *f* / **tactual ~** taktile Informationsdarbietung *f* / **visual ~** visuelle Informationsdarbietung *f*, Werbeauslage *f*

displeasure Unlust *f*, Missfallen *n*, Verdruss *m*

disposal Verfügung *f*

disposition Disposition *f*, Veranlagung *f*, Anlage *f*, Neigung *f*, Tendenz *f*, Hang *m* / **~ to learn** Lernvermögen *n*, Lernfähigkeit *f* / **~ of mind** Gemütsverfassung *f*, Temperament *n* / **~ to neurosis** neurotische Disposition *f*, neurotische Veranlagung *f* / **~ to rigidity** dispositionelle Rigidität *f* / **behavioural ~** Verhaltensdisposition *f* / **cycloid ~** zykloide Veranlagung *f* / **eidetic ~** eidetische Anlage *f* / **expressive ~** Ausdruckstendenz *f*, expressive Disposition *f* / **hereditary ~** Erbanlage *f* / **innate ~** angeborene Veranlagung *f* / **mental ~** geistige Veranlagung *f* / **nervous ~** nervöse Veranlagung *f* / **psychic ~** psychische Disposition *f* / **total ~** Gemütsverfassung *f*

dispossession Beraubung *f*, Enteignung *f*

dispraise tadeln

disproportion Missverhältnis *n*

disproportionate unverhältnismäßig

disputatious, disputative streitsüchtig

dispute Kontroverse *f*, Debatte *f*, Streit *m* / **industrial ~** Arbeitskonflikt *m*, Streik *m*, Tarifauseinandersetzung *f* / **matrimonial ~s** Ehestreitigkeiten *fpl*

disqualification Untauglichkeit *f*

disquiet unruhig / Unruhe *f*, Angst *f*

disremember vergessen

disruption Spaltung *f*, Zerreißung *f*

disruptive spaltend, disruptiv

dissatisfaction Unzufriedenheit *f*

dissatisfactory unbefriedigend

dissatisfied unzufrieden

dissatisfier Hygienefaktor *m*

dissect sezieren, auseinandernehmen

dissent Meinungsverschiedenheit *f* / nicht übereinstimmen

dissertation wissenschaftliche Abhandlung *f*, Dissertation *f*

dissident abweichend / Dissident *m*, Andersdenkender *m*

dissimilarity Verschiedenartigkeit *f*, Ungleichheit *f*

dissimilation Abbau *m*, Dissimilation *f*

dissimulate verbergen, sich verstellen, dissimulieren

dissimulation Verstellung *f*, Verheimlichung *f*, Heuchelei *f*, Dissimulation *f*

dissipation Vergeudung *f*, Verschwendung *f*, Ausschweifung *f*

dissociable unsozial

dissociated dissoziiert, abgespalten

dissociation Dissoziation *f*, Spaltung *f*, Trennung *f*, Auflösung *f*, Assoziationszerfall *m* / **~ amnesia** Dissoziationsamnesie *f* / **~ of consciousness** Bewusstseinsspaltung *f* / **~ of the ego** Ich–Spaltung *f* / **~ of ideas** Ideendissoziation *f* / **~ of personality** Persönlichkeitsspaltung *f* / **~ reaction** Spaltungsreaktion *f* / **~ of sensations** Empfindungsdissoziation *f* / **emotional ~** Empfindungsdissoziation *f*, Affektspaltung *f* / **mental ~** Bewusstseinsspaltung *f* / **sensory ~** Empfindungsdissoziation *f*

dissociative dissoziativ

dissofrustrance dissoziierte Frustration *f*

dissolution Auflösung *f*, Zersetzung *f*

dissonance Dissonanz *f* / **cognitive ~** kognitive Dissonanz *f*

dissymmetry Asymmetrie *f*

distal distal, von der Körpermitte abgewandt

distance Entfernung *f*, Distanz *f* / **~ between eyes** Augenabstand *m* / **~ discrimination** Unterscheidung *f* von Entfernungen / **~ estimate** Entfernungsschätzung *f* / **~ perception** Entfernungswahrnehmung *f* / **~ receptor** Fernempfangsorgan *n* / **~ sense** Fernsinn *m* / **~ type** Distanztyp *m* / **~ vision** Fernsicht *f* / **apparent ~** scheinbare Entfernung *f* / **focal ~** Brennweite *f* / **interocular ~** Augenabstand *m* / **long–~** Fern–, Weit–, über eine weite Entfernung / **psychic ~** seelische Distanz *f*, psychische Distanz *f* /

social ~ soziale Distanz *f*, sozialer Abstand *m* / ~ **scale** soziale Distanz–Skala *f* / **social–visual** ~ Sehabstand *m*

distant entfernt, zurückhaltend, kalt, distanziert

distaste Widerwille *m*, Abscheu *f*

distemper Verstimmung *f*

distension, distention Ausdehnung *f*, Streckung *f*, Weite *f*

disthymia Verstimmung *f*, Melancholie *f*

distinct getrennt, einzeln, deutlich, klar, ausgeprägt

distinction Unterscheidung *f*, ausgezeichnete Leistung *f*, Bedeutung *f*, auszeichnende Eigenschaft *f*, Individualität *f* / **qualitative** ~ qualitative Unterscheidung *f*

distinctiveness charakteristische Eigentümlichkeit *f*, Ausgeprägtheit *f*, Besonderheit *f*

distinctness Deutlichkeit *f*, Klarheit *f*

distorted verzerrt, entstellt

distortion Entstellung *f*, Verzerrung *f*, Verdrehung *f* / ~ **in dreams** Traumentstellung *f* / ~ **of dreams** Traumentstellung *f* / **electrotonic** ~ elektrotonische Verzerrung *f* / **parataxic** ~ parataktische Verzerrungen *fpl* / **perceptual** ~ Wahrnehmungsverzerrung *f*, Wahrnehmungsstörung *f* / **spatial** ~ räumliche Verzerrung *f* / **systematic** ~ systematische Verzerrung *f* / **unconscious** ~ unbewusste Verfälschung *f*

distract ablenken, verwirren, wahnsinnig machen

distractable ablenkbar

distracted verstört, zerstreut, unaufmerksam

distractibility Ablenkbarkeit *f*, Unachtsamkeit *f*

distraction Ablenkung *f*, Zerstreuung *f*, Verwirrtheit *f* / **drive to** ~ zum Wahnsinn treiben

distraught verzweifelt

distress Not *f*, Elend *n*, Kummer *m*, Qual *f* / ~ **call** Notschrei *m* / **dire** ~ schlimme Not *f* / **respiratory** ~ Atemnot *f*

distressing quälend, beunruhigend, schmerzlich

distributed verteilt

distribution Verteilung *f* / ~ **curve** Verteilungskurve *f* / ~**–free** verteilungsfrei / **asymmetrical** ~ asymmetrische Verteilung *f* / **asymptotic** ~ asymptotische Verteilung *f* / **bimodal** ~ zweigipflige Verteilung *f*, bimodale Verteilung *f* / **binomial** ~ Binomialverteilung *f* / **bivariate** ~ bivariate Verteilung *f* / **cumulative** ~ Häufigkeitsverteilung *f* / **cumulative** ~ **function** kumulative Häufigkeitsfunktion *f* / **exponential** ~ Exponentialverteilung *f* / **forced** ~ vorgegebene Verteilung *f* / **Gaussian** ~ Gauß'sche Verteilung *f*, Normalverteilung *f* / **grouped** ~ klassifizierte Verteilung *f* / **hypergeometric** ~ hypergeometrische Verteilung *f* / **leptokurtic** ~ steilgipflige Verteilung *f* / **mesokurtic** ~ normalgipflige Verteilung *f* / **multimodal** ~ mehrgipflige Verteilung *f* / **normal** ~ Normalverteilung *f* / **platykurtic** ~ abgeflachte Verteilung *f*, flachgipflige Verteilung *f* / **punctiform** ~ Punkteverteilung *f* / **rectilinear** ~ lineare Verteilung *f* / **skewed** ~ asymmetrische Verteilung *f*, schiefe Verteilung *f* / **symmetrical** ~ symmetrische Verteilung *f* / **unimodal** ~ eingipflige Verteilung *f*, unimodale Verteilungf / **U–shaped** ~ U–förmige Verteilung *f*

distributional Verteilungs–

distrust Misstrauen *n* / misstrauen

disturb stören, aufregen

disturbance Störung *f* / ~ **in associations** Lockerung *f* der Assoziation / ~ **in judgement** Urteilsstörung *f* / ~ **in regulation** Regulationsstörung *f* / ~ **in speech** Sprachstörung *f* / ~ **of accommodation** Akkomodationsstörung *f* / ~ **of activity and attention** einfache Aktivitäts– und Aufmerksamkeitsstörung *f* / ~ **of association** Assoziationsstörung *f* / ~ **of body image** Körperschemastörung *f* / ~ **of conduct** Störung *f* des Sozialverhaltens / ~ **of consciousness** Bewusstseinsstörung *f* / ~ **of development** Entwicklungsstörung *f* / ~ **of gait** Gehstörung *f* / ~ **of micturition** Blasenentleerungsstörung *f* / ~ **of mind** Geistesstörung *f* / ~ **of potency** Potenzstörung *f* / ~ **of smell** Geruchsstörung *f* / ~ **variable** Störgröße *f* / **affective** ~ Affektstörung *f* / **behavioural** ~ Verhaltensstörung *f* / **developmental** ~ Entwicklungsstörung *f* / **early** ~ frühe Störung *f* / **emotional** ~ Affektstörung *f*, Gefühlsstörung *f*, emotionale Störung *f* / **functional** ~ Funktionsstörung *f* / **gastrointestinal** ~ Magen–Darm–Störung *f* / **mental** ~ Geistesstörung *f*, psychische Störung *f* / **nervous** ~ nervöse Störung *f* / **perceptual** ~ Wahrnehmungsstörung *f* / **psychic** ~ psychische Störung *f* / **psychological** ~ psychische Störung *f* / **psychomotoric** ~ psychomotorische Störung *f* / **sensory** ~ sensorische Störung *f* / **situational** ~ situative Störung *f* / **visual** ~ Sehstörung *f*

disturbed gestört / **emotionally** ~ gemütskrank, emotional gestört / **mentally** ~ geistesgestört

disulfiram Disulfiram *n*, Tetraethylthiuramdisulfid *n*

disunion Trennung *f*

disuse Entwöhnung *f*, Absetzen *n*

ditention Aufmerksamkeitsspaltung *f*, geteilte Aufmerksamkeit *f*

diuresis Diurese *f*, Harnausscheidung *f*, Wasserlassen *n*

diuretic diuretisch, die Harnausscheidung betreffend / harntreibendes Mittel *n*, Diuretikum *n*

diurnal diurnal, tageszyklisch, Tages–

divagation Zerfahrenheit *f*, unzusammenhängende Sprache *f*, unzusammenhängendes Denken *n*, Divagation *f*

divergence, divergency Divergenz *f*, Abweichung *f*

divergent divergierend, abweichend, divergent

diversification Veränderung *f*, Abwechslung *f* / **verbal** ~ sprachliche Abwechslung *f*

diversiform verschiedenartig, vielgestaltig

diversion Ablenkung *f*, Zerstreuung *f*

diversity Verschiedenheit *f*, Mannigfaltigkeit *f*

divination Weissagung *f*, Prophezeiung *f*

divine, divining rod Wünschelrute *f*

diviner Wahrsager *m*, Wünschelrutengänger *m*

divinity Gott *m*, Gottheit *f*

divisibility Teilbarkeit *f*

division Teilung *f*, Spaltung *f*, Abteilung *f* / ~ **of the ego** Ich–Spaltung *f*, Spaltung *f* des Ichs / ~ **of labour** Arbeitsteilung *f* / **nuclear** ~ Kernteilung *f*

divorce Ehescheidung *f*, Scheidung *f*, Trennung *f*

dizygotic zweieiig, dizygot

dizziness Schwindel *m*, Vertigo *m* / **psychogenic** ~ Pseudoschwindel *m*

dizzy schwindelig

docile fügsam, gelehrig

docility Fügsamkeit *f*, Gelehrigkeit *f*

docimasia, docimasy Untersuchung *f*, Prüfung *f*

docimastic Untersuchungs–, Prüfungs–

doctrine Lehre *f*, Lehrmeinung *f*, Doktrin *f* / ~ **of centres** Zentrenlehre *f* / ~ **of chances** Wahrscheinlichkeitsrechnung *f* / ~ **of evolution** Evolutionstheorie *f* / ~ **of recapitulation** biogenetisches Grundgesetz *n*

document Schriftstück *n*, Akte *f*, Dokument *n* / **personal** ~ persönliche Unterlagen *fpl*, Personaldokument *n*

documentation Dokumentation *f*

dogma Dogma *n*, Lehrsatz *m*, Lehrmeinung *f*

dogmatic dogmatisch

dogmatism Dogmatismus *m* / ~ **scale** Dogmatismus–Skala *f*

dol Dol *n*, Einheit *f* der Schmerzintensität

dolichocephal Langköpfiger *m*, Dolichozephaler *m*

dolichocephalia, dolichocephalism, dolichocephaly Langköpfigkeit *f*, Dolichozephalie *f*

dolichocephalic, dolichocephalous langköpfig, dolichozephal

dolichocranial langköpfig, dolichozephal

dolichofacial langgesichtig, dolichofazial

dolichomorphic dolichomorph, lang und dünn, asthenisch

doll play Puppenspiel *n*

dolor Dolor *m*, Schmerz

dolorimetry Messung *f* der Schmerzintensität

dolorous schmerzhaft, schmerzlich

dolphin Delphin *m*

domatophobia Domatophobie *f*

domain Domain *f*, Kennung *f* einer Internetadresse / **public ~** Public Domain *f*

domestic zahm, Haus–

domesticate zähmen, domestizieren

domestication Eingewöhnung *f*, Zähmung *f*, Domestikation *f*

domesticity Familienleben *n*, häusliches Leben *n*, Neigung *f* zu Haus und Familie

dominance Dominanz *f*, Vorherrschaft *f* / **~ hierarchy** Dominanzhierarchie *f* / **~ level** Dominanzniveau *n* / **~ need** Dominanzstreben *n*, Streben *n* nach Überlegenheit / **cerebral ~** zerebrale Dominanz *f*, Hemisphärendominanz *f* / **genetic ~** genetische Dominanz *f* / **hemispherical ~** Hemisphärendominanz *f* / **imperfect ~** unvollkommene Dominanz *f* / **lateral ~** Seitendominanz *f*, laterale Dominanz *f* / **manual ~** Dominanz *f* einer Hand / **ocular ~** okulare Dominanz *f*, Dominanz *f* eines Auges / **repressed ~** verdrängtes Dominanzstreben *n*

dominant dominant, dominierend / Dominante *f*

dominate beherrschen

dominating dominierend, vorherrschend, beherrschend

domination Herrschaft *f*, Beherrschung *f*, Vorherrschaft *f*, Dominanz *f*

dominator modulator theory Dominator–Modulator–Theorie *f*

domineering dominierend, herrisch, herrschsüchtig

dominoes test Dominotest *m*

donation Gabe *f*, Spende *f*

donatism Donatismus *m*, tranceähnliche Faszination *f*

Donders law Donders Gesetz *n* der konstanten Orientierung

Don–Juanism Don–Juanismus *m*

Donnan| equilibrium Donnangleichgewicht *n* / **~ potential** Donnanpotenzial *n* / **~ system** Donnansystem *n*

dopa Dopa *n*, Dioxyphenylalanin *n*

dopamine Dopamin *n* / **~ agonist** Dopaminagonist *m* / **~ antagonist** Dopaminantagonist *m* / **~ hypothesis of schizophrenia** Dopaminhypothese *f* / **~ metabolite** Dopaminmetabolit *m* / **~ system** Dopaminsystem *n*

dopaminergic dopaminerg

dope betäuben, dopen, aufputschen / Rauschgift *n*, Aufputschmittel *n*, Betäubungsmittel *n*

Doppler| effect Doppler–Effekt *m* / **~ shift** Dopplerverschiebung *f* / **~ ultrasonography** Doppler–Sonographie *f*

doraphobia Doraphobie *f*, krankhafte Angst *f* vor Pelzen und Tieren

dorm Schlaf *m*

dormancy Ruhezustand *m*, Schlafzustand *m*, Inaktivität *f*, Latenz *f*

dormant schlafend, inaktiv, latent, im Unterbewusstsein vorhanden

doromania krankhafte Sucht *f* Geschenke zu machen

dorsad nach dem Rücken zu, rückenwärts

dorsal dorsal

dorsiflexion Dorsalflexion *f*

dorsoventral vom Rücken zum Bauch zu, dorsoventral

dose, dosis Gabe *f*, Dosis *f*

dotage geistige Altersschwäche *f*, Senilität *f*

dotard kindischer Greis *m*, kindischer alter Mensch *m*, seniler Mensch *m*

dotting test Punktiertest *m*

double doppelt, zweifach / verdoppeln / **~–alteration problem** Versuchsanordnung *f* mit Doppelalternativen / **~–aspect theory** Identitätsauffassung *f*, Einheitsauffassung *f* / **~–bind hypothesis** Double–bind–Hypothese *f* / **~–bind interaction** Double–bind–Interaktion *f*, Double–bind–Beziehung *f* / **~–blind technique** Doppelblindversuch *m* / **~ blind theory** Theorie *f* des Doppelblindversuchs / **~–entry table** bivariate Tabelle *f*, Tabelle *f* mit zwei Dimensionen / **~–frequency table** Punktediagramm *n*, Streudiagramm *n* / **~ helix** Doppelhelix *f* / **~–language theory** Identitätslehre *f* / **~–step device** Zweiphasentechnik *f* / **~–test technique** Doppeltestmethode *f*

doubt Zweifel *m*, Bedenken *n* / **obsessive ~s** zwanghafte Zweifel *mpl*

doubtful zweifelhaft, unsicher, unentschieden

doubting zweifelnd, Zweifel–

dousing, dowsing Wünschelrutengehen *n* / **~ rod** Wünschelrute *f*

dove Taube *f*

down–hearted deprimiert, verstimmt

Down's syndrome Down–Syndrom *n*, Mongolismus *m*, Langdon–Down–Krankheit *f*

doxepine Doxepin *n*

drainage Drainage *f*, Dränage *f*, Kanalisierung *f* / **~ hypothesis** Kanalisierungshypothese *f* / **~ theory** Kanalisierungstheorie *f* / **postural ~** Haltungskanalisierung *f*

dramamine Dimenhydrinat *n*

drama theory Psychodrama *n*

dramatism Dramatismus *m*

dramatization Dramatisierung *f*

drapetomania pathologischer Wandertrieb *m*, Sucht *f* zu vagabundieren, Drapetomanie *f*

drawing Zeichnung *f* Skizze *f* / **~–board** Zeichenbrett *n* / **~–book** Zeichenheft *n* / **~ completion test** Zeichenergänzungstest *m* / **~–paper** Zeichenpapier *n* / **~ scale** Zeichenskala *f* / **~ test** Zeichentest *m* / **pictorial ~** Zeichnung *f*

dread Furcht *f*, Schrecken *m*, Phobie *f* / **~ of disease** Krankheitsfurcht *f* / **~ of eating** krankhafte Nahrungsverweigerung *f*, Sitophobie *f* / **~ of glass objects** Angst *f* vor Glasgegenständen / **~ of open spaces** Platzangst *f*, Agoraphobie *f*

dream Traum *m* / träumen / **~ analysis** Traumanalyse *f* / **~ of being punished** Straftraum *m* / **~ censor** Traumzensor *m* / **~ censorship** Traumzensur *f* / **~ condensation** Traumverdichtung *f* / **~ content** Trauminhalt *m* / **~ determinant** Traumdeterminante *f* / **~ displacement** Traumverschiebung *f* / **~ distortion** Traumentstellung *f* / **~ ego** Traum–Ich *n* / **~ elements** Traumelemente *npl* / **~ formation** Traumbildung *f* / **~ instigators** Tagesreste *mpl* / **~ interpretation** Traumdeutung *f*, Traumauslegung *f* / **~–life** Traumleben *n* / **~ material** Traumstoff *m*, Trauminhalt *m* / **~ motive** Traummotiv *n* / **~ recall** Traumerinnerung *f* / **~ repression** Traumverdrängung *f* / **~ screen** Traumhintergrund *m* / **~ sensation** Traumempfinden *n* / **~ state** Traumzustand *m* / **~ structure** Traumstruktur *f* / **~ symbol** Traumsymbol *n* / **~ symbolism** Traumsymbolik *f* / **~ theory** Traumtheorie *f*, Traumlehre *f* / **~–thinking** Traumdenken *n* / **~ thought** Traumgedanke *m* / **~ wish** Traumwunsch *m* / **~ as wish fulfilment** Wunscherfüllung *f* im Traum / **~ work** Traumarbeit *f* / **absurd ~** absurder Traum *m* / **artificial ~** künstlicher Traum *m* (in Hypnose) / **hypnagogic ~** Einschlaftraum *m* / **hypnopompic ~** Traum *m* vor dem Erwachen / **latent ~ thought** latenter Trauminhalt *m*, Traumgedanke *m* / **manifest ~** manifester Traum *m* / **manifest ~ content** manifester Trauminhalt *m* / **prophetic ~** Wahrtraum *m* / **recurrent ~** sich wiederholender Traum *m* / **typical ~** typischer Traum *m* / **waking ~** Wachtraum *m*, Illusion *f* / **wet ~** nächtliche Pollution *f*, nächtlicher Samenerguss *m*

dreamer Träumer *m*, Phantast *m*

dreaminess Verträumtheit *f*

dreaming verträumt, Traum– / Träumen *n* / **lucid ~** Klarträumen *n*

dreamlike traumartig, wie im Traum

dreamy träumerisch, verträumt

drill Drill *m*, strenge Schulung *f*, Dressur *f* / abrichten, eindrillen, dressieren

drink–driving offence Trunkenheitsdelikt *n*

drinker Trinker *m* / **hard ~** Säufer *m* / **situational ~** Gelegenheitstrinker *m*

drinking Trinken *n*, Alkoholgenuss *m* / **~ behaviour** Trinkverhalten *n* / **excessive ~** übermäßiger Alkoholgenuss *m* / **social ~** Geselligkeitstrinken *n*, soziales Trinken *n*

drive Trieb *m*, Antrieb *m*, Drang *m*, Motiv *n* / **~ affect** Triebaffekt *m* / **~ arousal** Trieberregung *f* / **~ condition** Triebzustand *m* / **~ conversion** Triebverschiebung *f* / **~–determined** triebbestimmt, triebdeterminiert / **~ discrimination** Triebunterscheidung *f* / **~ displacement** Triebverschiebung *f*, Triebverdrängung *f* / **~–inducing operation** triebauslösender Vorgang *m* / **~ level** Triebniveau *n*, Triebspiegel *m* / **~ reduction** Triebreduktion *f*, Triebminderung *f* / **~–reduction theory** Triebreduktionstheorie *f* / **~ specificity** Triebspezifizierung *f* / **~ state** Triebzustand *m* / **~ stimulus** Triebreiz *m* / **~–stimulus reduction theory** Triebreduktionstheorie *f* / **~ strength** Triebstärke *f* / **acquired ~** erworbener Trieb *m* / **aesthetic ~** ästhetische Tendenz *f* / **affectional ~** affektiver Trieb *m* / **alien ~** irrelevanter Trieb *m* / **appetitive ~** Appetenztrieb *m*, Triebverlangen *n* / **carrying ~** durchgehender Trieb *m* / **esthetic ~** ästhetische Tendenz *f* / **excessive sexual ~** gesteigertes sexuelles Verlangen *n* / **exploratory ~** Entdeckungstrieb *m* / **general ~** allgemeiner Drang *m* / **instinctual ~** Primärtrieb *m*, physiologischer Trieb *m* / **irrelevant ~** irrelevanter Trieb *m* / **learnable ~** erlernbarer Trieb *m* / **learned ~** erworbener Trieb *m* / **manipulative ~** Untersuchungsdrang *m*, Neugierde *f* / **maternal ~** Mutterinstinkt *m*, Muttertrieb *m* / **motor ~** Bewegungsdrang *m* / **oral ~** oraler Trieb *m* / **partial ~** Partialtrieb *m* / **primary ~** angeborener Trieb *m*, Primärtrieb *m*, Urtrieb *m* / **respiratory ~** Atemantrieb *m* / **secondary ~** erworbener Trieb *m* / **securing ~** Schutzbedürfnis *n*, Sicherheitsbedürfnis *n* / **self–assertive ~** Selbstbehauptungstrieb *m* / **sensory ~** sinnlicher Trieb *m* / **sexual ~** Sexualtrieb *m*, Geschlechtstrieb *m*, sexueller Trieb *m* / **social ~** Gesellschaftstrieb *m*, Sozialtrieb *m* / **socialized ~** sozial akzeptabler Trieb *m* / **stimulated ~** stimulierter Trieb *m* / **visceral ~** physiologischer Trieb *m* / **viscerogenic ~** physiologischer Trieb *m* / **vital ~s** Lebenstriebe *mpl*, physiologische Triebe *mpl*

drivelling Faselei *f*, Vielrederei *f*, Geschwätzigkeit *f*

driver Fahrer *m* / **~ behaviour** Fahrverhalten *n* / **~ education** Fahrschulausbildung *f*, Fahrausbildung *f*, Fahrerschulung *f*

driving Synchronsteuerung *f*, Fahren *n* / **~ behaviour** Fahrverhalten *n* / **~ under the influence of drugs** Fahren *n* unter Rauschmitteleinfluss / **drunken ~** Fahren *n* unter Alkoholeinfluss

dromo|mania Dromomanie *f*, Wandertrieb *m* / **~phobia** Dromophobie *f*

dropping out of movements Bewegungselimination *f*

dropout Schulversager *m*, Studienabbrecher *m* / (aus der Gesellschaft) ausgeflippt / **potential ~** potenzieller Versager *m*, potenzieller Abbrecher *m*

Drosophila Fruchtfliege *f*, Drosophila *f*

drowsiness Schläfrigkeit *f*, Schlaftrunkenheit *f*, Somnolenz *f*, Schlummer *m*

drowsy somnolent, benommen, schläfrig

drug Droge *f*, Medikament *n*, Arzneimittel *n*, Rauschgift *n*, Rauschdroge *f* / ~ **abstinence** Drogenabstinenz *f* / ~ **abuse** Drogenmissbrauch *m*, Arzneimittelmissbrauch *m* / ~ **abuse liability** Suchtpotential *n* / ~ **abuse prevention** Suchtprävention *f* / ~ **abuser** Drogensüchtige(r) *m,f* / ~ **addict** Drogenabhängige(r) *m,f* Drogensüchtige(r) *m,f* Rauschgiftsüchtige(r) *m,f* Arzneimittelsüchtige(r) *m,f* / ~ **addict** rauschgiftsüchtig, arzneimittelsüchtig / ~ **addiction** Rauschmittelsucht *f*, Drogensucht *f*, Drogenabhängigkeit *f*, Arzneimittelsucht *f* / ~ **administration methods** Darreichungsformen *fpl* von Medikamenten / **adverse** ~ **reaction** Nebenwirkung *f* von Medikamenten / ~ **allergy** Medikamentenallergie *f*, Arzneimittelallergie *f* / ~ **dependence** Drogenabhängigkeit *f*, Arzneimittelabhängigkeit *f* / ~ **dependency** Drogenabhängigkeit *f*, Arzneimittelabhängigkeit *f* / **multiple** ~ **dependence** Polytoxikomanie *f* / ~ **distribution** Drogenhandel *m* / ~ **dosage** Dosierung *f* von Arzneien / ~ **education** Arzneimittelaufklärung *f* / ~ **effect** Medikamentenwirkung *f* / ~ **habituation** Drogengewöhnung *f* / ~**–induced congenital disorders** Geburtsschäden *mpl* durch Medikamentenabhängigkeit, drogeninduzierte angeborene Störungen *fpl* / ~**–induced hallucinations** durch Drogen hervorgerufene Halluzinationen *fpl*, drogeninduzierte Halluzinationen *fpl* / ~ **interaction** Arzneimittelwechselwirkung *f* / ~ **intoxication** Drogenrausch *m*, Arzneimittelvergiftung *f* / ~ **law** Arzneimittelgesetz *n* / ~ **legalization** Legalisierung *f* von Drogen / ~ **overdose** Überdosis *f* von Medikamenten, Drogenüberdosis *f* / ~ **potentiation** Arzneimittelpotenzierung *f* / ~ **psychosis** Suchtpsychose *f*, Rauschgiftpsychose *f* / ~ **rehabilitation** Drogenentwöhnung *f*, Drogenentziehungskur *f*, Drogenrehabilitation *f* / ~ **research** Arzneimittelforschung *f* / ~ **scene** Drogenszene *f* / ~ **self–administration** Selbstverabreichung *f* von Drogen / ~ **sensitivity** Arzneimittelsensibilisierung *f* / ~ **syndrome** Drogensyndrom *n* / ~ **synergism** Zusammenwirken *n* von Arzneimitteln, Synergismus *m* von Medikamenten / ~**–taking** Doping *n* / ~ **therapy** Behandlung *f* mit Arzneimitteln, medikamentöse Therapie *f* / ~ **tolerance** Medikamentenverträglichkeit *f*, Arzneimitteltoleranz *f* / ~ **trafficker** Rauschgifthändler *m*, Drogendealer *m* / ~ **trafficking** Rauschgifthandel *m* / ~ **usage** Medikamentenverbrauch *m*, Drogeneinnahme *f*, Drogengebrauch *m*, Drogenkonsum *m* / ~ **usage attitude** Einstellung *f* zum Drogenkonsum / ~ **usage screening** Drogentest *m* / **intravenous** ~ **usage** intravenöser Drogenkonsum *m* / ~ **withdrawal** Drogenentzug *m* / ~ **withdrawal effects** Entzugserscheinungen *fpl* bei der Drogenentwöhnung / **addictive** ~ Suchtmittel *n* / **adrenergic** ~**s** Sympathikomimetika *npl* / **adrenergic blocking** ~**s** Sympathikolytika *npl*, adrenerger Hemmstoff *m* / **adrenolytic** ~**s** Sympathikolytika *npl* / **anaesthetic** ~ Betäubungsmittel *n*, Anästhetikum *n*, Narkosemittel *n* / **analeptic** ~**s** Analeptika *npl*, zentralerregende Mittel *npl* / **analgesic** ~**s** Analgetika *npl*, schmerzstillende Mittel *npl* / **anorexigenic** ~ Appetithemmer *m* / **anticholinergic** ~ Anticholinergikum *n* / **anticoagulant** ~ gerinnungshemmende Substanz *f*, Antikoagulans *n* / **anticonvulsive** ~ krampflösendes Mittel *n* / **antidepressant** ~ Antidepressivum *n* / **antidiabetic** ~ Antidiabetikum *n* / **antiemetic**~ Mittel *n* gegen Erbrechen, Antiemetikum *n* / **antiepileptic** ~ Mittel *n* gegen Epilepsie, Antiepileptikum *n* / **antihistaminic** ~ Antihistaminikum *n* / **antihypertensive** ~ blutdrucksenkendes Mittel *n*, Antihypertonikum *n* / **anti–inflammatory** ~ entzündungshemmendes Arzneimittel *n* / **antinauseant** ~ Mittel *n* gegen Erbrechen, Antiemetikum *n* / **antineoplastic** ~ antineoplastische Substanz *f*, Antineoplastikum *n* / **antiparkinsonian**

~ Antiparkinsonmittel *n* / **antipsychotic ~** Mittel *n* gegen Psychosen / **antipyretic ~** Antipyretikum *n* / **antischizophrenic ~** Mittel *n* gegen Schizophrenie / **antispasmodic ~** krampflösendes Mittel *n*, Spasmolytikum *n* / **antitremor ~** Mittel *n* gegen Tremor / **antitubercular ~** Tuberkulosemittel *n* / **antitubocurarine ~** Gegenmittel *n* gegen Tubokurarin / **antiviral ~** virustatische Substanz *f*, antivirale Substanz *f* / **anxiolytic ~** Anxiolytikum *n*, Mittel *n* gegen Angst / **ataractic ~** Ataraktikum *n*, mildes Psychosedativum *n* / **ataraxic ~** Ataraktikum *n*, mildes Psychosedativum *n* / **cholinergic ~** Cholinergikum *n*, cholinerge Substanz *f* / **cholinergic blocking ~** Anticholinergikum *n*, cholinerge Hemmsubstanz *f* / **cholinolytic ~** Anticholinergikum *n* / **cholinomimetic ~** Parasympathikomimetikum *n*, Cholinomimetikum *n* / **CNS–affecting ~** ZNS–beeinflussende Substanz *f* / **CNS–depressant ~** ZNS–dämpfende Substanz *f* / **CNS–stimulating ~** ZNS–stimulierende Substanz *f* / **emetic ~** Brechmittel *n*, Emetikum *n* / **hallucinogenic ~** Halluzinogen *n* / **hard ~** harte Droge *f* / **hypnotic ~** Schlafmittel *n*, Hypnotikum *n* / **mydriatic ~**pupillenerweiterndes Mittel *n*, Mydriaticum *n* / **narcoanalytic ~** narkoanalytisches Mittel *n*, leichtes Schlafmittel *n* / **narcotic ~** Betäubungsmittel *n*, Narkotikum *n*, Schlafmittel *n* / **neuroleptic ~** Neuroleptikum *n* / **neuromuscular blocking ~** muskelrelaxierendes Mittel *n* / **nootropic ~** Nootropikum *n* / **oxytocic ~** wehenanregendes Mittel *n* / **parasympatholytic ~** Parasympatholytikum *n*, Cholinolytikum *n* / **psychedelic ~** psychedelische Droge *f* / **psychoactive ~** Psychopharmakon *n* / **psychoanaleptic ~** Psychoanaleptikum *n* / **psychodysleptic ~s** Psycholytika *npl* / **psycholytic ~s** Psycholytika *npl* / **psychotherapeutic ~** Psychopharmakon *n* / **psychotogenic ~s** Psychotogene *npl*, Psychotomimetika *npl* / **psychotomimetic ~s** Psychotomimetika *npl*, Psychotika *npl*, Psycholytika *npl* / **psychotonic ~** Psychotonikum *n* / **psychotropic ~** Psychopharmakon *n*, psychotroper Stoff *m* / **soft ~** weiche Droge *f* / **soporific ~** Schlafmittel *n* / **sympatholytic ~** Sympatholytikum *n* / **sympathomimetic ~** Sympathomimetikum *n* / **talk–out ~** Wahrheitsdroge *f* / **tranquilizing ~** Beruhigungsmittel *n*, Tranquilizer *m*, Sedativum *n* / **tricyclic antidepressant ~** trizyklisches Antidepressivum *n* / **true ~** Wahrheitsdroge *f*, Plauderdroge *f* / **vasopressor ~** blutdrucksteigerndes Mittel *n* / **vomit–inducing ~** Brechmittel *n*

drum Trommel *f* / **~–head** Trommelfell *n* / **~ membrane** Trommelfell *n* / **~ skin** Trommelfell *n* / **magnetic–~ storage** Magnettrommel–Speicher *m* / **smoked ~** Rußtrommel *f*

drunk betrunken

drunkard Trinker *m*, Säufer *m*, Trunkenbold *m* / **confirmed ~** Gewohnheitstrinker *m*, bekannter Trinker *m* / **habitual ~** Gewohnheitstrinker *m*

drunkenness Trunkenheit *f*, Trunksucht *f*, Dipsomanie *f*, Rauschzustand *m* / **pathological ~** pathologischer Rausch *m*

drying–out Alkohlentzug *m*

dryness Gefühlskälte *f*, Trockenheit *f*

dual doppelt, zweifach

dualism Dualismus *m* / **psychophysical ~** psychophysischer Parallelismus *m*, Leib–Seele–Dualismus *m*

Du Bois–Reymond's law Du Bois–Reymond–Gesetz *n*

duct Gang *m*, Kanal *m*, Ductus *m* / **~ of the cochlea** Schneckengang *m*, Ductus cochlearis *m* / **acoustic ~** äußerer Gehörgang *m* / **auditory ~** Gehörgang *m* / **cochlear ~** Ductus cochlearis *m*, Schneckengang *m* / **endolymphatic ~** Endolymphschlauch *m* / **semicircular ~s** Bogengänge *mpl*

ductless innersekretorisch

dull stumpfsinnig, dumpf, niedergeschlagen, monoton

dullard Dummkopf *m*

dullness Dummheit *f*, Dumpfheit *f* / Stumpfheit *f*, Teilnahmslosigkeit *f* / **mental ~** Stumpfsinn *m*, geistige Stumpfheit *f*

dumb stumm / **deaf and ~** taubstumm

dumbness Stummheit *f*, Mutismus *m*

dummy Attrappe *f*, Plazebo *n*, Babyschnuller *m*

duodenal duodenal, Zwölffingerdarm–

duodenum Zwölffingerdarm *m*, Duodenum *n*

duplication Verdopplung *f* / **~ of personality** Persönlichkeitsverdopplung *f*

duplicity zweifaches Vorhandensein *n*, Duplizität *f*, Doppelzüngigkeit *f*, Falschheit *f* / **~ of cases** Duplizität *f* der Fälle / **~ theory** Duplizitätstheorie *f*, duale Sehtheorie *f*

dura (mater) Dura mater *f*, harte Hirnhaut *f*

durables, durable goods Gebrauchsgüter *npl* / **~ expenditure** Ausgaben *fpl* für Gebrauchsgüter

dural dural, harte Hirnhaut betreffend

durance Zeiteinheit *f*, Lebensabschnitt *m*

duration Dauer *f* / **~ of action** Wirkungsdauer *f* / **~ of life** Lebensdauer *f* / **~ of sleep** Schlafdauer *f* / **least–perceptible ~** eben merkliche Dauer *f*

durative dauernd, andauernd, anhaltend

Durham rule Durham–Entscheidung *f*

duty Pflicht *f* / **off ~** außerhalb der Arbeitszeit, dienstfrei / **on ~** bei der Arbeit, diensttuend

dwarfish zwerghaft, zwergwüchsig, unterentwickelt

dwarfishness Zwergwuchs *m*, Unterentwicklung *f*

dwarfism Zwergwuchs *m*, Nanismus *m*, Nanosomie *f* / **hypophyseal ~** hypophysärer Zwergwuchs *m* / **pituitary ~** hypophysärer Zwergwuchs *m*, hypophysärer Infantilismus *m*

dyad Dyade *f*, Zweier–Verbindung *f* / **social ~** Zweiergruppe *f*

dyadic dyadisch, doppelt, paarweise

dying Sterben *n* / sterbend

dynamaesthesia, dynamesthesia Dynamästhesie *f*, Kraftempfindung *f*

dynamic dynamisch / Dynamik *f*

dynamics Dynamik *f* / **~ of repression** Verdrängungsdynamik *f* / **~ of transference** Übertragungsdynamik *f* / **allochthonous ~** allochthone Dynamik *f* / **autochthonous ~** autochthone Dynamik *f* / **behavioural ~** Verhaltensdynamik *f* / **intergroup ~** Dynamik *f* zwischen Gruppen, Intergruppendynamik *f* / **social ~** soziale Dynamik *f*

dynamis Dynamis *f*

dynamism Dynamismus *m*, dynamisches Prinzip *n* / **conjunctive ~** verbindendes, dynamisches Prinzip *n* / **disjunctive ~** trennendes, dynamisches Prinzip *n* / **psychic ~** dynamische Theorie *f*

dynamogenesis, dynamogeny Dynamogenese *f*

dynamogenic dynamogenetisch

dynamograph Dynamograph *m*

dynamometer, dynameter Dynamometer *n*, Kraftmesser *m*

dyne Dyn *n*, Einheit *f* der Kraft

dynorphin Dynorphin *n*

dysacousia, dysacousis, dysacousma Dysakusis *f*, Störung *f* der Gehörempfindlichkeit

dysadaptation, dysaptation mangelnde Adaptationsfähigeit *f*, Dysadaptation *f*

dysaesthesia verfälschte Sinneswahrnehmung *f*, Empfindungsstörung *f*, Dysästhesie *f*

dysaesthetic empfindungsgestört

dysantigraphia Dysantigraphie *f*

dysaphia Störung *f* des Tastsinnes

dysarthria Dysarthrie *f*, Bulbärsprache *f*, gestörte Lautbildung *f*, unartikuliertes Sprechen *n* / **~ literalis** Stammeln *n* / **~ syllabaris** Stottern *n*

dysarthric sprachgestört, artikulationsgestört

dysautonomia Dysautonomie *f*

dysbasia Gehstörung *f*, erschwertes Gehen *n*, Dysbasie *f*

dysbulia Willenshemmung *f*, gestörte Willenskraft *f*, Dysbulie *f*

dysbulic willensgestört, willensschwach

dyscalculia Rechenstörung *f*, Dyskalkulie *f*, Rechenschwäche *f*

dyschesia, dyschezia Dyschezie *f*

dyschiria ausgeprägte manuelle Ungeschicklichkeit *f*, Dyschirie *f*

dyschromasia, dyschromatopsia partielle Farbenblindheit *f*, Farbenfehlsichtigkeit *f*, Dyschromatopsie *f*

dyschromatope Farbenfehlsichtiger *m*

dyscinesia motorische Fehlfunktion *f*, Störung *f* im geordneten Bewegungsablauf, Dyskinesie *f*

dyscoimesis Dyskoimesis *f*, erschwertes Einschlafen *n*

dyscrasia Dyskrasie *f*, physiologisches Ungleichgewicht *n*

dysdiadochokinesia Dysdiadochokinese *f*, Störung *f* im geordneten Bewegungsablauf

dyseneia Artikulationsstörung *f* aufgrund von Taubheit

dysergasia abnorme Reaktionsweise *f*, toxische Psychose *f*, Dysergasie *f*

dysergastic abnorm, psychotisch

dysergia fehlende Muskelkoordination *f*, motorische Koordinationsstörung *f*, Dysergie *f*

dysesthesia verfälschte Sinneswahrnehmung *f*, Empfindungsstörung *f*, Dysästhesie *f*

dysesthetic empfindungsgestört

dysfunction Funktionsstörung *f*, Dysfunktion *f* / **amphetamine–induced sexual ~** amphetamininduzierte sexuelle Funktionsstörung *f* / **cerebellar ~** zerebellare Störung *f* / **cerebral ~** zerebrale Fehlfunktion *f* / **hormonal ~** hormonale Dysfunktion *f* / **hysterical ~** hysterische Funktionsstörung *f* / **minimal cerebral ~** minimale zerebrale Dysfunktion *f* / **orgasmic ~** Orgasmusstörung *f* / **sensory ~** Funktionsstörung *f* der Sinneswahrnehmung / **sexual ~ due to a general medical condition** sexuelle Funktionsstörungen *fpl* aufgrund eines medizinischen Krankheitsfaktors / **sexual ~, not caused by organic disorder or disease** nichtorganische sexuelle Funktionsstörung *f* / **somatoform autonomic ~** somatoforme autonome Funktionsstörung *f* / **substance–induced sexual ~** substanzinduzierte sexuelle Funktionsstörungen *fpl* / **vegetative ~** vegetative Funktionsstörung *f*

dysgenic erbschädigend

dysgenics Erforschung *f* von Erbschädigungen

dysgeusia Geschmacksstörung *f*, Geschmacksanomalie *f*, Dysgeusie *f*

dysglandular hormonal gestört, dysglandular

dysgnosia Intelligenzstörung *f*, geistiger Defekt *m*

dysgrammataxis Störung *f* in der Schreibbewegung

dasgrammatism Dysgrammatismus *m*

dysgraphia Schreibstörung *f*, Dysgraphie *f*

dyskinesia Dyskinesie *f*, motorische Fehlfunktion *f* / **tardive ~** tardive Dyskinesie *f*

dyskinetic dyskinetisch, fehlfunktionierend

dyskoimesis Dyskoimesis *f*, erschwertes Einschlafen *n*

dyslalia Sprachstörung *f*, Artikulationsstörung *f*, Stammeln *n*, Dyslalie *f*

dyslexia Lesestörung *f*, Störung *f* des Lesens, Dyslexie *f*

dyslogia sprachliche Ausdrucksstörung *f*, Dyslogie *f*

dysmenorrhoea, dysmenorrhea Dysmenorrhoe *f*, schmerzhafte Menstruation *f*, schmerzhafte Regel *f* / **psychogenic ~** psychogene Dysmenorrhoe *f*

dysmenorrhoeal, dysmenorrheal, dysmenorrhoeic, dysmenorrheic dysmenorrhoisch

dysmetria fehlerhaft regulierte Zielbewegungen *fpl*, Dysmetrie *f*

dysmimia Störung *f* von Mimik und Gestik, Störung *f* der Gebärdensprache, Dysmimie *f*

dysmnesia Gedächtnisstörung *f*

dysmorphophobia Angst *f* vor Missgestaltigkeit, Angst *f* vor missgestalteten Menschen, Dysmorphophobie *f*

dysmorphosis Missbildung *f*, Missgestalt *f*, Fehlbildung *f*, Dysmorphie *f*

dysnoesis Dysnoesis *f*

dysnoia Dysnoia *f*

dysopia, dysopsia Sehstörung *f*, Dysopie *f*, Dysopsie *f*

dysorexia gestörter Appetit *m*, Dysorexie *f*

dysorthography fehlerhafte Rechtschreibung *f*

dysosmia Geruchsstörung *f*, Dysosmie *f*

dysosphresia Störung *f* des Geruchssinnes, Dysosphresie *f*

dyspareunia Fehlen *n* des Wollustgefühls beim Geschlechtsakt, Schmerz *m* beim Koitus, Dyspareunie *f*

dyspepsia Dyspepsie *f*, Verdauungsstörung *f*, schlechte Verdauung *f* / **nervous ~** Magenneurose *f*

dyspeptic dyspeptisch, magenkrank

dysphagia, dysphagy Schluckstörung *f*, Dysphagie *f*

dysphasia Sprachstörung *f*, Aphasie *f*, Dysphasie *f*

dysphemia Sprachstörung *f*, Dysphemie *f*, Stottern *n*

dysphonia Dysphonie *f*, heisere Sprache *f*, Phonationsstörung *f*

dysphoria Unruhe *f*, gedrückte Stimmungslage *f*, Unbehagen *n*

dysphoric dysphorisch, nervös, unruhig

dysphrasia Sprachhemmung *f*, Sprachstörung *f*, Dysphrasie *f*

dysphrenia seelische Störung *f* aufgrund körperlicher Anomalien, Dysphrenie *f*

dysphylaxia Dysphylaxie *f*, Durchschlafstörung *f*

dyspituitarism gestörte Hypophysentätigkeit *f*

dysplasia Fehlbildung *f*, Missgestalt *f*, Wachstumsstörung *f*, Dysplasie *f*

dysplastic fehlentwickelt, dysplastisch

dyspnoea, dyspnea Atemnot *f*, Kurzatmigkeit *f*, Dyspnoe *f*

dyspnoeic, dyspneic dyspnoisch, schweratmig

dyspraxia Dyspraxie *f*, leichte Apraxie *f*

dysregulation Fehlsteuerung *f*, Fehlregulation *f*

dysrhythmia Rhythmusstörung *f* / **cerebral ~** Rhythmusstörung *f* der Gehirnwellen, zerebrale Dysrhythmie *f*

dyssomnia Schlafstörung *f*, Dyssomnie *f*

dysstasia Unsicherheit *f* beim Stehen

dysstatic nicht normal stehen bleibend

dyssyllabia Silbenstolpern *n*

dystaxia leichte Form *f* der Ataxie, partielle Ataxie *f*

dysteleology fehlende Zielausrichtung *f* in der Natur

dysthymia Dysthymie *f*, krankhafte Verstimmung *f*, Melancholie *f*, zyklothyme Depression *f*

dysthymic dysthym

dystonia Dystonie *f*, Tonusstörung *f*, fehlerhafter Tonus *m* von Muskeln und Geweben / **neurovegetative ~** vegetative Dystonie *f*

dystonic dystonisch / Dystoniker *m*

dystrophia, dystrophy Dystrophie *f*, Ernährungsstörung *f* / **adiposogenital ~** Dystrophia adiposogenitalis *f*, Fröhlich–Syndrom *n*, Fröhlich'sche Krankheit *f* / **muscular ~** Muskeldystrophie *f*

dysuria Beschwerden *fpl* beim Wasserlassen / **psychic ~** Unvermögen *n* in Gegenwart anderer Personen zu urinieren

E

eager eifrig, begierig

eagerness Begierde *f*, Verlangen *n* / ~ **to get personal importance** Geltungsstreben *n*, Geltungsdrang *m*

ear Ohr *n* / ~ **bone** Gehörknöchelchen *n* / ~ **canal** äußerer Gehörgang *m* / ~ **disorder** Ohrenkrankheit *f* / ~ **drum** Trommelfell *n*, Paukenhöhle *f* / ~ **guard** Ohrenschützer *m* / **~–minded** auditiv, akustisch ausgerichtet / ~ **plug** Ohrstöpsel *m* / ~ **speculum** Ohrspiegel *m* / ~ **tingling** Ohrensausen *n* / **external** ~ äußeres Ohr *n* / **humming** ~ Ohrensausen *n* / **inner** ~ Innenohr *n* / **internal** ~ Innenohr *n* / **middle** ~ Mittelohr *n* / **middle** ~ **deafness** Mittelohrschwerhörigkeit *f* / **sharp** ~ scharfes Gehör *n*, gutes Gehör *n*

earth–eating Erdessen *n*, Geophagie *f*

eating Nahrungsaufnahme *f*, Essen *n* / ~ **attitude** Einstellung *f* zum Essen / ~ **behaviour** Essgewohnheit *f* / ~ **disorder** Essstörung *f* / ~ **instinct** Nahrungstrieb *m* / ~ **of excrements** Kotessen *n*, Koprophagie *f* / ~ **pattern** Essgewohnheit *f* / **compulsive** ~ Esszwang *m*

Ebbinghaus| curve Ebbinghaus'sche Lernkurve *f*, Ebbinghaus–Kurve *f* / ~ **curve of retention** Ebbinghaus–Vergessenskurve *f*, Ebbinghaus–Behaltenskurve *f* / ~ **law of learning** Ebbinghaus–Gesetz *n*, Ebbinghaus'sches Gesetz *n* der Lernzeit / ~ **test** Ebbinghaustest *m*, Ergänzungstest *m*, Lückentest *m*

ebolo|lalia Ebololalie *f* / ~ **phrasia** Ebolophrasie *f*

ebriety Trunkenheit *f*, Ebrietas *f*

ebrious betrunken, trunken, volltrunken

eccentric exzentrisch, überspannt / exzentrischer Mensch *m*, Sonderling *m*

eccentricity Exzentrizität *f*, Überspanntheit *f*, Sonderlichkeit *f* / **retinal** ~ retinale Exzentrizität *f*

ecco analysis Ecco–Analyse *f*

ecdemomania Wanderlust *f*, Wandertrieb *m*, Ekdemomanie *f*

E–chart Snellen–Sehtafel *f*, Tafel *f* zur Prüfung der Sehschärfe

echo Echo *n*, Widerhall *m*, Nachklingen *n*, Resonanz *f* / ~ **encephalogram** Echoenzephalogramm *n* / ~ **encephalography** Echoenzephalographie *f* / ~ **principle** Nachahmungsprinzip *n* / ~ **reaction** Echoästhesie *f*

echoing widerhallende Nachahmung *f*

echo–acousia Echohören *n*

echoaesthesia, echoesthesia Nachempfindung

echographia Nachschreiben *n*, Echographie *f*

echokinesis, echokinesia Echokinese *f*, Echokinesie *f*, sinnloses Nachahmen *n* von gesehenen Bewegungen

echolalia Echolalie *f*, Echophrasie *f*, sinnloses Wiederholen *n* von Wörtern und Sätzen, Echosprache *f*

echolocation Echoortung *f*, Schalllokalisation *f*

echomatism Echoerscheinungen *fpl*, Echomatismus *m*

echomimia Echomimie *f*, sinnloses Nachahmen *n* von gesehenen Gebärden

echomotism sinnloses Nachahmen *n* von Bewegungen

echopathy krankhafter Nachahmungstrieb *m*, automatischer Nachahmungstrieb *m*

echophenomena Echoerscheinungen *fpl*, Echomatismus *m*, Echopathie *f*

echophototony Echophototonie *f*

echophrasia Echolalie *f*, Echophrasie *f*, sinnloses Wiederholen *n* von Wörtern und Sätzen

echopraxia, exhopraxis Echopraxie *f*, Echokinese *f*, sinnloses Nachahmen *n* von Bewegungen

echospeech Echosprache *f*, Echolalie *f*, Echophrasie *f*

echothymia Gefühlsansteckung *f*, Echothymie *f*, Massenhysterie *f*

E/C intervening variable intervenierende Variable *f* zwischen Kontroll– und Experimentalgruppe

eclampsia Eklampsie *f*, eklamptische Krämpfe *fpl*

eclamptic eklamptisch

eclamptogenetic, eclamptogenic, eclamptogenous krampfartig, krampfauslösend

eclectic eklektisch, aus verschiedenen Quellen zusammengestellt

eclecticism Eklektizismus *m*

eclimia krankhafter Heißhunger *m*, Bulimie *f*

ecmnesia Verlust *m* des Kurzzeitgedächtnisses, Ekmnesie *f*

ecological ökologisch

ecologist Ökologe *m*, Umweltforscher *m*

ecology Ökologie *f*, Umweltlehre *f* / **~ of social behaviour** Verhaltenstheorie *f* im sozialen Feld / **behavioural ~** Verhaltensökologie *f*

economic ökonomisch, wirtschaftlich, wirtschaftswissenschaftlich

economical sparsam, wirtschaftlich

economics Volkswirtschaft *f*, Wirtschaftswissenschaft *f*, Ökonomie *f* / **mental ~** geistige Ökonomie *f*

Economo's disease Economo–Krankheit *f*, Encephalitis epidemica *f*, Encephalitis lethargica *f*

economy Wirtschaft *f*, Wirtschaftlichkeit *f*, Sparsamkeit *f*, Ökonomie *f*

ecphoria, ecphory Wiedererinnerung *f*, Ekphorie *f*

ecphorize ekphorieren, eine Erinnerung wiederhervorrufen

ecstasise in Ekstase geraten, in Ekstase bringen

ecstasy Ekstase *f*, Verzückung *f*, fanatische Begeisterung *f*, Entrücktheit *f* / **manic ~** manische Ekstase *f*, ekstatischer Wahnsinn *m*

ecstatic ekstatisch, verzückt, entrückt

ectoblast Ektoblast *n*, äußeres Keimblatt *n*

ectoderm Ektoderm *n*, äußeres Keimblatt *n*

ectomia, ectomy Entfernung *f*, Resektion *f*, Exzision *f*

ectomorph, ectomorphic ektomorph

ectomorphy Ektomorphie *f*

ectoplasm Ektoplasma *f*, äußere Zytoplasmaschicht *f*

ectoplasmatic ektoplasmatisch

ectosuggestion Fremdsuggestion *f*, Suggestion *f* von außen

ectype Abweichungstyp *m*, Ektypus *m*

ectypia Abweichung *f* von der Norm, Typusabweichung *f*

eczema Ekzem *n*

edema Ödem *n*, Flüssigkeitsansammlung *f*, Wassersucht *f* / **angioneurotic ~** angioneurotisches Ödem *n*, Quincke–Ödem *n* / **cerebral ~** Hirnödem *n*, Hirnschwellung *f* / **hysterical ~** hysterisches Ödem *n* / **wandering ~** Wanderödem *n*, angioneurotisches Ödem *n*

edematous, edemic ödematös

edge detail Randdeutung *f*, Randdetail *n*

edging Betrachten *n* einer Rorschach–Tafel von einer Ecke aus

Edipus complex Ödipuskomplex *m*

educability Erziehbarkeit *f*, Bildsamkeit *f*, Lernfähigkeit *f*

educable erziehbar, lernfähig, bildungsfähig

education Erziehung *f*, Ausbildung *f*, Schulung *f* / **~ of mass** Volkserziehung *f* / **~ student** Pädagogikstudent *m* / **affective ~** affektive Erziehung *f* / **bilingual ~** zweisprachige Erziehung *f* / **compensatory ~** ausgleichende Erziehung *f*, kompensatorische Erziehung *f* / **compulsory ~** allgemeine Schulpflicht *f* / **continuing ~** weiterführende Ausbildung *f* / **continuous ~** ständige Weiterbildung *f* / **correctional ~** Fürsorgeerziehung *f* / **cultural ~** Allgemeinbildung *f*, geisteswissenschaftliche Ausbildung *f* / **cybernetic ~** kybernetische Pädagogik *f* / **elementary ~** Volksschulbildung *f*, Grundschulerziehung *f*, Grundschulausbildung *f* / **environmental ~** Umwelterziehung *f* / **equal ~** Bildungsgleichheit *f*, Chancengleichheit *f* im Bildungswesen / **experimental ~** Erziehungsexperiment *n*, Schulversuch *m* / **formal ~** schulische Bildung *f* / **higher ~** Hochschulausbildung *f* / **informal ~** Bildung *f* / **medical ~** medizinische Ausbildung *f* / **multicultural ~** multikulturelle Erziehung *f* / **musical ~** Musikerziehung *f* / **new ~** neue Ausbildung *f* / **nontraditional ~** alternative Pädagogik *f* / **paraprofessional ~** Ausbildung *f* nichtakademischen Fachpersonals / **permissive ~** antiautoritäre Erziehung *f* / **physical ~** Sportunterricht *m*, Sport *m* / **preschool ~** Vorschulerziehung *f*, Kindergartenerziehung *f* / **primary ~** Volksschulausbildung *f*, Volksschulwesen *n* / **private ~** Privatunterricht *m*, Privatschulunterricht *m* / **progressive ~** fortschrittliche Erziehung *f* / **religious ~** religiöse Erziehung *f*, Religionsunterricht *m* / **remedial ~** Heilpädagogik *f*, Förderunterricht *m* / **secondary ~** Sekundarstufenausbildung *f*, Gymnasialausbildung *f*, höhere Schulbildung *f* / **sexual ~** Sexualerziehung *f* / **social ~** Sozialpädagogik *f* / **special ~** Sonderpädagogik *f*, Sonderschulausbildung *f* / **special ~ student** Sonderschüler *m* / **special ~ teacher** Sonderschullehrer *m* / **supervised ~** kontrollierte Ausbildung *f* / **traditional ~** traditionelle Erziehung *f* / **visual ~** Anschauungsunterricht *m* / **vocational ~** Berufsausbildung *f*, Berufspädagogik *f* / **vocational ~ teacher** Berufsschullehrer *m*

educational erzieherisch, Erziehungs–, pädagogisch

educative erzieherisch, Erziehungs–

educator Erzieher *m*, Lehrer *m* / **specialized ~** Fachlehrer *m*

eduction Ableitung *f* / **~ of relations and of correlates** Beziehungserfassung *f*

edutainment unterhaltsame Vermittlung *f* von Lerninhalten, Infotainment *n*

effect Wirkung *f*, Effekt *m* / **~ of colours** Farbenwirkung *f* / **~ pleasure** Effektlust *f* / **~ of surroundings** Umgebungseinfluss *m* / **~ size** Effektgröße *f* / **accompanying ~** Begleiterscheinung *f* / **adverse ~s of medication** ungünstige Wirkungen *fpl* einer Medikation / **aural ~** Mikrophoneffekt *m* / **autokinetic ~** autokinetisches Phänomen *n* / **bipolar ~** gegensätzliche Wirkung *f* / **cochlear ~** Mikrophoneffekt *m* / **contrary ~** Gegenwirkung *f* / **cumulative ~** Kumulationswirkung *f*, kumulative Wirkung *f* / **delayed ~** verzögerte Wirkung *f*, Spätwirkung *f* / **differential ~** Differenzeffekt *m* / **distal ~** Entfernungswirkung *f* / **electrophonic ~** Elektrophoneffekt *m* / **environmental ~** Umwelteinfluss *m*, Milieuwirkung *f* / **gravitational ~** Wirkung *f* der Schwerkraft, Gravitationswirkung *f* / **iatrogenic ~** iatrogene Wirkung *f* / **inhibitory ~** Hemmwirkung *f* / **main ~** Hauptwirkung *f* / **off ~** Aus–Effekt *m* / **on ~** Ein–Effekt *m*, An–Reaktion *f* / **on–off~** An–Aus–Reaktion *f* / **permanent ~** Dauerwirkung *f* / **proactive ~** proaktive Wirkung *f* / **progestational ~** Gestagenwirkung *f* / **reactive ~** reaktiver Effekt *m* / **reciprocal ~** Wechselwirkung *f* / **relaxing ~** entspannende Wirkung *f* / **secondary ~** Nebenwirkung *f* / **sedative ~** sedierende Wirkung *f*, dämpfende Wirkung *f* / **side–~** Nebenwirkung *f* / **stimulating ~** Reizwirkung *f* / **stroboscopic ~** stroboskopische Erscheinung *f*, stroboskopisches Phänomen *n* / **subsequent ~** Nachwirkung *f*, Folgewirkung *f* / **tranquilizing ~** beruhigende Wirkung *f*

effective effektiv, wirksam

effectiveness Wirksamkeit *f* / **~ of groups** Gruppeneffizienz *f* / **organizational ~** Organisationseffektivität *f*

effector Effektor *m*, Erfolgsorgan *n*, Nervenendorgan *n* / **~ organs** Erfolgsorgane *npl*

effectuate bewirken, bewerkstelligen

effeminacy Weichlichkeit *f*, Verweichlichung *f*, unmännliches Wesen *n*

effeminate verweichlicht, weibisch / verweichlichte Person *f*, Muttersöhnchen *n*

effemination Effemination *f*, Verweiblichung *f*

efference Efferenz *f* / **~ copy** Efferenzkopie *f*

efferent efferent, nach außen führend, herausführend, effektorisch

efferential herausführend, nach außen führend

effervescence Aufbrausen *n*

efficacious wirksam

efficacy Wirksamkeit *f*, Wirkungsgrad *m*

efficiency Wirkungsgrad *m*, Leistungsgrad *m*, Leistungsfähigkeit *f*, Wirksamkeit *f* / **~ at work** berufliche Leistungsfähigkeit / **~ engineering** wissenschaftliche Betriebsführung *f*, Taylorismus *m* / **~ index** Index *m* des Wirkungsgrades / **~ quotient** Effizienzquotient *m* / **impaired visual ~** Sehuntüchtigkeit *f* / **industrial ~** industrielle Produktivität *f* / **predictive ~** Vorhersageleistung *f*, Vorhersagegenauigkeit *f* / **visual ~** Sehtüchtigkeit *f*

efficient wirksam, leistungsfähig, tüchtig, effizient

effluvium Körpergeruch *m*, Körperausdunstung *f*

effort Anstrengung *f*, Mühe *f* / **~ experience** Anstrengungsgefühl *n* / **~ syndrome** Anstrengungssyndrom *n* / **~ tolerance** Belastungstoleranz *f* / **~ tolerance test** Arbeitsbelastungsprobe *f* / **least ~ principle** Gesetz *n* der geringsten Anstrengung

egalitarism Gleichheitsstreben *n*

egg Ei *n*, Eizelle *f* / **one–~ twins** eineiige Zwillinge *mpl* / **two–~ twins** zweieiige Zwillinge *mpl*

ego Ich *n*, Ego *n* / **two–~–alien** ichfremd / **~–alter theory** Theorie *f* der Ich–Du–Beziehung / **~ anachoresis** Ich–Anachorese *f* / **~ analysis** Ich–Analyse *f* / **~ anxiety** Ich–Angst *f* / **~ attitudes** Ich–Einstellungen *fpl*, Ich–Haltungen *fpl* / **~ autonomy** Autonomie *f* des Ichs / **~ block** Ich–Blockierung *f* / **~ boundary** Ich–Grenze *f* / **~ cathexis** Ich–Besetzung *f* / **~ complex** Ich–Komplex *m* / **~ consciousness** Ich–Bewusstsein *n* / **~ defense** Ich–Abwehr *f* / **~ defense mechanism** Abwehrmechanismus *f* des Ichs / **~ defense reaction** Abwehrreaktion *f* des Ichs / **~ defensiveness** Ich–Abwehr *f*, Ich–Verteidigung *f* / **~ development** Ich–Entwicklung *f* / **~ discovery** Ich–Findung *f* / **~ drive** Ich–Trieb *m* / **~ dynamism** Ich–Dynamik *f* / **~ dystonia** fehlende Harmonie *f* mit dem Ich / **~–dystonic** ichfremd, ichwidrig / **~ erotism** Ichliebe *f*, Narzissmus *m* / **~ extension** Ich–Ausweitung *f* / **~ failure** Ich–Versagen *n* / **~ feeling** Ichgefühl *n* / **~ function** Ich–Funktion *f* / **~ goal** persönliches Ziel *n* / **~ growth** Ich–Entwicklung *f* / **~–id conflict** Konflikt *m* zwischen Ich und Es / **~ ideal** Ich–Ideal *n* / **~ identity** Ich–Identität *f* / **~ inflation** Ich–Aufbauschung *f* / **~ instinct** Ich–Trieb *m* / **~–integrative** ichintegrierend / **~ interest** Ich–Interesse *n* / **~–involved** ichbeteiligt, engagiert / **~ involvement** Ich–Beteiligung *f* / **~ level** Ich–Niveau *n*, Aktualniveau *n* / **~ libido** Ich–Libido *f*, narzisstische Libido *f* / **~ neurosis** Ich–Neurose *f* / **~–object polarity** Subjekt–Objekt–Polarität *f* / **~ organization** Ich–Organisation *f* / **~ psychology** Ich–Psychologie *f* / **~ regression** Ich–Regression *f* / **~ relevance** Ich–Bezug *m* / **~ resistance** Ich–Widerstand *m* / **~ strength**

Ich–Stärke *f* / ~ **structure** Ich–Struktur *f*, Ich–Gefüge *n* / ~ **synthesis** Ich–Synthese *f* / ~ **syntonia** Harmonie *f* mit dem Ich / ~**–syntonic** ichgerecht, ichentsprechend / ~ **threat** Ich–Bedrohung *f* / ~ **weakness** Ich–Schwäche *f* / **alien to the** ~ ichfremd / **archaic** ~ archaisches Ich *n* / **auxiliary** ~ Hilfsich *n* / **bound disciplined** ~ mangelnde Selbstbehauptung *f* / **collective** ~ kollektives Ich *n* / **dreaming** ~ Traum–Ich *n* / **duplicated** ~ Doppel–Ich *n*, Verdopplung *f* der Persönlichkeit / **foreign to the** ~ ichfremd / **hedonic** ~ Lust–Ich *n* / **ideal** ~ Ideal–Ich *n* / **narcissistic** ~ narzisstische Ich–Bezogenheit *f* / **narcistic** ~ **ideal** narzisstisches Ich–Ideal *n* / **phenomenal** ~ phänomenales Ich *n* / **supportive** ~ therapiefördernde Person *f* / **unbound assertive** ~ starke Selbstbehauptung *f*

egocentric egozentrisch, ichbezogen

egocentrism, egocentricity Egozentrismus *m*

egoism Egoismus *m*

egoist Egoist *m*

egoistic egoistisch

egomania krankhafte Selbstsucht *f*, Selbstüberschätzung *f*

egomorph Egomorpher *m*, Autist *m*

egomorphism Egomorphismus *m*, Autismus *m*, ichbezogene Interpretation *f* der Handlungen anderer

egopathy Egopathie *f*

egophilia Egophilie *f*, Selbstliebe *f*, Narzissmus *m*

egotic ichbezogen, eingebildet, eitel

egotism Egotismus *m*, Geltungsbedürfnis *n*

egotistic egoistisch, sich selbst in den Vordergrund stellend

egotize immer nur von sich sprechen, alles über Gebühr auf sich selbst beziehen

egotropic egozentrisch, ichbezogen

egregorsis Schlaflosigkeit *f*, Insomnie *f*, Unfähigkeit *f* zu schlafen

eidetic eidetisch / Eidetiker *m*

eidetics Eidetik *f*

eidotropic eidotrop

eisoptrophobia abnorme Furcht *f* vor Spiegeln, Eisoptrophobia *f*

ejaculate ejakulieren

ejaculatio Ejakulation *f*, Samenerguss *m* / ~ **praecox** vorzeitiger Samenerguss *m* / ~ **retarda** verzögerter Samenerguss *m*

ejaculation Ejakulation *f*, Samenerguss *m* / **nocturnal** ~ nächtlicher Samenerguss *m* / **premature** ~ vorzeitiger Samenerguss *m*, Ejaculatio praecox *f* / **retarded** ~ verzögerter Samenerguss *m*, Ejaculatio retarda *f*

eject projizieren, übertragen, auf eine andere Person verlagern

ejection Verlagerung *f*, Übertragung *f*, Projektion *f*

ejective übertragen, projiziert

elaborate ausarbeiten, bearbeiten

elaboration Bearbeitung *f* / ~ **of dreams** Traumbearbeitung *f*, Traumarbeit *f* / ~ **of physical symptoms for psychological reasons** Entwicklung *f* körperlicher Symptome aus psychischen Gründen / **secondary** ~ sekundäre Bearbeitung *f* im Traum

élan Begierde *f*, heftiges Verlangen *n* / ~ **vital** Elan vital *m*, Lebensschwungkraft *f*

elasticity Spannkraft *f*, Elastizität *f*

elation freudige Erregung *f*, Stolz *m*, gehobene Stimmung *f*, Hochstimmung *f*

elated in gehobener Stimmung, gut gelaunt

Elavil Amitriptylin *n*

Elberfeld horses Elberfeld–Pferde *npl*

elbow Ellbogen *m* / ~ **jerk** Ellbogenreflex *m*

elder| abuse Misshandlung *f* alter Menschen / ~ **care** Altenpflege *f*

elections, political politische Wahlen *fpl*

Electra complex Elektrakomplex *m*, weiblicher Ödipuskomplex *m*

electric, electrical elektrisch

electricity Elektrizität *f* / **static** ~ statische Elektrizität *f*

electroacoustic elektroakustisch

electroacupuncture Elektroakupunktur *f*

electroaesthesiometer Elektroästhesiometer *n*

electrobiology Elektrophysiologie *f*, Elektrobiologie *f*

electrocardiogram Elektrokardiogramm *n*, EKG

electrocardiograph Elektrokardiograph *m*, EKG–Apparat *m*

electrocardiography Elektrokardiographie *f*

electrochronogram elektrische Zeitaufschreibung *f*

electrochronograph Elektrochronograph *m*, elektrischer Zeitmesser *m*

electroconvulsive Elektrokrampf *m*

electrocorticogram Elektrokortikogramm *n*

electrode Elektrode *f* / ~ **impedance** Elektrodenwiderstand *m*, Elektrodenimpedanz *f* / ~ **potential** Elektrodenpotenzial *n* / ~ **resistance** Elektrodenwiderstand *m*

electrodiagnosis, electrodiagnostics Elektrodiagnostik *f*

electrodiagnostic elektrodiagnostisch

electroencephalogram EEG *n*, Elektroenzephalogramm *n*

electroencephalograph Elektroenzephalograph *m*

electroencephalographic elektroenzephalographisch

electroencephalography Elektroenzephalographie *f*

electroencephalophony Elektroenzephalophonie *f*

electroesthesiometer Elektroästhesiometer *n*

electrogastrogram Elektrogastrogramm *n*

electrogastrography Elektrogastrographie *f*

electrogenesis Elektrogenese *f*, Entstehung *f* eines elektrischen Potenzials

electrographic elektrographisch

electrography Elektrographie *f*

electrokymography Elektrokymographie *f*

electrolyte Elektrolyt *m*

electrolytic elektrolytisch

electromagnetic elektromagnetisch

electrometer Elektrometer *n*, Strommesser *m*

electromotive, electromotor elektromotorisch

electromyogram Elektromyogramm *n*

electromyograph Elektromyograph *m*, Gerät *n* zur Aufzeichnung von Muskelaktionsströmen

electromyography Elektromyographie *f*

electronarcosis Elektronarkose *f*

electron–proton theory Elektronen–Protonen–Theorie *f*

electronystagmography Elektronystagmographie *f*

electrooculogram Elektrookulogramm *n*

electrooculograph Elektrookulograph *m*

electrooculography Elektrookulographie *f*

electroolfactogram Elektroolfaktogramm *n*

electroosmosis Elektro–Osmose *f*

electropherogram Elektropherogramm *n*

electrophobia krankhafte Furcht *f* vor elektrischen Apparaten, Elektrophobie *f*

electrophone Elektrophon *n*

electrophoresis Elektrophorese *f*

electrophysiological elektrophysiologisch

electrophysiology Elektrophysiologie *f*, Elektrobiologie *f*

electropism Galvanotropismus *m*

electroplethysmography Elektroplethysmographie *f*, elektrische Aufzeichnung *f* der Blutvolumenschwankungen in einem Organ

electroretinogram Elektroretinogramm *n*

electroretinography Elektroretinographie *f*

electroscriptogram Elektroskriptogramm *n*

electroscriptograph Elektroskriptograph *m*

electroshock Elektroschock *m* / ~ **therapy** Elektroschocktherapie *f* / ~ **treatment** Elektroschockbehandlung *f*

electrosleep treatment Elektroschlafbehandlung *f*

electrosuggestion therapy Elektrosuggestivbehandlung *f*

electrotaxis Galvanotaxis *f*, Reagieren *n* von Lebewesen auf den elektrischen Strom

electrotherapeutic elektrotherapeutisch

electrotherapist Elektrotherapeut *m*

electrotherapy Elektrotherapie *f*

electrotonic elektrotonisch

electrotonus Elektrotonus *m*

electrotropism Galvanotropismus *m*

element Element *n* / **~s of consciousness** Elemente *npl* des Bewusstseins / **~s in the dream** Traumelemente *npl* / **~s of the dream** Traumelemente *npl* / **~ of a matrix** Element *n* einer Matrix / **binary ~** binäres Element *n* / **chemical ~** chemische Element *n* / **controlling ~** Stellglied *n* / **genetic ~s** genetische Elemente *npl* / **graphological ~s** Formelemente *npl* der Schrift / **identical ~s** identische Elemente *npl* / **mental ~s** psychische Elemente *npl* / **metallic ~** metallisches Element *n* / **nervous ~** nervöses Element *n* / **on/off ~** Ein/Aus–Element *n* / **retinal ~s** Netzhautteile *mpl* / **single ~** Einzelelement *n* / **social ~s** sozial mittelbare Verhaltenselemente *npl* / **statistical ~s** Einheiten *fpl* der Grundgesamtheit / **subconscious ~s** unterbewusste Elemente *npl*

elemental elementar, Elementar–

elementarism, elementalism Elementarismus *m*

elementary einfach, rudimentär, unentwickelt, elementar

Elgin check list Elgin'sche Prüfliste *f*

elicit hervorrufen, auslösen, hervorlocken

elimination Ausscheidung *f*, Absonderung *f*, Elimination *f* / **~ disorder** Störung *f* der Ausscheidung

elision Auslassen *n* phonetischer Einheiten, Elision *f*

elite Elite *f*, Oberschicht *f*

ellipsis Ellipse *f*, Unterdrückung *f* einzelner Wörter oder Wortgruppen

elocutionist Rhetoriklehrer *m*, Sprecherzieher *m*, erfahrener Rhetoriker *m*

elopement Entlaufen *n*, Durchgehen *n*, Durchbrennen *n*

elusion Ausweichen *n*

e–mail E–Mail *f*, elekronische Post *f*

emancipation Emanzipation *f*, Befreiung *f*, Gleichberechtigung *f* / **sexual ~** sexuelle Befreiung *f*

emasculate kastrieren, entmannen, verweichlichen / kastriert, entmannt, weibisch, weichlich

emasculation Entmannung *f*, Kastration *f*, Emasculatio *f*, Verweichlichung *f*

embarrassed außer Fassung, verwirrt, bestürzt, verlegen

embarrassment Verlegenheit *f*, Befangenheit *f*, Verwirrung *f*, Peinlichkeit *f*

embedded eingebettet

embeddedness, embedding Einbettung *f*, Einordnung *f*

embolalia, embololalia Embololalie *f*, Einschiebung *f* überflüssiger Laute oder Wörter

embolism Embolie *f* / **cerebral ~** Hirnembolie *f*

embololalia, embolophrasia Embololalie *f*, Gaxen *n*, Embolophrasie *f*, Einschiebung *f* überflüssiger Laute oder Wörter, Angophrasie *f*

embryo Embryo *m*, Keim *m*

embryogenesis, embryogeny Embryonalentwicklung *f*, Embryogenese *f*

embryology Embryologie *f*

embryonic, embryonal embryonal

emergence Auftreten *n*, Hervortreten *n*, Erscheinen *n*

emergency Not *f*, Notfall *m* / **~ arousal** Auslösen *n* der Notfallfunktion / **~ function** Notfallfunktion *f* / **~ reaction** Notfallreaktion *f* / ~ **service** Notdienst *m* / ~ **situation** Notfallsituation *f* / ~ **theory of emotions** Theorie *f* der Notfallfunktion

emergent auftauchend, entstehend

emergentism Theorie *f* der immanenten Evolution

emesia, emesis Erbrechen *n*

emetic Erbrechen verursachend

emetine treatment Emetinkur *f*

emetophobia krankhafte Angst *f* vor Erbrechen

emigrate emigrieren, auswandern

emigration Auswanderung *f*, Emigration *f*

emission Ausfließen *n*, Ausströmen *n*, Ejakulation *f* / ~ **of semen** Samenentleerung *f* / **nocturnal** ~ nächtlicher Samenerguss *m*, Pollution *f* / **seminal** ~ Samenerguss *m*

emit aussenden, hervorbringen

Emmert's law Emmert'sches Gesetz *n*

emmetrope Normalsichtiger *m*, Emmetroper *m*

emmetropia Normalsichtigkeit *f*, Emmetropie *f*

emmetropic normalsichtig, emmetrop

emote emotional reagieren, Emotionen zeigen

emoticon Smiley *n*, Emoticon *n*

emotion Emotion *f*, Gefühl *n*, Affekt *m*, Gemütsbewegung *f* / ~ **stupidity** Emotionsstupidität *f* / **cold** ~ kaltes Gefühl *n* / **conditioned** ~ bedingte Emotion *f*, konditionierte Emotion *f* / **derived** ~ abgeleitete Gemütsbewegung *f* / **induced** ~ induzierte Gemütsbewegung *f* / **primary** ~ Primärgefühl *n*, Urgefühl *n* / **protopathic** ~ idiopathische Emotion *f*, Primäremotion *f* / **unconscious** ~ unbewusstes Gefühl *n*

emotional emotional, gefühlsmäßig, leicht erregbar, affektiv

emotionalism emotionale Betrachtungsweise *f*, übermäßige Gefühlsbetonung *f*

emotionality gefühlsmäßige Veranlagung *f*, Emotionalität *f*, Affektivität *f* / **animal** ~ tierische Affektivität *f* / **general** ~ allgemeine Emotionalität *f*

emotive gefühlsmäßig, Gefühls–

emotivity Fähigkeit *f* zu emotionalen Reaktionen, Fähigkeit *f* zur Gefühlserregung, Gefühlserregbarkeit *f*, Affektivität *f*

empathic empathisch, einfühlend

empathicability Einfühlbarkeit *f*

empathize sich einfühlen, Empathie empfinden

empathy Empathie *f*, Einfühlung *f* / ~ **theory** Einfühlungstheorie *f* / **negative** ~ Einfühlung *f* trotz Widerstand

emphasis Nachdruck *m*, Betonung *f*, Emphase *f* / ~ **principle** Akzentuierungsprinzip *n*

emphysema, pulmonary Lungenemphysem *n*

empiric, empirical empirisch, auf Erfahrung beruhend, experimentell / **~–statistical** empirisch–statistisch

empiricism, empirism Empirismus *m*, Empirie *f*, Erfahrungswissenschaft *f* / **logical** ~ logischer Empirismus *m*, logischer Positivismus; *m* / **scientific** ~ empirische Erkenntnistheorie *f*, logischer Positivismus *m*

empiricist, empiric Empiriker *m*

employability Verwendungsfähigkeit *f*, Arbeitstauglichkeit *f*

employee Arbeitnehmer *m*, Angestellter *m*, Mitarbeiter *m*, Beschäftigter *m* / ~ **absenteeism** Arbeitsversäumnis *n*, Fehlzeiten *fpl* eines Mitarbeiters / ~ **assistance programme** betriebliches Hilfsprogramm *n* / ~ **attitudes** Arbeitnehmereinstellungen *fpl*, Mitarbeiterattitüden *fpl*, Betriebsklima *n* / ~ **benefit** Sozialleistung *f* für Arbeitnehmer / ~ **characteristics** Arbeitnehmermerkmale *npl* / ~ **efficiency** Leistungsfähigkeit *f* von Arbeitnehmern / ~ **evaluation form** Mitarbeiter–Beurteilungsformular *n* / ~ **health insurance** Krankenversicherung *f* der Arbeitnehmer

/ ~ **interaction** betriebliche Interaktion *f* / ~ **leave benefit** Urlaubsgeld *n*, Lohn- und Gehaltsfortzahlung *f* / ~ **motivation** Arbeitsmotivation *f* / ~ **pension plan** Altersversorgung *f* für die Arbeitnehmer, Firmenpensionsplan *m* / ~ **performance appraisal** Mitarbeiterbeurteilung *f* / ~ **productivity** Arbeitsproduktivität *f* / ~ **satisfaction** Arbeitszufriedenheit *f* / ~ **selection** Personalauswahl *f*, Personalauslese *f* / ~ **skills** Fachkenntnisse *fpl* / ~ **termination** Entlassung *f*, Beendigung *f* des Arbeitsverhältnisses / ~ **turnover** Personalfluktuation *f*, Personalwechsel *m*

employer Arbeitgeber *m* / ~ **attitudes** Arbeitgeberverhalten *n*, Arbeitgebereinstellungen *fpl*

employment Beschäftigung *f*, Einsatz *m*, Dienst *m* / ~ **conditions** Beschäftigungsbedingungen *fpl* / ~ **contract** Arbeitsvertrag *m* / ~ **discrimination** berufliche Diskriminierung *f* / ~ **history** beruflicher Werdegang *m* / ~ **interview** Einstellungsgespräch *n*, Einstellungsinterview *n* / ~ **market** Stellenmarkt *m* / ~ **process** Einstellungsvorgang *m* / ~ **psychology** Berufspsychologie *f* / ~ **reference inquiry** Einholung *f* einer Referenz zu Einstellungszwecken / ~ **status** Personalstand *m*, Beschäftigungssituation *f* / ~ **test** Einstellungstest *m*, Einstellungsuntersuchung *f* / **full** ~ Vollbeschäftigung *f*

empowerment Verantwortungsübernahme *f*

emprosthotonos Emprosthotonus *m*, Krampf *m* des Körpers in vornübergebeugter Stellung

empyreumatic empyreumatisch, brenzlig

emulation Wetteifer *m*, Nacheifern *n*

enabling soziale Förderung *f* von Problemverhalten

enantiodromia Enantiodromie *f*, Übergang *m* der Gegensätze ineinander

encapsulate absondern, einkapseln

encapsulation Absonderung *f*, Einkapselung *f* / **psychological** ~ psychologische Abschirmung *f*, psychische Isolation *f*

encéphale isolé isoliertes Gehirn *n*

encephalitis Enzephalitis *f*, Gehirnentzündung *f* / **epidemic** ~ Encephalitis epidemica *f*, Economo–Krankheit *f* / **lethargic** ~ Encephalitis epidemica *f*, Economo–Krankheit *f*

encephalization Enzephalisation *f*, phylogenetische Differenzierung *f* des Gehirns, Kortikalisierung *f*

encephalogram Enzephalogramm *n*, Hirnkurvenbild *n*

encephalograph Enzephalograph *m*, Gerät *n* zur Aufzeichnung von Hirnkurvenbildern

encephalography Enzephalographie *f*

encephalomalacia, encephalomalacy Gehirnerweichung *f*, Enzephalomalazie *f*

encephalomyelitis Entzündung *f* von Gehirn und Rückenmark, Enzephalomyelitis *f*

encephalon Gehirn *n*, Hirn *n*, Enzephalon *n*

encephalopathy Enzephalopathie *f*, Gehirnerkrankung *f*, Hirnschädigung *f* / **alcoholic** ~ Wernicke'sche Krankheit *f* / **hyperammonemic** ~ hepatozerebrales Syndrom *n* / **posttraumatic** ~ Friedmann Syndrom *n* / **saturnine** ~ Bleienzaphalopathie *f* / **subcortical arteriosclerotic** ~ subkortikale progressive Enzephalopathie *f*, Binswanger–Enzephalopathie *f* / **toxic** ~ toxische Enzephalopathie *f*, toxische Hirnschädigung *f* / **traumatic** ~ Boxerenzephalopathie *f*, traumatische Enzephalopathie *f*, postkommotionelles Syndrom *n*

encephalopsychosis organisch verursachte Geistesstörung *f*

encephalosclerosis Zerebralsklerose *f*

encephalosis Gehirnleiden *n*, Hirnerkrankung *f*

encephalospinal zerebrospinal

encode kodieren, verschlüsseln

encoded kodiert, verschlüsselt

encoding Kodierung *f*, Verschlüsselung *f*

encopresis Enkopresis *f*, Einkoten *n* / ~ **with (without) constipation and overflow incontinence** Enkopresis *f* mit (ohne) Verstopfung und Überlaufinkontinenz / **functional ~** funktionelle Enkopresis *f* / **nonorganic ~** nichtorganische Enkopresis *f*

encorticalization Kortikalisierung *f*, ontogenetische Differenzierung *f* des Gehirns

encounter treffen, begegnen / Begegnung *f*, Zusammentreffen *n* / ~ **group** Trainingsgruppe *f*, T–Gruppe *f*, Encounter–Gruppe *f*, Selbsterfahrungsgruppe *f*

encouragement Ermutigung *f*, Förderung *f*, Unterstützung *f*

enculturation Akkulturation *f*, Eingewöhnung *f* in eine neue Kultur

encystment Einkapselung *f*, Abschirmung *f* / ~ **of the self** psychische Abschirmung *f*, psychische Isolierung *f*

end Ziel *n*, Zielvorstellung *f*, Absicht *f*, Intention *f*, Ende *n* / aufhören, beenden / **~–brain** Endhirn *n*, Telenzephalon *n* / ~ **brush** Endbüschel *n* / **~–bud** Endkolben *m*, Endknötchen *n* / **~–bulb** Endkolben *m*, Nervenendknospe *f* / ~ **buttons** Endknöpfe *mpl* / **~–flake** Nervenendplatte *f* / ~ **foot** Endknopf *m* / ~ **item** Endprodukt *n* / **~–organ** Endorgan *n* / **~–path** Endweg *m* / **~–plate** Endplatte *f*, Nervenendplatte *f* / **~–plate potential** Endplattenpotenzial *n* / **~–pleasure** Orgasmus *m* / ~ **spurt** Endspurt *m*, Schlussantrieb *m* / **motor ~ plate** motorische Endplatte *f*

endeavour Anstrengung *f*, Bemühung *f*, Bestrebung *f*

endemic endemisch

ending Endigung *f*

endoblast Entoblast *n*

endocardium Endokard *n*

endocathection Eigenkathexis *f*, Vorgang *m* der inneren Besetzung, Innenkathexis *f*

endocranial endokranial, im Innern des Schädels gelegen

endocranium harte Hirnhaut *f*, Dura mater *f*, Endokranium *n*

endocrine endokrin, innersekretorisch, mit innerer Sekretion

endocrinological endokrinologisch

endocrinologist Endokrinologe *m*

endocrinology Endokrinologie *f*, Lehre *f* von den endokrinen Drüsen

endocrinopath Endokrinopath *m*, Kranker *m* aufgrund von Störungen der endokrinen Drüsen

endocrinopathy Endokrinopathie *f*, Erkrankung *f* innersekretorischer Drüsen

endocrinotherapy Therapie *f* mit Hormonpräparaten

endoderm Entoderm *n*

endogamy Endogamie *f*, Verwandtenehe *f*

endogenic, endogenous endogen

endogeny Entstehen *n* von innen heraus, Endogenese *f*

endolymph Endolymphe *f*

endomorph Endomorpher *m*, endomorpher Typus *m*

endomorphic endomorph

endomorphy Endomorphie *f*

endomusia stummes Singen *n*, stille Wiederholung *f* einer Melodie

endoneurium Bindegewebe *n* der Nervenfasern, Endoneurium *n*

endophasia inneres Sprechen *n*, Endophasie *f*

endoplasm Endoplasma *n*

endopsychic endopsychisch, innerpsychisch, innerseelisch

endorphin Endorphin *n*

endoscopic endoskopisch

endoscopy Endoskopie *f*

endosecretory innersekretorisch, endokrin

endosomatic endosomatisch, innerorganisch

endothelium Endothel *n*

endothymic endothym

endowment Begabung *f* / **native ~** angeborene Veranlagung *f*, natürliche Begabung

endtest Nachtest *m*, Abschlusstest *m*, postexperimenteller Versuch *m*

endurance Ausdauer *f*, Aushalten *n* / **~ limit** Dauerleistungsgrenze *f* / **~ test** Ausdauertest *m*, Ermüdungstest *m* / **~ training** Ausdauertraining *n* / **physical ~** physische Ausdauer *f* / **psychological ~** psychologische Ausdauer *f*, psychologische Belastbarkeit *f*, Ausdauer *f* und Energie *f*

enelicomorphism Zuerkennung *f* von Erwachsenencharakteristika an Kinder, Enelikomorphismus *m*

energiser Energetikum *n* / **psychic ~** psychischer Energiespender *m*, Aufputschmittel *n*

energy Energie *f* / **~ charge** Besetzung *f* mit Energie, Energiegehalt *m* / **~ equivalent** Energieäquivalent *n* / **~ expenditure** Energieaufwand *m*, Energieeinsatz *m*, Energieverbrauch *m* / **~ mobilisation** Aktivation *f*, Energiemobilisierung *f* / **actonal ~** Anpassungsenergie *f* / **basic ~–level** Grundumsatz *m* / **bound ~** gebundene Energie *f*, kanalisierte Energie *f* / **cathectic ~** Besetzungsenergie *f* / **effective ~** Energie *f* zur Erledigung von Aufgaben / **free ~** freie Energie *f* / **intrinsic ~** Energie *f* zum Zusammenhalt einer Gruppe / **kinetic ~** kinetische Energie *f* Bewegungsenergie *f* / **least ~** geringster Energieaufwand *m* / **libidinal ~** Libido *f*, sexuelle Energie *f* / **mental ~** geistige Energie *f* / **metabolic ~** Stoffwechselenergie *f* / **muscular ~** Muskelenergie *f* / **nervous ~** Nervenkraft *f* / **psychic ~** psychische Energie *f*, geistige Kraft *f* / **psychic ~ hypothesis** Hypothese *f* von der psychischen Energie / **radiant ~** Strahlenenergie *f* / **specific–~ doctrine** Lehre *f* von den spezifischen Sinnesenergien / **specific ~ of nerves** spezifische Nervenkraft *f* / **specific ~ of senses** spezifische Sinnesenergie *f* / **spectral ~** Spektralenergie *f* / **vital ~** Lebenskraft *f*, Lebensenergie *f*

enervate entnerven, entkraften / entnervt, kraftlos

enervation Entnervung *f*, Entkraftung *f*, Schwäche *f*

engagement Verpflichtung *f*, Engagement *f*, Beschäftigung *f*

engineer Ingenieur *m* / **industrial ~** Arbeitsstudieningenieur *m*, Industrial Engineer *m*

engineering Ingenieurwesen *n* / technisch / **~ aptitude test** Test *m* der technischen Begabung / **~ psychology** Ingenieurpsychologie *f* / **genetic ~** Gentechnologie *f*, Genmanipulation *f* / **human ~** Ingenieurpsychologie *f*, Ergonomie *f*, human engineering *n* / **industrial ~** Arbeitswissenschaft *f*, industrial engineering *n* / **social ~** Ingenieursoziologie *f*, ingenieurmäßiges Behandeln *n*, sozialer Gegebenheiten

engram Engramm *n*, Gedächtnisspur *f*, Gedächtniseindruck *m*

engrammatic, engrammic engrammatisch

enhancement Erhöhung *f*, Steigerung *f*, Dosis–Vergrößerung *f*

enhancer, cognitive Nootropikum *n*

enjoyment Freude *f*, Genuss *m*

enkephalin Enkephalin *n*

enlargement Erweiterung *f*, Ausweitung *f*, Vergrößerung *f*

enomania Delirium tremens *n*

enophthalmos tiefliegendes Auge *n*, Enophthalmie *f*

enormity Ungeheuerlichkeit *f*, Abscheulichkeit *f*, Greuel *n* / **depressive ~ delirium** délire d'énormité

enraged wütend, rasend

enosimania Enosimanie *f*

enrichment Anreicherung *f*, Bereicherung *f*

ensemble Anhäufung *f*, Menge *f*, Grundgesamtheit *f*, Ensemble *n*

entelechy Entelechie *f*

enteramine Enteramin *n*, Serotonin *n*

enteroceptor Interozeptor *m*

enteroneurosis Enteroneurose *f*

enterprise Unternehmen *n* / **private ~** freie Wirtschaft *f*, Privatunternehmen *n* / **public ~** Staatsunternehmen *n*

entheomania religiöser Wahnsinn *m*

enthusiasm Begeisterung *f*, Enthusiasmus *m*

entity Wesen *n*, Wesenheit *f*, Sein *n*, Dasein *n*, Entität *f*, Einheit *f*

entoblast Entoblast *n*, inneres Keimblatt *n*

entocranial endokranial, im Innern des Schädels gelegen

entoderm Entoderm *n*, Entoblast *n*, inneres Keimblatt *n*

entomology Insektenkunde *f*, Entomologie *f*

entomophobia krankhafte Angst *f* vor Insekten, Entomophobie *f*

entoptic im Augeninnern gelegen, entoptisch

entoptoscope Augenspiegel *m*

entotic entotisch, Innenohr–

entourage Umgebung *f*

entraining agent Zeitgeber *m*

entrance examination Aufnahmeprüfung *f*, Prüfung *f* der Eingangsvoraussetzungen

entrapment game Fangaufgabe *f*, unlösbare Testaufgabe *f*

entrepreneurship Unternehmertum *n*

entropy Entropie *f* / **social ~** soziale Entropie *f*

entry Eintrag *m*, Eintritt *m*

enucleation Ausschalung *f*, Enukleation *f*

enumeration Aufzählung *f*, Auflistung *f* / **~ test** Aufzählversuch *m* / **complete ~** vollständige Aufzählung *f* / **incomplete ~** unvollständige Aufzählung *f*

enuresis Enuresis *f*, Bettnässen *n*, Einnässen *n* / **~ nocturna** Bettnässen *n*, Enuresis nocturna *f* / **nocturnal ~** Bettnässen *n*, Enuresis nocturna *f* / **nonorganic ~** nichtorganische Enuresis *f*

envenom verbittern, erbittert machen

envious neidisch

environment Umgebung *f*, Umwelt *f*, Milieu *n* / **~–folded traits** umweltgeprägte Eigenschaften *fpl* / **~–related** umweltbezogen / **academic ~** akademisches Milieu *n* / **behavioural ~** Verhaltensfeld *n*, psychologisches Feld *n*, Lebensraum *m* / **determined by ~** milieubedingt / **external ~** äußere Umgebung *f*, Umwelt *f* / **in a controlled ~** in kontrollierter Umgebung / **internal ~** Innenwelt *f* / **natural ~** natürliche Umwelt *f* / **natural ~ type** Umwelt–Typus *m* / **protected ~** beschützende Umgebung *f* / **psychological ~** psychologisches Umfeld *n* / **rural ~** ländliches Milieu *n*, ländliche Umwelt *f* / **social ~** Milieu *n*, gesellschaftliche Umwelt *f*, soziale Umwelt *f* / **suburban ~** Vorstadtmilieu *n* / **urban ~** städtische Umwelt *f*

environmental milieumäßig, milieubedingt, Umwelt–

environmentalism Milieutheorie *f*, Environmentalismus *m*

envy Neid *m* / **penis ~** Penisneid *m*

enzygotic eineiig, monozygot

enzymatic enzymatisch

enzyme Enzym *n*, Ferment *n*, Biokatalysator *m* / **~ inhibitor** Enzymhemmstoff *m*, Enzyminhibitor *m*

eonism Transvestie *f*, Transvestitismus *m*

epencephalon Kleinhirn *n*, Rhombenzephalon *n*

ependyma Ependym *n*, Auskleidung *f* der ZNS–Hohlräume

ephapse elektrische Synapse *f*, Ephapse *f*

ephaptic ephaptisch

ephedrine Ephedrin *n*

epiblast Ektoderm *n*, äußeres Keimblatt *n*

epicanthus Epikanthus *m*, Hautfalte *f* am Oberlid, Mongolenfalte *f*

epicardium Epikard *n*

epicranium Kopfschwarte *f*

epicritic epikritisch

epidemic epidemisch

epidemiology Epidemiologie *f* / **psychiatric ~** psychiatrische Epidemiologie *f*

epidermis Oberhaut *f*, Epidermis *f*

epidural außerhalb der Dura mater, epidural

epigastric epigastrisch, Oberbauch–

epigenesis Epigenese *f*

epigenetic epigenetisch, Epigenesis–

epiglottic epiglottisch, Kehldeckel

epiglottis Kehldeckel *m*, Epiglottis *f*

epilepsy Epilepsie *f*, Fallsucht *f* / **~ produced by alcohol** Alkoholepilepsie *f* / **~ with hallucinations** halluzinatorische Epilepsie *f* / **~ with visual manifestations** visuelle Epilepsie *f* / **abdominal ~** abdominale Epilepsie *f* / **acquired ~** erworbene Epilepsie *f*, erworbene Epilepsie *f* / **adversive ~** Adversivepilepsie *f*, Adversivkrämpfe *mpl* / **affect–induced ~** psychogene Epilepsie *f* / **affective ~** Affektepilepsie *f* / **akinetic ~** akinetische Epilepsie *f* / **atonic ~** atonische Epilepsie *f* / **audiogenic ~** audiogene Epilepsie *f* / **auditive–hallucinatory ~** auditive Epilepsie *f* / **autonomic ~** autonome Epilepsie *f* / **centrencephalic ~** zentrenzephale Epilepsie *f* / **cerebellar ~** zerebellare Epilepsie *f* / **cortical ~** Rindenepilepsie *f*, Jackson–Epilepsie *f* / **cryptogenic ~** idiopathische Epilepsie *f*, endogene Epilepsie *f*, genuine Epilepsie *f* / **diencephalic ~** autonome Epilepsie *f*, Epilepsie *f* mit autonomen Symptomen / **elementary partial ~** epileptischer Elementaranfall *m*, Elementarepilepsie *f* / **essential ~** genuine Epilepsie *f*, idiopathische Epilepsie *f* / **experimental ~** experimentelle Epilepsie *f* / **focal ~** fokale Epilepsie *f*, Herdepilepsie *f*, Jackson–Epilepsie *f* / **genuine ~** genuine Epilepsie *f*, idiopathische Epilepsie *f* / **hereditary ~** angeborene Epilepsie *f*, hereditäre Epilepsie / **idiopathic ~** genuine Epilepsie *f*, idiopathische Epilepsie *f* / **Jacksonian ~** Jackson–Epilepsie *f*, Rindenepilepsie *f*, Jackson'sche Epilepsie *f*, kortikale Epilepsie *f* / **larval ~** larvierte Epilepsie *f* / **laryngeal ~** Kehlkopfschlag *m* / **latent ~** latente Epilepsie *f*, larvierte Epilepsie *f* / **limbic ~** limbische Epilepsie *f* / **masked ~** larvierte Epilepsie *f* / **matutinal ~** Aufwachepilepsie *f* / **metabolically induced ~** metabolische Epilepsie *f* / **minor ~** Petit mal *n* / **musicogenic ~** musikogene Epilepsie *f* / **myoclonic ~** Myoklonusepilepsie *f*, Unverricht Syndrom *n* / **nocturnal ~** Nachtepilepsie *f* / **nonconvulsive ~** nicht–konvulsive Epilepsie *f* / **old age ~** senile Epilepsie *f* / **organic ~** organische Epilepsie *f*, symptomatische Epilepsie *f* / **partial ~** fokale Epilepsie *f*, Herdepilepsie *f*, Jackson–Epilepsie *f* / **photogenic ~** photogene Epilepsie *f*, photosensible Epilepsie *f* / **photosensitive ~** photosensible Epilepsie *f*, photogene Epilepsie *f* / **post–work ~** Feierabendepilepsie *f* / **psychic ~** psychogene Epilepsie *f* / **psychomotor ~** psychomotorische Epilepsie *f* / **reactive ~** reaktive Epilepsie *f* / **residual ~** Residualepilepsie *f* / **sensory ~** sensorische Epilepsie *f* / **symptomatic ~** symptomatische Epilepsie *f* / **tardive ~** Spätepilepsie *f* / **traumatic ~** traumatische Epilepsie *f* / **temporal lobe ~** psychomotorische Epilepsie *f* / **versive ~** versive Epilepsie *f*

epileptic epileptisch / Epileptiker *m*

epileptiform epileptiform, epilepsieartig

epileptogenic, epileptogenous Epilepsie erzeugend, epileptogen

epileptoid epileptoid, epilepsieähnlich

epileptologist Fachmann *m* für Epilepsiefragen, Epilepsiespezialist *m*

epileptology Epilepsieforschung *f*, Lehre *f* von der Epilepsie, Epileptologie *f*

epiloia hypertrophische tuberöse Hirnsklerose *f*, Bourneville'sche Krankheit *f*

epinephrinaemia Adrenalinämie *f*

epinephrine Adrenalin *n*, Epinephrin *n*

epineurium Nervenscheide *f*, Epineurium *n*

epinosic mit einer Krankheit zusammenhängend

epiperiphal von der Körperoberflache herrührend

epiphenomenal begleitend, sekundär

epiphenomenalism Epiphänomenalismus *m*

epiphenomenon Epiphänomen *n*, Begleiterscheinung *f* ohne kausalen Zusammenhang

epiphora Tränenträufeln *n*, Epiphora *f*

epiphysis Epiphyse *f*, Zirbeldrüse *f* / **~ cerebri** Epiphyse *f*, Zirbeldrüse *f*

episcotister, episkotister Episkotister *n*

episode Episode *f*, vorübergehende, rückbildungsfähige Störung *f*, Ereigniszeitraum *m*, molarer Zeitabschnitt *m* / **acute psychotic ~** akute psychotische Episode, akuter psychotischer Schub *m* / **depressive ~** depressive Episode *f* / **depressive ~, unspecified** nicht näher bezeichnete depressive Episode *f* / **hypomanic ~** hypomanische Episode *f* / **interactive ~** Interaktionszeitraum *m* / **major depressive ~** Episode *f* einer Major Depression, typische depressive Episode *f* / **manic ~** manische Episode *f* / **manic ~, unspecified** nicht näher bezeichnete manische Episode *f* / **mixed ~** gemischte Episode *f* / **moderate depressive ~** mittelgradige depressive Episode *f* / **most recent ~, hypomanic** letzte Episode *f*, hypoman / **other depressive ~s** sonstige depressive Episoden *fpl* / **other manic ~s** sonstige manische Episoden *fpl* / **psychogenic psychotic ~** psychogene psychotische Episode *f* / **severe depressive ~ with psychotic symptoms** schwere depressive Episode *f* mit psychotischen Symptomen / **single manic ~** einzelne manische Episode *f*

epistemic erkenntnistheoretisch, epistemisch

epistemology Erkenntnistheorie *f*, Erkenntnislehre *f*, Epistemologie *f* / **genetic ~** genetische Epistemologie *f*

epistemophilia Genuss *m* in der Befriedigung des Wissensdurstes

epithalamic epithalamisch, auf dem Thalamus liegend

epithalamus Epithalamus *m*

epithelium Epithel *n* / **olfactory ~** Riechepithel *n*

epsilon–movement Epsilon–Bewegung *f*

Epstein–Barr viral disorder Epstein–Barr Virusinfektion *f*

equal gleich, gleichmäßig / **~ appearing** gleicherscheinend

equality Gleichheit *f*, Gleichmäßigkeit *f* / **~ judgment** Urteil *n* über die Gleichheit / **social ~** soziale Gleichstellung *f*, Gleichberechtigung *f*, soziale Gleichheit *f*

equalization Ausgleich *m*, Gleichmachung *f* / **~ of excitation** Erregungsausgleich *m*

equalize ausgleichen, gleichmachen

equanimity Gleichmut *m*

equation Gleichung *f* / **~ method** Herstellungsmethode *f* / **structural ~ modeling** Strukturgleichungsmodelle *npl* / **behavioural ~** Verhaltensformel *f* / **empirical ~** empirische Gleichung *f*, empirische Formel *f* / **linear ~** lineare Gleichung *f*, Gleichung *f* erster Ordnung / **normal ~** Formel *f* der Normalverteilung / **personal ~** persönliche Gleichung *f* / **quadratic ~** quadratische Gleichung *f* / **rational ~** Rationalgleichung *f*

equidiscriminating in gleichem Maße diskriminierend

equidistance gleicher Abstand *m*

equidistant in gleichem Abstand, gleich weit entfernt

equifinality Gleichgerichtetheit *f*, gleiche Zielausrichtung *f*

equilibrate kalibrieren, ins Gleichgewicht bringen

equilibrated ausgeglichen

equilibration Kalibrierung *f*, Aufrechterhaltung *f* des Gleichgewichts, Äquilibration *f*

equilibrium Gleichgewicht *n* / **~ potential** Gleichgewichtspotenzial *n* / **~ reflex** Gleichgewichtsreflex *m* / **~ sense** Gleichgewichtssinn *m* / **dynamic ~** Gleichgewichtszustand *m* / **ideal ~** ideales Gleichgewicht *n* / **psychic ~** seelisches Gleichgewicht *n* / **psychological**

~ psychologisches Gleichgewicht *n* / **static ~** Gleichgewichtszustand *m*, statisches Gleichgewicht *n*

equimax rotation Equimax–Rotation *f*

equipment Ausstattung *f*, geistiges Rüstzeug *n*

equipoise Gleichgewicht *n*, Zustand *m* der Balance

equipotential äquipotenziell, gleichgewichtig

equipotentiality Gleichgewichtigkeit *f*, gleiche Bedeutsamkeit *f*, Äquipotenzialität *f* / **~ of cues** Reizsubstitution *f* mittels gleichwertiger Reize / **cerebral ~** zerebrale Äquipotenzialität *f*

equity Billigkeit *f*, Gerechtigkeit *f*, Fairness *f*

equivalence Äquivalenz *f*, Gleichwertigkeit *f* / **~ belief** Äquivalenzglaube *m*, Äquivalenzannahme *f* / **~ coefficient** Äquivalenzkoeffizient *m*, Stabilitätskoeffizient *m* / **~ method** Paralleltest–Methode *f* / **~ relation** Äquivalenzrelation *f* / **~ test** Äquivalenzprüfung *f* / **behavioural ~** Verhaltensäquivalenz *f*, Reaktionsäquivalenz *f* / **motor ~** motorische Äquivalenz *f* / **neural ~** neurale Äquivalenz *f*

equivalent äquivalent, gleichwertig, gleichbedeutend / Äquivalent *n*, Gegenstück *n* / **epileptic ~** epileptisches Äquivalent *n* / **psychic ~** psychisches Äquivalent *n*

equivocal zweideutig, mehrdeutig

equivocality Zweideutigkeit *f*, Mehrdeutigkeit *f*

equivocation Zweideutigkeit *f*, Ausflucht *f*, nominelle Begriffsgleichheit *f*, Äquivokation *f*, fehlübertragene Information *f* in einem System

erectile anschwellend, anschwellbar, erektil

erection Erektion *f*

eremophobia Furcht *f* vor Einsamkeit, Furcht *f* vor dem Alleingelassenwerden

erethism Erregbarkeit *f*, Reizbarkeit *f*, Erethismus *m*

erethismic, erethistic, erethitic erregbar, reizbar, erethisch

ereutophobia, ereutrophobia Ereutophobie *f*, Furcht *f* zu erröten, Erythrophobie *f*

erg Erg *n*, Arbeitseinheit *f*, natürliches Bedürfnis *n*, Motiv *n* / **assertive ~** Selbstbehauptungsmotiv *n* / **gregarious ~** Geselligkeitsmotiv *n* / **narcistic ~** narzisstisches Motiv *n* / **protective ~** Schutzmotiv *n*

ergasia Totalität *f* der psychischen Funktionen

ergasiology, ergasiologia Ergasiologie *f*, Psychobiologie *f*

ergasiomania Beschäftigungsdrang *m*, Ergasiomanie *f*, Arbeitsbesessenheit *f*, Arbeitssucht *f*, krankhafte Arbeitswut *f*

ergasiophobia Arbeitsangst *f*, Bewegungsangst *f*, Ergasiophobie *f*

ergasthenia Erschöpfung *f* durch Arbeit

ergic ergisch, zielstrebig, Ziel–

ergodic ergodisch

ergogram Kurvenaufzeichnung *f* der Muskeltätigkeit, Ergogramm *n*

ergograph Kraftmesser *m*, Gerät *n* zur Messung der körperlichen Leistungsfähigkeit, Ergograph *m*

ergomania Beschäftigungsdrang *m*, krankhafte Arbeitswut *f*, Ergomanie *f*

ergomaniac an Beschäftigungsdrang Leidender *m*

ergometer Ergometer *n*, Dynamometer *n*

ergometric ergometrisch

ergometry Ergometrie *f*, Messung *f* der Arbeitsleistung

ergonomy, ergonomics, ergology Ergonomie *f*, Arbeitswissenschaft *f*

ergophobia Arbeitsangst *f*, Bewegungsangst *f*, Ergophobie *f*

ergostat Ergostat *m*, Gerät *n* zur Messung der Muskelkraft

ergotamine Ergotamin *n*

ergot derivative Mutterkornderivat *n*

ergotherapy Arbeitstherapie *f*

ergotropic ergotrop

erogeneity Erogeneität *f*, erotische Erregbarkeit *f*

erogenous erogen, erotogen

eromania, erotomania, eroticomania übersteigerter Geschlechtstrieb *m*, Liebeswahn *m*, Erotomanie *f*

Eros Eros *m*, Libido *f*, Lebenstrieb *m*, Liebestrieb *m* / **~ instinct** Lebenstrieb *m*

erotic erotisch

eroticism Erotik *f*, Geschlechtslust *f*, Erotizismus *m* / **anal ~** Analerotik *f* / **genital ~** Genitalerotik *f* / **oral ~** Oralerotik *f* / **urethral ~** Urethralerotik *f*

erotise erotisieren

erotism Erotik *f*, Geschlechtslust *f*, Erotismus *m* / **anal ~** Analerotik *f* / **buccal ~** Munderotik *f*, orale Erotik *f* / **dermal ~** Hauterotik *f* / **genital ~** Genitalerotik *f* / **olfactory ~** Geruchserotik *f* / **oral ~** Oralerotik *f* / **urethral ~** Urethralerotik *f*

erotization Erotisierung *f*, Libidinisierung *f*

erotogenic, erotogenetic erogen, erotogen, die Geschlechtslust erregend

erotogenicity, erotogeneity erotische Erregung *f*

erotographomania krankhafter Drang *m* Liebesbriefe zu schreiben, Erotographomanie *f*

erotomania, eroticomania übersteigerter Geschlechtstrieb *m*, Liebeswahn *m*, Erotomanie *f*, Liebessucht *f*, Liebeszwang *m*

erotomaniac liebestoll / Liebestoller *m*

erotopath sexuell anomal Veranlagter *m*, Erotopath *m*

erotopathic erotisch anomal, pervers

erotopathy Störung *f* im Sexualempfinden, sexuelle Perversion *f*

erotophobia Angst *f* vor erotischen Dingen, Erotophobie *f*

erotopsychic erotopsychisch

erotosexual erotisch–sexuell

erratic launenhaft, sprunghaft, unberechenbar, unregelmäßig

error Fehler *m*, Irrtum *m* / **~ of accommodation** Akkommodationsfehler *m* / **~ analysis** Fehleranalyse *f* / **~ of bias** systematischer Fehler *m*, Fehler *m* aufgrund eines konstanten Vorurteils / **~–choice technique** Fehler–Wahl–Verfahren *n* / **~ curve** Fehlerkurve *f* / **~ of estimate** Schätzfehler *m* / **~ in estimating** Schätzfehler *m* / **~ of expectation** Erwartungsfehler *m* / **~ of first kind** Fehler *m* erster Art, Typ–I–Fehler *m*, Alpha–Fehler *m* / **~ gradient** Fehlerquotient *m* / **~ of habituation** Gewohnheitsfehler *m* / **~ less** fehlerfrei / **~ of measurement** Messfehler *m*, Beobachtungsfehler *n* / **~ method** Fehlermethode *f*, Herstellungsverfahren *n* / **~ of observation** Beobachtungsfehler *m*, Messfehler *m* / **~ quotient** Fehlerquotient *m* / **~ of recognition** Erinnerungstäuschung *f*, Erinnerungsfälschung *f*, Paramnesie *f*, Bekanntheitstäuschung *f* / **~ of refraction** Brechungsfehler *m*, Refraktionsanomalie *f* / **~ of sampling** Stichprobenfehler *m* / **~ of second kind** Fehler *m* zweiter Art, Typ–II–Fehler *m*, Beta–Fehler *m* / **~ variance** Fehlervarianz *f* / **absolute ~** absoluter Fehler *m*, absolute Abweichung *f* / **accidental ~** Fehlerfaktor *m*, Zufallsfehler *m* / **anticipatory ~** Erwartungsfehler *m* / **average ~** durchschnittlicher Fehler *m* / **biased ~** systematischer Fehler *m* / **compensating ~** kompensatorischer Fehler *m* / **constant ~** systematischer Fehler *m*, konstanter Fehler *m* / **cumulating ~** systematischer Fehler *m* / **cumulative ~** systematischer Fehler *m* / **educative ~** Erziehungsfehler *m* / **experimental ~** Versuchsfehler *m* / **fortuitous ~** Zufallsfehler *m* / **incidental ~ of observation** zufälliger Beobachtungsfehler *m* / **instrumental ~** Messfehler *m* / **linguistic ~** sprachliche Fehlleistung *f* / **mean ~** mittlerer Fehler *m*, Standardfehler *m* / **median ~** Medianabweichung *f* / **motivated ~** motivierter Fehler *m* / **perceptual ~** Wahrnehmungsfehler *m* / **perseverative ~** perseverierender Fehler *m* / **persistent ~** systematischer Fehler *m* / **probable ~** wahrscheinlicher

Fehler *m* / **processing ~** Verfahrensfehler *m* / **random ~** Zufallsfehler *m* / **refractive ~** Brechungsfehler *m* / **relative ~** relativer Fehler *m* / **statistical ~** statistischer Fehler *m* / **subjective ~** subjektiver Fehler *m* / **systematic ~** systematischer Fehler *m* / **unbiased ~** reiner Zufallsfehler *m* / **unconscious ~** unbewusster Fehler *m* / **variable ~** Zufallsfehler *m*, Fehlerschwankung *f*

eructation Aufstoßen *n*, Rülpsen *n*

erythema Erythem *n*, Hautrötung *f*

erythrochloropia Blaugelbblindheit *f*, Erythrochloropie *f*

erythrocyte Erythrozyt *m*, rotes Blutkörperchen *n*

erythrocythemia Polyzythämie *f*, Erythrozytose *f*

erythrogenic, erythrogenetic rot werdend

erythromania Sucht *f* nach roten Gegenständen

erythrophobia Erythrophobie *f*, Ereutophobie *f*, Furcht *f* vor Erröten, krankhafte Angst *f* beim Sehen der Farbe „rot"

erythropoietin Erythropoetin *n*

erythroprosopalgia Erythroprosopalgie *f*, Cluster–Kopfschmerz *m*, Horton–Syndrom *n*

erythropsia, erythropia Erythropsie *f*, Rotsichtigkeit *f*

erythropsin Sehpurpur *m*, Rhodopsin *n*

escape fliehen / Flucht *f*, Entkommen *n* / **~ activity** Fluchtaktivität *f* / **~ behaviour** Fluchtverhalten *n* / **~ conditioning** Konditionieren *n* einer Fluchtreaktion / **~ from the ego** Flucht *f* vor dem Ich / **~ into fantasy** Flucht *f* in die Fantasie / **~ learning** Erlernen *n* einer Fluchtreaktion / **~ mechanism** Fluchtmechanismus *m*, Abwehrmechanismus *m* / **~ reaction** Fluchtreaktion *f* / **~ from reality** Flucht *f* vor der Realität *f* / **~ reflex** Fluchtreflex *m* / **~ response** Fluchtreaktion *f* / **~ tendency** Fluchttendenz *f* / **~ training** Konditionieren *n* einer Fluchtreaktion, Fluchttraining *n*

escapism neurotische Fluchttendenz *f*

escapist fliehend / Fliehender *m*

eserine Eserin *n*, Physostigmin *n*

esophageal Ösophagus–

esophagus Ösophagus *m*, Speiseröhre *f*, Schlund *m*

esophoria Esophorie *f*, latentes Einwärtsschielen *n*

esoteric esoterisch, nur für Auserwählte bestimmt

esotropia konvergierender Strabismus *m*

esprit de corps Korpsgeist *m*, Gruppengeist *m*, Gruppenmoral *f*

essay examination, essay testing Essay–Test *m*, Test *m* mit freier Aufgabenbeantwortung

essence Wesentliches *n*, Kern *n*, Extrakt *m*

essential wesentlich, wichtig, essenziell, idiopathisch, ohne bekannte Ätiologie

establishment Einrichtung *f*, Anstalt *f*, Institut *n*, Aufgliederung *f* der Persönlichkeit / **private ~** private Anstalt *f*, privates Institut *n* / **public ~** öffentliche Einrichtung *f*, Staatsinstitut *n*

esteem achten, hochschätzen / Wertschätzung *f*, Achtung *f* / **~ need** Bedürfnis *n* geachtet und geschätzt zu werden

esterase Esterase *f*

esthesia Empfindung *f*, Empfindlichkeit *f*

esthesiology Lehre *f* von den Empfindungen und Empfindungsorganen

esthesiometer Empfindlichkeitsmesser *m*, Tasterzirkel *m*, Ästhesiometer *n*

esthesiometry Empfindlichkeitsmessung *f*

esthesiophysiology Sinnesphysiologie *f*

esthete Ästhet *m*, Ästhetiker *m*

esthetic ästhetisch

esthetics Ästhetik *f*

estimate schätzen, abschätzen, bestimmen

estimation Schätzung *f*, Bestimmung *f* / ~ **difference** Schätzfehler *m*, Schätzdifferenz *f* / ~ **error** Schätzfehler *m* / ~ **value** Schätzwert *m* / **statistical** ~ statistische Schätzung *f*

estimative abschätzbar, Schätz–

estimator Schätzer *m*, Schätzmethode *f* / **unbiased** ~ erwartungstreue Schätzung *f*, fehlerfreie Schätzung *f*

estradiol Östradiol *n*

estral Brunst–

estrangement Entfremdung *f*

estrogen Östrogen *n*

estrogenic, estrogenous östruserzeugend, östrogen

estromania Östromanie *f*, Nymphomanie *f*

estrone Östron *n*

estrus, estrum Östrus *m*, Brunst *f*, Brunstzeit *f*

eta coefficient Korrelationskoeffizient Eta *m*

ethanol Äthanol *n*, Äthylalkohol *m*

ether Äther *m* / **anaesthetic** ~ Narkoseäther *m* / **ethyl** ~ Äthyläther *m*, Äther *m*

ethereal, etherial ätherisch, ätherartig

ethernet Ethernet *n*, lokales Netzwerk *n*

etheromania Ätherismus *m*

ethical, ethic ethisch, sittlich, moralisch

ethics Ethik *f*, Sittenlehre *f*, Moral *f* / **experimental** ~ Ethik *f* des Experimentierens / **professional** ~ Berufsethik *f*, Standesethik *f*

ethnic ethnisch, rassisch

ethnics Ethnologie *f*

ethnocentric ethnozentrisch

ethnocentrism Ethnozentrik *f*, Ethnozentrismus *m*

ethnogram Ethnogramm *n*, Volksbeschreibung *f*

ethnography Ethnographie *f*, Völkerkunde *f*, Völkerbeschreibung *f*

ethnolinguistics vergleichende Sprachwissenschaft *f*

ethnological ethnologisch

ethnology Ethnologie *f*, Völkerkunde *f*

ethnopsychology Völkerpsychologie *f*, Ethnopsychologie *f*

ethogram Ethogramm *n*, Beschreibung *f* aller Verhaltensweisen einer Tierart

ethological ethologisch

ethology Ethologie *f*, Verhaltensforschung *f*

ethos Ethos *n*, moralische Grundhaltungf

etiological ätiologisch

etiology Ätiologie *f*, Lehre *f* von den Ursachen

etymology Etymologie *f*, Lehre *f* von der Wortherkunft

euchromatopsy normales Farbsehen *n*, Euchromatopsie *f*

eudaemonism Eudamonismus *m*, Lehre *f* vom glückseligen Leben

eugenic eugenisch, erbhygienisch

eugenics, eugenism Eugenik *f*, Erbhygiene *f*

eugenol Eugenol *n*

eumorphic gut gebaut, normal gewachsen, von guter Gestalt

eunoia normale Geistestätigkeit *f*

eunuch Eunuch *m*

eunuchism Eunuchismus *m*

eunuchoid eunuchoid, eunuchenähnlich

eunuchoidismus Eunuchoidismus *m*

euosmia normaler Geruchssinn *m*

eupareunia normaler Koitus *m*, normaler Geschlechtsverkehr *m*, Koitus *m* mit Orgasmus

eupathia Eupathie *f*

euphemism Euphemismus *m*, beschönigender Ausdruck *m*

euphonic wohlklingend

euphony Wohlklang *m*, wohlklingende Stimme *f*

euphoretic euphorieerzeugend

euphoria Euphorie *f*, gesteigertes Lebensgefühl *n*, Glücksgefühl *n*, Wohlbefinden *n*, Hochstimmung *f* / **hypochondriac ~** hypochondrische Euphorie *f*

euphoriant Euphorikum *n*, euphorieerzeugendes Mittel *n*

euphoric euphorisch, glückselig

eupnea, eupnoea Eupnoe *f*, normale Ruheatmung *f*

eupraxia Ausführen *n* koordinierter Bewegungen, normaler Bewegungsablauf *m*, Eupraxie *f*

eupraxic koordiniert bewegend

eurhythmia regelmäßiger Pulsschlag *m*, normaler Rhythmus *m*, Eurhythmie *f*

eurhythmics rhythmische Gymnastik *f*, Eurhythmik *f*

eurotophobia Angst *f* vor weiblichen Geschlechtsorganen

eurycephalic, eurycranial euryzephal, breitschädelig

eurycephaly Breitschädeligkeit *f*, Euryzephalie *f*

eurymorph, eurysomatic eurymorph, eurysom, breitwüchsig

eurysomia Breitwuchs *m*

euthanasia Euthanasie *f*, Sterbehilfe *f*, schmerzloser Tod *m*

euthenics Euthenik *f*, Lehre *f* von der Verbesserung des Menschen durch Verbesserung seiner Umwelt

euthymia frohe Stimmungslage *f*, Tendenz *f* zu positiver Stimmungslage

eutony ausgeglichene Spannung *f*, Spannungsbalance *f*

evacuation Entleerung *f* / **~ reflex** Entleerungsreflex *m*

evaluate bewerten

evaluation Bewertung *f*, Wertung *f*, Beurteilung *f*, Evaluation *f* / **~ apprehension** wertende Versuchsinterpretation *f* / **~ of tests** Testauswertung *f*, Versuchsauswertung *f* / **forensic ~** forensische Begutachtung *f* / **personal ~** persönliche Bewertung *f* / **psychiatric ~** psychiatrische Beurteilung *f* / **psychological ~** psychologische Beurteilung *f* / **social ~ theory** soziale Bewertungstheorie *f* / **subjective ~** subjektive Bewertung *f* / **vocational ~** Berufseignungsdiagnostik *f*

even gleich, gleichmäßig, gleichmütig, ausgeglichen / **~ tempered** gleichmütig, gelassen

evenness Gleichmut *m*, Ausgeglichenheit *f*, Gelassenheit *f*

event Ereignis *n*, Vorfall *m*, Phänomen *n* / **~–related** ereigniskorreliert / **~ sampling** ereignisbezogene Zufallsauswahl *f* / **~ system** zielgerichtetes Interaktionssystem *n* / **independent ~s** unabhängige Ereignisse *npl* / **reinforcing ~** verstärkendes Ereignis *n* / **traumatic ~** traumatisches Ereignis *n*, psychische Traumatisierung *f*

evidence Beweis *m*, Klarheit *f*, Offenkundigkeit *f*, Evidenz *f* / **anecdotal ~** gelegentlicher Befund *m*, gelegentlich beobachteter Vorfall *m* / **circumstantial ~** Indizienbeweis *m* / **legal ~** gerichtlicher Beweis *m* / **palaeontological ~** paläontologischer Beweis *m*, vorgeschichtlicher Beweis *m* / **presumptive ~** mutmaßlicher Beweis *m*

evident augenscheinlich, offenkundig, evident

evil schlecht, böse

eviration Eviration *f*, Verlust *m* der Männlichkeit

evocation Geisterbeschwörung *f*, Heraufbeschwören *n*

evocative Erinnerungs–, hervorrufend, evokativ

evoke hervorrufen, auslösen

evolution Entwicklung *f*, Evolution *f* / **~ theory** Evolutionstheorie *f* / **essential ~** wesentliche Weiterentwicklung *f* / **mental ~** geistige Entwicklung *f* / **organic ~** organische Entwicklung *f* / **social ~** soziale Entwicklung *f*, soziale Veränderungen *fpl* / **spontaneous ~** Selbstentfaltung *f*

evolutionary Entwicklungs–, Evolutions–

evolutionism Evolutionismus *m*

Ewald|'s sound pattern theory Ewalds Schallbildertheorie *f* / **~ types** Ewald'sche Typen *mpl*

exacerbate erbittern, reizen

exacerbation Erbitterung *f*

exactitude Genauigkeit *f*

exactness Genauigkeit *f*, Richtigkeit *f*

exaggerated übertrieben

exaggeration Übertreibung *f* / **~ of a symptom** Symptomverstärkung *f*

exalt preisen, in Verzückung geraten, verherrlichen, schwärmen

exaltation Überschwänglichkeit *f*, Verzückung *f*, Exaltation *f*, Überspanntheit *f* / **~ state** Zustand *m* der Verzückung

exalted exaltiert, überschwänglich, verzückt

examination, exam Untersuchung *f*, Prüfung *f*, Test *m*, Examen *n* / **~ dream** Prüfungstraum *m* / **~ findings** Untersuchungsbefund *m* / **~ stupor** Examensstupor / **academic ~** Schulprüfung *f* / **comprehensive ~** Abschlussprüfung *f* / **mental ~** psychologische Untersuchung *f* / **neurological ~** neurologische Untersuchung *f* / **objective ~** objektiver Test *m*, objektives Prüfverfahren *n* / **ophthalmological ~** Augenuntersuchung *f*, ophthalmologische Untersuchung *f* / **physical ~** körperliche Untersuchung *f* / **propaedeutic ~** Vorexamen *n*, propädeutisches Examen *n* / **professional ~** berufliche Qualifikationsprüfung *f* / **psychiatric ~** psychiatrische Untersuchung *f* / **psychological ~** psychologische Untersuchung *f* / **subjective ~** subjektiver Test *m*, subjektives Prüfverfahren *n*

examine untersuchen, prüfen, testen

examinee Prüfling *m*, Proband *m*, Versuchsperson *f*

examiner Versuchsleiter *m*, Prüfer *m*, Testleiter *m*

exanthropia Exanthropie *f*

excentric exzentrisch, überspannt / exzentrischer Mensch *m*, Sonderling *m*

excentricity Exzentrizität *f*, exzentrisches Verhalten *n*, Überspanntheit *f*

exceptional außergewöhnlich

excerebration Enthirnung *f*, Exzerebration *f*

excess Kurtosis *f*, Steilheitsgrad *m* einer Verteilung, Übermaß *n*, Exzess *m* / **~ behaviour** exzessives Verhalten *n* / **~ sound pressure** Schallüberdruck *m* / **sexual ~** sexuelle Ausschweifung *f*

excessive übermäßig, überstark

exchange Austausch *m* / **~ theory** Austauschtheorie *f* / **social ~ theories** Theorien *fpl* des sozialen Austauschs

excision Ausscheidung *f*, Exzision *f*, Entfernung *f*

excitability Erregbarkeit *f*, Reizbarkeit *f*, Iritabilität *f* / **~ curve** Erregungskurve *f* / **cortical ~** kortikale Erregbarkeit *f*

excitable erregbar, reizbar, reizempfänglich, reizempfindlich, nervös

excitableness Reizbarkeit *f*, Erregbarkeit *f*, Nervosität *f*

excitant Reizmittel *n*, Stimulans *n*, Excitans *n*

excitation Erregung *f*, Reizung *f* Reiz *m*, Angeregtheit *f* / **~–contraction coupling** elektromechanische Kopplung *f* / **~–contraction uncoupling** elektromechanische Entkopplung *f* / **~ gradient** Erregungsgradient *m* / **~–inhibition theory** Theorie *f* der Erregungshemmung / **~ pattern** Erregungsmuster *n* / **~ process** Erregungsvorgang *m* / **~ quantity** Erregungsgröße *f* / **~ state** Reizzustand *m*, Erregungszustand *m* / **~ tendency** Erregungstendenz *f* / **~ therapy** Reiztherapie *f* / **~ time** Erregungszeit *f* / **all–or–none ~** Alles–oder–Nichts–Erregung *f* / **conducted ~** fortgeleitete Erregung *f* / **electric ~** elektrischer Reiz *m* / **local ~** lokale Erregung *f* / **maintained ~** Dauererregung *f* / **nervous ~** Nervenerregung *f* / **neural ~** Nervenerregung *f* / **primary ~** primäre Erregung *f* / **sensory ~** Sinnesreizung *f*

excitatory exzitatorisch, Erregungs–

excite erregen

excited erregt

excitement Erregung *f*, Alteration *f* / **~ phase** Erregungsphase *f* / **~–quiescence** Erregung–Ruhe *f* / **reactive ~** reaktive Erregung *f* / **sexual ~** geschlechtliche Erregung *f*

exciting erregend, aufregend

exclude ausschließen

exclusion Ausschluss *m*, Ausgrenzung *f* / **~ of reality** Realitätsabsperrung *f* / **false ~** falscher Ausschluss *m*, Fehler *m* Typ I / **valid ~** begründeter Ausschluss *m*

exclusive ausschließlich, Allein–

exclusiveness Ausschließlichkeit *f* / **~ of mind** Schubladendenken *n*

excrement Kot *m*, Exkremente *npl*, Faeces *pl*

excrescence Auswuchs *m*

excretion Ausscheidung *f*, Exkretion *f* / **~ of urine** Harnabsonderung *f*, Harnlassen *n*, Miktion *f*

execution Ausführung *f*

executive ausführend / leitender Angestellter *m*, Führungskraft *f*, Staatsgewalt *f* / **~ development** Weiterbildung *f* von Führungskräften / **~ search consultant** Personalberater *m*, Headhunter *m* / **senior ~** leitender Angestellter *m*, Top–Manager *m*

exercise üben, ausüben / Übung *f*, Training *n* / **~ response** Übungsreaktion *f* / **~ therapy** Übungstherapie *f* / **bodily ~s** Leibesübungen *fpl* / **formal ~** formale Übung *f* / **physical ~s** Leibesübungen *fpl* / **remedial ~s** Beschäftigungstherapie *f*

exertion Ausübung *f*, Anstrengung *f*

exertional Anstrengungs–, Arbeits–

exhalation Ausatmung *f*, Exspiration *f*

exhaustion Erschöpfung *f*, Ermüdung *f* / **~ delirium** Erschöpfungsdelirium *n* / **~ depression** Erschöpfungsdepression *f* / **~ psychosis** Erschöpfungspsychose *f*, Zusammenbruch *m* / **~ stage** Erschöpfungsphase *f* / **mental ~** mentale Erschöpfung *f*

exhaustive erschöpfend, vollständig

exhibit exhibieren

exhibition need Bedürfnis *n* die Aufmerksamkeit anderer auf sich zu lenken

exhibitionism Exhibitionismus *m*, Zeigelust *f* / **repressed ~** verdrängter Exhibitionismus *m*

exhibitionist Exhibitionist *m*

exhibitionistic exhibitionistisch

existence Existenz *f*, Dasein *n* / **human ~** menschliche Existenz *f*

existential existenziell

existentialism Existenzialismus *m*

existing bestehend, vorhanden

exit interview Austrittsinterview *n*, Abgangsgespräch *n*, Gespräch *n* über die Kündigungsgründe

Exner|'s disk Exner–Scheibe *f*, Exner–Spirale *f* / **~'s spiral** Exner–Spirale *f*, Exner–Scheibe *f*

exocathection Kathexis *f*, Vorgang *m* der Besetzung (nach außen)

exocathexis Besetzung *f*

exocentric exozentrisch

exodus Abwanderung *f*, Auswanderung *f* / **rural ~** Landflucht *f*

exogamy Exogamie *f*, Ehe *f* außerhalb des eigenen Clans

exogenetic, exogenic, exogenous exogen, von außen kommend, aufgrund äußerer Ursachen

exolinguistics Metalinguistik *f*

exophoria Exophorie *f*, latentes Auswärtsschielen *n*

exophoric auswärts schielend

exophthalmia Glotzäugigkeit *f*, Exophthalmie *f*

exophthalmos, exophthalmus Exophthalmus *m*, Glotzauge *n*, Hervortreten *n* des Augapfels

exopsychic außerpsychisch, exopsychisch

exorcism Exorzismus *m*, Austreiben *n* böser Geister aus Besessenen

exosomatic exosomatisch

exosomaesthesia Empfindung *f* außerhalb des Körpers

exoteric exoterisch, für Außenstehende bestimmt, gemeinverständlich

exotropia Auswärtsschielen *n*, Strabismus divergens *m*

expansion Ausdehung *f*, Ausbreitung *f*, Erweiterung *f* / **binomial ~** Binomialverteilung *f*, höherer Ordnung

expansive expansiv, überschwänglich, größenwahnsinnig

expansiveness Mitteilsamkeit *f*, Großsprecherei *f*, Größenwahn *m*

expectancy Erwartung *f* / **~ chart** Tabelle *f* der Erwartungswerte / **~ hypothesis** Erwartungshypothese *f* / **~ table** Tabelle *f* der Erwartungswerte / **~ theory** Erwartungstheorie *f* / **generalized ~** generalisierte Erwartung *f*

expectant Erwartungs–

expectation Erwartung *f*, Antizipation *f* / **~ neurosis** Erwartungsneurose *f* / **~ value** Erwartungswert *m* / **anxious ~** Erwartungsangst *f* / **mathematical ~** mathematische Erwartung *f* / **parental ~s** Elternerwartungen *fpl* / **statistical ~** statistische Erwartung *f*

expenditure Ausgabe *f*, Aufwand *m*, Verbrauch *m* / **~ of energy in abstract thought** Energieaufwand *m* beim abstrakten Denken

experience Erfahrung *f*, Erlebnis *n* / erfahren, lernen / **~ balance** Erlebnistyp *m* / **~ of conversion** Bekehrungserlebnis *n* / **~ of dislike** Unlusterlebnis *n* / **~ of enlightenment** Erleuchtungserlebnis *n*, Erweckungserlebnis *n* / **~ error** Erfahrungstrugschluss *m* / **~ level** Erfahrungsniveau *n* / **~ of failure** Misserfolgserlebnis *n* / **~ of pain** Schmerzerleben *n* / **~ of satisfaction** Befriedigungserlebnis *n* / **~–type** Erlebnistyp *m* / **affective ~** gefühlsbetontes Erlebnis *n* / **conscious ~** bewusstes Erleben *n* / **corrective emotional ~** korrigierend wirkende emotionale Erfahrung *f* / **determining ~** determinierendes Erlebnis *n* / **early ~** frühkindliche Erfahrungen *f* / **frustrating ~** frustrierendes Erlebnis *n* / **immediate ~** unmittelbare Erfahrung *f* / **mystical ~** mystische Erfahrung *f* / **personal ~** persönliche Erfahrung *f*, eigene Erfahrung *f* / **psychedelic ~s** psychedelische Erlebnisse *npl* / **religious ~** religiöse Erfahrung *f* / **traumatic ~** traumatisches Erlebnis *n* / **vicarious ~** substitutives Erlebnis *n*, stellvertretende Erfahrung *f*

experienced erfahren, sachkundig

experiencer Erfahrender *m*, Erlebender *m*

experiential Erfahrungs–, empirisch

experiment Experiment *n*, Versuch *m*, Probe *f* / experimentieren, versuchen, erproben / **~ control** Versuchskontrolle *f*, experimentelle Kontrolle *f* / **~ volunteer** freiwillige Versuchsperson *f* / **biotic ~** biotisches Experiment *n* / **blank ~** Leerversuch *m*, Kontrollexperiment *n* / **chronic ~** Dauerversuch *m* / **comparative ~** Vergleichsexperiment *n* / **controlled ~** exakt kontrolliertes Experiment *n* / **critical ~** Entscheidungsexperiment *n* / **crucial ~** Entscheidungsexperiment *n* / **decisive ~** Entscheidungsexperiment *n* / **double–blind ~** Doppelblindversuch *m* / **exploratory ~** Erkundungsexperiment *n*, Vorversuch *m*, Voruntersuchung *f* / **parallel ~** Parallelversuch *m* / **preliminary ~** Voruntersuchung *f*, Vorversuch *m*

experimental experimentell, Versuchs–, Experimental–

experimentalist Experimentator *m*

experimentation Experimentieren *n*, Versuchen *n*, experimentelle Untersuchung *f*, experimentelle Forschung *f*

experimenter, experimentor Experimentator *m*, Versuchsleiter *m* / **~ bias** Versuchsleitererwartungseffekt *m*, Versuchsleiterfehler *m* / **~ effect** Versuchsleitereffekt *m* / **~ expectation** Versuchsleitererwartung *f*

experimentum Experiment *n*, Versuch *m* / **~ crucis** Entscheidungsversuch *m*, Entscheidungsexperiment *n*

expert erfahren, fachkundig / Experte *m*, Fachmann *m*, Gutachter *m* / ~ **adviser** Fachberater *m* / ~ **evidence** Sachverständigengutachten *n* / ~ **opinion** Gutachten *n* / ~ **power** Fachautorität *f* / ~ **system** Expertensystem *n* / ~ **testimony** Gutachten *n*, Expertengutachten *n*, gerichtliches Sachverständigengutachten *n* / **psychological** ~ psychologischer Sachverständiger *m*

expiation Buße *f*, Sühne *f*

expiration Ausatmen *n*, Ablauf *m*

explain auslegen, erklären

explanation Auslegung *f*, Deutung *f*, Erklärung *f*, Interpretation *f* / **causal** ~ Kausalerklärung *f* / **historical** ~ historische Deutung *f* / **spatial** ~ Erklärung *f* des Raumes / **theoretical** ~ theoretische Erklärung, spekulative Deutung *f*

explication ausführliche Darlegung *f*, Explikation *f*, Erklärung *f*

explicit explizit, ausdrücklich, deutlich

exploitation Ausbeutung *f*, Ausnützung *f* / **parental** ~ elterliche Ausbeutung *f*, Ausbeutung *f* durch die Eltern

exploitive ausbeutend, ausnützend

exploration Exploration *f*, Anamnese *f*, Befragung *f*, Interview *n* / **free** ~ freies Suchverhalten *n* / **mental** ~ psychodiagnostische Befragung *f* / **serial** ~ **method** Methode *f* der eben merklichen Unterschiede

exploratory Erkundungs–, explorativ

explore untersuchen, erkunden, explorieren

exploring Untersuchungs–, untersuchend

explosiveness Veranlagung *f* zu Explosivreaktionen, Explosivität

exponent Exponent *m*

exponential exponentiell

exposition Erklärung *f*, Ausstellung *f* / ~ **attitude** Erklärungstendenz *f*, explikative Tendenz *f* / ~ **need** Erklärungsbedürfnis *n*

ex post facto rückwirkend, im Nachhinein getan, retrospektiv

exposure Darbietung *f*, Exposition *f* / ~ **field** Expositionsfeld *n*, Darbietungsfeld *n* / ~ **period** Expositionszeit *f*, Darbietungszeit *f* / ~ **therapy** Expositionstherapie *f* / ~ **time** Expositionszeit *f*, Darbietungszeit *f* / **indecent** ~ Exhibitionismus *m* / **occupational** ~ Gesundheitsrisiken *npl* am Arbeitsplatz / **prenatal** ~ pränatale Gefährdung *f*

expression Ausdruck *m*, Äußerung *f* / ~ **of affect** Affektausdruck *m* / ~ **of the face** Gesichtsausdruck *m*, Mimik *f* / ~ **method** Ausdrucksmethode *f* / ~ **test** Ausdruckstest *m* / **emotional** ~ Gemütsausdruck *m* / **facial** ~ Gesichtsausdruck *m*, Mimik *f* / **listless** ~ teilnahmsloser Ausdruck *m* / **vacant** ~ Ausdrucksstarre *f* / **verbal** ~ mündlicher Ausdruck *m*

expressionless ausdruckslos

expressionlessness Ausdrucksstarre *f*

expressive Ausdrucks–, ausdrucksvoll

expressiveness, expressivity Ausdruckskraft *f* des Mienenspiels, Ausdrucksfähigkeit *f*

extend ausdehnen, strecken, erweitern

extension Ausdehnung *f*, Erweiterung *f*, Extension *f* / ~ **of a muscle** Extension *f* eines Muskels / ~ **reflex** Extensionsreflex *m* / ~ **tendency** Streckungstendenz *f*

extensional erweitert

extensionalization semantische Begriffsbestimmung *f*, Extensionalisierung *f*

extensity Extensität *f*, Gefühl *n* der Weite / ~ **of a mood** Extensität *f* einer Stimmung

extensive ausgedehnt, umfassend, extensiv

extensor Streckmuskel *m*, Strecker *m*, Extensor *m* / ~ **muscle** Strecker *m*, Streckmuskel *m* / ~ **thrust** Streckmuskelreflex *m* / **crossed** ~ **reflex** gekreuzter Streckreflex *m*

extent Ausdehnung *f*, Umfang *m*, Ausmaß *n*

exteriorisation Projektion *f* nach außen, Exteriorisation *f*

external extern, äußere(r, s) / ~ **auditory** Außenohr–

externalisation Exteriorisation *f*, Externalisation *f*, Projektion *f* nach außen

externalize nach außen projizieren, nach außen verlegen, externalisieren

exteroceptive exterozeptiv, augenreizempfänglich

exteroceptor Exterozeptor *m*, Oberflächenendnerv *m*

exterofective auf äußere Reize reagierend, exterofektiv

exterosystem angeborenes System *n* für Außenweltbeziehungen, Exterosystem *n*, Ich–Funktionen *fpl*

extinction Auslöschung *f*, Löschung *f*, Schwächung *f*, Extinktion *f* / **~ of the conditioned response** Auslöschung *f* der bedingten Reaktion / **~ curve** Extinktionskurve *f* / **~ of the ego** Auslöschung *f* des Ichs / **~ ratio** Verhältnis *n* der nicht–verstärkten zu den verstärkten Reaktionen / **covert ~** latentes Auslöschen *n* / **differential ~** differentielles Auslöschen *n* / **experimental ~** experimentelles Auslöschen *n* / **latent ~** latentes Auslöschen *n*, latente Abschwächung *f* / **partial ~** Teilabschwächung *f* / **secondary ~** sekundäres Auslöschen *n*

extinguish auslöschen, beseitigen, ausrotten

extirpate exstirpieren, herausschneiden

extirpation Exstirpation *f*, völliges Ausschneiden *n*

extracellular extrazellulär

extraception Extrazeption *f*

extracerebral außerhalb des Gehirns

extrachance außerhalb des Zufalls liegend

extracranial außerhalb des Schädels

extracurricular außerschulisch, außerhalb der Schule oder Universität, außerhalb des Lehrplans

extradural außerhalb der Dura gelegen

extrajection Projektion *f*, Hinausverlagerung *f*, Hinausverlegen *n*

extramarginal außerhalb des Bewusstseins liegend, außersinnlich

extramarital außerehelich

extramural extramural, außerhalb der Mauern gelegen, außerhalb einer Institution

extraneous fremd, Außen–

extrapolate extrapolieren

extrapolation Extrapolation *f*

extrapsychotic extrapsychotisch

extrapunitive extrapunitiv

extrapunitiveness extrapunitive Haltung *f*

extrapyramidal extrapyramidal, außerhalb der Pyramidenbahn gelegen

extrasensory außersinnlich, hellseherisch

extrasocial ohne soziale Beziehung, ohne soziale Bindung

extraspectral außerhalb des Spektrums

extrasystole Extrasystole *f*, Extraschlag *m* des Herzens

extratensive extratensiv

extratensivity Extratension *f*, Extratensivität *f*

extravagance Überspanntheit *f*, Zügellosigkeit *f*, Extravaganz *f*

extravagant übertrieben, überspannt, extravagant

extraversion, extroversion Extraversion *f*, nach außen gerichtetes Interesse *n*

extravert, extrovert extravertiert sein, extrovertiert sein / Extravertierter *m*, Extrovertierter *m*

extravert, extrovert, extroverted, extroversive extravertiert, extrovertiert

extrinsic exogen, extrinsic, von außen wirkend

extrojection Projektion *f*, Hinausverlagerung *f*, Hinausverlegen *n*

extrospection Fremdbeobachtung *f*, Extrospektion *f*

extrospective extrospektiv, Fremdbeobachtung betreibend

exuberance Überschwänglichkeit *f*

exvia Extraversion *f*

eye Auge *n* / **~ appeal** Blickfang *m* / **~–brain** Ophthalmenzephalon *n* / **~ catcher** Blickfang *m* / **~ chart** Sehtafel *f* / **~ col-**

our Augenfarbe *f* / ~ **contact** Sichtkontakt *m*, Blickkontakt *m* / ~ **convergence** Augenkonvergenz *f* / ~ **coordination** Augenkoordination *f* / ~ **disorder** Augenleiden *n*, Augenerkrankung *f* / ~ **dominance** Augendominanz *f* / ~ **fixation** Blickfixierung *f* / ~ **ground** Augenhintergrund *m* / **~–hand coordination** Auge–Hand–Koordination *f* / **~–level** Augenhöhe *f* / **~–minded** mit visueller Erinnerung begabt / **~–mindedness** visuelle Dominanz *f* / ~ **movement** Augenbewegung *f* / ~ **movement desensitization therapy** Augenbewegungsdesensibilisierung *f* / ~ **muscles** Augenmuskeln *mpl* / ~ **pause** Augenstillstand *m* / **~–shaped** augenförmig / ~ **socket** Augenhöhle *f* / ~ **span** Blickspanne *f*, Blickumfang *m* / ~ **speculum** Augenspiegel *m* / **~–voice span** Distanz *f* welche das Auge im gelesenen Text dem gerade vorgelesenen Text voraus ist / ~ **witness** Augenzeuge *m* / **compound** ~ Insektenauge *n*, Facettenauge *n* / **consensual** ~ **reflex** unwillkürlicher Pupillenreflex *m* / **crossed** **~s** Schielen *n*, Strabismus *m* / **cyclopean** ~ Zyklopenauge *n* / **dark–adapted** ~ an die Dunkelheit angepasstes Auge *n* / **emmetropic** ~ normalsichtiges Auge *n* / **evil** ~ böser Blick *m* / **extrinsic** ~ **muscle** äußerer Augenmuskel *m* / **intrinsic** ~ **muscle** innerer Augenmuskel *m* / **nonrapid** ~ **movement** langsame Augenbewegung *f* / **parallel** ~ **movement** parallele Augenbewegung *f* / **rapid** ~ **movement** schnelle Augenbewegung *f*, Rapid Eye Movement *n* / **reduced** ~ reduziertes Auge *n* / **rolling** ~ **movement** Augenrollen *n* / **schematic** ~ schematisches Auge *n*

eyeball Augapfel *m*

eyeblink Augenblinzeln *n*, Lidschlag *m* / ~ **conditioning** Konditionierung *f* des Lidschlagreflexes / ~ **reflex** Lidschlussreflex *m*, Lidschlagreflex *m*

eyedness, eyeness Augendominanz *f*

eyelid Augenlid *n* / ~ **closure reflex** Lidschlussreflex *m* / ~ **conditioning** Lidschlusskonditionierung *f* / ~ **reflex** Lidschlussreflex *m* / **conditioned** ~ **response** bedingter Lidschlagreflex *m*

eyesight Sehkraft *f*, Sehen *n*

eyewink reflex Lidschlagreflex *m*

F

fabrication Erdichtung *f*, Fabulieren *n*

fabulation Erdichtung *f*, Fabulieren *n*

face Gesicht *n*, Ausdruck *m*, Mimik *f* / **~ perception** Gesichterwahrnehmung *f* / **~ saving** den Anschein wahrend / **~ sheet** Deckblatt *n* / **~–to–back position** Position *f* von hinten, Koitus *m* von hinten / **~–to–face group** Intimgruppe *f*, Gruppe *f* mit unmittelbarem Kontakt / **~–to–face position** von Angesicht zu Angesicht *n*, Koitus *m* von vorn / **~ validity** Scheinvalidität *f*, Scheingültigkeit *f* / **~ value** Mitte *f* eines Klassenintervalls, Nominalwert *m*, scheinbarer Wert *m* / **Parkinsonian ~** Maskengesicht *n* bei Parkinson'scher Krankheit

facetious witzig, spaßig, drollig

facial Gesichts–

facies Fazies *f*, Gesicht *n*

facilitation Bahnung *f*, Erleichterung *f* / **~ of conductibility** Bahnung *f* / **~ of transmission** Bahnung *f* der Übertragung / **associative ~** assoziative Bahnung *f* / **heterosynaptic ~** heterosynaptische Bahnung *f* / **neural ~** Bahnung *f* / **parasympathetic ~** parasympathische Bahnung *f* / **postsynaptic ~** postsynaptische Bahnung *f* / **presynaptic ~** präsynaptische Bahnung *f* / **reproductive ~** reproduktive Bahnung *f* / **retroactive ~** retroaktive Bahnung *f* / **social ~** soziale Förderung *f*, soziale Erleichterung *f*, soziale Aktivierung *f* / **spatial ~** räumliche Bahnung *f* / **synaptic ~** synaptische Bahnung *f* / **temporal ~** zeitliche Bahnung *f*

facility Einrichtung *f*, Institution *f* / **~ admission** Aufnahme *f* in eine Institution / **~ discharge** Entlassung *f* aus einer Institution / **~ environment** institutionelle Umgebung *f*

facioplegia Gesichtslähmung *f*, Fazialisparese *f*

facsimile Faksimile *n*, Nachbildung *f* / **~ copy** Faksimile *n* / **~ data transmission** Bildfunk *m*

fact Tatsache *f* / **social ~** soziales Phänomen *n*

factfinding question Frage *f* zur Ermittlung des Sachverhalts

factitious künstlich, nachgemacht

factor Faktor *m* / **~ analysis** Faktorenanalyse *f* / **~ axes** Faktorenachsen *fpl* / **~ coefficient** Faktorenladung *f* / **~ configuration** Faktorenstellung *f*, Faktorenkonfiguration *f* / **~ covariance matrix** Faktorenkorrelationsmatrix *f* / **~ efficiency** Faktorenwirksamkeit *f*, faktorieller Einfluss *m* / **~ fixation** Faktorenbestimmung *f*, Faktorenfestlegung *f* / **~ invariance** Unveränderlichkeit *f* der Faktoren / **~ loading** Faktorenladung *f* / **~ matrix** Faktorenmatrix *f* / **~ reflection** Umkehrung *f* der Vorzeichen, Faktorenumkehrung *f* / **~ resolution** Faktoreninterpretation *f*, Faktorenzerlegung *f* / **~ rotation** Achsendrehung *f*, Rotation *f* / **~ space** faktorieller Raum *m* / **~–specification equation** Faktorengleichung *f* / **~ structure** Faktorenstruktur *f* / **~ theory** Faktorentheorie *f* / **~ theories of intelligence** faktorielle Intelligenztheorien *fpl* / **~ theories of learning** faktorielle Lerntheorien *fpl* / **~ weight** Faktorengewicht *n*, Faktorenladung *f* / **areal ~** Raumfaktor *m* / **balancing ~** Gegengewicht *n*, Gegenfaktor *m* / **bionomic ~** bionomischer Faktor *m*, ökologischer Faktor *m* / **bipolar ~** bipolarer Faktor *m* / **common ~** gemeinsamer Faktor *m* / **confounding ~** Störfaktor *m* / **contributing**

~ Begleitumstand *m* / **determining ~** determinierender Faktor *m*, bestimmender Faktor *m* / **disturbing ~** Störfaktor *m* / **ecological ~** Umweltfaktor *m*, ökologischer Faktor *m* / **emotional ~** emotioneller Faktor *m* / **environmental ~s** Milieufaktoren *mpl*, Umgebungsfaktoren *mpl*, Umweltbedingungen *fpl* / **extrinsic ~** „extrinsic factor" *m*, extrinsischer Faktor *m* / **five ~ personality model** Fünffaktorenmodell *n* der Persönlichkeit / **general ~** G–Faktor *m*, gemeinsamer Faktor *m* / **genetic ~** Erbfaktor *m* / **germinal ~** Keimfaktor *m* / **hereditary ~** Erbfaktor *m* / **human ~s engineering** Ergonomie *f* / **intrinsic ~** „intrinsic factor" *m*, intrinsischer Faktor *m* / **inverse ~ analysis** Q–Technik *f* / **inverted ~ analysis** Q–Technik *f* / **moral ~** moralischer Faktor *m* / **multiple ~ analysis** multiple Faktorenanalyse *f* / **multiple–~ inheritance** multifaktorielle Vererbung *f* / **nonspecific ~** unspezifischer Faktor *m* / **numerical ~** numerischer Faktor *m*, N–Faktor *m* / **primary ~** Grundfaktor *m* / **psychological ~** psychischer Faktor *m* / **psychological ~s affecting medical condition** psychische Faktoren *mpl*, die medizinische Krankheitsfaktoren beeinflussen / **psychological ~s affecting physical condition** psychische Faktoren *mpl* mit Einfluss auf den körperlichen Zustand / **psychological and behavioural ~s associated with disorders or diseases classified elsewhere** psychologische Faktoren *mpl* und Verhaltensfaktoren *mpl* bei andernorts klassifizierten Störungen und Krankheiten / **psychosocial ~** psychosozialer Faktor *m* / **representative ~s** repräsentative Faktoren *mpl* / **rotated ~ matrix** rotierte Faktorenmatrix *f* / **simple ~** Bezugsvektor *m* / **situational ~** Situationsfaktor *m* / **social ~s** soziale Faktoren *mpl*, soziale Phänomene *npl* / **sociocultural ~** soziokultureller Faktor *m* / **spatial ~** Faktor *m* der räumlichen Vorstellung / **specific ~** spezifischer Faktor *m*, S–Faktor *m* / **two–~ theory** Zwei–Faktoren–Theorie *f* / **unique ~** spezifischer Faktor *m* / **verbal ~** sprachlicher Faktor *m*, verbaler Faktor *m* / **visual–spatial ~** visuell–räumlicher Faktor *m*

factorial Faktoren–, Faktor–

factoring, factorization Faktorenextraktion *f*, Durchführung *f* einer Faktorenanalyse / **ad–lib ~** Faktorenextraktion *f* unter gleichzeitiger Verwendung verschiedener Methoden

factorist Anhänger *m* der Faktorentheorie der Intelligenz

factorize eine Faktorenanalyse durchführen, Faktoren extrahieren

factory Fabrik *f*, Werk *n* / **~ environment** Arbeitsbedingungen *fpl* in einer Fabrik

factual tatsächlich, Tatsachen–

factuality Tatsächlichkeit *f*, tatsächliches Vorhandensein *n*

faculty Fähigkeit *f*, Vermögen *n*, Talent *n*, Fakultät *f*, Fachrichtung *f* / **~ of hearing** Hörfähigkeit *f* / **~ of imagination** Vorstellungsvermögen *n* / **~ psychology** Vermögenspsychologie *f* / **~ of speech** Sprechfähigkeit *f* / **~ of thought** Denkfähigkeit *f* / **~ of vision** Sehvermögen *n* / **critical ~** Kritikfähigkeit *f* / **imaginative ~** Vorstellungsvermögen *n* / **intuitive ~** Anschauungsvermögen *n*, Intuitionsvermögen *n* / **mental ~** geistige Fähigkeit *f*, geistiges Vermögen *n* / **mental ~ theory** Theorie *f* des geistigen Vermögens, Theorie *f* der formellen Bildung / **moral ~** Sittlichkeitsempfinden *n*

fad Liebhaberei *f*, Marotte *f* / **~s and fashions** Modeerscheinungen *fpl*

fading Ausschleichen *n*, Abschwächung *f*, Fading *n*, Abklingen *n*, Nachlassen *n*, Prinzip *n* abnehmender Lernhilfen / **~ in** Einblenden *n* / **~ out** Ausblenden *n* / **~ technique** allmähliches Nachlassen *n*, Fading–Technik *f*, Schwund–Technik *f*

faecal kotig, fäkal, Kot–

faeces Exkremente *npl*, Kot *m*, Faeces *pl*

failure Misserfolg *m*, Fehlschlag *m*, Fehlen *n* / ~ **motivation** Misserfolgsmotivation *f* / ~ **neurosis** Misserfolgsneurose *f* / ~ **of action** Fehlleistung *f* / ~ **of appetite** Appetitlosigkeit *f* / ~ **of compensation** Kompensationsschwäche *f* / ~ **of genital response** Versagen *n* genitaler Reaktionen / ~ **rate** Misserfolgsrate *f*, Prozentsatz *m* der Misserfolge / ~ **to thrive** Wachstumsstörung *f* / **academic** ~ Schulversagen *n* / **cardiac** ~ Herzinsuffizienz *f*, Herzversagen *n*, Myokardinsuffizienz *f* / **renal** ~ Nierenversagen *n*

faint in Ohnmacht fallen, ohnmächtig werden

fainting Ohnmacht *f*

faintness Schwäche *f*, Ohnmachtsgefühl *n*

fairness Ehrlichkeit *f*, Gerechtigkeit *f*, Fairness *f*

faith Vertrauen *n*, Glaube *m* / **~–cure** Gesundbeten *n*, Glaubensheilung *f* / **~–healing** Gesundbeten *n*, Glaubensheilung *f* / **~–healer** Gesundbeter *m*

fakability Verfälschbarkeit *f*

faking Täuschung *f*, Fälschung *f*, Vortäuschen *n*

fall chronometer Fallchronometer *n*, Fallapparat *m*

fallacy Trugschluss *m*, Irrtum *m*, Sophisterei *f* / **biological** ~ biologischer Trugschluss *m* / **historical** ~ historischer Trugschluss *m* / **pathetic** ~ Vermenschlichung *f*, Anthropomorphismus *m* / **pathological** ~ pathologische Sophisterei *f*

falling Fall *m* / ~ **dream** Falltraum *m* / ~ **reflex** Fallreflex *m* / ~ **sickness** Fallsucht *f*, Epilepsie *f*

false falsch / **~–negative** fälschlicherweise negativ / **~–positive** fälschlicherweise positiv / **~–valid** fälschlicherweise richtig

falseness Falschheit *f*, Unaufrichtigkeit *f*

falsification Fälschung *f*, Verfälschung *f* / ~ **of memory** Gedächtnisillusion *f* / **retrospective** ~ Erinnerungsfälschung *f*, Paramnesie *f*

falsity Falschheit *f*, Unaufrichtigkeit *f*

fame Ruf *m*, Ruhm *m*

familial familiär, Familien–

familiarity Vertrautheit *f*, Bekanntheit *f* / ~ **factor** Bekanntheitsfaktor *m* / ~ **feeling** Bekanntheitsgefühl *n*

family Familie *f* / ~ **affairs** Familienverhältnisse *npl* / ~ **atmosphere** Nestwärme *f*, Familienatmosphäre *f* / ~ **background** familiärer Hintergrund *m*, Familienverhältnisse *npl* / ~ **breakdown** Auseinanderbrechen *n* der Familie / ~ **caregiver** pflegender Familienangehöriger *m* / ~ **climate** Familienatmosphäre *f* / ~ **complex** Familienkomplex *m* / ~ **constellation** Familienkonstellation *f* / ~ **council** Familienrat *m* / ~ **counseling** Familienberatung *f* / ~ **crisis** Familienkrise *f*, Familienkrach *m* / ~ **discord** Familienstreit *m*, Familienkrach *m* / ~ **environment** Familienmilieu *n* / ~ **history** Familienanamnese *f* / ~ **idiocy** amaurotische Idiotie *f* / ~ **life** Familienleben *n* / ~ **life education** Familienerziehung *f*, Familienbildung *f* / ~ **limitation** Beschränkung *f* der Kinderzahl, Geburtenbeschränkung *f* / ~ **medicine** Familienmedizin *f* / ~ **member** Familienmitglied *n* / ~ **neurosis** Familienneurose *f* / ~ **norm** Familiennorm *f* / ~ **of origin** Herkunftsfamilie *f* / ~ **physician** Hausarzt *m* / ~ **planning** Familienplanung *f* / ~ **psychotherapy** Familienpsychotherapie *f* / ~ **relations** familiäre Beziehungen *fpl*, Familienleben *n* / ~ **relationships** familiäre Beziehungen *fpl*, interne Familienbeziehungen *fpl* / ~ **resemblance** familiäre Ähnlichkeit *f*, Ähnlichkeit *f* der Familienmitglieder untereinander / ~ **role** Familienrolle *f* / ~ **romance** Familienroman *m* / ~ **setting** familiärer Hintergrund *m* / ~ **size** Familiengröße *f* / ~ **social work** Familientherapie *f* / ~ **socioeconomic level** sozioökonomischer Status *m* der Familie / ~ **structure** Familienstruktur *f* / ~ **therapy** Familientherapie *f* / ~ **violence** Gewalt *f* in der Familie / **~–work relationship** Koordination *f* von Familie und Beruf /

amaurotic ~ idiocy amaurotische Idiotie *f*, Tay–Sachs–Krankheit *f* / **broken ~** zerrüttete Familienverhältnisse *npl* / **dysfunctional ~** gestörte Familie *f* / **extended ~** Familienverband *m*, Großfamilie *f* / **human ~** Menschheit *f*, menschliche Gesellschaft *f* / **interethnic ~** ethnisch gemischte Familie *f* / **interracial ~** rassisch gemischte Familie *f* / **nuclear ~** Kernfamilie *f* / **occupational ~** Berufsgruppe *f* / **schizophrenogenic ~** schizophrenogene Familie *f*

fan Verehrer *m*, leidenschaftlicher Anhänger *m*

fanatic fanatisch, enthusiastisch / Fanatiker *m*, Eiferer *m*

fanaticism, fanatism Fanatismus *m*

fancy Phantasie–, Einbildungs– / Phantasie *f*, Einbildung *f* / sich vorstellen, sich einbilden

fancyful launisch, kapriziös

fantasm Phantasma *n*, Trugbild *n*, Sinnestäuschung *f*, Phantasiegebilde *n*

fantastic phantastisch, eingebildet

fantasy Phantasie *f*, Vorstellung *f*, Einbildung *f* / **~ formation** Phantasieentfaltung *f* / **~ life** Phantasieleben *n* / **~ making** Phantasieentfaltung *f* / **~ stage** Phantasiestadium *n* / **~ thinking** Tagträumerei *f* / **active ~** aktive Phantasie *f* / **creative ~** schöpferische Phantasie *f* / **determined by ~** phantasiegetragen / **forced ~** provozierte Phantasie *f* / **parthogenic ~** Phantasie *f* von einer Jungfrau geboren zu sein / **passive ~** passive Phantasie *f* / **sexual ~** sexuelle Phantasie *f*

fantom Phantom *n*, Sinnestäuschung *f*, Scheinbild *n*

faradic faradisch, Faraday'sche (r, s)

faradisation Faraday'sche Reizung *f*

far–field Feldpotential *n* / **~ sightedness** Weitsichtigkeit *f*, Hypermetropie *f*

fascia Faszie *f*, Muskelhülle *f*

fascicle Bündel *n*, Faszikel *m*, Faserstrang *m*

fascicular, fasciculate büschelförmig, faszikulär

fasciculation Bündelbildung *f*, Faszikelbildung *f*

fasciculus Bündel *n*, Büschel *n*, Faszikel *m* / **~ cuneatus** Burdach–Strang *m* / **~ gracilis** Goll'scher Strang *m* / **~ of nerve fibres** Nervenfaserbündel *n* / **lateral ~** Seitenstrang *m*

fascinate bezaubern, faszinieren, verlocken

fascination Faszination *f*, Bezauberung *f*

fashion Mode *f*

fastidium Ekel *m*, Abscheu *m*

fat| cell Fettzelle *f* / **~ deposition** Fettspeicherung *f* / **~ metabolism** Fettstoffwechsel *m*

fatal tödlich, verhängnisvoll, gefährlich

fatalism Fatalismus *m*

fate Schicksal *n* / **~ neurosis** Schicksalsneurose *f* / **common ~** gemeinsames Schicksal *n*

fatality tödlicher Unfall *m*, Todesfall *m*

father Vater *m* / **~ absence** Abwesenheit *f* des Vaters, Vaterlosigkeit *f* / **~–child communication** Vater–Kind–Kommunikation *f* / **~–child relation** Vater–Kind–Beziehung *f* / **~ complex** Vaterkomplex *m*, Elektrakomplex *m*, weiblicher Ödipuskomplex *m* / **~ figure** Vaterimago *f* / **~ fixation** extreme Vaterbindung *f*, Vaterfixierung *f* / **~ imago** Vaterimago *f*, Vaterbild *n* / **~ right** Vaterrecht *n* / **~ substitute** Vaterersatz *m* / **~ surrogate** Vaterersatz *m*, Vatersurrogat *n* / **adolescent ~** jugendlicher Vater *m* / **castrating ~** kastrierender Vater *m* / **expectant ~** werdender Vater *m* / **primal ~** Urvater *m* / **single ~** alleinerziehender Vater *m* / **teenage ~** minderjähriger Vater *m*

fatiguability, fatigability Ermüdbarkeit *f*

fatigue Ermüdung *f*, Müdigkeit *f* / ermüden / **~ disease** Erschöpfungszustand *m* / **~ effect** Ermüdungseffekt *m* / **~ neurosis** Nervenzusammenbruch *m*, Kampfneurose *f*, Ermüdungsneurose *f* / **~ syndrome** Erschöpfungssyndrom *n* / **chronic ~ syn-**

drome chronisches Müdigkeitssyndrom *n* / ~ **test** Ermüdungstest *m* / **afferent** ~ afferente Drosselung *f* / **auditory** ~ Ermüdung *f* des Gehörs / **chromatic** ~ Farbermüdung *f* / **cerebral** ~ zentrale Ermüdung *f* / **cumulative** ~ kumulative Ermüdung *f* / **flying–**~ Fliegerneurose *f* / **mental** ~ geistige Ermüdung *f*, zentrale Ermüdung *f* / **muscular** ~ Muskelermüdung *f*, körperliche Ermüdung *f* / **nervous** ~ Ermüdung *f* der Nerven, Erholungsphase *f* der Nerven / **perstimulatory** ~ Ermüdung *f* aufgrund einer Dauerreizung / **physical** ~ körperliche Ermüdung *f*, muskuläre Ermüdung *f* / **retinal** ~ Ermüdung *f* der Sehsubstanz / **visual** ~ visuelle Ermüdung *f*

fatiguing ermüdend, anstrengend

fatuity Einfältigkeit *f*, Dummheit *f*

fault Fehler *m* / ~**–finding** tadelnd, kritisierend

faulty fehlerhaft, unvollkommen

fear Furcht *f*, Angst *f* / ~ **of animals** Tierangst *f* / ~ **of bearing a monster** Angst *f* vor einer Missgeburt / ~ **of bees** Angst *f* vor Bienen / ~ **of being touched** Berührungsangst *f* / ~ **of blood** Blutangst *f*, Blutscheu *f* / ~ **of blushing** Furcht *f* zu erröten, Erythrophobie *f* / ~ **of cats** Katzenangst *f* / ~ **of childbirth** Geburtsangst *f* / ~ **of comets** Kometenangst *f* / ~ **commitment** Bindungsangst *f* / ~ **of contamination** Furcht *f* vor Verunreinigung / ~ **of crowds** Massenangst *f* / ~ **of darkness** Dunkelangst *f* / ~ **of death** Todesfurcht *f* / ~ **of demons** Furcht *f* vor bösen Geistern / ~ **of the devil** Angst *f* vor dem Teufel / **irrational** ~ **of disease** Krankheitsfurcht *f* / ~ **of dogs** Hundeangst *f* / ~ **of enclosed places** Angst *f* vor geschlossenen Räumen, Klaustrophobie / ~ **of an examination** Examensangst *f*, Prüfungsangst *f* / ~ **of failure** Misserfolgsangst *f* / ~ **of fire** Furcht *f* vor Feuer / ~ **of flying** Flugangst *f* / ~ **of ghosts** Gespensterfurcht *f* / ~ **of God** Gottesfurcht *f* / ~ **of heart disease** Herzangst *f* / ~ **of height** Höhenangst *f*, Dinophobie *f* / ~ **of hell** Höllenangst *f* / ~ **of the id** Es–Angst *f* / ~ **of incest** Inzestangst *f*, Inzestscheu *f* / ~ **of insects** Insektenangst *f* / ~ **of life** Lebensangst *f* / ~ **of lightnings** Angst *f* vor Blitzen, Gewitterangst *f* / ~ **of losing love** Angst *f* vor Liebesverlust / ~ **of marriage** Angst *f* vor der Ehe / ~ **of masturbation** Onaniefurcht *f*, Masturbationsangst *f* / ~ **of mice** Furcht *f* vor Mäusen / ~ **of open places** Platzangst *f*, Agoraphobie *f* / ~ **of people** Menschenscheu *f* / ~ **of punishment** Furcht *f* vor Strafe / ~ **of the sea** Angst *f* vor dem Meer / ~ **of semen** Spermatophobie *f*, Furcht *f* vor dem Samenerguss / ~ **of sexual intercourse** Angst *f* vor dem Koitus / ~ **of sinning** Furcht *f* vor Versündigung / ~ **of snakes** Schlangenfurcht *f* / ~ **of solitude** Angst *f* vor dem Alleinsein, Monophobie *f* / ~ **of sounds** Angst *f* vor Geräuschen / ~ **of spiders** Angst *f* vor Spinnen / ~ **of strangers** Furcht *f* vor Fremden / ~ **of success** Erfolgsangst *f* / ~ **survey schedule** Angstfragebogen *m* / ~ **of thirteen** Angst *f* vor der Zahl „dreizehn" / ~ **of thunder** Gewitterangst *f*, Gewitterfurcht *f* / ~ **of vaccination** Impfangst *f* / ~ **of venereal diseases** Angst *f* vor Geschlechtskrankheiten / ~ **of water** Wasserscheu *f* / ~ **of women** Angst *f* vor Frauen / ~ **of work** Arbeitsangst *f*

feasibility Durchführbarkeit *f*

feasible durchführbar

feature Merkmal *n*, Charakteristikum *n*, Erscheinungsbild *n*, Gesichtszug *m* / **atypical** ~ atypisches Merkmal *n* / **auditory** ~**s** Hörcharakteristika *npl* / **binary** ~ **system** binäres Merkmalsystem *n* / **distinctive** ~ distinktives Merkmal *n* / **facial** ~**s** Gesichtszüge *mpl* / **prodromal** ~ Frühsymptom *n*, Vorzeichen *n* / **semantic** ~ semantisches Merkmal *n* / **with atypical** ~**s** mit atypischen Merkmalen / **with catatonic** ~**s** mit katatonen Merkmalen / **with depressive** ~**s** mit depressiven Merkmalen / **with manic** ~**s** mit manischen Merkmalen / **with melancholic ~s** mit melancholischen Merkmalen / **with mixed ~s** mit gemischten Merkmalen

featureless konturlos, nichtssagend

febrile fiebrig, fiebernd

feces Exkremente *npl*, Kot *m*, Faeces *pl*

Fechner|'s cloud experiment Fechners Wolkenexperiment *n* / **~'s colours** Fechner–Benham–Farben *fpl* / **~–Helmholtz law** Gesetz *n* von Fechner und Helmholtz / **~'s law** Fechner'sches Gesetz *n* / **~'s paradox** Fechner'sches Paradox *n* / **~'s shadow experiment** Fechners Schattenexperiment *n* / **~'s weight holders** Fechners Gewichtsvergleich *m*

Fechnerian Fechner'sche(r, s)

fecund fruchtbar

fecundate befruchten

fecundation Befruchtung *f*, Schwängerung *f*

fecundity Fruchtbarkeit *f*, Fertilität *f*, Zeugungskraft *f*

feebleminded schwachsinnig, geistesschwach, geistig minderbegabt

feeble–mindedness Schwachsinn *m*, Geistesschwäche *f*, geistige Zurückgebliebenheit *f*, Hypophrenose *f* / **high–grade ~** hochgradiger Schwachsinn *m* / **primary ~** angeborener Schwachsinn *m* / **secondary ~** erworbener Schwachsinn *m* / **slight ~** leichte Debilität *f*

feebleness Schwäche *f*, Debilität *f*

feedback Rückkopplung *f*, Rückmeldung *f*, Feedback *n* / **~ circuit** Rückkopplungskreislauf *m* / **~ control** Regelung *f* / **~ control system** Regelkreis *m* / **~ inhibition** Feedbackhemmung *f*, Rückwärtshemmung *f* / **~ loop** Rückkopplungsschleife *f* / **~ mechanism** Regelkreis *m*, Rückkopplungsmechanismus *m* / **~ mechanism theory** Regelkreislehre *f* / **~ system** Regelsystem *n*, Regelkreis *m* / **auditory ~** akustische Rückkopplung *f*, auditive Rückmeldung *f* / **delayed ~** verzögerte Rückmeldung *f* / **delayed auditory ~** verzögerte auditive Rückmeldung *f* / **immediate ~** sofortige Rückmeldung *f* / **negative ~** negative Rückkopplung *f* / **positive ~** positives Feedback *n*, Regelung *f* / **sensory ~** sensorische Rückmeldung *f* / **visual ~** visuelle Rückkopplung *f*, visuelles Feedback *n*

feed–forward Vorwärtssteuerung *f*, Vorwärtsregelung *f* / **~–inhibition** Feedforwardhemmung *f*

feeding Fütterung *f*, Ernährung *f*, Stillen *n* / **~ disorder of infancy and childhood** Fütterstörung *f* im frühen Kindesalter / **~ disorder of infancy or early childhood** Fütterstörung *f* im Säuglings– oder Kleinkindalter / **~ and eating disorders of infancy or early childhood** Fütter– und Essstörungen *fpl* im Säuglings– oder Kleinkindalter / **~–experiment** Fütterungsversuch *m* / **~ inhibition** Fütterungshemmung *f* / **~ instinct** Nahrungsinstinkt *m* / **~ practice** Ernährungsgewohnheit *f* / **~ problem** Essschwierigkeit *f* / **artificial ~** künstliche Ernährung *f* / **forced ~** Zwangsernährung *f*

feel fühlen, empfinden, betasten

feeling Gefühl *n*, Empfinden *n*, Fühlen *n* / **~ of anxiety** Angstgefühl *n* / **~ of belongingness** Zugehörigkeitsgefühl *n* / **~ of comfort** Wohlbehagen *n* / **~ of difference** Gefühl *n* des Andersseins / **~ of discomfort** Unbehaglichkeitsgefühl *n* / **~ of elation** Beglückungsgefühl *n* / **~ of emptiness** Gefühl *n* der Leere / **~ of fatigue** Müdigkeitsgefühl *n* / **~ of fitness** Gefühl *n* der Übereinstimmung / **~ of guilt** Schuldgefühl *n*, Schuldbewusstsein *n* / **~ of hunger** Hungergefühl *n* / **~ of ill–health** Befindlichkeitsstörung *f* / **~ of impending death** Todesahnung *f* / **~ of inadequacy** Unzulänglichkeitsgefühl *n* / **~ of indifference** Gefühl *m* der Gefühllosigkeit / **~ of inferiority** Minderwertigkeitsgefühl *n* / **~ of insufficiency** Unzulänglichkeitsgefühl *n* / **~–into** Einfühlung *f* / **~ of omnipotence** Allmachtsgefühl *n* / **~ of pain** Schmerzgefühl *n* / **~ of persecution** Verfolgungsgefühl *n* / **~ of reality** Wirklichkeitsgefühl *n*, Realitätsempfinden *n* / **~ of responsibility** Verantwortungsgefühl *n* / ~ **of satiation** Sättigungsgefühl *n* / ~ **of security** Sicherheitsgefühl *n*, Geborgenheitsgefühl *n* / ~ **of tiredness** Müdigkeitsgefühl *n* / ~ **tone** Gefühlston *m* / ~ **type** Empfindungstypus *m* / ~**–type personality** gefühlsbetonte Persönlichkeit *f* / ~ **of uneasiness** unbehagliches Gefühl *n* / ~ **of unreality** Unwirklichkeitsgefühl *n* / **aesthetic** ~ ästhetisches Empfinden *n* / **ambivalent** ~**s** ambivalente Gefühle *npl*, affektive Ambivalenz *f* / **asthenic** ~ schwacher Gefühlsausdruck *m* / **esthetic** ~ ästhetisches Empfinden *n* / **floating** ~ freiflottierender Affekt *m* / **guilty** ~ Schuldgefühl *n*, Schuldbewusstsein *n* / **oceanic** ~ ozeanisches Gefühl *n* / **social** ~ Sozialgefühl *n* / **tired** ~ Müdigkeitsgefühl *n*

feign heucheln

feint, feigning Simulation *f*, Vortäuschung *f*

fellatio Genitalkuss *m*, Fellatio *f*

fellow resident Mitpatient *m*, Mitbewohner *m*

felony Verbrechen *n*, schweres Verbrechen *n*

female weiblich / weibliches Wesen *n* / **battered** ~ misshandelte Frau *f* / **human** ~ Frau *f*

feminine feminin, weiblich

femininity, feminity Weiblichkeit *f* / ~ **complex** Weiblichkeitskomplex *m*

feminisation Feminierung *f*, Verweiblichung *f* / **testicular** ~ **syndrome** Gonadendysgenesie *f*, Hairless–women–Syndrom *n*, testikuläre Femininisierung *f*

feminism Verweiblichung *f*, Feminismus *m*

feminist Feminist *m* / ~ **therapy** feministische Therapie *f*

fenestra Fenster *n* / ~ **ovalis** ovales Fenster *n*, Vorhoffenster *n* / ~ **rotunda** rundes Fenster *n*

fenestration Fensterungsoperation *f*, Fensterung *f*

fenfluramine Fenfluramin *n*

fentanyl Fentanyl *n*

feral wild, unkultiviert

Féré| method Féré–Methode *f* / ~ **phenomenon** Féré –Phänomen *n*

Ferguson's reflex Ferguson–Reflex *m*

ferment gären / Ferment *n*

fermentation Vergärung *f*

Ferry–Porter law Ferry–Porter–Gesetz *n*, Porter–Gesetz *n*

fertile fruchtbar

fertilisation Befruchtung *f*, Schwängerung *f*

fertilise befruchten

fertility Fertilität *f*, Fruchtbarkeit *f* / ~ **enhancement** Fertilitätssteigerung *f*, Erhöhung *f* der Fruchtbarkeit, Fertilitätsbehandlung *f*

fertilisation Befruchtung *f*

festination Trippelgang *m*, trippelnder Gang *m*

fetal fötal, Fötus–

fetid schlecht riechend, stinkend

fetish Fetisch *m*

fetishism Fetischismus *m* / **olfactory** ~ Geruchsfetischismus *m* / **sexual** ~ sexueller Fetischismus *m* / **transvestitic** ~ transvestitischer Fetischismus *m*

fetishist Fetischist *m*

fetor Gestank *m* / ~ **ex ore** Mundgeruch *m*

fetus Fetus *m*, Foetus *m*

fever Fieber *n* / **psychogenic** ~ psychogenes Fieber *m* / **rheumatic** ~ rheumatisches Fieber *n* / **therapeutic** ~ Heilfieber *n*, künstlich erzeugte Hyperthermie *f* / **traumatic** ~ Unfallfieber *n*

***F* distribution** *F*–Verteilung *f*

***F* factor** *F*–Faktor *m*

fiat Erlaubnis *f*, Zustimmung *f*, Bestätigung *f* / ~ **of the will** Einwilligung *f*

fiber, fibre Faser *f* / ~**s of Corti** Cortische Zellen *fpl* / ~ **diameter** Faserdurchmesser *m* / ~ **spectrum** Faserspektrum *n* / **afferent** ~ afferente Faser *f* / **cholinergic** ~ cholinerge Faser *f* / **climbing** ~ Kletterfaser *f* / **collateral** ~ Kollaterale *f* / **commissural** ~ Kommissurenfaser *f* / **corti-**

cofugal ~ efferente Faser *f* / **corticopetal** ~ afferente Faser *f* / **efferent** ~ efferente Faser *f* / **extrafusal** ~ extrafusale Muskelfaser *f* / **fast** ~ schnelle Faser *f*, „fast fiber" *f* / **histaminergic** ~**s** histaminerge Fasern *fpl* / **intrafusal** ~ intrafusale Muskelfaser *f* / **medullated** ~ markhaltige Faser *f* / **mossy** ~**s** Moosfasern *fpl* / **myelinated** ~ markhaltige Faser *f* / **myocardial** ~ Herzmuskelfaser *f* / **nonmedullated** ~ marklose Faser *f* / **nonmyelinated** ~ marklose Faser *f* / **postganglionic** ~ postganglionäre Faser *f* / **preganglionic** ~ präganglionäre Faser *f* / **single** ~ Einzelfaser *f* / **slow** ~ langsame Faser *f*, „slow fiber" *f* / **sympathetic** ~ Sympathikusfaser *f*

fibril Fibrille *f*, kleine Faser *f*, dünne Faser *f* / **protoplasmic** ~ Protoplasmafibrille *f*

fibrillary, fibrillar feinfaserig, fibrillär

fibrillate feinfaserig, fibrillär / auffasern, in Fasern spalten

fibrillation Aufspaltung *f* in kleine Fasern, Fibrillation *f*, Flimmern *n* / **auricular** ~ Vorhofflimmern *n* / **ventricular** ~ Kammerflimmern *n*

fibrosis, cystic zystische Fibrose *f*

Fick|'s method Fick'sche Methode *f* / ~**'s principle** Fick'sches Prinzip *n*

fiction Fiktion *f*, Erdichtung *f*, Annahme *f* / **directive** ~ leitende Fiktion *f* / **guiding** ~ leitende Fiktion *f* / **institutional** ~ institutionelle Erfindung *f* / **neurotic** ~ neurotische Fiktion *f*

fictitious fiktiv, erfunden

fidelity Treue *f*, Wiedergabegenauigkeit *f*, Genauigkeit *f* / **marital** ~ eheliche Treue *f*

fidgets Nervosität *f*, nervöse Unruhe *f*, Zappeligkeit *f*

fidgety unruhig, nervös, zappelig

FidoNet Fidonet *n*, weltumspannendes, nicht–kommerzielles Rechnernetz *n*

fiducial, fiduciary Vertrauens–, treuhänderisch

field Feld *n*, Bereich *m*, Region *f* / ~ **of attention** Aufmerksamkeitsbereich *m* / ~ **of behaviour** Verhaltensfeld *n* / ~ **cognition mode** Felderkenntnisweise *f* / ~ **of consciousness** Bewusstseinsfeld *n*, Bewusstseinsumfang *m* / ~ **dependence** Feldabhängigkeit *f* / ~ **education** praktische Ausbildung *f*, Feldausbildung *f* / ~ **effect** Feldwirkung *f* / ~ **emphasis** Feldbetonung *f* / ~ **expectancy** Felderwartung *f* / ~ **of experience** Erlebnisfeld *n* / ~ **experiment** Feldexperiment *n*, Feldversuch *m*, Anwendungsexperiment *n* / **curricular** ~ **experience** Praxisfeld–Curriculum *n* / ~ **of fixation** zentrales Sehfeld *n* / ~ **force** Feldkraft *f* / ~ **of force** Kraftfeld *n* / ~ **independence** Feldunabhängigkeit *f* / ~**–interview method** Methode *f* der Felduntersuchung / ~ **investigation** Felduntersuchung *f*, Feldforschung *f* / ~ **investigator** Feldforscher *m*, Interviewer *m* / ~ **method** Methode *f* der Felduntersuchung / ~ **observation** Feldbeobachtung *f* / ~**s of psychology** Bereiche *mpl* der Psychologie / ~ **of regard** Blickfeld *n* / ~ **research** Feldforschung *f* / ~ **of research** Forschungsbereich *m* / ~ **structure** Feldstruktur *f* / ~ **study** Felduntersuchung *f*, Feldstudie *f* / ~**–theoretical** feldtheoretisch / ~ **theory** Feldtheorie *f* / ~ **of touch** Tastbereich *m* / ~ **vector** Feldvektor *m* / ~ **of vision** Gesichtsfeld *n*, Sehfeld *n* / ~ **of work** Arbeitsbereich *m*, Forschungsbereich *m* / ~ **worker** Feldforscher *m*, Interviewer *m* / **auditory** ~ Hörbereich *m*, Hörbreite *f* / **cortical** ~ Rindenregion *f*, Rindenfeld *n* / **cutaneous receptive** ~ Hautrezeptorfeld *n* / **dark** ~ Dunkelfeld *n* / **educational** ~ **trip** Exkursion *f* / **excitatory** ~ Erregungsfeld *n* / **exteroceptive** ~ Exterozeptorenfeld *n* / **homogeneous** ~ Ganzfeld *n* / **inhibitory receptive** ~ inhibitorisches rezeptives Feld *n* / **interoceptive** ~ Interozeptorenfeld *n* / **marginal** ~ Marginalfeld *n*, Randfeld *n* / **mathematical** ~ mathematisches Feld *n* / **minimal audible** ~ unterer Hörbereich *m* / **occupational** ~ Tätigkeitsbereich *m* / **olfactory** ~ Riechfeld *n* /

open ~ behaviour Verhalten *n* in freier Wildbahn / **perceptual ~** Wahrnehmungsfeld *n* / **phenomenal ~** phänomenales Feld *n* / **phenomenological ~** phänomenales Feld *n* / **proprioceptive ~** Propriozeptorenfeld *n* / **psychological ~** psychologisches Feld *n*, Lebensraum *m* / **psychophysical ~** Lebensraum *m*, psychologisches Feld *n* / **psychophysiological ~** Lebensraum *m*, psychologisches Feld *n* / **receptive ~** Rezeptorfeld *n* / **retinal ~** Netzhautbereich *m* / **reversed ~** umgekehrtes Feld *n* / **scalar ~** skalares Feld *n* / **sensoritonic ~** Feld *n* der Empfindungsspannung / **sensory ~** Wahrnehmungsfeld *n*, sensorisches Feld *n* / **social ~** soziales Feld *n*, Sozialstruktur *f* / **spatial ~** Raumfeld *n* / **structured ~** strukturiertes Feld *n*, organisiertes Feld *n* / **temporal ~** augenblicklich, plötzlich / **tilting–~** Kippfeld *n*, Kippbrett *n* / **visual ~** Gesichtsfeld *n*, Sehfeld *n* / **visual receptive ~** visuelles Rezeptorfeld *n* / **visual ~ defect** Sehfeldausfall *m*

fighting Kampf *m*

figment Erdichtung *f*, Einbildung *f*, Wahnvorstellung *f*

figural figural

figure Figur *f* / **~ and ground** Figur *f* und Grund *m* / **~–ground** Figur–Grund *m*, Figur–Grund–Verhältnis *n* / **~–ground differentiation** Figur–Grund–Differenzierung *f* / **~–ground discrimination** Figur–Grund–Differenzierung *f*, Figur–Grund–Diskrimination *f* / **~–ground experience** Figur–Grund–Erfahrung *f* / **~–ground perception** Figur–Grund–Wahrnehmung *f* / **ambiguous ~** mehrdeutige Figur *f*, Kippfigur *f* / **composite ~** zusammengesetztes Traumbild *n*, Urbild *n* / **congruent ~s** kongruente Bilder *npl*, deckungsgleiche Abbildungen *fpl* / **embedded ~** eingebettete Figur *f*, Vexierbild *n* / **good ~** gute Gestalt *f*, gute Form *f* / **good–~ theory** Theorie *f* der guten Gestalt / **hidden ~** eingebettete Figur *f*, Vexierbild *n*, Suchbild *n* / **human ~** menschliche Gestalt *f*, menschliche Deutung *f* / **inverted ~** Umkehrfigur *f*, Kippfigur *f* / **public ~** bekannte Persönlichkeit *f*, Persönlichkeit *f* des öffentlichen Lebens / **reversible ~** Reversionsfigur *f*, Kippfigur *f* / **significant ~** signifikante Zahl *f*

filament, filamentum Filament *n*

file Akte *f*, Ablage *f*, Registratur *f* / **~ allocation table** Dateizuornungstabelle *f* / **~ medium** Registraturmethode *f* / **~ server** Zentralrechner *m* eines Netzwerks / **~ transfer protocol** Dateitransferprotokoll *n* / **rotary ~** drehbare Aktenablage *f*

filial kindlich

filiation Kindschaft *f*, Abstammung *f*

filiform fadenförmig

fillet Schleife *f* / **acoustic ~** akustische Schleife *f*, seitliche untere Schleifenbahn *f* / **medial ~** mediale Schleife *f*

film Film *m* / **~ colour** Flächenfarbe *f* / **~ strip** Filmstreifen *m* / **educational ~** Lehrfilm *m*

filter Filter *m oder n* / **acoustic ~** akustisches Filter *n*

filtering Filtern *n* / **selective ~** Selektieren *n*, Auswählen *n*, Zensieren *n*

filtration rate, glomerular glomeruläre Filtrationsrate *f*

final final, endgültig, letzte(r, s)

finalism Lehre *f* von der Zweckmäßigkeit allen Handelns, Lehre *f* von der Zweckbestimmtheit allen Geschehens, Teleologie *f* / **stubborn ~** sturer Finalismus *m*

finality Finalität *f*, Zweckbestimmtheit *f*, Zweckgerichtetheit *f*

finding Befund *m* / **abnormal ~** abnormer Befund *m* / **normal ~s** Normalbefund *m* / **objective ~s** objektiver Befund *m* / **pathological ~s** pathologischer Befund *m*

finger Finger *m* / **~ agnosia** Fingeragnosie *f*, Tastblindheit *f*, Stereoagnosie *f* / **~ alphabet** Fingersprache *f*, Zeichensprache *f* / **~ dexterity** Fingerfertigkeit *f*, manuelle Geschicklichkeit *f* / **~–nail** Fingernagel *m* / **~–nose test** Fingernasenprobe *f* / **~**

painting Fingermalen *n* / **~-print** Fingerabdruck *m* / **~-print identification** Erkennung *f* aufgrund des Fingerabdrucks, Daktyloskopie *f* / **~ spelling** Fingersprache *f*, Daktylologie *f*, Cheirologie *f* / **~ tapping** schnelles Klopfen *n* mit den Fingern auf eine Unterlage, Fingerklopfen *n*

finite endlich, begrenzt

fire Feuer *n* / **pathological ~-setting** pathologische Brandstiftung *f* / **~ wall** Firewall *f*, Internet–Schutzmauer *f* / **~-worship** Feuerkult *m*

firing Feuern *n*, Entladung *f* / **~ level** Schwellendepolarisation *f*, „firing level" *n*

first–order erste Ordnung *f* / **~ correlation coefficient** Korrelationskoeffizient *m* erster Ordnung / **~ factor** Faktor *m* erster Ordnung

Fisher's test Fisher–Test *m*, Signifikanztest *m* nach Fisher

fissible, fissile teilungsfähig, spaltbar

fissility Teilbarkeit *f*, Spaltbarkeit *f*

fission Spaltung *f*, Teilung *f*, Mitose *f* / **cellular ~** Zellteilung *f* / **nuclear ~** Kernteilung *f*, Kernspaltung *f* / **social ~** Trennung *f*

fissural Spalt–, Spaltungs–

fissure Spalt *m*, Fissur *f*, Sulcus *m* / **~ of Rolando** Rolando–Furche *f* / **calcarine ~** Fissura calcarina *f*, Sulcus calcarinus *m* / **central ~** Rolando–Furche *f*, Sulcus centralis Rolandi *m* / **cerebellar ~** Kleinhirnfurche *f* / **cerebral ~** Sylvius–Furche *f* / **lateral ~** Sylvius–Furche *f* / **longitudinal cerebral ~** Fissura interhemisphaerica *f*, Fissura longitudinalis cerebri *f* / **sagittal ~** Fissura interhemisphaerica *f* / **Sylvian ~** Sylvius–Furche *f*

fistula Fistel *f*

fistular, fistulate, fistulous fistulös

fit Anfall *m*, Attacke *f*, Anpassung *f* / passend, tauglich, verwendbar / passen, geeignet sein / **~ of anger** Wutanfall *m*, Zornesausbruch *m* / **~ of rage** Wutanfall *m* / **~ of temper** Zornesausbruch *m* / **best ~** beste Anpassung *f* / **catatonic ~** Katatonieanfall *m* / **convulsive ~** Krampfanfall *m* / **crying ~** Schreikrampf *m* / **epileptic ~** epileptischer Anfall *m* / **epileptic ~s of laughter** epileptischer Lachanfall *m*, epileptisches Lachen *n* / **generalized ~** generalisierter Anfall *m* / **hysterical ~** hysterischer Anfall *m* / **Jacksonian ~** Anfall *m* bei Jackson–Epilepsie, fokaler Anfall *m* / **laughing ~** Lachanfall *m* / **nervous ~** Nervenzusammenbruch *m* / **uncinate ~** Uncinatusanfall *m*

fitful unbeständig, launenhaft

fitness Tauglichkeit *f* / **~ for work** Arbeitsfähigkeit *f* / **~ to plead** Verhandlungsfähigkeit *f* / **physical ~** körperliche Fitness *f*, körperliche Leistungsfähigkeit *f*

fittingness Einpassung *f*

five–track plan Aufteilung *f* einer Schulklasse in fünf unterschiedliche Leistungsgruppen

fixated fixiert, unveränderlich

fixation Fixation *f*, Fixierung *f*, Bindung *f*, Festigung *f* / **~ of affect** Affektbindung *f*, Fixierung *f* von Gefühlen / **~ upon the father** extreme Vaterbindung *f*, Fixierung *f* auf den Vater / **~ frequency** Häufigkeit *f* der Fixationspausen / **~ line** Fixationslinie *f* / **~ movement** Fixationsbewegung *f* / **~ pause** Fixationspause *f*, Fixationsdauer *f* / **~ period** Fixationsperiode *f* / **~ point** Fixationspunkt *m*, Zeitpunkt *m* / **~ reaction time** Reaktionszeit *f* bis zur Fixation / **~ time** Fixationszeit *f* / **abnormal ~** abnorme Fixierung *f* / **affective ~** Affektbindung *f*, Fixierung *f* von Gefühlen / **anal ~** Fixierung *f* auf der analen Stufe / **binocular ~** Fixation *f* mit beiden Augen / **infantile ~ experiences** Fixierung *f* auf frühkindlichen Erfahrungen / **libidinal ~** Libidobindung *f*, Libidofixierung *f*, libidinöse Bindung *f* / **moving ~** bewegende Fixation *f* / **negative ~** negative Fixierung *f*, Vermeidungslernen *n* / **parental ~** Elternbindung *f*, Fixierung *f* an die Eltern

/ **positive ~** positive Fixierung *f*, Kanalisierung *f* / **pregenital ~** prägenitale Fixierung *f* / **visual ~** Fixation *f* des Auges

fixed festgelegt, festgefügt, eingeschliffen, fix

fixed–alternative mit vorgegebenen Alternativantworten

fixed–class mit fester Klassenzugehörigkeit, mit fester Kastenzuordnung

fixed–interval mit gleicher Zeitspanne, mit konstantem Intervall

fixedness Starre *f*, Rigidität *f*, Fixierung *f*, Mangel *m* an Flexibilität / **functional ~** funktionale Fixierung *f*

fixed–ratio in gleichem Verhältnis

fixity Festigkeit *f*, Stabilität *f* / **~ of purpose** Zielsicherheit *f*

flaccid entspannt, weich, schlaff

flagellate geißeln / Geißeltierchen *n*

flagellation Geißelung *f*, Flagellantismus *m*, Flagellation *f* / **~ of children** Prügeln *n* von Kindern, Dippoldismus *m*

flagellomania krankhafter Trieb *m* sich selbst oder andere zu geißeln

flash Blitz *m* / **~ back** Nachhallzustand *m* / **~ card** kurzzeitig dargebotene Karte *f*, Lernkarte *f* / **~ device** Tachistoskop *n*, Blitzgerät *n* / **~ light** Blitzlicht *n*

flashmeter Blitzgerät *n* mit Zeitverschluss

flat flach, eintönig, langweilig, monoton

flattening Verflachung *f* / **~ of affect** Affektverflachung *f* / **~ of emotion** Gefühlsverflachung *f* / **affective ~** affektive Verarmung *f*, Affektverflachung *f* / **emotional~** Gefühlsverarmung *f*, Gefühlsverflachung *f*, Gefühlsverödung *f*, Gemütsverödung *f*

flavour Geschmack *m*

flexibilitas cerea Flexibilitas cerea *f*, wachsartige Biegsamkeit *f*

flexibility Flexibilität *f*, Anpassungsfähigkeit *f*, Fügsamkeit *f*, Lenkbarkeit *f* / **~ of closure** Flexibilität *f* bei der Strukturierung / **adaptive ~** Anpassungsfähigkeit *f* / **mental ~** Umstellbarkeit *f*, Anpassungsfähigkeit *f* / **waxy ~** wachsartige Biegsamkeit *f*, Flexibilitas cerea *f*

flexible anpassungsfähig, fügsam, flexibel

flexion Beugung *f*, Flexion *f*, Ablenkung *f* / **~ reflex** Beugereflex *m*

flexor Beugemuskel *m*, Flexor *m* / **~ muscle** Beuger *m*, Beugemuskel *m* / **~ reflex** Beugereflex *m* / **~ tonus** Beugetonus *m*

flextime flexible Arbeitszeit *f*

flexure Flexur *f*, Biegung *f*

flicker Flimmern *n* / **~ discrimination** Unterscheidung *f* des Flimmerns / **~ fusion** Flimmerverschmelzung *f* / **~ fusion frequency** Flimmerverschmelzungsfrequenz *f* / **~ fusion point** Flimmerverschmelzungsgrenze *f* / **~ and fusion** Flimmern *n* und Verschmelzen *n* / **~ interval** Flimmerintervall *n* / **~ phenomenon** Flimmern *n*, Flimmererscheinung *f* / **~ photometry** Flimmerphotometrie *f* / **auditory ~** Tonflimmern *n*, Tonvibration *f* / **binocular ~** alternierendes Flimmern *n* vor den beiden Augen / **chromatic ~** farbiges Flimmern *n* / **critical ~ frequency** kritische Flimmerfrequenz *f*, Flimmergrenze *f*, Flimmerverschmelzungsfrequenz *f* / **critical ~ fusion frequency** kritische Flimmerfrequenz *f* / **critical ~ fusion threshold** Flimmergrenze *f* / **critical ~ interval** kritisches Flimmerintervall *n*

flight Flucht *f* / **~ behaviour** Fluchtverhalten *n* / **~ from reality** Flucht *f* vor der Realität / **~ instrumentation** Fluginstrumente *npl* / **~ into dreams** Flucht *f* in eine Phantasiewelt / **~ into illness** Flucht *f* in die Krankheit / **~ of colours** schnelle Folge *f* farbiger Nachbilder / **~ of ideas** Ideenflucht *f* / **~ reaction** Fluchtreaktion *f* / **~ simulation** Flugsimulation *f*

flipped–out ausgeflippt

flirtation Flirt *m*, Liebelei *f*

floating flottierend

flooding Reizüberflutung *f*

floor of a test unteres Differenzierungsniveau *n* eines Tests

flop Misserfolg *m*, Versager *m*, Nicte *f*

flow fließen / Fließen *n*, Flow–Erleben *n*, Monatsblutung *f* / **~ chart** Flussdiagramm *n* / **~ process charts** Flussdiagramm *n* / **cerebral blood ~** Hirndurchblutung *f*

flower child Blumenkind *n*, Hippie *m*

flowery blumig, geziert

fluctuate fluktuieren, schwanken, zögern

fluctuation Schwankung *f*, Veränderung *f*, Fluktuation *f* / **~s** Variationen *fpl*, Schwankungen *fpl* / **~ of attention** Aufmerksamkeitsschwankung *f*, fluktuierende Aufmerksamkeit *f* / **~s of consciousness** fluktuierendes Bewusstsein *n* / **~ of sample** Stichprobenschwankung *f* / **~ of sampling** Stichprobenschwankung *f* / **~ theory** Theorie *f* von der Signalwahrnehmung

fluency Flüssigkeit *f*, Geläufigkeit *f* / **~ test** Test *m* der Sprachflüssigkeit / **associational ~** Assoziationsflüssigkeit *f* / **expressional ~** Ausdrucksflüssigkeit *f* / **ideational ~** Gedankenflüssigkeit *f* / **verbal ~** Wortflüssigkeit *f*, Sprachgewandtheit *f*, Flüssigkeit *f* des sprachlichen Ausdrucks

fluid flüssig, fließend / Flüssigkeit *f*, Liquor *m* / **~ electrode** Flüssigkeitselektrode *f* / **~ intake** Flüssigkeitsaufnahme *f* / **amniotic ~** Fruchtwasser *n* / **cerebrospinal ~** Hirnflüssigkeit *f*, Zerebrospinalflüssigkeit *f*, Liquor cerebrospinalis *m* / **labyrinthine ~** Labyrinthflüssigkeit *f*, Perilymphe *f* / **spinal ~** Rückenmarksflüssigkeit *f*

fluidity Flüssigkeit *f*

fluorescence Fluoreszenz *f*

fluoxetine Fluoxetin *n*

fluphenazine Fluphenazin *n*

flurazepam Flurazepam *n*

flurried aufgeregt

flurry nervöse Erregung *f*, Unruhe *f*, Aufregung *f*

flush Erröten *n*

fluster aufgeregt sein, sich aufregen / Aufregung *f*

flutter Flattern *n*, Flimmern *n*, Aufregung *f*, Unruhe *f* / **auditory ~** Tonvibration *f* / **sound ~** Tonvibration *f* / **ventricular ~** Kammerflattern *n*

fluttering Flattern *n* / **~ of the heart** Herzflattern *n*

fluvoxamine Fluvoxamin *n*

flux Fluss *m*, Strom *m* / **luminous ~** Lichtstrom *m*, Lichtenergie *f* / **radiant ~** Lichtstrahlung *f*

focal fokal, herdförmig

focalisation Fokalisation *f*, Zusammenfassung *f* in einem Brennpunkt

focus Herd *m*, Fokus *m*, Brennpunkt *m* / **~ of attention** Aufmerksamkeitsfokus *m*, Aufmerksamkeitszentrum *n* / **cerebral ~** Gehirnherd *m* / **conjugate ~** Herdpaare *npl* / **irritable ~** Reizungsherd *m* / **principal ~** Hauptherd *m*

focusing Zusammenfassung *f* in einem Brennpunkt, Zentrieren *n*, Fokussieren *n*

foetal fetal, Fetus–

foetus Fötus *m*, Fetus *m*, Frucht *f*

foible Schwäche *f*, schwache Seite *f*, Eigenheit *f*, Marotte *f*

folie Irresein *n* / **~ à deux** induziertes Irresein *n*, Induktionspsychose *f* / **~ du doute** krankhafte Unentschlossenheit *f*, Zweifelsucht *f*, Folie du doute *f* / **~ de toucher** Kontrektationszwang *m*, Berührungszwang *m*

folium Blatt *n*

folk Volk *n*, Leute *pl*, Nation *f*, Volks– / **~ medicine** Volksmedizin *f* / **~ mind** Volksseele *f*, Volksgeist *m*, Gruppenseele *f* / **~ psychology** Völkerpsychologie *f*, Ethnopsychologie *f* / **~–tale** Sage *f*, Volkserzählung *f*

folklore Folklore *f*, Volkskunde *f*, Volkstumskunde *f*

folkloric volkskundlich, Folklore–

folkways Volksbrauch *m*, Denkungsweise *f* des Volkes

follicle–stimulating hormone follikelstimulierendes Hormon *n*, Follikelreifungshormon *n*

folliculin Follikudin *n*, Alpha–Follikelhormon *n*, Östron *n*

follow folgen, sich anschließen, verfolgen

follower Anhänger *m*, Begleiter *m*, Mitläufer *m*, Verfolger *m*

followership Anhängerschaft *f*, Nachfolge *f*

following Anhang *m* / folgend, Folge–

follow–up Nachuntersuchung *f*, Katamnese *f* / **~ history** Katamnese *f* / **~ study** Nachuntersuchung *f*, Katamnese *f*

fontanel, fontanelle Fontanelle *f*

food Nahrung *f*, Futter *n* / **~ additive** Nahrungsmittelzusatz *m* / **~ allergy** Nahrungsmittelallergie *f* / **~ deprivation** Nahrungsentzug *m* / **~–getting behaviour** Futtersuchverhalten *n*, Fütterungsverhalten *n* / **~–getting response** Fütterungsverhalten *n* / **~ intake** Nahrungsaufnahme *f* / **~ magazine** Futtermagazin *n* / **~ preference** Nahrungspräferenz *f* / **~ response** Fütterungsverhalten *n*

fooling Zerstreuung *f*, Ausschweifung *f*

foot Fuß *m* / **~ anaesthesia** Fußunempfindlichkeit *f* / **~–candle** Foot–Kerze *f* / **~–drawing** Fußzeichnung *f*, Zeichnen *n* mit den Füßen / **~ fetishism** Fußfetischismus *m* / **~–lambert** Foot–Lambert *m* / **~–writing** Schreiben *n* mit den Füßen

footedness Dominanz *f* eines Fußes, bevorzugter Gebrauch *m* eines Fußes

footrule correlation Spearmans–Korrelation *f*

foramen Loch *n*, Foramen *n* / **interventricular ~** Foramen interventriculare *n*

forbidden verboten, untersagt

force Kraft *f*, Stärke *f*, Macht *f*, Einfluss *m* / **~ of attraction** Anziehungskraft *f* / **~ of expression** Ausdruckskraft *f*, Aussagekraft *f* / **~ of habit** Macht *f* der Gewohnheit / **autochthonous ~** autochthone Kraft *f* / **driving ~** Triebkraft *f* / **dynamic ~** psychische Kraft *f* / **expressive ~** Ausdruckskraft *f* / **gravitational ~** Schwerkraft *f* / **instinctual ~** Triebkraft *f* / **magnetic ~** Magnetismus *m*, magnetische Kraft *f* / **muscular ~** Muskelkraft *f* / **odylic ~** Od *n*, angeblich vom Menschen ausstrahlende Kraft *f* / **psychic ~** psychische Energie *f* / **vital ~** Lebenskraft *f*

forced erzwungen, gezwungen, Zwangs–

forceps delivery Zangengeburt *f*

forcing Erzwingen *n*, Forcieren *n*, Vorantreiben *n*

forebrain Vorderhirn *n*, Prosenzephalon *n* / **medial ~ bundle** mediales Vorderhirnbündel *n*

forecast Vorhersage *f*, Prognose *f*

foreconscious vorbewusst / Vorbewusstes *n*

foreconsciousness Vorbewusstsein *n*

fore–exercise Vorübung *f*

foreign fremd, ausländisch, nicht passend / **~ to the ego** ichfremd

foreigner Ausländer *m*, Fremder *m*

foreman Vorarbeiter *m*, Meister *m* / **industrial ~** Vorarbeiter *m*, Industriemeister *m*

forensic forensisch, gerichtlich

foreperiod Vorphase *f*, Vorzeitraum *m*

foreplay Vorspiel *m*, Liebesspiel *m* / **coital ~** Liebesspiel *n* vor dem Koitus, Vorspiel *n*

forepleasure Vorlust *f*, Lust *f* beim sexuellen Vorspiel

forerunner Wegbereiter *m*, Vorläufer *m*

foreshortening Verkürzung *f*

foresight Vorhersehen *n*, Vorsicht *f*, Vorsorge *f*

forethought Vorsorge *f*, Vorbedacht *m*

forgetful vergesslich

forgetfulness Vergesslichkeit *f*

forgetting Vergessen *n* / **~ curve** Vergessenskurve *f* / **~ rate** Schnelligkeit *f* des Vergessens / **intentional ~** Vergessen *n* durch Verdrängen

forgiveness Verzeihen *n*, Vergeben *n*

form Form *f*, Gestalt *f*, Muster *n*, Gebilde *n*, Anordnung *f*, Struktur *f*, Konfiguration *f* / **~s of association** Assoziationsformen *fpl* / **~ blindness** Formblindheit *f* / **~ board** Formenbrett *n* / **~ class** Wortstrukturklasse *f*, Wortart *f* / **~–colour response** Form–Farb–Antwort *f* / **~ constancy** Formkonstanz *f*, Gestaltkonstanz *f* / **~ determinant** formdeterminiert / Formdeterminante *f* / **~ of expression** Ausdrucksform *f* / **~–level** Formniveau *n* / **~ perception** Gestaltwahrnehmung *f* / **~ psychology** Gestaltpsychologie *f* / **~–quality** Gestaltqualität *f*, Formqualität *f* / **~s register** Formelverzeichnis *n* / **~ response** Formantwort *f* / **~ and shape perception** Form– und Gestaltwahrnehmung *f* / **alternate ~** Parallelform *f* / **closed ~** geschlossene Form *f* / **comparable ~** Parallelform *f* vergleichbare Form *f* / **correlated ~** Parallelform *f* / **down–to–earth ~** praxisnahe Form *f*, bodenständige Form *f* / **duplicate ~** Duplikat *n* / **equal ~** gleiche Form *f*, Parallelform *f* / **equivalent ~** Äquivalenzform *f*, Parallelform *f* / **good ~s** gute Formen *fpl* / **intermediate ~** Übergangsform *f*, Zwischenform *f* / **matched ~** zugeordnete Form *f*, Äquivalenzform *f* / **open ~** offene Form *f* / **original ~** Grundform *f* / **parallel ~** Parallelform *f* / **primitive ~** Urform *f*, Grundform *f* / **similar ~** entsprechende Form *f* / **standard ~** Standardform *f*, Normalform *f*

formal formal, formell

formalism Formalismus *m*

formant Formant *m*

formation Bildung *f*, Entstehung *f* / **~ of analogies** Analogiebildung *f* / **~ of complex** Komplexbildung *f* / **~ of the superego** Über–Ich–Bildung *f* / **~ of symptoms** Symptombildung *f* / **genetic ~** genetische Ausprägung *f* / **hippocampal ~** Hippocampusformation *f* / **reticular ~** Formatio reticularis *f*, Retikulärformation *f* / **substitutive ~** Ersatzbildung *f*

formative bildend, formend

formboard Formenbrett *n* / **~ test** Formlegetest *m*, Formenbrett *n*

formication Ameisenlaufen *n*, Kribbeln *n*

formula Formel *f* / **~ translation** Programmsprache FORTRAN *f* / **fundamental ~** Grundformel *f*

fornicate außerehelichen Beischlaf ausüben, Unzucht *f* treiben

fornication außerehelicher Beischlaf *m*

fornix Fornix *f*, Gewölbe *n*, Scheidengewölbe *n*

fortify ermutigen, stärken, seelisch stützen

fortuitous zufällig, Zufalls–

forward vorne, vorwärts gerichtet, in der Zukunft

foster Pflege– / aufziehen, pflegen, fördern / **~–care** Versorgung *f* in Pflegefamilien / **~ child** Pflegekind *n* / **~–child fantasy** Einbildung *f* nur ein Pflegekind seiner Eltern zu sein / **~–father** Pflegevater *m* / **~–home** Pflegeheim *n* / **~–mother** Pflegemutter *f* / **~–parents** Pflegeeltern pl

foul faul, schmutzig, zotig

founded begründet, fundiert

founding begründend, konstituierend

four–colour theory Vierfarbentheorie *f*

fourfold vierfach, vierteilig, aus vier Einheiten bestehend

Fourier| analysis Fourier'sche Analyse *f* / **~'s law** Fourier'sches Gesetz *n* / **~'s series** Fourier–Serien *fpl*

fovea centralis Fovea centralis *f*, Netzhautgrube *f*, Sehgrube *f*

foveal zur Fovea gehörig

fraction Fraktion *f*

fractional fraktioniert, bruchstückweise, minimal

fractionation Fraktionierung *f*, Gliederung *f*, Fraktionieren *n*, Gliedern *n*

fragmentation Gedankenzerfall *m*, Gedankenflucht *f*

fragrant duftend

frame Rahmen *m*, Gefüge *n*, Verfassung *f*, Lernschritt *m* in einem Lernprogramm / ~ **frequency** Bildfolgefrequenz *f*, Bildwiederholrate *f* / ~ **of mind** Gemütsverfassung *f*, geistige Verfassung *f* / ~ **of reference** Bezugssystem *n*, Bezugsrahmen *m* / ~ **repetition rate** Bildwiederholrate *f*

framework System *n*, Bezugssystem *n* / ~ **of thinking** Denkrahmen *m* / **dyadic** ~ dyadisches Bezugssystem *n*

frank offen, aufrichtig

frankness Offenheit *f*, Aufrichtigkeit *f*, Wahrhaftigkeit *f*

Frank–Starling mechanism Frank–Starling–Mechanismus *m*

frantic wahnsinnig, toll, rasend

fraternal brüderlich

fraternity Bruderschaft *f*, Studentenverbindung *f* / ~ **membership** Mitgliedschaft *f* in einer Studentenverbindung

***F* ratio** *F*–Wert *m*

fraud Betrug *m*

freak Laune *f*, Launenhaftigkeit *f*

freaky ausgeflippt

free frei, ungebunden / **~–answer** mit offener Antwort

freedom Freiheit *f* / ~ **of movement** Bewegungsfreiheit *f* / ~ **reflex** Freiheitsreflex *m* / **psychological** ~ psychologische Freiheit *f*

free|–floating frei–flottierend / **~–handed** freigebig / **~–response** mit offener Antwort, mit ungebundener Aufgabenbeantwortung / **~–spoken** offen, leutselig / **~–thinking** Freidenkerei *f*, freidenkend / **~–thought** Freidenkerei *f*, freidenkend / ~ **ware** kostenlose Software *f*, Freeware *f* / **~–will** Willensfreiheit *f*, freiwillig / **~–will doctrine** Lehre *f* von der Willensfreiheit

freezing Schreckstarre *f*

frenetic rasend, tobend, toll, wahnsinnig

Frenzel's| glasses *or* spectacles Frenzel–Brille *f*, Frenzel–Leuchtbrille *f*

frenzy Toben *n*, Koller *m*, Raserei *f*, Wahnsinn *m*

frequency Häufigkeit *f*, Frequenz *f* / ~ **analysis** Fourier–Analyse *f* / **configural** ~ **analysis** Konfigurationsfrequenzanalyse *f* / ~ **of attacks** Anfallshäufigkeit *f* / ~ **characteristic** Frequenzgang *m* / ~ **chart** Häufigkeitsdiagramm *n* / ~ **curve** Häufigkeitskurve *f*, Häufigkeitsverteilung *f* / ~ **diagram** Häufigkeitsdiagramm *n* / **~–difference threshold** Frequenzunterschiedsschwelle *f* / ~ **of disease** Erkrankungshäufigkeit *f* / ~ **distribution** Häufigkeitsverteilung *f* / ~ **function** Häufigkeitsfunktion *f* / ~ **graph** Häufigkeitsdiagramm *n* / ~ **of incidence** Häufigkeit *f* des Auftretens, Häufigkeit *f* des Vorkommens / ~ **law** Häufigkeitsgesetz *n*, Wiederholungsgesetz *n* / ~ **level** Frequenzniveau *n*, Frequenzhöhe *f* / ~ **method** Frequenzmethode *f* / ~ **modulation** Frequenzmodulation *f* / ~ **polygon** Häufigkeitspolygon *n*, Häufigkeitsdiagramm *n* / ~ **of responding** Reaktionshäufigkeit *f* / ~ **response** Frequenzgang *m* / ~ **of stimulation** Reizfrequenz *f* / ~ **surface** Fläche *f* unter der Häufigkeitsverteilung / ~ **spectrum** Frequenzspektrum *n* / ~ **table** Häufigkeitstabelle *f* / ~ **theories of hearing** Frequenztheorien *fpl* des Hörens / **absolute** ~ absolute Häufigkeit *f* / **acoustic** ~ Schallfrequenz *f* / **basic** ~ Grundfrequenz *f* / **critical** ~ kritische Frequenz *f* / **critical** ~ **of fusion** Flimmerverschmelzungsfrequenz *f* / **cumulative** ~ kumulative Häufigkeit *f*, kumulierte Häufigkeit *f* / **cumulative** ~ **curve** kumulative Häufigkeitskurve *f*, kumulative Häufigkeitsverteilung *f* / **cumulative** ~ **distribution** kumulative Häufigkeitsverteilung *f* / **cumulative** ~ **function** kumulative Verteilungsfunktion *f* / **cumulative** ~ **graph** kumulative Häufigkeitskurve *f*, Ogive *f* / **cut–off** ~ Grenzfrequenz *f* / **expected** ~ erwartete Häufigkeit *f* / **fundamental** ~ Grundfrequenz *f* / **high** ~

Hochfrequenz *f* hohe Frequenz *f* / **J–shaped ~ curve** J–förmige Häufigkeitsverteilung *f* / **low ~ current** Schwachstrom *m* / **marginal ~** Zeilenhäufigkeit *f*, Spaltenhäufigkeit *f* / **modal ~** modale Häufigkeit *f*, Modalwert *m* / **multimodal ~ curve** mehrgipflige Häufigkeitskurve *f* / **natural ~** Eigenfrequenz *f* / **normal ~ curve** Normalverteilungskurve *f*, Gauß–Kurve *f* / **normal ~ curve equation** Gleichung *f* der Normalverteilungskurve / **observed ~** beobachtete Häufigkeit *f* / **rectangular ~ polygon** Histogramm *n* / **relative ~** relative Häufigkeit *f* / **spatial ~** räumliche Frequenz *f* / **theoretical ~** theoretische Häufigkeit *f* / **temporal ~** temporale Frequenz *f* / **U–shaped ~ curve** U–förmige Häufigkeitsverteilung *f*

Freudian Freud'sche(r, s)

Freudianism, Freudism Lehre *f* von Sigmund Freud

friction Reibung *f*, Friktion *f*

Friedman test Friedman–Test *m*, Rangvarianzanalyse *f*

Friedmann's disease Narkolepsie *f*

friendship Freundschaft *f* / **~ group** Freundeskreis *m*, Freundesgruppe *f* / **platonic ~** platonische Liebe *f*

fright Schreck *m*, Schrecken *m* / **~ neurosis** Schreckneurose *f*

frigid gefühlsarm, kalt, frigide

frigidity Gefühlskälte *f*, Frigidität *f*

fringe Rand *m*, Grenze *f* / **~ benefit** Sozialleistung *f*, Nebenleistung *f*, Zusatzleistung *f* / **~ of consciousness** Bewusstseinsrand *m*

fringer Randfigur *f*, Randperson *f*

Froehlich's syndrome Fröhlich–Krankheit *f*, Dystrophia adiposogenitalis *f*

frog Frosch *m*

frontal frontal, Stirn–

frottage Frottage *f*, Massage *f* der Geschlechtsorgane

frotteur Frotteur *m*

frotteurism Frotteurismus *m*

fruit fly Fruchtfliege *f*, Drosophila *f*

fruity fruchtig

frustrate frustrieren

frustrated frustriert

frustration Frustration *f* / **~–aggression hypothesis** Frustrations–Aggressionshypothese *f* / **~ reaction test** Frustrations–Reaktionstest *m* / **~ response** Reaktion *f* auf Frustration / **~ test** Frustrationstest *m* / **~ tolerance** Frustrationstoleranz *f* / **conditioned ~** konditionierte Frustration *f* / **external ~** Frustration *f* von außen / **internal ~** innere Frustration *f*

***F* scale** *F*–Skala *f*, Faschismus–Skala *f*

***F* score** *F*–Wert *m*

***F* test** *F*–Test *m*

fuel Brennstoff *m*

fugue Fugue *f*, Dämmerzustand *m* / Verlassen *n* der gewohnten Umgebung im Dämmerzustand, amnesieartiger Zustand *m* / **~ reaction** amnestische Handlung *f*, Fugue–Reaktion *f* / **dissociative ~** dissoziative Fugue *f* / **epileptic ~** epileptische Amnesie *f* / **hysterical ~** Wandertrieb *m*, Poriomanie *f*

fulfilment, fulfillment Erfüllung *f*

Fullerton–Cattell law Fullerton–Cattell'sches Gesetz *n*

fullness Fülle *f*, Klangfülle *f*, Weite *f*

fumble–and–success Versuch *m* und Irrtum *m*

function Funktion *f* / funktionieren / **~ of the ego** Ich–Funktion *f* / **~ engram** Funktionsengramm *n* / **~ fluctuation** Funktionsfluktuation *f* / **~ pleasure** Funktionslust *f* / **~ psychology** Funktionspsychologie *f* / **~ types** Funktionstypen *mpl* / **~ unit** Funktionseinheit *f*, funktionelle Einheit *f* / **~ word** Funktionswort *n* / **anticipatory ~** antizipatorische Funktion *f* / **automatic ~ of spinal cord** Reflexautomatismus *m* / **autonomous ~** autonome Funktion *f* / **cerebral ~** Gehirnfunktion *f*, Gehirntätigkeit *f* / **cerebral motor ~s** motorische Gehirnfunktionen *fpl* / **characteristic ~** charakteristische Funktion *f* / **cognitive ~** kognitive Funktion *f* / **cortical ~** Hirnrindenfunktion *f* / **cumulative ~** additive Funktion *f* kumulative Funktion *f* / **defective ~** Fehlfunktion *f* / **discriminant ~** Unterscheidungsfunktion *f* / **double ~ term** bifunktioneller Begriff *m* / **elementary ~** Elementarfunktion *f*, Grundfunktion *f* / **epicritic ~** epikritische Funktion *f* / **exponential ~** Exponentialfunktion *f* / **full ~** Funktionstüchtigkeit *f* / **higher mental ~** Abstraktionsleistung *f* / **homeostatic ~s** homeostatische Funktionen *fpl* / **intellectual ~** geistige Funktion *f* / **linear ~** lineare Funktion *f* / **mental ~** psychische Funktion *f* / **motor ~s** motorische Funktionen *fpl* / **nervous ~** Nerventätigkeit *f*, Nervenfunktion *f* / **partial ~** Teilfunktion *f* / **primary ~** Primärfunktion *f* / **psychic ~** psychische Funktion *f* / **psychometric ~** psychometrische Funktion *f* / **quadratic ~** quadratische Funktion *f* / **reproductive ~** Fortpflanzungsfunktion *f* / **secondary~** Nebenfunktion *f*, sekundäre Funktion *f* / **semiotic ~** semiotische Funktion *f*, Zeichenfunktion *f* / **sensory–motor ~s** sensumotorische Funktionen *fpl* / **sexual ~** sexuelle Funktion *f*, Sexualfunktion *f* / **sexual ~ disturbance** sexuelle Funktionsstörung *f* / **sudomotor ~** Sudomotorik *f* / **symbolic ~** Symbolfunktion *f* / **tactile ~** Tastfunktion *f* / **trophic ~** Ernährungsfunktion *f* / **urinary ~ disorder** Funktionsstörung *f* der Harnblase / **vicarious ~** substitutive Funktion *f*, Ersatzfunktion / **weak ~** Unterfunktion *f* / **weak cerebral ~** Hirnleistungsschwäche *f*

functional funktionell, Funktions–

functionalisation Aufgliederung *f* in Funktionseinheiten

functionalism Funktionalismus *m*, funktionelle Psychologie *f* / **probabilistic ~** probabilistischer Funktionalismus *m*

functionalistic funktionalistisch, funktionsbezogen

functioning Funktionieren *n* / **social ~** angemessenes Sozialverhalten *n* / **vicarious ~** Übernahme *f* einer Ersatzfunktion

fundament Grundlage *f*, Anlage *f*, Fundament *n*

fundamental grundlegend, fundamental, Grundlagen–

fundamentalism Fundamentalismus *m*

fundamentalist Dogmatiker *m*

funneling, funnelling Kanalisierung *f*, Hineinfügen *n*, Übertragung *f*

furious rasend, wütend

furor Wutanfall *m*, Anfall *m*, Furor *m* / **epileptic ~** Furor epilepticus *m*, Raserei *f* am Ende des epileptischen Anfalls

fury Raserei *f*, Wut *f* / **maniacal ~** Tobsucht *f*

fusion Verschmelzung *f*, Mischung *f* / **~ of chromosomes** Chromosomenverschmelzung *f* / **~–defusion** Verschmelzung *f*, Entmischung *f* / **~ frequency** Verschmelzungsfrequenz *f* / **~ of instincts** Triebmischung *f* / **~ of stimuli** Reizverschmelzung / **binaural ~** binaurale Lautverschmelzung *f* / **binocular ~** binokulare Verschmelzung *f* / **instinctual ~** Triebverschmelzung *f* / **partial ~** Triebverschmelzung *f* / **tonal ~** Tonverschmelzung *f*

future Zukunft *f* / zukünftig

futorologist Zukunftsforscher *m*, Futurologe *m*

futurology Zukunftsforschung *f*, Futurologie *f*

fuzziness of peripheral vision Undeutlichkeit *f* des peripheren Sehens

G

gag ungewöhnlicher Einfall *m*, Gag *m* / **~ reflex** Würgereflex *m*, Rachenreflex *m*

gaga verrückt, schwachsinnig, kindisch

gage eichen, kalibrieren

gain Gewinn *m*, Zunahme *f*, Nutzen *m* / **~ from illness** Krankheitsgewinn *m* / **episonic ~** Krankheitsgewinn *m* / **morbid ~** Erlangung *f* von Vorteilen aufgrund krankhaften Verhaltens / **negative ~** Abnahme *f* / **primary ~** Primärgewinn *m* / **primary ~ from illness** primärer Krankheitsgewinn *m* / **positive ~** Zunahme *f* / **secondary ~ from illness** sekundärer Krankheitsgewinn *m*

gait Gang *m*, Gangart *f*

galeanthropy Galeanthropie *f*, krankhafte Vorstellung *f* eine Katze zu sein

galeophobia Angst *f* vor Katzen, Galeophobie *f*

gall| bladder Gallenblase *f* / **~ stone** Gallenstein *m*

Gall's craniology Gall'sche Schädellehre *f*, Phrenologie *f*

Galton| bar Galton–Stab *m* / **~'s law** Galton–Gesetz *n* / **~'s questionary** Galtons Fragebogen *m* / **~ whistle** Galton–Pfeife *f*

galvanic galvanisch

galvanisation Gleichstrombehandlung *f*, Galvanisation *f*

galvanometer Galvanometer *n*

galvanotaxis Galvanotaxis *f*

galvanotonus Galvanotonus *m*, galvanisch bedingte Muskelspannung *f*

galvanotropism Galvanotropismus *m*, Galvanotaxis *f*

gamble Glücksspiel betreiben, hoch spielen, spekulieren

gambling Glücksspiel *n*, Spielen *n* / **pathological ~** pathologisches Glücksspiel *n*, pathologisches Spielen *n*, Spielsucht *f*

game Spiel *n* / **~ theory** Spieltheorie *f*

gamete Gamet *m* / **~–producing cell** Keimzelle *f*

gametogenesis Gametenbildung *f*

gamma Gamma *n* / **~–aminobutyric acid** Gamma–Aminobuttersäure *f* / **~–aminobutyric acid agonist** Gamma–Aminobuttersäure–Agonist *m* / **~–aminobutyric acid antagonist** Gamma–Aminobuttersäure–Antagonist *m* / **~ globulin** Gammaglobulin *n* / **~ loop** Gamma–Schleife *f* / **~ movement** Gamma–Bewegung *f* / **~ radiation** Gamma–Strahlung *f* / **~ rhythm** Gamma–Rhythmus *m*

gammacism fehlende Artikulation *f* der g–Laute, Gammazismus *m*, Kehlstammeln *n*

gamogenesis geschlechtliche Fortpflanzung *f*

gamone Gamon *n*, Befruchtungshormon *n*

gamonomania Heiratssucht *f*, Gamomanie *f*

gamophobia Heiratsangst *f*, Gamophobie *f*

gang Bande *f* / **~ membership** Bandenmitgliedschaft *f* / **juvenile ~** Jugendbande *f*, Bande *f* von Jugendlichen

ganglia Ganglien *npl* / **~ blocking** Ganglienblockade *f*

gangliar, ganglionic, ganglionary Ganglien–

gangliated, ganglionated mit Ganglien versehen

ganglion Ganglion *n* / **~ blocking drug** Ganglienblocker *m* / **~ cell** Ganglienzelle *f* / **~ cell group** Ganglienzellgruppe *f* / **~ of Corti** Corti–Ganglion *n*, Hörsinneszelle *f* / ~ **of glossopharyngeal nerve** Glossopharyngeusganglion *n* / ~ **potentials** Ganglienpotentiale *npl* / **autonomic** ~ vegetatives Grenzstrangganglion *n* / **basal** ~ Großhirnganglion *n*, Basalganglion *n* / **cerebral** ~ Zerebralganglion *n* / **Gasserian** ~ Gasser'sches Ganglion *n* / **midget** ~ **cell** Miniaturganglienzelle *f* / **spinal** ~ Spinalganglion *n*, Intervertebralganglion *n* / **spiral** ~ Ganglion spirale cochleae *n* / **stellate** ~ Sternganglion *n* / **sympathetic** ~ Sympathikusganglion *n* / **visceral** ~ Eingeweideganglion *n*

gangliosidosis Gangliosidose *f*

Ganser's syndrome Ganser–Syndrom *n*, Pseudodemenz *f*, vorgetäuschte Geistesstörung *f*, Scheinblödsinn *m*

gap Lücke *f* / ~ **junction** offener Zellkontakt *m*, Nexus *m* / ~ **of memory** Gedächtnislücke *f*, amnestische Lücke *f* / **tonal** ~ Hörlücke *f*

gargalaesthesis, gargalesthesis Kitzelempfindung *f*

gargalanaesthesia Unempfindlichkeit *f* gegenüber Kitzeln

gargalhyperaesthesia Überempfindlichkeit *f* gegenüber Kitzeln

gargoylism Gargoylismus *m*, Dysostosis multiplex *f*, Pfaundler–Hurler–Krankheit *f*, Hurler–Syndrom *n*

garrulity, garrulousness Geschwätzigkeit *f*

garrulous geschwätzig

gas, respiratory Atemgas *n*

gasoline sniffing Benzinismus *m*, Benzinsucht *f*, Benzinomanie *f*

gastrectomy Magenentfernung *f*

gastric Magen–, gastrisch

gastrin Gastrin *n*

gastrocolic gastrokolisch

gastro–intestinal gastrointestinal, Magen–Darm–

gastropod Schnecke *f*, Gastropode *m*

gastrula Gastrula *f*, Becherkeim *m*

gastrulation Gastrulation *f*, Gastrulabildung *f*

gate Pforte *f*, Eingang *m* / ~**–frame** Zugangseinheit *f* / ~**–keeper** Person *f* die Nachrichten und Informationen vor der Weitergabe an den Empfänger selektiert und manipuliert / ~ **way** Netzkoppler *m*, Überleiteinrichtung *f*, Gateway *n*

gatophobia Angst *f* vor Katzen

gauge eichen, kalibrieren

gauging Eichung *f*, Kalibration *f*

Gaussian Gauß'sche (r, s)

gavage Mästen *n*, Vollfüttern *n*, Zwangsernährung *f* mittels Magensonde

gay Homosexueller *m* / ~ **liberation movement** Bürgerrechtsbewegung *f* für die gesellschaftliche Anerkennung der Homosexuellen

gaze starrer Blick *m*

geese Gänse *fpl*

gelasma, gelasmus Lachkrampf *m*, krampfhaftes Lachen *n*, Gelasma *n*

geloplegia Geleoplegie *f*, Gelolepsie *f*, Lachschlag *m*

gemellary Zwillings–

gemmule Gemmula *f*, kleinstes Erbteilchen *n*

gender Geschlecht *n* / ~ **identity disorder** Geschlechtsidentitätsstörung *f* / ~ **identity disorder in adolescents or adults** Geschlechtsidentitätsstörung *f* bei Jugendlichen oder Erwachsenen / ~ **identity disorder (of childhood)** Störung *f* der Geschlechtsidentität (in der Kindheit) / **atypical** ~ **identity disorder** atypische Störung *f* der Geschlechtsidentität / ~ **role** Geschlechtsrolle *f*

gene Gen *n*, Erbfaktor *m*, Erbanlage *f* / ~ **activation** Genaktivierung *f* / ~ **expression** Genexpression *f* / ~ **pair** Genpaar *n* / ~ **regulation** Genregulation *f* / **allele** ~**s** Allele *npl*, allele Gene *npl* / **allelomorphic** ~**s** Allelogene *npl*, allelomorphe Gene *npl* / **dominant** ~ dominantes Gen *n*, dominanter Erbfaktor *m* / **major** ~ bedeutendes Gen *n* / **mutated** ~ mutiertes

Gen *n* / **recessive ~** rezessives Gen *n*, rezessiver Erbfaktor *m* / **sex–linked ~** Geschlechtsgen *n*

genealogy Genealogie *f*, Familienkunde *f*

genera Gattungen *fpl*

general allgemein, generell

generalisation Generalisation *f*, Generalisierung *f*, Verallgemeinerung *f* / **~ curve** Generalisationskurve *f* / **~ extinction** Auslöschung *f* einer Generalisierung / **~ of fear** Angstgeneralisierung *f* / **~ gradient** Generalisationsgradient *m* / **associative ~** Reizgeneralisation *f*, Reaktionsgeneralisation *f* / **cognitive ~** kognitive Generalisation *f* / **mediate ~** mittelbare Generalisation *f*, semantische Konditionierung *f* / **perceptual ~** Wahrnehmungsgeneralisierung *f* / **semantic ~** Verallgemeinerung *f* von Bedeutungen, semantische Generalisierung *f* / **verbal ~** Wortgeneralisation *f*

generality Allgemeinheit *f*, allgemeine Äußerung *f* / **interorgan ~** gemeinsame Organeigenschaft *f*

generalize generalisieren, verallgemeinern

generating Erzeugung *f*, Hervorbringen *n* / **~ of anxiety** Angstentwicklung *f*

generation Zeugung *f*, Fortpflanzung *f*, Entstehung *f*, Erzeugung *f*, Generation *f* / **~ effect** Generierungseffekt *m* / **~ gap** Generationenunterschied *m* / **~ of anxiety** Angsterzeugung *f*, Angstentwicklung *f* / **filial ~** Filialgeneration *f* / **parental ~** Elterngeneration *f* / **spontaneous ~** Urzeugung *f*, Abiogenese *f*

generator potential Generatorpotential *n*

generic generisch, allgemein, Gattungs–

generosity Großzügigkeit *f* / **~ error** Fehler *m* der zu großzügigen Beurteilung, Milde–Effekt *m*

genesis Genese *f*, Entstehung *f* / **actual ~** Aktualgenese *f*

genetic genetisch, entwicklungsgeschichtlich, ontogenetisch

genetics Genetik *f*, Erblehre *f*, Vererbungslehre *f* / **behavioural ~** Genetik *f*, Verhaltensgenetik *f* / **classical ~** klassische Genetik *f* / **human ~** Humangenetik *f* / **molecular ~** Molekulargenetik *f*, molekulare Genetik *f*

genic genbedingt

genidentic mit identischen Genen

genital genital, geschlechtlich

genitalia Genitalien *npl*, äußere Geschlechtsorgane *npl*, Geschlechtsteile *npl* / **female ~** weibliche Genitalien *npl*, weibliche Geschlechtsorgane *npl* / **male ~** männliche Genitalien *npl*, männliche Geschlechtsorgane *npl*

genitality Genitalität *f*

genitals Genitalien *npl*, Geschlechtsapparat *m*, Geschlechtsorgane *npl*, Geschlechtsteile *npl*

genius Genie *n*, schöpferische Fähigkeit *f*

genocide Genozid *m*, Völkermord *m*

genome Genbestand *m*, Genom *n*, Erbgut *n*, haploider Chromosomensatz *m*

genomotive Geno–Motiv *n*

genophobia krankhafte Angst *f* vor allem Geschlechtlichem, Genophobie *f*

genotype Genotypus *m*, Erbbild *n*

genotypic, genotypical genotypisch

gens genealogische Linie *f*, Familienstamm *m*, Geschlecht *n*, patrilinearer Volksstamm *m*

genuine echt, genuin, angeboren

genuineness Echtheit *f*

genus Art *f*, Gattung *f*, Geschlecht *n*

geocentric geozentrisch

geography response Geographie–Deutung *f*, Kartendeutung *f*

geometric, geometrical geometrisch

geophagia, geophagism, geophagy Erdessen *n*, Geophagie *f*

geophagist Erdesser *m*, Geophag *m*

geophagous erdessend, geophag

geopsychical geopsychisch

geopsychology Geopsychologie *f*

geotaxis Geotaxis *f*, Geotropismus *m*

geotropic geotropisch

geotropism Geotropismus *m*

gephyrophobia Brückenangst *f*, Angst *f* vor Abgründen, Gephyrophobie *f*

geriatric geriatrisch

geriatrics Geriatrie *f*, Lehre *f* von den Krankheiten des Alters

geriopsychosis Alterspsychose *f*

germ Keim *m* / ~ **cell** Keimzelle *f* / ~ **gland** Keimdrüse *f* / ~ **layer** Keimblatt *n* / ~ **plasm** Keimplasma *n*

germinal germinal, Keim–

geroderma, gerodermia Greisenhaut *f*, Geroderma *f*

geromorphism greisenhaftes Aussehen *n* jüngerer Leute, Geromorphismus *m*

gerontocracy Gerontokratie *f*, Herrschaft *f* der Stammesältesten

geronto|logy Gerontologie *f*, Alterskunde *f* / ~ **philia** Gerontophilie *f* / ~ **phobia** Angst *f* vor dem Alter, Angst *f* vor dem Altern, Gerontophobie *f* / ~ **psychiatry** Gerontopsychiatrie *f*, Alterspsychiatrie *f*, geriatrische Psychiatrie *f*

Gerstmann's syndrome Gerstmann'sches Syndrom *n*

Gesell| developmental norms Entwicklungsnormen *fpl* nach Gesell / ~ **developmental scales** Entwicklungsstufen *fpl* nach Gesell / ~ **developmental schedule** Entwicklungsnormen *fpl* nach Gesell

gestagen Gestagen *n*

Gestalt, gestalt Gestalt *f*, Form *f*, Gebilde *n*, Anordnung *f*, Konfiguration *f* / ~ **completion test** Gestaltergänzungstest *m* / ~ **of curve** Kurvenform *f*, Kurvengestalt *f* / ~ **factor** Gestaltfaktor *m*, Gestaltgesetz *n* / ~ **homology** Gleichartigkeit *f* der Gestalt / ~ **law** Gestaltgesetz *n* / ~ **learning** Gestaltlernen *n* / ~ **principle** Gestaltprinzip *n* / ~ **psychology** Gestaltpsychologie *f* / ~ **psychotherapy** Gestaltpsychotherapie *f* / ~ **quality** Gestaltqualität *f* / ~ **theory** Gestaltheorie *f* / ~ **therapy** Gestalttherapie *f* / **autochthonous** ~ autochthone Gestalt *f* / **good** ~ gute Gestalt *f* / **temporal** ~ Zeitgestalt *f*

gestalting Gestaltung *f*, Verstärken *n* der Prägnanz

Gestaltism Gestaltpsychologie *f*

Gestaltist Gestaltpsychologe *m*

gestation Gestation *f*, Schwangerschaft *f*, Gravidität *f*

gestational Schwangerschafts–

gesticulate gestikulieren, durch Gesten ausdrücken

gesticulation Gestikulation *f*, Gebärdenspiel *n*

gesture Geste *f*, Gebärde *f*, Ausdrucksbewegung *f* / ~ **language** Gebärdensprache *f* / **expressive** ~ Ausdrucksgeste *f* / **magic** ~ magische Gebärde *f* / **plus** ~ Überkompensationsverhalten *n*

g factor g–Faktor *m*, G–Faktor *m*, gemeinsamer Faktor *m*, Generalfaktor *m*

geusis Schmecken *n*

ghost Geist *m* / ~ **theory** animistische Theorie *f*, Animismus *m*, Geistertheorie *f*

giant Riese *m* / ~ **synapsis** Riesensynapse *f*

giantism Riesenwuchs *m*, Gigantismus *m*

gibberish Kauderwelsch *n*, dummes Geschwätz *n*

Gibson effect Gibson–Effekt *m*, Gibson–Gradient *m*

giddiness Schwindel *m*, Schwindelgefühl *n*, Vertigo *m*, Leichtsinn *m*, Unbesonnenheit *f* / **free from** ~ schwindelfrei

gift Begabung *f*, Talent *n*

gifted begabt, talentiert / Hochbegabte *m,f* / **intellectually** ~ geistig begabt, hochbegabt / **mentally** ~ geistig begabt, hochbegabt

giftedness Begabung *f*

gigantism Riesenwuchs *m*, Gigantismus *m* / **acromegalic** ~ akromegalischer Riesenwuchs *m* / **cerebral** ~ Sotos–Syndrom *n* / **eunuchoid** ~ eunuchoider Hochwuchs *m*

Gilbreth chronoscope Gilbreth–Uhr *f*

Gilles de la Tourette| disorder Gilles de la Tourette Krankheit *f*, Maladie des tics *f* / **~ disease** Gilles de la Tourette Krankheit *f*, Maladie des tics *f*

girdle sensation Gürtelschmerz *m*, Gürtelgefühl *n*

given bestimmt, gegeben, vorhanden

gland Drüse *f* / **~s of internal secretion** Drüsen *fpl* mit innerer Sekretion / **accessory thyroid ~** Nebenschilddrüse *f*, Epithelkörperchen *n* / **adrenal ~** Nebenniere *f* / **adrenal ~ disorder** Nebennierenerkrankung *f* / **adrenal ~ secretion** Nebennierensekretion *f* / **anterior pituitary ~** vordere Hypophyse *f* / **closed ~** innersekretorische Drüse *f* / **convoluted ~** Schweißdrüse *f* / **digestive ~** Verdauungsdrüse *f* / **ductless ~** innersekretorische Drüse *f*, Drüse *f* ohne Ausführungsgang / **endocrine ~** endokrine Drüse *f* / **endocrine ~ secretion** Sekretion *f* der endokrinen Drüsen / **exocrine ~** exokrine Drüse *f*, Drüse *f* mit Ausführungsgang / **gastric ~** Magendrüse *f* / **genital ~** Geschlechtsdrüse *f* / **lacrimal ~** Tränendrüse *f* / **mammary ~** Brustdrüse *f*, Milchdrüse *f* / **mandibular ~** Unterkieferdrüse *f* / **mucous ~** Schleimdrüse *f* / **open ~** exokrine Drüse *f* / **parathyroid ~** Nebenschilddrüse *f*, Epithelkörperchen *n* / **parotid ~** Ohrspeicheldrüse *f*, Parotis *f* / **perspiratory ~** Schweißdrüse *f* / **pineal ~** Epiphyse *f*, Zirbeldrüse *f* / **pituitary ~** Hypophyse *f* / **preputial ~** Vorhautdrüse *f* / **reproductive ~** Geschlechtsdrüse *f* / **rinsing ~** Spüldrüse *f* / **salivary ~** Speicheldrüse *f* / **sebaceous ~** Talgdrüse *f* / **seromucous ~** seromuköse Drüse *f* / **sexual ~** Geschlechtsdrüse *f* / **sublingual ~** Unterzungendrüse *f* / **submandibular ~** Unterkieferdrüse *f* / **sudoriferous ~** Schweißdrüse *f* / **sudoriparous ~** Schweißdrüse *f* / **suprarenal ~** Nebenniere *f* / **thyroid ~** Schilddrüse *f* / **vaginal ~s** Vaginaldrüsen *fpl*, Scheidendrüsen *fpl*

glandular glandulär, Drüsen–, drüsenartig

glandule kleine Drüse *f*

glans Glans *f*, Eichel *f*

glare Blendung *f* / **~ effect** Blendwirkung *f*

glass sensation Glasempfindung *f*

glassiness Durchsichtigkeit *f*

glaucoma Glaukom *n*, grüner Star *m*

glia Glia *f*, Neuroglia *f*

glioma Gliom *n*

gliosis Gliose *f*, Gliawucherung *f*

glittering glänzend, glitzernd

global global, Gesamt–, umfassend, gesamt

globulin Globulin *n*, Eiweiß *n*

globus Globus *m*, Kugel *f* / **~ hystericus** Globus hystericus *m*, Globusgefühl *n* / **~ pallidus** Globus pallidus *m*

glomerular glomerulär

glomerulonephritis Glomerulonephritis *f*

glomerulus Glomerulus *m*

glomus Gefäßknäuel *n,m*, Glomus *m*

gloss Glanz *m*, Erläuterung *f*, Anmerkung *f*, Fußnote *f*

glossa Zunge *f*

glossal Zungen–

glossary Wörterbuch *n*, Glossar *n*

glossiness Glanz *m*

glossolalia Glossolalie *f*, Zungenreden *n*

glossomania Glossomanie *f*, Schwatzsucht *f*

glossophobia Glossophobie *f*, Lalophobie *f*, Sprechangst *f*

glossosynthesis Wortneubildung *f*, Neologismus *m*

glossy glänzend

glottal Stimmritzen–

glottis Stimmritze *f*, Glottis *f*

glove anaesthesia Handschuhanästhesie *f*

glow Glut *f*, Glühen *n*

glucagon Glukagon *n*

glucocorticoid Glukokortikoid *n* / **~ hormone** Glukokortikoid *n*

glucogenic glukogen

gluconeogenesis Glukoneogenese *f*

glucoreceptor Glukorezeptor *m*

glucose Traubenzucker *m*, Glukose *f*, Dextrose *f*, Fruchtzucker *m* / **~ level** Glukosespiegel *m* / **~ metabolism** Glukosestoffwechsel *m* / **~ value** Glukosewert *m*, Glukosespiegel *m*

glue sniffing Leimschnüffeln *n*, Inhalieren *n* von Klebstoffdünsten, Trichloräthylen–Sucht *f*

glutamate Glutamat *n*

glutamic, glutaminic glutaminsauer, Glutamin–

glutamine Glutamin *n*

glutathione Glutathion *n*

glutethimide Glutethimid *n*

glutton Vielfraß *m*, Unersättlicher *m*

gluttonous gefräßig, gierig

gluttony Gefräßigkeit *f*, krankhafter Appetit *m*

glycaemia, glycemia Glykämie *f*, Glykose *f* im Blut

glycine Glyzin *n*, Glykokoll *n*, Aminoessigsäure *f*

glycogen Glykogen *n*, Leberstärke *f* / **~ storage** Glykogenspeicher *m*

glycogenolysis Glykogenolyse *f*

glycolipid Glykolipid *n*

glycolysis Glykolyse *f*

glycometabolism Zuckerstoffwechsel *m*

glycopexis Glykogenspeicherung *f*

glycoprotein Glykoprotein *n*

glycoregulation Blutzuckerregulation *f*

glycosuria Glykosurie *f*, Glykoseausscheidung *f* im Urin

gnash mit den Zähnen knirschen

gnome Gnom *m*, Erdgeist *m* / Denkspruch *m*, Sinnspruch *m*, Aphorismus *m*

gnosiology Erkenntnislehre *f*, Erkenntnistheorie *f*

gnosis Gnosis *f*

gnostic gnostisch

gnosticism Gnostizismus *m*

goal Ziel *n*, Zweck *m*, Absicht *f*, Intention *f* / **~ behaviour** zielgerichtetes Verhalten *n* / **~–directed** zielgerichtet / **~–directed behaviour** zielgerichtetes Verhalten *n*, Zielverhalten *n* / **~–directed motivation** zielgerichtete Motivation *f*, Zielmotivation *f* / **~–directed movement** zielgerichtete Bewegung *f*, Zielbewegung *f* / **~–directedness** Zielgerichtetheit *f* / **~ discrepancy** Zieldiskrepanz *f* / **~ distance** Zieldistanz *f* / **~ gradient** Zielgradient *m* / **~ image** Zielvorstellung *f* / **~–inhibited drive** zielgehemmter Trieb *m* / **~ object** Ziel *n*, Zielobjekt *n* / **~ orientation** Zielorientierung *f*, Zielgerichtetheit *f* / **~–oriented behaviour** zielgerichtetes Verhalten *n* / **~ reaction** Zielreaktion *f* / **~ response** Zielreaktion *f* / **~–seeking behaviour** zielstrebiges Verhalten *n* / **~ set** Zieleinstellung *f*, Zielantizipation *f* / **~ setting** Zielsetzung *f* / **~ situation** Ziel *n* / **~ stimulus** propriozeptiver Zielreiz *m* / **~ tension** Zielspannung *f* / **achieved ~** erreichtes Ziel *n* / **antedating ~ reaction** antizipatorische Zielreaktion *f* / **antedating ~ response** antizipatorische Zielreaktion *f* / **anticipatory ~ reaction** antizipatorische Zielreaktion *f* / **anticipatory ~ response** antizipatorische Zielreaktion *f* / **collective ~** gemeinsames Ziel *n* / **common ~** gemeinsames Ziel *n* / **conscious ~ setting** bewusste Zielsetzung *f* / **directional ~ process** gerichteter Zielprozess *m* / **educational ~** Lernziel *n*, Erziehungsziel *n* / **ergic ~** Triebziel *n*, Handlungsziel *n* / **final ~** Endziel *n* / **fractional antedating ~ response** fraktionelle antizipatorische Zielreaktion *f* / **fractional anticipatory ~ response** fraktionelle antizipatorische Zielreaktion *f* / **intermediate ~** Zwischenziel *n* / **learned ~** sekundäres Ziel *n*, erlerntes Motiv *n* / **organizational ~** Organisationsziel *n*, Organisationszweck *m* / **primary ~** Urziel *n*, angeborenes Triebziel *n*, allgemeiner Beweggrund *m* / **secondary ~** sekundäres Ziel *n*, erworbenes Motiv *n* / **subsidiary ~** Ersatzziel *n*

goat Ziege *f*, Ziegenbock *m*

god Gott *m* / **~ concept** Gottesbegriff *m*, Gottesvorstellung *f* / **belief in ~** Gottesglaube *m*

goiter, goitre Kropf *m*, Struma *n* / **exophthalmic ~** Basedow–Krankheit *f*, Glotzaugenkrankheit *f*

goitrous kropfartig, strumaartig

Golgi| apparatus Golgi–Apparat *m* / **~ cells** Golgi–Zellen *fpl* / **~–Mazzoni bodies** Golgi–Mazzoni–Körperchen *n* / **~–Mazzoni corpuscle** Golgi–Mazzoni–Körperchen *n* / **~ tendon organ** Golgi–Sehnenorgan *n*, Golgi–Sehnenspindel *f*

Goll|'s column Goll–Strang *m* / **~'s nucleus** Goll–Kern *m* / **~'s tract** Goll–Strang *m*

Gompertz curve Gompertz–Kurve *f*

gonad Gonade *f*, Geschlechtsdrüse *f*, Keimdrüse *f* / **female ~** Eierstock *m* / **male ~** Hoden *m*

gonadal, gonadial, gonadic Gonaden–, Geschlechtsdrüsen–

gonadotrophic, gonadotropic gonadotrop, die Geschlechtsdrüsen anregend

gonadotrophin, gonadotropin Gonadotropin *n*

goniometer Winkelmesser *m*, Goniometer *n*

gonochorism Geschlechtsentwicklung *f*

gonorrhoea, gonorrhea Gonorrhoe *f*, Tripper *m*

good–humoured gutmütig, gut gelaunt

goodness of fit Güte *f* der Anpassung

goose Gans *f* / **~–pimples** Gänsehaut *f*

Gordon's reflex Gordon–Reflex *m*

gorilla Gorilla *m*

gossip Klatsch *m*

Gottschaldt figures Gottschaldt–Figuren *fpl*

gradate langsam übergehen, abstufen

gradated abgestuft

gradation Abstufung *f*, Stufenfolge *f*, Gradation *f* / **~ of colour** Farbabstufung *f* / **~ method** Stufenmethode *f*

gradational stufenweise fortschreitend, stufenartig

grade Grad *m*, Rang *m*, Stufe *f*, Masse *f* / **~ acceleration** Überspringen *n* von Schulklassen / **~ equivalent** Klassenäquivalent *n* / **~ level** Klassenstufe *f* / **~ norm** Klassennorm *f* / **~–point average** Durchschnitt *m* der erzielten Klassennoten / **~ scale** Skala *f* nach Klassenstufen / **~ score** Klassenwert *m*, Klassenpunktzahl *f* / **~ skipping** Auslassen *n* von Klassen, Überspringen *n* von Klassen / **high–~** hochgradig / **low–~** in geringem Maße

graded eingeteilt, eingestuft, klassifiziert

gradient Gradient *m* / **~ of delay** Verzögerungsgradient *m* / **~ of effect** Wirkungsgradient *m* / **~ of generalization** Generalisationsgradient *m* / **~ of reinforcement** Verstärkungsgradient *m* / **~ of response generalization** Gradient *m* der Reaktionsgeneralisation / **~ of stimulus generalization** Gradient *m* der Reizgeneralisation / **~ of texture** Gradient *m* der visuellen Strukturwahrnehmung / **~ theory** Gradiententheorie *f* / **anterior–posterior ~** zephalokaudaler Entwicklungsgradient *m* / **axial ~** Achsengradient *m*, axialer Gradient *m*, Axialgradient *m* / **electrical ~** elektrischer Gradient *m* / **electrochemical ~** elektrochemischer Gradient *m* / **neural ~** Neurogradient *m*, Nervengradient *m* / **physiological ~** physiologischer Gradient *m*, Stoffwechselgradient *m*

grading Eingruppierung *f*, Einstufung *f*, Einordnung *f*, Benotung *f* / **educational ~** Benotung *f* in der Schule, Notengebung *f*

gradualism Theorie *f* der allmählichen stufenlosen Entwicklung, Gradualismus *m*

graduate Hochschulabsolvent *m*, Fachhochschulabsolvent *m* / **~ education** akademische Ausbildung *f* / **~ psychology education** Psychologiestudium *n* / **~ re-**

cord examination schriftliche Hochschulprüfung *f* / ~ **school** Hochschule *f* / ~ **student** Hochschulstudent *m*

graduation Glättung *f* / Hochschulabschluss *m*, Fachhochschulabschluss *m* / ~ **curve** geglättete Verteilungskurve *f*

grain Korn *n*, Körnung *f*

graininess Körnigkeit *f*

grammar Grammatik *f* / **formal** ~ Formalgrammatik *f* / **generative transformational** ~ generative Transformationsgrammatik *f*

grandchild Enkelkind *n*, Enkel *n*

grand mal großer epileptischer Anfall *m*, Grand mal *n*, Haut–mal–Epilepsie *f*

grandeur Größenidee *f*

grandiose großartig, imposant, größenwahnsinnig

grandiosity Größenwahn *m*

grandparents Großeltern *pl* / **great** ~ Urgroßeltern *pl*

granularity Körnigkeit *f*, körnige Beschaffenheit *f*

granulocyte Granulozyt *m*

graph graphische Darstellung *f*, Kurve *f*, Diagramm *n* / ~ **paper** kariertes Papier *n* / **rectangular** ~ Histogramm *n*, Stabdiagramm *n*

grapheme Graphem *n*, Buchstabe *m*, geschriebenes Phonem *n*

graphic graphisch, anschaulich, lebhaft, genau

graphical graphisch, zeichnerisch

grapho|analysis Charakterbeurteilung *f* anhand der Schrift / **~dyne** Schriftdruckmesser *m* / **~logist** Graphologe *m*, Schriftdeuter *m*, Schriftanalytiker *m* / **~logy** Graphologie *f*, Schriftbeurteilung *f*, Schriftdeutung *f*, Lehre *f* von der Handschriftendeutung / **~mania** Schreibwut *f* / **~metry** Graphometrie *f* / **~pathology** Handschriftenbeurteilung *f* zur Diagnosestellung, Graphopathologie *f* / **~phobia** Graphophobie *f* / **~psychology** Schriftpsychologie *f* / **~rrhoea** Kritzelsucht *f*, unkontrollierte Schreibsucht *f*, Graphorrhoe *f* / **~spasm** Schreibkrampf *m*, Graphospasmus *m* / **~therapy** Graphotherapie *f*, Schreibtherapie *f* / **~typology** Schrifttypologie *f*

grapho|kinaesthetic Schreibbewegungs– / **~logical** graphologisch, schriftanalytisch / **~motor** Schreibbewegungs–, graphomotorisch

grasp reflex, grasping reflex Greifreflex *m* / **visual** ~ Seh–Greifreflex *m*

grass Haschisch *n oder* Marihuana *n*

Grassmann laws Grassmann'sche Gesetze *npl*

gratification Belohnung *f*, Befriedigung *f* / ~ **of instinct** Triebbefriedigung *f* / **instinctual** ~ Triebbefriedigung *f* / **substitute** ~ Ersatzbefriedigung *f*

gratitude Dankbarkeit *f*

grave schwerwiegend, gewichtig, ernst

graveness Schwere *f*, Wichtigkeit *f*, Ernst *m*

Graves' disease Basedow'sche Krankheit *f* / Glotzaugenkrankheit *f*

gravid gravid, schwanger

gravidity Gravidität *f*, Schwangerschaft *f*

gravimeter Gravimeter *n*

gravity Schwere *f*, Wichtigkeit *f*, Ernst *m*, Schwerkraft *f*

gray grau / Grau *n* / **cortical** ~ Rindengrau *n* / **median** ~ mittleres Grau *n*, mittelgrau / **middle** ~ mittelgrau / **periaqueductal** ~ zentrales Höhlengrau *n*, Griseum centrale *n*, Substantia grisea centralis cerebri *f*

great–man theory Theorie *f* der großen Persönlichkeiten

greediness Gier *f*, Habsucht *f*, Vielfresserei *f*

greedy gierig, habgierig, gefräßig

green grün / **~–blind** grünblind / **~–blindness** Grünblindheit *f* / **~–violet–white syndrome** Grün–Violett–Weiß–Syndrom *n*

greenness Grün *n*, grüne Farbe *f*, Unreife *f*, Naivität *f*

gregarious Herden–, in Herden lebend, gesellig

gregariousness Herdentrieb *m*, Herdeninstinkt *m*, sozialer Instinkt *m*, Geselligkeitsstreben *n*

grey grau / Grau *n* / **cortical ~** Höhlengrau *n* / **median ~** mittelgrau / **middle ~** mittelgrau

grid Gitter *n* / **~ current** Gitterstrom *m* / **electrical ~** elektrisches Gitter *n* / **managerial ~** Management–Verhaltensgitter *n*

grief Schmerz *m*, Kummer *m*, Trauer *f*

grimace Grimasse *f*, Fratze *f*

grip Griff *m* / **~ pressure** Greifdruck *m* / **~ time** Greifzeit *f*

Griselda complex Griselda–Komplex *m*

groan stöhnen, ächzen / Stöhnen *n*, Ächzen *n*

groggy angschlagen, torkelig, taumelnd, betrunken

grooming Elegantmachen *n*, Herausputzen *n*, Säubern *n* / **animal ~ behaviour** tierisches Putzverhalten *n*

groove Furche *f*, Rinne *f* / **medullary ~** Markfurche *f* / **neural ~** Markfurche *f*

grope tasten, tastend suchen

gross ungewöhnlich dick, korpulent, sehr fett, grob / **~ motor** grobmotorisch

grossness Grobheit *f*, Dummheit *f*

grotesque grotesk, übersteigert, absurd

ground Grund *m*, Beweggrund *m*, Hintergrund *m* / **anterior ~ bundle** Vorderstranggrundbündel *n* / l/ **ateral ~ bundle** Seitenstranggrundbündel *n*

group Gruppe *f* / **~ absolutism** Gruppenintoleranz *f*, Gruppenabsolutismus *m* / **~ acceptance** Gruppenakzeptanz *f*, Aufnahme *f* in die Gruppe / **~ achievement** Gruppenleistung *f* / **~ analysis** Gruppenanalyse *f* / **~ atmosphere** Gruppenatmosphäre *f* / **~ behaviour** Gruppenverhalten *n*, kollektives Verhalten *n* / **~ beliefs** Gruppenmeinungen *fpl*, Gruppenüberzeugungen *fpl* / **~ boundary** Gruppengrenze *f* / **~–centered** gruppenzentriert, gruppenorientiert / **~–centered leadership** gruppenzentrierte Führung *f*, demokratische Führung *f* / **~ climate** Gruppenatmosphäre *f* / **~ cohesion** Gruppenkohäsion *f*, Gruppenzusammenhalt *m* / **~ cohesiveness** Gruppenzusammenhalt *m*, Gruppenzusammenhang *m* / **~ communication** Kommunikation *f* in der Gruppe / **~ conformity** Gruppenkonformität *f* / **~ consciousness** Gruppenbewusstsein *n*, Kollektivbewusstsein *n*, Wir–Bewusstsein *n* / **~ consensus** Gruppenkonsens *m* / **~ contagion** Ausbreitung *f* in der Gruppe / **~ counseling** Gruppenberatung *f* / **~ decision** Gruppenentscheidung *f* / **~ decision making** Entscheidungsfindung *f* in der Gruppe / **~ development** Gruppenbildung *f*, Gruppenentwicklung *f* / **~ differences** Gruppenunterschiede *mpl* / **~ dimension** Gruppendimension *f*, Gruppencharakteristik *f* / **~ discussion** Gruppendiskussion *f* / **~ dynamics** Gruppendynamik *f* / **~ effect** Gruppenwirkung *f* / **~ effectiveness** Gruppeneffizienz *f* / **~ evolution** Gruppenevolution *f* / **~ expectations** Gruppenerwartungen *fpl* / **~ experiment** Gruppenversuch *m*, Gruppenexperiment *n* / **~ factor** Gruppenfaktor *m* / **~ fallacy** Gruppentäuschung *f* / **~ fission** Gruppenspaltung *f*, Gruppenteilung *f* / **~ formation** Gruppenbildung *f* / **~ forming** Gruppenbildung *f* / **~ function** Gruppenfunktion *f* / **~ fusion** Gruppenfusion *f*, Gruppenverschmelzung *f* / **~ goal** Gruppenziel *n* / **~ head** Gruppenleiter *n* / **~ homes** Wohngruppen *fpl* / **~ identification** Gruppenidentifikation *f* / **~ identity** Gruppenidentität *f* / **~ ideology** Gruppenideologie *f* / **~ instruction** Gruppenunterricht *m* / **~ intelligence test** Gruppen–Intelligenztest *m* / **~ interval** Klassenintervall *n* / **~ interview** Gruppeninterview *n* / **~ leader** Gruppenführer *m* / **~ leadership** Gruppenführung *f* / **~ maintenance synergy** Energie *f* zur Sicherung des Gruppenzusammenhalts / **~**

marriage Gruppenehe *f* / ~ **median** Klassenmedian *m* / ~ **member** Gruppenmitglied *n* / ~ **membership** Gruppenmitgliedschaft *f* / ~ **method of factorization** Methode *f* der gruppenweisen Faktorenextraktion / ~ **mind** Gruppengeist *m*, Gruppenseele *f*, Kollektivseele *f*, Massengeist *m*, Massenseele *f* / ~ **morale** Gruppenmoral *f*, Gruppengeist *m* / ~ **norm** Gruppennorm *f* / ~**–oriented leadership** gruppenorientierte Führung *f*, demokratische Leitung *f* / ~ **participation** Gruppenteilnahme *f* / ~ **performance** Gruppenleistung *f* / ~ **piecework** Gruppenakkord *m* / ~ **pressure** Gruppendruck *m*, Gruppenzwang *m* / ~ **problem solving** Problemlösen *n* in der Gruppe / ~ **process** Gruppenprozess *m* / ~ **productivity** Gruppenleistung *f*, Produktivitat *f* in der Gruppe / ~ **properties** Gruppeneigenschaften *fpl* / ~ **psychoanalysis** Gruppenpsychoanalyse *f* / ~ **psychology** Gruppenpsychologie *f* / ~ **psychotherapy** Gruppenpsychotherapie *f*, Gruppentherapie *f* / **directive** ~ **psychotherapy** direktiv–suggestive Gruppenpsychotherapie *f* / ~ **rigidity** Gruppenrigidität *f* / ~ **situation** Gruppensituation *f* / ~ **size** Gruppengröße *f* / ~ **solidarity** Gruppensolidarität *f* / ~**–specific** gruppenspezifisch / ~ **spirit** Gruppengeist *m*, Gruppenmoral *f*, Korpsgeist *m* / ~ **standard** Gruppennorm *f* / ~ **structure** Gruppenstruktur *f* / ~ **superego** Gruppen–Überich *n* / ~ **symbol** Gruppenzeichen *n*, Gruppensymbol *n* / ~ **syntality** Syntalität *f*, „Persönlichkeit" *f* einer Gruppe / ~ **test** Gruppentest *m* / ~ **testing** Gruppentestung *f*, Durchführen *n* eines Gruppentests / ~ **theory** Gruppentheorie *f* / ~ **therapist** Gruppentherapeut *m* / ~ **therapy** Gruppentherapie *f* / **bifocal** ~ **therapy** bifokale Gruppenpsychotherapie *f* / ~ **treatment methods** gruppentherapeutische Methoden *fpl* / ~ **values** Gruppenwerte *mpl*, Gruppenideale *npl* / ~ **work** Arbeit *f* in Freizeitgruppen, Gruppenarbeit *f* / **analytic** ~ Analysegruppe *f* / **allopatric** ~ geographisch isolierte Gruppe *f*, allopatrische Gruppe *f* / **artificial** ~ künstliche Gruppe *f* / **autonomous** ~ autonome Gruppe *f* / **between** ~**s design** Intergruppendesign *n* / **closed** ~ geschlossene Gruppe *f* / **co–acting** ~ nebeneinander arbeitende Gruppe *f* / **comparable** ~**s** Vergleichsgruppe *f* / **compound** ~ aus Untergruppen zusammengesetzte Gruppe *f* / **contrived** ~ zusammengestellte Versuchsgruppe *f* / **cultural** ~ Kulturgruppe *f* / **direct–contact** ~ Intimgruppe *f*, Gruppe *f* mit unmittelbarem Kontakt / **equivalent** ~**s** gleichwertige Gruppen *fpl*, äquivalente Gruppen *fpl* / **ethnic** ~ ethnische Gruppe *f*, Völkergruppe *f* / **experimental** ~ Versuchsgruppe *f*, Experimentalgruppe *f* / **formal** ~ formelle Gruppe *f* / **frozen** ~ stationäre Gruppe *f* / **functional** ~ funktionale Gruppe *f* / **horizontal** ~ Gruppe *f* mit Mitgliedern der gleichen sozialen Schicht / **informal** ~ informelle Gruppe *f* / **leaderless** ~ führerlose Gruppe *f* / **leaderless** ~ **discussion** Gruppendiskussion *f* ohne Leiter / **marathon** ~ **therapy** Marathon–Gruppentherapie *f* / **marginal** ~ Randgruppe *f* / **matched** ~**s** Vergleichsgruppen *fpl*, angeglichene Gruppen *fpl*, entsprechende Gruppen *fpl*, gleichwertige Gruppen *fpl* / **motor** ~**s** motorische Gruppen *fpl* / **multiple–**~ **method** multiple Gruppenmethode *f* / **natural** ~ natürliche Gruppe *f* / **normal** ~ Normalgruppe *f*, Normgruppe *f* / **occupational** ~ Berufsgruppe *f* / **open** ~ offene Gruppe *f* / **organized** ~ organisierte Gruppe *f* / **primary** ~ Primärgruppe *f* / **psychological** ~ psychologische Gruppe *f* / **random** ~ Zufallsgruppe *f* / **religious** ~ Religionsgemeinschaft *f*, Orden *m* / **secondary** ~ Sekundärgruppe *f* / **selected** ~ ausgewählte Gruppe *f* / **small** ~ Kleingruppe *f* / **small** ~ **research** Kleingruppenforschung *f* / **social** ~ soziale Gruppe *f*, soziale Gemeinschaft *f* / **standard** ~ Normalgruppe *f*, Standardgruppe *f* Normgruppe *f* / **territorial** ~ Territorialgruppe *f* / **therapeutic** ~ therapeutische Gruppe *f* / **unitary** ~ einheitliche Gruppe *f* / **vertical** ~ Gruppe *f* mit Mitgliedern unterschiedlicher sozialer Schichten / **we–~** Wir–Gruppe *f* / **working ~** Arbeitsgemeinschaft *f*

grouping Gruppierung *f*, Einordnen *n* in Gruppen / **~ error** Klassenaufteilungsfehler *m* / **homogeneous ~** Einteilung *f* in homogene Gruppen / **operational ~** operationale Gruppierung *f* / **perceptual ~** Wahrnehmungsgruppierung *f* / **spatial ~** räumliche Aufteilung *f*

grown–up Erwachsener *m*

growth Wachstum *n*, Entfaltung *f* / **~ curve** Wachstumskurve *f* / **~ deformity** Wachstumsdeformität *f* / **~ differential** Entwicklungsunterschied *m*, Wachstumsdifferenzial *n* / **~ disk** Wachstumsfuge *f* / **~ gradient** Wachstumsgradient *m* / **~ hormone** Wachstumshormon *n*, Somatotropin *n* / **~ hormone inhibiting hormone** Somatostatin *n* / **~ hormone releasing hormone** Somatoliberin *n*, Somatotropin–releasing–Faktor *m* / **~ motive** Selbstentfaltungsmotiv *n* / **~ need** Entfaltungsbedürfnis *n*, Selbstaktualisationsbedürfnis *n* / **~ plate** Wachstumsfuge *f* / **~ principle** Entfaltungsprinzip *n* / **~ spurt** Wachstumsschub *m* / **accretionary ~** Wachstum *n* / **anatomical ~** Körperwachstum *n*, anatomisches Wachstum *n* / **areal ~** Zunahme *f* des Körpervolumens / **developmental ~** Entwicklung *f* / **differential ~** unterschiedliches Wachstum *n* / **educational ~** Erziehungsergebnis *n* / **horizontal ~** Erweiterung *f* gleichartiger Fertigkeiten / **lineal ~** Längenwachstum *n* / **mental ~** geistige Entwicklung *f*, Intelligenzzunahme *f* / **physical ~** Körperwachstum *n*, Längenwachstum *n* / **physiological ~** physiologische Reifung *f* / **ponderal ~** Gewichtszunahme *f* / **saltatory ~** sprunghaftes Wachstum *n* / **skeletal ~** Skelettwachstum *n* / **social ~** soziale Entwicklung *f*, soziale Reifung *f* / **split ~** ungleiches Wachstum *n*, unterschiedliches Wachstum *n* / **vertical ~** Erwerb *n* komplexerer Fertigkeiten

gruff mürrisch, verdrießlich, barsch, schroff

grumble murren, nörgeln

grumbler Querulant *m*, Nörgler *m*

guanethidine Guanethidin *n*

guanine Guanin *n*

guanosine Guanosin *n*

guardian Hüter *m*, Schützer *m* / **~ship** Vormundschaft *f*, Pflegschaft *f* / **public ~ship** Amtsbetreuung *f*, Amtsvormundschaft *f*

guarding Abwehrspannung *f*

guessing Vermuten *n*, Schätzen *n* / **~ game** Ratespiel *n* / **~ sequence** sequentielle Schätztendenz *f*

guidance Beratung *f*, Führung *f*, Lenkung *f* / **~ clinic** Beratungsstelle *f*, Erziehungsberatungsstelle *f* / **educational ~** schulpsychologische Beratung *f*, pädagogische Beratung *f* / **occupational ~** Berufsberatung *f* / **professional ~** Berufsberatung *f* / **vocational ~** Berufsberatung *f*

guilt Schuld *f* / **~ culture** Kultur *f* auf individuellem Schuldgefühl basierend / **~ feeling** Schuldgefühl *n*, Schuldbewusstsein *n* / **imagined ~** eingebildete Schuld *f* / **unconscious ~ feeling** unbewusstes Schuldgefühl *n*

guinea pig Meerschweinchen *n*

gullibility Leichtgläubigkeit *f*

Gulliver complex Gulliver–Komplex *m*

gust Gust *n*, Geschmackseinheit *f*

gustation Geschmack *m*, Geschmackssinn *m*, Geschmacksvermögen *n*

gustative, gustatory geschmacklich, gustativ, Geschmacks–

gustometry Gustometrie *f*, Geschmacksprüfung *f*

gutterophonia Sprache *f* durchsetzt mit Kehlkopflauten, gutturale Sprache *f*

Guttman scale Guttman–Skala *f*

guttural guttural, Kehl–

gymnasium Turnhalle *f*, Turnplatz *m*

gymnastic Gymnastik *f*, Übung *f* / **logopaedic ~** Sprachheilübung *f* / **orthopaedic ~** Heilgymnastik *f*

gymnophobia krankhafte Angst *f* vor nackten Körpern, Gymnophobie *f*

gymnosophy Nacktkultur *f*, Freikörperkultur *f*, Nudismus *m*

gynaecocracy, gynecocracy Frauenherrschaft *f*, matriarchalische Herrschaft *f*, Gynäkokratie *f*

gynaecologist, gynecologist Gynäkologe *m*, Frauenarzt *m*

gynaecology, gynecology Gynäkologie *f*, Frauenheilkunde *f*

gynaecomania, gynecomania Satyriasis *f*, krankhaft gesteigerter männlicher Geschlechtstrieb *m*, Geilheit *f*

gynaecomastia, gynaecomasty, gynaecomastism Gynäkomastie *f*, Brustentwicklung *f* bei Männern

gynaecophobia, gynecophobia, gynaephobia, gynephobia krankhafte Angst *f* vor Frauen, Gynäkophobie *f*

gynagogy Gynagogie *f*, psychotherapeutische Behandlung *f* von geschlechtsspezifischen psychischen Störungen bei Frauen

gynander Mannweib *n*, Virago *f*

gynandria, gynandry, gynandrism, gynanthropism, gynanthropia Gynandrie *f*, weiblicher Pseudohermaphroditismus *m*

gynandromorphism Gynandromorphismus *m*, zwitterhaftes Auftreten *n* gegengeschlechtlicher Körpermerkmale

gynandromorphous gynandromorph, gynandrisch

gynandromorphy Gynandromorphie *f*

gynandrous gynandrisch

gyration Drehung *f*, Wendung *f*

gyrencephala Gehirnwindungen *fpl*

gyrus Gyrus *m*, Gehirnwindung *f* / **angular ~** Gyrus angularis *m* / **cingular ~** Gyrus cinguli *m* / **cingulate ~** Gyrus cinguli *m* / **occipital ~** Hinterhauptwindung *f* / **post central ~** Gyrus postcentralis *m* / **precentral ~** Gyrus praecentralis *m* / **transverse anterior temporal ~** Heschl–Querwindung *f* / **uncinate ~** Uncus gyri parahippocampalis *m*

H

Haab|'s pupil reflex Haab'scher Reflex *m*, Haab'scher Pupillenreflex *m* / **~'s pupillary reflex** Haab'scher Reflex *m*, Haab'scher Pupillenreflex *m* / **~'s reflex** Haab'scher Reflex *m*

hab Einheit *f* der Gewohnheitsstärke, Hab *n*

habenula Epiphysenstiel *m*, Habenula *f*

habit Gewohnheit *f*, Angewohnheit *f*, Habit *m* / **~ and impulse disorders** abnorme Gewohnheiten *fpl* und Störungen *fpl* der Impulskontrolle / **~ contraction** Tic *m*, Tick *m*, ticartige Zuckungen *fpl* / **~ deterioration** Verfall *m* der Gewohnheiten / **~ family** Gewohnheitshierarchie *f* / **~ family hierarchy** hierarchische Gruppierung *f* der Gewohnheiten, Gewohnheitshierarchie *f* / **~ formation** Gewohnheitsbildung *f*, Gewöhnung *f*, Suchtentstehung *f* / **~–forming** Sucht erzeugend, Gewohnheit bildend / **~ hierarchy** Gewohnheitshierarchie *f* / **~ interference** Hemmung *f* von Gewohnheiten / **~ of mind** geistige Verfassung *f* / **~ pattern** Gewohnheitsmuster *n*, Gewohnheitsstruktur *f* / **~ progression** Weiterentwicklung *f* von Gewohnheiten / **~ spasm** Tic *m*, ticartiger Manierismus *m* / **~ strength** Gewohnheitsstärke *f*, Kraft *f* der Gewohnheit / **~ structure** Gewohnheitsstruktur *f* / **~ training** Gewohnheitstraining *n* / **bad ~** schlechte Angewohnheit *f* / **consuming ~s** Verbrauchsgewohnheiten *fpl* / **eating ~s** Essgewohnheiten *fpl* / **laryngeal ~** Sprechgewohnheit *f* / **motor ~** motorische Gewohnheit *f* / **nervous ~** nervöse Gewohnheit *f* / **obsessional ~** Zwangsgewohnheit *f* / **sensory ~** sensorische Gewohnheit *f* / **social ~** soziale Gewohnheit *f*

habitat Lebensraum *m*, natürlicher Wohnort *m*, Habitat *n* / **~ selection** Auswahl *f* des Wohnbereichs

habitual gewöhnlich, Gewohnheits–, habituell

habituate gewöhnen

habituation Gewöhnung *f*, Habituation *f* / **~ training** Gewohnheitstraining *n*

habitude Gewohnheit *f*, Praxis *f*

habitus Habitus *m*, äußere Erscheinung *f* / **~ apoplecticus** apoplektischer Habitus *m* / **~ phtisicus** phtisischer Habitus *m*

habromania euphorische Demenz *f*

Haeckel's law Haeckel'sches Gesetz *n*, biogenetisches Grundgesetz *n*

haematophobia, haemophobia Angst *f* vor Blut, Hämatophobie *f*, Blutscheu *f*

haemodialysis Blutwäsche *f*, Hämodialyse *f*

haemorrhage Blutung *f* / **cerebral ~** Hirnblutung *f*, Apoplexie *f* / **intracerebral ~** Gehirnblutung *f*, Hirnblutung *f* / **intracranial ~** Blutung *f* im Schädel, intrakranielle Blutung *f* / **subdural ~** Gehirnblutung *f*, subdurale Blutung *f*

haemotherapeutics, haemotherapy Bluttherapie *f*, Behandlung *f* mit Blutpräparaten

hagiotherapy Glaubensheilung *f*

hair Haar *n* / **~ aesthesiometer** Haarästhesiometer *n*, Haarempfindlichkeitsmesser *m* / **~ cell** Haarzelle *f*, Sinneshaar *n* / **~ eating** Haarkauen *n*, Trichophagie *f* / **~ esthesiometer** Haarästhesiometer *n*, Haarempfindlichkeitsmesser *m* / **~ fetishism** Haarfetischismus *m* / **~ follicle** Haarfollikel *m*, Haarbalg *m* / **~ loss** Haarausfall *m* / **~ pulling** Haareausreißen *n*, Trichotillomanie *f* / ~ **sensibility** Haarempfindlichkeit *f* / **auditory** ~ Hörhaar *n* / **sensory** ~ Sinneshaar *n*

half halb / **~–asleep** im Halbschlaf / **~–awake** halbwach / **~–blind** halbblind / **~–blood** Halbblut– / **~–bred** Mischlings– / **~–breed** Mischling *m* / **~–brother** Stiefbruder *m*, Halbbruder *m* / **~–cast** Mischling *m*, Halbblut *n* / **~–conscious** halbbewusst / **~–consciousness** Dämmerzustand *m* / **~–deaf** halbtaub / **~–educated** halbgebildet / **~–shadow polariscope** Halbschattenapparat *m* / **~–sister** Stiefschwester *f*, Halbschwester *f* / **~–term** Halbsemester *n* / **~–truth** Halbwahrheit *f* / **~–way house** Zwischenstation *f*, Übergangseinrichtung *f*

hallucinate Halluzinationen haben, halluzinieren

hallucination Halluzination *f*, Sinnestäuschung *f* / ~ **of sight** Gesichtshalluzination *f* / ~ **of taste** Geschmackshalluzination *f*, gustatorische Halluzination *f* / **apperceptive** ~ apperzeptive Halluzination *f* / **auditive** ~ akustische Halluzination *f* / **auditory** ~ akustische Halluzination *f* / **cenesthesic** ~ Leibhalluzination *f* / **elementary** ~ elementare Halluzination *f* / **endoscopic** ~ endoskopische Halluzination *f* / **extracampine** ~ extrakampine Halluzination *f* / **gustatory** ~ Geschmackshalluzination *f*, gustatorische Halluzination *f* / **haptic** ~ Tasthalluzination *f*, haptische Halluzination *f*, taktile Halluzination *f* / **hypnagogic** ~ Halbschlafhalluzination *f*, hypnagoge Halluzination *f* / **hypnopompic** **~s** hypnopompische Visionen *fpl*, hypnopompische Halluzinationen *fpl* / **induced** ~ induzierte Halluzination *f* / **kinesthetic** ~ Bewegungshalluzination *f*, kinästhetische Halluzination *f* / **lilliputian** ~ Liliputanerhalluzination *f* / **macroptic** ~ Gulliverhalluzination *f* / **musical** ~ Klanghalluzination *f* / **negative** ~ negative Halluzination *f* / **olfactive** ~ Geruchshalluzination *f* / **olfactory** ~ Geruchshalluzination *f* / **oneiroid** ~ oneiroide Halluzination *f* / **peripheral** ~ periphere Halluzination *f* / **pontine visual** **~s** Pick Vision *f* / **psychic** ~ psychische Halluzination *f* / **psychomotor** ~ psychomotorische Halluzination *f* / **sensory** ~ Empfindungshalluzination *f* / **somatic** ~ körperlicher Beeinflussungswahn *m*, leibliches Beeinflussungserlebnis *n* / **tactile** ~ Gefühlshalluzination *f*, Tasthalluzination *f*, taktile Halluzination *f* / **teleologic** ~ teleologische Halluzination *f* / **unilateral** ~ unilaterale Halluzination *f* / **vestibular** ~ vestibuläre Halluzination *f* / **visual** ~ Vision *f*, Gesichtshalluzination *f*, visuelle Halluzination *f*

hallucinative, hallucinatory halluzinatorisch

hallucinogen Halluzination auslösendes Mittel *n*, Halluzinogen *n* / ~ **abuse** Halluzinogenmissbrauch *m* / ~ **dependence** Halluzinogenabhängigkeit *f* / ~ **intoxication** Halluzinogenintoxikation *f*, Halluzinogenrausch *m* / ~ **intoxication delirium** Halluzinogenintoxikationsdelir *n* / ~ **persisting perception disorder** persistierende Wahrnehmungsstörung *f* im Zusammenhang mit Halluzinogenen / ~ **use** Halluzinogenkonsum *m*

hallucinogen|–induced halluzinogeninduziert / **~–related** im Zusammenhang mit Halluzinogenen

hallucinolytic halluzinolytisch

hallucinosis Halluzinose *f* / **acute** ~ akute Halluzinose *f*, Alkoholhalluzinose *f* / **alcoholic** ~ Trinkerhalluzinose *f*, Alkoholhalluzinose *f* / **organic** ~ organische Halluzinose *f* / **periodic** ~ periodische Halluzinose *f*

hallucinotic halluzinatorisch

halo Halo *m*, Hof *m*, Heiligenschein *m* / ~ **effect** Halo–Effekt *m*

haloperidol Haloperidol *n*

halving method Halbierungsmethode *f*

hamartophobia Angst *f* vor Fehlhandlungen

hammer Hammer *m*

Hampton Court maze Hampton–Court–Labyrinth *n*

hamster Hamster *m*

hand Hand *f* / **~–tool dexterity test** handwerklicher Geschicklichkeitstest *m*

handedness Händigkeit *f* / **~ classification** Klassifikation *f* nach Händigkeit

handgrip Handgriff *m*, Händedruck *m*

handicap Behinderung *f* / **auditory ~** Hörbehinderung *f* / **physical ~** Körperbehinderung *f* / **sensory ~** Behinderung *f* einer Sinnesfunktion

handicapped behindert / **adventitiously ~** behindert aufgrund äußerer Einwirkung / **aurally ~** hörbehindert / **congenitally ~** mit angeborener Behinderung / **mentally ~** geistig behindert / **multiply ~** mehrfachbehindert / Mehrfachbehinsderte *m,f* / **orthopaedically ~** körperbehindert / **physically ~** körperbehindert / **severely ~** schwerbehindert / **visually ~** sehbehindert

handicraft Handwerk *n*, Handarbeit *f*

handiness Gewandtheit *f*, Handlichkeit *f*

handiwork Handarbeit *f*, manuelle Arbeit *f*

handle handhaben, hantieren, umgehen / Griff *m*, Hebel *m*, Arm *m* / **movable ~** Kurbel *f*, Dreharm *m*

handling Handhabung *f*

handwriting Handschrift *f* / **~ analyst** Graphologe *m*, Schriftanalytiker *m* / **~ legibility** Lesbarkeit *f* der Handschrift / **~ scale** Handschriftenskala *f* / **~ system** Schriftsystem *n* / **slanting ~** Schrägschrift *f*, stark geneigte Schrift *f*

hangover Nachwirkungen *fpl*, Hangover–Effekt *m*, Kater *m*

haphalgesia Berührungsschmerz *m*, Haphalgesie *f*

haphephobia Haphephobie *f*, Haptophobie *f*, Furcht *f* vor Berührungen

haploid mit einfachem Chromosomensatz, haploid

haplology Silbenverschlucken *n*

haploscope Haploskop *n*

happening Geschehen *n*, Ereignis *n*, Happening *n* / **compulsive ~** Zwangsgeschehen *n*

happiness Glück *n*, Freude *f*, Glückseligkeit *f* / **~ pills** Glückspillen *fpl*, Psychopharmaka *npl*

haptephobia Berührungsangst *f*

haptic haptisch, Berührungs–

haptics Lehre *f* von den Tastempfindungen, Haptik *f*

haptodysphoria Berührungsunbehagen *n*, Haptodysphorie *f*

haptometer Haptometer *n*, Gerät *n* zur Messung von Berührungsreizen

haptophobia Berührungsangst *f*, Haptophobie *f*

haptotaxis, haptotropism Thigmotaxis *f*, Orientierungsreaktion *f* nach Berührung

harassment, sexual sexuelle Belästigung *f*

hard–of–hearing schwerhörig

hardiness Widerstandsfähigkeit *f*

hardness of hearing Schwerhörigkeit *f*

hardware Hardware *f*, Datenerfassungs– und –verarbeitungsanlagen *fpl*, Computeranlage *f*

harm Schaden *m* / schädigen, verletzen

harm–avoidance need Bedürfnis *n* zur Schadenvermeidung, Bedürfnis *n* der Gefahr zu entfliehen

harmful schädlich, nachteilig

harmless unschädlich, harmlos

harmonic harmonisch / Oberton *m* / **aural ~** Oberton *m*

harmonize übereinstimmen, harmonieren, in Einklang bringen

harmony Einklang *m*, Eintracht *f*, Harmonie *f* / **aural ~** Gehörharmonie *f* / **pre–established ~** prästabilierte Harmonie *f*

harp theory Harfentheorie *f*

harpaxophobia Harpaxophobie *f*, Furcht *f* vor Dieben

harshness Rauheit *f*, Härte *f*

hashish Haschisch *m*, indischer Hanf *m* / **~ intoxication** Haschischvergiftung *f*, Haschischrausch *m* / **~ psychosis** Haschischpsychose *f*

hate Hass *m* / hassen

hatred Hass *m* / **~ of one's brother** Bruderhass *m* / **~ of mankind** Menschenhass *m*, Misanthropie *f* / **unreasoning ~** blinder Hass *m*

haunted–swing illusion Schaukelillusion *f*, Hexenschaukel *f*

haut mal großer epileptischer Anfall *m*, Grand mal *n*

Hawthorne experiment Hawthorne–Untersuchung *f* / **~ effect** Hawthorne–Effekt *m*

hay fever Heufieber *n*, Heuschnupfen *m*

hazard Zufall *m*, Gefahr *f*, Risiko *n* / **occupational ~** Unfallgefahr *f* am Arbeitsplatz, Berufsrisiko *n*

hazardous gefährlich, gewagt, gefahrvoll

haze Nebel *m*, Unklarheit *f*

head Kopf *m* / **~ banging** Kopfstoßen *n*, Schlagen *n* mit dem Kopf, autoaggressives Kopfanschlagen *n* / **~–eye coordination** Kopf–Auge–Koordination *f* / **~ injury** Kopfverletzung *f*, Schädel–Hirn–Trauma *n* / **~ nystagmus** Kopfnystagmus *m* / **~'s shadow** Kopfschatten *m* / **~ start** Anlauf *m* / **~ trauma** Schädeltrauma *n* / **closed ~ injury** geschlossene Hirnverletzung *f* / **dolichocephalic ~** Langschädel *m*

headache Kopfschmerzen *mpl* / **~ in neurasthenia** Kopfschmerz *m* als neurasthenischer Schutz / **functional ~** psychogener Kopfschmerz *m* / **hysteric ~** hysterischer Kopfschmerz *m* / **migrainous ~** Migräne *f* / **nervous ~** psychisch bedingter Spannungskopfschmerz *m* / **psychogenic ~** psychogener Kopfschmerz *m*, psychisch bedingter Spannungskopfschmerz *m* / **sick ~** Migräne *f*, Hemikranie *f*

headhunter Personalberater *m*, „Kopfjäger“ *m*

headship Führung *f*, Leitung *f*

Head's zones Head–Zonen *fpl*

headstrong eigensinnig, eigenwillig, halsstarrig

heal heilen

healing Heilung *f* / **mental ~** Geistheilung *f*

health Gesundheit *f* / **~ attitude** Einstellung *f* zur Gesundheit / **~ behaviour** Gesundheitsverhalten *n* / **maladaptive ~ behaviour** gesundheitsgefährdendes Verhalten *n*

health care Gesundheitsversorgung *f* / **~ costs** Kosten *pl* im Gesundheitswesen / **~ policy** Gesundheitspolitik *f* / **~ psychology** Psychologie *f* im Gesundheitswesen / **~ seeking behaviour** Aufsuchen *n* von Gesundheitseinrichtungen / **~ services** Gesundheitsdienste *mpl* / **~ utilization** Inanspruchnahme *f* von Gesundheitseinrichtungen

health| complaints Gesundheitsbeschwerden *fpl* / **~ education** Gesundheitserziehung *f* / **~–impaired** gesundheitlich beeinträchtigt, krank / **~ insurance** Krankenversicherung *f* / **~ knowledge** Gesundheitswissen *n* / **~ promotion** Gesundheitsförderung *f* / **~ psychology** Gesundheitspsychologie *f* / **~ screening** Gesundheits–Screening *n* / **holistic ~** ganzheitliches Behandlungskonzept *n* / **mental ~** psychische Gesundheit *f*, seelische Gesundheit *f*, Psychohygiene *f* / **mental ~ inservice training** Weiterbildung *f* für psychosoziale Berufe / **mental ~ personnel** psychosoziales Personal *n* / **mental ~ programme** psychosoziales Gesundheitsprogramm *n* / **mental ~ services** psychosoziale Dienste *mpl* / **preventive mental ~** präventive psychiatrische Gesundheitsfürsorge *f* / **public ~ services** öffentliches Gesundheitswesen *n*

hear hören, zuhören

hearer Hörer *m*, Zuhörer *m*

hearing Hören *n*, Gehör *n* / **~ acuity** Hörschärfe *f* / **~ aid** Hörgerät *n*, Hörhilfe *f* / **~ contact** Hörkontakt *m* / **~ defect** Hörfehler *m*, Hörstörung *f* / **~ disorder** Hörstörung *f* / **~–impaired** hörbehindert / **~ loss** Hörverlust *m* / **perceptive ~ loss** Schallempfindungsschwerhörigkeit *f*, Schallempfindungsstörung *f* / **~ measures** Hörtest *m* / **~–mute** hörstumm / **~ muteness** Hörstummheit *f* / **~ mutism** Hörstummheit *f* / **~ ossicle** Gehörknöchelchen *n* / **~ range** Hörbereich *m*, Hörfeld *n* / **~ theories** Hörtheorien *fpl* / **~ of voices** Stimmenhören *n* / **binaural ~** beidohriges Hören *n*, binaurales Hören *n* / **coloured ~** Farbenhören *n* / **defective ~** Hörfehler *m* / **hard of ~** schwerhörig / **monaural ~** einohriges Hören *n*, monaurales Hören *n* / **partially ~ impaired** partiell Hörgeschädigte *m,f* / **residual ~** Hörreste *mpl* / **uniaural ~** einohriges Hören *n*, monaurales Hören *n* / **visual ~** Lippenlesen *n*

heart Herz *n* / **~ action** Herztätigkeit *f* / **~ attack** Herzanfall *m* / **~ auricle** Vorhofohr *n*, Herzohr *n* / **~beat** Herzschlag *m* / **~ complaint** Herzbeschwerden *fpl* / **~–consciousness** Herzklopfen *n* / **~ disease** Herzkrankheit *f* / **~ disorder** Herzleiden *n* / **~ failure** Herzschwäche *f*, Herzfehler *m* / **~ insufficiency** Herzinsuffizienz *f* / **~ murmur** Herzgeräusch *n* / **~ neurosis** Herzneurose *f* / **~ pain** Herzschmerz *m* / **~rate** Herzfrequenz *f* / **~rate–affecting drug** Herzfrequenz beeinflussendes Medikament *n* / **~ surgery** Herzchirurgie *f* / **~ transplant** Herzverpflanzung *f*, Herztransplantation *f* / **~ trouble** Herzleiden *n*, Herzkrankheit *f* / **~ valve** Herzklappe *f* / **stenotic ~ valve** Herzklappenstenose *f* / **~ ventricle** Herzkammer *f* / **broken ~** tiefe Depression *f* / **irritable ~** nervöses Herz *n*, Herzneurose *f* / **learn by ~** auswendig lernen

heat Hitze *f*, Leidenschaft *f*, Brunst *f* / **~ adaptation** Hitzeadaptation *f* / **~ collapse** Hitzekollaps *m* / **~ effect** Wärmewirkung *f*, Hitzewirkung *f* / **~ loss** Wärmeabgabe *f* / **evaporative ~ loss** evaporative Wärmeabgabe *f* / **~ perception** Thermoperzeption *f* / **~ radiation** Wärmestrahlung *f* / **~–regulator** Wärmeregulator *m*, Thermostat *m* / **~ sensation** Hitzeempfindung *f* / **~–spectrum** Wärmebereich *m* / **~ spot** Wärmepunkt *m* / **~ stress** Wärmebelastung *f*, Hitzebelastung *f* / **~ stroke** Hitzschlag *m* / **~ syncope** Hitzekollaps *m* / **~–treatment** Wärmebehandlung *f*, Thermotherapie *f*

heat–avoidance need Bedürfnis *n* nach Vermeidung von Hitze

heautoscopia Doppelgängerphänomen *n*

heaviness Schwere *f*, Schwerfälligkeit *f*

Hebb's theory of perceptual learning Hebbs Theorie *f* des Wahrnehmungslernens

hebephrenia Hebephrenie *f*, Jugendirresein *n* / **degenerative ~** Defekthebephrenie *f*

hebephreniac Hebephrener *m*

hebephrenic hebephren

hebetated abgestumpft, empfindungslos, torpid

hebetic, heboid heboid, Pubertäts–

hebetude Abstumpfung *f*, geistige Stumpfheit *f*, Stumpfsinnigkeit *f*, Lethargie *f*, Erstarrung *f*

hebetudinous stumpfsinnig, abgestumpft, lethargisch

heboidophrenia Heboidophrenie *f*

hectic hektisch

hedonia Hedonie *f*, Lust *f*

hedonic hedonisch, Lust–, lustvoll

hedonics Hedonik *f*, Lehre *f* von der Psychologie der Lust und ihren physiologischen Korrelaten

hedonism Hedonismus *m*, Lehre *f* von der Lust / **psychological ~** Theorie *f* des Lustprinzips

hedonist Hedenonist *m*, Anhänger *m* des Hedonismus

hedonistic hedonistisch

heed Aufmerksamkeit *f* / beachten, Acht geben

heedful aufmerksam

heedfulness Achtsamkeit *f*, Aufmerksamkeit *f*

heedless unachtsam

heedlessness Unachtsamkeit *f*

Heinis| constant persönliche Konstante *f*, Heinis–Konstante *f* / **~ law of mental growth** Heinis' Gesetz *n* des Intelligenzwachstums

helicoid spiralförmig

helicotrema Helikotrema *n*, Schneckenloch *n*

heliophobia Heliophobie *f*, Lichtscheu *f*, Angst *f* vor Sonnenlicht, Photophobie *f*

heliotaxis Heliotaxis *f*, Phototropismus *m*

heliotropic heliotropisch

heliotropism Heliotropismus *m*

helix Teil *m* der Ohrmuschel, Ohrleiste *f*, Helix *f*

Hellin's law Hellin'sches Gesetz *n*

Helmholtz|–Kohlrausch effect Helmholtz–Kohlrausch–Effekt *m* / **~ squares** Helmholtz–Quadrate *npl* / **~ theory** Helmholtz–Resonanztheorie *f* / **~ theory of hearing** Helmholtz'sche Hörtheorie *f* / **~ theory of vision** Helmholtz'sche Sehtheorie *f*

helminthophobia Helminthophobie *f*, Angst *f* vor parasitischen Würmern

helper cell T–Helfer–Zelle *f*

helpful hilfreich, nützlich

helpless hilflos

helplessness Hilflosigkeit *f*, Ratlosigkeit *f* / **learned ~** gelernte Hilflosigkeit *f*

help–seeking hilfesuchend

hematoma Bluterguss *m*, Hämatom *n*

hematophobia Angst *f* vor Blut, Hämatophobie *f*, Blutscheu *f*

hematopoietin Erythropoetin *n*

hemeralopia, hemeralopsia, hemeranopia, hemeranopsia Tagblindheit *f*, Nachtsichtigkeit *f*, Nachtblindheit *f*, Hemeralopie *f*

hemiablepsia Halbsichtigkeit *f*, Halbblindheit *f*, Hemianopsie *f*

hemiachromatopsia halbseitige Farbenblindheit *f*

hemiageusia einseitiger Geschmacksverlust *m*, Hemiageusie *f*

hemialgia Halbseitenschmerz *m*, Hemialgie *f*

hemiamaurosis Halbsichtigkeit *f*, Hemianopsie *f*

hemianaesthesia, hemianesthesia Hemianästhesie *f*, Halbseitenanästhesie *f*

hemianalgesia halbseitige Schmerzunempfindlichkeit *f*, Hemianalgesie *f*

hemianacusia einseitige Taubheit *f*

hemianopia, hemianopsia, hemianopsy Halbblindheit *f*, Halbsichtigkeit *f*, Hemianopsie *f*

hemianopic, hemianoptic hemianopisch, halbsichtig

hemianosmia einseitige Geruchsstörung *f*

hemiataxia halbseitige Ataxie *f*

hemiballism einseitige Schleuderbewegungen *fpl*, Hemiballismus *m*

hemichromatopsia halbseitige Farbenblindheit *f*

hemicrania Migräne *f*, Hemikranie *f*, halbseitiger Kopfschmerz *m*

hemidecortication halbseitige Enthirnung *f*, Abtragen *n* einer Hirnhälfte

hemidesmosome Halbdesmosom *n*

hemiepilepsy Hemiepilepsie *f*

hemihypaesthesia, hemihypoaesthesia halbseitige Gefühlsstörung *f*

hemihyperaesthesia, hemihyperesthesia halbseitige Hautüberempfindlichkeit *f*, Hemihyperästhesie *f*

hemilateral halbseitig

hemiopia Halbsichtigkeit *f*, Halbblindheit *f*, Hemianopsie *f*

hemiparesis halbseitige Lähmung *f*, Hemiparese *f*

hemiplegia halbseitige Lähmung *f*, Hemiplegie *f*

hemiplegic halbseitengelähmt, hemiplegisch

hemispasm Halbseitenkrampf *m*

hemisphere Hemisphäre *f*, Halbkugel *f* / **cerebral ~** Großhirnhemisphäre *f* / **cerebellar ~** Kleinhirnhemisphäre *f* / **dominant ~** dominante Hirnhemisphäre *f*

hemispherectomy Entfernung *f* einer Hirnhälfte, Hemisphärektomie *f*

hemispherical Hirnhemisphären–

hemocrinia Hämokrinie *f*, Hormontransport *m* auf dem Blutwege

hemodialysis Hämodialyse *f*

hemoglobin Blutfarbstoff *m*, Hämoglobin *n*

hemolysis Hämolyse *f*

hemophilia Bluterkrankheit *f*, Hämophilie *f*

hemophobia Angst *f* vor Blut, Hämatophobie *f*

hemorrhage Blutung *f* / **cerebral ~** Gehirnblutung *f*, Apoplexie *f* / **intracerebral ~** Gehirnblutung *f*, Hirnblutung *f* / **intracranial ~** Blutung *f* im Schädel, intrakranielle Blutung *f* / **subdural ~** Gehirnblutung *f*, subdurale Blutung *f*

hemotherapeutics, hemotherapy Bluttherapie *f*, Behandlung *f* mit Blutpräparaten

hemothymia Hämothymie *f*, krankhafte Erregung *f* beim Anblick von Blut

hemp Hanf *m*, Cannabis *f*

Henle's| canal Henle–Schleife *f* / **~ loop** Henle–Schleife *f*

heparin Heparin *n*

hepatic hepatisch, Leber–

hepatitis Leberentzündung *f*, Hepatitis *f* / **toxic ~** toxische Hepatitis *f*

Herbartianism, Herbartism Herbart'sche Psychologie *f*

herd Herde *f* / **~ conformity** kulturelle Konformität *f* / **~ instinct** Herdentrieb *m*, Herdeninstinkt *m*, sozialer Instinkt *m*

hereditarianism Lehre *f* von der Erbbedingtheit des Verhaltens

hereditary erblich, hereditär

heredity Vererbung *f*, Erblichkeit *f*, Erbgang *m* / **~–environment controversy** Anlage–Umwelt–Kontroverse *f* / **~–predisposition theory** Theorie *f* von der erblichen Veranlagung negativer Eigenschaften / **biological ~** biologische Vererbung *f* / **social ~** soziale Vererbung *f*, soziale Übermittlung *f*

Hering|afterimage Hering'sches Nachbild *n* / **~ aftersensation** Hering'sches Nachbild *n* / **~–Breuer reflex** Hering–Breuer–Reflex *m* / **~ grays** Hering'sche Grauskala *f* / **~ greys** Hering'sche Grauskala *f* / **~ illusion** Hering'sche Täuschung *f* / **~ theory of vision** Hering'sche Gegenfarbentheorie *f* / **~ window** Hering'sches Fenster *n*

heritability Erblichkeit *f*, Vererbbarkeit *f*

heritage Erbe *n*, Erbgut *n* / **social ~** soziales Erbe *n*

Hermann's local circuit theory Hermann'sche Strömchentheorie *f*

hermaphrodism Zwitterbildung *f*, Zwittertum *n*, Hermaphroditismus *m* / **spurious ~** Scheinzwittertum *n*, Pseudohermaphroditismus *m*

hermaphrodite Zwitter *m*, Hermaphrodit *m* / zwitterig, hermaphroditisch / **psychosexual ~** psychosexueller Hermaphrodit *m*

hermaphroditic zwitterig, hermaphroditisch

hermaphroditism Zwitterbildung *f*, Zwittertum *n*, Hermaphroditismus *m* / **psychosexual ~** psychosexueller Hermaphroditismus *m*

hermeneutics Hermeneutik *f*

hermetic magisch

hermetics Magie *f*, Okkultismus *m*

hero Held *m*, Heroe *m*

heroin Heroin *n* / ~ **addiction** Heroinabhängigkeit *f*

heroinomania Heroinsucht *f*, Heroinismus *m*

herpes| encephalitis Herpesenzephalitis *f* / ~ **genitalis** Herpes genitalis *m* / ~ **simplex** Herpes simplex *m* / ~ **simplex encephalitis** Herpesenzephalitis *f* / ~ **zoster** Gürtelrose *f*, Herpes zoster *m*

hesitant zögernd, unschlüssig

hesitate zögern, zaudern

hesitating zögernd, zaudernd

hesitation, hesitance, hesitancy Zögern *n*, Unschlüssigkeit *f*

hesperanopia Nachtblindheit *f*, Tagsichtigkeit *f*, Hemeralopie *f*

Heschl's convolution Heschl–Querwindung *f*

heterocentric auf den Andern ausgerichtet, altruistisch

heterochromia Heterochromie *f*, verschiedenartige Färbung *f*

heterochromosome Geschlechtschromosom *n*, Allosom *n*

heterochronia, heterochrony, heterochronism Heterochronie *f*, Zeitverschiebung *f*, Zeitdifferenz *f*

heterochronic abweichend in der zeitlichen Reihenfolge, heterochron

heterodox andersgläubig, unorthodox

heteroerotic alloerotisch

heteroerotism, heteroeroticism Alloerotik *f*, Alloerotismus *m*

heterofacilitation Fremdbahnung *f*

heterogamete Gamet *m* eines ungleichen Gametenpaares, Heterogamet *m*

heterogametic mit verschiedenen Gameten

heterogamy Heterogamie *f*, charakterliche Ungleichheit *f* zwischen Ehepartnern

heterogeneity, heterogenicity Verschiedenartigkeit *f*, Heterogenität *f*

heterogeneous, heterogenic, heterogenous heterogen, verschiedenartig

heterogenesis, heterogony Heterogenese *f*, Heterogonie *f*, Entwicklung *f* von Neuem, Nichtangelegtem

heterogenital andersgeschlechtlich

heterokinesia Allokinese *f*

heterokinetic allokinetisch

heterolalia Heterolalie *f*, Heterophasie *f*

heterologous heterolog, abweichend

heterology Abweichen *n*, Heterologie *f*

heterometropia Heterometropie *f*, unterschiedliches Sehen *n* beider Augen

heteromorph, heteromorphic, heteromorphous heteromorph, verschieden gestaltig

heteromorphosis Heteromorphose *f*

heteroneurosis Fremdneurose *f*

heteronomous heteronom, fremdbestimmt

heteronomy Heteronomie *f*, Fremdgesetzlichkeit *f*

heterophasia Heterophasie *f*, Heterolalie *f*

heterophemy Heterolalie *f*, Heterophasie *f*, Versprechen *n*, Lapsus linguae *m*

heterophil, heterophilic heterophil, gegengeschlechtlich ausgerichtet

heterophilia Heterophilie *f*, gegengeschlechtliche Anziehung *f*

heterophoria latentes Schielen *n*, Heterophorie *f*

heterophthalmia Verschiedenheit *f* beider Augen

heteropolar heteropolar

heterorexia anomale Essgelüste *npl*, Verlangen *n* nach ungewöhnlichen Speisen, Parorexie *f*

heteroscedastic heteroscedastisch, heteroskedastisch

heteroscedasticity Heteroscedastizität *f*, Heteroskedastizität *f*

heteroscope Heteroskop *n*, Apparat *m* zur Messung des Schielwinkels

heterosexual heterosexuell, andersgeschlechtlich

heterosexuality Heterosexualität *f*

heterosmia Heterosmie *f*, Geruchshalluzination *f*

heterosociality Sozialbeziehungen *fpl* zwischen gegengeschlechtlichen Partnern

heterosuggestibility Beeinflussbarkeit *f* durch andere Personen

heterosuggestion Fremdsuggestion *f*

heterotropia Schielen *n*, Strabismus *m*

heterozygosity Mischerblichkeit *f*

heterozygote Heterozygot *m*, mischerbiges Individuum *n*

heterozygous, heterozygotic heterozygot, mischerbig

heuristic heuristisch, erfinderisch / heuristische Methode *f*

hexamethonium Hexamethonium *n*

hexis konstante Verhaltensweise *f*, habituelle Reaktion *f*

hexobarbital Hexobarbital *n*

Heymans' law of inhibition Heymann'sches Hemmungsgesetz *n*

hibernate Winterschlaf halten

hibernation Winterschlaf *m*, Überwinterung *f*

hidrosis übermäßiges Schwitzen *n*, Hidrose *f*, Schweißabsonderung *f*, Schweißsekretion *f*

hierarchic, hierarchical hierarchisch

hierarchy Hierarchie *f* / **~ of habits** Gewohnheitshierarchie *f* / **~ of needs** Bedürfnishierarchie *f* / **motivational ~** Bedürfnishierarchie *f*, Motivationshierarchie *f* / **occupational ~** Stellenhierarchie *f*, berufliche Rangordnung *f* / **social ~** soziale Hierarchie *f*, soziale Rangordnung *f*

hieroglyphic hieroglyphisch

hiero|glyphics Hieroglyphen *fpl*, ägyptische Bilderschrift *f* / **~mania** religiöser Wahnsinn *m* / **~phobia** Hierophobie *f*

hilus of kidney Nierenhilus *m*

hindbrain Rautenhirn *n*, Rhombenzephalon *n*, Hinterhirn *n*, Metenzephalon *n*

hindsight nachträglich, im nach hinein

hint Wink *m*, Anspielung *f*, Lernhilfe *f*

Hipp chronoscope Hipp–Chronoskop *n*

hippanthropia Wahn *m* ein Pferd zu sein, Hippanthropie *f*

hippie, hippy Hippie *m*, Blumenkind *n*

hippocampus Hippocampus *m*, Ammonshorn *n*

hippus Hippus *m*, Pupillenathetose *f*

hircine bockartig riechend, nach Bock stinkend

hircismus Bocksgeruch *m*, Schweißgeruch *m*

hiring Personaleinstellen *n*, Einstellung *f*, Anstellen *n*

hirsutism abnorme Körperbehaarung *f* [bei Frauen], übermäßiger Haarwuchs *m*, Hirsutismus *m*

histamine Histamin *n* / **~ headache** Histaminkopfschmerz *m*, Cluster–Kopfschmerz *m*, Horton–Syndrom *n* / **~ receptor** Histaminrezeptor *m*

histaminergic histaminerg

histanoxia Gewebeanoxie *f*

histidine Histidin *n*

histodifferentiation Gewebsdifferenzierung *f*

histogenesis, histogeny Gewebebildung *f*, Histogenese *f*

histogenetic, histogenic histogenetisch, Gewebebildung betreffend

histogram Säulendiagramm *n*, Histogramm *n*

histography Gewebsbeschreibung *f*

histology Gewebelehre *f*, Histologie *f*

histophysiology Gewebsphysiologie *f*

historical geschichtlich, entwicklungsgeschichtlich, anamnestisch

historigram Verlaufskurve *f*

history Geschichte *f*, Anamnese *f* / **~ of psychology** Geschichte *f* der Psychologie / **medical ~** Krankengeschichte *f* / **prior ~** in der Vorgeschichte

histotome Mikrotom *n*

histrionic theatralisch, schauspielerisch

hitch festmachen, anbinden / Schwierigkeit *f*, Problem *n*

Hitzig girdle Hitzig–Gürtel *m*

HIV| infection HIV–Infektion *f* / **~ testing** HIV–Test *m*

hoarding Hamstern *n*

hoarse rauh, heiser

hoarseness Rauheit *f*, Heiserkeit *f*

hobby Steckenpferd *n*, Liebhaberei *f*, Hobby *n*

Hodgkin–Huxley model Ionentheorie *f* der Erregung

hodological hodologisch

hodology Hodologie *f*

Hoffmann's reflex Hoffmann–Reflex *m*

Höfler illusion Höfler'sche Täuschung *f*

hold Macht *f*, Einfluss *m* / **limited ~** Zeitkontingent *n*, Zeiteinschränkung *f*

hole screen Reduktionsschirm *m*

holergasia Holergasie *f*, Persönlichkeitspsychose *f*

holergastic holergastisch, psychotisch

holiday Feiertag *m*, Urlaub *m*

holism Ganzheitsauffassung *f*, Ganzheits– und Zweckbetrachtung *f*, Holismus *m*

holistic holistisch, ganzheitlich

Hollerith machine Hollerithmaschine *f*

Holmgren| test Holmgren'sches Verfahren *n* / **~ wools** Holmgren'sche Wollfäden *mpl*

holograph eigenhändig geschriebene Urkunde *f*

holoism Holoismus *m*, Philosophie *f* der ganzheitlichen Erziehung

holophrase, holophrasis Holophrase *f*, Ein–Wort–Satz *m*

holophrastic Ein–Wort–Satz betreffend, holophrastisch

homatropine Homatropin *n*, Atropin *n* und Mandelöl *n*, Phenylglykoltropinum *n*

home Heim *n*, Anstalt *f* / **~ accident** Haushaltsunfall *m* / **~ care** häusliche Pflege *f* / **~ care personnel** Personal *n* in der häuslichen Pflege / **~ environment** häusliches Milieu *n* / **~ for the blind** Blindenanstalt *f* / **~–reared** zu Hause erzogen / **~ schooling** Hausunterricht *m* / **~ visiting programme** Hausbesuchsprogramm *n* / **broken ~** gestörte Familienverhältnisse *npl*, zerstörte Familie *f* / **eventide ~** Altersheim *n* / **mental ~** geschlossene Anstalt *f* / **old people's ~** Altersheim *n*

homebound häuslich gebunden, ans Haus gefesselt, Heim–, auf dem Heimweg / häuslich gebundener behinderter oder älterer Mensch *m*

homeless heimatlos, obdachlos / Obdachlose *m,f*

homelessness Heimatlosigkeit *f*

homeopathy Homöopathie *f*

homeostasis Homöostase *f*, Konstanz *f* des Organismus, physiologisches Gleichgewicht *n*, homöostatisches Gleichgewicht *n*

homeostatic homöostatisch

homeothermism, homeothermy Homöothermie, Warmblütigkeit *f*

homepage Homepage *f*

homesickness Heimweh *n*

homespunness Hausbackenheit *f*

homework Hausaufgaben *fpl*

homeyness Behaglichkeit *f*

homicidal mörderisch, Tötungs–

homicide Mord *m*, Tötung *f*, Totschlag *m*

homicidology Homizidologie *f*

homicidomania Mordsucht *f*, Homizidomanie *f*

homilophobia Homilophobie *f*, Angst *f* öffentlich zu sprechen oder aufzutreten

homing Heimkehr *f* / ~ **instinct** Heimatsinn *m*, Heimkehrtrieb *m*

hominids Hominiden *mpl*, Familie *f* der Primaten

homo Mensch *m* / ~ **sapiens** Homo sapiens *m*

homochromy Gleichfarbigkeit *f*, Einfarbigkeit *f*

homocystinuria Homocystinurie *f*

homoeopathy Homöopathie *f*

homoerotic homoerotisch, homosexuell, homophil

homoerotism, homeroticism Homoerotik *f*, Homoerotismus *m*, Homophilie *f*, Homosexualität *f*

homogamete Gamet *m* eines gleichartigen Gametenpaares, Homogamet *m*

homogametic gleicherbig, homogametisch

homogamy Homogamie *f*, charakterliche Gleichheit *f* zwischen Ehepartnern

homogeneity Homogenität *f*, Gleichartigkeit *f* / ~ **index** Homogenitätsindex *m* / ~ **of variance** Varianzhomogenität *f*

homogeneous, homogenous homogen, gleichartig

homogenital gleichgeschlechtlich, homosexuell

homogenitalism Homosexualität *f*

homogenitality Homogenitalität *f*, ausgeübte Homosexualität *f*

homogeny Homogenität *f*, Gleichartigkeit *f*

homograph Wort *n* mit Mehrfachbedeutung, Homograph *m* / ~ **test** Wortbedeutungstest *m*

homolateral gleichseitig, homolateral, auf der gleichen Körperseite

homologous homolog, übereinstimmend

homologue entsprechender Körperteil *m*, homologes Organ *n*

homology Entsprechung *f*, Übereinstimmung *f*, Homologie *f* / **behavioural** ~ Verhaltensentsprechung *f*

homonomous homonom, gleichwertig

homonomy Homonomie *f* / ~ **drive** Homonomietrieb *m*,Trieb *m* sich gesellschaftlichen und kulturellen Kategorien anzupassen

homonym Homonym *n*, gleichnamiges Wort *n*

homonymous homonym, gleichnamig

homonymy Homonymie *f*, Gleichnamigkeit *f*

homophonic, homophonous homophon, gleichlautend

homophony Homophonie *f*, Gleichklang *m*

homoplastic homoplastisch

homoscedastic homoscedastisch, homoskedastisch

homoscedasticity Homoscedastizität *f*, Homoskedastizität *f*

homosexual homosexuell / homophil / Homosexueller *m* / **male** ~ männlicher Homosexueller *m*

homosexuality Homosexualität *f*, Homophilie *f* / **female** ~ weibliche Homosexualität *f* / **latent** ~ latente Homosexualität *f* / **male** ~ männliche Homosexualität *f* / **repressed** ~ verdrängte Homosexualität *f*

homosociality Sozialbeziehungen *fpl* zwischen Gleichgeschlechtlichen

homotopic gleichartig, am gleichen Ort

homotypy Entsprechung *f*, Homologie *f*

homozygosis Gleicherbigkeit *f*, Homozygotie *f*

homozygote Homozygot *m*

homozygous, homozygotic gleicherbig, homozygot, reinrassig

homunculus Homunkulus *m*, künstlich erzeugter Mensch *m*

honesty Ehrlichkeit *f*

Honi phenomenon Honi–Phänomen *n*

hope Hoffnung *f*

hopelessness Hoffnungslosigkeit *f*

hopping reaction Sprungreaktion *f*

horde Horde *f* / **~ of brothers** Brüderhorde *f* / **primal ~** Urhorde *f* / **primal–~ stage** Stadium *n* der Urhorde

horizontal horizontal

horme Horme *f*, zielgerichtetes Streben *n*

hormic hormisch

hormonal hormonal

hormone Hormon *n* / **~ receptor** Hormonrezeptor *m* / **~ therapy** Hormonbehandlung *f*, Hormontherapie *f* / **adrenocorticotropic ~** ACTH *n*, Kortikotropin *n* / **adrenotropic ~** Kortikotropin *n* / **anterior pituitary ~** Hypophysenvorderlappenhormon *n* / **antidiuretic ~** antidiuretisches Hormon *n*, Vasopressin *n*, Adiuretin *n* / **cortical ~** Rindenhormon *n* / **corticotropic ~** Kortikotropin *n* / **follicular ~** Follikelhormon *n* / **glandotropic ~** glandotropes Hormon *n* / **gonadotropic ~** Gonadotropin *n* / **lactogenic ~** laktogenes Hormon *n*, Prolaktin *n*, / **luteinising ~** Luteinisierungshormon *n* / **luteinising ~–releasing hormone** Lutiliberin *n* / **luteotropic ~** luteotropes Hormon *n*, Luteotropin *n* / **metabolic ~** Stoffwechselhormon *n* / **oestrogenic ~** Östrogen *n* / **parathyroid ~** Nebenschilddrüsenhormon *n* / **pituitary ~** Hypophysenhormon *n* / **placental ~** Plazenta–Hormon *n* / **posterior pituitary ~** Hypophysenhinterlappenhormon *n*, Neurohypophysenhormon *n* / **progestational ~** Gelbkörperhormon *n*, Progesteron *n* / **regulatory ~** Regulationshormon *n* / **releasing ~** Releasinghormon *n* / **somatotropic ~** Wachstumshormon *n* / **thyreotropic ~** thyreotropes Hormon *n* / **thyroid ~** Schilddrüsenhormon *n* / **thyroid stimulating ~** Thyreotropin *n*, thyreotropes Hormon *n*

hormonotherapy Hormonbehandlung *f*, Hormontherapie *f*

horn Horn *n* / **~ of Ammon** Ammonshorn *n* / **anterior ~** Vorderhorn *n* / **anterior ~ cell** Vorderhornzelle *f* / **dorsal ~** Hinterhorn *n*, Dorsalhorn *n* / **lateral ~** Seitenhorn *n* / **posterior ~** Hinterhorn *n* / **ventral ~** Vorderhorn *n*

horncell Ganglienzelle *f* eines Horns / **anterior ~** Vorderhornzelle *f*

Horner|'s law Horner'sches Gesetz *n* / **~ syndrome** Horner'scher Symptomenkomplex *m*, Horner–Trias *f*

horny geil, hornartig

horopter Horopter *m*, Sehgrenze *f*

horoscope Horoskop *n*

horripilation Haarsträuben *n*

horror Entsetzen *n*, Abscheu *f*, Schrecken *m* / **the ~s** Angstzustand *m* bei Delirium tremens

Horton's syndrome Horton–Syndrom *n*, Histaminkopfschmerz *m*, Cluster–Kopfschmerz *m*

hospice Hospiz *n*

hospital Krankenhaus *n*, Klinik *f*, Anstalt *f* / **~ accreditation** Krankenhauszulassung *f* / **~ administration** Krankenhausverwaltung *f* / **~ admission** Aufnahme *f* ins Krankenhaus, Einweisung *f* ins Krankenhaus / **~ care** Krankenhausbehandlung *f* / **~ discharge** Entlassung *f* aus dem Krankenhaus / **~ environment** Krankenhausumfeld *n* / **~ programme** klinisches Therapieprogramm *n* / **~ readmission** Wiederaufnahme *f* in einem Krankenhaus / **~ staff** Krankenhauspersonal *n* / **general ~ psychiatric unit** psychiatrische Station *f* eines Allgemeinkrankenhauses / **mental ~** Irrenanstalt *f* / **psychiatric ~** psychiatrisches Krankenhaus *n*, Nervenklinik *f*, Nervenheilanstalt *f* / **receiving ~** Aufnahmeklinik *f*, Aufnahmekrankenhaus *n*

hospitalisation Unterbringung *f* in einem Krankenhaus, Krankenhausaufenthalt *m*, Hospitalisierung *f* / **partial ~** teilstationäre Unterbringung *f* / **psychiatric ~** Unterbringung *f* in einer Nervenklinik, psychiatrischer Krankenhausaufenthalt *m*

hospitalise in ein Krankenhaus unterbringen, hospitalisieren

hospitalism Hospitalismus *m*

host Gastgeber *m*

hostage Geisel *f*

hostile feindlich, feindselig / **~ to society** gesellschaftsfeindlich, antisozial

hostility Feindschaft *f*, Feindseligkeit *f*, Feindlichkeit *f* / **displaced ~** verschobene Aggression *f*

hot heiß, warm, geil / **~-headed** jähzornig, cholerisch / **~-tempered** cholerisch, aufbrausend, jähzornig

hours of work Arbeitszeit *f*, Arbeitsstunden *fpl*

Hoyt formula Hoyt–Formel *f*

hue Farbton *m* / **extraspectral ~** außerhalb des Spektrums liegender Farbton *m* / **invariable ~s** invariante Farbtöne *npl* / **primary ~** Primärfarbe *f* / **spectral ~** Farbton *m* einer Spektralfarbe *f*

hull Hülle *f* / **foreign ~** äußere Hülle *f*

human menschlich

humane human, menschenfreundlich, humanistisch

humanisation Humanisierung *f*, Vermenschlichung *f*, menschliche Gestaltung *f*

humanism Humanismus *m*

humanistic humanistisch

humanitarian Menschenfreund *m* / menschenfreundlich

humanities Geisteswissenschaften *fpl*

humanity Menschheit *f*, Menschlichkeit *f*, Humanität *f*

humanness Menschlichkeit *f*

humidity Feuchtigkeit *f*

humiliate erniedrigen, demütigen

humiliation Erniedrigung *f*, Demütigung *f*

humility Demut *f*

humoral humoral

humorous humorvoll, lustig, spaßig

humour, humor Humor *m*, Stimmung *f*, Temperament *n*, Gemütsart *f*, Körperflüssigkeit *f* / **aqueous ~** Augenflüssigkeit *f* / **good ~** gute Laune *f* / **vitreous ~** Glaskörperflüssigkeit *f*, Glaskörper *m*

Humphrey|'s effect Humphreys Effekt *m*, Partialverstärkungseffekt *m* / **~'s paradox** Humphreys Paradox *n*

hunger Hunger *m* / **~ complex** Hungerkomplex *m* / **~ contraction** Hungerkontraktion *f* / **~ drive** Hungertrieb *m* / **~ pangs** Hungerschmerz *m*, Hungerstiche *mpl* / **excessive ~** Fresssucht *f*, Sitomanie *f* / **morbid ~** krankhafter Heißhunger *m*, Bulimie *f* / **ravenous ~** Heißhunger *m* / **specific ~** spezifischer Hunger *m* / **wolfish ~** Wolfshunger *m*, Heißhunger *m*

hunting Jagen *n*

Huntington's chorea, Huntington's disease Chorea Huntington *f*, Erbchorea *f*

Hunt's neuralgia Ramsey Hunt–Syndrom *n*

Hurler's syndrome Hurler–Syndrom *n*, Gargoylismus *m*, Hurler–Krankheit *f*

hyalophagia Hyalophagie *f*

hybrid Hybrid *m*, Mischling *m* / hybrid, mischerbig

hybridisation Kreuzung *f*, Bastardierung *f*, Hybridisation *f*

hybridism Hybridismus *m*, Vermischung *f* von Kulturen

hybridity Mischbildung *f*

hydantoin Hydantoin *n*

hydralazine Hydralazin *n*

hydrazine Hydrazin *n*

hydrencephalus Wasserkopf *m*, Hydrozephalus *m*

hydrocarbon Kohlenwasserstoff *m*

hydrocephalic, hydrocephalous wasserköpfig, hydrozephal

hydrocephalus Wasserkopf *m*, Hydrozephalus *m*

hydrocephaly Wasserkopf *m*, Gehirnwassersucht *f*

hydrocortisone Hydrocortison *n*, Kortisol *n*

hydrodipsomania Hydrodipsomanie *f*, plötzlich auftretender Durst *m*

hydrogen Wasserstoff *m*

hydromancy Wahrsagen *n* aus den Formen der Wasserbewegungen

hydromania unstillbarer Durst *m*, krankhafter Drang *m* zum Selbstmord durch Ertränken

hydrophobia Wasserscheu *f*, Hydrophobie *f*, Tollwut *f*

hydrophobic wasserscheu, hydrophob

hydrophobophobia krankhafte Angst *f* vor Tollwut

hydrotaxis, hydrotropism Hydrotaxis *f*, Hydrotropismus *m*

hydrotherapeutics, hydrotherapy Hydrotherapie *f*, Wasserheilkunde *f*

hydroxydopamine Hydroxydopamin *n*

hydroxylamine Hydroxylamin *n*

hydroxylase Hydroxylase *f* / **~ inhibitor** Hydroxylase–Hemmer *m*

hydroxyprolinemia Hydroxyprolinämie *f*

5–hydroxytryptamine Serotonin *n*, Enteramin *n*, 5–Hydroxytryptamin *n*

5–hydroxytryptophan 5–Hydroxytryptophan *n*

hydroxyzine Hydroxyzin *n*

hygiene Hygiene *f* / **~ factor** Hygienefaktor *m*, Erhaltungsfaktor *m* / **mental ~** Psychohygiene *f* / **racial ~** Rassenhygiene *f* / **social ~** Sozialhygiene *f*

hygienic hygienisch

hygrophobia krankhafte Angst *f* vor Feuchtigkeit

hymen Jungfernhäutchen *n*, Hymen *n*

hyoid Zungenbein *n* / **~ bone** Zungenbeinknochen *m*

hyoscine Skopolamin *n*

hyoscyamine Hyoszyamin *n*

hypacousia, hypacousis, hypacusia, hypacusis Schwerhörigkeit *f*, Hörstörung *f*, Hypakusis *f*

hypaesthesia herabgesetzter Tastsinn *f*, verminderte Empfindung *f*, Hypästhesie *f*

hypalgesia, hypalgia Hypalgesie, verminderte Schmerzempfindlichkeit *f*

hypalgesic, hypalgetic hypalgetisch, mit verminderter Schmerzempfindlichkeit

hypaphrodisia herabgesetztes Sexualempfinden *n*, mangelnde Geschlechtslust *f*

hyperacidity Übersäuerung *f*

hyperactive hyperaktiv, überaktiv

hyperactivity Überaktivität *f*, Bewegungsdrang *m* / **disorganized ~** Handlungszerfall *m*

hyperacuity übergroße Hör– und/oder Sehschärfe *f*

hyperacusia, hyperacusis übergroße Hörschärfe *f*, übergroße Schallempfindlichkeit *f*, Hyperakusie *f*

hyperaemia Blutüberfülle *f*, Hyperämie *f*

hyperaesthesia Überempfindlichkeit *f* / **acoustic ~** Hyperakusis *f* / **auditory ~** Hyperakusis *f* / **gustatory ~** Geschmacksüberempfindlichkeit *f*, Hypergeusie *f* / **olfactory ~** Geruchsüberempfindlichkeit *f*

hyperaesthetic überempfindlich

hyperaffective stark erregbar

hyperaffectivity überstarke Erregbarkeit *f*, Überempfindlichkeit *f*, Hyperaffektivität *f*

hyperalgesia, hyperalgia Hyperalgesie *f*, Schmerzüberempfindlichkeit *f*

hyperammonemia Hyperammonämie *f*

hyperattentionality übermäßige Aufmerksamkeitszuwendung *f*

hyperbilirubinemia Hyperbilirubinämie *f*

hyperbola Hyperbel *f*

hyperbulia krankhafter Betätigungsdrang *m*, Hyperbulie *f*, krankhafte Aktivität *f*

hypercalcemia Hyperkalzämie *f*

hypercapnia erhöhter Kohlensäuregehalt *m* im Blut, Hyperkapnie *f*

hypercathexis Überbesetzung *f*, Hyperkathexis *f*

hypercholesterolemia erhöhter Cholesteringehalt *m* des Blutes, Hypercholesterinämie *f*

hyperchromatosis Hyperchromatose *f*, Hyperchromasie *f*

hypercinesia, hypercinesis Hyperkinese *f*, übermäßige Bewegungen *fpl*

hypercoenaesthesia, hypercenesthesia Euphorie *f*

hypercritical überkritisch

hypercryaesthesia Überempfindlichkeit *f* gegen Kälte

hyperemotional übererregbar, stark erregbar

hyperemotivity Übererregbarkeit *f*, Überempfindlichkeit *f*

hyperenergia, hyperenergy übermäßige Energie *f*

hyperephidrosis übermäßiges Schwitzen *n*, vermehrte Schweißabsonderung *f*, Hyperhidrosis *f*

hyperergasia manische Überaktivität *f*, übermäßiger Arbeitsdrang *m*, Hyperergasie *f*

hyperergastic manisch überaktiv

hyperesophoria Hyperesophorie *f*

hyperesthesia Überempfindlichkeit *f* / **acoustic ~** Hyperakusis *f* / **auditory ~** Hyperakusis *f* / **gustatory ~** Hypergeusie *f* / **olfactory ~** Geruchsüberempfindlichkeit *f*

hyperexcitability Übererregbarkeit *f*

hyperexcitable übererregbar

hyperexophoria Hyperesophorie *f*

hyperfeminisation übertriebene Verweiblichung *f* / Vorhandensein *n* übermäßiger weiblicher Charakteristika

hyperfunction Überfunktion *f*

hypergenesis Überentwicklung *f*, Hyperplasie *f*

hypergenetic überentwickelt, hypertroph

hypergenitalism übermäßige Entwicklung *f* der Geschlechtsteile, Hypergenitalismus *m*

hypergeusia überfeiner Geschmack *m*, Hypergeusie *f*

hypergia Überempfindlichkeit *f*

hyperglycaemia, hyperglycosaemia Hyperglykämie *f*, erhöhter Blutzuckerspiegel *m*

hyperglycaemic hyperglykämisch

hyperglykaemia, hyperglycemia Hyperglykämie *f*, Blutzuckererhöhung *f*

hypergnosis, hypergnosia Projektion *f* innerer Konflikte auf die Umwelt, Hypergnosis *f*

hypergonadism Hypergonadismus *m*, Überfunktion *f* der Geschlechtsdrüsen

hyperhedonia gesteigertes Lustgefühl *n*, Hyperhedonie *f*

hyperhidrosis, hyperidrosis übermäßige Schweißproduktion *f*

hyperinsulinism Hyperinsulinismus *m*

hyperkinaesthesia, hyperkinesthesia Überempfindlichkeit *f* auf Bewegungsreize, Hyperkinästhesie *f*

hyperkinesis, hyperkinesia Hyperkinese *f*, Bewegungsunruhe *f* / **professional ~** Beschäftigungsneurose *f*

hyperkinetic hyperkinetisch

hyperlink Hyperlink *m*, Link *m*

hyperlogia abnormer Redefluss *m*, Hyperlogie *f*, Logorrhoe *f*, Polyphrasie *f*, krankhafte Geschwätzigkeit *f*, Zungendelirium *n*, Logomanie *f*

hypermania schwere Manie *f*

hypermasculinisation abnorme Vermännlichung *f*

hypermature überentwickelt, überreif

hypermedia Hypermedien *npl*, Multimedia *npl*

hypermetrope Übersichtige *m,f*

hypermetropia Übersichtigkeit *f*, Hypermetropie *f*

hypermetropic übersichtig, hypermetrop

hypermimia übertriebene Mimik *f*, Hypermimie *f*

hypermnesia, hypermnesis ungewöhnlich gutes Gedächtnis *n*

hypermotility abnorm gesteigerter Bewegungsdrang *m*, übermäßige Beweglichkeit *f*, Hypermotilität *f*, Hyperkinese *f*

hypernormal übernormal

hyperopia Übersichtigkeit *f*, Hypermetropie *f*

hyperopic übersichtig, hypermetrop

hyperorexia Heißhunger *m*, Bulimie *f*

hyperosmia Hyperosmie *f*, krankhaft gesteigertes Geruchsvermögen *n*

hyperparathyroidism Überfunktion *f* der Nebenschilddrüsen, Hyperparathyreoidismus *m*

hyperpathia Hyperpathie *f*

hyperphagia Hyperphagie *f*, übermäßige Nahrungsaufnahme *f*, Polyphagie *f* / **nocturnal ~** Nachtesser–Syndrom *n*

hyperphasia unzusammenhängender schneller Wortwirrwarr *m*, Hyperphasie *f*

hyperphoria latentes Höhenschielen *n*

hyperphrasia abnormer Redefluss *m*, Logorrhoe *f*, Polyphrasie *f*

hyperphrenia manische Geistesstörung *f*, Hyperphrenie *f*

hyperpituitarism Hypophysenüberfunktion *f*

hyperplasia Hyperplasie *f*, Gewebsvergrößerung *f* durch Zellvermehrung

hyperplastic hyperplastisch

hyperpnoea, hyperpnea vermehrte Atmung *f*, Hyperpnoe *f*

hyperpolarisation Hyperpolarisation *f*, Zunahme *f* des Membranpotentials über den normalen Wert

hyperprosexia übermäßige Aufmerksamkeitsfixierung *f* auf ein Reizobjekt, Hyperprosexie *f*

hyperprotection Überbesorgtheit *f*, übermäßiger Schutz *m*

hyperpyrexia extrem hohes Fieber *n*, Hyperpyrexie *f*

hyperreactive hyperreaktiv

hyperreflexia Hyperreflexie *f*

hypersensibility, hypersensitiveness, hypersensitivity Überempfindlichkeit *f*

hypersensitive überempfindlich

hypersexuality übermäßige sexuelle Aktivität *f*, abnorm gesteigerte Sexualität *f*, Hypersexualität *f*

hypersomnia Schlafsucht *f*, Hypersomnie *f* / **nonorganic ~** nichtorganische Hypersomnie *f* / **primary ~** primäre Hypersomnie *f*

hyperspace *n*–dimensionaler Raum *m*, Hyperspace *m*

hypersthenia überhöhter Tonus *m*, Hypersthenie *f*

hypersusceptibility Überempfindlichkeit *f*

hypersusceptible überempfindlich

hypertelorism Hypertelorismus *m*, Vergrößerung *f* des Abstandes der inneren Augenwinkel

hypertension hoher Blutdruck *m*, Bluthochdruck *m*, Hypertonie *f* / **arterial ~** arterieller Hochdruck *m* / **essential ~** essenzieller Bluthochdruck *m* / **senile ~** Altershochdruck *m*

hypertensive hypertonisch

hypertext Hypertext *m*, nicht–linearer Bildschirmtext *m*

hyperthermia, hyperthermy Wärmestauung *f*, Überwärmung *f*, Hyperthermie *f*

hyperthymia Hyperthymie *f*, gesteigerte Affektivität *f*, hypomanischer Erregungszustand *m*

hyperthymic hyperthym, leicht erregbar, zu gesteigerter Affektivität neigend

hyperthyroidism Schilddrüsenüberfunktion *f*, Hyperthyreose *f*, Hyperthyreoidismus *m*

hypertonia Hypertonus *m*, Hypertonie *f* / **muscular ~** Muskelstarre *f*, Muskelrigidität *f*

hypertonic hypertonisch

hypertonicity Hypertonie *f*, Hypertonus *m*

hypertonus Hypertonus *m*, Hochdruck *m*, gesteigerter Druck *m* / **~ of muscles** hohe Muskelspannung *f*

hypertrophy, hypertrophia Hypertrophie *f*, Vergrößerung *f*

hypertropia Begleitschielen *n*

hyperventilation Hyperventilation *f*, Hyperpnoe *f* / **~ syndrome** Hyperventilationssyndrom *n* / **~ tetany** Hyperventilationstetanie *f*

hypesthesia herabgesetzter Tastsinn *m*, verminderte Empfindung *f*, Hypästhesie *f* / **olfactory ~** Hyposmie *f*, abnormal geringe Geruchsempfindlichkeit *f*

hyphedonia krankhaft vermindertes Lustgefühl *n*, Hyphedonie *f*

hyphenated mit Bindestrich geschrieben

hyphidrosis verminderte Schweißabsonderung *f*

hypnaesthesia Schläfrigkeit *f*, Schlafgefühl *n*

hypnagogic einschläfernd, hypnagogisch, beim Einschlafen auftretend

hypnagogue Schlafmittel *n* / schlafbringend, hypnagog

hypnoanalysis Hypnoanalyse *f*

hypnocatharsis Hypnokatharsis *f*

hypnogenesis Hypnoseerzeugung *f*, Schlaferzeugung *f*

hypnogenic, hypnogenetic, hypnogenous einschläfernd, Hypnose erzeugend

hypnoid, hypnoidal, hypnoid hypnoseähnlich, schlafähnlich

hypnoidisation Erzeugen *n* von Hypnose

hypnolepsy Schlafsucht *f*, Hypnolepsie *f*

hypnology Wissenschaft *f* von der Hypnose, Lehre *f* von den hypnotischen Vorgängen, Hypnologie *f*

hypnonarco–analysis Narkoanalyse *f*

hypnopathy Hypnopathie *f*, Narkolepsie *f*

hypnophobia Angst *f* vor dem Einschlafen

hypnopompic Halbschlaf–, Aufwach–

hypnosis Hypnose *f* / **active ~** Aktivhypnose *f* / **graduated active ~** gestufte Aktivhypnose *f*

hypnosuggestive hypnosuggestiv

hypnotherapist Hypnotherapeut *m*, therapeutischer Hypnotiseur *m*

hypnotherapy Hypnotherapie *f*, Heilschlaf *m*

hypnotic hypnotisch

hypnotisability Hypnotisierbarkeit *f*

hypnotisable hypnotisierbar

hypnotisation Hypnotisieren *n*, Durchführen *n* von Hypnose

hypnotise hypnotisieren

hypnotism Hypnotismus *m*, Hypnose *f* / **self–induced ~** Selbsthypnose *f*

hypnotist Hypnotiseur *m*

hypnotoid hypnoseähnlich

hypnotoxin Hypnotoxin *n*, (hypothetisches) schlafauslösendes Hormon *n*

hypoacousis, hypoacusis Hypoakusie *f*, Schwerhörigkeit *f*

hypoaesthesia, hypoesthesia herabgesetztes Tastgefühl *n*, verminderte Schmerzempfindlichkeit *f*, Hypästhesie *f*

hypoaffective gefühlsarm, wenig emotional

hypoalgesia verminderte Schmerzempfindlichkeit *f*, Hypalgesie *f*

hypoblast Entoblast *n*, Entoderm *n*, inneres Keimblatt *n*

hypoblastic zum inneren Keimblatt gehörig, entodermal

hypobulia Willensschwäche *f*, Hypobulie *f*, herabgesetzte Willenskraft *f*

hypocapnia Kohlensäuremangel *m* im Blut, Hypokapnie *f*

hypochondria, hypochondry Krankheitseinbildung *f*, Hypochondrie *f*

hypochondriac Hypochonder *m* / hypochondrisch

hypochondriasis Krankheitswahn *m*, Hypochondrie *f*

hypochondriast Hypochonder *m*

hypocinesia, hypocinesis Bewegungsmangel *m*, Hypokinese *f*

hypocrisy Hypokrisie *f*, Heuchelei *f*

hypocrite Heuchler *m*

hypocritical heuchlerisch

hypodermic subkutan, unter die Haut

hypoemotional gefühlsarm, wenig emotional

hypoergasia psychobiologische Unterfunktion *f*, Depression *f*

hypoesthesia herabgesetztes Tastgefühl *n*, verminderte Schmerzempfindlichkeit *f*, Hypästhesie *f*

hypofunction Unterfunktion *f*, Hypofunktion *f*

hypogenitalism Unterentwicklung *f* der Geschlechtsmerkmale, Hypogenitalismus *m*

hypogeusia herabgesetzte Geschmacksempfindung *f*, Hypogeusie *f*

hypoglossal sublingual, unter der Zunge gelegen

hypoglycaemia, hypoglycemia verminderter Blutzuckerspiegel *m*, Hypoglykämie *f*

hypoglycaemic, hypoglycemic blutzuckersenkend, hypoglykämisch

hypognathous mit zu kleinem Unterkiefer, mit unterentwickeltem Unterkiefer, hypognath

hypogonadism Unterfunktion *f* der Geschlechtsdrüsen, Hypogonadismus *m* / **pituitary ~** hypophysärer Infantilismus *m*

hypohormonism hormonale Unterfunktion *f*

hypokinesis, hypokinesia Bewegungsmangel *m*, Hypokinesie *f*

hypokinetic bewegungsarm, hypokinetisch

hypologia stark verminderte Sprechfähigkeit *f*, Hypologie *f*

hypomania Hypomanie *f*, leichte Manie *f*

hypomaniac Hypomaner *m*

hypomanic hypomanisch

hypometropia Kurzsichtigkeit *f*

hypomimia Verminderung *f* der Mimik, Hypomimie *f*, herabgesetzte mimische Ausdruckskraft *f*

hypomimic mit verminderter Mimik, hypomimisch

hypomnesis, hypomnesia Gedächtnisschwäche *f*, mangelhafte Erinnerung *f*, Hypomnesie *f*

hypomotility Bewegungsschwäche *f*, Hypomotilität *f*

hyponoia Hyponoia *f*

hypoparathyroidism Unterfunktion *f* der Nebenschilddrüsen, Unterfunktion *f* der Epithelkörperchen, Hypoparathyreoidismus *m*

hypophonia verminderte Sprechfähigkeit *f*, verminderte Fähigkeit *f* zur Lautbildung

hypophoria nach unten gerichtetes Schielen *n*

hypophrasia verminderte sprachliche Ausdrucksfähigkeit *f*, Sprechunwilligkeit *f*, Hypophrasie *f*

hypophrenia Geistesschwäche *f*, Oligophrenie *f*, Schwachsinn *m*, Hypophrenie *f*

hypophrenic geistesschwach, geistig minderbegabt, geistig zurückgeblieben, schwachsinnig / Schwachsinniger *m*, Geistesschwacher *m*

hypophrenosis Hypophrenose *f*, Schwachsinn *m*

hypophyseal hypophysär

hypophysectomise die Hypophyse operativ entfernen

hypophysectomy Hypophysenentfernung *f*, Hypophysektomie *f*

hypophysis Hypophyse *f*, Hirnanhang *m*, Hirnanhangdrüse *f* / **~ cerebri** Hirnanhang *m*, Hypophyse *f* / **~ disorder** Hypophysenstörung *f*

hypopituitarism Unterfunktion *f* der Hypophyse, Hypopituitarismus *m*

hypoplasia, hypoplasty Unterentwicklung *f*, Hypoplasie *f*

hypoplastic unterentwickelt, hypoplastisch

hypopraxia mangelnde Aktivität *f*, Inaktivität *f*, Hypopraxie *f*

hypoprosexia unangemessen verminderte Aufmerksamkeit *f*, Hypoprosexie *f*

hyposecretion verminderte Sekretion *f*

hyposensitive von verminderter Empfindlichkeit, unterempfindlich

hyposensitivity, hyposensitiveness verminderte Empfindlichkeit *f*, herabgesetzte Sensibilität *f*

hyposexuality verminderte Geschlechtslust *f*, Hyposexualität *f*, Anerotismus *m*

hyposmia mangelhafter Geruchssinn *m*, Hyposmie *f*

hypostasis Grundlage *f*, Wesen *n*, Hypostase *f*

hypostatization Verdinglichung *f*, Vergegenständlichung *f*, Hypostasierung *f*

hypostatize verdinglichen, vergegenständlichen, hypostasieren

hyposynergia Koordinationsstörung *f*

hypotaxia, hypotaxis mittlerer Grad *m* der Hypnose, Hypotaxie *f*, Hypotaxis *f*

hypotension niedriger Blutdruck *m*, Hypotonie *f*

hypotensive mit niedrigem Blutdruck, hypotonisch / Hypotoniker *m*

hypothalamic hypothalamisch

hypothalamus Hypothalamus *m* / ~ **lesion** Hypothalamusschädigung *f*, Hypothalamusläsion *f* / **medial** ~ medialer Hypothalamus *m*

hypothermia passive Unterkühlung *f*, Hypothermie *f*

hypothesis Hypothese *f*, Annahme *f* / ~ **of constancy** Konstanzannahme *f* / ~ **of neurohumoral transmission** chemische Theorie *f* der Erregungsübertragung / ~ **testing** Hypothesenüberprüfung *f* / **cognitive** ~ **testing** kognitive Hypothesentestung *f* / ~ **theory** Hypothesentheorie *f* / **all–or–none** ~ Alles–oder–Nichts–Hypothese *f* / **alternative** ~ Alternativhypothese *f* / **and–summation** ~ Und–Summenhypothese *f* / **deterministic** ~ deterministische Hypothese *f* / **falsifiable** ~ falsifizierbare Hypothese *f* / **functional** ~ Funktionshypothese *f* / **fundamental** ~ Grundhypothese *f* / **probabilistic** ~ Wahrscheinlichkeitshypothese *f*, probabilistische Hypothese *f* / **triadic** ~ Triadenhypothese *f* / **working** ~ Arbeitshypothese *f*

hypothesize eine Hypothese aufstellen, annehmen

hypothesizing Bildung *f* einer Hypothese, Aufstellen *n* einer Hypothese

hypothetical hypothetisch

hypothetico–deductive hypothetisch–deduktiv

hypothymia mangelnde affektive Ansprechbarkeit *f*, Niedergeschlagenheit *f*, Depression *f*, Hypothymie *f*

hypothyroid hypothyreoid, mit Schilddrüsenunterfunktion

hypothyroidism, hypothyreosis Schilddrüsenunterfunktion *f*, Hypothyreose *f*, Hypothyreoidismus *m*

hypotonia, hypotony Hypotonie *f*, niedriger Blutdruck *m*

hypotonic hypotonisch, mit niedrigem Blutdruck

hypotonicity Tonusverminderung *f*

hypotrophic unterernährt, hypotroph

hypotrophy Unterernährung *f*, Hypotrophie *f*

hypoxaemia, hypoxemia Sauerstoffmangel *m* im Blut, Hypoxämie *f*

hypoxaemic, hypoxemic hypoxämisch

hypoxia Hypoxie *f*, Sauerstoffmangel *m* in den Körpergeweben

hypoxyphilia Hypoxyphilie *f*

hypoventilation Hypoventilation *f*

hypsarrhythmia Hypsarrhythmie *f*, Arrhythmie *f* hoher EEG–Wellen

hypsophobia, hypsiphobia Höhenschwindel *m*, Höhenangst *f*, Hypsophobie *f*, Dinophobie *f*

hysterectomy Entfernung *f* der Gebärmutter, Hysterektomie *f*

hysteria Hysterie *f* / **hypnoid ~** Hypnoidhysterie *f* / **traumatic ~** traumatische Hysterie *f*

hysteriac Hysteriker *m*

hysteric, hysterical hysterisch

hystericism, hysterism hysterische Veranlagung *f*

hysterics hysterischer Anfall *m*

hysteriform hystericahnlich, hysteriform

hystero–epilepsy Hysteroepilepsie *f*

hysterogenic, hysterogenetic, hysterogenous hysterogen, Hysterie erzeugend

hysteroid hysteroid

hysteromania hysterische Manie *f*, Hysteromanie *f*

hysteroneurasthenia hysterisch gefärbte Neurasthenie *f*

hysteropia hysterisch bedingte Sehstörung *f*

hysterospasm Uteruskrampf *m*

I

iatric ärztlich

iatrogenic durch den Arzt ausgelöst, durch ärztliche Einwirkung entstanden, iatrogen

iatrogeny Iatrogenie *f*

icebreaker Eisbrecher *m*

ichthyophobia Ichthyophobie *f*, Angst *f* vor Fischen

icon Bild *n*, Vorstellungsbild *n*, Piktogramm *n*

iconic bildlich, vorstellungsmäßig

iconolagny Wollustempfinden *n* beim Betrachten von Bildern / Ikonolagnie *f*

iconolatry Bilderanbetung *f*

iconomania Ikonomanie *f*, Vernarrtheit *f* in Bilder

iconomaniac Bildernarr *m*

iconometer Rahmensucher *m*

iconoscope Bildspeicherröhre *f*, Elektronenstrahlabtaster *m*, Ikonoskop *n*

icterus Gelbsucht *f*, Ikterus *m* / **nuclear ~** Kernikterus *m*

ictus Akzentuierung *f*, Akzent *m*, plötzlicher Anfall *m*, Iktus *m*, Ictus *m*

I curve I–Kurve *f*

id Es *n* / **~–ego conflict** Ich–Es–Konflikt *m* / **~ function** Es–Instanz *f* / **~ resistance** Es–Widerstand *m*

idea Idee *f*, Vorstellung *f*, Gedanke *m*, kognitiver Prozess *m* / **~ of insufficiency** Insuffizienzvorstellung *f* / **~ of reference** Beziehungsidee *f* / **abstract ~** abstrakte Vorstellung *f* / **autochthonous ~** autochthone Idee *f*, Wahnidee *f* / **basic ~** Grundidee *f* / **collective ~** Kollektivvorstellung *f* / **compulsive ~** Zwangsidee *f*, Zwangsvorstellung *f* / **controlling ~** dominierender Gedanke in, leitende Idee *f* / **delusional ~** Wahnidee *f*, Wahnvorstellung *f* / **expiatory ~** Sühneidee *f* / **fixed ~** fixe Idee *f*, Monoideismus *m* / **generalized ~** Allgemeinvorstellung *f* / **guiding ~** Leitvorstellung *f*, Leitidee *f* / **hypochondriac ~** hypochondrische Idee *f* / **ideomotor ~** ideomotorische Vorstellung *f* / **imaginary ~** Phantasievorstellung *f* / **imperative ~** Zwangsidee *f*, fixe Idee *f* / **innate ~** angeborene Vorstellung *f* / **insistent ~** persistierende Idee *f*, fixe Idee *f* / **latent ~** latenter Gedanke *m* / **obsessional ~** Zwangsgedanke *m*, Zwangsidee *f* / **obsessive ~** Zwangsgedanke *m*, Zwangsidee *f* / **overcharged ~** überwertige Idee *f* / **persistent ~** persistierende Idee *f*, fixe Idee *f* / **purposive ~** Zielvorstellung *f*

ideal ideal, ideell, eingebildet, Ideen–, Gedanken– / Ideal *n*, Wunschbild *n*, Leitbild *n*, Vorbild *n*

idealisation Idealisierung *f*

idealise idealisieren

idealised idealisiert, Ideal–

idealism Idealismus *m*

idealist Idealist *m*

idealistic idealistisch

ideation Ideenbildung *f*, Ideation *f*, Gedankenbildung *f* / **suicidal ~** Suizidgedanken *mpl*

ideational, ideative ideatorisch, Ideen–, konzeptionell, Begriffs–

idée fixe fixe Idee *f*, Zwangsidee *f*, Zwangsgedanke *m*

idée–force Gedankendynamik *f*, Aktualisierungstendenz *f* von Ideen

identical identisch

identifiability Identifizierbarkeit *f* / ~ **principle** Prinzip *n* der Reizunterscheidung

identification Identifikation *f*, Identifizierung *f* / ~ **test** Identifikationstest *m* / ~ **with the aggressor** Identifikation *f* mit dem Angreifer / ~ **with the conquered** Identifikation *f* mit dem Besiegten / **crossparental** ~ Identifikation *f* mit dem gegengeschlechtlichen Elternteil / **faulty sexual** ~ geschlechtliche Fehlidentifizierung *f* / **primary** ~ primäre Identifikation *f* / **projective** ~ projektive Identifikation *f* / **secondary** ~ sekundäre Identifikation *f* / **transferred** ~ übertragene Identifikation *f*, Übertragung *f*, Projektion *f*

identify identifizieren

identity Identität *f*, Individualität *f*, Persönlichkeit *f* / ~ **crisis** Identitätskrise *f* / ~ **hypothesis** Identitätshypothese *f* / ~ **problem** Identitätsproblem *n* / **ethnic** ~ ethnische Identität *f* / **dissociative** ~ **disorder** dissoziative Identitätsstörung *f* / **formal** ~ formale Identität *f* / **perceptual** ~ Wahrnehmungsidentität *f* / **personal** ~ persönliche Identität *f*, Identität *f* der Persönlichkeit / **professional** ~ berufliche Identität *f* / **psychosocial** ~ psychosoziale Identität *f* / **sexual** ~ sexuelle Identität *f* / **social** ~ soziale Identität *f*

ideodynamics Ideodynamik *f*

ideogenous, ideogenetic ideogen, aus einer Idee entstanden

ideogram, ideograph Begriffszeichen *n*, Ideogramm *n*

ideographic ideographisch

ideokinetic ideokinetisch, ideomotorisch, psychomotorisch

ideological ideologisch

ideology Ideologie *f*, Begriffslehre *f* / **anti-democratic** ~ antidemokratische Ideologie *f*

ideomotor ideomotorisch, psychomotorisch, ideokinetisch

idiocrasy Idiosynkrasie *f*, charakteristische Eigenart *f*, Besonderheit *f*

idiocratic idiosynkratisch

idiocy Idiotie *f*, Schwachsinn *m* stärksten Grades, hochgradiger Schwachsinn *m* / **absolute** ~ völliger Schwachsinn *m* / **amaurotic** ~ amaurotische Idiotie *f*, Tay–Sachs–Krankheit *f* / **cretoid**~ Idiotie *f* bei Kretinismus / **epileptic** ~ Schwachsinn *m* aufgrund einer Epilepsie / **hydrocephalic** ~ Idiotie *f* bei Wasserkopf / **infantile amaurotic familial** ~ infantile amaurotische familiäre Idiotie *f* / **intrasocial** ~ Idiotie *f*, die eine Eingliederung in die Gesellschaft zulässt / **late infantile amaurotic** ~ spätinfantile amaurotische Idiotie *f* / Dollinger–Bielschowsky Syndrom *n*, Bielschowsky–Jansky–Schob Syndrom *n* / **mongolian** ~ Mongolismus *m*, Down–Syndrom *n* / **mongoloid** ~ Mongolismus *m*, Down–Syndrom *n* / **traumatic** ~ Schwachsinn *m* nach Schädelverletzungen

idiodynamics Eigendynamik *f*

idiogamia Idiogamie *f*

idioglossia Idioglossie *f*, unverständliche Sprache *f*

idiographic idiographisch

idiohypnotism Selbsthypnose *f*

idiokinetic ideokinetisch, ideomotorisch, psychomotorisch

idiolalia Idiolalie *f*, erfundene Sprache *f*

idiolect Idiolekt *m*, Privatsprache *f*

idiom Idiom *n*, Spracheigentümlichkeit *f* / **personal** ~ persönliche Ausdrucksweise *f*, persönlicher Stil *m*

idioneurosis idiopathische Neurose *f*

idiopathic, idiopathetic idiopathisch, essenziell

idiopathy Krankheit *f* aus eigenem Ursprung, Krankheit *f* ohne feststellbare Ursache

idiophrenia Idiophrenie *f*, Störung *f* aufgrund einer organischen Gehirnerkrankung

idiophrenic idiophren, geistesgestört aufgrund einer Gehirnerkrankung

idioplasm Keimplasma *n*, Erbsubstanz *f*, Idioplasma *n*

idioretinal retinaeigen

idiosyncrasy, idiosyncracy Idiosynkrasie *f*, charakteristische Eigenart *f*, Besonderheit *f*, Exzentrizität *f*

idiosyncratic idiosynkratisch

idiot Idiot *m*, Schwachsinniger *m* / ~ **savant** Idiot–Savant *m*, geistig Behinderte *m,f* mit Spezialbegabung

idiotic idiotisch, blödsinnig, schwachsinnig

idiotism Idiotie *f*, Idiotismus *m*

idiotropic idiotrop, auf das eigene Selbst gerichtet, vegetativ, den eigenen Körper betreffend

idiotype Idiotypus *m*, Genotypus *m*, Erbbild *n*

idiotypic idiotypisch, erblich

idioverse Lebensraum *m*, Erfahrungsraum *m*, eigener Mikrokosmos *m*

idol Idol *n*

ignorance Unwissen *n*, Ignoranz *f* / **pluralistic** ~ vermeintliches Wissen *n* über die Anschauungen der Anderen

ileum Krummdarm *m*, unterer Teil *m* des Dünndarms, Ileum *n*

ill krank / Kranke *m,f* / **homeless mentally** ~ nichtsesshafte psychisch Kranke *m,f*

illata gefolgerte Dinge *npl*, Konstrukte *npl*

illegitimate illegitim, unehelich, unrechtmäßig

illicit unerlaubt, verboten, rechtswidrig

illiteracy Analphabetentum *n*

illiterate ungebildet / Analphabet *m*

illness Krankheit *f* / ~ **behaviour** Krankheitsverhalten *n* / **accompanying** ~ Begleitkrankheit *f* / **chronic** ~ chronische Krankheit *f* / **chronic mental** ~ chronische psychische Krankheit *f* / **feigned** ~ Scheinkrankheit *f* / **iatrogenic** ~ durch ärztliche Einwirkung ausgelöste Krankheit *f* / **manic–depressive** ~ manisch–depressive Erkrankung *f* / **mental** ~ Geisteskrankheit *f* / **physical** ~ körperliche Krankheit *f* / **psychosomatic** ~ psychosomatische Krankheit *f*

illogical unlogisch

illuminance Beleuchtungsintensität *f*

illuminant leuchtend, erleuchtend

illumination Beleuchtung *f*, Illumination *f*, Erleuchtung *f* / ~ **colours** Leuchtfarbe *f* / ~ **flicker** Beleuchtungsflimmern *n*

illuminometer Photometer *n*

illusion Illusion *f*, Täuschung *f*, Sinnestäuschung *f* / ~ **of déjà–vu** Déjà–vu–Illusion *f*, Bekanntheitstäuschung *f* / ~ **of doubles** Doppelgänger–Illusion *f* / ~ **of hearing** Hörtäuschung *f* / ~ **of memory** Erinnerungstäuschung *f*, Erinnerungsillusion *f*, Pseudomnesie *f* / ~ **of motion** Scheinbewegung *f* / ~ **of movement** kinästhetische Täuschung *f*, Bewegungstäuschung *f* / ~ **of smell** Geruchstäuschung *f*, Geruchsillusion *f* / **acoustic** ~ Hörtäuschung *f* / **assimilative** ~ Assimilationsillusion *f* / **associative** ~ Assoziationsillusion *f* / **autokinetic** ~ autokinetische Illusion *f*, autokinetisches Phänomen *n* / **conscious** ~ **theory** Theorie *f* der bewussten Täuschung *f* / **geometrical** ~ geometrische Täuschung *f* / **geometrical–optical** ~ geometrisch–optische Täuschung *f* / **haptic** ~ haptische Täuschung *f* / **horizontal–vertical** ~ Vertikal–Horizontal–Täuschung *f* / **interpretative** ~ Bedeutungswahn *m* / **kinaesthetic** ~ kinästhetische Täuschung *f* / **kinehaptic** ~ kinehaptische Täuschung *f* / **mnesic** ~ Erinnerungstäuschung *f*, Pseudomnesie *f* / **oculogyral** ~ **movement** Augenbewegungsillusion *f* / **olfactory** ~ Geruchsillusion *f*, Geruchstäuschung *f* / **optical** ~ optische Täuschung *f*, Gesichtstäuschung *f* / **perceptual** ~ Wahrnehmungstäuschung *f* / **sensory** ~ Empfindungstäuschung *f*, Pseudoästhesie *f* / **stroboscopic** ~ stroboskopische Täuschung *f* / **tactual** ~ Tasttäuschung *f*

illusional, illusionary Illusions–, Täuschungs–

illusionism Illusionismus *m*

illusive trügerisch, täuschend, Schein–

illusiveness Schein *m*, Täuschung *f*

illusory Schein–

illustriousness Berühmtheit *f*

image Bild *n*, Vorstellungsbild *n*, Vorstellung *f*, Image *n* / **~ agglutination** Bildagglutination *f* / **~ analysis** Imageanalyse *f* / **~ building** Imagebildung *f* / **~ cathexis** Bildbesetzung *f* / **~ contrast** Bildkontrast *m* / **~ rater system** Verfahren *n* zur systematischen Untersuchung des Images / **after-~** Nachbild *n* / **auditory ~** Klangbild *n* / **catathymic ~ perception** katathymes Bilderleben *n* / **collective ~** Kollektivvorstellung *f* / **composite ~** zusammengesetztes Bild *n*, zusammengesetztes Vorstellungsbild *n*, Urbild *n* / **concrete ~** konkretes Vorstellungsbild *n* / **delusional ~** Wahnbild *n* / **eidetic ~** eidetisches Anschauungsbild *n*, eidetische Vorstellung *f* / **enacted ~** Handlungsvorstellung *f* / **general ~** allgemeine Vorstellung *f* / **generic ~** zusammengesetztes Vorstellungsbild *n* / **hallucinatory ~** Trugbild *n* / **hypnagogic ~** schlaffördernde Vorstellung *f* / **idealized ~** Idealbild *n*, idealisierte Vorstellung *f* / **ideational ~** Vorstellungsbild *n* / **inner ~** Leitbild *n* / **inverted ~** umgekehrtes Bild *n* / **mental ~** Anschauungsbild *n*, Vorstellung *n* / **negative ~** negatives Bild *n*, negatives Image *n* / **oneiric ~** Traumbild *n* / **optical ~** optisches Bild *n* / **perceived ~** wahrgenommenes Bild *n* / **perceptual ~** Wahrnehmungsbild *n* / **personal ~** persönliches Vorstellungsbild *n* / **positive ~** positives Bild *n*, positives Image *n* / **primordial ~** Urbild *n*, Archetyp *m* / **psychovisual ~** Erscheinungsbild *n* / **recurrent ~** sich ständig wiederholendes Vorstellungsbild *n* / **retinal ~** Netzhautbild *n* / **schematic ~** schematisches Bild *n*/ **secondary ~** sekundäres Bild *n* / **spatial ~** Raumbild *n*, räumliches Bild *n* / **stereoscopic ~** Raumbild *n*, stereoskopisches Bild *n* / **symbolic ~** symbolisches Bild *n*, symbolische Vorstellung *f* / **tied ~** assoziative Vorstellung *f* / **verbal ~** Wortbild *n* / **virtual ~** virtuelle Vorstellung *f*, tatsächliche Vorstellung *f* / **visual ~** Bild *n*, optisches Vorstellungsbild *n*

imageless ohne bildliche Vorstellung, vorstellungslos

imagery Vorstellung *f*, bildhafte Vorstellung *f* / **~ type** Vorstellungstypus *m* / **auditive ~** akustischer Vorstellungstypus *m* / **conceptual ~** Begriffsvorstellung *f*, begriffliche Vorstellung *f* / **eidetic ~** eidetische Bildvorstellung *f*, eidetischer Vorstellungstypus *m* / **emotive ~** emotionale Gegenvorstellung *f* / **guided affective ~** katathymes Bilderleben *n* / **kinaesthetic ~** kinästhetischer Vorstellungstypus *m* / **mental ~** geistige Vorstellung *f* / **spatial ~** räumliche Bildvorstellung *f* / **visual ~** visueller Vorstellungstypus *m*, optischer Vorstellungstypus *m*

imaginal bildlich, vorgestellt

imaginary imaginär, eingebildet, nur in der Einbildung vorhanden, fiktiv / Imaginäre *n*

imagination Einbildungskraft *f*, Einbildung *f*, Phantasie *f*, Vorstellung *f*,Vorstellen *n*, Imagination *f* / **anticipatory ~** Zielvorstellung *f* / **constructive ~** konstruktive Vorstellung *f* / **creative ~** schöpferische Vorstellung *f* / **fanciful ~** Phantasievorstellung *f* / **reproductive ~** Erinnerungsvorstellung *f*, Erinnerungsbild *n*

imaginative phantasievoll, Einbildungs–, schöpferisch, erfinderisch

imagine sich vorstellen, sich einbilden

imago Imago *f*, Urbild *n* / **~ of the father** Vaterimago *f* / **~ of the mother** Mutterimago *f* / **maternal ~** Mutterimago *f* / **parental ~** Elternimago *f* / **paternal ~** Vaterimago *f*

imbalance Ungleichgewicht *n*, gestörtes Gleichgewicht *n*, Gleichgewichtsstörung *f* / **hormonal ~** Hormonstörung *f* / **intellectual ~** unterschiedlich stark ausgeprägte intellektuelle Fähigkeiten *fpl* / **muscular ~** Muskelschwäche *f* / **oculo-**

motor ~ gestörtes okulomotorisches Gleichgewicht *n* / **sympathetic ~** Vagotomie *f*, Übererregbarkeit *f* des parasympathischen Nervensystems / **vasomotor ~** vasomotorische Ataxie *f*, Gefäßataxie *f*

imbecile imbezill, schwachsinnig, geistig zurückgeblieben / Imbeziller *m*, Schwachsinniger *m*, Geistesschwacher *m* / **mongoloid ~** Mongoloider *m*

imbecility Imbezillität *f*, mittelgradiger Schwachsinn *m* / **mongolian ~** Mongolismus *m*, Down–Syndrom *n* / **mongoloid ~** Mongolismus *m*, Down–Syndrom *n* / **moral ~** moralischer Schwachsinn *m*, Gemütlosigkeit *f*

imipramine Imipramin *n*, Tofranil *n*

imitate nachahmen, imitieren

imitation Nachahmung *f*, Imitation *f* / **~ learning** Imitationslernen *n* / **delayed ~** verzögerte Nachahmung *f* / **hysterical ~** hysterische Imitation *f* / **reciprocal ~** gegenseitige Nachahmung *f* / **servile ~** sklavische Nachahmung *f*

imitative nachgemacht, nachahmend

imitativeness Nachahmungstendenz *f*

immanence, immanency Inhärenz *f*, Immanenz *f*

immanent inhärent, immanent

immaterial immateriell, geistig, unwichtig, nebensächlich

immateriality Geistigkeit *f*, Unkörperlichkeit *f*

immature unreif, unentwickelt

immaturity Unreife *f* / **~ reaction** Reaktion *f* aufgrund von Unreife / **emotional ~** emotionale Unreife *f* / **sexual ~** Geschlechtsunreife *f*

immediate unmittelbare (r, s), sofortige (r, s)

immersion course Intensivkurs *m*

immigrant Einwanderer *m*

immigration Einwanderung *f*

imminent imminent, drohend, unmittelbar bevorstehend

immobilisation Immobilisierung *f*, Ruhigstellung *f*

immobility Unbeweglichkeit *f* / **catatonic ~** Attonität *f* / **social ~** soziale Immobilität *f* / **tonic ~** tonische Immobilität *f*, Spannungsunbeweglichkeit *f*, Totstellen *n*

immoral unmoralisch, unsittlich

immorality Unsittlichkeit *f*, Sittenlosigkeit *f*

immortality Unsterblichkeit *f*

immune| complex Antigen–Antikörperkomplex *m* / **~ system** Immunsystem *n*

immunohistochemical immunhistochemisch

immunisation Immunisierung *f*

immunise immunisieren, immun machen

immunity Immunität *f*, Unempfindlichkeit *f* / **acquired ~** erworbene Immunität *f* / **cell–mediated ~** zelluläre Immunität *f*, zellvermittelte Immunität *f* / **cellular ~** zelluläre Immunität *f* / **humoral ~** humorale Immunität *f* / **innate ~** angeborene Immunität *f*

immuno|globuline Immunoglobulin *n*, Immunglobulin *n* / **~competence** Immunkompetenz *f* / **~deficiency** Immundefekt *m*, Immunmangelkrankheit *f*, Defektimmunopathie *f* / **~fluorescence** Immunfluoreszenz *f* / **~histochemistry** Immunhistochemie *f* / **~logy** Lehre *f* von den spezifischen Abwehrreaktionen, Immunologie *f* / **~pathology** Immunpathologie *f*, Lehre *f* von den fehlgesteuerten Immunmechanismen / **~reaction** Immunreaktion *f* / **~reactivity** Immunreaktivität *f* / **~ stimulant** Immunstimulans *n* / **~suppression** Immunsuppression *f*

impact Einwirkung *f*, Einfluss *m*, Wirkung *f*, Werbewirkung *f* / **~ test** Wirkungstest *m* / **long–range ~** Langzeitwirkung *f*

impairment Beeinträchtigung *f*, Schädigung *f*, Schwächung *f* / **~ of hearing** Hörschaden *m*, Schwerhörigkeit *f*, Hörbehinderung *f* / **~ of learning faculty** Lernbehinderung *f*, Lernstörung *f* / **~ index** Schädigungsindex *m* / **~ in speech** Sprachstörung *f*, Sprachfehler *m* / **~ of vi-**

sion Sehbehinderung *f* / **cognitive ~** kognitive Beeinträchtigung *f* / **functional ~** Funktionsstörung *f* / **mental ~** psychische Störung *f*

impaludation Malariakur *f*, Fieberkur *f*

impartial unparteiisch, vorurteilsfrei

impassiveness, impassivity Unempfindlichkeit *f*

impatient ungeduldig, unzufrieden, unduldsam

impedance Wellenwiderstand *m*, Impedanz *f*, Wechselstromwiderstand *m*

impediment Behinderung *f*, Fehler *m*, Hindernis *n* / **~ in speech** Sprachfehler *m*

imperative Imperativ *m*, Gebot *n* / **categorical ~** kategorischer Imperativ *m*

imperceptible nicht wahrnehmbar, unmerklich, verschwindend klein

imperception mangelnde Wahrnehmungsfähigkeit *f*, Seelenblindheit *f*, optische Agnosie *f*

impermeability Undurchdringlichkeit *f*, Impermeabilität *f*

impersonal unpersönlich, objektiv

impersonation Personifizierung *f*, Verkörperung *f*

impertinent ungehörig, unverschämt, impertinent

imperviousness Undurchdringlichkeit *f*, Unzugänglichkeit *f*

impetus Triebkraft *f*, Impuls *m*

implant, cochlear Cochlea–Implantat *n*

implantation Einpflanzung *f*, Einnistung *f*, Nidation *f*

implementation Einführung *f*, Ausführung *f*, Durchführung *f*

implication Implikation *f*, stillschweigende Folgerung *f*

implicit implizit, inbegriffen

implosion therapy Überflutungstherapie *f*

import Bedeutung *f*, Sinn *m*

impotence, impotency Impotenz *f*, Zeugungsunfähigkeit *f*, Unvermögen *n*, Schwäche *f* / **anal ~** psychogene Obstipation *f*, psychisch bedingte Verstopfung *f* / **erective ~** erektive Impotenz *f*, erektile Dysfunktion *f* / **orgastic ~** Orgasmus–Impotenz *f* / **psychic ~** psychische Impotenz *f*, funktionelle Impotenz *f* / **sexual ~** Impotenz *f*, Zeugungsunfähigkeit *f*

impoverishment Verarmung *f*, Erschöpfung *f*

impracticalness Unbrauchbarkeit *f*, unpraktische Art *f*

impregnation Schwängerung *f*, Befruchtung *f*

impress Prägung *f*, Stempel *m*, Auswirkung *f*

impressibility Empfänglichkeit *f*, Eindrucksfähigkeit *f*

impressible leicht zu beeindrucken, empfänglich

impression Eindruck *m*, Sinnesempfindung *f*, Impression *f* / **~ formation** Eindrucksbildung *f* / **~ management** Eindrucksverarbeitung *f*, Eindruckssteuerung *f* / **~ method** Eindrucksmethode *f* / **absolute ~** absoluter Eindruck *m* / **direct ~** unmittelbarer Eindruck *m* / **first ~** erster Eindruck *m* / **maternal ~** Eindruck *m* von der Mutter / **novel ~** neuer Eindruck *m* / **sensory ~** Sinneseindruck *m* / **sensual ~** Sinneseindruck *m* / **visual ~** Gesichtseindruck *m*, optischer Eindruck *m*

impressionability Beeindruckbarkeit *f*, Beeinflussbarkeit *f*, Zugänglichkeit *f*

impressionable beeindruckbar, leicht beeinflussbar

impressive eindrucksvoll, imponierend

impressiveness Wirksamkeit *f*

imprint prägen, einprägen / Prägung *f*

imprinting Prägung *f*

Improbable unwahrscheinlich

improve verbessern, besser werden, Fortschritte machen

improvement Verbesserung *f*, Fortschritt *m* / **~ over chance** über der Zufallswahrscheinlichkeit liegende Verbesserung *f*

impuberal, impubic präpubertär, geschlechtsunreif, ohne Schamhaare

impuberism, impuberty Präpubertät *f*, Vorpubertät *f*

impudence Unverschämtheit *f*, Frechheit *f*, Vermessenheit *f*

impulse Impuls *m*, Antrieb *m*, Trieb *m* / **~ buying** Impulskauf *m* / **~-conducting** reizleitend / **~ of contrectation** Kontrektationstrieb *m*, Berührungstrieb *m* / **~ control** Impulskontrolle *f* / **~-control disorder** Störung *f* der Impulskontrolle / **~ debilitation** Antriebsverarmung *f* / **~ discharge** Impulsentladung *f*, Triebentladung *f* / **~ generator** Impulsgenerator *m*, Taktgeber *m* / **~ meter** Impulsmesser *m* / **~ presentation** Triebvorstellung *f* / **abortive ~** abortiver Impuls *m* / **afferent ~** zentripetaler Reiz *m* / **aggressive ~** Aggressionstrieb *m* / **antidromic ~** gegenläufiger Impuls *m* / **apical ~** Herzspitzenstoß *m* / **congenital ~** Instinkt *m*, Primärtrieb *m* / **creative ~** Schaffensdrang *m* / **destructive ~** Zerstörungstrieb *m*, zerstörerischer Impuls *m* / **efferent ~** zentrifugaler Reiz *m* / **excitatory ~** Erregungsimpuls *m* / **imitative ~** Nachahmungstrieb *m* / **instinctive ~** Triebregung *f* / **instinctual ~** Triebregung *f* / **irresistible ~** unwiderstehlicher Drang *m* / **morbid ~** krankhafter Trieb *m* / **motor ~** Bewegungsdrang *m* / **natural ~** Grundtrieb *m* / **nervous ~** Nervenimpuls *m* / **neural ~** Nervenimpuls *m* / **obsessional ~** Zwangsimpuls *m* / **psychooptical ~** Fusionszwang *m* / **psychosexual ~** psychosexueller Trieb *m* / **repressed ~** vedrängter Impuls *m*, verdrängte Regung *f* / **sadistic ~** sadistischer Impuls *m* / **sensory ~** Sinnesimpuls *m* / **sexual ~** Geschlechtstrieb *m* / **vital ~** Lebenstrieb *m*

impulsion Impuls *m*, Drang *m*, Antrieb *m*, Trieb *m*, Anreiz *m*, Anstoß *m* / **repressed ~** verdrängter Impuls *m* / **voluntary ~** Willensimpuls *m* / **wandering ~** Wandertrieb *m*

impulsive impulsiv, triebhaft, leicht erregbar

impulsiveness, impulsivity Impulsivität *f*, Neigung *f* zu raschem Handeln, impulsives Verhalten *n*

impunitive impunitiv, straffrei

impunitiveness impunitive Haltung *f*

imputability Zurechnungsfähigkeit *f*, Imputabilität *f*

inability Unfähigkeit *f*, Unvermögen *n* / **~ to concentrate** Konzentrationsschwäche *f* / **~ to establish contact** Kontaktmangel *m*, Bindungsunfähigkeit *f* / **~ to modify** Verarbeitungsschwäche *f* / **~ to work** Arbeitsunfähigkeit *f* / **~ to write** Agraphie *f*

inaccessibility Unzugänglichkeit *f*, Verschlossenheit *f*, Unerreichbarkeit *f*

inaccessible verschlossen, unnahbar, unzugänglich, unerreichbar, gesperrt

inaccuracy Ungenauigkeit *f*, Fehler *m*, Irrtum *m*

inaction, inactivity Untätigkeit *f*, Ruhe *f*, Trägheit *f*, Gleichgültigkeit *f*

inactivation Inaktivierung *f*

inactive inaktiv, passiv, in Ruhe, untätig

inadaptation mangelnde Anpassung *f*, Fehlanpassung *f*

inadequacy Unzulänglichkeit *f*, Unangemessenheit *f* / **personal ~** persönliche Unzulänglichkeit *f*, Untüchtigkeit *f* / **psychic ~** psychische Minderwertigkeit *f*

inadequate unzulänglich, unangemessen, inadäquat

inadmissible unzulässig, unstatthaft

inadvertently versehentlich, unbeabsichtigterweise

inane leer, hohl, albern, sinnlos

inanition Leere *f*, Entkräftung *f*, Schwäche *f* vor Hunger, Inanition *f*, seelische Verkümmerung *f*, Ermüdung *f*, Erschöpfung *f*

inanity Albernheit *f* / **~** leeres Geschwätz *n*

inappetence Appetitlosigkeit *f*, Anorexie *f*, Inappetenz *f*, fehlendes Sexualverlangen *n*, erotische Kälte *f*

inapt untauglich, ungeeignet, unfähig

inaptitude, inaptness Untauglichkeit *f*, Ungeeignetheit *f*, Unfähigkeit *f*

inarticulate unartikuliert, undeutlich

inattention Unaufmerksamkeit *f* / **selective ~** selektive Aufmerksamkeit *f*

in–basket technique Postkorbübung *f*

inborn ererbt, angeboren

inbreeding Inzucht *f*

incantation Beschwörung *f*, Zauberformel *f*

incapability Unfähigkeit *f*

incapable unfähig

incapacitating stark beeinträchtigend, stark behindernd

incapacitation through anxiety Angstlähmung *f*

incapacity Unfähigkeit *f*, Unvermögen *n* / **legal ~** Geschäftsunfähigkeit *f* / **mental ~** Unzurechnungsfähigkeit *f* / **senile ~** altersbedingte Unzurechnungsfähigkeit *f*

incarceration Einkerkerung *f*, Strafvollzug *m*, Einklemmung *f*

incendiarism Brandstiftungstrieb *m*, Pyromanie *f*, Aufwiegelung *f*

incendiary Brandstifter *m* / durch Brandstiftung verursacht, brandstifterisch, aufwieglerisch

incentive Anreiz *m*, Anreizmittel *n*, Ansporn *m*, Motivationsfaktor *m*, Lockmittel *n* / **~ motivation theory** Anreiz–Motivationstheorie *f* / **~ plan** Leistungsanreizplan *m* / **~ reinforcement** Anreizverstärkung *f* / **~ salience** Anreizhervorhebung *f* / **~ system** leistungsbezogenes Entlohnungssystem *n* / **~ value** Reizwert *m*, Anreizwert *m* / **educational ~s** Bildungsanreize *mpl* / **monetary ~** finanzieller Anreiz *m*, Geldprämie *f* / **negative ~** Strafe *f* negativer Anreiz *m* / **secondary ~** sekundärer Anreiz *m*

incest Inzest *m*, Blutschande *f*, Inzucht *f* / **~ barrier** Inzestschranke *f* / **~ complex** Inzestkomplex *m* / **~ dream** Inzesttraum *m* / **~ prohibition** Inzestverbot *n* / **~ taboo** Inzesttabu *n*

incestuous Inzest–

incidence Häufigkeit *f*, Vorkommen *n*, Auftreten *n*, Inzidenz *f* / **~–rate** Häufigkeit *f* des Auftretens

incident Vorfall *m*, Zwischenfall *m*, Ereignis *n* / **critical ~** kritischer Fall *m* / **critical ~ technique** Methode *f* der kritischen Fälle

incidental zufällig, nebensächlich

incipient anfänglich, beginnend, zu Beginn

incite anregen, anreizen, motivieren, stimulieren, animieren, aufhetzen

incitement Anregung *f*, Ansporn *m*, Anreiz *m*

incivism fehlende staatsbürgerliche Gesinnung *f*

inclination Neigung *f*, Hang *m*, Disposition *f* / **~ toward aggressiveness** Aggressionsneigung *f*

inclusion Einschluss *m* / **false ~** falscher Einschluss *m* / **valid ~** richtiger Einschluss *m*

incoherence Inkohärenz *f*, Zusammenhanglosigkeit *f*

incoherent zusammenhanglos, inkohärent

income Einkommen *n* / **~ level** Einkommensniveau *n*, Einkommensstufe *f*, Gehaltsstufe *f*

incommensurable unvergleichbar, untereinander nicht messbar, inkommensurabel, unvereinbar

incommunicative zurückhaltend, verschlossen, nicht mitteilsam, verschwiegen

incompatibility Unverträglichkeit *f*, Unvereinbarkeit *f*, Inkompatibilität *f* / **~ of roles** Unvereinbarkeit *f* von Rollen / **Rh–~** Rh–Unverträglichkeit *f*

incompatible unvereinbar, unverträglich, inkompatibel

incompetence Unfähigkeit *f*, Untauglich keit *f*, Unzulänglichkeit *f*, Inkompetenz *f* / **legal ~** Geschäftsunfähigkeit *f*

incompetency Geschäftsunfähigkeit *f*

incompetent unfähig, unzulänglich, inkompetent

incomplete unvollständig, Lücken–

incomprehensible unbegreiflich, unverständlich

inconceivable unbegreiflich, unverständlich, unfassbar, unvorstellbar

incongruent, incongruous nicht übereinstimmend, unvereinbar, widerspruchsvoll, inkongruent

incongruity, incongruence fehlende Übereinstimmung *f*, Missverhältnis *n*, Unvereinbarkeit *f*, Deckungsungleichheit *f*, Inkongruenz *f*

inconsequence Inkonsequenz *f*, Folgewidrigkeit *f*

inconsequent inkonsequent, folgewidrig, unzusammenhängend

inconsiderate unbedachtsam, unüberlegt, rücksichtslos

inconsistency Inkonsistenz *f*, Unstetigkeit *f*, innerer Widerspruch *m*, Unvereinbarkeit *f*

inconsistent inkonsistent, unstetig, widerspruchsvoll, sich widersprechend, inkonsequent, unvereinbar

incontinence Unenthaltsamkeit *f*, sexuelle Unmäßigkeit *f*, Inkontinenz *f* / **~ of the faeces** unfreiwilliger Abgang *m* von Stuhl, Enkopresis *f*, fäkale Inkontinenz *f* / **~ of speech** Geschwätzigkeit *f* / **~ of urine** Blaseninkontinenz *f*, Harninkontinenz *f*, unwillkürliches Harnlassen *n* / **faecal ~** unfreiwilliger Abgang *m* von Stuhl, Enkopresis *f*, fäkale Inkontinenz *f* / **urinary ~** Harninkontinenz *f*, Blaseninkontinenz *f*, unwillkürliches Harnlassen *n*

incontinent unmäßig, ohne Selbstbeherrschung, nicht enthaltsam

incoordination fehlende Koordination *f*, mangelndes Zusammenspiel *n*, Inkoordination *f* / **~ test** Test *m* zur Feststellung von Koordinationsstörungen / **motor ~** fehlende motorische Koordination *f*

incorporation Inkorporation *f*, Einverleibung *f* / **oral ~** orale Einverleibung *f*

incorrigible unverbesserlich

increment Zuwachs *m*, Zunahme *f* / **~ of intensity** Intensitätsanstieg *m* / **~ of stimulus strength** Zunahme *f* der Reizstärke / **~ threshold** Unterschiedsschwelle *f* / **social ~** sozial bedingte Leistungssteigerung *f*

incremental Steigerungs–, Zuwachs–

incretion innere Sekretion *f*, Inkretion *f*

incubation Inkubation *f*

incubator Brutkasten *m*, Wärmebett *n*, Inkubator *m*

incubus Inkubus *m*, männlicher Dämon *m* der mit schlafenden Frauen geschlechtlich verkehrt, Alptraum *m*

inculcation Einschärfung *f*, drillmäßiges Einüben *n*

inculpation Beschuldigung *f*, Vorwurf *m*, Tadel *m*

incurable unheilbar

incus Amboss *m*

indecency Unanständigkeit *f*, Unschicklichkeit *f*, Unzucht *f* / **~ with dependants** Unzucht *f* mit Abhängigen

indecent unschicklich, unanständig, ungehörig

indecision Unentschlossenheit *f*, Unschlüssigkeit *f*

indefinite unbestimmt, unklar, undeutlich

indefinitive unbestimmt, indeterminiert

indemnity Entschädigung *f*, Schadenersatz *m*, Abfindung *f* / **~ neurosis** Entschädigungsneurose *f*, Assekurose *f*

independence Unabhängigkeit *f*

independent unabhängig, selbständig / Unabhängiger *m*, Selbständiger *m*

indeterminate unbestimmt, unbestimmbar, indeterminiert

indeterminism Indeterminismus *m*

index Index *m*, Kennziffer *f* / **~ of consistency** Konsistenzindex *m* / **~ of determination** Determinationsindex *m*, Determinationskoeffizient *m* / **~ of discrimination** Diskriminationsindex *m* / **~ of dispersion** Streuungsindex *m* / **~ of flexibil-**

ity Flexibilitätsindex *m* / ~ **of forcasting efficiency** Index *m* der Vorhersagegenauigkeit / ~ **of independence** Homogenitätsindex *m* / ~ **of precision** Genauigkeitsindex *m* / ~ **of refraction** Brechungsindex *m* / ~ **of reliability** Reliabilitätsindex *m* / ~ **of responsiveness** Sensibilitätsindex *m* / ~ **of sinistrality** Index *m* der Linkshändigkeit / **anatomical** ~ Knochenbildungsindex *m* / **cephalic** ~ Schädelindex *m* / **cranial** ~ Schädelindex *m* / **morphological** ~ morphologischer Index *m* / **orbital** ~ Index *m* der Augenhöhle (Länge zu Höhe) / **predictive** ~ Index *m* der Vorhersagegenauigkeit / **refractive** ~ Brechungsindex *m* / **therapeutic** ~ therapeutische Breite *f*

indicant Indikator *m*, Anzeichen *n*, Symptom *n*

indicate anzeigen, hinweisen

indication Indikation *f*, Hinweis *m*, Zeichen *n*

indicator Indikator *m*, Zeichen *n*, Anzeichen *n* / ~ **of a complex** Komplexanzeichen *n* / ~ **yellow** Indikatorgelb *n* / **mechanical** ~ mechanisches Messgerät *n*

indices Indizes *mpl*, Kennziffern *fpl*

indifference Indifferenz *f*, Gleichgültigkeit *f*, Teilnahmslosigkeit *f*, Gefühlsleere *f* / ~ **point** Indifferenzpunkt *m* / ~ **zone** Indifferenzbereich *m* / **sexual** ~ Frigidität *f*, Geschlechtskälte *f*

indifferent gleichgültig, gemütlos, neutral, indifferent

indigenous eingeboren, einheimisch / Eingeborene(r) *m,f*

indirect indirekt, mittelbar

indirection Umweg *m*, List *f*

indiscipline Mangel *m* an Disziplin

indisposition Unpässlichkeit *f*, Abgeneigtheit *f*, Abneigung *f*

indissociation Undifferenziertheit *f*, undifferenzierte Wahrnehmung *f*

indistinct ungegliedert, undifferenziert

indistinctness Undeutlichkeit *f*, mangelnde Gliederung *f*

individual Individuum *n* / individuell, einzeln, Persönlichkeits–

individualisation Individualisierung *f*

individualism Individualismus *m*

individualist Individualist *m*

individualistic individualistisch

individuality Individualität *f*, Persönlichkeit *f* / **graphic** ~ Schriftpersönlichkeit *f*, individuelle Eigenart *f* der Schrift

individualize individualisieren

individuation Individuation *f*, Entfaltung *f* der Persönlichkeit / ~ **process** Prozess *m* der Persönlichkeitsentfaltung

indoctrination Unterweisung *f*, Belehrung *f*, Indoktrination *f*

indolence Indolenz *f*, Trägheit *f*, Schmerzlosigkeit *f*

indolent indolent, träge, unempfindlich, schmerzlos

indomitable unbezähmbar

induce veranlassen, verursachen, überreden, induzieren, durch Induktion ableiten, schließen

induced erzeugt, induziert

inducement Anreiz *m*, Beweggrund *m*, Lockmittel *n*

induction Induktion *f*, Einführung *f* / ~ **coil** Induktionsspule *f* / ~ **of sleep** Schlaferzeugung *f* / ~ **test** Induktionstest *m* / **cortical** ~ Großhirnrindeninduktion *f*, kortikale Induktion *f* / **direct spinal** ~ direkte Rückenmarksinduktion *f* / **immediate spinal** ~ unmittelbare Rückenmarksinduktion *f* / **mathematical** ~ mathematische Schlussfolgerung *f* / **negative** ~ negative Induktion *f* / **neural** ~ neurale Induktion *f* / **perceptual** ~ Wahrnehmungsinduktion *f* / **positive** ~ positive Induktion *f* / **reciprocal** ~ reziproke Induktion *f* / **simultaneous** ~ gleichzeitige Induktion *f* / **sympathetic** ~ Sympathie–Induktion *f*, Handlungsangleichung *f* / **visual** ~ optische Induktion *f*

inductive induktiv, Induktions–

indulgence Nachsicht *f*, Gewährenlassen *n*, Toleranz *f* / **parental ~** Nachsicht *f* von Seiten der Eltern

indulgent nachsichtig, schonend

industrial industriell, Industrie–, Arbeits–, Betriebs–

industrialisation Industrialisierung *f*

industrious fleißig

inebriate betrunken, berauscht / betrunken machen / Betrunkener *m*, Trunkenbold *m*

inebriation Trunkenheit *f*, Rausch *m*, Rauschzustand *m*

inebriety Trunksucht *f*, Trunkenheit *f*, Alkoholismus *m*

ineducability Unerziehbarkeit *f*

ineducable unerziehbar

ineffable unsagbar, unaussprechlich

ineffective wirkungslos, unwirksam

ineffectiveness Unwirksamkeit *f*, Wirkungslosigkeit *f*

inefficacy Unwirksamkeit *f*, Erfolglosigkeit *f*

inefficiency Leistungsschwäche *f*, Unwirtschaftlichkeit *f*, Ineffizienz *f*

inefficient unfähig, untauglich, ineffizient

inequality Ungleichheit *f*, Verschiedenheit *f* / **educational ~** ungleiche Bildung *f*

inert träge, inaktiv, untätig

inertia, inertness Trägheit *f*, Untätigkeit *f*, Arbeitsunlust *f* / **general mental ~~** allgemeine Denkfaulheit *f*, Perseverationstendenz *f* / **mental ~** Denkfaulheit *f*

inexcitability Unerregbarkeit *f*

inexcitable unerregbar, nicht erregbar

inexperienced unerfahren, nicht geübt

inexpressive ausdruckslos, nichtssagend

infancy Säuglingsalter *n*, Säuglingsperiode *f*, Säuglingszeit *f*, frühes Kindesalter *n*

infant Säugling *m*, Kleinkind *n*, Baby *n* / kindlich, jung / **~ behaviour** frühkindliches Verhalten *n* / **~ development** Entwicklung *f* des Kleinkindes, frühkindliche Entwicklung *f*, Entwicklung *f* im Säuglings– und Kleinkindalter / **~ intelligence scale** Intelligenzskala *f* für Kleinkinder / **~ psychology** Psychologie *f* des Kleinkindes / **~ test** Entwicklungstest *m* für Kleinkinder / **~ vocalisation** Kleinkindersprache *f* / **new–born ~** Neugeborenes *n* / **premature ~** Frühgeburt *f* / **sudden ~ death** plötzlicher Säuglingstod *m*

infanticide Kindestötung *f*

infantile infantil, Kleinkind–, Kindheits–

infantilism Infantilismus *m*, Entwicklungshemmung *f*, Stehenbleiben *n* auf kindlicher Entwicklungsstufe / **late ~** Späteunuchoidismus *m* / **sexual ~** sexueller Infantilismus *m*

infantility Kindlichkeit *f*

infarction, infarct Infarkt *m* / **myocardial ~** Myokardinfarkt *m*, Herzinfarkt *m*

infatuation erotische Zuneigung *f* von kurzer Dauer, Vernarrtheit *f*, Schwärmerei *f*

infavoidance need Bedürfnis *n* Demütigungen zu vermeiden

infection Infektion *f*, Entzündung *f* / **cerebral ~** zerebrale Infektion *f* / **psychic ~** Induktionskrankheit *f*

infecund steril, unfruchtbar

infecundity Sterilität *f*, Unfruchtbarkeit *f*

infer schließen, folgern, ableiten

inference Folgerung *f*, Schluss, Inferenz *f*, Schlussfolgerung *f* / **statistical ~** statistische Inferenz *f* / **unconscious ~** unbewusste Folgerung *f*

inferior untergeordnet, gering, minderwertig, untere (r, s) / **~ oblique** musculus obliquus inferior *m* / **~ rectus** musculus rectus inferior *m* / **constitutionally ~** konstitutionell minderwertig

inferiority Minderwertigkeit *f*, Unterlegenheit *f* / **~ complex** Minderwertigkeitskomplex *m* / **~ feeling** Minderwertigkeitsgefühl *n*, Minderwertigkeitskomplex *m* / **emotional ~** emotionale Minderwertigkeit *f* / **functional ~** minderwertige Funktion *f* / **general ~** allgemeine Minderwertigkeit *f* / **morphological ~** Minderwertigkeit *f* von Organen, körperliche Unzulänglichkeiten *fpl* / **organic ~** Organminderwertigkeit *f*, Minderwertigkeit *f* von Organen

infertile unfruchtbar, infertil, steril

infertility Unfruchtbarkeit *f*, Infertilität, Sterilität *f*

infibulation Verschluss *m* der Genitalöffnung, Genitalienverschluss *m*, Infibulation *f*

infinite Unendlichkeit *f* / unendlich, endlos

infinitesimal Infinitesimal–, unendlich klein

infinity Unendlichkeit *f*, unendliche Menge *f*

infirm schwach, kränklich, hinfällig

infirmity Schwäche *f*, Gebrechlichkeit *f*, Hinfälligkeit *f* / **~ of purpose** Unentschlossenheit *f*

inflated aufgeblasen

inflation Inflation *f*, Aufgeblasenheit *f* / **ego ~** Inflation *f* des Ichs

inflection, inflexion Biegung *f*, Flexion *f*, Modulation *f*

inflexible starr, inflexibel, rigide

inflexidia Starrheit *f* / **tense ~** angespannte Starrheit *f*

inflow of stimulus Reizzufuhr *f*

influence Einfluss *m*, Einwirkung *f*, Beeinflussung *f*, Einflusnahme *f*, Macht *f* / beeinflussen, einwirken / **~ delusion** Beeinflussungswahn *m* / **cultural ~** kultureller Einfluss *m* / **environmental ~** Umgebungseinfluss *m*, Milieuwirkung *f*, Umwelteinfluss *m* / **hormonal~** Hormoneinwirkung *f* / **interpersonal ~** interpersonaler Einfluss *m* / **mutual ~** gegenseitige Beeinflussung *f* / **parental ~** elterlicher Einfluss *m* / **personal ~** persönlicher Einfluss *m* / **prenatal ~** pränataler Einfluss *m* / **social ~** sozialer Einfluss *m*, Einfluss *m* aufgrund von Status oder Position / **stimulating ~** Reizeinfluss *m*, Reizeinwirkung *f*

influential einflussreich, von Einfluss

influenza Grippe *f*

influx Zufluss *m*, Zufuhr *f* / **~ of stimuli** Reizzufuhr *f* / **continuous ~ of impulses** Dauerreizüberflutung *f* / **luminous ~** Lichtstrom *m*

inform unterrichten, informieren, benachrichtigen

informal informell, formlos

informant Informant *m*, Gewährsmann *m*, Berichterstatter *m*

information Information *f*, Nachricht *f*, Mitteilung *f*, Informationsgehalt *m* / **~ coding** Informationsverschlüsselung *f* / **~ density** Informationsdichte *f* / **~ exchange** Informationsaustausch *m* / **~ feedback** Informationsrückfluss *m* / **~ flow** Informationsfluss *m* / **~ pedagogics** Informationspädagogik *f* / **~ processing** Informationsverarbeitung *f*, Nachrichtenverarbeitung *f* / **~ psychology** Informationspsychologie *f* / **~ seeking** Informationssuche *f* / **~ service** Informationsdienst *m* / **~ storage** Informationsspeicher *m* / **~ system** Informationssystem *n* / **~ test** Informationstest *m* / **~ theory** Informationstheorie *f* / **~ transfer** Informationsübertragung *f* / **adapted ~** angepasste Information *f* / **automated ~ coding** vollautomatische Kodierung *f*, automatisierte Informationskodierung *f* / **automated ~ processing** automatische Informationsverarbeitung *f* / **automated ~ retrieval** automatische Informationsgewinnung *f* / **automated ~ storage** automatische Informationsspeicherung *f* / **cognitive ~** kognitive Information *f* / **genetic ~** genetische Information *f*, Erbinformation *f*, Erbsubstanz *f* / **human ~ process** kognitiver Prozess *m* / **human ~ storage** Informationsspeicher *m* des Menschen, menschliches Gedächtnis *n* / **memorial ~** Gedächtnisinformation *f* / **selective ~** selektive Information *f* / **semantical ~** semantische Information *f* / **transient ~** Momentaninformation *f*, flüchtige Information *f*

informational Informations–, informatorisch

infraaudible unterhalb der Hörgrenze

infraconscious unterbewusst

infraction Übertretung *f*, Verletzung *f* / **minor ~** geringfügige Übertretung *f*

infrahuman infrahuman, tierisch

infraliminary unterschwellig

infralogical prälogisch, vorlogisch

infrapsychic unterhalb der Bewusstseinsschwelle

infrared infrarot

infrasonic unter der Hörgrenze

infravertive infravertiv, nach unten gerichtet

infundibulum Infundibulum *n*

ingestion Aufnahme *f*, Einnehmen *n*

ingoing introvertiert

ingoingness introversive Haltung *f*, Introversion *f*

ingratiation Einschmeicheln *n*, Gewinnen *n* von Gunst, Sich–Beliebtmachen *n*, Ingratiation *f*

ingratitude Undankbarkeit *f*

in–group Eigengruppe *f*, Wir–Gruppe *f*, In–Group *f*

inhalant Inhalationsmittel *n*, Inhalans *n* / **~ abuse** Inhalantienmissbrauch *m*, Schnüffelsucht *f* / **~ dependence** Inhalantienabhängigkeit *f* / **~–induced** inhalantieninduziert / **~ intoxication** Inhalantienintoxikation *f* / **~ intoxication delirium** Inhalantienintoxikationsdelir *n* / **~–related** im Zusammenhang mit Inhalantien / **~ use** Inhalantienkonsum *m*

inhalation Einatmung *f*, Inhalation *f*

inherence, inherency Inhärenz *f*, Immanenz *f* / **~ effect** Immanenzgesetz *n*

inherent inhärent

inherit erben, ererben

inheritance Vererbung *f*, Heredität *f* / **biparental ~** Vererbung *f* von beiden Elternteilen / **blending ~** Mischerbigkeit *f* / **Mendelian ~** Vererbung *f* nach den Mendel'schen Gesetzen / **nulliplex ~** Vererbung *f* zweier gleicherbig rezessiver Merkmale / **simplex ~** einfache Vererbung *f*

inherited vererbt, angeboren

inhibit hemmen, inhibieren, unterbinden

inhibitable hemmbar

inhibited gehemmt

inhibitedness Hemmung *f*, Inhibition *f* / **timid ~** schüchterne Gehemmtheit *f*

inhibiting hemmend

inhibition Hemmung *f*, Inhibition *f* / **~ of delay** Verzögerungshemmung *f* / **~ of expression** Ausdruckshemmung *f* / **~ neurosis** Hemmungsneurose *f* / **~ potential** Hemmungspotenzial *n* / **~ reinforcement** Hemmungsverstärkung *f* / **~ of thinking** Denkhemmung *f* / **~ of thought** Hemmung *f* des Gedankenganges / **~ zone** Hemmzone *f* / **affective ~** affektive Hemmung *f* / **associative ~** assoziative Hemmung *f* / **autogenic ~** interne Hemmung *f*, autogene Hemmung *f*, Selbsthemmung *f* / **behavioural ~ system** Verhaltenshemmsystem *n* / **central ~** zentrale Hemmung *f* / **conditioned ~** konditionierte Hemmung *f* / **conditioned reactive ~** konditionierte reaktive Hemmung *f* / **connective ~** Beziehungshemmung *f* / **cortical ~** kortikale Hemmung *f* / **descending ~** absteigende Hemmung *f* / **differential ~** Differenzierung *f*, Unterscheidungshemmung *f* / **ecphoric ~** Erinnerungshemmung *f* / **external ~** externe Hemmung *f*, äußere Hemmung *f* / **extinctive ~** Löschungshemmung *f*, experimentelle Löschung *f* / **internal ~** interne Hemmung *f*, innere Hemmung *f* / **intrinsic ~** innere Hemmung *f* / **latent ~** latente Hemmung *f* / **lateral ~** Seitenhemmung *f*, Umfeldhemmung *f* / **motor ~** motorische Hemmung *f* / **nervous ~** nervöse Hemmung *f* / **postexcitatory ~** Hemmung *f* nach einer Reizung / **postsynaptic ~** postsynaptische Hemmung *f* / **presynaptic ~** präsynaptische Hemmung *f* / **proactive ~** proaktive Hemmung *f* / **protective ~** Schutzhemmung *f* / **reactive ~** reaktive Hemmung *f* / **reciprocal ~** reziproke Hemmung *f* / **reciprocal ~ therapy** Verhaltenstherapie *f* durch reziproke Hemmung *f* / **reproductive ~** reproduktive Hemmung *f*, rückwirkende Hemmung *f* / **retroactive ~** retroaktive Hemmung *f*, negative Hemmung *f*, rückwirkende Hemmung *f* / **social ~** soziale Hemmung *f* / **terminal ~** höchster Hemmgrad *m* / **vocational ~** berufliche Hemmung *f*

inhibitive, inhibitory hemmend, Hemmungs–

inhibitor Inhibitor *m*, Hemmungsnerv *m*, Hemmer *m*, Hemmstoff *m*

inion Protuberanz *f* des Hinterhauptbeines

initial anfänglich, Anfangs–, Initial–

initiate beginnen, in Gang setzen, einweihen / eingeführt, eingeweiht / Eingeweihter *m*, Anfänger *m*

initiation Einweihung *f*, Einführung *f*, Initiation *f* / **~ ceremony** Initiationszeremonie *f*, Reifeweihe *f*, Initien *fpl* / **~ rites** Initiationsriten *fpl*, Initien *fpl*

initiative Initiative *f*, Entschlusskraft *f*, Anstoß *m*, Anregung *f*

initiator Initiator *m*, Urheber *m*, Anreger *m*, Sender *m*

initiatory beginnend, einführend, zur Einweihung dienend

injection Injektion *f*, Spritze *f* / **hypodermic ~** subkutane Injektion *f* / **intracutancous ~** intrakutane Injektion *f* / **intramuscular ~** intramuskuläre Injektion *f* / **intraperitoneal ~** intraperitoneale Injektion *f*, Spritze *f* in den Bauchraum / **intraspinal ~** lumbale Injektion *f* / **intravenous ~** intravenöse Injektion *f* / **sedative ~** Beruhigungsspritze *f* / **subcutaneous ~** subkutane Injektion *f*

injury Verletzung *f*, Schadigung *f*, Schaden *m*, Trauma *n* / **~ to the head** Kopfverletzung *f* / **~ due to light** Lichtschädigung *f* / **cerebral ~** Gehirnschädigung *f* / **electrical ~** Verletzung *f* durch elektrischen Strom / **industrial ~** Betriebsunfall *m*, Berufsschädigung *f*

injustice Ungerechtigkeit *f*, Unrecht *n*

inkblot test Tintenklecks–Test *m*

inlaw angeheirateter Verwandter *m*

inlooking introspektiv

inmate Insasse *m*, Mitbewohner *m*, Sträfling *m*

innate angeboren

inner inner, Innen– / **~–directed** innengeleitet

innervate innervieren, anregen

innervation Innervation *f*, Erregung *f* / **~ apraxia** Innervationsapraxie *f* / **~ ratio** Innervationsquotient *m* / **inhibitory ~** hemmende Innervation *f* / **motor ~** motorische Innervation *f* / **multiple ~** multiple Innervation *f* / **reciprocal ~** reziproke Innervation *f* / **segmental ~** segmentäre Innervation *f* / **sensory ~** sensorische Innervation *f*

innovation Neuerung *f*, Erfindung *f*, Innovation *f*

innovative Innovations–, Neuerungs–

innovativeness Neuerungsverhalten *n*, Innovationsverhalten *n*

inoculation Impfung *f*, Impfmethode *f*

inositol triphosphate Phosphoinositol *n*

in–patient Krankenhauspatient *m*, stationärer Patient *m*

in–phase Phasengleichklang *m*

input Eingangsenergie *f*, Eingangsinformation *f*, Eingangsvariable *f*, Eingabe *f*, Input *m* / **~ channel** Eingabekanal *m* / **~ data** Eingabedaten *npl* / **~ equivocation** Sendeäquivokation *f* / **~ impedance** Eingangswiderstand *m*, Eingangsimpedanz *f* / **~–output** Eingabe *f* –Ausgabe *f* / **~ quantity** Eingangsgröße *f* / **~ rate** Lerngeschwindigkeit *f* / **~ resistance** Eingangswiderstand *m* / **~ signal** Eingangsgröße *f*, Eingabesignal *n* / **~ stimulus** Eingangsreiz *m* / **afferent ~** afferenter Einstrom *m*

inquilinism Schmarotzertum *n*, Symbiose *f*

inquire erforschen

inquirer Untersucher *m*, Forscher *m*

inquiry, inquest Erforschung *f*, Forschung *f*, Untersuchung *f*, Befragung *f* / ~ **method** Befragungsmethode *f*, Erhebungsmethode *f*

inquisitiveness Neugierde *f*

insane geisteskrank, verrückt, irrsinnig, wahnsinnig

insanity Geisteskrankheit *f*, Geistesstörung *f*, Psychose *f*, Irresein *n*, Wahnsinn *m*, Insania *f* / ~ **of grandeur** Größenwahn *m*, Megalomanie *f* / **adolescent~** Jugendirresein *n*, Hebephrenie *f* / **affective** ~ Affektpsychose *f* / **alcoholic** ~ Alkoholpsychose *f* / **alternating** ~ manisch– depressives Irresein *n* / **circular** ~ zirkuläres Irresein *n*, manisch–depressives Irresein *n* / **compound** ~ Mischpsychose *f* / **compulsive** ~ Zwangspsychose *f* / **cyclic** ~ zyklische Psychose *f*, zirkuläres Irresein *n* / **depressive** ~ Depression *f*, Depressionszustand *m* / **developmental** ~ Entwicklungspsychose *f* / **emotional** ~ Affektpsychose *f* / **hebephrenic** ~ Hebephrenie *f*, Jugendirresein *n* / **hereditary** ~ erbliche Psychose *f* / **induced** ~ induziertes Irresein *n*, Folie à deux *f* / **lactational** ~ Schwangerschaftspsychose *f* / **manic–depressive** ~ manisch–depressives Irresein *n* / **melancholic** ~ Melancholie *f*, Depression *f* / **moral** ~ moralischer Schwachsinn *n*, „moral insanity" *f* / **perceptual** ~ halluzinatorische Psychose *f* / **periodic** ~ zirkuläres Irresein *n*, zyklische Psychose *f*, periodisches Irresein *n* / **polyneuritic** ~ Korsakow–Psychose *f* / **puerperal** ~ Wochenbettpsychose *f*, Puerperalpsychose *f* / **recurrent** ~ rezidivierende Psychose *f* / **religious** ~ Religionswahn *m*, religioser Wahnsinn *m*, Theomanie *f* / **senile** ~ Alterspsychose *f* / **suicidal** ~ Selbstmordwahn *m* / **toxic** ~ Intoxikationspsychose *f*

insect Insekt *n* / **social** ~ Staaten bildendes Insekt *n*

insecure unsicher

insecurity Unsicherheit *f* / **emotional** ~ emotionale Unsicherheit *f*

insemination Befruchtung *f*, Besamung *f* / **artificial** ~ künstliche Befruchtung *f*

insenescence Altwerden *n*, Altern *n*, Alterungsprozess *m*

insensibility, insensitivity Unempfindlichkeit *f*, Gleichgültigkeit *f*, Gefühllosigkeit *f*

insensible, insensitive unempfindlich, gleichgültig, gefühllos, besinnungslos

inservice berufsbegleitend

insight Einsicht *f*, Einsichtsvermögen *n* / ~ **learning** Lernen *n* durch Einsicht / ~ **therapy** Einsichtstherapie *f*

insightful einsichtig

insignificance Bedeutungslosigkeit *f*

insincerity Unaufrichtigkeit *f*, Falschheit *f*

insistence Beharren *n*, Nachdruck *m*, Eindringlichkeit *f* / ~ **of a colour** Anziehungskraft *f* einer Farbe

insistent beharrlich, eindringlich, nachdrucksvoll, stark

in situ an Ort und Stelle, in seiner (ihrer) natürlichen Lage

insobriety Unmäßigkeit *f*, Trunkenheit *f*

insociable nicht umgänglich, ungesellig

insolence Unverschämtheit *f*, Frechheit *f*

insolent anmaßend, unverschämt, frech

insomnia Schlaflosigkeit *f*, Asomnie *f* / ~ **type** Insomnie–Typus *m* / **fatal familial** ~ fatale familiäre Schlaflosigkeit *f* / **intermittent** ~ Durchschlafstörung *f* / **mild** ~ leichte Schlaflosigkeit *f* / **nonorganic** ~ nichtorganische Insomnie *f* / **primary** ~ primäre Insomnie *f*

inspection Untersuchung *f*, Beobachtung *f*, Introspektion *f* / ~ **mode** Modalwert *m* / **~–technique** Auswertungsmethode *f*

inspiration Einatmung *f*, Inspiration *f*, Eingebung *f*, plötzlicher Einfall *m* / **~–expiration ratio** Verhältnis *n* von Einatmungsdauer zu Ausatmungsdauer

inspire einatmen, veranlassen, begeistern, inspirieren

instability Unbeständigkeit *f*, Unstetigkeit *f*, Labilität *f*, Unausgeglichenheit *f*, Unsicherheit *f* / **affective ~** Affektlabilität *f* / **emotional ~** emotionale Labilität *f*, Affektlabilität *f*

instable unbeständig, unstetig, labil

instance Beispiel *n*, Instanz *f*

instant Augenblick *m*, Moment *m* / unmittelbar, sofortig

instantaneous augenblicklich, sofortig

instigate anreizen, anregen, motivieren, stimulieren

instigation Anregung *f*, Motivierung *f*, Stimulierung *f*

instigator treibende Kraft *f*, motivierende Person *f*

instinct Instinkt *m*, Trieb *m* / **~ of construction** Bautrieb *m* / **~ derivate** Instinktderivat *n* / **~ of destruction** Destruktionstrieb *m* / **~ disturbance** Triebstörung *f* / **~ of dominance** Machttrieb *m* / **~ to master** Machttrieb *m* / **~ of nutrition** Nahrungstrieb *m* / **~ of play** Spieltrieb *m* / **~ of self–destruction** Selbstzerstörungstrieb *m* / **~ of self–preservation** Selbsterhaltungstrieb *m* / **acquisitive ~** Sammeltrieb *m*, Erwerbssucht *f* / **aggressive ~** Aggressionstrieb *m* / **collecting ~** Sammeltrieb *m* / **complementary ~s** Komplementartriebe *mpl* / **delayed ~** spätentwickelter Instinkt *m* / **derivative ~** Instinktabkömmling *m* / **destructive ~** Destruktionstrieb *m* / **fundamental ~** Grundtrieb *m* / **generative ~** Fortpflanzungstrieb *m* / **gregarious ~** Herdentrieb *m* / **imitative ~** Nachahmungstrieb *m* / **investigatory ~** Forschungstrieb *m* / **maternal ~** Mutterinstinkt *m* / **natural ~** Naturtrieb *m* / **nutritional ~** Nahrungstrieb *m* / **partial ~** Partialtrieb *m* / **passive ~** passiver Trieb *m* / **possessive ~** Machttrieb *m*, Besitzstreben *n* / **primal ~** Urtrieb *m*, Grundtrieb *m* / **procreative ~** Fortpflanzungstrieb *m* / **protective ~** Schutztrieb *m* / **religious ~** religiöser Trieb *m* / **sexual ~** Sexualtrieb *m*, Geschlechtstrieb *m* / **social ~** Geselligkeitstrieb *m*, sozialer Trieb *m* / **unsatisfied ~s** unbefriedigte Triebe *mpl*

instinctive instinktiv, instinktmäßig

instinctivist Anhänger *m* der Instinkttheorie

instinctivity Triebhaftigkeit *f*

instinctoid triebartig, fundamental

instinctual triebhaft, triebmäßig

institution Institution *f*, Einrichtung *f* / **~ visitation** Besuch *m* bei Häftlingen / **correctional ~** Besserungsanstalt *f*, Strafanstalt *f*, Strafvollzugseinrichtung *f* / **social ~** soziale Institution *f*

institutional institutionell, institutionalisiert, festgelegt

institutionalisation Institutionalisierung *f*, Einrichtung *f*, Anstaltsunterbringung *f*

institutionalise institutionalisieren, in einer Anstalt unterbringen, verwahren

institutionalism Institutionalismus *m*

instruct unterrichten, unterweisen, lehren, informieren, anweisen

instruction Unterweisung *f*, Unterricht *m*, Anweisung *f*, Ausbildung *f*, Instruktion *f* / **~ manual** Testanweisung *f* / **~ test** Schultest *m*, Schulleistungstest *m* / **~ for use** Gebrauchsanweisung *f* / **audio–visual ~** audiovisueller Unterricht *m*, audiovisuelle Unterweisung *f*, Unterricht *m* mit Lehrtonfilmen / **experimental ~** Versuchsanweisung *f*, Versuchsinstruktion *f* / **individualised ~** Einzelunterricht *m*, individualisierter Unterricht *m* / **programmed ~** programmierte Unterweisung *f*, programmierte Instruktion *f*, programmierter Unterricht *m* / **remedial ~** Sonderunterricht *m* / **televised ~** Fernsehunterricht *m*, fernsehunterstützter Unterricht *m*, Schulfernsehen *n* / **visual ~** Anschauungsunterricht *m*

instructional Unterrichts–, Erziehungs–, Lehr–, Unterweisungs–

instructive lehrreich

instructor Unterweiser *m*, Ausbilder *m*, Lehrer *m*, Dozent *m*

instrument Werkzeug *n*, Instrument *n*, Hilfsmittel *n* / **~ control** Instrumentensteuerung *f* / **~ of precision** Präzisionsinstrument *n* / **musical ~** Musikinstrument *n* / **scientific ~** wissenschaftliches Verfahren *n*, wissenschaftliche Methode *f*, wissenschaftliches Hilfsmittel *n* / **stereotactic ~** stereotaktisches Instrument *n*

instrumental instrumentell, mit einem Hilfsmittel, als Werkzeug dienend

instrumentality Instrumentalität *f*

insufficiency Unzulänglichkeit *f*, Untauglichkeit *f*, Minderwertigkeit *f*, Insuffizienz *f* / **~ feeling** Minderwertigkeitsgefühl *n*, Insuffizienzgefühl *n* / **coronary ~** Koronarinsuffizienz *f*

insufficient unzulänglich, untauglich, insuffizient

insula Insula *f*, Insula Reili *f*, Insel *f*

insulation Isolierung *f* / **emotional ~** Affektisolierung *f*

insulin Insulin *n* / **~-antagonistic** Insulin antagonistisch / **~ coma** hypoglykämisches Koma *n* / **~ coma therapy** Insulinkomabehandlung *f* / **~ deficiency** Insulinmangel *m* / **~ shock** Insulinschock *m* / **~-shock therapy** Insulintherapie *f*, Insulinschocktherapie *f*

insulinisation Insulinbehandlung *f*, Insulintherapie *f*

insult Beleidigung *f*, Insult *m* / beleidigen, beschimpfen

insulting beleidigend, Schmäh–

insupportable unerträglich, unausstehlich

insurance Versicherung *f* / **~ neurosis** Rentenneurose *f* / **social ~** Sozialversicherung *f*

insurgent aufrührerisch / Aufrührer *m*, Rebell *m*

insurmountable unüberwindbar

insusceptibility Unempfindlichkeit *f*, Unempfänglichkeit *f*

insusceptible unempfindlich, unzugänglich

intact unbeschädigt, funktionierend, intakt

intake Aufnahme *f*, Einlass *m* / **~ interview** Erstinterview *n* / **~-rejection hypothesis** Hypothese *f* von der Abhängigkeit der Reizverarbeitung von der Herzleistung

integer ganze Zahl *f* / ganzzahlig

integral vollständig, Integral– / Integral *n*

integrality Vollständigkeit *f*

integrant integrierend, wesentlich, notwendig

integrate vervollständigen, integrieren, ergänzen

integrating integrierend, wesentlich, wichtig

integration Integration *f*, Eingliederung *f*, Assimilation *f* / **~ of behaviour** Verhaltensintegration *f* / **~ of personality** Integration *f* der Persönlichkeit / **binocular ~** binokulare Verschmelzung *f* / **cerebral ~** Integration *f* im Gehirn / **educational ~** schulische Integration *f* / **primary ~** primäre Integration *f* / **racial ~** Aufhebung *f* der Rassentrennung / **secondary ~** sekundäre Integration *f* / **sensory ~** sensorische Integration *f* / **social ~** soziale Integration *f*, Eingliederung *f* in die Gesellschaft

integrative integrierend, Integrations–

integrity Vollständigkeit *f*, Unversehrtheit *f*, Integrität *f*, Rechtschaffenheit *f* / **~ testing** Testung *f* der Ehrlichkeit

intellect Intellekt *m*, Verstand *m*, Denkfähigkeit *f* / **passive ~** passiver Verstand *m*

intellection Verstehen *n*, Begreifen *n*, Gedanke *m*, Begriff *m*

intellective verstandesmäßig, Verstandes–, denkend

intellectual verstandesmäßig, gedanklich, geistig, intellektuell, intelligent, begabt, vernünftig, gebildet, klug

intellectualism Intellektualismus *m*, Idealismus *m*, Rationalismus *m*

intellectualistic intellektualistisch

intellectualisation Intellektualisierung *f*

intellectuality Verstandeskraft *f*, Intellektualität *f*, Intelligenz *f*

intelligence Intelligenz *f*, Denkfähigkeit *f*, Verstand *m* / **~ coefficient** Intelligenzkoeffizient *m* / **~ level** Intelligenzniveau *n* / **~ measure** Intelligenzmaß *n*, Intelligenzwert *m* / **~ quotient** Intelligenzquotient *m* / **~ scale** Intelligenzskala *f*, Messverfahren *n* zur Bestimmung der Intelligenz / **~ test** Intelligenztest *m* / **~ testing** Intelligenzmessung *f* / **abstract ~** theoretische Intelligenz *f* / **academic ~** hohe theoretische Denkfähigkeit *f*, akademische Intelligenz *f* / **aesthetic ~** ästhetische Intelligenz *f*, künstlerische Befähigung *f* / **artificial ~** künstliche Intelligenz *f* / **biological ~** biologische Intelligenz *f* / **borderline ~** Intelligenz *f* im Grenzbereich zur Debilität / **conceptual ~** begriffliche Intelligenz *f*, abstrakte Intelligenz *f* / **concrete ~** praktische Intelligenz *f* / **defective ~** Intelligenzdefekt *m*, Intelligenzmangel *m* / **esthetic ~** ästhetische Intelligenz *f* / **functional ~ level** Funktionsebene *f* der Intelligenz / **general ~** Intelligenz *f*, allgemeine Intelligenz *f* / **innate ~** angeborene Intelligenz *f* / **marginal ~** Intelligenz *f* im Grenzbereich zur Debilität / **measured ~** gemessene Intelligenz *f* / **mechanical ~** mechanisch–technische Intelligenz *f* / **mechanical ~ test** Test *m* der technischen Begabung / **nonverbal ~** nicht–verbale Intelligenz *f*, sprachfreie Intelligenz *f* / **psychometric ~** Intelligenzrohwert *m* / **reproductive ~** reproduktive Intelligenz *f* / **sensorimotor ~** sensumotorische Intelligenz *f* / **social ~** soziale Intelligenz *f* / **superior ~** höhere Intelligenz *f* / **verbal ~** verbale Intelligenz *f*, sprachliche Intelligenz *f*

intelligent intelligent, verständig

intelligibility Verständlichkeit *f*, Klarheit *f* des Ausdrucks

intelligible verständlich, klar

intemperance Unmäßigkeit *f*, Unbeherrschtheit *f*, Trunksucht *f*

intend beabsichtigen

intensification Intensivierung *f*, Verstärkung *f*

intension Begriffsinhalt *m*, Bedeutung *f*

intensity Stärke *f*, Intensität *f*, Stärkegrad *m* / **~ of action** Handlungsstärke *f*, Aktionsintensität *f*, Wirkungsstärke *f* / **~ of affect** Affektbetrag *m* / **~–difference limen** Intensitätsunterschiedsschwelle *f* / **~–difference threshold** Intensitätsunterschiedsschwelle *f* / **~ discrimination** Intensitätsunterscheidung *f* / **~ level** Pegel *m*, Intensitätsniveau *n* / **~ of smell** Geruchsintensität *f* / **~ of stimulus** Reizintensität *f* / **~ of sound** Schallintensität *f* / **~ sensor** Intensitätssensor *m* / **~ theory** Intensitätstheorie *f* / **~ threshold** Intensitätsschwelle *f* / **acoustic ~ level** Schallstärkepegel *m* / **luminous ~** Lichtstärke *f* / **radiant ~** Strahlungsintensität *f*, Leuchtdichte *f* / **total ~** Gesamtintensität *f*

intensive, intense intensiv, stark

intent Absicht *f*, Vorhaben *n*, Ziel *n* / gerichtet, gespannt / **~ analysis** Bedeutungsanalyse *f*

intention Absicht *f*, Vorhaben *n*, Intention *f*, Streben *n* / **~ movement** Intentionsbewegung *f* / **~ tremor** Intentionstremor *m*, Intentionszittern *n*

intentional absichtlich, planmäßig, intentional

intentionalism Intentionalismus *m*

intentionality Gerichtetsein *n*, Intentionalität *f* / **objective ~** Objektgerichtetheit *f* / **unconscious ~** unbewusste Intentionalität *f*

intentness gespannte Aufmerksamkeit *f*, Entschlossenheit *f*/ **~ of purpose** Zielstrebigkeit *f*

interact aufeinander einwirken, wechselseitig beeinflussen, interagieren

interaction Interaktion *f*, Wechselwirkung *f*, Zusammenspiel *n*, interindividuelles Verhalten *n* / **~ analysis** Interaktionsanalyse *f* / **~–influence theory** Theorie *f* der Führung durch Interaktionswirkung / **~ ma-**

trix Interaktionsmatrix *f* / ~ **principle** Interaktionsprinzip *n* / ~ **process** Interaktionsprozess *m* / ~ **process analysis** Interaktionsprozessanalyse *f* / ~ **recorder** Gerät *n* zur Erfassung von Interaktionen / ~ **training** Interaktionstraining *n* / ~ **variance** Interaktionsvarianz *f* / **interhaemispheric** ~ Hemisphäreninteraktion *f* / **interpersonal** ~ interpersonale Interaktion *f* / **interspecies** ~ Interspeziesinteraktion *f* / **sensory** ~ Interaktion *f* der Sinne / **social** ~ soziale Interaktion *f* / **tonal** ~ Klanggestalt *f*, Zusammenspiel *n* der Klänge

interactionism Interaktionismus *m*, Wechselwirkungslehre *f* / **symbolic** ~ symbolischer Interaktionismus *m*

interactive wechselseitig beeinflussend, interaktiv

interbehaviour interindividuelles Verhalten *n*, sich gegenseitig beeinflussendes Verhalten *n*, Interaktion *f*

interbehavioural wechselwirkend, Interaktions–

interbehaviouralism Interaktionspsychologie *f*

interbrain Zwischenhirn *n*

interbreeding Kreuzung *f*, Kreuzen *n*

intercalate einschalten, einschieben, interpolieren

intercalation Einschaltung *f*, Interpolation *f*

intercept Koordinatenabschnitt *m*, Axenabschnitt *m* / abschneiden, unterbrechen, abstellen

interception Hemmung *f*, Unterbrechung *f*, Aufhalten *n*

intercerebral zwischen den Hirnhälften liegend, interhemisphärisch

intercession Fürsprache *f*, Fürbitte *f*, Vermittlung *f*

intercommunication gegenseitige Kommunikation *f*, wechselseitige Verständigung *f*, Interkommunikation *f*

intercommunicator Gerät *n* zur gegenseitigen Kommunikation

intercomportment interindividuelles Verhalten *n*, Interaktion *f*

interconnected untereinander verknüpft, miteinander verbunden

interconnection Verbindung *f*, wechselseitige Verknüpfung *f*, Wechselbeziehung *f*

intercorrelate interkorrelieren

intercorrelation Interkorrelation *f*, Korrelation *f* zwischen den Variablen einer Gruppe

intercourse Umgang *m*, Verkehr *m*, Beischlaf *m* / **anal** ~ analer Geschlechtsverkehr *m*, Analverkehr *m* / **extramarital** ~ außerehelicher Geschlechtsverkehr *m* / **premarital** ~ vorehelicher Geschlechtsverkehr *m* / **sexual** ~ Geschlechtsverkehr *m*, Beischlaf *m*, Koitus *m*

intercrossing Kreuzung *f* / **racial** ~ Rassenmischung *f*

interdependence, interdependency gegenseitige Abhängigkeit *f*, Interdependenz *f*

interdependent voneinander abhängig, interdependent

interdiction Verbot *n*, Untersagung *f*

interest Interesse *n* / sich interessieren / ~ **blank** Interessenfragebogen *m* / ~ **group** Interessengemeinschaft *f* / ~ **inventory** Interessenfragebogen *m* / ~ **pattern** Interessenstruktur *f* / ~ **questionary** Interessenfragebogen *m* / ~ **scale** Interessenskala *f* / ~ **schedule** Interessenliste *f* / ~ **situation** zielgerichtete Situation *f* / ~ **survey** Interessentest *m* / ~ **test** Interessentest *m* / **educational** ~ **inventory** Schulinteressenfragebogen *m* / **extrinsic** ~ Sekundärinteresse *n* / **intrinsic** ~ Primärinteresse *n* / **manifest** ~ offenkundiges Interesse *n* / **occupational** ~ Berufsinteresse *n* / **occupational** ~ **inventory** Berufsinteressenfragebogen *m* / **occupational** ~ **measure** Berufsinteressenmaß *n* / **vocational** ~ Berufsinteresse *n* / **vocational** ~ **inventory** Berufsinteressenfragebogen *m*

interface Schnittstelle *f*

interfere sich überlagern, beeinträchtigen, hemmen, stören, behindern

interference Interferenz *f*, Störung *f*, Beeinträchtigung *f* / ~ **theory** Interferenztheorie *f* / ~ **tube** Interferenzapparat *m* / **cognitive** ~ kognitive Interferenz *f* / **proactive** ~ proaktive Hemmung *f* / **reproductive** ~ rückwirkende Hemmung *f* / **retroactive** ~ retroaktive Hemmung *f*

interferential Interferenz–, Hemmungs–

interferon Interferon *n*

intergrade Zwischenform *f*

intergroup zwischen Gruppen existierend

interhemispheric zwischen den Hirnhemisphären gelegen

interior innen, Innen– / Innere *n*, Seele *f*

interiorisation Internalisieren *n*, Verinnerlichen *n*, Verinnerlichung *f*

interiorize internalisieren, verinnerlichen

interjection Ausruf *m*, Interjektion *f* / ~ **theory** Interjektionstheorie *f*

interjudge zwischen Beurteilern

interleukin Interleukin *n*

interlocking Verzahnung *f*, Verschachtelung *f*

intermarriage Heirat *f* zwischen Blutsverwandten, Heirat *f* zwischen Partnern sozial oder rassisch verschiedener Gruppen

intermediary, intermediate intermediär, vermittelnd, Zwischen–

intermedin Zwischenlappenhormon *n*, Intermedin *n*

intermission Intervall *n*, krankheitsfreie Zeit *f*, Intermission *f*, Intermittenz *f*, Unterbrechung *f*

intermit unterbrechen, intermittieren

intermittence Aussetzen *n*, Unterbrechung *f*, Intermittenz *f* / ~ **tone** unterbrochener Ton *m* / **tonal** ~ auditorisches Flimmern *n*

intermittent intermittierend, diskontinuierlich

intern, interne Assistenzarzt *m*, Praktikant *m*

internal innerlich, inner, intern

internalisation Verinnerlichung *f*, Introjektion *f*, Internalisierung *f*

internalise verinnerlichen, internalisieren

interned interniert, eingesperrt

internet Internet *n*, internationales Computernetzwerk *n* / ~ **address** Internetadresse *f* / ~ **protocol** Internet–Protokoll *n*

interneuron, interneurone Interneuron *n*, Zwischenneuron *n*, Schaltneuron *n*

internment Internierung *f*

internodium, internode Internodium *n*, internodales Segment *n*

internship Assistentenzeit *f*, Assistentenjahr *n* / **medical** ~ Medizinalassistentenzeit *f*, assistenzärztliche Ausbildungszeit *f*

interoception Interozeption *f*

interoceptive innenreizempfänglich, interozeptiv

interoceptor Interorezeptor *m*, Interozeptor *m*

interocular zwischen den Pupillenmittelpunkten, interokular

interorgan generality gemeinsame Eigenschaft *f* aller Organe

interosystem inneres System *n*, interne Einheit *f*

interparoxysmal zwischen Krampfanfällen auftretend

interpenetration gegenseitige Durchdringung *f*

interpersonal zwischenmenschlich

interpolate interpolieren

interpolation Interpolation *f* / ~ **formula** Interpolationsformel *f* / **linear** ~ lineare Interpolation *f*

interpose dazwischenstellen, dazwischenlegen

interposition Zwischenstellung *f*

interpret interpretieren, auslegen, deuten, erklären

interpretation Interpretation *f*, Auslegung *f*, Deutung *f*, Erklärung *f* / ~ **of dreams** Traumdeutung *f*, Traumauslegung *f*,

Trauminterpretation *f*, Traumausdeuten *n* / **allegoric ~** allegorische Deutung *f* / **anagogic ~** anagogische Deutung *f*, anagogische Interpretation *f*, psychoanalytische Interpretation *f* / **over-~** Überdeutung *f*, Überinterpretation *f* / **psychoanalytic ~** psychoanalytische Deutung *f* / **reductive ~** reduktive Deutung *f* / **rich ~** umfassende Deutung *f* / **serial ~** Deutung *f* von Traumserien / **theoretical ~** theoretische Interpretation *f*

interpretative auslegend, deutend

interpreter Traumdeuter *m*, Ausleger *m*, Dolmetscher *m*

interpsychology Interpsychologie *f*, Wissenschaft *f* vom zwischenmenschlichen Verhalten, Sozialpsychologie *f*

interquartile zwischen den Quartilen, Interquartil–

interrelate in Wechselbeziehung treten, untereinander zusammenhängen

interrelatedness wechselseitiger Zusammenhang *m*

interresponse zwischen den Reaktionen gelegen

interrogation Befragung *f* / **legal ~** Verhör *n*

interrogatory, interrogative fragend, Frage– / Befragung *f*

interruption Unterbrechung *f* / **~ beat** unterbrochener Taktschlag *m* / **~ tone** unterbrochener Ton *m*

intersection Nervenkreuzung *f*, Schnittpunkt *m* / **~ of events** Zusammentreffen *n* von Ereignissen

intersensory unter gleichzeitiger Beteiligung mehrerer Sinnesorgane

intersex Hermaphrodit *m*, Intersex *m*, Zwischenform *f*

intersexual hermaphroditisch, intersexuell, mit Merkmalen beider Geschlechter versehen

intersexuality Intersexualität *f*, zwischengeschlechtlicher Zustand *m*

intersocial zwischenmenschlich, sozial

interspace, interstice Zwischenraum *m*, Intervall *n*, Spalte *f*

interstimulation gegenseitige Beeinflussung *f* des Verhaltens, Verhaltensänderung *f* bei der Wahrnehmung anderer Personen

interstimulus zwischen zwei Reizen gelegen, reizfrei

interstitium Interstitium *n*

intersubjective intersubjektiv

intersubjectivity Intersubjektivität *f*

intertone Zwischenton *m*, Unterton *m*

intertrial zwischen zwei Versuchen

interval Intervall *n*, Zwischenraum *m*, Zwischenzeit *f*, Tonabstand *m* / **~ distribution** Intervallverteilung *f* / **~ estimation** Intervallschätzung *f* / **~ reinforcement** Intervallverstärkung *f* / **~ scale** Intervallskala *f* / **~ schedule** Intervallprogramm *n*, Zeitspannenfolge *f* / **~ training** Intervalltraining *n* / **~ of uncertainty** Unsicherheitsbereich *m* / **colourless ~** farbloser Bereich *m* / **equal-appearing ~s** gleicherscheinende Intervalle *npl* / **equal-~ scale** Skala *f* gleicher Intervalle / **fiducial ~** Vertrauensintervall *n* / **fixed ~** gleiche Zeitspanne. *f* / **fixed-~ reinforcement** feste Intervallverstärkung *f*, Verstärkung *f* in festgelegten Intervallen, gleiche Zeitspannenfolge *f* / **interresponse-~** Intervall *n* zwischen zwei Reaktionen / **interstimulus-~** Intervall *n* zwischen zwei Reizen, reizfreies Intervall *n*, Interstimulusintervall *n* / **intertrial-~** Intervall *n* zwischen zwei Versuchen / **lucid ~** lichter Augenblick *m* / **median ~** Medianintervall *n* / **modal ~** Modalintervall *n* / **photochromatic ~** farbloser Bereich *m*, photochromatisches Intervall *n* / **preparatory ~** Vorbereitungszeitspanne *f*, Intervall *n* zwischen „Achtung"–Signal und Reizdarbietung / **successive ~s method** Methode *f* der sukzessiven Intervalle / **variable ~** veränderliche Zeitspanne *f*, variables Intervall *n* / **variable-~ reinforcement** variable Intervallverstärkung *f*, Verstärkung *f* mit variablen Zeitspannen / **variable-~ schedule** veränderliche Zeitspannenfolge *f*, variabler Intervallverstärkungsplan *m*

intervening intervenierend, vermittelnd, Zwischen–

intervention Intervention *f*, Eingriff *m* / **early ~** Frühförderung *f* / **paradoxical ~** paradoxe Intervention *f* / **psychotherapeutic ~ technique** psychotherapeutische Interventionsmethode *f*

interview Interview *n*, Befragung *f*, psychodiagnostisches Gespräch *n* / **~ clinic** Interviewerschulung *f* / **~ schedule** Interviewplan *m* / **diagnostic ~** diagnostisches Interview *n* / **focused ~** thematisches Interview *n* / **nondirective ~** ungelenktes Interview *n*, freies Interview *n* / **personal ~** mündliche Befragung *f* / **psychodiagnostic ~** psychodiagnostisches Gespräch *n*, psychodiagnostisches Interview *n* / **structured ~** strukturiertes Interview *n*, gelenktes Interview *n* / **unstructured ~** unstrukturiertes Interview *n*, freies Interview *n*

interviewee Befragte (r) *f,m*, Interviewte (r) *f,m*

interviewer Befrager *m*, Interviewer *m* / **~ bias** Interviewerfehler *m*, Voreingenommenheit *f* des Interviewers, Verzerrung *f* durch Interviewereinfluss

interviewing Interviewen *n*

intestinal Darm–, intestinal

intestine Darm *m*, Eingeweiden / **small ~** Dünndarm *m* / **straight ~** Enddarm *m*

intimacy Intimität *f*, Vertrautheit *f* / **~ principle** Prinzip *n* der Vertrautheit / **physical ~** Geschlechtsverkehr *m*, Koitus *m*

intolerable unerträglich

intolerance Intoleranz *f*, Unverträglichkeit *f* / **~ of ambiguity** Unfähigkeit *f* mehrdeutige Situationen zu ertragen, Intoleranz *f* gegenüber Mehrdeutigkeit

intolerant unduldsam, unnachsichtig, intolerant

intonation Intonation *f*, Tonfall *m*, Betonung *f* / **~ contour** Intonationskontur *f*

intoxicant Rauschmittel *n*, Rauschdroge *f*, Gift *n* / berauschend, vergiftend

intoxication Vergiftung *f*, Intoxikation *f*, Rauschzustand *m*, Trunkenheit *f* / **~ psychosis** Alkoholpsychose *f* / **acute ~** akute Intoxikation *f* / **alcoholic ~** Alkoholvergiftung *f*, Alkoholrausch *m* / **chronic alcoholic ~** chronische Alkoholvergiftung *f* / **pathological ~** pathologischer Rausch *m*

intraception Intrazeption *f*

intracerebellar im Kleinhirn gelegen

intracerebral im Großhirn gelegen, intrazerebral

intraconscious im Bewusstsein befindlich, mitbewusst

intracortical innerhalb der Hirnrinde gelegen, intrakortikal

intracranial im Schädelinnern gelegen, intrazephal, intrakranial

intractability Störrigkeit *f*, Halsstarrigkeit *f*, Widerspenstigkeit *f*

intrafamiliar innerhalb der Familie, intrafamiliär

intragression Autoaggression *f*, Tendenz *f* zur Selbstzüchtigung

intraindividual intraindividuell, innerhalb des gleichen Individuums

intramural innerhalb einer Institution stattfindend, intramural

intranet Intranet *n*, firmeninternes Computernetzwerk *n*

intraneural im Nerv gelegen, endoneural

intraocular im Innern des Augapfels gelegen, intraokulär

intraorganismal innerhalb des Organismus entstehend, im Organismus gelegen

intrapsychic, intrapsychical intrapsychisch, im Psychischen begründet

intrapunitive intrapunitiv

intratensive intratensiv

intrauterine intrauterin, in der Gebärmutter gelegen, im Uterusinnern gelegen

intraversion Introversion *f*

intravital intravital, während des Lebens

intrication of drives Triebmischung *f*, Triebverschmelzung *f*

intrinsic, intrinsical immanent, intrinsisch, innere(r, s), Eigen–

introception Introzeption *f*, Internalisierung *f*, Verinnerlichung *f*

introject introjizieren

introjected introjiziert

introjection Introjektion *f*, Personifizierung *f*, Identifizierung *f*

intromission Einführung *f* / **~–copulation–ejaculation mechanism** Begattungsmechanismus *m*, Ablauf *m* der Begattung mit Einführung des Penis, Kopulation *f* und Ejakulation *f*

intromittent einführend

intropunitive intropunitiv, Selbststrafungs–

intropunitiveness Selbstbestrafung *f*, Selbstbeschuldigung *f*

introspection Selbstbeobachtung *f*, Introspektion *f*, innere Wahrnehmung *f*, Erlebnisbeobachtung *f*

introspectionism Betonung *f* der Introspektion, auf Introspektion gegründete Psychologie *f*, Introspektionismus *m*

introspective introspektiv, nach innen gerichtet

introspectiveness Ausgerichtetsein *n* nach innen, introspektive Haltung *f*

introversion Introversion *f* / **active ~** aktive Introversion *f* / **passive ~** passive Introversion *f*

introversive introversiv, introvertiert

introversiveness Introversivität *f*, Introversion *f*, introversive Tendenz *f*

introvert Introvertierter *m*, Introvertierte *f* / introvertiert, nach innen gerichtet

introverted introvertiert, nach innen gerichtet

intrusion störendes Eindringen *n*, Beeinträchtigung *f*

intuition Intuition *f*, Anschauung *f*, unmittelbares Erkennen *n*, unmittelbare Einsicht *f* / **articulated ~** klar erkenntliche Intuition *f*

intuitionism, intuitivism, intuitionalism Lehre *f* vom anschaulichen Denken, Intuitionalismus *m*

intuitive, intuitional intuitiv

intumescence Schwellung *f*, Anschwellung *f*

invagination Einstülpung *f*, Invagination *f*

invalid ungültig, nicht valid, invalid

invalidate ungültig machen, entkräften

invalidation Ungültigmachen *n*, Entkräftung *f*

invalidism Invalidität *f* / **early ~** Frühinvalidität *f*

invalidity Ungültigkeit *f*, fehlende Validität *f*, Invalidität *f* / **~ of marriage** Nichtigkeit *f* der Ehe

invariability Unveränderlichkeit *f*, Konstanz *f*, Beständigkeit *f*, Invarianz *f*

invariable unveränderlich, beständig, invariabel, konstant

invariance Invarianz *f*, Beständigkeit *f*, Konstanz *f*, Unveränderlichkeit *f* / **factorial ~** Faktorenkonstanz *f*

invariant invariabel, beständig, konstant, unveränderlich

inventiveness Erfindungsgabe *f*, Einfallsreichtum *m*, Kreativität *f*

inventory Fragebogen *m*, Frageliste *f*, Inventar *n* / **~ test** Fragebogentest *m* / **biographical ~** biographischer Fragebogen *m*, Fragebogen *m* zum Lebenslauf / **horizontal ~** Querschnittsfragebogen *m* / **neurotic ~** Neurosenfragebogen *m* / **personal ~** Persönlichkeitsfragebogen *m* / **psychoneurotic ~** Fragebogen *m* zur Feststellung von Psychoneurosen

inverse umgekehrt, invertiert, entgegengesetzt / Gegenteil *n*

inversion Umkehrung *f*, Inversion *f*, Vertäuschung *f* / **~ of affect** Affektumkehr *f* / **amphigenous ~** gleichzeitig vorhandene

Homo– und Heterosexualität *f* / **sexoaesthetic ~** Transvestitismus *m* / **sexual ~** Homosexualität *f*, sexuelle Inversion *f* / **visceral ~** Verlagerung *f* der Eingeweide

invert umkehren, invertieren / Homosexueller *m*, Lesbierin *f*, Invertierter *m*, Invertierte *f*

invertebrate wirbelloses Tier *n*

inverted umgekehrt, invertiert, homosexuell

investigate erforschen

investigation Untersuchung *f*, Erforschung *f*, Forschung *f* / **~ of behaviour** Verhaltensforschung *f* / **~ method** Untersuchungsmethode *f* / **controlled ~** gezielte Untersuchung *f* / **experimental ~** experimentelle Untersuchung *f*, Experiment *n* / **preliminary ~** Voruntersuchung *f*, Vorversuch *m*

investigator Forscher *m*

investigatory Forschungs–

investment Besetzung *f*, Kathexis *f* / **cognitive–dynamic ~ strain** Spannung *f* der kognitiv–dynamischen Besetzung / **parental ~** elterliches Engagement *n*

invia Introversion *f*

invigilation Aufsichtführung *f*

inviolacy need Bedürfnis *n* nach Unversehrtheit

invirility Unmännlichkeit *f*, Impotenz *f*, Zeugungsunfähigkeit *f*

in vitro fertilisation In–vitro–Fertilisation *f*

involuntariness Unwillkürlichkeit *f*, Unabsichtlichkeit *f*, Unfreiwilligkeit *f*

involuntary unwillkürlich, unfreiwillig, unabsichtlich, nicht–willensmäßig, automatisch

involution Rückbildung *f*, Involution *f* / **~ melancholia** Involutionspsychose *f*, Rückbildungspsychose *f* / **senile ~** Altersrückbildung *f*, Altersinvolution *f* / **sexual ~** Menopause *f*

involutional Rückbildungs–, Involutions–, rückbildend

involve enthalten, mit sich bringen, beteiligt sein, umfassen

involvement Beteiligung *f*, Engagement *n* / **ungrudging ~** Engagiertheit *f*

iodine Jod *n* / **~ deficiency** Jodmangel *m*

iodopsin Iodopsin *n*

ion Ion *n* / **~ concentration** Ionenkonzentration *f*

ionisation Ionisation *f*, Ionisierung *f*

ionise ionisieren

ioniser Ionisator *m*

iophobia Furcht *f* vor Vergiftung

iproniazid Iproniazid *n*

ipsation Selbstbefriedigung *f*, Masturbation *f*, Ipsation *f*

ipsative ipsativ, auf sich selbst bezogen

ipseity personales Selbst *n*, eigentliches Selbst *n*, Proprium *n*

ipsilateral gleichseitig, auf der gleichen Seite gelegen, ipsilateral

ipsism Onanie *f*, Masturbation *f*, Selbstbefriedigung *f*, Ipsation *f*, Ipsismus *m*

irascibility starke Reizbarkeit *f*, Jähzorn *m*

irascible stark reizbar, jähzornig

irides Irides *fpl*, Regenbogenhäute *fpl*

iridial Iris–, Regenbogenhaut–

iridocele Irisvorfall *m*, Iridozele *f*

iridodiagnosis Augendiagnose *f*, Irisdiagnose *f*

iridokinesia, iridokinesis Irisbewegung *f*

iridologist Augendiagnostiker *m*

iridology Lehre *f* von der Augendiagnose, Iriskunde *f*

iris Iris *f*, Regenbogenhaut *f* / **~ reflex** Pupillenreflex *m*, Irisreflex *m*

irradiance, irradiancy Ausstrahlung *f*, Strahlung *f*

irradiate ausstrahlen

irradiation Strahlung *f*, Ausstrahlung *f*, Irradiation *f*, Ausbreitung *f* / **~ of inhibition** Hemmungsirradiation *f* / **~ pattern** Ausbreiten *n* eines Verhaltensmusters / **~ of reflexes** Reflexausbreitung *f*, Reflexirradiation *f* / ~ **theory of learning** Irradiationstheorie *f* des Lernens / **excitatory** ~ Erregungsausbreitung *f*

irrational irrational, unlogisch, unvernünftig

irrationalism Irrationalismus *m*, irrationales Verhalten *n*

irrationality Irrationalität *f*, Vernunftwidrigkeit *f*

irreality Irrealität *f* / ~ **feeling** Gefühl *n* der Unwirklichkeit / ~ **level** Irrealitätsebene *f* / **~–reality dimension** Irrealitäts–Realitätsdimension *f*

irregular unregelmäßig, irregulär

irregularity Unregelmäßigkeit *f*, Abweichung *f* von der Norm, Irregularität *f*

irrelevant nicht zur Sache gehörig, belanglos, unerheblich, irrelevant

irresistibility Unwiderstehlichkeit *f*

irresistible unwiderstehlich

irresolute unentschlossen, unschlüssig, entschlussunsicher

irresoluteness Unentschlossenheit *f*, Entschlusslosigkeit *f*, mangelnde Entschlusskraft *f*

irresponsibility Unzurechnungsfähigkeit *f*

irresponsible unzurechnungsfähig, nicht verantwortlich

irresponsive unempfänglich

irretentiveness Gedächtnisschwäche *f*

irreverence Respektlosigkeit *f*, Verachtung *f*

irreversibility Irreversibilität *f* / ~ **of conduction** Leitungsfähigkeit *f* nur in einer Richtung

irreversible irreversibel, nicht umkehrbar

irritability Erregbarkeit *f*, Reizbarkeit *f*, Irritabilität *f* / **neural** ~ Erregbarkeit *f* der Nerven

irritable erregbar, reizbar

irritant Reizmittel *n*, Irritans *n*

irritate irritieren, erregen, reizen, stimulieren

irritating reizend, störend

irritation Reizung *f*, Reizzustand *m*, Erregung *f*, Irritation *f*, Entzündung *f* / **cerebral** ~ Gehirnreizung *f* / **excessive** ~ übermäßige Reizung *f*, Überreizung *f* / **mechanical** ~ mechanische Reizung *f*

irrumation Fellatio *f*, Genitalkuss *m*, Coitus in os *m*

irruption Durchbruch *m*

ischaemia, ischemia Ischämie *f*, Blutleere *f* / **cerebral** ~ Gehirnischämie *f*, zerebrale Ischämie *f*

Ishihara| colour plates Farbtafeln *fpl* nach Ishihara, isochromatische Tafeln *fpl* / ~ **test** Farbenprobe *f* nach Ishihara

island Insel *f* / ~ **deafness** Tontaubheit *f* / ~ **of hearing** Hörinsel *f* / **~s of Langerhans** Langerhans'sche Inseln *fpl* / ~ **of memory** Erinnerungsinsel *f* / ~ **of Reil** Insula Reili *f*, Reil'sche Insel *f* / **tonal** ~ Hörinsel *f*

isocarboxazid Isocarboxazid *n*, Isokarbonsäure *f*

isochromatic gleichmäßig gefärbt, isochromatisch

isochronal, isochronic, isochronous isochron, in gleichen Intervallen, bei gleicher Zeitdauer, gleichzeitig

isochrone Isochron *n*, Zeitlinie *f*

isochronia, isochronism Isochronie *f*, Isochronismus *m*, Gleichzeitigkeit *f*

isoenzyme Isoenzym *n*

isogenous isogen, mit gleichen Erbanlagen, der Entstehung nach gleich

isokurtic normalgipflig, isokurtisch

isolable isolierbar

isolate isolieren, absondern

isolated isoliert, Einzel–

isolation Absonderung *f*, Isolation *f*, Isolierung *f* / ~ **of affect** Affektisolierung *f* / ~ **amentia** Isolationsamentia *f* / ~ **defense** Isolationsabwehr *f* / ~ **effect** Isolationseffekt *m* / ~ **mechanism** Isolierungsmechanismus *m* / ~ **psychosis** Einsamkeitspsychose *f* / **artificial** ~ künstliche Isolierung *f* / **compulsive** ~ Zwangsisolierung *f*, erzwungene Isolierung *f* / **psychic ~** psychische Isolierung *f* / **sensory ~** experimentelle Isolation / **social ~** gesellschaftliche Isolierung *f*, soziale Isolation *f*

isometric isometrisch, bei gleicher Muskellänge

isometropia Isometropie *f*, gleiche Refraktion *f* beider Augen

isometropic isometrop, auf beiden Augen gleichermaßen brechend

isometry Isometrie *f*

isomorphic isomorph, gleichförmig

isomorphism Isomorphismus *m* / **~ hypothesis** Isomorphieprinzip *n*

isomorphy Isomorphie *f*

isoniazid Isoniazid *n*, Isonikotinsäurehydrazid *n*

isopia gleiche Sehschärfe *f* auf beiden Augen

isoplastic aus gleichem Gewebe, isoplastisch

isoproterenol Isoproterenol *n*, Isoprenalin *n*

isostere Verbindungslinie *f* zwischen Punkten gleicher Dichte

isotonic isotonisch, mit gleicher Spannung

isotropic isotrop, mit gleicher Richtungsausdehnung

isotypical typengleich, vom gleichen Typus

isozyme Isoenzym *n*

issue Ergebnis *n*, Resultat *n*, Folge *f*, Nachkommenschaft *f*, Thema *n*, entscheidende Frage *f* / **political ~** politische Streitfrage *f*, politisches Thema *n* / **social ~** soziales Problem *n* / **social ~ poll** Sozialumfrage *f*

issueless ohne Nachkommen

isthmus Verengung *f*, enge Stelle *f*, Einmündung *f*, Isthmus *m*

It Es *n*

itch jucken / Jucken *n*, Ekzem *n*

itchiness, itching Jucken *n*, Juckreiz *m*

itchy juckend

item Item *n*, Einzelaufgabe *f*, einzelner Gegenstand *m*, Lehreinheit *f* / **~ analysis** Itemanalyse *f*, Aufgabenanalyse *f* / **~ content** Aufgabeninhalt *m*, Iteminhalt *m* / **~ difficulty** Aufgabenschwierigkeit *f* / **~–difficulty index** Schwierigkeitsindex *m* / **~–discrimination index** Trennschärfeindex *m* / **~–reponse curve** Item–Response–Kurve *f* / **~ scalability** Eindimensionalität *f* der Aufgaben, Skalierbarkeit *f* der Aufgaben / **~ scaling** Schwierigkeitsgraduierung *f*, Aufgabenreihung *f* / **~ selection** Aufgabenselektion *f* / **~ validity** Aufgabengültigkeit *f*, Validität *f* einer Aufgabe / **~ weighting** Aufgabengewichtung *f* / **critical ~** äußerst wichtige Aufgabe *f* / **cultural ~** kultureller Gegenstand *m* / **inter–~ coefficient** Konsistenzkoeffizient *m*

itemization Aufgliederung *f*

iteration Wiederholung *f*, Iteration *f* / **~ method** Iterationsmethode *f*

iterative sich wiederholend, iterativ

J

Jackson|'s law Jackson–Gesetz *n* / **~'s membrane** Jackson–Membran *f* / **~'s syndrome** Jackson–Syndrom *n*

Jacobson's organ Jacobson–Organ *n*

jactation, jactitation Hin– und Herwerfen *n* des Körpers, Jaktation *f*, Körperkrämpfe *mpl*

jail Gefängnis *n*, Untersuchungsgefängnis *n*, Strafanstalt *f*

jamais vu Jamais–vu–Erlebnis *n*

James–Lange theory of emotions James–Lange'sche Gefühlstheorie *f*

jargon Kauderwelsch *n*, Berufssprache *f*, Standessprache *f*, Zunftsprache *f*, Jargon *m* / **~ aphasia** Jargonaphasie *f*, semantische Aphasie *f*, Kauderwelschaphasie *f* / **~ apraxia** Jargonapraxie *f* / **~ stage** Kauderwelsch–Phase *f* / **neologistic ~** Kunstsprache *f*

Jastrow| cylinders Jastrow–Zylinder *mpl* / **~ illusion** Jastrow'sche Täuschung *f*, Kreisring–Sektorentäuschung *f*

jaundice Gelbsucht *f*

Java Java *n (plattformunabhängige Programmiersprache)*/ **~ applet** Java–Applet *n*, Kleinprogramm *n* in Java / **~ man** Java–Mensch *m*, Pithekanthropus *m* / **~ Script** JavaScript *n*

jaw Kiefer *m* / **~ jerk** Kieferreflex *m*/ **~ reflex** Kieferreflex *m*

J coefficient J–Koeffizient *m*

J curve J–Kurve *f* / **~ of conforming behaviour** J–Kurve *f* des konformen Verhaltens

jealous eifersüchtig

jealousy Eifersucht *f* / **delusional ~** Eifersuchtswahn *m* / **sibling ~** Geschwisterrivalität *f*, Geschwistereifersucht *f*

jellyfish Qualle *f*

Jendrassik's| manoeuvre Jendrassik'scher Handgriff *m* / **~ reinforcement of reflexes** Jendrassik'scher Handgriff *m*

jerk Zuckung *f*, Reflex *m* / **nervous ~** nervöses Zucken *n*, Tic nerveux *m* / **plantar ~** Fußsohlenreflex *m*

job Arbeit *f*, Arbeitsplatz *m*, Tätigkeit *f*, Beruf *m* / **~ analysis** Arbeitsplatzanalyse *f*, Arbeitsanalyse *f*, Berufsbild *n*, Analyse *f* der Berufsarbeit / **~ applicant** Stellenbewerber *m*, Arbeitssuchender *m* / **~ applicant attitude** Stellenbewerbereinstellung *f* / **~ applicant interview** Einstellungsgespräch *n*, Vorstellungsgespräch *n*, Bewerbungsgespräch *n* / **~ applicant screening** Bewerberauswahl *f*, Bewerberauslese *f*, Personalauslese *f* / **~ attitude** Arbeitseinstellung *f* / **~ characteristics** Arbeitsplatzmerkmale *npl* / **~ classification** Berufsklassifikation *f* / **~ content** Aufgabenbereich *m*, Tätigkeitsinhalt *m* / **~ description** Stellenbeschreibung *f* / **~ design** Arbeitsgestaltung *f*, Arbeitsplatzgestaltung *f* / **~ discrimination** Benachteiligung *f* im Arbeitsleben / **~ enlargement** „Job Enlargement“ *n*, Aufgabenvergrößerung *f*, horizontale Aufgabenausweitung *f* / **~ enrichment** „Job Enrichment“ *n*, Arbeitsplatzbereicherung *f*, Erweiterung *f* des Verantwortungsbereichs, Übernahme *f* zusätzlicher höherer Verantwortlichkeiten / **~ evaluation** Arbeitsbewertung *f*, Arbeitsplatzbewertung *f*, Stellenbewertung *f* / **~ experience** Berufserfahrung *f* / **~ experience level** Berufserfahrung *f* / **~ holder** Stelleninhaber *m* / **~ hopping** häufiger Stellenwechsel *m* zur Einkommenssteigerung / **~ instruction training** Arbeitsunterweisung *f* / **~ invol-**

vement berufliches Engagement *n*, Arbeitseinsatz *m* / ~ **knowledge** berufsbezogenes Wissen *n* / ~ **level** Tätigkeitseinstufung *f* / ~ **mobility** berufliche Mobilität *f* / ~ **performance** Arbeitsleistung *f*, berufliche Leistung *f* / ~ **performance evaluation** Mitarbeiterbeurteilung *f*, Leistungsbeurteilung *f* / ~ **placement** Zuweisung *f* einer Arbeitsstelle, Arbeitseinsatz *m* / ~ **psychograph** psychologisches Profil *n* eines Arbeitsplatzes, Anforderungsprofil *n* / ~ **rating** Arbeitsbewertung *f* / ~ **requirement** Arbeitsplatzanforderung *f* / ~ **rotation** Stellenwechsel *m*, Job Rotation *f* / ~ **satisfaction** Arbeitszufriedenheit *f* / ~ **search** Stellensuche *f* / ~ **security** Sicherheit *f* des Arbeitsplatzes, Arbeitsplatzrisiko *n* / ~ **selection** Arbeitsplatzwahl *f* / ~ **sharing** Arbeitsplatzteilung *f* / ~ **specification** Berufsbild *n*, Anforderungsprofil *n* / **horizontal ~ loading** horizontale Aufgabenerweiterung *f*, Erweiterung *f* des Aufgabenbereichs durch Hinzufügen ähnlicher Aufgaben / **off the ~ training** Seminartraining *n*, Schulung *f* / **on the ~ training** praktische Ausbildung *f* am Arbeitsplatz / **vertical ~ loading** Übernahme *f* höherwertiger Aufgaben zu den vorhandenen

Jocasta complex Jokastakomplex *m*

jocularity Heiterkeit *f*, Fröhlichkeit *f*, Spaß *m*

joie de vivre Lebensfreude *f*, Wohlbehagen *n*

joint Verbindung *f*, Gelenk *n* / verbunden, vereint, gemeinschaftlich, gemeinsam / ~ **disorder** Gelenkerkrankung *f* / ~ **sensor** Gelenksensor *m*

joke Witz *m*

Jordan curve Jordan–Kurve *f*

Jost's law Jost'sche Sätze *mpl*, Jost'sche Regeln *fpl*

joule Joule *n*

journeyman Gehilfe *m*, Geselle *m*

joy Freude *f* / ~ **of living** Lebensfreude *f*

judge beurteilen, entscheiden, urteilen / Richter *m*, Kenner *m*, Sachverständiger *m* / **independent ~** unabhängiger Beurteiler *m* / **juvenile ~** Jugendrichter *m* / **unprejudiced ~** neutraler Richter *m*

judgement, judgment Urteil *n*, Beurteilung *f* / ~ **of condemnation** Verurteilung *f* / ~ **discrepancy** Diskrepanz *f* des Urteils / ~ **disturbance** Störung *f* der Urteilskraft, Urteilsstörung *f* / ~ **rating** Beurteilung *f*, Bewertung *f*, Schätzung *f* / **absolute ~** absolutes Urteil *n*, absolute Urteilsabgabe *f* / **clinical ~** klinische Beurteilung *f* / **comparative ~** vergleichende Beurteilung *f*, vergleichendes Urteil *n* / **deficient ~** Urteilsschwäche *f* / **doubtful ~** unsicheres Urteil *n* / **impaired ~** Urteilsstörung *f* / **moral ~** moralisches Urteil *n* / **psychophysical ~** psychophysische Beurteilung *f*

juggins Trottel *m*, Dummkopf *m*

juice, gastric Magensaft *m*

jumping Springen *f*

junction Verbindung *f* / **myoneural ~** neuromuskuläre Synapse *f* / **neuromuscular ~** neuromuskuläre Verbindung *f*, neuromuskuläre Synapse *f* / **synaptic ~** Synapse *f*

Jung association test Jung'scher Assoziationstest *m*

Jungian Jung'sche(r, s), nach C.G.Jung

jurisdiction Rechtsprechung *f*, Gerichtsbarkeit *f*

jurisprudence Rechtswissenschaft *f*

just gerecht, unparteiisch, gerade, soeben, richtig, genau

justice Gerechtigkeit *f*, Recht *n* / **criminal ~** Strafjustiz *f*

justification Rechtfertigung *f*, Berechtigung *f*, Grund *m*

juvenile jugendlich, Jugend–, juvenil, jung, Jugendlicher *m* / ~ **court** Jugendgericht *n* / ~ **delinquency** Jugendkriminalität *f*, jugendliche Delinquenz *f* / ~ **demoralization** Jugendverwahrlosung *f* / ~ **judge** Jugendrichter *m* / ~ **paresis** jugendliche Parese *f*

juvenilism Juvenilismus *m*

juvenility Jugendlichkeit *f*, jugendliche Unreife *f*

juxtapose nebeneinanderstellen

juxtaposition Juxtaposition *f*, Nebeneinanderstellung *f*

K

Kahn's test Kahn–Reaktion *f*

kaid Kaid *m*, arabischer Stammeshäuptling *m*

kainophobia, kainotophobia krankhafte Angst *f* vor Neuem

Kanner's syndrome Kanner–Syndrom *n*, frühkindlicher Autismus *m*

Kantianism, Kantism Kantianismus *m*

karyochrome kernfärbend

karyogamy Kernverschmelzung *f*, Kernfusion *f*

karyogenesis Kernentwicklung *f*

karyokinesis indirekte Zellteilung *f*, Mitose *f*, mitotische Zellteilung *f*, Karyokinese *f*

karyoplasm Kernplasma *n*, Karyoplasma *n*

karyotype disorder Chromosomenstörung *f*

katabolism Katabolismus *m*, Abbau *m* im Stoffwechsel

katalepsis Katalepsie *f*, Starrsucht *f*

katasexual nekrophil, sodomistisch

katasexuality Nekrophilie *f* Vampirismus *m*, Sodomie *f*

katatonia Katatome *f*

kation Kation *n*

Kaufmann's treatment Kaufmann'sche Methode *f*, Kaufmann–Verfahren *n*

Keeler polygraph Keeler–Polygraph *m*, Lügendetektor *m* nach Keeler

keirospasmus Schreibkrampf *m*, Handkrampf *m*

Kelley's| constant process Kelley's Konstanzverfahren *n* / **~ iteration method** Kelley's Wiederholungsverfahren *n*

Kelvin scale Kelvinskala *f*, absolute Temperaturskala *f* / **~ of temperature** Kelvin–Temperaturskala *f*

kenophobia Kenophobie *f*, Angst *f* vor leeren Räumen und Plätzen

kenotoxin Ermüdungsstoff *m*

keratometer Keratometer *n*, Hornhautkrümmungsmesser *m*, Hornhautmesser *m*

keratoplasty Hornhauttransplantation *f*

keratoscope Keratoskop *n*

keratoscopy Keratoskopie *f*

keraunoneurosis traumatische Neurose *f* nach Blitzschlag, Keraunoneurose *f*

keraunophobia krankhafte Furcht *f* vor Blitzen, Keraunophobie *f*

kernel sentence Kernsatz *m*

Kernig's sign Kernig–Zeichen *n*

ketamine Ketamin *n*

ketogenic ketonbildend, ketogen

ketone bodies Ketonkörper *mpl*

ketosteroid Ketosteroid *n*

key Schlüssel *m*, Taste *f*, Hebel *m*, Manipulandum *n*, Pickscheibchen *n*, Auswertungsschablone *f* / **~ board** Tastatur *f* / **~–punch** Locher *m* / **~ stimulus** Auslöser *m* / **~–verifier** Prüfer *m* / **~–word** Schlüsselwort *n*

kidnapping Entführung *f*

kidney Niere *f* / **~ disease** Nierenerkrankung *f* / **~ stones** Nierensteine *mpl* / **~ transplantation** Nierentransplantation *f*

Kiesow's painless cheek area Kiesows schmerzloser Backenbereich *m*

killer cell, natural natürliche Killerzelle *f*

kilo Kilo *n*, Kilogramm *n*

kin Familie *f*, Sippe *f*, Geschlecht *n*

kinaesthesia, kinaesthesis, kinesthesia, kinesthesis Bewegungsempfindung *f*, Kinästhesie *f*, Muskelsinn *m*

kinaesthesiometer, kinesthesiometer Kinästhesiometer *n*, Vorrichtung *f* zur Prüfung der Empfindlichkeit des Muskelsinnes

kinaesthetic, kinesthetic kinästhetisch

kinase Kinase *f*

kindergarten Kindergarten *m* / ~ **teacher** Erzieherin *f*, Kindergärtnerin *f*

kindness Freundlichkeit *f*, Güte *f*

kinehaptic kinehaptisch, Bewegungstast–

kinematograph Kinematograph *m*

kinemia Herzzeitvolumen *n*

kinephantom Bewegungsrichtungstäuschung *f*

kinesia, kinesis Kinesie *f*, Bewegung *f*

kinesics Kinesik *f*, Lehre *f* von der Körperkommunikation

kinesimeter Bewegungsmesser *m*, Kinesimeter *n*

kinesiology Lehre *f* von den körperlichen Bewegungen, Bewegungstherapie *f*

kinesitherapy, kinesiotherapy Bewegungstherapie *f*, Kinesiotherapie *f*

kinesophobia Furcht *f* vor Bewegungen, Kinesophobie *f*

kinetic kinetisch

kinetics Bewegungslehre *f*

kinetoscope Kinetoskop *n*

kinetosis Kinetose *f*, Reisekrankheit *f*

kinocilium Kinozilie *f*

Kinsey report Kinsey–Report *m*

kinship Blutsverwandtschaft *f*, nahe Verwandtschaft *f*, Sippe *f* / ~ **recognition** Verwandtschaftserkennung *f* / ~ **system** Verwandtschaftssystem *n* / ~ **structure** Verwandtschaftsstruktur *f*, Sippenstruktur *f*

Kirschmann| law Kirschmann–Gesetz *n* / **~'s contrast law** Kirschmann'sches Kontrastgesetz *n*

Kjersted–Robinson law Kjersted–Robinson'sches Gesetz *n*

Kleine–Levin syndrome Kleine–Levin Syndrom *n*

kleptolagnia Kleptolagnie *f*, sexuelle Erregung *f* beim Stehlen

kleptomania Kleptomanie *f*, pathologisches Stehlen *n*, Stehlsucht *f*

kleptomaniac Kleptomaner *m*

kleptophobia Angst *f* vor Dieben, Kleptophobie *f*

Kline| reaction Kline–Reaktion *f* / ~ **test** Kline–Test *m*

Klinefelter's syndrome Klinefelter–Syndrom *n*

klinotaxis Klinotaxis *f*, Hinwendung *f* zur Reizquelle

Klüver–Bucy syndrome Klüver–Bucy–Syndrom *n*, neuropsychiatrische Ausfälle *mpl* bei doppelseitiger Temporalhirnläsion

knee Knie *n* / ~ **jerk** Patellarreflex *m*, Kniesehnenreflex *m* / ~ **reflex** Kniesehnenreflex *m*, Patellarreflex *m*

knob Knopf *m*, Vorsprung *m*, Höcker *m* / **synaptic ~s** Endknöpfe *mpl*, Held–Auerbach'sche Endknöpfchen *npl*

know wissen, erkennen, kennen / **~–how** Erfahrung *f*, Wissen *n*

knower Erkennender *m*

knowledge Kenntnis *f*, Erkenntnis *f*, Wissen *n*, Kenntnisse *fpl* / ~ **level** Wissensstand *m* / ~ **memory** Wissensgedächtnis *n* / ~ **of human nature** Menschenkenntnis *f* / ~ **of results** Kenntnis *f* der Ergebnisse, Ergebnismitteilung *f*, Information *f* über die Ergebnisse / ~ **seeking** Wissensdrang *m*, Wissensdurst *m* / **carnal ~** Geschlechtsverkehr *m* / **common ~** Allgemeinwissen *n* / **declarative ~** deklaratives Wissen *n* / **functional ~** funktionelles Wissen *n* / **immediate ~ of results** sofortige Erfolgsmitteilung *f* / **ontological ~** ontologische Erkenntnis *f* / **procedural ~** prozedurales Wissen *n*

Koenig| cylinders König'sche Zylinder *mpl* / **~'s symptom** König–Symptom *n*

Köhler| after–effect Köhler'scher Nacheffekt *m* / **~ effect** Köhler–Effekt *m*

Kohler–Restorff phenomenon Kohler–Restorff–Phänomen *n*

koinotropic auf Gruppen ausgerichtet

Kolmer| reaction Kolmer–Reaktion *f* / **~ test** Kolmer–Test *m*

kolytic hemmend, auflösend

Korsakoff's| psychosis Korsakow–Psychose *f* / **~ syndrome** Korsakow–Syndrom *n*, Korsakow–Psychose *f*

Korte's laws Korte'sche Gesetze *npl*

Kozhevnikov|'s disease Kojewnikow–Epilepsie *f* / **~ epilepsy** Kojewnikow–Epilepsie *f*

Krabbe's disease Krabbe–Syndrom *n*

Kraepelin ergograph Kraepelin'scher Ergograph *m*

krauomania Krauomanie *f*

Krause's| bulbs Krause–Endkolben *mpl* / **~ corpuscule** Krause–Endkolben *m* / **~ endbulbs** Krause–Endkolben *mpl* / **~ ending** Krause–Endkolben *m*

Kretschmer type Kretschmer–Körperbautyp *m*

K–R formulas Kuder–Richardson–Formeln *fpl*

kryptomnesic unterbewusst

K scale K–Skala *f*

K spike K–Spitze *f*

kteis Darstellung *f* der weiblichen Sexualorgane

kubisagari Kubisagarikrankheit *f*, japanische Schwindelkrankheit *f*

Kuder preference record Kuder–Interessenfragebogen *m*

Kuder–Richardson| coefficients of equivalence Kuder–Richardson–Aquivalenzkoeffizienten *mpl* / **~ formula** Kuder–Richardson–Formel *f*

Kufs' disease Kufs Syndrom *n*

Kundt's rule Kundt'sche Regel *f*

Kussmaul|'s aphasia Kussmaul Aphasie *f* / **~ breathing** Lufthunger *m*, Kussmaul–Atmung *f* / **~'s coma** diabetisches Koma *n*, Kussmaul–Koma *n*

kurtosis Kurtosis *f*, Exzess *m*, Steilheit *f* einer Verteilung, Krümmung *f* einer Verteilungskurve

kwashiorkor Kwashiorkor *n*

kybernetics Kybernetik *f*

kymograph Kymograph *m*, Kymographion *n*

kymographic kymographisch

kymography Kymographie *f*

kynophobia krankhafte Angst *f* vor Hunden, Furcht *f* an Tollwut zu erkranken

kyphosis Kyphose *f* / **juvenile ~** Scheuermann'sche Krankheit *f*, Adoleszentenkyphose *f* / **senile ~** Alterskyphose *f*, Altersrundrücken *m*

kyphotic kyphotisch

L

label Bezeichnung *f*; Kennzeichen *n*, Produktname *m* / benennen, abstempeln

labeling Benennung *f*, Bezeichnen *n*, Labeling *n*

labia Lippen *fpl*, Schamlippen *fpl*

labial labial, Lippen– / Labiallaut *m*, Lippenlaut *m*

labile labil, unbeständig, unsicher

lability Labilität *f*, Unbeständigkeit *f*, Unsicherheit *f* / **~ of affects** Affektlabilität *f* / **~ of mood** Stimmungslabilität *f* / **affective ~** affektive Labilität *f*, Labilität *f* der Affekte / **emotional ~** emotionelle Labilität *f* / **mental ~** psychische Labilität *f*

labiograph Gerät *n* zur Aufzeichnung von Lippenbewegungen

labiomancy Lippenlesen *n*, Ablesen *n* von den Lippen

labium Lippe *f*, Schamlippe *f*

laboratory Versuchsraum *m*, Experimentierraum *m*, Laboratorium *n*, Labor *n* / **~ animal** Versuchstier *n* / **~ assistant** Laborant *m*, Laborantin *f* / **~ findings** Versuchsergebnisse *npl* / **~ investigation** experimentelle Untersuchung *f* / **~ simulation** Planspiel *n* / **educational ~** Schullabor *n*, Experimentierraum *m* / **experimental ~** Versuchsraum *m*, Versuchslabor *n*, Experimentierraum *m*

labour, labor Arbeit *f*, Wehen *pl* / **~ act** Arbeitsgesetz *n* / **~ dispute** Arbeitskampf *m*, Streik *m* / **~ grading system** Arbeitsbewertungssystem *n* / **~ legislation** Arbeitsrechtsgesetzgebung *f* / **~ management relations** Arbeitgeber–Arbeitnehmer–Verhältnis *n* / **~ market** Arbeitsmarkt *m* / **~ mobility** Arbeitskräftemobilität *f* / **~ output** Arbeitsleistung *f* / **~ pains** Geburtswehen *fpl* / **~ relations** Arbeitnehmer–Arbeitgeber–Verhältnis *n* / **~ turnover** Personalfluktuation *f* / **~ turnover rate** Fluktuationsrate *f* der Belegschaft / **~ union** Gewerkschaft *f* / **~ union member** Gewerkschaftsmitglied *n* / **manual ~** Handarbeit *f*, körperliche Arbeit *f*

labourer Arbeiter *m* / **skilled ~** Facharbeiter *m*

labyrinth Labyrinth *n*, Innenohr *n*, Irrgarten *m*, Irrgang *m* / **~ disorder** Labyrinthstörung *f* / **~ reflex** Labyrinthreflex *m* / **auditory ~** Labyrinth *n* / **bony ~** knöchernes Labyrinth *n* / **membranous ~** häutiges Labyrinth *n* / **tonic ~–eye reflex** tonischer Labyrinthreflex *m* der Augäpfel

labyrinthine labyrinthisch

laceration Riss *m*, Fleischwunde *f*

lachrymal Tränen–

lacinia Franse *f*

lack Mangel *m*, Fehlen *n* / **~ of affiliative bond** Bindungslosigkeit *f* / **~ of appetite** Appetitlosigkeit *f* / **~ of concentration** Konzentrationsschwäche *f* / **~ of deep sensibility** Tiefenanästhesie *f*, Bathyanästhesie *f* / **~ of discrimination** Kritikschwäche *f* / **~ of drive** Antriebsmangel *m*, Antriebsarmut *f* / **~ of emotional bond** Bindungslosigkeit *f* / **~ of energy** mangelnde Energie *f* / **~ of growth** Wachstumsstörung *f* / **~ of ideas** Ideenarmut *f* / **~ of inhibition** Hemmungslosigkeit *f* / **~ of initiative** Mangel *m* an Initiative, Antriebslosigkeit *f* / **~ of interest** Interesselosigkeit *f* / **~ of self–confidence** mangelndes Selbstvertrauen *n* / **~ of self–control** mangelnde Selbstkontrolle *f*, Unbeherrschtheit *f* / **~ of tact** Taktlosigkeit *f* / **~ of tone** Tonusmangel *m* / **~ of will power** Willensschwäche *f*, Entschlusslosigkeit *f* / ~ **or loss of sexual desire** Mangel *m* oder Verlust *m* von sexuellem Verlangen

lacrimal Tränen–

lactate dehydrogenase Laktatdehydrogenase *f*

lactation Stillen *n*, Laktation *f*, Milchbildung *f* / ~ **psychosis** Laktationspsychose *f*

lactic Milch–

lacuna Lücke *f* / **tonal** ~ Tonlücke *f*, Hörlücke *f*

lacunar, lacunary mit Lücken versehen, lakunar

Ladd–Franklin theory of colour vision Ladd–Franklin–Theorie *f* des Farbensehens

ladder Leiter *f* / ~ **of success** Erfolgsleiter *f*, Weg *m* zum Erfolg / **social** ~ soziale Hierarchie *f*, Statusgradient *m*

lag Verzögerung *f*, zeitlicher Abstand *m* / ~ **of sensation** Nachdauer *f* der Empfindung / **cultural** ~ kultureller Rückstand *m* / **social** ~ soziale Rückständigkeit *f*

lagena Lagena *f*, Ende *n* der Innenohrschnecke

lagophthalmos, lagophthalmia Hasenauge *n*, Lagophthalmus *m*

laissez–faire „laissez faire" *n*, Gewährenlassen *n*, Gehenlassen *n* / ~ **atmosphere** „laissez faire"–Atmosphäre *f*, antiautoritäre Atmosphäre *f* / ~ **leadership** „laissez faire"–Führung *f*

laliatry Phoniatrie *f*, Stimmheilkunde *f*

lallation Lallen *n*

lalling Lallen *n* / lallend

laloneurosis nervöse Sprachstörung *f*, Sprechneurose *f*

lalopathy Sprachstörung *f*, Lalopathie *f*

lalophobia Sprechangst *f*, Lalophobie *f*, Glossophobie *f*

laloplegia Sprachlähmung *f*

lalorrhoea, lalorrhea Schwatzsucht *f*, Lalorrhoe *f*, Logorrhoe *f*, Logomanie *f*, Polyphrasie *f*

Lamarckianism, Lamarckism Lamarckismus *m*

lambda Lambda / ~ **index** Lambda–Index *m*

lambert Lambert *n*

Lambert–Beer law Lambert–Beer–Gesetz *n*

lamella Lamelle *f*, Plättchen *n*

lancination stechender Schmerz *m*, ziehender Schmerz *m*

Landau–Kleffner syndrome Landau–Kleffner Syndrom *n*

landmark Anhaltspunkt *m*

Landolt| circles Landolt–Ringe *mpl* / ~ **rings** Landolt–Ringe *mpl*

Langerhans|' cell Langerhans–Zelle *f* / **islands of** ~ Langerhans–Inseln *fpl* / **islets of** ~ Langerhans–Inseln *fpl*

language Sprache *f* / ~ **and speech disorders** Sprach– und Sprechstörungen *fpl* / ~ **ability** Sprachbegabung *f*, Sprachbeherrschung *f* / ~ **acquisition** Spracherwerb *m* / ~ **arts education** Spracherziehung *f*, Sprachausbildung *f*, muttersprachlicher Unterricht *m* / ~ **behaviour** Sprachverhalten *n* / ~ **centre** Sprachzentrum *n* / ~ **of colour** Farbensprache *f* / ~ **deafness** sensorische Aphasie *f*, Worttaubheit *f* / ~ **delay** Sprachverzögerung *f* / ~ **development** Sprachentwicklung *f* / ~ **disorder** Sprachstörung *f*, Sprachschwäche *f* / ~ **function** Sprachfunktion *f* / ~ **laboratory** Sprachlabor *n* / ~ **method** sprachliche Methode *f*, verbale Methode *f* / ~ **proficiency** Sprachtüchtigkeit *f* / ~ **trouble** Sprachfehler *m*, Sprachstörung *f* / ~ **usage** Sprachgebrauch *m* / ~ **zone** Sprachzentrum *n* des Gehirns / **active** ~ aktive Sprache *f*, aktive Sprachbeherrschung *f* / **algorithmic** ~ ALGOL *n*, algorithmische Sprache *f* / **artificial** ~ Kunstsprache *f* / **autistic** ~ autistischer Sprachgebrauch *m* / **colloquial** ~ Umgangssprache *f* / **deaf–and–dumb** ~

Taubstummensprache *f* / **egocentric ~** egozentrisches Sprechen *n* / **expressive ~ disorder** expressive Sprachstörung *f* / **figurative ~** bildhafte Sprache *f* / **foreign ~** Fremdsprache *f* / **foreign ~ education** Fremdsprachenausbildung *f*, Fremdsprachenunterricht *m*, Sprachenausbildung *f* / **foreign ~ learning** Erlernen *n* von Fremdsprachen, Fremdsprachenlernen *n* / **foreign ~ translation** Übersetzung *f*, fremdsprachliche Übersetzung *f*, Fremdsprachenübersetzung *f* / **graphic ~** Schriftsprache *f* / **mixed receptive–expressive ~ disorder** kombinierte rezeptiv–expressive Sprachstörung *f* / **native ~** Muttersprache *f* / **passive ~** passive Sprache *f*, passive Sprachbeherrschung *f* / **receptive ~ disorder** rezeptive Sprachstörung *f* / **symbolic ~** Symbolsprache *f* / **universal ~** Welthilfssprache *f* / **written ~** geschriebene Sprache *f*, Schriftsprache *f*, Schriftzeichensystem *n*

languid, languorous matt, schlaff, abgeschlagen

languish erschlaffen, ermatten, schwach werden

languor, languidness Mattigkeit *f*, Schlaffheit *f*, Apathie *f*

lanuginous lanugoartig, lanuginös, weichhaarig

lanugo Lanugohaar *n*

Laplacian Laplace'sche (r, s)

lapse Versehen *n*, Fehler *m*, Entgleisung *f*, Abweichen *n*, Petit mal *n*, leichter epileptischer Anfall *m* / **~ of memory** Erinnerungstäuschung *f* / **~ of the tongue** Versprechen *n*

lapsus Versehen *n*, Fehler *m* / **~ calami** Verschreiben *n* / **~ linguae** Versprechen *n*, Lapsus linguae *m* / **~ memoriae** Vergessen *n*

larva Larve *f*, Puppe *f*, Raupe *f*

larval Larven–, Raupen–, larviert

laryngeal Kehlkopf–, Larynx–, laryngeal

laryngograph Laryngograph *m*, Kehltonschreiber *m*, Gerät *n* zur Aufzeichnung von Kehlkopfbewegungen

laryngographical laryngographisch

laryngoscope Kehlkopfspiegel *m*, Laryngoskop *n*

laryngoscopy Laryngoskopie *f*, Kehlkopfspiegelung *f*

larynx Kehlkopf *m*, Laryrix *m*

lascivia Nymphomanie *f*

lascivious geil, lüstern

lasciviousness Geilheit *f*, Lüsternheit *f*

Lasègue's sign Lasègue Zeichen *n*

Laser irridiation Laserstrahlung *f*, Laserstrahl *m*

Lashley| jumping apparatus Lashley–Sprungapparat *m* / **~ jumping box** Lashley–Sprungkasten *m* / **~ jumping stand** Lashley–Sprungstand *m*

lassitude Müdigkeit *f*, Mattigkeit *f*, Erschöpfung *f*, Abspannung *f*

lasting anhaltend, dauernd, beständig

lata, latah, lattah Latah *f*, vorübergehende anfallartige psychotische Veränderung *f*

late–onset verzögernd auftretend

latency Latenz *f* / **~ period** Latenzperiode *f*, Latenzphase *f* / **~ stage** Latenzphase *f*, Latenzperiode *f* / **sexual ~** geschlechtliche Latenzphase *f* / **sexual ~ period** geschlechtliche Latenzphase *f*

latent latent, verborgen

laterad zur Seite hin

lateral seitlich, lateral

laterality Lateralität *f*, Seitendominanz *f*, Seitenbevorzugung *f*

lateralization Lateralisierung *f*, Lateralisation *f*

laterophobia Angst *f* vor seitlichem Liegen, Laterophobie *f*

lateropulsion Lateropulsion *f*, Neigung *f* zum Seitwärtsfallen

latitude Breite *f*, Spielraum *m* / **~ of acceptance** Akzeptanzbereich *m*, Zone *f* der Zustimmung / **~ of noncommitment** Bereich *m* der Indifferenz / **~ of rejection** Ablehnungsbereich *m*

lattice Gitter *n*, Gefüge *n* / **dynamic ~** dynamisches Gefüge *n* / **neurofibril ~** Neurofibrillengitter *n* / **square ~** quadratisches Gitter *n*

laugh lachen / Lachen *n*, Gelächter *n* / **hysterical ~** hysterisches Lachen *n*

laughable lächerlich

laughing lachend / Lachen *n* / **~-gas** Lachgas *n* / **~ seizure** epileptisches Lachen *n* / **hysterical ~ fit** hysterischer Lachkrampf *m* / **spasmodic ~** Lachkrampf *m*

laughter Gelächter *n*, Lachen *n* / **compulsive ~** Zwangslachen *n* / **convulsive ~** Lachkrampf *m* / **epileptic ~** epileptisches Lachen *n*, epileptischer Lachanfall *m* / **forced ~** Zwangslachen *n* / **gelastic ~** epileptisches Lachen *n* / **obsessive ~** Zwangslachen *n*

law Gesetz *n*, Prinzip *n* / **~-abiding** gesetzestreu, friedlich / **~ enforcement** Gesetzesvollzug *m* / **~ of advantage** Gesetz *n* des Vorteils / **~ of analogy** Analogiegesetz *n* / **~ of assimilation** Assimilationsgesetz *n* / **~ of association** Assoziationsgesetz *n* / **~ of associative shifting** Prinzip *n* der Assoziationsverschiebung / **~ of averages** Gesetz *n* der Durchschnittswerte / **~ of biogenesis** Gesetz *n* der Biogenese / **~-breaker** Gesetzesbrecher *m*, Gesetzesübertreter *m* / **~ of closure** Gesetz *n* der Geschlossenheit / **~ of coalescence** Gesetz *n* der Verschmelzung / **~ of cohesion** Kohäsionsgesetz *n* / **~ of colour mixture** Farbenmischgesetz *n* / **~ of combination** Kombinationsgesetz *n* / **~ of common fate** Gesetz *n* des gemeinsamen Schicksals / **~ of comparative judgment** Gesetz *n* des Vergleichsurteils / **~ of compensation** Kompensationsprinzip *n* / **~ of configuration** Gestaltgesetz *n* / **~ of conflicting associations** Gesetz *n* der widerstreitenden Assoziationen / **~ of context** Gesetz *n* des Kontextes, Kontextprinzip *n* / **~ of contiguity** Kontiguitätsgesetz *n*, Gesetz *n* der Berührungsassoziation / **~ of continuity** Gesetz *n* der guten Kurve / **~ of contradiction** Gesetz *n* des Widerspruchs / **~ of contrast** Kontrastgesetz *n* / **~ of degradation** Entartungsgesetz *n* / **~ of diminishing returns** Gesetz *n* des abnehmenden Lernfortschrittes / **~ of disuse** Gesetz *n* des Nichtgebrauchs / **~ of effect** Gesetz *n* der Wirkung, Erfolgsgesetz *n*, Effektgesetz *n* / **~ of equality** Gesetz *n* der Gleichheit / **~ of errors** Fehlergesetz *n* / **~ of exercise** Gesetz *n* der Übung, Übungsgesetz *n* / **~ of facilitation** Bahnungsgesetz *n*, Bahnungsprinzip *n* / **~ of filial regression** Regressionsgesetz *n*, Rückschlagsgesetz *n*, Gesetz *n* der Generationsregression / **~ of fittingness** Gesetz *n* der Zusammengehörigkeit / **~ of fixation** Gesetz *n* des Einprägens / **~ of frequency** Häufigkeitsgesetz *n*, Wiederholungsgesetz *n* / **~ of good continuation** Gesetz *n* der guten Kurve, Gesetz *n* der guten Fortsetzung / **~ of habit** Gesetz *n* der Gewöhnung / **~ of identity** Identitätsgesetz *n* / **~ of illuminance** Beleuchtungsgesetz *n* / **~ of illumination** Beleuchtungsgesetz *n* / **~ of inheritance** Erbgesetz *n* / **~ of initial values** Ausgangswertgesetz *n* / **~ of irreversible solidarity** Fundierungsgesetz *n* / **~ of latency** Latenzgesetz *n* / **~s of learning** Lerngesetze *npl* / **~ of least action** Prinzip *n* der geringsten Anstrengung / **~ of least effort** Prinzip *n* der geringsten Anstrengung / **~ of least squares** Gesetz *n* der kleinsten Quadrate / **~ of maximum work** Gesetz *n* des Arbeitsmaximums, Gesetz *n* des maximalen Energieaufwandes / **~s of memory** Gedächtnisgesetze *npl* / **~ of nature** Naturgesetz *n* / **~ of parsimony** Ökonomieprinzip *n* / **~ of partial activity** Gesetz *n* der Teilhandlung / **~ of piecemeal activity** Gesetz *n* der Teilhandlung / **~ of precision** Präzisionsgesetz *n* / **~ of pregnance** Prägnanzgesetz *n* / **~ of primacy** Gesetz *n* des Vorrangs / **~ of primitivisa-**

tion Primitivierungsgesetz *n* / **~ of probability** Wahrscheinlichkeitsgesetz *n* / **~ of progression** Progressionsgesetz *n* / **~ of proximity** Gesetz *n* der Nähe / **~ of readiness** Gesetz *n* der Reaktionsbereitschaft / **~ of recency** Gesetz *n* der Neuheit / **~ of reflex fatigue** Gesetz *n* der Reflexermüdung / **~ of refraction** Brechungsgesetz *n* / **~ of regression** Regressionsgesetz *n*, Rückschlagsgesetz *n* / **~ of relative centrations** Gesetz *n* der relativen Zentrierungen, Gesetz *n* der Wahrnehmungszentrierungen / **~ of repetition** Wiederholungsgesetz *n*, Häufigkeitsgesetz *n* / **~ of segregation** Spaltungsgesetz *n* / **~ of shifting** Gesetz *n* der Verschiebung / **~ of short–circuiting** Gesetz *n* des Kurzschließens / **~ of similarity** Gesetz *n* der Ähnlichkeit / **~ of simplest path** Gesetz *n* des geringsten Widerstandes / **~ of simplicity** Ökonomieprinzip *n* / **~ of spatial summation** Gesetz *n* der räumlichen Summation / **~ of specific sense energies** Gesetz *n* der spezifischen Sinnesenergien / **~ of sufficient reason** Gesetz *n* des hinreichenden Grundes / **~ of temporal summation** Gesetz *n* der zeitlichen Summation / **~ of tension** Spannungsgesetz *n* / **~s of thought** Denkgesetze *npl* / **~ of use** Übungsgesetz *n* / **~ of use and disuse** Gesetz *n* des Gebrauchs und Nichtgebrauchs / **all–or–none ~** Alles–oder–Nichts–Gesetz *n* / **biogenetic ~** biogenetisches Grundgesetz *n*, Rekapitulationstheorie *f*, Wiederholungsprinzip *n* / **civil ~** Zivilrecht *n*, bürgerliches Recht *n* / **criminal ~** Strafgesetz *n* / **distributive ~** Streuungsgesetz *n* / **empirical ~** empirisches Gesetz *n* / **fundamental ~** Grundgesetz *n* / **ideomotor ~** Ideo–Realgesetz *n*, Carpenter–Effekt *m* / **Mendelian ~** Mendel'sches Gesetz *n* / **myelinogenetic ~** Gesetz *n* der Myelinbildung / **natural ~** Naturgesetz *n* / **parallel ~** Parallelitätsgesetz *n* / **phonetic ~** Lautgesetz *n* / **psychophysical~** psychophysisches Gesetz *n*

lawful gesetzlich

lawfulness Rechtmäßigkeit *f*, Gesetzlichkeit *f*, Rechtsgültigkeit *f*

lawgiver Gesetzgeber *m*

lawlessness Gesetzlosigkeit *f*, Zügellosigkeit *f*

lay Laien–, nicht fachmännisch

layer Lage *f*, Schicht *f*, Stratum *n* / **~s of character** Schichten *fpl* des Charakters / **~ of cones** Zapfenschicht *f* / **~ of ganglion cells** Schicht *f* der Ganglienzellen / **~ of rods** Stäbchenschicht *f* / **bacillary ~** Bazillenschicht *f* / **basal ~** Basalschicht *f* / **blastodermic ~** Keimblatt *n* / **cerebral ~** Gehirnschicht *f* / **cerebellar granular ~** Kleinhirnkörnerschicht *f* / **cortical ~** Rindenschicht *f* / **fibrous ~** Faserschicht *f* / **granular ~** Körnerschicht *f* / **inner granular ~** innere Körnerschicht *f* / **Malpighian ~** malpighische Schicht *f* / **marginal ~** Randschicht *f* / **medullary ~** Markschicht *f* / **nuclear ~s** Kernschichten *fpl* / **reticular ~** Retikulärschicht *f* / **retinal ~** Netzhautschicht *f* / **vesicular ~** Bläschenschicht *f*, Ganglienschicht *f*

layman Laie *m*, Nichtfachmann *m*

laziness Faulheit *f*, Trägheit *f* / **mental ~** Denkfaulheit *f*

lazy faul, träge

L–Dopa L–Dopa *f*, Levodopum *n*

lead führen, leiten, hinführen, anführen / Führung *f*, Leitung *f*, Vorangehen *n*, Blei *n* / **~ delirium** Bleidelirium *n* / **~ encephalitis** Bleienzephalopathie *f* / **~ encephalopathy** Bleienzephalopathie *f* / **~ neuritis** Bleineuropathie *f* / **~ neuropathy** Bleineuropathie *f* / **~ poisoning** Bleivergiftung *f* / **~ time** Anlaufzeit *f* / **different ~** differente Elektrode *f* / **indifferent ~** indifferente Elektrode *f*

leader Führer *m*, Anführer *m*, Leiter *m* / **~–centered** führerzentriert, auf den Leiter ausgerichtet / **~ status** Führungsstatus *m*, Status *m* eines Leiters / **appointed ~** formeller Führer *m* / **authoritarian ~** autoritärer Führer *m* / **emergent ~** natürlicher Führer *m*, informeller Führer *m* / **formal**

~ formeller Führer *m* / **informal ~** informeller Führer *m* / **positional ~** Führer *m* aufgrund seiner Position / **religious ~** religiöser Führer *m*

leadership Führerschaft *f*, Führertum *n*, Führung *f*, Leitung *f* / **~ effectiveness** Führungseffektivität *f* / **~ function** Führungsfunktion *f* / **~ qualities** Führungsqualitäten *fpl*, Führungseigenschaften *fpl* / **~ principle** Führerprinzip *n* / **~ style** Führungsstil *m* / **attempted ~** Führungsversuch *m* / **authoritarian ~** autoritäre Führung *f* / **autocratic ~** autokratische Führung *f* / **charismatic ~** charismatische Führung *f* / **democratic ~** demokratische Führung *f* / **formal ~** institutionalisierte Führung *f*, formelle Leitung *f* / **informal ~** informelle Leitung *f*, informelle Führerschaft *f* / **laissez–faire ~** laissez–faire Führung *f* / **participative ~** Mitbestimmung *f* in der Leitung, partizipierende Führerschaft *f* / **permissive ~** liberale Führung *f*, tolerante Führung *f* / **punitive ~** Führung *f* mittels Strafe / **task–oriented ~** aufgabenbezogene Führung *f*

leading führend, Haupt–, erste (r, s) / **~ off** Abgriff *m*, Ableitung *f*

leakage Ausfließen *n*, Spannungsreduktion *f*

leaning upon Anlehnung *f*

learn lernen

learnable erlernbar, lernbar

learned erworben, erlernt, sekundär

learner Lernender *m* / **slow ~** Lernbehinderter *m*

learning Lernen *n*, Erwerb *m*, Aneignung *f* / **~ ability** Lernvermögen *n*, Lernfähigkeit *f* / **~ activity** Lernvorgang *m*, Lernfunktion *f* / **~ awareness** Lernbewusstsein *n* / **~ capacity** Lernfähigkeit *f*, Aufnahmekapazität *f* / **~ centre** Lernzentrum *n* / **~ coefficient** Lernkoeffizient *m* / **~ crutch** Lernhilfe *f*, Gedächtnisstütze *f*, mnemotechnisches Hilfsmittel *n* / **~ curve** Lernkurve *f* / **~ difficulty** Lernbehinderung *f* / **~ dilemma** Lerndilemma *n* / **~ disability** Lernbehinderung *f*, Lernunvermögen *n* / **~ disorder** Lernstörung *f* / **~ disorder not otherwise specified** nicht näher bezeichnete Lernstörung *f* / **~ by doing** Lernen *n* in der Praxis / **~ to learn** positiver Lerntransfer *m* / **~ machine** lernender Automat *m*, Lehrmaschine *f* / **~ material** Lernstoff *m* / **~ matrix** Lernmatrix *f* / **~ method** Lernmethode *f*, Lernverfahren *n* / **~ model** Lernmodell *n* / **~ motivation** Lernmotivation *f* / **~ process** Lernprozess *m* / **~ psychology** Lernpsychologie *f* / **~ rate** Lerngeschwindigkeit *f*, Lerntempo *n* / **~ result** Lernergebnis *n*, Lernleistung *f* / **~ schedule** Lernplan *m* / **~ by selecting and connecting** selektiv–strukturelles Lernen *n* / **~ set** Lerneinstellung *f*, Lernhaltung *f* / **~ strategy** Lernstrategie *f* / **~ system** Lernsystem *n* / **~ test** Lerntest *m* / **~ theory** Lerntheorie *f* / **~ by wholes** Ganzheitslernen *n* / **active ~** aktives Lernen *n* / **associative ~** Assoziationslernen *n*, assoziatives Lernen *n* / **automatic ~** antomatisches Lernen *n* / **aversive ~** Lernen *n* von Vermeidungsverhalten / **blind ~** Auswendiglernen *n* / **cognitive ~** kognitives Lernen *n* / **co–~** gemeinsames Lernen *n* / **collateral ~** zufälliges Lernen *n* / **complete ~ method** Erlernungsmethode *f* / **conceptual ~** Begriffelernen *n*, konzeptionelles Lernen *n* / **concomitant ~** zufälliges Lernen *n* / **conscious ~** bewusstes Lernen *n* / **cooperative ~** kooperatives Lernen *n* / **directed ~** gelenktes Lernen *n*, Lernen *n* unter Aufsicht / **discriminative ~** Unterscheidungslernen *n* / **distributed ~** verteiltes Lernen *n* / **experiential ~** Erfahrungslernen *n* / **fractionated ~** fraktioniertes Lernen *n*, Lernen *n* von untergliederten Einheiten / **ideational ~** sinnvolles Lernen *n* / **identificatory ~** Imitationslernen *n* / **imitative ~** Imitationslernen *n*, Beobachtungslernen *n* / **implicit ~** implizites Lernen *n* / **incidental ~** zufälliges Lernen *n*, inzidentelles Lernen *n* / **incremental ~** additiv–schrittweises Lernen *n* / **insightful ~** Lernen *n* durch Einsicht / **instrumental ~** instrumentelles Lernen *n*, instrumentelles Bedingen *n* / **intentional ~** Lernen *n* mit Lernabsicht, intentionales Lernen *n* / **intraserial ~** Lernen *n* von Reihenfolgen / **latent ~** latentes Lernen *n* / **logical ~** Bedeutungslernen *n*, logisches Lernen *n* / **massed ~** massiertes Lernen *n* / **meaningful ~** Bedeutungslernen *n* / **mechanical ~** Auswendiglernen *n* / **mnemonic ~** Lernen *n* mit mnemotechnischen Hilfsmitteln, mnemotechnisches Lernen *n* / **motor ~** motorisches Lernen *n*, Bewegungslernen *n* / **nonverbal ~** nichtverbales Lernen *n* / **observational ~** Beobachtungslernen *n*, Lernen *n* durch Beobachten / **one–trial ~** Lernen *n* bei einem Lerndurchgang / **operant ~** operantes Lernen *n* / **passive ~** zufälliges Lernen *n*, passives Lernen *n* / **perceptual ~** Wahrnehmungslernen *n* / **perceptual–motor ~** sensumotorisches Lernen *n*, perzeptiv–motorisches Lernen *n* / **programmed ~** programmiertes Lernen *n*, programmierter Unterricht *m* / **purposive ~** zielgerichtetes Lernen *n* / **rational ~** logisches Lernen *n*, Bedeutungslernen *n* / **relational ~** Beziehungslernen *n*, Lernen *n* von Relationen / **rote ~** Auswendiglernen *n*, Memorieren *n*, Wort–für–Wort–Lernen *n*, mechanisches Lernen *n* / **selective ~** selektives Lernen *n* / **sensumotor ~** sensumotorisches Lernen *n* / **sequential ~** sequentielles Lernen *n* / **serial ~** Reihenlernen *n*, Serienlernen *n*, serielles Lernen *n* / **social ~** soziales Lernen *n* / **spaced ~** verteiltes Lernen *n* / **spatial ~** räumliches Lernen *n* / **statistical ~ theory** statistische Lerntheorie / **subliminal ~** unterschwelliges Lernen *n* / **verbal ~** verbales Lernen *n* / **verbatim ~** auswendig lernen / **vicarious ~** stellvertretendes Lernen *n*, Modelllernen *n* / **whole ~** ganzheitliches Lernen *n*

least kleinste (r, s), geringste (r, s) / **~–noticeable** eben merklich, kleinste(r, s) wahrnehmbare / **~–perceptible** eben wahrnehmbar, geringste(r, s) wahrnehmbare

leaving the field Aus–dem–Felde–Gehen *n*

lecanomancy Wahrsagen *n* aus einem Wasserbecken

lecherous wollüstig, geil

lechery Wollust *f*, Geilheit *f*

lecithin Lezithin *n*

lecture Vortrag *m*, Vorlesung *f* / **~ method** Vortragsmethode *f*, Vortragstechnik *f*

Lee effect Lee–Effekt *m*, fehlerhaftes und verlangsamtes Sprechen *n* bei verzögerter akustischer Rückkopplung

left links / **~–handed** linkshändig / **~–handedness** Linkshändigkeit *f* / **~–hander** Linkshänder *m*

leg Bein *n*

legal juristisch, Rechts–, forensisch

legalisation Legalisierung *f*

legend Legende *f*, Mythos *m*, Sage *f*, Zeichenerklärung *f*, Bildunterschrift *f*

legibility Leserlichkeit *f*

legitimacy Legitimität *f*, Rechtmäßigkeit *f*, Echtheit *f*, eheliche Geburt *f*

legitimate legitim, rechtmäßig, berechtigt, folgerichtig, ehelich

legitimation Legitimation *f*, Gültigkeitserklärung *f*

legs, restless Restless–legs–Syndrom *n*, Wittmaack–Ekbom Syndrom *n*

leisure Freizeit *f*, Muße *f* / **~ class** wohlhabende Klasse *f*, nichtarbeitende Klasse *f* / **~ time** Freizeit *f*

lemniscus Lemniscus *m*, Schleife *f* / **acoustic ~** akustische Schleife *f*, Lemniscus lateralis *m* / **lateral ~** seitliche untere Schleifenbahn *f*, Lemniscus lateralis *m* / **medial ~** mediale Schleife *f*, Lemniscus medialis *m*

lemur Lemure *f*

length Länge *f* / **~–breadth index** Längen–Breiten–Index *m*, Schädelindex *m* / **~ of stay** Aufenthaltsdauer *f*, Behandlungsdauer *f* / **cranial ~** Schädellänge *f* / **focal ~** Brennweite *f*

lengthening Verlängerung *f* / **~ reaction** Verlängerungsreaktion *f* / **~ of a test** Testverlängerung *f*

leniency, lenience Milde *f*, Nachsicht *f* / **~ effect** Milde–Effekt *m* / **~ error** Beurteilungsfehler *m* aufgrund zu großer Nachsicht

lenient mild, nachsichtig

lenitive lindernd / Linderungsmittel *n*

Lennox–Gastaut's syndrome Lennox Syndrom *n*

lens Linse *f* / **achromatic ~es** Linsen *fpl* ohne chromatische Aberration / **collecting ~** Sammellinse *f* / **concave ~** Zerstreuungslinse *f* / **corneal ~** Hornhautlinse *f*, Kontaktlinse *f* / **crystalline ~** Linse *f*, Augenlinse *f* / **cylindrical ~** zylindrische Linse *f*, Zylinderglas *n* / **focusing ~** Sammellinse *f* / **negative ~** Zerstreuungslinse *f* / **punctual ~** Punktalglas *n* / **spheric ~** sphärische Linse *f* / **toric ~** torisches Brillenglas *n*

lenticular, lenticulate, lentiform linsenförmig, lentikulär

leptocephalic, leptocephalous schmalköpfig, leptozephal

leptocephalus Schmalkopf *m*, Leptozephalus *m*

leptokurtic schmalgipflig, leptokurtisch

leptomeninx weiche Hirnhaut *f*, Leptomeninx *f*, Pia mater *f* und Arachnoidea *f*

leptomorph, leptomorphic leptomorph

leptomorphy Leptomorphie *f*

leptosomatic, leptosomic leptosom

leptosome Leptosomer *m*, leptosomer Typ *m*

leptosomia leptosomer Körperbau *m*, Leptosomie *f*

lerema, leresis Altersschwatzhaftigkeit *f*

lesbian lesbisch / Lesbierin *f*, Tribade *f*, Invertierte *f*

lesbianism lesbische Liebe *f* / weibliche Homosexualität *f*, Tribadie *f*

lesion Verletzung *f*, Schädigung *f*, Schaden *m*, Läsion *f* / **~ of the brain** Gehirnschädigung *f* / **cerebral ~** Gehirnverletzung *f*, Hirnschaden *m* / **cortical ~** Rindenläsion *f* / **focal ~** Schädigung *f* eines Gehirnzentrums, Herdläsion *f* / **nervous ~** Nervenschädigung *f* / **neural ~** Nervenläsion *f* / **subcortical ~** subkortikale Schädigung *f* / **traumatic ~** Verletzung *f*, Wunde *f*, Schädigung *f*

lesson Unterrichtsstunde *f*, Lehrstunde *f*, Lektion *f*, Aufgabe *f* / **~ plan** Stundenplan *m*, Unterrichtsplan *m*

lethal tödlich, letal

lethality Sterblichkeit *f*, Letalität *f*

lethargic lethargisch, stumpf, abgestumpft

lethargy Lethargie *f*, Abstumpfung *f*

lethe Gedächtnisverlust *m*, Vergesslichkeit *f*

letter recognition Buchstabenerkennen *n*

leucine Leuzin *n*, Leucin *n*

leucocyte, leukocyte Leukozyt *m*, weißes Blutkörperchen *n* / **~ count** Leukozytenzahl *f* / **granular ~** Granulozyt *m*

leucocytosis, leukocytosis Leukozytose *f*

leucotomy, leukotomy Leukotomie *f*, Lobotomie *f* / **frontal ~** frontale Leukotomie *f*, Lobotomie *f* / **prefrontal ~** Lobotomice *f*, frontale Leukotomie *f*

leukaemia, leukemia Leukämie *f*

level Niveau *n*, Stufe *f*, Grad *m*, Stand *m* / nivellieren, ausgleichen / **~ of adaptation** Adaptationsniveau *n*, Anpassungsniveau *n* / **~ of anxiety** Angststärke *f*, Angstniveau *n* / **~ of aspiration** Anspruchsniveau *n*, Aspirationsniveau *n* / **~ of attention** Aufmerksamkeitsgrad *m* / **~s of character** Charakterschichten *fpl* / **~ of confidence** Vertrauensniveau *n*, Konfidenzniveau *n* / **~ of consciousness** Bewusstseinsstufe *f*, Bewusstseinsgrad *m* / **~ of development** Entwicklungsstufe *f*, Entwicklungsgrad *m*, Entwicklungsabschnitt *m* / **~s of factuality** Objektivitätsstufen *fpl* / **~ of fusion** Grad *m* der Verschmelzung / **~–headed** ausgeglichen, ruhig / **~ of intelligence** Intelligenzniveau *n*, Intelligenzstufe *f* / **~ of management** Leitungsebene *f*, Führungsebene *f* / **~ of motivation** Motivationsstufe *f* / **~ of performance** Leistungsstufe *f*, Leistungsgrad *m* / **~ of reality** Realitätsniveau *n* / ~ **of significance** Signifikanzniveau *n*, Signifikanzgrenze *f* / ~ **test** Niveautest *m* / **common ~ traits** miteinander korrelierende Eigenschaften *fpl* / **concrete ~** konkretes Niveau *n* / **critical ~** kritischer Wert *n* / **developmental ~** Entwicklungsstufe *f* / **educational ~** Schulstufe *f* / **emotional ~** Gefühlsniveau *n*, Gemütsebene *f* / **firing ~** Schwellendepolarisation *f* / **genital ~** genitale Stufe *f*, genitale Phase *f* / **mental ~** geistiges Niveau *n*, geistige Stufe *f* / **middle ~ managers** mittlere Führungskräfte *fpl* / **occupational ~** Berufsebene *f*, berufliches Niveau *n* / **operant ~** Spontanrate *f*, Ausgangsniveau *n* / **socioeconomic ~** sozio–ökonomisches Niveau *n*, Status *m*

leveling, levelling Gleichmachen *n*, Nivellierung *f*, Glättung *f*, Ausgleich *m* / ~ **effect** Nivellierungseffekt *m* / **~–sharpening dimension** Dimension *f* der Nivellierung vs. Akzentuierung

leveller, leveler Nivellierer *m*, Gleichmacher *m*

levelness Gleichheit *f*, Ausgeglichenheit *f*

lever Hebel *m*, Manipulandum *n*, Taste *f* / **~–pressing** Hebelbetätigung *f*, Hebeldrücken *n*

levitation Levitation *f*

levodopa L–Dopa *n*, Levodopa *n*

levophobia Linksangst *f*

lewd geil, unzüchtig

lewdness Geilheit *f*, Unzucht *f*

Lewinian Lewinscher, von Lewin

lexicology Lexikologie *f*, Lehre *f* von den Wortbedeutungen

lexicon Lexikon *n*, Wörterbuch *n*

liability Hang *m*, Verantwortung *f*, Haftbarkeit *f*, Verbindlichkeit *f*, Verpflichtung *f*

liable verantwortlich, haftbar, verpflichtet

liar Lügner *m*, Lügnerin *f* / **pathological ~** pathologischer Lügner *m*

liberalism Liberalismus *m*

liberate befreien, entbinden, entlassen

liberation Befreiung *f*, Entlassung *f* / ~ **from anxiety** Angstentbindung *f* / **homosexual ~ movement** homosexuelle Emanzipationsbewegung *f*, Bürgerrechtsbewegung *f* für die gesellschaftliche Anerkennung der Homosexuellen

libertarian Anhänger *m* der Lehre von der Willensfreiheit

libertarianism Lehre *f* von der Willensfreiheit

libertine Wüstling *m*, Lüstling *m*, Libertin *m*

libertinism, libertinage Zügellosigkeit *f*

liberty Freiheit *f*

libidinal libidinös, Libido–

libidinisation Libidobesetzung *f*, Erotisierung *f*

libidinize mit Libido besetzen, erotisieren

libidinous wollüstig, sexuell hochaktiv

libido Libido *f* Geschlechtstrieb *m*, sexuelle Energie *f* / ~ **analog** Libidoanalogon *n* / ~ **arrest** Libidofixierung *f* / ~ **fixation** Libidofixierung *f*, libidinöse Bindung *f*, Fixierung *f* / ~ **object** Libidoobjekt *n* / ~ **theory** Libidotheorie *f* / **bisexual ~** bisexuelle Libidobindung *f*, psychosexueller Hermaphroditismus *m* / **bound ~** gebundene Libido *f*, fixierte Libido *f* / **narcistic ~** narzisstische Libido *f*, Subjektlibido *f* / **objectual ~** Objektlibido *f* / **sexual ~** Geschlechtslust *f*

licence Erlaubnis *f*, Genehmigung *f*, Lizenz *f*

licensing Erteilung *f* einer Genehmigung, Zulassung *f* / **professional ~** Berechtigung *f* zur Berufsausübung, berufliche Zulassung *f*

licensure Verleihung *f* einer Lizenz, Verleihung *f* eines Diploms, Erteilung *f* einer Genehmigung

licentiate Lizenziat *m*, Inhaber *m* eines Diploms

licentious ausschweifend, zügellos

licentiousness Ausschweifung *f*, Zügellosigkeit *f*

licking Lecken *n*

lidocaine Lidocain *n*, Xylocitin *n*

lie lügen / Lüge *f* / **~ detector** Lügendetektor *m*

Liebmann effect Liebmann–Effekt *m*

life Leben *n* / **~ age** Lebensalter *n* / **~ cycle** Lebenszyklus *m*, Lebensphase *f* / **~ cycle analysis** Lebenslaufanalyse *f* / **~ event** Lebensereignis *n* / **~ expectancy** Lebenserwartung *f* / **~ experience** Lebenserfahrung *f*, Lebensereignis *n* / **~ goal** Lebensziel *n* / **~ history** Lebensgeschichte *f*, Biographie *f*, Lebensbeschreibung *f*, Lebensdarstellung *f* / **~ impulse** Lebensdrang *m* / **~ instinct** Lebenstrieb *m*, Eros *m* / **~ lie** Lebenslüge *f* / **~ line** Lebenslinie *f*, Leitlinie *f* / **~–organisation pattern** Lebensstil *m* / **~ panorama** Lebensbilderschau *f* / **~ plan** Lebensplan *m* / **~ record** Lebensbeschreibung *f*, Biographie *f*, Lebensgeschichte *f* / **~ review** Lebensrückblick *m* / **~ satisfaction** Lebenszufriedenheit *f* / **~ space** Lebensraum *m*, psychologisches Feld *n*, Verhaltensfeld *n* / **~ span** Lebensdauer *f*, Lebensspanne *f* / **~–span psychology** Psychologie *f* der Lebensphasen / **~ style** Lifestyle *m*, Lebensstil *m* / **~–style changes** Lebensstilwandel *m* / **~–sustaining treatment** lebenserhaltende Behandlung *f* / **~–table** Sterblichkeitstabelle *f* / **~–time** Lebenszeit *f* / **affective ~** Gefühlsleben *n*, Affektleben *n* / **autistic ~** autistisches Verhalten *n* / **early ~** Kindheit *f* / **emotional ~** Gefühlsleben *n* / **foetal *od.* fetal ~** Fetalleben *n* / **inner ~** Gefühlsleben *n*, Innenleben *n* / **instinctual ~** Triebleben *n* / **intellectual ~** Verstandesleben *n* / **married ~** Eheleben *n* / **mental ~** Geistesleben *n*, Seelenleben *n* / **psychical ~** Seelenleben *n* / **sexual ~** Geschlechtsleben *n* / **social ~** soziales Leben *n* / **tired of ~** lebensmüde / **uterine ~** Intrauterinleben *n* / **weary of ~** lebensmüde

lifetime personality unveränderliche Persönlichkeitsmerkmale *npl*, Kernpersönlichkeit *f*

ligament Band *n*, Muskelband *n*, Ligament *n* / **round ~** rundes Muskelband *n*

ligand Ligand *m*

ligation Unterbinden *n*, Ligatur *f* / **tubal ~** Tubenligatur *f*

light Licht *n*, Beleuchtung *f* / hell / **~–adapted** an Helligkeit adaptiert / **~ adaptation** Lichtadaptation *f*, Helladaptation *f* / **~ compass reaction** Licht–Kompass–Reaktion *f* / **~ dread** Lichtscheu *f*, Photophobie *f* / **~–headed** unbesonnen, leichtsinnig, unbedacht / **~–heartedness** Frohsinn *m*, Leichtherzigkeit *f* / **~ induction** Lichtinduktion *f* / **~ microscope** Lichtmikroskop *n* / **~ quantum** Lichtquant *n* / **~ reflex** Lichtreflex *m*, Pupillenreflex *m* / **~ refraction** Lichtbrechung *f* / **~ response** Lichtreaktion *f* / **~ sensation** Lichtempfindung *f* / **~ sense** Lichtsinn *m* / **~–sensitive** lichtempfindlich / **~ sensitivity** Lichtempfindlichkeit *f* / **~ stimulus** Lichtreiz *m* / **~ wave** Lichtwelle *f* / **consensual ~ reflex** unwillkürlicher Pupillenreflex *m* / **idioretinal ~** Eigengrau *n*, Eigenlicht *n*, Augengrau *n* / **monochromatic ~** einfarbiges Licht *n*, monochromatisches Licht *n* / **reflected ~** reflektiertes Licht *n* / **retinal ~** Eigenlicht *n*, Eigengrau *n*, Augengrau *n*

lighting Beleuchtung *f*

lightness Helligkeit *f*, Licht *n*, Helligkeitsempfindung *f*

likability, likeability sympathische Erscheinung *f*

like–dislike Anziehung — Abneigung *f*

likelihood Wahrscheinlichkeit *f* / **~ function** Wahrscheinlichkeitsfunktion *f* / **~ ratio** Wahrscheinlichkeitsquotient *m* / **maximum ~** maximale Wahrscheinlichkeit *f*, Maximum–Likelihood *f*

like–mindedness Geistesverwandtschaft *f*

likeness Ähnlichkeit *f*, Gleichartigkeit *f*

Likert| attitude scale Likert'sche Einstellungsskala *f*, Likert–Attitüdenskala *f* / **~ procedure** Likert–Skala *f* / **~ scale** Likert–Skala *f*

liking Neigung *f*, Gefallen *m*, Geschmack *m*

limb Glied *n* / **artificial ~** künstliches Glied *n*, Prothese *f*

limbic limbisch

limen Grenze *f*, Schwelle *f*, Reizschwelle *f* / **differential ~** Unterschiedsschwelle *f* / **spatial ~** Raumschwelle *f*

liminal Schwellen–, Grenz–

limit Grenze *f* / begrenzen, beschränken / **~ of error** Fehlergrenze *f* / **~s method** Grenzmethode *f*, Methode *f* der eben merklichen Unterschiede / **~ of perception** Wahrnehmungsgrenze *f* / **critical ~** kritische Grenze *f* / **fiducial ~** Vertrauensgrenze *f* / **functional ~** Lähmungszeit *f* / **lower fiducial ~** untere Vertrauensgrenze *f* / **physiological ~** physiologische Grenze *f* / **tonal ~** Klanggrenze *f* / **upper ~** Leistungsgrenze *f* / **upper fiducial ~** obere Vertrauensgrenze *f*

limitation Begrenzung *f*, Einschränkung *f*

limited begrenzt, eng umschrieben

line Linie *f* / **~s of association** Assoziationsbahnen *fpl*, assoziative Verbindungen *fpl* / **~s of connection** Verbindungsbahnen *fpl*, Assoziationsbahnen *fpl* / **~ of direction** Sehlinie *f* Richtungslinie *f* / **~ of fixation** Fixierlinie *f*, Blicklinie *f* / **~ function** Linienfunktion *f* / **~ of least resistance** Weg *m* des geringsten Widerstandes / **~ of reasoning** Denkweise *f*, Denkrichtung *f* / **~ of regard** Blicklinie *f* / **~ of sight** Sehlinie *f*, Sehachse *f*, Visierlinie *f* / **~ of thought** Denkweise *f*, Denkrichtung *f* / **~ of vision** Visierlinie *f*, Sehlinie *f* / **arithmetic ~** arithmetische Kurve *f* / **hot–~ services** Telefonseelsorge *f*, Notrufdienste *mpl*, telefonische Hilfsdienste *mpl* / **primary ~ of sight** primäre Sehlinie *f* / **separating ~** Trennlinie *f* / **spectral ~** Spektrallinie *f* / **straight ~** gerade Linie *f* / **visual ~** Sehlinie *f*, Visierlinie *f*

lineal Längen–, in direkter Linie abstammend, direkt, geradlinig

linear linear, geradlinig

linearity Geradlinigkeit *f*, Linearität *f*

lingam Lingam *m*, Phallus *m*

lingual Zungen–, lingual / Zungenlaut *m*, Lingual *m*, Linguallaut *m*

linguistic sprachwissenschaftlich

linguistics Sprachwissenschaft *f*, Linguistik *f*

link Verbindung *f*, Bindeglied *n*, Link *m* / verbinden, verketten, verknüpfen / **~ analysis** Arbeitsablaufanalyse *f* / **connecting ~** Bindeglied *n* / **spiritual ~** geistiges Band *n*

Link Instrument Trainer Link–Trainer *m*, Flugsimulator *m*

linkage Verbindung *f*, Verkettung *f*, Verknüpfung *f* / **genetic ~** Erbbindung *f*, Genkoppelung *f*

linked verbunden, verkettet

linking Verbindung *f*, Assoziation *f* / **mental ~** geistige Verbindung *f*

lip Lippe *f* / **~ eroticism** Lippenerotik *f* / **~ erotism** Lippenerotik *f* / **~ key** Lippenschlüssel *m* / **~–read** von den Lippen ablesen / **~–reading** Lippenlesen *n* / **~–smacking automatism** Schmatzautomatismus *m*

lipase Lipase *f*

lipid, lipide Lipid *n*, Fett *n* / **~ membrane** Lipidmembran *f* / **~ metabolism** Fettstoffwechsel *m*, Lipidstoffwechsel *m* / **~ metabolism disorder** Fettstoffwechselstörung *f*, Lipidstoffwechselstörung *f*

lipocyte Fettzelle *f*

lipoidosis Störung *f* des Lipoidstoffwechsels, Lipoidspeicherkrankheit *f*, Lipoidose *f* / **ganglioside ~** Tay–Sachs–Krankheit *f*, infantile amaurotische Idiotie *f*

lipolysis Lipolyse *f*

lipopexia Fettspeicherung *f*, Fetteinlagerung *f*

lipoprotein Lipoprotein *n*

lipothymia Ohnmacht *f*

Lipp's illusion Lipp'sche Richtungstäuschung *f*

liquidation Liquidation *f*, Auflösung *f*

liquor Flüssigkeit *f*, Liquor *m* / Branntwein *m* / **cerebral ~** Hirnwasser *n*, Liquor cerebrospinalis *m*

lisp lispeln / Lispeln *n*

lisping Lispeln *n* / lispelnd

Lissajou's figures Lissajous–Figuren *fpl*

lissencephalous lissenzephal, mit windungslosem glatten Gehirn versehen

lissencephalus Lissenzephaler *m*, Säugetier *n* mit windungslosem glatten Gehirn

listening Zuhören *n* / **~ comprehension** Hörverständnis *n* / **~ exercise** Hörübung *f* / **binaural ~** Zuhören *n* mit beiden Ohren

listing Aufzählung *f*, Auflistung *f*

Listing's law Listingsches Gesetz *n*

listless teilnahmslos, gleichgültig, apathisch

listlessness Lustlosigkeit *f*, Teilnahmslosigkeit *f*, Apathie *f*

literacy Bildung *f*, Alphabetisierungsniveau *n* / **~ programme** Alphabetisierungsprogramm *n* / **~ test** Schreib– und Lesetest *m*

literal wörtlich, buchstabengetreu

literary Literatur–, Schrift–, gelehrt

literate gebildet, gelehrt / Gebildeter *m*, Gelehrter *m*

literature Literatur *f*, Schrifttum *n* / **~ review** Literaturübersicht *f* / **religious ~** religiöse Literatur *f*

lithium Lithium *n* / **~ carbonate** Lithiumkarbonat *n* / **~ therapy** Lithiumtherapie *f*

litigation Rechtsstreit *m*, Streit *m* / **~ mania** Querulantentum *n*, Querulantenwahn *m* / **~ neurosis** querulatorische Reaktion *f*, „Rechtsneurose" *f*

litigious streitsüchtig

litigiousness Streitsucht *f*, Prozesssucht *f*, Querulantentum *n*

litter size Brut– und Wurfgröße *f*

Little's disease Little'sche Krankheit *f*, zerebrale Kinderlähmung *f*

live leben, wohnen / lebend, lebendig

liveness Klangtreue *f*, naturgetreue Resonanz *f*

liver Leber *f* / **~ disorder** Leberleiden *n*, Lebererkrankung *f*

living| alone Alleinleben *n* / **~ arrangement** Form *f* des Zusammenlebens / **~ will** Lebenswille *m*

Lloyd Morgan's canon Morgans Kanon *m*

load Belastung *f*, Gewichtung *f*, Faktorenladung *f* / **~ capacity** Belastbarkeit *f*, Belastungsfähigkeit *f* / **continuous ~** Dauerbelastung *f* / **environmental ~** Umweltbelastung *f* / **full ~** Vollbelastung *f* / **maximum ~** Höchstbelastung *f* / **permanent ~** Dauerbelastung *f*

loading Ladung *f*, Faktorenladung *f*, Gewichtszahl *f*

loathe verabscheuen, Ekel empfinden

loathing Widerwille *m*, Ekel *m*

lobe Lappen *m* / **~s of the brain** Gehirnlappen *m* / **~ of the cerebellum** Kleinhirnlappen *m* / **~ of the cerebrum** Gehirnlappen *m* / **anterior ~ of the hypophysis** Hypophysenvorderlappen *m* / **anterior pituitary ~** Hypophysenvorderlappen *m* / **central ~** Stammlappen *m* / **cerebellar ~** Kleinhirnlappen *m* / **frontal ~** Stirnlappen *m*, Frontallappen *m*, Stirnhirn *n* / **limbic ~** limbischer Cortex *m* / **occipital ~** Hinterhauptlappen *m*, Okzipitallappen *m* / **olfactory ~** Riechlappen *m* / **optic ~s** Sehsphäre *f*, Sehzentrum *n* / **parietal ~** Scheitellappen *m* / **posterior ~** Hinterlappen *m* / **posterior ~ of the hypophysis** Hypophysenhinterlappen *m* / **posterior pituitary ~** Hypophysenhinterlappen *m* / **pyramidal ~** Pyramidenlappen *m* / **temporal ~** Schläfenlappen *m*, Temporallappen *m* / **temporal ~ epilepsy** Schläfenlappenepilepsie *f*, Temporallappenepilepsie *f* / **temporal ~ seizure** psychomotorischer Anfall *m*

lobectomy Lobektomie *f*, Lappenresektion *f* / **prefrontal ~** Resektion *f* des vorderen Teils des Lobus frontalis

lobopodium Pseudopodium *n*

lobotomy Lobotomie *f*, Leukotomie *f* / **prefrontal ~** Lobotomie *f*, frontale Leukotomie *f*

lobular lappig, lobulär

lobus Lappen *m*, Lobus *m*

local lokal, örtlich

localisation Lokalisation *f*, Lokalisierung *f* / **~ of sound** Schallokalisierung *f* / **auditory ~** Schallokalisierung *f*, auditive Lokalisation *f* / **cerebral ~** zerebrale Lokalisation *f* / **cortical ~** Lokalisation *f* im Gehirn / **perceptual ~** Lokalisierung *f* einer Wahrnehmung, perzeptive Lokalisierung *f*

localise lokalisieren, beschränken

localised lokalisiert, herdförmig

locality Lage *f* / **~ memory** Ortsgedächtnis *n* / **~ sign** Lokalzeichen *n* / **~ survey** Überprüfung *f* der Örtlichkeit

location chart Tafel *f* für die Lokalisierung

lock–and–key model Schlüssel–Schloss–Modell *n*

locked eingesperrt, eingeschlossen, verriegelt

locking Starre *f* / **autonomic ~** tonische Muskelstarre *f*

lockjaw Kiefersperre *f*, Tetanus *m*

lock mechanism Verschlussmechanismus *m*

lockout Aussperrung *f*

locomote fortbewegen, bewegen

locomotion Fortbewegung *f*, Ortsveränderung *f*, Lokomotion *f* / **intellectual ~** intellektuelle Lokomotion *f*, geistige Fortentwicklung *f* / **physical ~** räumliche Fortbewegung *f* / **psychological ~** psychologische Lokomotion *f* / **social ~** sozialer Fortschritt *m*, soziale Lokomotion *f*, Aufrücken *m*

locomotive Bewegungs–, Fortbewegungs–

locomotor lokomotorisch, fortbewegend

locus Ort *m*, Stelle *f*, geometrischer Ort *m* / **~ of control** Ort *m* der Steuerung (des Denkens) / **internal external ~ of control** Kontrollüberzeugungen *fpl*

locutor Sprecher *m*, Sprechender *m*

lodging Wohnung *f*, Wohnort *m*, Einquartierung *f*

logagnosia, logagnosis sensorische Aphasie *f*, Worttaubheit *f*, Wortblindheit *f*

logagraphia Agraphie *f*, Schreibunfähigkeit *f*

logamnesia sensorische Aphasie *f*, amnestische Aphasie *f*, Worttaubheit *f*

logaphasia motorische Aphasie *f*, Worttaubheit *f*

logarithm Logarithmus *m* / **natural ~** natürlicher Logarithmus *m*

logarithmic logarithmisch

logasthenia Logasthenie *f*, Wortvergessen *n*, Denkstörung *f* bei Aphasie

logic Logik *f* / **affective ~** affektive Logik *f*

logical logisch, folgerichtig

logician Logiker *m*

log–log paper Papier *n* mit horizontalen und vertikalen Logarithmusskalen

logoclonia Logoklonie *f*, krankhafte Wiederholung *f* von Wortendsilben

logogram Wortzeichen *n*, Logogramm *n*

logomania Logorrhoe *f*, Redezwang *m*, Redesucht *f*, Polyphrasie *f*

logoneurosis Sprachneurose *f*, Logoneurose *f*

logopaedia, logopedia, logopaedics, logopedics Sprachheilkunde *f*, Logopädie *f*

logopaedic, logopedic logopädisch, Sprachheil–

logopaedist, logopedist Sprachheilkundler *m*, Logopäde *m*

logopathy Sprachstörung *f*, Logopathie *f*

logophasia Artikulationsstörung *f*

logophobia Sprechangst *f* Logophobie *f*

logorrhoea, logorrhea Logorrhoe *f*, Redezwang *m*, Schwatzsucht *f*, Schwatzhaftigkeit *f*

logospasm krampfartiges Sprechen *n*, Logospasmus *m*, Stottern *n*

logotherapy Logotherapie *f*

loneliness Einsamkeit *f*

long lang / **~-headed** langköpfig / **~-headedness** Langköpfigkeit *f* / **~-range** auf lange Sicht / **~-sighted** weitsichtig, hypermetrop / **~-sightedness** Weitsichtigkeit *f*, Hypermetropie *f*, Hyperopie *f* / **~-term** Langzeit–, auf weite Sicht

longevity Langlebigkeit *f*

longevous langlebig

longilineal lang und dünn, lang aufgeschossen, asthenisch

longing sehnsüchtig / Sehnsucht *f*, Verlangen *n*

longitudinal Längs–, Längsschnitt

longitype langwüchsiger Typ *m*

longitypical lang aufgeschossen, lang wüchsig, lang und dünn

looking–glass| self Spiegel–Selbst *n*, reflektiertes Selbst *n* / **~ theory** Spiegeltheorie *f*

loop Schleife *f* / **open ~ control** Steuerung *f* / **explanatory ~** Erläuterungsschleife *f* / **nephronic ~** Henle–Schleife *f* / **remedial ~** Korrekturschleife *f*

loquacious schwatzhaft, geschwätzig

loquaciousness Schwatzhaftigkeit *f*

loquacity Schwatzhaftigkeit *f*, Geschwätzigkeit *f* / **senile ~** Altersschwatzhaftigkeit *f*

lorazepam Lorazepam *n*

lordosis Lordose *f*, Wirbelsäulenverkrümmung *f*

loss Verlust *m*, Ausfall *m* / **~ of accomodation** Akkomodationsverlust *m* / **~ of appetite** Appetitlosigkeit *f*, Anorexie *f* / **~ of attachment** Verlust von Bindung / **~ of concentration** Konzentrationsverlust *m* / **~ of consciousness** Bewusstloswerden *n* / **~ of consciousness of a part of the body** Orientierungsstörung *f* am Körperschema / **~ of contact** Kontaktverlust *m* / **~ of female sexual characteristics** Defemination *f* / **~ of hearing** Gehörverlust *m* / **~ of identity** Identitätsverlust *m* / **~ of logical thinking** alogische Denkstörung *f* / **~ of love** Liebesverlust *m* / **~ of memory** Gedächtnisverlust *m* / **~ of orientation** Orientierungsstörung *f* / **~ of reality** Realitatsverlust *m* / **~ of a reflex** Reflexverlust *m* / **~ of sensation** Gefühlsverlust *m* / **~ of the sense of smell** Geruchsverlust *m*, Anosmie *f* / **~ of sight** Erblindung *f* / **~ of will power** Abulie *f*, Willensschwache *f*

loudness Lautstärke *f* Lautheit *f* / **~ discrimination** Lautstärkenunterscheidung *f*, Lautstärkediskrimination *f* / **~ level** Lautstärke *f*, Lautstärkepegel *m*, Lautstärkeniveau *n* / **~ perception** Lautstärkewahrnehmung *f* / **~ scale** Lautstärkeskala *f*, Phonskala *f* / **~ threshold** Lautstärkeschwelle *f* / **~ unit** Lautstärkeeinheit *f* / **equal ~** gleiche Lautstärke *f* / **equal ~ contour** Linie *f* der gleichen Lautstärke / **equal ~ level** Niveau *n* gleicher Lautstärke / **equivalent ~** gleiche Lautstärke *f*

love Liebe *f*, Zuneigung *f* / lieben / **~ life** Liebesleben *n*, Geschlechtsleben *n* / **~-match** Liebesehe *f* / **~ object** Libidoobjekt *n*, Liebesobjekt *n* / **~ play** Liebesspiel *n* / **~ relationship** Liebesbeziehung *f* / **genital ~** genitale Liebe *f* / **Greek ~** Homosexualität *f* / **maternal ~** Mutterliebe *f* / **parental ~** Elternliebe *f* / **partial ~** Liebe *f* gegenüber einem Teil einer Person / **platonic ~** platonische Liebe *f*, unsinnliche Liebe *f* / **puppy ~** erste heiße Jugendliebe *f* / **phallic ~** phallische Liebe *f*

loveless lieblos, ungeliebt

loving liebevoll, zärtlich, zugetan

low niedrig, gering, niedergeschlagen / **~ grade** sehr niedrig / **~-spirited** niedergeschlagen, depressiv, bedrückt

lower unter, niedriger, tiefer / abschwächen, erniedrigen, herabsetzen

lowness of spirit Niedergeschlagenheit *f*, depressive Verstimmung *f*

loxapine Loxapin *n*

loxophthalmus Schielen *n*

loyal loyal, treu, redlich

loyalty Loyalität *f*, Treue *f*, Redlichkeit *f*

lubrication Lubrikation *f*

lucid klar, bei Bewusstsein

lucidity Klarheit *f*

ludic spielend, im Spiel

ludicrous lächerlich, lachhaft, grotesk

lues Lues *f*, Syphilis *f*

luetic, luic luisch, syphilitisch, luetisch

lumbar Lenden–, Lumbal–, lumbal

lumber Gerümpel *n* / **neurotic ~** neurotisches Gerümpel *n*

lumen Lumen *n*

luminance Leuchtkraft *f*, Strahlungsintensität *f*, Lumineszenz *f* / **~ factor** Faktor *m* der Leuchtdichte / **~ threshhold** Schwelle *f* der Leuchtkraft

luminosity Strahlung *f* Leuchtkraft *f*, Helligkeit *f* / **~ coefficient** Strahlungskoeffizient *m* / **~ curve** Kurve *f* der Strahlungsstärken / **absolute ~** absolute Helligkeit *f*, absolute Leuchtkraft *f* / **relative ~ factor** Faktor *m* der relativen Helligkeit

luminous leuchtend, hell, strahlend

lumper grobklassifizierender Systematiker *m*

lunacy Geistesstörung *f*, Irrsinn *m*, Wahnsinn *m*

lunatic geißstesgestört, irrsinnig, wahnsinnig, psychotisch / Wahnsinniger *m*, Irrer *m*, Geistesgestörter *m*

lunatism Mondsüchtigkeit *f*, Lunatismus *m*

lung Lunge *f* / **~ disorder** Lungenerkrankung *f*, Lungenleiden *n* / **~ perfusion** Lungenperfusion *f* / **~ volumes** Lungenvolumina

Luria technique Luria–Technik *f*, Luria–Test *m*

lust Begierde *f*, Wollust *f*, starkes Verlangen *n* / **~ murder** Lustmord *m* / **sexual ~** sexuelle Begierde *f*

luster, lustre Glanz *m*, Schein *m*, Schimmer *m*

lustful wollüstig, geil

lustration Lustration *f*, Reinigungsopfer *n*, Reinigung *f*

lustrous glänzend, strahlend

lutin Progesteron *n*

lux Lux *n*

luxmeter, luxometer Lux–Photometer *n*, Gerät *n* zur Messung der Lichtstärke in Lux

Luys' body Luy'scher Körper *m*

lycanthrope Geisteskranker *m* der glaubt ein Tier zu sein

lycanthropic lykanthrop

lycanthropy, lycomania Vorstellung *f* Geisteskranker, ein Tier zu sein

lycorexia Heißhunger *m*, Wolfshunger *m*

lying Lügen *n* / lügenhaft, lügnerisch / **pathological ~** pathologisches Lügen *n*

lymph Lymphe *f* / **~ adenopathy** Lymphadenopathie *f* / **~ cell** Lymphzelle *f* / **~ edema** Lymphödem *n* / **~ node** Lymphknoten *m* / **~ vessel** Lymphgefäß *n*

lymphatic lymphatisch, Lymph–

lymphatism Lymphatismus *m*, lymphatische Konstitution *f*

lymphocyte Lymphozyt *m*, Lymphzelle *f*

lymphocytosis Lymphozytose *f*, krankhafte Vermehrung *f* der Lymphozyten

lymphokine Lymphokin *n*

lynching Lynchen *n*, Ausübung *f* von Volksjustiz

lypemania Lipemanie *f*, Melancholie *f*, Schwermut *f*

lypothymia Melancholie *f*, Lypothymie *f*

lysis Auflösung *f*, Lysis *f*

lysosome Lysosom *n*

lyssophobia krankhafte Angst *f* vor Tollwut, Lyssophobie *f*

M

Mach| band Mach–Band *n* / **~ rotation frame** Mach'sche Trommel *f*

Machiavellianism Machiavellismus *m*

machine Maschine *f*, Rechenanlage *f* / **~ code** Maschinensprache *f* / **~ language** Maschinensprache *f* / **~ scoring** maschinelle Testauswertung *f* / **human ~ system** Mensch–Maschine–System *n* / **human ~ system design** Mensch–Maschine–System–Gestaltung *f* / **~ theory** Maschinentheorie *f* / **verifying ~** Prüfmaschine *f* / **xerographic ~** Fotokopierer *m*

macrencephalia, macrencephaly Gehirnhypertrophie *f*, Megalenzephalie *f*, abnorm großes Gehirn *n*

macroaesthesia, macroesthesia Makroästhesie *f*, Gefühlstäuschung *f* bei der alle betasteten Gegenstände größer erscheinen

macrobiosis Langlebigkeit *f*

macrobiotic langlebig

macrobiotics Makrobiotik *f*

macrocephalia, macrocephaly abnorme Kopfgröße *f*, Großköpfigkeit *f*, Makrozephalie *f*

macrocephalic, macrocephalous großköpfig, makrozephal

macrocheilia abnorme Lippenvergrößerung *f*

macrocosm Weltall *n*, Makrokosmos *m*

macrocosmic makrokosmisch

macrodactylia, macrodactyly, macrodactylism Langfingerigkeit *f*, übermäßig lange Finger *fpl*, Makrodaktylie *f*

macrogenitosomia vorzeitige krankhafte Körper– und Geschlechtsentwicklung *f* / **~ praecox** krankhafte Frühreife *f*

macroglossia vergrößerte Zunge *f*, Makroglossie *f*

macrognathia Vergrößerung *f* des Oberkiefers, Makrognathie *f*

macrognathic mit vergrößertem Kiefer

macrographia Schreiben *n* mit übermäßig großen Buchstaben

macromania Größenwahn *m*, krankhafte Überschätzung *f* der Größenverhältnisse

macromolecule Makromolekül *n*, Riesenmolekül *n*

macrophage, macrophagocyte Makrophage *m*

macrophallus abnorm langer Penis *m*

macropia, macropsia, macropsy Größersehen *n* von Gegenständen, Megalopsie *f*, Makropsie *f*

macropodia, macropody Riesenwuchs *m* der Füsse, Makropodie *f*

macroscopic mit bloßem Auge sichtbar, makroskopisch

macroscopy Untersuchung *f* mit bloßem Auge

macrosociology Makro–Soziologie *f*

macrosomatia, macrosomia Riesenwuchs *m*, Gigantismus *m*, Makrosomie *f*

macrosomatic mit Riesenwuchs, makrosomatisch

macrosplanchnic mit großen Eingeweiden, mit großem Bauch

macula Macula *f*, Fleck *m* / **~ acustica** Macula acustica *f* / **~ lutea** gelber Fleck *m*, Macula lutea *f* / **~ organ** Makulaorgan *n*

macular fleckig, gefleckt, makulär

mad verrückt, wahnsinnig, toll, wütend / **the ~** die Verrückten *mpl*, die Irren *mpl* / **~ genius hypothesis** Hypothese *f* von der Nachbarschaft von Genialität und Wahnsinn

madcap toller Kerl *m*

Maddox| prism Maddox–Prisma *n* / **~ rod** Maddox–Stäbchen *n*

madhouse Irrenhaus *n*

madman Verrückter *m*, Wahnsinniger *m*

madness Wahnsinn *m*, Verrücktheit *f*, Irrsinn *m*, Ekstase *f*

magazine Magazin *n*, Zeitschrift *f* / **electronic ~** elektronische Zeitschrift *f*, E–Zine *f*

magenta Magentarot *n* / purpurfarbig

magic magisch, Zauber– / Magie *f*, Zauberei *f*

magico–phenomenalistic magisch–phänomenal

magistral Herren–, Lehrer–, Meister

magnanimity Großmut *f*, Großzügigkeit *f*

magnesium Magnesium *n* / **~ ion** Magnesiumion *n*

magnetic magnetisch

magnetics Lehre *f* vom Magnetismus

magnetisable magnetisierbar

magnetisation Magnetisierung *f*

magnetise magnetisieren

magnetiser Magnetiseur *m*

magnetism Magnetismus *m* / **animal ~** tierischer Magnetismus *m*, Mesmerismus *m*, Magnetotherapie *f*

magnetoencephalography Magnetoenzephalographie *f*

magnetophone Magnetophon *n*

magnetotaxis, magnetotropism Magnetotaxis *f*, Magnetotropismus *m*

magnetotherapy Magnetotherapie *f*

magniloquence Großsprecherei *f*

magniloquent großsprecherisch, prahlerisch

magnitude Größe *f*, Umfang *m* / **~ estimation** Größenschätzung *f* / **~ of effect** Effektgröße *f* / **apparent ~** scheinbare Größe *f*, Sehgröße *f*

maidenhood Jungfräulichkeit *f*, Virginität *f*

maieusiophobia Geburtsangst *f*, Angst *f* vor der Geburt, Maieusiophobie *f*

maieutic mäeutisch, ausfragend

maieutics Mäeutik *f*

mail survey schriftliche Umfrage *f*

mailbox Mailbox *f*, elektronischer Briefkasten *m*

mailing Mailing *n*, Verschicken *n* von Nachrichten als E–Mail / **~ list** Mailing–Liste *f*, Liste *f* mit E–Mail–Adressen

main–line shooter Person *f* die sich Drogen intravenös spritzt

mainspring Haupttriebfeder *f*

mainstreaming Hauptausrichtung *f*, Hauptrichtung *f* / Integration *f* Behinderter

maintenance Erhaltung *f*, Instandhaltung *f* / **~ dose** Erhaltungsdosis *f* / **~ energy** Energie *f* zum Zusammenhalten einer Gruppe / **~ factor** Erhaltungsfaktor *m*, Hygienefaktor *m* / **~ functions** homeostatische Funktionen *fpl* / **~ heat** Erhaltungswärme *f* / **~ level** Erhaltungsniveau *n* / **clinically supervised ~ or replacement regime** ärztlich überwachtes Ersatzdrogenprogramm *n* / **~ schedule** Erhaltungsprogramm *n* / **~ therapy** Erhaltungstherapie *f*, Dauertherapie *f*, Stabilisierungsbehandlung *f* / **low ~** pflegeleicht / **high ~** pflegebedürftig

major größer, älter / **~ depression** Major Depression *f*

majority Mehrheit *f* / **~ group** Mehrheitsgruppe *f* / **~ opinion** Mehrheitsmeinung *f*

make–believe, make–belief Schein *m*, Vorwand *m*, Spiegelfechterei *f*

mal Leiden *n*, Anfall *m* / **grand ~** großer epileptischer Anfall *m* / **petit ~** Petit mal *m*, leichter epileptischer Anfall *m*

malacia Malazie *f*, Erweichung *f*

maladaptation Fehlanpassung *f*, mangelhafte Anpassung *f*

maladjusted nicht angepasst

maladjustment Fehlanpassung *f*, schlechte Anpassung *f*, ungenügende Anpassung *f*, Fehlhaltung *f* der Persönlichkeit / **emotional ~** emotionale Fehlanpassung *f* / **general neurotic ~ factor** allgemeiner Faktor *m* der neurotischen Fehlanpassung / **situational ~** situative Fehlanpassung *f* / **social ~** mangelnde soziale Anpassung *f*, soziale Fehlanpassung *f* / **vocational ~** mangelnde berufliche Anpassung *f*, Berufsverfehlung *f*

maladroit ungeschickt

maladroitness Ungeschicklichkeit *f*

malady Krankheit *f*

malaise Unwohlsein *n*

malapert unverschämt, frech, naseweis

malaria Malaria *f*, Sumpffieber *n*, Paludismus *m* / **tertian ~** Malaria tertiana *f*, Drittetagsfieber *n*

malarialisation Malariakur *f*, Malariatherapie *f*

malarialise Malariakur machen lassen, mit Fiebertherapie behandeln

malariatherapy Malariatherapie *f*, Malariakur *f*

malassimilation Assimilationsstörung *f*

malconformation Missbildung *f*, Misswuchs *m*

maldevelopment Entwicklungsstörung *f*, Fehlentwicklung *f*

male männlich / Mann *m* / **human ~** Mann *m*

malevolence Missgunst *f*, böser Wille *m*

malevolent böswillig, missgünstig

malfeasance gesetzwidrige Handlung *f*, Übeltat *f*

malfeasant gesetzwidrig, kriminell

malformation Missbildung *f* Misswuchs *m*, Fehlbildung *f*, Deformation *f* / **congenital ~** angeborene Missbildung *f*

malformed fehlgebildet, verkrüppelt, missgestaltet

malfunction Funktionsstörung *f*, Dysfunktion *f*

malice Bosheit *f*, Bösartigkeit *f*, Arglist *f*

malign bösartig, boshaft, verleumderisch / verleumden, herabsetzen

malignancy, malignity Bösartigkeit *f*, Bosheit *f*, Feindseligkeit *f*

malignant bösartig, boshaft, feindselig

malinger simulieren, sich krank stellen, eine Krankheit vortäuschen

malingerer Simulant *m*

malingering Simulation *f*, Simulieren *n*, Vortäuschen *n* eines Leidens

malleability Anpassungsfähigkeit *f*, Flexibilität *f*, Gefügigkeit *f*, Umstellungsfähigkeit *f*

malleable anpassungsfähig, flexibel, gefügig

malleus Hammer *m*, Malleus *m*

malnutrition Unterernährung *f*, schlechte Ernährung *f*

malobservation fehlerhafte Beobachtung *f*, schlechte Beobachtung *f*

malodorous übelriechend

malpractice falsche Behandlung *f*, Kunstfehler *m*

Malthus' theory Malthus'sches Gesetz *n*

Malthusianism Malthusianismus *m*

maltreatment Misshandlung *f*

mamma weibliche Brust *f*, Mamma *f*

mammal, mammalian Säugetier *n*, Sänger *m*

Mammalia Säugetiere *npl*, Klasse *f* der Säugetiere

mammary Mamma–, weibliche Brust–

mammilla Brustwarze *f*

mammography Mammographie *f*

man Mensch *m*, Mann *m* / **~–machine simulation** Mensch–Maschine–Simulation *f*, Planspiel *n* / **~–machine system** Mensch Maschine–System *n* / **~–to–man**

rating interindividuell–vergleichende Beurteilung *f* / **marginal ~** Randpersönlichkeit *f*, Randfigur *f* / **odd ~** Original *n*, Taglöhner *m* / **one–dimensional ~** eindimensionaler Mensch *m* / **primitive ~** Urmensch *m* / **unworthy of ~** menschenunwürdig

mana Mana *f*

manageable fügsam, lenksam

management Führung *f*, Leitung *f*, Management *n* / **~ by communication and participation** kooperative Führung *f* / **~ by control and direction** autoritäre Führung *f* / **~ decision** Führungsentscheidung *f* / **~ decision making** Entscheidungsfindung *f* im Management / **~ by delegation** Führung *f* durch Delegation von Verantwortung / **~ development** Förderung *f* und Entwicklung *f* von Führungskräften / **~ engineer** Arbeitsstudieningenieur *m*, Industrial Engineer *m* / **~ by exception** Führung *f* durch Eingreifen in Ausnahmesituationen / **~ games** Unternehmensplanspiele *npl* / **~ information system** Managementinformationssystem *n* / **~ method** Managementmethode *f*, Führungsmethode *f* / **~ by motivation** Führung *f* durch Motivation / **~ by objectives** Fürung *f* durch Zielsetzung / **~ personnell** Führungskräfte *fpl* / **~ planning** Managementplanung *f*, Unternehmensplanung *f* / **~ potential** Führungspotenzial *n* / **~ responsibility** Führungsverantwortung *f* / **~ by results** ergebnisorientierte Unternehmensführung *f* / **~ science** Lehre *f* von der Unternehmensführung / **~ by systems** Führung *f* durch Systematisierung / **~ according to task** aufgabenbezogenes Management *n* / **~ training** Führungskräfteschulung *f*, Managementtraining *n* / **~ tools** Instrumente *npl* der Unternehmensführung / **lower ~** untere Leitungsebene *f*, untere Führungskrafte *fpl* / **middle ~** mittlere Führungsebene *f* / **participative ~** partizipative Führung *f*, kooperative Führung *f*, partizipatives Management *n* / **scientific ~** wissenschaftliche Betriebsführung *f* / **top ~** Geschäftsleitung *f*, oberste Unternehmensleitung *f* / **traditional ~ theory** traditionelle Führungstheorie *f*

manager Führungskraft *f*, Manager *m* / **~ disease** Managerkrankheit *f*

managerial Leitungs–, Führungs–

mancinism Linkshandigkeit *f*

mand sprachlich unvollständige Forderung *f* / **~ function** Ruffunktion *f*

mandala Mandala *n*

mandible, mandibula Unterkiefer *m*, Mandibula *f*

mania Manie *f*, Sucht *f*, Wahnsinn *m* / **~ of being noticed** Beobachtungswahn *m* / **~ of business** Beschäftigungsdelir *n* / **~ with psychotic symptoms** Manie *f* mit psychotischen Symptomen / **~ without psychotic symptoms** Manie *f* ohne psychotische Symptome / **acute ~** akute Manie *f*, akutes Delirium *n* / **akinetic ~** akinetische Manie *f* / **anxious ~** ängstliche Manie *f*, Angstpsychose *f* / **chronic ~** chronische Manie *f* / **collecting ~** Sammelsucht *f*, Sammelwut *f*, Sammelwahn *m* / **dancing ~** Tanzwut *f* / **destructive ~** Zerstörungswut *f* / **doubting ~** Zweifelsucht *f* / **homicidal ~** Mordmanie *f* / **inhibited ~** gehemmte Manie *f* / **puerperal ~** Wochenbettmanie *f*, Mania puerperalis *f* / **recurrent ~** periodische Manie *f*, remittierende Manie *f* / **religious ~** Mania religiosa *f*, religiöser Wahn *m* / **suicidal ~** Selbstmordsacht *f*, Autophonomanie *f* / **touching ~** Sucht *f* alles anzufassen / **unproductive ~** stumme Manie *f*, unproduktive Manie *f*

maniac manisch, wahnsinnig, verrückt / Verrückter *m*, Wahnsinniger *m*, Besessener *m*

maniacal manisch, wahnsinnig, verrückt

maniaphobia krankhafte Angst *f* verrückt zu werden, Lyssophobie *f*

manic manisch / **~–depressive** manisch–depressiv / Manischdepressiver *m*

manifest manifest, offenkundig, deutlich hervortretend / sich manifestieren, zutage treten, in Erscheinung treten

manifestation Manifestation *f*, Auftreten *n*, Zutagetreten *n*, Äußerung *f*, Symptom *n* / **~ rate** Auftretenshäufigkeit *f* / **early ~** Frühform *f* / **neurological ~** neurologisches Symptom *n*

manifold mannigfach, zahlreich

manikin menschliches Modell *n* / **~ test** Gliederpuppenlegetest *m*

Manila hemp Manilahanf *m*

maniloquism Zeichensprache *f*, Fingersprache *f*

manipulandum Manipulandum *n*, Pickscheibchen *n*

manipulate manipulieren, geschickt beeinflussen, handhaben

manipulation Manipulation *f*, Handhabung *f* / **~ technique** Manipulationstechnik *f*, Manipulationsmethode *f*

manipulative manipulatorisch

manitou Manitou *m*, Gottheit *f* der Indianer, mächtige überirdische Person *f*

mankind Menschheit *f*, Menschen *mpl*, Menschengeschlecht *n*

manlike, manly mannhaft, männlich, wie ein Mann

manliness Männlichkeit *f*, Mannhaftigkeit *f*

manner Art *f*, Weise *f* / **~ of behaviour** Verhaltensweise *f*

mannered manieriert, gekünstelt

mannerism Manieriertheit *f*, Manierismus *m*, gekünstelte Angewohnheit *f*, unnatürliches Ausdrucksverhalten *n*

mannerliness Höflichkeit *f*, Manierlichkeit *f*, gute Kinderstube *f*

manning Personalaufstockung *f* / **~ table** Personalanforderungsplan *m*, Personaleinstellungsplan *m*

mannish männisch, unweiblich

manometer Druckmesser *m*, Manometer *n*

manometric manometrisch

manoptoscope Gerät *n* zur Bestimmung der Augendominanz

manpower Arbeitskräfte *fpl*, Personal *n*, Belegschaft *f* / **~ allocation** Personalzuweisung *f* / **~ planning** Personalplanung *f*, Personaleinsatzplanung *f*

manslaughter Totschlag *m*, fahrlässige Tötung *f*

manual manuell / Handbuch *n*, Leitfaden *m* / **Diagnostic and Statistical ~ of Mental Disorders (DSM)** diagnostisches und statistisches Manual *n* psychischer Störungen

manuscript handschriftlich / Manuskript *n* / **~ writing** Manuskriptschreiben *n*, Manuskripterstellung *f*

map Karte *f* / **cognitive ~** kognitive Karte *f*, kognitive Landkarte *f*

maple syrup urine disease Ahornsirupkrankheit *f*

mapping Kartierung *f*

maprotiline Maprotilin *n*

marantic, marasmic marastisch, Verfall–

marasmus Verfall *m*, Entkräftung *f*, Marasmus *m* / **senile ~** Altersverfall *m*, Altersschwäche *f*

marathon group therapy Marathonselbsterfahrungsgruppe *f*

Marbe effect Marbe–Effekt *m*

Marburg school Marburger Schule *f*

Marchiafava–Bignami Disease Marchiafava–Bignami Syndrom *n*

Marcuse's| teaching Marcuse'sche Lehre *f* / **~ theory** Marcuse'sche Theorie *f*

Marey tambour Marey'sche Trommel *f*, Marey'scher Tambour *m*

margin Rand *m*, Grenze *f* / **~ of attention** Aufmerksamkeitsgrenze *f* / **~ of consciousness** Marginalbewusstsein *n* / **~ of error** Fehlerbreite *f*

marginal Rand–, Grenz–, marginal

Marie's disease Marie Syndrom *n*, Marie'sche Krankheit *f*, Akromegalie *f*

marihuana, marijuana Marihuana *n*, getrocknete Hanfblätter *npl*, Cannabis *m*, Hanf *m* / **~ laws** Marihuanagesetzgebung *f* / **~ legalisation** Marihuanalegalisierung *f* / **~ usage** Marihuanaeinnahme *f*, Marihuanakonsum *m*

Mariotte's| blind spot blinder Fleck *m*, Mariotte'scher Fleck *m* / **~ experiment** Mariotte–Versuch *m* / **~ law** Boyle–Mariotte–Gesetz *n*

marital ehelich, Ehe–

mark Kennzeichen *n*, Merkmal *n*, Zensur *f*, Schulnote *f* / **~ sensing** Markierung *f* mit Graphitstift

marked deutlich, markant, ausgeprägt, auffallend, markiert, gezeichnet, merklich

marker Markierung *f*, Marker *m* / **~ test** Bezugstest *m* / **biological ~** biologischer Marker *m*

market Markt *m* / **~ analysis** Marktanalyse *f* / **~ investigation** Marktuntersuchung *f* / **~ observation** Marktbeobachtung *f* / **~ penetration** Marktdurchdringung / **~ psychology** Marktpsychologie *f* / **~ research** Marktforschung *f* / **~ share** Marktanteil *m* / **~ survey** Marktuntersuchung *f* / **psychological ~ research** psychologische Marktforschung *f*

marketing Vertrieb *m*, Marketing *n*, Absatzlehre *f*, Absatzbemühungen *fpl* / **~ executive** Vertriebsleiter *m*, Marketingdirektor *m* / **~ management** Absatzmanagement *n* / **~–mix** Marketingplan *m* / **~ research** Absatzforschung *f*, Marketingforschung *f*, Marktforschung *f*

Markov| chain Markoff–Kette *f* / **~ process** Markoff–Prozess *m*

marriage Heirat *f*, Ehe *f*, Eheschließung *f* / **~ attitude** Einstellung *f* zur Ehe / **~ clinic** Eheberatungsstelle *f* / **~ counseling** Eheberatung *f*, Partnerberatung *f* / **~ counseling agency** Eheberatungsstelle *f* / **~ rite** Hochzeitsbrauch *m*, Eheschließungsritus *m* / **~ therapy** Eheberatung *f* / **consanguineous ~** Heirat *f* zwischen Blutsverwandten / **endogamous ~** Verwandtenheirat *f*, endogame Ehe *f*, Endogamie *f* / **exogamous ~** Exogamie *f*, Ehe *f* mit einem Mitglied eines anderen Clans / **interfaith ~** religiöse Mischehe *f*, Ehe *f* zwischen Partnern verschiedenen Glaubens / **interracial ~** Ehe *f* zwischen verschiedenen Rassen *n*, rassische Mischehe *f* / **miscegenous ~** gemischtrassische Ehe *f* / **plural ~** Polygamie *f*

married verheiratet

marrow Mark *n*, Medulla *f* / **~–brain** Medulla oblongata *f*, Nachhirn *n* / **cerebral~** Marklager *n* / **spinal ~** Rückenmark *n*

marsupial Beuteltier *n*

Martius disk Martius–Scheibe *f*

masculine männlich, viril

masculinisation Vermännlichung *f*, Virilisierung *f*

masculinise vermännlichen, virilisieren, maskulinisieren

masculinism Maskulinismus *m*, Virilismus *m*, Mannweibtum *n*

masculinity Männlichkeit *f*, Maskulinität *f* / **~ complex** Männlichkeitskomplex *m* / **~–femininity** männlich–weiblich / **~–femininity stereotypy** Männlichkeits–Weiblichkeits–Stereotypie *f*

maser Maser *m*

mask Maske *f* / maskieren, verdecken, verbergen

masked maskiert, verdeckt, larviert, verborgen

masking Maskierung *f*, Überlagerung *f* / **~ audiogram** Lärmaudiogramm *n* / **~ effect of a sound** Überlagerungseffekt *m* eines Tones / **~ method** Überlagerungsverfahren *n* / **~ of odours** Geruchsüberlagerung *f* / **auditory ~** akustische Überlagerung *f*, auditive Maskierung *f* / **backward ~** retroaktive Maskierung *f*, rückwirkende Maskierung *f* / **foreward ~** proaktive Maskierung *f* / **visual ~** visuelle Maskierung *f*

masochism Masochismus *m* / **erotogenic ~** erotogener Masochismus *m*, primärer Masochismus *m* / **female ~** weiblicher Masochismus *m*, femininer Masochismus *m* / **ideal ~** idealer Masochismus *m* / **moral ~** moralischer Masochismus *m* / **primary ~** primärer Masochismus *m*, erotogener Masochismus *m* / **psychic ~** psychischer Masochismus *m* / **sexual ~** sexueller Masochismus *m*

masochist Masochist *m*

masochistic masochistisch

mass Masse *f*, Menge *f* / **~ action** Massenwirkung *f*, gehäufte Reaktion *f* / **~ action principle** Prinzip *n* der Massenwirkung / **~ action theory** Theorie *f* der Massenwirkung / **~ activity** Massenwirkung *f* / **~ audience** Massenpublikum *n* / **~ behaviour** Massenverhalten *n* / **~ communication** Massenkommunikation *f* / **~ concentration** Massenkonzentration *f* / **~ contagion** Massenansteckung *f* / **~ discharge** Summenentladung *f* / **~ effect** Masseneffekt *m*, Summationseffekt *m* / **~ hysteria** Massenhysterie *f* / **~ masochism** Massenmasochismus *m* / **~ media** Massenmedien *npl* / **~ media of communication** Massenkommunikationsmittel *npl* / **~ meeting** Massenversammlung *f* / **~ method** Massenmethode *f* / **~ mind** Massengeist *m*, Gruppengeist *m*, Gruppenseele *f*, Kollektivseele *f* / **~ movement** Massenbewegung *f* / **~ observation** Massenbeobachtung *f*, soziale Feldforschung *f* / **~ polarisation** Konzentration *f* der Aufmerksamkeit einer Masse / **~ produce** in Serie fertigen / **~ production** Serienfertigung *f*, Massenfertigung *f* / **~ protest** massiver Protest *m*, Massenprotest *m* / **~ psychology** Massenpsychologie *f* / **~–psychosis** Massenpsychose *f* / **~–reaction** gehäufte Reaktion *f* / **~ reflex** Summenerregung *f* / **~ response** Summenerregung *f*, Summenaktionspotenzial *n* / **~ society** Massengesellschaft *f* / **~ suggestion** Massensuggestion *f* / **~ tourism** Massentourismus *m* / **apperceptive ~** Apperzeptionsmasse *f* / **dispersed ~** abstrakte Masse *f*, Masse *f* ohne Beieinandersein der Mitglieder / **~es** die niedere Masse *f*, das gemeine Volk *n*

massed massiert, konzentriert

massiveness, massivity das Schwere *n*, das Massive *n*, Massivität *f*

Masson disk Masson'sche Scheibe *f*

massotherapy Massagebehandlung *f*

mast cell Mastzelle *f*

mastectomy Brustamputation *f*, Mastektomie *f*

master beherrschen / Meister *m*, Lehrer *m* / Haupt– / **~ record** Hauptunterlage *f*, Hauptakte *f* / **~ scale** Hauptskala *f*

mastery Beherrschung *f* / **~ of anxiety** Angstbewältigung *f* / **~ motive** Streben *n* nach Perfektion, Streben *n* nach Meisterschaft / **~ need** Perfektionsbedürfnis *n*, Streben *n* nach Perfektion / **active ~** aktive Beherrschung *f*

mastication Kauakt *m*, Kauvorgang *m*

mastocyte Mastzelle *f*

masturbate masturbieren, onanieren, sich selbst befriedigen

masturbation Selbstbefriedigung *f*, Masturbation *f*, Onanie *f* / **~ anxiety** Masturbationsangst *f* / **~ phantasy** Masturbationsphantasie *f* / **~ substitute** Masturbationsersatz *m*, Onanieersatz *m* / **automatic ~** mechanische Masturbation *f* / **compulsive ~** Zwangsonanie *f* / **psychic ~** psychische Masturbation *f*

masturbator Onanist *m*, Masturbator *m*

mat matt

matched zugeordnet, entsprechend, Vergleichs–

matching Zuordnen *n* / passend / **~ method** Zuordnungsmethode *f* / **~ to sample** Zuordnungsleistung *f* / **~ to sample test** Zuordnungstest *m* / **~ technique** Zuordnungstechnik *f*, Zuordnungsmethode *f* / **~ test** Zuordnungstest *m* / **associative ~** Zuordnen *n* von Assoziationen / **blind–~ technique** Methode *f* der Blindzuordnung

mate paaren, sich paaren, geschlechtlich verkehren / Gefährte *m*, Gatte *m*, Gattin *f* / **human ~ selection** Partnerwahl *f* beim Menschen / **~ swapping** Partnertausch *m*

mater Mutter *f* / **dura ~** Dura mater *f*, harte Hirnhaut *f* / **pia ~** Pia mater *f*, weiche Hirnhaut *f*

material Stoff *m*, Material *n* / materiell, stofflich, wichtig / **~ of dreams** Traummaterial *n*, Traumstoff *m* / **analytic ~** analytisches Material *n* / **hazardous ~** gesundheitsgefährdender Stoff *m* / **memorized ~** auswendig gelerntes Material *n*, im Gedächtnis eingeprägtes Material *n* / **raw ~** Rohmaterial *n*, Rohstoff *m*

materialisation Materialisation *f*, Verkörperung *f*

materialism Materialismus *m*

materialist Materialist *m*

materialistic materialistisch

materialize materialisieren, verwirklichen

maternal mütterlich, Mutter–

maternity Mutterschaft *f* / **~ home** Entbindungsanstalt *f* / **~ hospital** Entbindungsklinik *f* / **~ nurse** Hebamme *f*

mathematical mathematisch

mathematico–deductive mathematisch–deduktiv

mathematics, maths Mathematik *f* / **~ achievement** Mathematikleistung *f* / **~ anxiety** Mathematikangst *f* / **~ disorder** Rechenstörung *f* / **~ education** Mathematikausbildung *f*, Mathematikunterricht *m*

mating Paarung *f*, Begattung *f*, geschlechtliche Vereinigung *f*, Beischlaf *m*, Geschlechtsakt *m* / **assortiveness ~** Partnerübereinstimmung *f* / **~ behaviour** Paarungsverhalten *n* / **~ instinct** Paarungstrieb *m*, Begattungstrieb *m* / **~ period** Brunstperiode *f*, Brunstzeit *f* / **~ season** Brunstzeit *f*, Brunstperiode *f* / **assortative ~** Partnerwahl *f* nach übereinstimmenden Merkmalen, Partnerwahl *f* nach Ähnlichkeitsgesichtspunkten / **class–assortative ~** Heirat *f* innerhalb der eigenen Klasse

matriarchal matriarchalisch, mutterrechtlich

matriarchy, matriarchate Matriarchat *n*, Mutterherrschaft *f*

matrices Matrizen *fpl*

matricide Muttermord *m*, Muttermörder *m*

matriculation Immatrikulation *f*, Einschreibung *f*, Aufnahmeprüfung *f*

matrilineal matrilinear, der mütterlichen Linie zugehörig

matriliny mütterliche Linie *f*, Familie *f* mütterlicherseits

matrimonial ehelich, Ehe–

matrimony Ehe *f*, Ehestand *m*

matrix Matrix *f* / **conceptual ~** konzeptionelle Matrix *f* / **residual ~** Residualmatrix *f*, Restmatrix *f*

matt matt, glanzlos, unpoliert

matter Substanz *f*, Materie *f*, Sache *f*, Angelegenheit *f* / **central gray ~** zentrales Höhlengrau *n* / **cerebral ~** Hirnsubstanz *f* / **cortical ~** Rindensubstanz *f* / **fecal ~** Fäzes *pl*, Exkremente *npl* / **gray ~** graue Substanz *f* / **grey ~** graue Substanz *f* / **psychic ~** seelischer Stoff *m* / **white ~** weiße Gehirnsubstanz *f*

mattoid Paranoiker *m*

maturation Reifung *f* / **~ arrest** Reifungshemmung *f* / **~–degeneration hypothesis** Hypothese *f* von der Reifung und Entartung / **~ hypothesis** Reifungshypothese *f* / **~ of ovum** Eireifung *f* / **~ process** Reifeprozess *m*, Reifungsprozess *m*, Reifungsvorgang *m* / **~ theory** Reifungstheorie *f* / **anticipatory ~** vorweggenommene Reifung *f* / **ergic ~** ergische Reifung *f* / **physical ~** körperliche Reifung *f* / **sexual ~** Geschlechtsreifung *f* / **sexual ~ disorder** sexuelle Reifungskrise *f*, sexuelle Reifungsstörung *f*

mature reif, entwickelt / reifen, reif werden / **sexually ~** geschlechtsreif

maturity Reife *f* / **~ rating** Reifeschätzung *f*, Reifebeurteilung *f* / **early ~** Frühreife *f* / **emotional ~** emotionale Reife *f* / **genital ~** Geschlechtsreife *f* / **intellectual ~** intellektuelle Reife *f* / **mental ~** geistige Reife *f* / **physical ~** körperliche Reife *f*, physische Reife *f* / **psychosexual ~** psychosexuelle Reife *f* / **social ~** soziale

Reife *f* / **sexual ~** Geschlechtsreife *f*, sexuelle Reife *f* / **vocational ~** Berufsreife *f*

maxilla Oberkiefer *m*

maxillary Kiefer–, maxillar

maxim Maxime *f*, Grundsatz *m*

maximal maximal, höchst, größt

maximation Steigerung *f* / **reciprocal ~** reziproke Verstärkung *f*

maximum Maximum *n*, größte Menge *f* / Höchst–, größt, Maximal– / **~ sensation** maximale Empfindung *f*

Maxwell| disks Maxwell'sche Scheiben *fpl* / **~'s demons** Maxwellsche Dämonen *mpl* / **~ triangle** Maxwell–Dreieck *n*

Mayer's waves Mayer'sche Wellen *fpl*, Mayer–Blutdruckwellen *fpl*

maze Labyrinth *n*, Irrgarten *m*, Irrgang *m* / **~ experiment** Labyrinthversuch *m* / **~ learning** Labyrinthlernen *n* / **~ learning ability** Fähigkeit *f* zum Erlernen eines Labyrinthweges / **~ pathway** Labyrinthgang *m* / **~ running** Durchlaufen *n* eines Labyrinths / **~ runway** Weg *m* durch ein Labyrinth / **~ test** Labyrinth–Test *m* / **elevated ~** erhöhtes Labyrinth *n* / **enclosed–alley ~** Labyrinth *n* mit überdeckten Gängen / **mental ~ learning** Labyrinthlernen *n*, Lernen *n* durch mentales Training / **open ~** offenes Labyrinth *n* / **temporal ~** Wiederholungslabyrinth *n* / **verbal ~** Wortlabyrinth *n*

M'Naghten rules M'Naghten–Gesetz *n*

me mich / Ich *n*, Selbst *n* / **bodily ~** Körper Ich *n* / **empirical ~** wahrgenommenes Ich *n*, Ich–Erfahrung *f* / **psychological ~** Selbstbild *n*, Selbstwahrnehmung *f*

mealtime behaviour Essverhalten *n* bei Tisch

mean durchschnittlich, Mittel– / Mittelwert *m*, Durchschnitt *m* / beabsichtigen, bedeuten, sagen wollen / **~s activity** zweckgerichtete Aktivität *f* / **~s of communication** Kommunikationsmittel *npl* / **~s–end capacity** Fähigkeit *f* die Mittel–Zweckrelation zu erfassen / **~s–end expectation** Mittel–Zweck–Erwartung *f* / **~s–end readiness** Mittel–Zweck–Erwartung *f*, zweckgerichtete Erwartungsbereitschaft *f* / **~s–end relation** Mittel–Zweck–Relation *f*, Mittel–Zweck–Beziehung *f* / **~–error procedure** Herstellungsmethode *f*, Methode *f* des mittleren Fehlers / **~s of expression** Ausdrucksmittel *npl* / **~s object** Mittel *n*, Hilfsmittel *n* / **~s of power** Machtmittel *npl* / **arithmetic ~** arithmetisches Mittel *n* / **assumed ~** angenommener Mittelwert *m*, festgelegter Mittelwert *m* / **coercive ~s** Zwangsmittel *n* / **geometric ~** geometrisches Mittel *n* / **golden ~** goldener Mittelweg *m* / **guessed ~** angenommener Mittelwert *m* / **harmonic ~** harmonisches Mittel *n* / **logarithmic ~** geometrisches Mittel *n* / **obtained ~** empirisch erhaltener Mittelwert *m* / **true ~** wahrer Mittelwert *m* / **weighted ~** gewogenes Mittel *n*, gewichteter Mittelwert *m* / **working ~** angenommener Mittelwert *m*, festgelegter Mittelwert *m*

meaning Sinn *m*, Bedeutung *f* / **antithetic ~ of primal words** Gegensinn *m* der Urworte / **associative ~** assoziative Bedeutung *f* / **connotative ~** konnotative Bedeutung *f* / **denotative ~** denotative Bedeutung *f* / **extensional ~** extensive Bedeutung *f* / **intentional ~** beabsichtigte Bedeutung *f*, gewollte Bedeutung *f* / **nonverbal ~** nichtverbale Bedeutung *f* / **verbal ~** verbale Bedeutung *f*, sprachliche Bedeutung *f*, Wortbedeutung *f*

meaningful bedeutungsvoll

meaningfulness Bedeutungshaltigkeit *f*

meaningless bedeutungslos, sinnlos

measles Masern *pl*

measurability Messbarkeit *f* / **objective ~** objektive Messbarkeit *f*

measure messen / Maß *n*, Maßstab *m*, Maßnahme *f*, Test *m* / **~ of central tendency** Maß *n* der zentralen Tendenz / **~ of contingency** Kontingenzmaß *n* / **~ of precision** Feinmessung *f* / **~ of relation** Beziehungsmaß *n* / **comparable ~s** vergleichbare Messungen *fpl* / **correctional ~** Besserungsmaßregel *f* / **derived ~** abgeleitetes Maß *n*, Sekundärscore *m* / **developmental ~** Entwicklungstest *m* / **disciplinary ~** Disziplinarmaßnahme *f* / **discrete ~** diskrete Messzahl *f*, Einzelmaßnahme *f* / **perceptual ~** Wahrnehmungsmessverfahren *n* / **photometric ~s** lichttechnische Maße *npl* / **precautionary~** Vorsichtsmaßnahme *f* / **reformatory ~** Besserungsmaßregel *f* / **repeated ~** wiederholte Messung *f* / **representative ~** repräsentativer Wert *m* / **sensorimotor ~** sensumotorischer Test *m* / **standard ~** Normalmaß *n*, Normalmaßstab *m* / **true ~** wahre Messung *f* / **weighted ~** gewichtetes Maß *n*

measurement Messung *f*, Messen *n*, Maß *n* / **~ of abilities** Messung *f* von Fähigkeiten / **~ of change** Veränderungsmessung *f* / **~ of intelligence** Intelligenzmessung *f* / **absolute ~** Messung *f* in absoluten Werten / **additive conjoint ~** additive verbundene Messung *f* / **auditory ~** Hörmessung *f*, Audiometrie *f* / **conjoint ~** verbundene Messung *f* / **direct ~** direkte Messung *f*, direkte Skalierung *f* / **educational ~** Schulmessung *f*, pädagogische Diagnostik *f* / **indirect ~** indirekte Messung *f*, indirekte Skalierung *f* / **interactive ~** Interaktionsmaß *n* / **ipsative ~** ipsative Messung *f* / **mental ~** psychologische Messung *f* / **psychophysical ~** psychophysikalische Messung *f* / **relative ~** Messung *f* in relativen Werten / **statistical ~** statistische Messung *f*

measuring Messung *f*, Messen *n* / **~-apparatus** Messgerät *n*, Messapparat *m* / **~-device** Messvorrichtung *f* / **~ of fatigue** Ermüdungsmessung *f* / **~-instrument** Messgerät *n*, Messinstrument *n* / **~ method** Messmethode *f*

meatus Gang *m*, Kanal *m*, Meatus *m* / **external auditory ~** äußerer Gehörgang *m* / **internal auditory ~** innerer Gehörgang *m*

mecamylamine Mecamylamin *n*

mechanical mechanisch

mechanics Mechanik *f* / **psychic ~** Seelenmechanik *f*

mechanic's visual keenness test Test *m* der technischen Sehschärfe

mechanism Mechanismus *m* / **~ of action** Wirkungsweise *f*, Wirkmechanismus *m* / **~ of development** Entstehungsmechanismus *m* / **acquired releasing ~** erworbener Auslösemechanismus *m* / **coping ~** Verarbeitungsmechanismus *m* / **inhibiting ~** Hemmungsmechanismus *m* / **innate releasing ~** angeborener Auslösemechanismus *m* / **Mendelian ~s** Mendel'sche Vererbungsmechanismen *mpl* / **mental ~** psychische Struktur *f* / **neurotic ~** neurotischer Mechanismus *m* / **releasing ~** Auslösemechanismus *m* / **undoing ~** Ungeschehenmachen *n* / **working-off ~s** Abarbeitungsmechanismen *mpl*

mechanistic mechanistisch

mechanomorphism mechanistische Theorie *f*, mechanistische Betrachtungsweise *f*, Mechanomorphismus *m*

mechanoperception Mechanoperzeption *f*

mechanoreception Mechanorezeption *f*

mechanoreceptor Mechanorezeptor *m*

mechanosensor Mechanosensor *m*

mechanotherapy Mechanotherapie *f*

meconeuropathia nervöse Störungen *fpl* bei Morphinismus, Rauschgiftneurose *f*

meconism Morphinismus *m*, Morphiumsucht *f*, Opiumvergiftung *f*

media Medien *npl* / **~ analysis** Werbeträgeranalyse *f* / **~ man** Werbeplaner *m* / **~ plan** Mediaplan *m*, Streuplan *m* / **~ planning** Mediaplanung *f* / **~ research** Mediaforschung *f*, Werbeträgerforschung *f* / **~ survey** Werbeträgerforschung *f* / **educational ~** Unterrichtsmedien *npl* / **instructional ~** Unterrichtsmedien *npl*, Lehrmedien *npl* / **news ~** Nachrichtenmedien *npl* / **refracting ~** Brechungsmedien *npl*

medial mittler, media

median Median *m*, Zentralwert *m* / in der Mitte liegend, mittler, Median– / **~ gray** mittelgrau / **~ grey** mittelgrau

mediate mittelbar, indirekt / vermitteln

mediating vermittelnd

mediation Vermittlung *f* / **~ hypothesis** Vermittlungstheorie *f* / **~–integration model** Vermittlungs– und Integrationsmodell *n* / **~ theory** Theorie *f* der vermittelnden Prozesse, Vermittlungstheorie *f*, Mediationstheorie *f* / **cognitive ~** kognitive Strukturierung *f*, kognitive Mediation *f* / **representational ~ process** vorstellungsmäßiger Vermittlungsprozess *m*

mediator intervenierendes System *n*, Vermittler *m*, Schaltneuron *n*, Mediator *m*

medic Mediziner *m*, Medizinstudent *m*

medical medizinisch, ärztlich

medicament Medikament *n*, Heilmitteln, Arznei *f* / **calming ~** Beruhigungsmittel *n*

medication Medikament *n*, Medikation *f*, Verordnung *f* / **~–induced disorder** medikamenteninduzierte Störung *f* / **~–induced movement disorder** medikamenteninduzierte Bewegungsstörung *f* / **~–induced postural tremor** medikamenteninduzierter Haltetremor *f*

medicine Medizin *f* / **~–man** Medizinmann *m* / **alternative ~** Alternativmedizin *f* / **forensic ~** Gerichtsmedizin *f*, forensische Medizin *f* / **geriatric ~** Geriatric *f*, Lehre *f* von den Alterskrankheiten / **legal ~** Gerichtsmedizin *f* / **mental ~** Psychiatrie *f* / **preventive ~** Präventivmedizin *f* / **psychological ~** Psychosomatik *f*, Psychiatrie *f* / **psychosomatic ~** psychosomatische Medizin *f*, Psychosomatik *f* / **social ~** Sozialmedizin *f* / **socialized ~** staatlicher Gesundheitsdienst *m* / **soothing ~** Beruhigungsmittel *n* / **suggestive ~** Suggestivbehandlung *f* / **veterinary ~** Veterinärmedizin *f*, Tiermedizin *f*

medico– medizinisch / **~ legal** gerichtsmedizinisch / **~ pedagogical** medizinisch–pädagogisch / **~ psychological** medizinisch–psychologisch / **~ psychology** medizinische Psychologie *f* / **~ social** sozialmedizinisch

meditation Meditation *f*, Nachdenken *n*

medium Medium *n*

mediumise in Trance versetzen

mediumistic Medium–, als Medium

mediumship Eigenschaft *f* als Medium zu fungieren

medroxyprogesterone Medroxyprogesteron *n*

medulla Rückenmark *n*, Medulla *f* / **~ dorsalis** Dorsalmark *n* / **~ oblongata** Nachhirn *n*, Medulla oblongata *f* / **~ spinalis** Rückenmark *n* / **~ of the spine** Rückenmark *n* / **adrenal ~** Nebennierenmark *n* / **adrenal ~ hormone** Nebennierenmarkhormon *n* / **cerebral ~** Marklager *n* des Hirns

medullary markartig, Mark–, Knochenmark–

medullated mit Markscheide versehen, markhaltig

medusa Meduse *f*, Qualle *f*

medullo–adrenal Nebennierenmark–

meeting Besprechung *f*, Konferenz *f*, Treffen *n*, Zusammenkunft *f*, Tagung *f* / **stormy~** stürmische Sitzung *f* / **professional ~** Fachtagung *f*

megacephalic, megacephalous großköpfig, makrozephal

megacephaly, megalencephaly, megalocephalia, megalocephaly Großköpfigkeit *f*, Megalozephalie *f*

megalocephalic großköpfig

megalographia Makrographie *f*, Megalographie *f*

megalomania Größenwahn *m*, Megalomanie *f*

megalomaniac Größenwahnsinniger *m*, Megalomaner *m*

megalopia, megalopsia Größersehen *n* von Gegenständen, Makropsie *f*, Megalopsie *f*

megalosplanchnic mit sehr großen Eingeweiden versehen, pyknisch, untersetzt

megrim Migräne *f*, Hemikranie *f* / **the ~s** Depression *f*, Schwermut *f*, Melancholie *f*

meiosis Meiose *f*, Reifeteilung *f*

Meissner's corpuscle Meissner'sches Tastkörperchen *n*

mel Mel *n*, Honig *m*

melancholia Melancholie *f*, Schwermut *f*, Depression *f* / **agitated ~** agitierte Melancholie *f* / **climacteric ~** klimakterische Melancholie *f*, Wechseljahrmelancholie *f* / **involutional ~** Involutionsmelancholie *f*, Altersmelancholie *f* / **recurrent ~** schubweise wiederkehrende Melancholie *f*

melancholiac Melancholiker *m*, Depressiver *m*, Schwermütiger *m*

melancholic melancholisch, depressiv, schwermütig / Melancholiker *m*, Depressiver *m*, Schwermütiger *m*

melancholy Melancholie *f*, Depression *f*, Schwermut *f* / schwermütig, traurig, depressiv / **climacteric ~** klimakterische Melancholie *f*, Wechseljahrmelancholie *f* / **puerperal ~** Wochenbettdepression *f*

melanin Melanin *n*, dunkles Pigment *n*

melanism Schwarzsucht *f*, Melanismus *m*, dunkle Pigmentbildung *f* der Haut

melanocyte Pigmentzelle *f*, Melanozyt *m* / **~ stimulating hormone** Melanozyten stimulierendes Hormon *n*

melatonin Melatonin *n* / **~ test** Melatonin–Test *m*

meliorism Meliorismus *m*

melioristic melioristisch

melissophobia krankhafte Angst *f* vor Bienen und Wespen, Melissophobie *f*

melody Melodie *f*

melomania Melomanie *f*

member Mitglied *n*, Glied *n* / **controlled ~** Regelstrecke *f* / **retained–~s method** Treffermethode *f*

membership Mitgliedschaft *f* / **~ character** Gliedcharakter *m* / **~ group** Zugehörigkeitsgruppe *f*, Mitgliedsgruppe *f*

membrane Membran *f*, Haut *f* Häutchen *n* / **~ action potential** Membran–Aktionspotenzial *n* / **~ of the brain** Hirnhaut *f* / **~ capacity** Membrankapazität *f* / **~ charge** Membranladung *f* / **~ conductance** Membranleitfähigkeit *f* / **~ of Corti** Corti'sche Membran *f* / **~ impedance** Membranwiderstand *m*, Membranimpedanz *f* / **~ patch clamp** Membranfleckklemme *f* / **~ permeability** Membranpermeabilität *f*, Membrandurchlässigkeit *f* / **~ potential** Membranspannung *f*, Membranpotenzial *n* / **~ protein** Membranprotein *n* / **~ resistance** Membranwiderstand *m* / **~ resting potential** Membran–Ruhepotenzial *n* / **~ theory of conduction** Theorie *f* der Membranleitung / **~ time constant** Membran–Zeitkonstante *f* / **~ transport system** Membrantransportsystem *n* / **basilar ~** Basilarmembran *f* / **buccal mucous ~** Mundschleimhaut *f*, Wangenschleimhaut *f* / **conductible ~** leitfähige Membran *f* / **excitable ~** erregbare Membran *f* / **gastric mucous ~** Magenschleimhaut *f* / **limiting ~** Grenzmembran *f* / **mucous ~** Schleimhaut *f* / **mucous ~ of the mouth** Mundschleimhaut *f* / **nictating ~** Nickhaut *f* / **nodal ~** nodale Membran *f* / **olfactory ~** Riechschleimhaut *f* / **polarized ~** polarisierte Membran *f* / **postsynaptic ~** postsynaptische Membran *f* / **presynaptic ~** präsynaptische Membran *f* / **reticular ~** Membrana reticularis *f* / **semipermeable ~** semipermeable Membran *f*, halbdurchlässige Membran *f* / **sensitive ~ of the eye** Netzhaut *f* / **synaptic ~** synaptische Membran *f* / **tectorial ~** Membrana tectoria *f* / **tympanic ~** Trommelfell *n* / **virginal ~** Jungfernhäutchen *n*, Hymen *n*

memorability Denkwürdigkeit *f*, Erinnerungsfähigkeit *f*, Erinnerungswürdigkeit *f*

memorable der Erinnerung wert, denkwürdig

memorandum Lernstoff *m*, einzuprägender Stoff *m*

memoric Gedächtnis–, Erinnerungs–

memoriter auswendig, Pauk–

memorization Einprägung *f* im Gedächtnis, Vorgang *m* der Gedächtnisprägung / **serial ~** Reihenlernen *n*

memorize einprägen, auswendig lernen, erinnern

memorizing Einprägen *n*, Memorieren *n*, Auswendiglernen *n* / **~ method** Memoriermethode *f*, Methode *f* des Auswendiglernens / **~ technique** Mnemotechnik *f*, Technik *f* des Einprägens

memory Gedächtnis *n*, Erinnerung *f* / **~ afterimage** Erinnerungsnachbild *n* / **~ apparatus** Gedächtnisapparat *m*, Gedächtnistrommel *f* / **~ colour** Gedächtnisfarbe *f* / **~ curve** Gedächtniskurve *f* / **~ decay** Gedächtnisschwund *m* / **~ disorder** Gedächtnisstörung *f* / **~ drawing** Gedächtnisbild *n* / **~ drum** Gedächtnistrommel *f* / **~ experiment** Gedächtnisexperiment *n* / **~ factor** Gedächtnisfaktor *m* / **~ function** Gedächtnisfunktion *f* / **~ gap** Gedächtnislücke *f*, Amnesie *f* / **~ hallucination** Gedächtnishalluzination *f*, Erinnerungsverfälschung *f* / **~ illusion** Erinnerungsillusion *f*, Erinnerungstäuschung *f*, Gedächtnistäuschung *f*, Paramnesie *f* / **~ image** Erinnerungsvorstellung *f*, Gedächtnisbild *n* / **~ level** Erinnerungsebene *f* / **~ location** Erinnerungsfeld *n* / **~ for past events** Altgedächtnis *n* / **~ pattern** Gedächtnisstruktur *f* / **~–retention** Behalten *n* im Gedächtnis / **~ span** Gedächtnisspanne *f*, Gegenwartsdauer *f* / **~ system** Erinnerungssystem *n* / **~ test** Gedächtnistest *m* / **~ trace** Gedächtnisspur *f*, Erinnerungsspur *f*, Erinnerungselement *n*, Erinnerungsrest *m*, Engramm *n* / **~ training** Gedächtnistraining *n* / **~ type** Gedächtnistypus *m* / **abstract ~** abstrakte Erinnerung *f* / **affective ~** Gefühlserinnerung *f* / **associative ~** semantisches Assoziationsgedächtnis, mechanisches Gedächtnis *n*, assoziatives Gedächtnis *n*, Erinnerungsassoziation *f* / **auditory ~** akustisches Gedächtnis *n* / **autistic ~** autistische Erinnerung *f* / **autobiographical ~** autobiographisches Gedächtnis *n* / **behavioral ~** Verhaltensgedächtnis *n* / **biological ~** biologisches Gedächtnis *n* / **collective ~** Kollektivgedächtnis *n* / **concrete ~** konkretes Gedächtnis *n* / **deceptive ~** Erinnerungstäuschung *f* / **defective ~** Gedächtnisschwäche *f* / **early ~** frühe Erinnerung *f* / **echoic ~** echoisches Gedächtnis *n* / **eidetic ~** eidetisches Gedächtnis *n* / **episodic ~** episodisches Gedächtnis *n* / **explicit ~** explizites Gedächtnis *n* / **false ~** Gedächtnistäuschung *f* / **feeble ~** Gedächtnisschwäche *f* / **iconic ~** ikonisches Gedächtnis *n* / **immediate ~** unmittelbares Behalten *n*, Kurzzeitgedächtnis *n*, Kurzzeitspeicher *m* / **impaired ~** Gedächtnisstörung *f* / **inaccessible ~** unzugängliche Erinnerung *f* / **incidental ~** Zufallsgedächtnis *n* / **individual ~** Detailgedächtnis *n* / **integral ~** gesamtes Gedächtnis *n* / **logical ~** Erinnerung *f* von Bedeutungen / **long–term ~** Langzeitgedächtnis *n* / **musical ~** musikalisches Gedächtnis *n* / **organic ~** Organerinnerung *f* / **phylogenetic ~** phylogenetisches Gedächtnis *n* / **productive ~** produktives Gedächtnis *n* / **racial ~** biologisches Gedächtnis *n*, Kollektivgedächtnis *n* / **repressed ~** unterdrückte Erinnerung *f* / **reproductive ~** reproduktives Gedächtnis *n* / **retentive ~** Erinnerungsschärfe *f*, gutes Gedächtnis *n* / **selective ~** selektives Gedächtnis *n* / **semantic ~** semantisches Gedächtnis *n* / **sensory ~** sensorisches Gedächtnis *n* / **sensorimotor ~** sensumotorisches Gedächtnis *n* / **short–term ~** Kurzzeitgedächtnis *n*, Fluoreszenzgedächtnis *n* / **spatial ~** räumliches Gedächtnis *n* / **traumatic ~** Unfallerinnerung *f*, traumatische Erinnerung *f* / **unconscious ~** unbewusste Erinnerung *f*, verdrängte Erinnerung *f* / **unintentional ~** Zufallsgedächtnis *n* / **verbal ~** Wortgedächtnis *n*, verbales Gedächtnis *n* / **visual ~** visuelles Gedächtnis *n* / **visuospatial ~** visuell–räumliches Gedächtnis *n* / **working ~** Arbeitsspeicher *m*

menace Drohung *f*, Bedrohung *f* / drohen, bedrohen

menacme Menakme *f*, Zeitraum *m* der weiblichen Geschlechtstätigkeit zwischen Pubertät und Menopause

menarche Menarche *f*, Eintritt *m* der ersten Regelblutung *f*, Auftreten *n* der ersten Menstruation

mendacious verlogen, lügnerisch, lügenhaft

mendacity Lügenhaftigkeit *f*, Verlogenheit *f* / **pathological ~** Lügensucht *f*, pathologisches Lügen *n*

Mendel| Bechterew's reflex Mendel–Bechterew'scher Reflex *m*, Fußrückenreflex *m* / **~'s law** Mendel'sches Gesetz *n*

Mendelian Mendel'sche (r, s), der Mendel'schen Regel entsprechend

Mendelism, Mendelianism Mendels Lehre *f*, Mendel'sche Regeln *fpl*, Mendel'sche Gesetze *npl*, Mendelismus *m*

Ménière's| disease Ménière'sche Krankheit *f* / **~ syndrome** Ménière'sche Symptomenkomplex *m*, Ménière–Syndrom *n*

meninges Hirnhäute *fpl*, Meningen *fpl* / **cerebral ~** Hirnhäute *fpl*

meningioma Gehirnhautgeschwulst *n*, Meningiom *n*

meningism Meningismus *m*, Pseudomeningitis *f*

meningitis Meningitis *f*, Hirnhautentzündung *f* / **bacterial ~** bakterielle Meningitis *f* / **spinal ~** Meningitis spinalis *f* / **viral ~** Virusmeningitis *f*

meningo|–encephalitis Entzündung *f* des Gehirns und der Häute, Meningoenzephalitis *f* / **~ myelocele** Meningomyelozele *f*

meningopathy Hirnhauterkrankung *f*

meningovascular Hirnhautgefäß—, meningovaskulär

meninx Hirnhaut *f*, Meninx *f*

meniscus Meniskus *m*, Halbmuschelglas *n*, konvex–konkave Linse *f*

menopausal klimakterisch

menopause Wechseljahre *npl*, Menopause *f*, Klimakterium *n*

menorrhagia abnorm starke Monatsblutung *f*, verlängerte Menstruation *f*

menorrhoea, menorrhea Monatsblutung Regel *f*, Menstruation *f*

menses Regel *f*, Menses *fpl*, Menstruation *f*, Monatsblutung *f*

menstrual Regel–, Menstruations–, menstruell

menstruant Menstruierende *f*

menstruate menstruieren, die Regel haben

menstruating menstruierend

menstruation Menstruation *f*, Regel *f*, Periode *f* / **delayed ~** verzögerte Menstruation *f* / **excessive ~** Menorrhagie *f*, abnorm starke Monatsblutung *f* / **painful ~** Dysmenorrhoe *f*, Menstruationsbeschwerden *fpl* / **white ~** Menstruation *f* ohne Blutung

mensurability Messbarkeit

mensurable messbar

mensuration Messung *f*

mental geistig, psychisch, seelisch, Geistes–, Gemüts–, mental

mentalism Mentalismus *m*, subjektivierende Psychologie *f*

mentalistic mentalistisch, psychologisch

mentality Mentalität *f*, Geisteshaltung *f*, Geistesart *f*, Denkart *f*

mentally geistig / **~ deficient** schwachsinnig, geistig minderbegabt, geistesschwach / **~ deranged** geisteskrank, psychotisch, verrückt, wahnsinnig / **~ disturbed** geistesgestört, psychotisch, verrückt / **~ handicapped** geistig behindert

mentation Geistesfunktion *f*, Geistestätigkeit *f*, geistige Prozesse *mpl*

menticide Tötung *f* des eigenen Willens, Gehirnwäsche *f*, Mentizid *n*

mentism Mentismus *m*

mentor Mentor *m*

meperidine Meperidin *n*, Pethidin *n*

mephenisin Mephenisin *n*

meprobamate Meprobamat *n*

meralgia paraesthetica Meralgia paraesthetica *f*, Bernhardt'sche Insel *f*

merchandising Verkaufsförderung *f*

mercury poisoning Merkurialismus *m*, chronische Quecksilbervergiftung *f*

mercy Barmherzigkeit *f*, Gnade *f* / **~ killing** Gnadentod *m*, Euthanasie *f*, aktive Sterbehilfe *f*

merge verschmelzen, ineinander aufgehen

merger Fusion *f*, Verschmelzung *f* / **organizational ~** organisatorischer Zusammenschluss *m*, Fusion *f* von Organisationen

meridian Meridian *m*

merit Verdienst *n*, Vorzug *m* / verdienen / **~ increase** leistungsbezogene Gehaltserhöhung *f* / **~ ranking** Rangreihenbildung *f* / **~ rating** Leistungsbeurteilung *f*, Personalbeurteilung *f* / **~ scale** Wertskala *f* Leistungsskala *f*

Merkel|–Ranvier cell Merkel–Zelle *f* / **~'s cell** Merkel–Zelle *f*/ **~'s corpuscule** Merkel'sche Tastzelle *f* / **~'s law** Merkel'sches Gesetz *n* / **~'s touch cells** Merkel Tastzellen *fpl*

meropia Teilblindheit *f*

merry–go–round phenomenon Karusselphänomen *n*

merycism, merycismus Meryzismus *m*, Rumination *f*, mit Lustgefühlen verbundenes Wiederkäuen *n*, Aufstoßen *n*

Merzbacher–Pelizaeus syndrome Pelizaeus–Merzbacher–Krankheit *f*

mesaticephalic, mesaticephalous Mittelhirn–, mittelköpfig, mesozephal

mescal Meskal *n*, Meskalin *n*

mescaline Meskalin *n*

mescalism Meskalinsucht *f*

mesencephalic Mittelhirn–, mesenzephal

mesencephalon Mittelhirn *n*, Mesenzephalon *n*

mesial medial, in der mittleren Linie eines Körpers gelegen

mesmeric heilmagnetisch, hypnotisch, mesmerisch

mesmerise magnetisieren, hypnotisieren, nach der Mesmer'schen Methode behandeln

mesmerism Mesmerismus *m*, tierischer Magnetismus *m*, Lehre *f* vom Heilmagnetismus, Hypnose *f*

mesmerist Anhänger *m* der Mesmer'schen Lehre, Heilmagnetiseur *m*, Hypnotiseur *m*

mesoblast Mesoblast *n*, mittleres Keimblatt *n*, Mesoderm *n*

mesocephal, mesocephalic Mittelhirn–, mesozephal, mittelköpfig

mesocephalon Mittelhirn *n*, Mesenzephalon *n*

mesocephaly, mesocephalism Mesozephalie *f*

mesoderm Mesoderm *n*, mittleres Keimblatt *n*, Mesoblast *n*

mesodermal mesodermal, das mittlere Keimblatt betreffend

mesokurtic normalgipflig, von normaler Krümmung

mesokurtosis Normalgipfligkeit *f*, normale Kurtosis *f*, mittlere Krümmung *f* einer Verteilungskurve

mesology Lehre *f* von der Umwelt, Milieulehre *f*, Mesologie *f*

mesomorphic, mesomorphous mesomorph

mesomorphy, mesomorphism Mesomorphie *f*

mesoridazine Mesoridazin *n*

mesosomatic, mesosomatous von mittlerer Körpergröße, mesosomatisch

message Botschaft *f*, Mitteilung *f*, Kommunikationsinhalt *m*, E–Mail *n*, Nachricht *f* in einer Newsgroup / **immediate ~** direkte Mitteilung *f* / **mediate ~** mittelbare Botschaft *f* / **sensory ~** Sinneseindruck *m*

messenger Bote *m* / **~ RNA** Boten–RNS *f*

messianism Sendungsbewusstsein *n*, Messianismus *m*

metabolic metabolisch, Stoffwechsel–

metabolism Stoffwechsel *m*, Metabolismus *m* / ~ **of activity** Betriebsstoffwechsel *m* / ~ **disorder** Stoffwechselstörung *f* / **basal** ~ Grundumsatz *m* / **developmental** ~ Aufbaustoffwechsel *m* / **disordered** ~ Stoffwechselstörung *f* / **disturbed** ~ Stoffwechselstörung *f* / **respiratory** ~ Gasaustausch *m* / **total** ~ Gesamtumsatz *m*, Gesamtstoffwechsel *m*

metabolite Stoffwechselprodukt *n*, Stoffwechselzwischenprodukt *n*, Metabolit *m*

metacarpal Mittelhand–, metakarpal / Mittelhandknochen *m*

metachronism Fehler *m* in der zeitlichen Reihenfolge

metachrosis Farbwechsel *m* bei Tieren

metacinesis Metakinese *f*

metacognition Metakognition *f*

metagenesis Generationswechsel *m*, Metagenese *f*

metagenital ohne Beteiligung der Genitalien, extragenital

metagnomy Hellsehen *n*

metagnosiometry Messung *f* der Meinungsänderungen

metagnosis Meinungsänderung *f*

metakinesis Metakinese *f*

metalanguage Metasprache *f*

metalinguistic metasprachlich, metalinguistisch

metalinguistics Metalinguistik *f*

metallic metallisch

metallophobia Metallangst *f*, Angst *f* vor der Berührung von Metallen, Metallophobie *f*

metallotherapy Behandlung *f* mit Metallen

metamemory Metagedächtnis *n*

metamere Körpersegmente *npl*, Metamere *npl*, Ursegmente *npl*

metameric metamer

metamerism metamerer Bau *m*, Metamerismus *m*, Metamerie *f*

metamorphic gestaltverändernd, veränderlich, metamorph

metamorphism Metamorphismus *m*

metamorphopsia Verzerrtsehen *n*, Metamorphopsie *f*

metamorphosis Umwandlung *f*, Umgestaltung *f*, Metamorphose *f* / **sexual** ~ Geschlechtsumwandlung *f*

metanerg Metanerg *n*, erworbene psychische Wurzeleigenschaft *f*

metanergic metanergisch

metaphor Metapher *f*, übertragener Ausdruck *m*

metaphysics Metaphysik *f*

metapsychical metapsychisch

metapsychics Parapsychologie *f*, Metapsychik *f*, Metapsychologie *f*

metapsychoanalysis Metapsychoanalyse *f*

metapsychology Metapsychologie *f*, Metapsychik *f*, Parapsychologie *f*

metascience wissenschaftlicher Empirismus *m*, wissenschaftliches Studium *n* der Wissenschaft

metastable metastabil, halbbeständig, labil

metastasis Tochtergeschwulst *f*, Metastase *f*

metathalamus Metathalamus *m*, Kniehökker *m*

metathesis Umstellung *f*, Metathesis *f*

metathetic metathetisch, Umstellungs–

metazoon Mehrzeller *m*, mehrzelliges Lebewesen *n*, Metazoon *n*

metedrine psychosis Weckaminpsychose *f*

metempiric, metempirical jenseits empirischer Überprüfung, außerhalb der empirischen Verifikation

metempsychosis Seelenwanderung *f*, Metempsychose *f*

metencephalic Hinterhirn

metencephalon Metenzephalon *n*, Hinterhirn *n*

metenym test Test *m* mit Mehrfachwortbedeutungen

meter Messgerät *n*, Messer *m* / ~ **angle** Messwinkel *m* / ~**–candle** Messkerze *f*, Lux *n*

methadone Methadon *n* / ~ **maintenance** Methadonbehandlung *f*, Aufrechterhaltung *f* des Methadonspiegels, Methadonerhaltungsdosis *f*

methamphetamine, methedrine Methamphetamin *n*

methanol Methanol *n*, Methylalkohol *m*

methaqualone Methaqualon *n*

methionine Methionin *n*

method Methode *f*, Verfahren *n* / ~ **of absolute judgments** Methode *f* der absoluten Urteile, Methode *f* der Einzelreize / ~ **of adjustment** Herstellungsmethode *f*, Methode *f* des mittleren Fehlers, Reproduktionsmethode *f* / ~ **of administration** Anwendungsweise *f* / ~ **of agreement** Methode *f* der Übereinstimmung / ~ **of average error** Methode *f* des mittleren Fehlers / ~ **of beats** Taktschlagmethode *f* / ~ **of concomitant variations** Methode *f* der gleichzeitigen Variationen / ~ **of constant stimuli** Methode *f* der konstanten Reize / ~ **of constant stimulus differences** Methode *f* der konstanten Reizunterschiede / ~ **of correct associates** Treffermethode *f* / ~ **of co–twin control** Zwillingskontrollmethode *f* / ~ **of dichotomic classification** Methode *f* der Zweiteilung / ~ **of differences** Unterschiedsregel *f* / ~ **of disappearing differences** Methode *f* der verschwindenden Unterschiede, Grenzmethode *f* / ~ **of double stimuli** Methode *f* der verdoppelten Reize / ~ **of elimination** Eliminationsmethode *f* / ~ **of equal and unequal cases** Methode *f* der gleichen und ungleichen Fälle / ~ **of equal–appearing intervals** Methode *f* der gleicherscheinenden Intervalle, Methode *f* der mittleren Abstufungen / ~ **of equal sense differences** Methode *f* der gleichmäßigen Abstufungen, Methode *f* der mittleren Abstufungen / ~ **of equal sense distances** Methode *f* der gleichmäßigen Abstufungen, Methode *f* der mittleren Abstufungen / ~ **of equation** Herstellungsmethode *f* / ~ **of equivalents** Methode *f* der Äquivalente / ~ **of examination** Untersuchungsmethode *f* / ~ **of exhaustion** Anpassungsmethode *f* / ~ **of expression** Ausdrucksmethode *f* / ~ **of graded dichotomies** Methode *f* der stufenweisen Zweiteilung / ~ **of groups of stimuli** Reizgruppenmethode *f* / ~ **of interference** Interferenzmethode *f* / ~ **of interpretation** Interpretationsmethode *f* / ~ **of investigation** Untersuchungsmethode *f* / ~ **of isolated stimuli** Methode *f* der Einzelreize / ~ **of just noticeable differences** Methode *f* der eben merklichen Unterschiede, Grenzmethode *f*, Grenzverfahren *n* / ~ **of least differences** Methode *f* der kleinsten Unterschiede, Methode *f* der eben merklichen Unterschiede, Grenzmethode *f*, Grenzverfahren *n* / ~ **of least perceptible differences** Methode *f* der eben merklichen Unterschiede, Methode *f* der kleinsten Unterschiede / ~ **of least squares** Methode *f* der kleinsten Quadrate / ~ **of limits** Grenzmethode *f*, Grenzverfahren *n* / ~ **of maximum–likelihood** Maximum–Likelihood–Methode *f* / ~ **of mean error** Methode *f* des mittleren Fehlers, Herstellungsmethode *f* / ~ **of mean gradations** Methode *f* der mittleren Abstufungen, Methode *f* der gleicherscheinenden Intervalle / ~ **of mean stimuli** Methode *f* der mittleren Abstufungen, Methode *f* der gleicherscheinenden Intervalle / ~ **of minimal changes** Methode *f* der Minimaländerungen, Grenzverfahren *n*, Grenzmethode *f* / ~ **of paired associates** Methode *f* des Paarvergleichs, Methode *f* des paarweisen Vergleichs / ~ **of paired comparison** Methode *f* des Paarvergleichs, Methode *f* des paarweisen Vergleichs / ~ **of positive and negative cases** Methode *f* der richtigen und falschen Fälle / ~ **of prompting** Antriebsmethode *f* / ~ **of rank order** Rangreihenmethode *f* / ~ **of rating** Beurteilungsmethode *f*, Bewertungsmethode *f* / ~ **of reproduction** Herstellungsmethode *f*,

Methode *f* des mittleren Fehlers, Reproduktionsmethode *f*, Gedächtnismethode *f* / ~ **of retained members** Treffermethode *f* / ~ **of right and wrong cases** Methode *f* der richtigen und falschen Fälle, Konstanzmethode *f* / ~ **of right and wrong judgments** Methode *f* der richtigen und falschen Fälle / ~ **of right associates** Treffermethode *f* / ~ **of sampling** Stichprobenmethode *f*, Stichprobenverfahren *n* / ~ **of selection** Auswahlmethode *f* / ~ **of serial exploration** Methode *f* der Reihenexploration / ~ **of single stimuli** Methode *f* der Einzelreize, Methode *f* der absoluten Urteile / ~ **of standardization** Standardisierungsmethode *f* / ~ **of successive approximation** Näherungsverfahren *n*, Approximationsverfahren *n* / ~ **of successive intervals** Methode *f* der sukzessiven Intervalle / ~ **of successive reproductions** Methode *f* der sukzessiven Reproduktionen / ~ **of supralinimal differences** Methode *f* der gleicherscheinenden Intervalle / ~ **of systemic observation** Methode *f* der systematischen Beobachtung / **~s time measurement** Methoden–Zeitmessung *f*, MTM–Verfahren *n* / ~ **of treatment** Behandlungsart *f* / ~ **of triads** Triadenmethode *f* / **ad–lib** ~ gleichzeitige Anwendung *f* verschiedener Analysemethoden / **analytical** ~ analytische Methode *f* / **anticipatory** ~ Antizipationsmethode *f* / **axiomatic** ~ axiomatische Methode *f* / **Baconian** ~ induktive Methode *f* / **bifactor** ~ Zweifaktorenmethode *f* / **biographical** ~ biographische Methode *f* / **catechetical** ~ Frage–Antwort–Methode *f*, Befragungsmethode *f* / **cathartic** ~ kathartische Methode *f* / **clinical** ~ klinische Methode *f* / **clinical ~s training** klinische Ausbildung *f* / **comparative** ~ Methode *f* des Paarvergleichs, Methode *f* des paarweisen Vergleichs / **constant** ~ Konstanzverfahren *n* / **contraceptive ~s** empfängnisverhütende Methoden *fpl* / **correlational** ~ Korrelationsverfahren *n* / **cross–cultural** ~ Methode *f* des Kulturvergleichs / **crosssectional** ~ Querschnittsmethode *f* / **descriptive** ~ Beschreibungsmethode *f*, deskriptive Methode *f* / **double blind** ~ Doppelblindmethode *f* / **dynamic** ~ dynamische Methode *f* / **empirical** ~ empirische Methode *f* / **endosomatic** ~ endosomatische Methode *f*, Tarchanoff–Methode *f* / **equipercentile** ~ Äquipercentilmethode *f* / **exosomatic** ~ exosomatische Methode *f*, Féré–Methode *f* / **experimental** ~ experimentelle Methode *f*, Versuch *m*, Experiment *n* / **Galilean** ~ Methode *f* des Galilei / **genetic** ~ genetische Methode *f* / **graphic** ~ graphische Auswertungsmethode *f* / **heuristic** ~ heuristische Methode *f* / **historico–critical** ~ historisch–kritische Methode *f* / **hypothetico–deductive** ~ hypothetisch–deduktive Methode *f*, mathematisch–deduktive Methode *f* / **imaging** ~ bildgebendes Verfahren *n* / **inductive** ~ induktive Methode *f* / **introspective** ~ Selbstbeobachtungsmethode *f* / **intuitive** ~ Resonanzmethode *f* / **logotherapeutic** ~ logotherapeutische Methode *f* / **longitudinal** ~ Längsschnittmethode *f* / **mathematico–deductive** ~ mathematisch–deduktive Methode *f*, Methode *f* der Postulate / **multifactorial** ~ multifaktorielles Verfahren *n* / **multivariate** ~ multivariate Methode *f* / **narrative** ~ Erzählmethode *f* / **new** ~ neue Methode *f*, neues Verfahren *n* / **objective** ~ objektive Methode *f* / **observational** ~ Beobachtungsmethode *f* / **operational** ~ operationale Methode *f* / **optokinetic** ~ optokinetisches Verfahren *n* / **oral** ~ orale Methode *f*, Methode *f* der Lautsprache / **organoleptic** ~ sinnliche Prüfmethode *f* / **pedagogic** ~ pädagogische Methode *f* / **phonetic** ~ phonetische Methode *f* / **postulational** ~ Methode *f* der Postulate, mathematisch–deduktive Methode *f* / **projective** ~ projektives Verfahren *n* / **psychophysical ~s** psychophysische Messmethoden *fpl* / **psychotherapeutic** ~ psychotherapeutische Methode *f* / **qualitative** ~ qualitative Methode *f* / **quantitative** ~ quantitative Methode *f* / **scientific** ~ wissenschaftliche Methode *f*, wissenschaftliches Verfahren *n* / **scopic** ~ skopische Methode *f*, Ablesemethode *f* / **serial ~** Reihenmethode *f* / **statistical ~** statistische Methode *f* / **stereotactic ~** stereotaktische Operationsmethode *f* / **subjective ~** subjektive Methode *f* / **subjective estimate ~** subjektives Schätzverfahren *n*, subjektives Beurteilungsverfahren *n* / **therapeutic ~** Behandlungsmethode *f* / **total ~** Ganzheitsmethode *f* / **traditional ~** traditionelle Methode *f*, herkömmliche Methode *f* / **verbal ~** mündliche Methode *f*

methodological methodologisch

methodology Methodenlehre *f*, Methodologie *f* / **experimental ~** experimentelle Methodenlehre *f*

methohexital, methohexitone Methohexital *n*

methoxamine Methoxamin *n*

methoxyhydroxyphenylglycol (3,4) Methoxyhydroxyphenylglycol (3,4) *n*

methyldopa Methyl–DOPA *f*

methylenedioxy–methamphetamine Methylendioxymethamphetamin *n*

methylmorphine Methylmorphin *n*, Kodein *n*

methylphenidate Methylphenidat *n*

methylphenyltetrahydropyridine Methylphenyltetrahydropyridin *n*

5–methyluracil Thymin *n*

meticulosity, meticulousness übergroße Genauigkeit *f*, peinliche Genauigkeit *f*, Pedanterie *f*

meticulous übergenau, peinlich genau

metonymical metonymisch

metonymy Metonymie *f*

Metrazol Pentamethylentetrazol *n*, Pentetrazol *n* / **~ shock therapy** Schockbehandlung *f* mit Pentetrazol

metrics Metrik *f*, Verslehre *f*

metromania Metromanie *f*, Reimsucht *f*

metron Metron *n*

metronome Taktmesser *m*, Tempogeber *m*, Metronom *n*

metronoscope Lesetachistoskop *n*

Meyer's contrast experiment Meyers Kontrastversuch *m*

mezcaline Meskalin *n*

mianserin Mianserin *n*

mice Mäuse *fpl*

micella, micelle Mizelle *f*

micrencephalia, micrencephaly abnorme Kleinheit *f* des Gehirns, Mikrenzephalie *f*

microbar Mikrobar *n*

microcephalia, microcephaly, microcephalism Kleinköpfigkeit *f*, Mikrozephalie *f*

microcephalic, microcephalous kleinköpfig, mikrozephal

microcomputer Mikrocomputer *m*

microcosm Mikrokosmos *m*

microcounseling Kurzberatung *f*, Microcounseling *n*

micro–electrode Mikroelektrode *f* / **capillary ~** Glaskapillarmikroelektrode *f*, Kapillarmikroelektrode *f*

microencephalous kleinhirnig

micro–encephaly Kleinhirnigkeit *f*

microfilm Mikrofilm *m*, Kleinstfilm *m* / **~ aperture card** Mikrofilm–Fensterkarte *f*

microglia Mikroglia *f*, Mikrogliazelle *f*

microgram, microgramme Mikrogramm *n*, Millionstel Gramm *n*

microgroup Kleinstgruppe *f*, Mikrogruppe *f*

microgyria Kleinheit *f* der Gehirnwindungen, Mikrogyrie *f*

micromania Kleinheitswahn *m*, Mikromanie *f*

micrometer millionster Teil *m* eines Meters, Mikrometer *n*

micromillimeter millionster Teil *m* eines Millimeters, Millimikron *n*

micron tausendstel Millimeter *n*, Mikron *n*, Mikrometer *n,m*

micro–organism Mikroorganismus *m*

microphobia Angst *f* vor Bazillen, krankhafte Furcht *f* vor kleinen Dingen

microphone Mikrophon *n*

microphonia, microphony Mikrophonie *f*, verringerte Stimmstärke *f*, schwache Stimme *f*

microphonic stimmlich schwach / **~s** Mikrophonpotenziale *npl* / **aural ~** Cochlea–Mikrophonpotenzial *n* / **cochlear ~** Cochlea–Mikrophonpotenzial *n*

microphthalmia Kleinheit *f* des Augapfels, Mikrophthalmie *f*

micropia, micropsia Kleinsehen *n*, Mikropsie *f*

microsecond millionster Teil *m* einer Sekunde

microsociology Mikrosoziologie *f*, Kleinstgruppenforschung *f*

microsomatic kleinwüchsig, von kleinem Körperwuchs / Kleinwüchsiger *m*, Zwerg *m*

microsomia, microsomatia Zwergwuchs *m*, Mikrosomie *f*

microsplanchnic, microsplanchnous schmalbäuchig

microstereognosis Fähigkeit *f* kleinste Gegenstände durch Tasten zu erkennen

microstructure Feinstruktur *f*, Mikrostruktur *f*

microteaching Training *n* des Lehrverhaltens mittels Video–Kontrolle, Microteaching *n*

microteleopsia Mikroteleopsie *f*

microtome Mikrotom *n*, Schneideapparat *m* für Gewebsschnitte

microtomic feine Gewebsschnitte betreffend

microtomy Herstellen *n* von feinen Gewebsschnitten, Mikrotomie *f*

microtubule Mikrotubulus *m*

microvillus Mikrovillus *m*

microwave Mikrowelle *f* / **~ communication** Mikrowellenübertragung *f*

miction Miktion *f*, Harnlassen *n*, Harnabsonderung *f*

micturate Wasser lassen, Harn lassen, urinieren

micturition Miktion *f*, Harnlassen *n*, Harnabsonderung *f*

midazolam Midazolam *n*

midbrain Mittelhirn *n*, Mesenzephalon *n* / **~ reflex** Mittelhirnreflex *m*

middle mittlere (r, s), Mittel– / Mitte *f* mittlerer Teil *m*

midget Zwerg *m* / Miniatur–, Kleinst–

mid–interval Medianintervall *n*

midlife crisis Krise *f* in der Lebensmitte

midparent Elterndurchschnitt *m*, Mittelwert *m* einer Variablen bei beiden Elternteilen gemessen

midperiod Halbzeit *f*

midpoint Mitte *f*, Mittelpunkt *m*

midrange Mittelbereich *m* / **~ value** Mittelbereichswert *m*

midscore Zentralwert *m*, Mittelwert *m*, Median *m*

midwifery Hebammendienst *m*

Mignon delusion Mignonwahn *m*

migraine Migräne *f*, Hemikranie *f*, Halbseitenkopfschmerz *m* / **~ headache** Migränekopfschmerz *m*, Migräne *f*

migrainous migräneartig

migration Wanderung *f* / **~ worker** Wanderarbeitnehmer *m* / **human ~** Migration *f*, menschliches Wanderverhalten *n* / **selective ~** selektive Wanderung *f*

migratory wandernd, Wander–

mild leicht, mild, sanft, mäßig

mildness Milde *f*, Sanftmut *f*

milieu Milieu *n*, Umwelt *f*, Umgebung *f* / **~ therapy** Milieutherapie *f*, Milieugestaltung *f*

militancy Kampfgeist *m*, Angriffslust *f*, Gewalttätigkeit *f*, Militanz *f*

militarism Militarismus *m*

military militärisch, Militär–, Wehr–

milk|–ejection reflex Milchejektionsreflex *m* / ~ **let–down reflex** Milchejektionsreflex *m*

millilambert Millilambert *n*

milimeter Millimeter *m*

millimicron Millimikron *n*, millionster Teil *m* eines Millimeters

millioctave Millioktav *f*

milliphot Milliphot *m*

millisecond tausendstel Sekunde *f*

Mill's canon Mills Kanon *m*, Induktionsregeln *fpl*

mimeograph Vervielfältigungsmaschine *f*, Vervielfältigung *f*

mimesis Nachahmen *n*, Nachäffen *n*, Mimikry *f*, biologische Tarnung *f*

mimetic nachahmend, nachgemacht, Schein–, Mimikry–

minimetism Mimikry *f*, Tarnverhalten *n*

mimic nachgeahmt, nachgemacht / Schauspieler *m*, Mimiker *m*, Imitator *m* / nachahmen, nachäffen

mimicry Mimikry *f*, biologische Tarnung *f*

miming Mimik *f*, Mienenspiel *n*

mimodrame Gebärdenspiel *n*, Mimik *f*, Pantomime *f*

mind Geist *m*, Seele *f*, Psyche *f*, Verstand *m*, Intellekt *m* / **~–blindness** zerebrale Blindheit *f*, optische Agnosie *f* / **~–body problem** Leib–Seele–Problem *n* / **~–cure** Psychotherapie *f*, psychotherapeutische Behandlung *f* / **~–curist** Psychotherapeut *m* / ~ **deafness** Seelentaubheit *f*, akustische Agnosie *f* / **~–dust theory** Theorie *f* der beseelten Materie, Monadenlehre *f* / ~ **pain** Seelenschmerz *m*, Seelenleiden *n*, Psychalgie *f* / ~ **reading** Gedankenlesen *n* / **~–stuff theory** Theorie *f* der beseelten Materie, Monadenlehre *f* / **~–twist hypothesis** Hypothese *f* über die funktionelle Natur psychogener Störungen / **~–wandering** gelegentliche Geistesabwesenheit *f*, Träumerei *f* / **clear** ~ klares Bewusstsein *n* / **dosed** ~ Voreingenommenheit *f* / **clouded** ~ getrübtes Bewusstsein *n* / **collective** ~ Kollektivseele *f*, Gruppengeist *m*, Gruppenseele *f*, Massenseele *f*, Konsensus *m* / **conscious** ~ Bewusstseinsinhalt *m* / **diacritic** ~ scharfsinniger Geist *m* / **dirty** ~ obszöne Gedanken *mpl* / **open** ~ geistige Offenheit *f*, Unvoreingenommenheit *f* / **plastic** ~ bildsamer Geist *m*, plastischer Verstand *m* / **social** ~ Gemeinschaftsgeist *m* / **subconscious** ~ Unterbewusstsein *n* / **unconscious** ~ Unbewusstes *n* / **versatile** ~ beweglicher Geist *m*, wendiger Geist *m*

mineralocorticoid Mineralokortikoid *n*

miniature Miniatur *f*, Kleinformat *n* / ~ **end–plate potential** Miniaturendplattenpotenzial *n* / ~ **life situation** lebensgetreue Miniatursituation *f* / ~ **situation test** Miniatursituation *f* / ~ **system** Miniaturmodel *n*, Miniatursystem *n*

minimal minimal, Minimal–, kleinst

minimax Minimax *n* / ~ **expected loss strategy** Minimax–Strategie *f* für einen erwarteten Verlust / ~ **principle** Minimax–Prinzip *n* / ~ **risk strategy** Minimax–Strategie *f* / ~ **solution** Minimax–Lösung *f* / ~ **theorem** Minimax–Theorem *n*

minimum Minimum *n*, Mindestmaß *n*, Minimal–, Mindest–, Kleinst– / ~ **audible field** untere Hörschwelle *f*, Hörbarkeitsschwelle *f* / ~ **audible pressure** unter Hördruck *m* / ~ **separable** Trennschärfe *f* des Sehens, Punktsehschärfe *f* / ~ **visible** Sichtbarkeitsschwelle *f*, sehbares Minimum *n*

minor kleiner, geringer, unbedeutend, geringfügig

minority Minderheit *f*, Minorität *f* / ~ **group** Minderheitsgruppe *f*, Minoritätsgruppe *f* / ~ **group discrimination** Minderheitendiskrimination *f*, Benachteiligung *f* von Minoritäten im gesellschaftlichen Leben

minute |ventilation Atemzeitvolumen *n* / ~ **volume** Atemzeitvolumen *n*, Herzminutenvolumen *n*

miosis Pupillenverengung *f*, Miosis *f*

miotic pupillenverengend, miotisch

mirror Spiegel *m* / ~ **drawing** Spiegelzeichnung *f*, Spiegelzeichnen *n* / ~ **image** Spiegelbild *n* / ~ **perception** spiegelverkehrte Wahrnehmung *f* von Gedrucktem / ~ **reading** Spiegellesen *n*, spiegelverkehrtes Lesen *n* / ~ **reversal** spiegelverkehrte Abbildung *f* / ~ **script** Spiegelschrift *f* / ~ **self** Spiegel–Ich *n* / ~ **sign** Spiegelzeichen *n* / ~ **stage** Spiegelstufe *f* / ~ **test** Spiegeltest *m* / ~ **tracing** Spiegelzeichnung *f* / ~ **writing** Spiegelschrift *f* / **reflecting** ~ Reflektor *m*, Reflexionsspiegel *m*

mirroring Spiegeln *n*

mirth Heiterkeit *f*, Fröhlichkeit *f*

misandria, misandry Männerhass *m*, Misandrie *f*

misanthrope, misanthropist Misanthrop *m*, Menschenfeind *m*

misanthropia, misanthropy Menschenhass *m*, Misanthropie *f*

misanthropic menschenfeindlich, misanthropisch

misapprehension falsche Auffassung *f*, Missverständnis *n*

misbegotten unehelich, unnatürlich

misbehaviour schlechtes Betragen *n*, Fehlverhalten *n*

misbelief Irrglaube *m*

miscalculation falsche Berechnung *f*, Rechenfehler *m*, falsches Urteil *n*

miscarriage Fehlgeburt *f*

miscegenation Rassenmischung *f*

miscellaneous Verschiedenes *n*

mischief Unheil *n*, Schaden *m*, Unfug *m*

mischievous schädlich, nachteilig, boshaft

misconception Missverständnis *n*, falsche Auffassung *f*

misconduct schlechtes Betragen *n*, Ehebruch *m*

misdemeanant Straffälliger *m*, Delinquent *m*

misdemeanour strafbares Vergehen *n*

misdiagnosis Fehldiagnose *f*

misdoing Übeltat *f*

miserable unglücklich, elend, kläglich

misery Elend *n*, Not *f*, Trübsal *f*, Schmerz *m*

misfit ungeeignete Person *f*

misfortune Unglück *n*, Missgeschick *n*

misidentification Fehlidentifizierung *f*, Personenverkennung *f*

misinterpretation Fehldeutung *f*, Missdeutung *f*

misjudgment Fehlurteil *n*

mismanagement Misswirtschaft *f*, schlechte Leitung *f*, schlechte Verwaltung *f*

mismatch nicht zusammenpassen

misogamist Ehefeind *m*

misogamy Misogamie *f*, krankhafte Ehescheu *f*

misogynist Frauenfeind *m*

misogynous frauenfeindlich

misogyny Misogynie *f*, Frauenhass *m*

misologia, misology Diskussionshass *m*, Abneigung *f* gegen Reden

misoneism Neuerungshass *m*, Abneigung *f* gegen Änderungen

misopaedia, misopedia krankhafte Abneigung *f* gegen Kinder, Misopädie *f*

misopsychia krankhafter Lebensüberdruss *m*

misperception Trugwahrnehmung *f*, fehlerhafte Wahrnehmung *f* / ~ **test** projektiver Test *m*, Apperzeptionstest *m*

misprint Druckfehler *m* / verdrucken

mispronunciation falsche Aussprache *f*, schlechte Aussprache *f*

misreading Verlesen *n*

misreckoning Fehlberechnung *f*, falsche Rechnung *f*

miss verfehlen, verpassen, versäumen, durchfallen / Verlust *m*, Verpassen *n*

missing fehlend

mistake Fehler *m*, Irrtum *m*

mistrust Misstrauen *n* / nicht trauen, misstrauen

mistuned verstimmt

misunderstand missverstehen, sich irren

misunderstanding Missverständnis *n*, Uneinigkeit *f*

misunderstood missverstanden

misuse Missbrauch *m* / falsch gebrauchen, missbrauchen

mitigate mildern, lindern

mitochondrion Mitochondrie *f*

mitosis Mitose *f*, Karyokinese *f*, indirekte Zellteilung *f*

mitotic mitotisch, indirekte Zellteilung betreffend

mix mischen, vermischen, vermengen

mixed kombinierte, gemischt, Misch–

mixoscopia Mixoskopie *f*, Voyeurtum *n*

mixoscopic mixoskopisch, voyeurhaft

mixture Mischung *f*, Gemisch *n* / **~ of colour** Farbenmischung *f*

mix–up Verwirrung *f*, Mischmasch *m*

mnemasthenia Gedächtnisschwäche *f*

mneme Gedächtnis *n*, Erinnerung *f*, Mneme *f*

mnemic Gedächtnis–, Erinnerungs–

mnemometer Gedächtnisapparat *m*, Mnemometer *n*

mnemonic mnemonisch, mnemotechnisch

mnemonics Mnemonik *f*, Mnemotechnik *f*

mnemonisation Memoriertechnik *f*

mnemotechnical mnemotechnisch

mnemotechnics Mnemotechnik *f*, Technik *f* der Benutzung von Gedächtnishilfsmitteln

mnesic mnestisch

moan Stöhnen *n*

mob Mob *m*, Auflauf *m*

mobile beweglich, mobil / Handy *n*

mobilisation Mobilisierung *f* / **~ of energy** Mobilisierung *f* von Energie / **high ~** Mobilisierung *f* von Energie

mobility Mobilität *f* / **~ aid** Bewegungshilfsmittel *npl* / **geographical ~** geographische Mobilität *f* / **horizontal ~** horizontale Mobilität *f* / **occupational ~** berufliche Mobilität *f* / **physical ~** physische Mobilität *f* / **social ~** soziale Mobilität *f* / **vertical ~** vertikale Mobilität *f* / **vocational ~** berufliche Mobilität *f*

moclobemide Moclobemid *n*

modal modal

modality Modalität *f*, Sinnesmodalität *f*, Art *f* und Weise *f* / **sensory ~** Sinnesmodalität *f*

mode Modus *m*, Modalwert *m*, häufigster Wert *m*, Art *f* und Weise *f*, Mode *f* / **~ of action** Wirkungsweise *f* / **~ of adjustment** Anpassungsart *f* / **~ of appearance** Erscheinungsweise *f* / **~ of behaviour** Verhaltensweise *f* / **~ of expression** Ausdrucksweise *f* / **~ of life** Lebensart *f*, Lebensweise *f* / **~ of manifestation** Erscheinungsart *f* / **~ of reaction** Reaktionsweise *f* / **apparent ~** offensichtlicher Modus *m*, empirischer Modalwert *m* / **computed ~** geschätzter Modus *m*, berechneter Modus *m* / **crude ~** offensichtlicher Modus *m* / **empirical ~** empirischer Modalwert *m* / **estimated ~** geschätzter Modalwert *m* / **parataxic ~** parataxische Vorgehensweise *f* / **refined ~** gebildeter Modus *m*, korrigierter Modus *m*, geschätzter Modus *m* / **theoretical ~** theoretischer Modalwert *m* / **true ~** wahrer Modalwert *m*

model Modell *n*, Vorbild *n*, Leitbild *n*, Denkmodell *n* / **~ psychosis** experimentelle Psychose *f* / **~ school** Modellschule *f* / **behavioural ~** Verhaltensmodell *n* / **bifactor ~** Zweifaktorenmodell *n* / **conceptual ~** Begriffsmodell *n*, konzeptionelles Schema *n* / **deterministic ~** deterministisches Modell *n* / **experimental ~** Versuchsmodell *n* / **hierarchical ~** hierarchisches Modell *n* / **hypothetico–deductive ~** hypothetisch–deduktives Modell *n* / **mathematical ~** mathematisches Modell *n* / **mathematical ~ psychology** mathematische Modellpsychologie *f* /

medical ~ medizinisches Modell *n*, Krankheitsmodell *n* / **statistical** ~ **of learning** statistisches Lernmodell *n* / **stochastic** ~ stochastisches Modell *n* / **theoretical** ~ theoretisches Modell *n*, Denkmodell *n*

modeling Modellbildung *f*, passives Lernen *n*, Imitationslernen *n* / ~ **behaviour** Imitationsverhalten *n*, Nachahmung *f* / **heuristic** ~ heuristische Modellbildung *f* / **mathematical** ~ mathematische Modellbildung *f* / **stochastic** ~ stochastische Modellbildung *f*

modem Modem *n*

moderate mittelgradig, mittelschwer, mäßig, gemäßigt

moderator variable Moderatorvariable *f*

modern neu, modern

modesty Bescheidenheit *f*, Sittsamkeit *f* / **sexual** ~ Scham *f*, Schamhaftigkeit *f*

modification Modifikation *f*, Änderung *f*, Abänderung *f*, Abwandlung *f* / ~ **of consciousness** Bewusstseinsänderung *f* / **adaptive** ~ Anpassungsmodifikation *f* / **behavioural** ~ Verhaltensmodifikation *f* / **intraocular** ~ Veränderung *f* des Innenauges

modifier modifizierende Variable *f*

modify modifizieren, abändern, abwandeln

modiolus Achse *f* der knöchernen Schnecke des Ohres, Modiolus *m*

modulate modulieren, die Tonart wechseln

modulation Modulation *f*, visueller Modulator *m* / ~ **capacity** Modulationskapazität *f*

modulator Modulator *m*, Regulator *m* / **visual** ~ visueller Modulator *m*, visuelles Rezeptorensystem *n*

modulus Modul *m*

modus Art *f* und Weise *f*, Methode *f*, Modus *m*

mogiarthria Sprachstörung *f*, Mogiarthrie *f*

mogigraphia Schreibkrampf *m*, Mogigraphie *f*, Graphospasmus *m*

mogilalia Sprachstörung *f*, erschwertes Sprechen *n*, Mogilalie *f*

mogiphonia Stimmschwäche *f*, Phonasthenie *f*, Mogiphonie *f*

mol, mole Mol *n*

molar molar, ganzheitlich, in einer Einheit

molarism Molarismus *m*, Molaranalyse *f*

molarity molare Konzentration *f*, Molarität *f*

molecular molekular

molecularism Molekularismus *m*, Atomismus *m*, Elementarismus *m*

molilalia Sprachstörung *f*, erschwertes Sprechen *n*, Mogilalie *f*

molimen Menstruationsschmerz *m* / **premenstrual** ~ prämenstruelle Beschwerde *f*

molindone Molindon *n*

mollusc, mollusk Molluske *f*, Weichtier *n*

moment Augenblick *m*, Merkmal *n*, Moment *n,m*, Messwertabweichung *f* / ~ **of a sample** Stichprobenabweichung *f* / **second–order** ~ Moment *n* zweiter Ordnung, zweites Moment *n*

momentary momentan, augenblicklich, vorübergehend

momentum Moment *n*, Antrieb *m*, Triebkraft *f*

momism übermäßige Mutterabhängigkeit *f*

monad Monade *f*, organische Einheit *f*

monadic monadisch

monadism Monadenlehre *f*

monaural einohrig, monaural, monotisch

mongolian mongoloid

mongolism, mongolianism Mongolismus *m*, mongoloide Idiotie *f*, Trisomie 21 *f*, Down–Syndrom *n* / **trisomic dysmorph** ~ trisomal dysmorphe Entwicklungsstörung *f*

mongoloid mongoloid / Mongoloider *m*

monism Monismus *m*

monitor Monitor *m*, Überwachungsgerät *n*, Tutor *m* / überwachen

monitoring Überwachung *f*, Beaufsichtigung *f*

monkey Affe *m*

monoamine oxidase Monoaminooxydase *f* / **~ inhibitor** Monoaminooxydase–Hemmer *m*, MAO–Hemmer *m*

monoblepsia Sehen *n* mit nur einem Auge

monochord mit nur einer Chorda versehen

monochorionic mit nur einem einzigen Chorion versehen, monochorionisch

monochromasia, monochromasy, monochromatism monochromatisches Sehen *n*, Einfarbensehen *n*, Monochromasie *f*, totale Farbenblindheit *f*

monochromat Farbenblinder *m*, Monochromat *m*

monochromatic, monochromic monochromatisch, einfarbig

monochromator Monochromator *m*, Gerät *n* zur Erzeugung einfarbigen Lichts

monocular einäugig, monokular

monocyte Monozyt *m*

monoecious, monecious monözisch, hermaphroditisch

monogamous monogam

monogamy Monogamie *f*, Einehe *f*

monogenesis, monogeny, monogony ungeschlechtliche Fortpflanzung *f*, Parthogenese *f*, Monogenie *f*

monogenism Theorie *f* von der Abstammung der Menschheit von einem gemeinsamen Urmenschen, Monogenismus *m*

monoglot einsprachig

monograph Monographie *f*

monographic monographisch

monoideism Monoideismus *m*, fixe Idee *f*, Zwangsidee *f*

monolingualism Beherrschung *f* einer Sprache, Einsprachigkeit *f*

monologue Monolog *m* / **collective ~** kollektiver Monolog *m* / **dual ~** Monolog *m* zu zweit

monomania Monomanie *f* Zwangsvorstellung *f*, Monopsychose *f* / **affective ~** Affektpsychose *f* / **ambitious ~** Größenwahn *m*

monomaniac monoman / Monomaner *m*

monophasia Monophasie *f*, Fähigkeit *f* nur ein Wort zu sprechen, Fähigkeit *f* nur einen Satz hervorzubringen

monophasic monophasisch, Monophasie–

monophobia Angst *f* vor dem Alleinsein, Monophobie *f*

monophthalmia Einäugigkeit *f*, Monophthalmie *f*

monoplegia Lähmung *f* eines einzelnen Gliedes, Monoplegie *f*

monopolar monopolar, unipolar, einpolig

monopsia einäugiges Sehen *n*, Monopsie *f*

monorhinic mit einem Nasenloch riechend, monorhin

monosaccharide Monosaccharid *n*, Einfachzucker *m*

monosexual eingeschlechtlich, monosexuell

monospasm lokaler Krampf *m*, Krampf *m* eines einzelnen Gliedes, Monospasmus *m*

monosynaptic monosynaptisch

monotic ein Ohr betreffend, monotisch, monaural

monotone eintönige Wiederholung *f*, Eintönigkeit *f*, Einerlei *n*

monotonic monoton, stetig, eintönig

monotonous monoton, eintönig, einförmig

monotony Monotonie *f*, Eintönigkeit *f*, Langeweile *f*

monotropic monotrop, aufgrund eines einzigen Merkmals anziehend

monovular eineiig

monozygotic monozygot, eineiig

monster Missbildung *f*, Missgestalt *f*, Monstrum *n*

monstrosity, monstrousness Missbildung *f*, angebotene Deformität *f*, Monstrosität *f*

monstrous missgestaltet, unförmig, ungeheuerlich, monströs

Montessori| method Montessori–Methode *f*, Montessori–Pädagogik *f* / **~ pegboard** Montessori–Steckbrett *n*

mood Stimmung *f*, Gemütslage *f*, Laune *f* / **~ disorder** affektive Störung *f* / **~ disorder due to a general medical condition** affektive Störung *f* aufgrund eines medizinischen Krankheitsfaktors / **amphetamine–induced ~ disorder** amphetamininduzierte affektive Störung *f* / **hallucinogen–induced ~ disorder** halluzinogeninduzierte affektive Störung *f* / **organic ~ disorder** organische affektive Störung *f* / **~ episode** Episode *f* einer affektiven Störung / **~ syndrome** affektives Syndrom *n* / **basic vital ~** Lebensgrundstimmung *f* / **~–congruent psychotic features** stimmungskongruente, psychotische Merkmale *npl* / **delusional ~** Wahnstimmung *f* / **depressive ~** depressive Verstimmung *f* / **~–incongruent psychotic features** stimmungsinkongruente, psychotische Merkmale *npl* / **organic ~ disorders** organische affektive Störungen *fpl* / **organic ~ syndrome** organisch bedingtes affektives Syndrom *n* / **persistent ~ disorders** anhaltende affektive Störungen *fpl* / **subdepressive ~** subdepressive Verstimmung *f*

moodiness Launenhaftigkeit *f*, schlechte Laune *f*

moody launenhaft, launisch, mürrisch

moon Mond *m* / **~ blindness** Mondblindheit *f*, Nachtblindheit *f* / **~ illusion** Mondtäuschung *f* / **~ walking** Mondsucht *f*, Lunatismus *m*, Somnambulismus *m*

moot strittig, zweifelhaft, hypothetisch / zur Debatte stellen

moral moralisch, sittlich, Moral– / Moral *f*, Ethik *f*, sittliches Verhalten *n* / **~s** sittliches Verhalten *n*, Tugend *f*

morale Kohäsion *f*, Gruppenklima *n*, Betriebsklima *n*

moralist Sittenprediger *m*, Moralist *m*

morality Sittlichkeit *f*, Ethik *f*, Moral *f*, sittliches Verhalten *n* / **double ~** doppelte Moral *f*

moramentia Schwachsinnigkeit *f* mit moralischen Defekten

morbid krankhaft, krank, morbid

morbidity Morbidität *f*, Krankhaftigkeit *f*, Krankheitsstand *m*, Erkrankungshäufigkeit *f*, Erkrankungsziffer *f*

morbidness Krankhaftigkeit *f*, krankhafter Zustand *m*

mores sittlicher Kodex *m* / **social ~** gesellschaftlicher Sittenkodex *m*, Sozialethik *f*

Morgan's| canon Morgans Kanon *m* / **~ principle** Morgans Kanon *m*

moria Moria *f*, Witzelsucht *f*

Morita therapy Morita–Therapie *f*

Moro reflex Moro–Reflex *m*, Umklammerungsreflex *m*

moron Debiler *m*, Schwachsinniger *m*

moronic schwachsinnig

moronity, moronism, morosis leichte Debilität *f*, Schwachsinn *m*

morpheme Morphem *n* / **lexical ~** lexikalisches Morphem *n* / **relational ~** referentielles Morphem *n*

morphia Morphium *n*

morphine Morphium *n*, Morphin *n* / **~ addict** Morphinsüchtige *m,f*, Morphiumsüchtige *m,f* / **~ addiction** Morphinsucht *f*, Morphiumsucht *f* / **~ habit** Morphiumsucht *f*, Morphinismus *m*

morphinism Morphinismus *m*, Morphiumsucht *f*

morphinist Morphinist *m*, Morphiumsüchtige *m,f*

morphinistic morphiumsüchtig

morphino|mania Morphinismus *m*, Morphiumsucht *f* / **~phagy** Morphinophagie *f*

morphinomaniac Morphiumsüchtiger *m*, Morphinist *m*

morpho|analysis Gestaltanalyse *f* / **~genesis** Morphogenese *f*, Gestaltbildung *f*, Formwerdung *f* / **~genesia** Morphogenese *f*, Gestaltbildung *f*, Formwerdung *f* / **~geny** Morphogenese *f*, Gestaltbildung *f*, Formwerdung *f* / **~genotype** Morphogenotypus *m* / **~logy** Morphologie *f*, Lehre *f* vom Körperbau / **~lysis** Gestaltzerfall *m* / **~phenotype** Morphophonotypus *m* / **~psia** Morphopsie *f*

morphological morphologisch

mortal tödlich, letal

mortality Sterblichkeit *f*, Sterblichkeitsziffer *f*, Mortalität *f* / **~ rate** Sterblichkeitsziffer *f*, Mortalitätsrate *f*

mortido Todestrieb *m*, Thanatos *m*

morula cell Blastomere *f*

mos Sitten *fpl*, sittlicher Kodex *m*

mosaic Mosaik *n* / **~ of the cortex** Rindenmosaik *n* / **~ eye** Mosaikauge *n* / **~ of functions** Funktionsbündel *n* / **~ hypothesis** Mosaikhypothese *f*, Mosaikauffassung *f* / **~ test** Mosaiktest *m*

moss fibers Moosfasern *fpl*

moth Nachtfalter *m*, Motte *f*

mother Mutter *f* / **~ absence** Abwesenheit *f* der Mutter, Mutterlosigkeit *f* / **~–child communication** Mutter–Kind–Kommunikation *f* / **~–child relation** Mutter–Kind–Beziehung *f* / **~ complex** Ödipuskomplex *m* / **~ figure** Mutterfigur *f*, Mutterbild *n* / **~ fixation** Mutterbindung *f* / **~ instinct** Muttertrieb *m*, mütterlicher Trieb *m* / **~ right** Mutterrecht *n* / **~ substitute** Mutterersatz *m* / **~ surrogate** Muttersurrogat *n*, Mutterersatz *m* / **~–tongue** Muttersprache *f* / **adolescent ~** jugendliche Mutter *f* / **domineering ~** dominierende Mutter *f* / **expectant ~** werdende Mutter *f* / **teenage ~** minderjährige Mutter *f* / **phallic ~** phallische Mutter *f* / **schizophrenogenic ~** schizophrenieverursachende Mutter *f*, schizophrenogene Mutter *f* / **single ~** alleinerziehende Mutter *f* / **unwed ~** ledige Mutter *f*

mothering Bemuttern *n*, mütterliche Betreuung *f*

motif Leitgedanke *m*, Leitmotiv *n*, Motiv *n*

motile beweglich, bewegungsfähig / motorischer Typus *m*

motility Motilität *f*, Bewegungsfähigkeit *f*, Beweglichkeit *f* / **intestinal ~** Darmmotilität *f*

motion Bewegung *f* / **~ illusion** Bewegungstäuchung *f* / **~ parallax** Bewegungsparallaxe *f* / **~ perception** Bewegungswahrnehmung *f* / **~ picture** Film *m* / **~ picture method** Filmmethode *f* / **~ sickness** Kinetose *f*, Reisekrankheit *f* / **~ study** Arbeitsablaufstudie *f*, Bewegungsstudie *f* / **apparent ~** Scheinbewegung *f* / **dimensional ~ system** System *n* vorbestimmter Bewegungszeiten / **educational ~ pictures** Unterrichtsfilm *m* / **goal–directed ~** Zielmotorik *f* / **illusory ~** Scheinbewegung *f* / **phenomenal ~** Scheinbewegung *f* / **rotary ~** Drehbewegung *f* / **slow ~** Zeitlupe *f* / **stereoscopic~ pictures** dreidimensionaler Film *m*, 3D–Film *m*

motionlessness Bewegungslosigkeit *f*, Unbeweglichkeit *f*

motivate motivieren, begründen, anregen, anreizen, stimulieren

motivation Motivation *f*, Antrieb *m*, Trieb *m*, Drang *m*, Triebfeder *f*, Motivierung *f*, Anregung *f* / **~ analysis** Motivationsanalyse *f* / **~ distortion scale** Motivationsverfälschungsskala *f*, Korrekturskala *f* / **~ research** Motivforschung *f*, Motivationsforschung *f* / **~ training** Motivationstraining *n* / **conditioned ~** bedingte Motivation *f* / **conjunctive ~** konjunktive Motivation *f* / **disjunctive ~** disjunktive Motivation *f* / **extrinsic ~** Anregung *f*, Motivierung *f* / **internal ~** physiologischer Trieb *m* / **intrinsic ~** intrinsische Motivation *f* / **primary ~** Urtrieb *m*, Instinkt *m*, Primärtrieb *m*, physiologischer Trieb *m* / **secondary ~** erworbene Motivation *f* / **social ~** soziale Motivation *f* / **unconscious ~** unbewusster Trieb *m*, unbewusste Motivation *f*

motivational Motiv–, Trieb–, Motivations–, motivational

motivator Trieb *m*, Motivationsfaktor *m*, autonomes Motiv *n*

motive Motiv *n*, Trieb *m*, Antrieb *m*, Drang *m*, Impuls *m*, Beweggrund *m*, Grund *m*, Motivation *f* / **~ force** Motivstärke *f* / **~ pattern** Motivkonstellation *f* / **~ power** Triebkraft *f* / **abient ~** Vermeidungstrieb *m* / **basic ~** Grundmotiv *n* / **dependable ~** zuverlässiger Beweggrund *m* / **extrinsic ~** extrinsisches Motiv *n* / **interested ~** eigennütziges Motiv *n* / **intrinsic ~** intrinsisches Motiv *n* / **leading ~** Leitmotiv *n* / **organic ~** physiologischer Trieb *m* / **physiological ~** physiologischer Trieb *m* / **sexual ~** sexuelles Motiv *n* / **social ~** soziales Bedürfnis *n*, soziales Motiv *n* / **sociogenic ~** soziogenes Motiv *n*, gesellschaftlich bedingtes Motiv *n* / **unconscious ~** unbewusster Trieb *m*

motoneuron, motoneurone Motoneuron *n*, motorische Vorderhornzelle *f*

motor, motorial motorisch, bewegend, Bewegungs–

motoricity Motorik *f* / **manual ~** Motorik *f* der Hände

motorium motorisches Zentrum *n*, motorisches Rindenfeld *n*

mouches volantes Mouches volantes *fpl*, Mückensehen *n*

mountain sickness Höhenkrankheit *f*

mourning Trauer *f*

mouth Mund *m* / **~ erotism** Oralerotik *f*, Munderotik *f* / **~–to–mouth advertising** Mundpropaganda *f* / **~ writing** Schreiben *n* mit dem Mund

movable beweglich

movement Bewegung *f*, Körperbewegung *f* / **~ determinant** Bewegungsdeterminante *f* / **~ disorder** Bewegungsstörung *f* / **atypical stereotypic ~ disorder** atypische stereotype Bewegungsstörung *f* / **stereotyped ~ disorders***(ICD 10)* stereotype Bewegungsstörungen *fpl* / **stereotypic ~ disorder***(DSM IV)* stereotype Bewegungsstörung *f* / **stereotypic ~ disorder with self–injurious behavior** stereotype Bewegungsstörung *f* mit selbstschädigendem Verhalten / **~ Gestalt** Bewegungsgestalt *f* / **~ image** Bewegungsvorstellung *f* / **~–produced stimulus** Bewegungsreiz *m*, somästhetischer Reiz *m* / **~ parallax** Bewegungsparallaxe *f* / **~ perception** Bewegungswahrnehmung *f* / **~ response** Bewegungsreaktion *f* / **~ storm** Bewegungssturm *m* / **~ therapy** Bewegungstherapie *f* / **active ~** aktive Bewegung *f* / **activist ~** Bürgerinitiative *f*, Aktivistenbewegung *f* / **antialcohol ~** Anti–Alkoholbewegung *f* / **apparent ~** Scheinbewegung *f* / **associated ~** Mitbewegung *f* / **automatic ~** unwillkürliche Bewegung *f* / **ballistic ~** ballistische Bewegung *f*, Schleuderbewegung *f* / **choreiform ~s** choreaartige Bewegungen *fpl* / **circus ~** Kreisbewegung *f* / **compensatory ~** Ausgleichsbewegung *f* / **conjugate ~s** paarweise Bewegung *f* der Augen, parallele Augenbewegungen *fpl* / **convulsive ~** krampfartige Bewegung *f* / **coordinated ~s** Bewegungsabläufe *mpl* / **defensive ~** Abwehrbewegung *f* / **expressive ~** Ausdrucksbewegung *f* / **forced ~** Tropismus *m* / **ideomotor ~** unwillkürliche Bewegung *f* / **illusory ~** Scheinbewegung *f* / **intentional ~** willkürliche Bewegung *f*, gerichtete Bewegung *f* / **involuntary ~** unwillkürliche Bewegung *f* / **nodding ~** Nickbewegung *f*, Kopfnicken *n* / **passive ~** passive Bewegung *f* / **phenomenal ~** Scheinbewegung *f* / **psychoanalytic ~** psychoanalytische Bewegung *f* / **radical ~** extremistische Bewegung *f*, radikale Bewegung *f* / **random ~** Zufallsbewegung *f* / **rapid eye ~** schnelle Augenbewegung *f* / **reflex ~** Reflexbewegung *f* / **restricted ~** Bewegungseinschränkung *f* / **rotary ~** Drehbewegung *f*, Rotationsbewegung *f* / **rotational ~** Rotationsbewegung *f* / **saccadic ~** ruckartige Bewegung *f* / **shaking ~** Schüttelbewegung *f* / **social ~** soziale Bewegung *f*, Bürgerinitiative *f* / **spastic ~** spastische Bewegung *f* / **stereotyped ~s** Bewegungsstereotypien *fpl* / **stroboscopic ~** stroboskopische Bewegung *f* /

sucking ~ Saugbewegung *f* / **torsional ~** Drehbewegung *f* / **useless ~** sinnlose Bewegung *f* / **voluntary ~** willkürliche Bewegung *f*, Willkürbewegung *f*

movies Film *m*, Kino *n*

moving bewegend, gleitend, ergreifend, rührend

mucin Muzin *n*

mucosa Schleimhaut *f* / **buccal ~** Mundschleimhaut *f* / **nasal ~** Nasenschleimhaut *f* / **olfactory ~** Riechschleimhaut *f* / **oral ~** Mundschleimhaut *f* / **vaginal ~** Vaginalschleimhaut *f*

mucous schleimig, Schleim–

mucus Schleim *m*

Müllerl–Lyer illusion Müller–Lyer'sche Täuschung *f* / **~'s fibers** Müller–Fasern *fpl* / **~'s law** Müller–Gesetz *n*, Gesetz *n* der spezifischen Sinnesenergien / **~–Schumann law** Müller–Schumann'sches Gesetz *n* / **~–Urban method** Müller–Urban–Methode *f* / **~–Urban weighting** Gewichtung *f* nach Müller–Urban

multicausal aufgrund mehrerer Ursachen, bedingt durch mehrere Ursachen

multicellular vielzellig, multizellulär

multiculturalism Multikulturalismus *m*

multidimensional multidimensional, aus mehreren Dimensionen bestehend

multifactorial durch mehrere Faktoren bedingt, multifaktoriell

multiform vielgestaltig

multigroup method Multigruppenmethode *f*, multiple Gruppenmethode *f*

multi–infarct dementia Multiinfarkt–Demenz *f*

multilingual mehrsprachig, multilingual

multilingualism Mehrsprachigkeit *f*, Multilingualismus *m*

multimeaning Mehrfachbedeutung *f* / **~ words test** Test *m* mit mehrdeutigen Wörtern

multimedia Multimedia *npl*

multimodal mehrgipflig

multiple mehrfach, vielfach, multipel

multiplexity Komplexität *f*, Vielgestaltigkeit *f* / **cognitive ~** kognitive Komplexität *f*

multiplicity Vielfälltigkeit *f*, Vielgestaltigkeit *f*

multiplier Multiplikator *m*, Verstärker *m*

multipolar multipolar, mit vielen Fortsätzen

multistage mehrstufig

multivalent mehrwertig, vielwertig, multivalent, polyvalent

multivariate multivariabel

mumbled speech Gemurmel *n*, Gemummel *n*

mumbling Gemurmel *n*, Gemummel *n*

Munsell colour system Munsell Farbsystem *n*

murder Mord *m*, Tötung *f* / **lustful ~** Lustmord *m* / **ritual ~** Ritualmord *m*

murderer Mörder *m*

murmur Geräusch *n*, Gemurmel *n* / **cardiac ~** Herzgeräusch *n* / **functional ~** funktionelles Geräusch *n*

muscae volitantes „mouches volantes" *fpl*, Mückensehen *n*

muscarine Muskarin *n*

muscimol Muscimol *n*

muscle Muskel *m* / **~s** Muskulatur *f*, Muskeln *mpl* / **~ action potential** Muskelaktionspotenzial *n* / **~ balance** Muskelgleichgewicht *n* / **~ cell** Muskelzelle *f* / **~ contraction** Muskelkontraktion *f* / **~ contraction headache** Muskelkontraktionskopfschmerz *m* / **~ cramp** Muskelkrampf *m* / **~ erotism** Muskelerotik *f* / **~ fibre** Muskelfaser *f* / **~ potential** Muskelaktionspotential *n* / **~ reading** Muskellesen *n*, Gedankenlesen *n* aus Muskelbewegungen / **~ relaxation** Muskelentspannung *f* / **progressive ~ relaxation** Jacobson Muskelrelaxation *f*, progressive Muskelrelaxation *f* / **~ relaxing drugs** Muskelrelaxantien *npl* / **~ sensation** Muskelempfindung *f* / **~ sense** Bewegungssinn *m* / **~ spasm** Muskelkrampf *m*, Muskelspasmus *m* / **~ spindle** Muskelspindel *f* /

~ tension Muskelspannung *f* / **~ tissue** Muskelgewebe *n* / **~ tone** Muskeltonus *m*, Tonus *m* / **~ tonus** Muskeltonus *m*, Tonus *m* / **~ twitch** Muskelzucken *n*, Muskelzuckung *f* / **accessory ~** Nebenmuskel *m* / **antagonistic ~** Antagonist *m*, antagonistischer Muskel *m* / **ciliary ~** Ziliarmuskel *m* / **extraocular ~s** äußere Augenmuskeln *mpl* / **facial ~** Gesichtsmuskel *m* / **involuntary ~** unwillkürlicher Muskel *m*, glatter Muskel *m* / **intrinsic ~ reflex** Muskeleigenreflex *m* / **masticatory ~** Kaumuskel *m* / **mimetic ~** Gesichtsmuskel *m*, mimischer Muskel *m* / **nonstriated ~** glatter Muskel *m*, unwillkürlicher Muskel *m* / **oblique ~** schräger Muskel *m* / **ocular ~** Augenmuskel *m* / **oculomotor ~** Augenbewegungsmuskel *m* / **orbicular ~** Ringmuskel *m* / **organic ~** Eingeweidemuskel *m* / **plain ~** glatter Muskel *m*, unwillkürlicher Muskel *m* / **pectoral ~** Brustmuskel *m* / **red ~** rotes Muskelgewebe *n*, rote Muskelfaser *f* / **skeletal ~** Skelettmuskel *m* / **smooth ~** glatter Muskel *m*, unwillkürlicher Muskel *m* / **spinal ~** Dornmuskel *m* / **striated ~** quergestreifter Muskel *m*, gestreifter Muskel *m* / **striped ~** quergestreifter Muskel *m*, gestreifter Muskel *m* / **synergistic ~** Synergist *m*, mitwirkender Muskel *m* / **ulnar ~** ulnarer Muskel *m* / **unstriated ~** glatter Muskel *m*, unwillkürlicher Muskel *m* / **unstriped ~** glatter Muskel *m*, unwillkürlicher Muskel *m* / **visceral ~** Eingeweidemuskel *m* / **voluntary ~** willkürlicher Muskel *m*, quergestreifter Muskel *m*, motorischer Muskel *m* / **white ~** weißes Muskelgewebe *n*, weiße Muskelfaser *f*

muscular muskulär, Muskel–

musculature Muskulatur *f* / **ventricular ~** Kammermuskulatur *f*

musculocutaneous Hautmuskel–

musculoskeletal Skelettmuskulatur betreffend

music Musik *f* / **~ education** Musikerziehung *f* / **~ perception** Musikwahrnehmung *f* / **~ therapy** Musiktherapie *f* / **serial ~** Zwölftonmusik *f*

musical musikalisch, Musik

musician Musiker *m* / **~'s cramp** Pianistenkrampf *m*, Musikerkrampf *m*

musicotherapy Musiktherapie *f*

musophobia krankhafte Angst *f* vor Musik

mussitation Gemurmel *n*, Lippenbewegen *n* ohne Lautbildung, Mussitation *f*

mutant mutiertes Gen *n* / mutierend

mutating mutierend

mutation Mutation *f*, Erbänderung *f*, Veränderung *f*, Wechsel *m* / **genetic ~** Genmutation *f*

mutationism Mutationstheorie *f*

mute stumm / Stummer *m* / **deaf ~** Taubstummer *m* / **deaf and ~** taubstumm

muteness Stummheit *f*

mutilation Verstümmelung *f*, Mutismus *m*, Stummheit *f*

mutism Mutismus *m*, krankhaftes Nichtsprechen *n*, Stummheit *f* trotz intakter Sprechwerkzeuge / **deaf-~** Taubstummheit *f* / **elective ~** elektiver Mutismus *m*, freiwilliger Mutismus *m* / **hysterical ~** hysterischer Mutismus *m* / **organic ~** organischer Mutismus *m*, Aglossie *f* / **schizophrenic ~** Mutismus *m* bei Schizophrenie / **selective ~** selektiver Mutismus *m*

mutitas Mutismus *m*, krankhaftes Nichtsprechen *n*, Stummheit *f* trotz intakter Sprechwerkzeuge

mutual gegenseitig, wechselseitig, reziprok

mutualism Theorie *f* von der gegenseitigen sozialen Abhängigkeit

mutuality Gegenseitigkeit *f*

myaesthesia Muskelsensibilität *f*, Muskelsinn *m*

myalgia Muskelschmerz *m*

myasthenia Muskelschwäche *f*, Myasthenie *f* / **~ gravis** Myasthenia gravis *f*

myasthenic myasthenisch, muskellschwach

myatonia, myatony Muskelatonie *f*, schlechter Muskeltonus *m*, schwache Muskulatur *f*

mydriasis Pupillenerweiterung *f* Mydriasis *f*

mydriatic pupillenerweiternd

myelencephalic, myelencephalous spinal, Rückenmarks–

myelencephalon Nachhirn *n*, verlängertes Mark *n*, Myelenzephalon *n*, Medulla oblongata *f*, Bulbus *m*

myelin Myelin *n*, Nervenmark *n* / ~ **sheath** Myelinscheide *f*, Markscheide *f*

myelinated markhaltig, myelinisiert

myelinic Myelin–

myelinisation, myelination Myelinbildung *f*, Markscheidenbildung *f*

myelinogenetic myelinbildend

myelitis Rückenmarksentzündung *f*, Myelitis *f*

myelon Rückenmark *n*, Medulla spinalis *f*

myesthesia Muskelsensibilität *f*, Muskelsinn *m*

myiodesopsia, myiodesopia Mückensehen *n*, „Mouches volantes“ *fpl*

myocardium Herzmuskel *m*, Myokard *n*

myoclonia Myoklonie *f*, rasche, blitzartige Zuckungen *fpl* in einzelnen Muskeln

myoclonic myoklonisch, Muskelkrampf–

myoclonus Muskelkrampf *m*, Myoklonus *m* / ~ **epilepsy** Myoklonusepilepsie *f*, Unverricht–Krankheit *f*

myocyte Muskelzelle *f*

myodesopsia Mückensehen *n*, „Mouches volantes“ *fpl*

myodystonic myodystonisch, gestört bezüglich des Muskeltonus

myodystony Störung *f* des Muskeltonus

myofibril Myofibrille *f*, Muskelfaser *f*

myogenetic, myogenic, myogenous vom Muskelgewebe stammend, muskulären Ursprungs, myogen

myoglobin Myoglobin *n*

myogram Myogramm *n*, Muskelkurve *f*

myograph Myograph *m*, Apparat *m* zur Registrierung der Muskeltätigkeit

myography Myographie *f*, graphische Darstellung *f* der Muskeltätigkeit

myokinesis Muskeltätigkeit *f*, Muskelarbeit *f*

myokinetic myokinetisch, myomotorisch, motorisch

myokymia Myokymie *f*, fibrilläre Zuckung *f*

myolemma Myolemm *n*, Sarkolemm *n*

myology Muskelkunde *f*, Myologie *f*

myoneural neuromuskulär

myope Kurzsichtiger *m*, Myoper *m*

myopia Myopie *f*, Kurzsichtigkeit *f*

myopic kurzsichtig, myop

myosin Myosin *n*, Muskeleiweiße *npl* / ~ **filament** Myosinfilament *n* / ~ **head** Myosinköpfchen *n*

myosis Pupillenverengung *f*, Miose *f*

myospasm Muskelkrampf *m*, Myospasmus *m*

myostatic koordiniert, zusammenwirkend

myotactic myotaktisch, Muskelberührungs–

myotic pupillenverengend, miotisch

myotome Myotom *n*

myotonia Myotonie *f*, Muskelkrampf *m*

myotonic myotonisch, Myotonie–

myotonometer Myotonometer *n*, Gerät *n* zur Messung der Muskelspannung

myringa, myrinx Trommelfell *n*

myrmeciasis Kribbeln *n*, Gekribbel *n*, Prickeln *n*, Jucken *n*, Ameisenlaufen *n*

mysophobia Mysophobie *f*, Berührungsangst *f*, krankhafte Angst *f* vor Beschmutzung

mysophilia pathologisches Interesse *n* am Schmutz

mystic mystisch, geheimnisvoll / Mystiker *m*

mysticism Mystizismus *m*, Mystik *f*

mystification Täuschung *f*, Irreführung *f*, Geheimnistuerei *f*, Mystifikation *f*

mytacism Mytazismus *m*, falsche Verwendung *f* des Buchstaben „m“

myth, mythos Mythos *m*, erfundene Geschichte *f* / **anthropogenetic ~s** anthropogene Mythen *mpl*

mythical mythisch, sagenhaft

mythography Aufzeichnung *f* von Mythen, beschreibende Mythologie *f*

mythological mythologisch

mythology Mythologie *f*

mythomania Lügensucht *f*, Prahlsucht *f*, Mythomanie *f*, Pseudologie *f*

mythomaniac Geschichtenerzähler *m*, Lügner *m*, Prahler *m*

myxidiocy Kretinismus *m*

myxoedema, myxedema Myxödem *n* / **~ madness** Myxödempsychose *f* / **congenital ~** Kretinismus *m*

N

n–achievement Leistungsbedürfnis *n*, Erfolgsbedürfnis *n*, Leistungsmotiv *n*

nadir tiefster Stand *m*, Tiefstand *m*, Nullpunkt *m*

naevus Muttermal *n*, Leberfleck *m*, Nävus *m*

n–affiliation Bedürfnis *n* nach Gruppenzugehörigkeit, Bedürfnis *n* nach freundlicher Interaktion mit anderen Menschen, Bedürfnis *n* geliebt zu werden, Geselligkeitsbedürfnis *n*, Gesellungsmotiv *n*

nail Nagel *m* / **~–biter** Nägelkauer *m* / **~–biting** Nägelkauen *n*, Nägelbeißen *n*

naïve, naive naiv, unbefangen, ungekünstelt

nalorphine Nalorphin *n*

naloxone Naloxon *n*

naltrexone Naltrexon *n*

naming Benennung *f*, Benennen *n*, Bezeichnen *n*

Nancy school Nancyer Schule *f*

nanism Zwergwuchs *m*, Nanismus *m* / **pituitary ~** hypophysärer Infantilismus *m*

nanoid zwergenhaft, sehr klein

nanosecond Nanosekunde *f*, milliardstel Sekunde *f*

nanosoma, nanosomia Zwergwuchs *m*

nanous zwerghaft, zwergartig, zwergwüchsig

nanus Zwerg *m*

nap Kurzschlaf *m*, Nickerchen *n*

naphthomania Naphthomanie *f*, Benzinismus *m*

narcism Narzissmus *m*, Autoerotismus *m* / **~ erg** narzisstisches Motiv *n*

narcissism Narzissmus *m*, Autoerotismus *m* / **negative ~** negativer Narzissmus *m* / **primal ~** primärer Narzissmus *m* / **primary ~** primärer Narzissmus *m* / **secondary ~** sekundärer Narzissmus *m*

narcissist Narzisst *m*, in sich selbst Verliebter *m*

narcissistic narzisstisch

narcoanalysis Narkoanalyse *f*, Psychoanalyse *f* mit Hilfe von Narkotika

narcocatharsis psychisches Abreagieren *n* unter Narkose

narcodiagnosis Narkodiagnose *f*, Diagnose *f* unter Narkose

narcohypnia, narcohypnosis hypnotischer Tiefschlaf *m*, tiefe Hypnose *f*, Narkohypnose *f*

narcolepsy Narkolepsie *f*, Schlummersucht *f* / **idiopathic ~** genuine Narkolepsie *f*, idiopathische Narkolepsie *f* / **symptomatic ~** symptomatische Narkolepsie *f*

narcoleptic narkoleptisch

narcoma narkotisch bedingtes Koma *n*

narcomania Rauschmittelsucht *f*, Trunksucht *f*, Narkomanie *f*

narcomaniac rauschmittelsüchtig, rauschgiftsüchtig / Rauschmittelsüchtiger *m*, Rauschgiftsüchtiger *m*

narcosis Narkose *f* / **~ therapy** Schlaftherapie *f*, Narkotherapie *f* / **prolonged ~** verlängerte Narkose *f*

narcosomania Schlafmittelsucht *f*, Rauschmittelsucht *f*

narcosuggestion Suggestionstherapie *f* unter Narkose

narcosynthesis Narkosynthese *f*

narcotherapist Psychotherapeut *m* der Narkotherapie praktiziert, Narkotherapeut *m*

narcotherapy Schlaftherapie *f*, Narkotherapie *f*

narcotic narkotisch, einschläfernd / Betäubungsmittel *n*, Narkosemittel *n*, Rauschgift *n* / **~ addict** Betäubungsmittelabhängige *m,f*, Betäubungsmittelsüchtige *m,f* / **~ addiction** Betäubungsmittelsucht *f*

narcotism, narcoticism Rauschmittelsucht *f*, Schlafmittelsucht *f*, Narkotismus *m*

naris Nasenloch *n*, Nasenöffnung *f*

narrative Erzählung *f*

narrowed eingeengt, verengt

narrowing Einengung *f*, Verengung *f*, Beschränkung *f*, Stenose *f* / **~ of the field of consciousness** Einengung *f* des Bewusstseinsfeldes / **~ of the pupils** Pupillenverengung *f*

nasal nasal, Nasen–

nasalism Näseln *n*

nasality Nasalität *f*

nascent im Entstehen begriffen, wachsend, entstehend

nasion Nasion *n*

nasopharyngeal Nasenrachen–

nasopharynx Nasenrachenraum *m*, Nasopharynx *f*, Epipharynx *f*

natal Geburts–

natality Geburtenziffer *f*, Geburtenhäufigkeit *f*, Geburtenzahl *f* auf tausend Einwohner

natimortality Geburtensterblichkeit *f*, perinatale Mortalität *f*

national National–, national / Staatsangehöriger *m*, Landsmann *m* / **foreign ~** Ausländer *m*

nationalism Nationalismus *m*, Nationalgefühl *n*, Nationalstolz *m*

native eingeboren, einheimisch, angeboren, von Natur aus eigen / Eingeborener *m*

nativism Nativismus *m*, Lehre *f* von der Naturanlage, Bevorzugung *f* Einheimischer gegenüber Immigranten

nativistic nativistisch, auf Naturanlage beruhend

natriuresis, natruresis Natriurese *f*, Natriumausscheidung *f* im Harn

natural natürlich, Natur–, naturbedingt, angeboren

naturalism Naturalismus *m*

naturalist Naturforscher *m*, Naturwissenschaftler *m*, Naturfreund *m*, Anhänger *m* des Naturalismus

naturalistic naturalistisch, naturgetreu

nature Natur *f*, Naturzustand *m*, Naturanlage *f*, natürliche Beschaffenheit *f* / **~ of neurosis** Art *f* der Neurose / **~–nurture** Anlage–Umwelt / **~–nurture controversy** Erbe–Umwelt–Streit *m*, Erbe–Umwelt–Problem *n*, Anlage–Umwelt–Problem *n* / **~–nurture problem** Erbe–Umwelt–Problem *n*, Anlage–Umwelt–Problem *n* / **~–nurture ratio** Anlage–Umwelt–Verhältnis *n* / **human ~** menschliche Natur *f* / **original ~** ursprüngliche Natur *f* / **second ~** zweite Natur *f*, Gewohnheit *f*, Über–Ich *n*

naturism Freikörperkultur *f*, Nudismus *m*

naughty frech, ungezogen, unartig

nausea Brechreiz *m*, Übelkeit *f*, Reisekrankheit *f*, Ekel *m*

nauseous ekelhaft, eklig, widerlich

Neanderthal man Neandertaler *m*

nearsight, nearsightedness Kurzsichtigkeit *f*, Myopie *f*

nearsighted kurzsichtig, myop

neatness Nettigkeit *f*, Sauberkeit *f*, Ordentlichkeit *f*

nebula Hornhauttrübung *f*

necessary notwendig, zwangsläufig, notgedrungen

necessity Notwendigkeit *f* / **dire ~** notgedrungen

neck Hals *m*, Nacken *m*, Genick *n* / **tonic ~ reflex** tonischer Halsreflex *m*, tonischer Nackenreflex *m*

Necker cube Necker–Würfel *m*

necking Knutschen *n*, Liebkosung *f*, Necking *n*

necromancer Geisterbeschwörer *m*, Magier *m*, Zauberer *m*, Hexer *m*

necromancy Nekromantik *f*, Geisterbeschwörung *f*, schwarze Kunst *f*, Hexerei *f*

necromania Nekrophilie *f*, Leichenschändung *f*, Vampirismus *m*

necrophagia Verspeisen *n* von Leichenteilen, Nekrophagie *f*

necrophile, necrophilous leichenschänderisch, sich an Leichen vergehend, nekrophil

necrophilia, necrophily, necrophilism Leichenschändung *f*, Nekrophilie *f*, Nekromanie *f*, sexuelle Handlung *f* an Leichen

necrophobia krankhafte Angst *f* vor Leichen, Nekrophobie *f*

necrosis Nekrose *f*, Gewebstod *m*

necrotic nekrotisch, gangränös

need Bedürfnis *n*, Bedürfnisspannung *f*, Motiv *n* / **~ assessment** Bedarfsanalyse *f* / **~–drive–incentive pattern** Bedürfnis–Trieb–Ziel–Gefüge *n* / **~ for acceptance** Bedürfnis *n* akzeptiert zu werden / **~–achievement** Leistungsmotiv *n*, Leistungsmotivation *f*, Leistungsbedürfnis *n* / **~ for affection** Zärtlichkeitsbedürfnis *n* / **~ for affiliation** Geselligkeitsbedürfnis *n* / **~ for approval** Anerkennungsmotivation *f*, Bedürfnis *n* nach Anerkennung / **~ for attention** Bedürfnis *n* nach Beachtung / **~ for belongingness and love** Zugehörigkeits– und Liebesbedürfnis *n* / **~ for cognition** Erkenntnisstreben *n* / **~ for dominance** Dominanzstreben *n*, Streben *n* nach Überlegenheit / **~ for esteem** Anerkennungsbedürfnis *n* / **~ for gratification** Bedürfnis *n* nach Befriedigung / **~ for punishment** Strafbedürfnis *n* / **~ for repression** Verdrängungsbedürfnis *n* / **~ for self–actualization** Bedürfnis *n* nach Selbstverwirklichung / **~ for superiority** Bedürfnis *n* nach Überlegenheit / **~ fulfillment** Bedürfnisbefriedigung *f* / **~ gratification** Bedürfnisbefriedigung *f* / **~–integrate** Bedürfnissystem *n* / **~ of leaning–upon** Anlehnungsbedürfnis *n* / **~ pattern** Bedürfnisgefüge *n*, Bedürfnissystem *n* / **~–power** Machtmotiv *n* / **~ reduction** Bedürfnisreduktion *f* / **~ satisfaction** Bedürfnisbefriedigung *f* / **~ state** Bedürfniszustand *m* / **~ system** Bedürfnissystem *n* / **~ tension** Bedürfnisspannung *f* / **~ to function** Funktionstrieb *m* / **acquired ~** erworbenes Bedürfnis *n*, sekundäres Bedürfnis *n* / **affiliative ~** Geselligkeitsbedürfnis *n* / **aware ~** bewusstes Bedürfnis *n* / **basic ~** Grundbedürfnis *n* / **biogenic ~** physiologisches Bedürfnis *n*, Primärbedürfnis *n* / **cognitive ~** geistiges Bedürfnis *n* / **conscious ~** bewusst wahrgenommenes Bedürfnis *n* / **covert ~** verstecktes Bedürfnis *n* / **dependable ~** zuverlässig vorhandenes Bedürfnis *n* / **derived ~** erworbenes Bedürfnis *n* / **economic ~** materielles Bedürfnis *n* / **endopsychic ~** inneres Bedürfnis *n* / **external ~** äußeres Bedürfnis *n* / **felt ~** empfundenes Bedürfnis *n*, Motiv *n*, bewusstes Bedürfnis *n* / **innate ~** Grundbedürfnis *n*, Primärbedürfnis *n*, physiologisches Bedürfnis *n* / **instinctoid ~** Grundbedürfnis *n* / **internal ~** physiologisches Bedürfnis *n*, Grundbedürfnis *n* / **manifest ~** sichtbares Bedürfnis *n*, offenes Bedürfnis *n*, manifestes Bedürfnis *n* / **mental ~** geistiges Bedürfnis *n* / **neurotic ~** neurotisches Bedürfnis *n* / **overt ~** manifestes Bedürfnis *n* / **primary ~** Primärbedürfnis *n*, Grundbedürfnis *n* / **psychological ~** psychisches Bedürfnis *n* / **quasi ~** Quasi–Bedürfnis *n* / **secondary ~** sekundäres Bedürfnis *n*, erworbenes Bedürfnis *n*, erlerntes Bedürfnis *n* / **self–oriented ~** ich–zentriertes Bedürfnis *n* / **social ~** soziales Bedürfnis *n*, Geselligkeitsbedürfnis *n* / **somagenic ~** physiologisches Bedürfnis *n* / **somatogenlc ~** physiologisches Bedürfnis *n* / **special ~ s** Sonderförderungsbedarf *m* / **universal ~** allgemeines Bedürfnis *n* / **viscerogenic ~** leibliches Bedürfnis *n*

needle Nadel *f* / ~ **electrode** Nadelelektrode *f* / ~ **sharing** Spritzentausch *m*

neencephalon Neenzephalon *n*, ontogenetisch neuere Gehirnteile *mpl*

negation Verneinung *f*, Negation *f* / ~ **of the ego** Verneinung *f* des Ich / **conducive** ~ förderliche Verneinung *f*

negative negativ, fehlend

negativism Negativismus *m* / **active** ~ aktiver Negativismus *m* / **internal** ~ Sperrung *f* / **passive** ~ passiver Negativismus *m*

negativistic negativistisch

neglect vernachlässigen, unterlassen / Vernachlässigung *f*, Verwahrlosung *f* / ~ **of child** Vernachlässigung *f* eines Kindes

neglectful nachlässig

negligence Nachlässigkeit *f*

negotiation Verhandlung *f*

neighbourhood Nachbarschaft *f*

neoanalysis Neoanalyse *f*

neoanalyst Neoanalytiker *m*, Anhänger *m* der neoanalytischen Schule

neoanalytic neoanalytisch

neobehaviorism Neobehaviorismus *m*

neocatharsis Neokatharsis *f*

neocerebellum phylogenetisch neuer Teil *m* des Kleinhirns, Neozerebellum *n*

neocortex Neokortex *m*

neo–Darwinism Neo–Darwinismus *m*

neoformation Neoplasie *f*, Gewebeneubildung *f*

neo–Freudian Neo–Freudianer *m*

neo–Freudianism Neo–Freudianismus *m*

neolalia Sprache *f* mit unverständlichen Wortneuschöpfungen bei Psychotikern, Neolalie *f*

neo–Lamarckism Neo–Lamarckismus *m*

neologism Neologismus *m*, Neubildung *f*, neuer Ausdruck *m*

neonatal neugeboren

neonate neugeboren / Neugeborenes *n*, neugeborenes Kind *n*

neonatus Neugeborenes *n*, neugeborenes Kind *n*

neonomadism modernes Nomadentum *n*, moderne Völkerwanderung *f*

neopallial Neopallium betreffend

neopallium Neopallium *n*

neophalism totale Alkoholabstinenz *f*

neophalist Antialkoholiker *m*, Abstinenzler *m*

neophasia Neophasie *f*

neophenomenology Neo–Phänomenologie *f*

neophilism Neuerungssucht *f*, Neuerungswut *f*

neophobia Angst *f* vor allem Neuen, Neophobie *f*

neophrenia Neophrenie *f*

neoplasia Neoplasie *f*, Gewebeneubildung *f*

neoplasm Neubildung *f*, Geschwulstbildung *f*, Tumor *m*, Neoplasma *n* / **benign** ~ gutartige Geschwulst *f* / **endocrine** ~ Drüsentumor *m* / **malignant** ~ bösartiger Tumor *m* / **mammary** ~ Brusttumor *m*

neopositivism Neopositivismus *m*

neopsychoanalysis Neopsychoanalyse *f*, Neoanalyse *f*, Neo–Freudianismus *m*

neostigmine Neostigmin *n*

neoteny unvollkommene Entwicklung *f* eines Organs, Neotenie *f*

neper Neper *n*, Maßeinheit *f* für die Dämpfungsgröße

Nernst's law Nernst–Gesetz *n* / **~–Lillie theory** Nernst–Lillie'sche Theorie *f* der Erregung

nerval zu einem Nerven gehörig, nerval, Nerven–

nerve Nerv *m* / ~ **arc** Nervenbogen *m*, Reflexbogen *m* / ~ **block** Leitungsanästhesie *f*, Nervenblockade *f* / ~ **blocking** Leitungsanästhesie *f* / ~ **bundle** Nervenbündel *n* / ~ **cell** Nervenzelle *f*, Neuron *n* / ~ **centre** Nervenzentrum *n*, Nervenkern *m* / ~ **conduction** Nervenleitung *f* / ~ **cord** Nervenstrang *n* / ~ **current** Nervenstrom *m*, Nervenimpuls *m* / ~ **deafness** nervös bedingte Schwerhörigkeit *f* / ~ **disorder** Neuropathie *f*, Nervenleiden *n* / **peripheral** ~ **disorder** Erkrankung *f* des peripheren Nervensystems / ~ **ending** Nervenendigung *f*, Nervenendfaser *f* / ~ **end–organ** Nervenendorgan *n*, Erfolgsorgan *n* / ~ **excitation** Nervenerregung *f* / ~ **of expression** Bewegungsnerv *m* / ~ **fascicle** Nervenbündel *n* / ~ **fatigue** Nervenermüdung *f* / ~ **fibre** Nervenfaser *f* / ~ **fibril** Nervenfibrille *f*, Neurofibrille *f* / ~ **force** Leistungskraft *f* der Nerven / ~ **function** Nerventätigkeit *f*, Nervenfunktion *f* / ~ **ganglion** Ganglion *n* / ~ **growth factor** Nervenwachstumsfaktor *m* / ~ **of hearing** Hörnerv *m*, Gehörnerv *m* / ~ **impulse** Nervenimpuls *m*, Nervenerregung *f*, Aktionspotenzial *n*, Spike *m* / ~ **irritation** Nervenreizung *f* / ~ **layer** Nervenschicht *f* / ~ **membrane** Nervenmembran *f* / ~–**muscle preparation** Nerven–Muskel–Päparat *n* / ~ **net** Nervennetz *n*, Ganglienkomplex *m* / ~ **pathway** Nervenbahn *f* / ~ **patient** Nervenkranker *m* / ~ **pattern** Nervenanordnung *f*, neurales Muster *n* / ~ **plexus** Nervengeflecht *n*, Nervenplexus *m* / ~ **process** Nervenfortsatz *m* / ~ **root** Nervenwurzel *f* / ~ **sheath** Nervenhülle *f*, Nervenscheide *f* / ~ **of smell** Geruchsnerv *m* / ~ **specialist** Neurologe *m*, Nervenfacharzt *m* / ~ **stem** Nervenstamm *m* / ~ **stimulus** Nervenreiz *m* / ~ **strain** nervöse Überanstrengung *f*, nervöse Überreizung *f* / ~ **supply** Nervenversorgung *f*, Innervierung *f* / ~ **termination** Nervenendigung *f* / ~ **tissue** Nervengewebe *n* / ~ **track** Nervenbahn *f*, Leitungsbahn *f* / ~ **tract** Nervenbahn *f* / ~ **trunk** Nervenstamm *m* / **abducens** ~ Abduzens *m*, Nervus abducens *m* / **abducent** ~ Abduzens *m*, Nervus abducens *m* / **accessory** ~ Beinerv *m*, Nervus accessorius *m* / **acoustic** ~ Hörnerv *m*, Gehörnerv *m*, Akustikus *m* / **adrenergic** ~ adrenergische Nervenfaser *f* / **afferent** ~ afferenter Nerv *m*, sensibler Nerv *m*, Sinnesnerv *m*, zentripetaler Nerv *m* / **auditory** ~ Gehörnerv *m*, Akustikus *m* / **autonomic** ~ autonomer Nerv *m* / **centrifugal** ~ efferenter Nerv *m*, motorischer Nerv *m*, zentrifugaler Nerv *m* / **centripetal** ~ afferenter Nerv *m*, sensibler Nerv *m*, Sinnesnerv *m*, zentripetaler Nerv *m* / **cerebral** ~ Gehirnnerv *m* / **cervical** ~ Halsnerv *m* / **cholinergic** ~ cholinerger Nerv *m* / **cochlear** ~ Schneckennerv *m* / **cranial** ~ Hirnnerv *m* / **cutaneous** ~ Hautnerv *m* / **efferent** ~ efferenter Nerv *m*, motorischer Nerv *m* / **esodic** ~ afferenter Nerv *m* / **exodic** ~ efferenter Nerv *m* / **facial** ~ Gesichtsnerv *m*, Fazialis *m* / **facial** ~ **canal** Fazialiskanal *m* / **femoral** ~ Oberschenkelnerv *m* / **free** ~ **ending** freie Nervenendigung *f* / **frontalis** ~ Nervus frontalis *m* / **gangliated** ~ sympathischer Nerv *m* / **glossopharyngeal** ~ Zungenschlundnerv *m*, Glossopharyngeus *m* / **gustatory** ~ Geschmacksnerv *m* / **hypoglossal** ~ Nervus hypoglossus *m* / **inhibitory** ~ Hemmungsnerv *m*, Hemmer *m* / **lingual** ~ Zungennerv *m* / **locomotor** ~ motorischer Nerv *m*, Bewegungsnerv *m* / **median** ~ Nervus medianus *m* / **medullary** ~ markhaltiger Nerv *m* / **medullated** ~ markhaltiger Nerv *m* / **mixed** ~ Nerv *m* mit sensiblen und motorischen Fasern / **motor** ~ motorischer Nerv *m*, efferenter Nerv *m*, zentrifugaler Nerv *m* / **multipolar** ~ **cell** multipolare Nervenzelle *f* / **nonmedullated** ~ markloser Nerv *m* / **obturator** ~ Nervus obturatorius *m* / **oculomotor** ~ Okulomotorius *m* / **olfactory** ~ Geruchsnerv *m*, Riechnerv *m*, Olfaktorius *m* / **ophthalmic** ~ Augennerv *m* / **optic** ~ Sehnerv *m*, Optikus *m* / **palatine** ~ Gaumennerv *m* / **pathetic** ~ Trochlearis *m* / **peripheral** ~ peripherer Nerv *m* / **phrenic** ~ Phrenikus *m*, Nervus phrenicus *m* / **pilomotor** ~ Arrector pili *m* / **pneumogastric** ~ Vagus *m* / **radial** ~ Speichennerv *m*, Nervus radialis *m* / **second** ~ Sehnerv *m*, Optikus *m* / **secretory** ~ sekretorischer Nerv *m* / **segmented** ~ **fibre** segmentierte Nervenfaser *f* / **sensory** ~ sensorischer Nerv *m*, Sinnesnerv *m*, Empfindungsnerv *m*, afferenter Nerv *m*, zentripetaler Nerv *m* / **sensory**

~ apparatus Sinnesapparat *m* / **somatic ~s** sensible und motorische Nerven *mpl* / **spinal ~** Rückenmarksnerv *m* / **spinal accessory ~** Beinerv *m* / **sudomotor ~s** sudomotorische Nerven *mpl* / **sympathetic ~** Sympathikus *m* / **sciatic ~** Ischiasnerv *m* / **terminal ~** Endnerv *m* / **thoracic ~** Dorsalnerv *m* / **trifacial ~** Trigeminus *m* / **trigeminal ~** Trigeminus *m* / **trochlear ~** Trochlearis *m* / **tympanic ~** Gehörnerv *m*, Hörnerv *m* / **ulnar ~** Ellennerv *m* / **vagus ~** Vagus *m* / **vasoconstrictor ~** gefäßverengender Nerv *m*, Vasokonstriktor *m* / **vasodilator ~** gefäßerweiternder Nerv *m*, Vasodilator *m* / **vasomotor ~** vasomotorischer Nerv *m* / **vestibular ~s** Gleichgewichtsnerven *mpl*

nerveless energielos, schlaff, schwach, kraftlos

nervelessness Energielosigkeit *f*, Schlaffheit *f*, Kraftlosigkeit *f*

nerviness Nervosität *f*

nervism Neurismus *m*

nervosism Nervenleiden *n*, Nervenkrankheit *f*, Nervenzusammenbruch *m*, Neuropathie *f*, Neurasthenie *f*

nervosity Nervosität *f*

nervous nervös, erregbar, Nerven–

nervousness Nervosität *f*, Nervenschwäche *f*, leichte Erregbarkeit *f*

nervus Nerv *m* / **~ acusticus** Gehörnerv *m*, Akustikus *m* / **~ axillaris** Nervus axillaris *m* / **~ patheticus** Augenrollnerv *m* / **~ staticus** Gleichgewichtsnerv *m* / **~ trochlearis** Trochlearis *m* / **~ vestibularis** Gleichgewichtsnerv *m*

nest Nest *n*, Brutstätte *f* / **~ building** Nestbau *m*

nesting Nisten *n*, Brüten *n* / **~ time** Brutzeit *f*

net Netz *n*, Gewebe *n* / **neural ~** Nervennetz *n*, Gangliennetz *n*

netiquette Benimmregeln *fpl* im Internet

network Netz *n*, Netzwerk *n*, Gefüge *n* / **~ therapy** Systemtherapie *f* / **nervous ~** Nervengeflecht *n* / **neuronal ~** neuronales Netzwerk *n* / **nomological ~** nomologisches Gefüge *n* / **social ~** soziales Gefüge *n*

neume Neume *f*

neuradynamia Neurasthenie *f*, Erschöpfungsneurasthenie *f*, Nervenschwäche *f*

neural neural, Nerven–

neuralgia Neuralgie *f*, Nervenschmerz *m*, neuralgischer Schmerz *m* / **ciliary ~** Ziliarneuralgie *f* / **trigeminal ~** Trigeminusneuralgie *f*

neuralgic neuralgisch

neurasthenia Neurasthenie *f*, Nervenschwäche *f* / **cardiovascular ~** Herzneurose *f* / **gastric ~** Magenneurose *f* / **postinfective ~** postinfektiöse Neurasthenie *f* / **professional ~** Berufsneurose *f* / **pulsating ~** Herzschlaghören *n* / **sexual ~** Sexualneurasthenie *f*

neurastheniac Neurastheniker *m*

neurasthenic neurasthenisch, nervenschwach

neurataxy Neurasthenie *f*

neuraxis Neuralachse *f*, zerebrospinale Achse *f*

neuraxon Achsenzylinder *m*, Achsenzylinderfortsatz *m*, Axon *n*, Neurit *m*

neure Neuron *n*

neurilemma Neurilemm *n*, Schwann'sche Scheide *f*

neurilemmoma Schwann–Tumor *m*

neurin, neurine Neurin *n*

neurit, neurite Neurit *m*, Achsenzylinder *m*, Axon *n*

neuritic neuritisch

neuritis Neuritis *f*, Nervenentzündung *f*

neuroanatomical neuroanatomisch

neuroanatomy Anatomie *f* des Nervensystems, Neuroanatomie *f*

neurobiology Neurobiologie *f*

neurobiotaxis Neurobiotaxis *f*, Neuroblast *m*, unausgereifte Nervenzelle *f*

neuroblast Neuroblast *n*, embryonale Nervenzelle *f*

neuroblastoma Geschwulst *f* aus Neuroblasten, Neuroblastom *n*, Neurozytom *n*

neurochemistry Neurochemie *f*

neurocirculatory neurozirkulatorisch, Nervenkreislauf–

neurocranium Gehirnschädel *m*, Neurokranium *n*

neurocrinia Neurokrinie *f*, Bildung *f* von Neurosekreten im Zwischenhirn

neurocyte Nervenzelle *f*, Neuron *n*, Neurozyt *m*

neurocytoma Geschwulst *f* aus Neuroblasten, Neurozytom *n*, Neuroblastom *n*

neurodendron, neurodendrite Dendrit *m*

neurodermatitis Neurodermatitis *f*

neurodynamic neurodynamisch

neurodystonia vegetative Dystonie *f*

neuroendocrine neuroendokrin

neuroendocrinology Lehre *f* von den Wechselbeziehungen zwischen Nerven– und Hormonsystem, Neuroendokrinologie *f*

neuroethology Verhaltensphysiologie *f*

neurofibril, neurofibrilla Neurofibrille *f*

neurofibrillar neurofibrillär

neurofilament Neurofilament *n*

neurogenetic, neurogenic, neurogenous nervlich bedingt, neurogen, von den Nerven ausgehend

neuroglia Nervengewebe *n*, Nervenkitt *m*, Neuroglia *f*, Glia *f* / ~ **cell** Neurogliazelle *f*, Gliazelle *f*, Neurogliozyt *m*

neurogram Neurogramm *n*

neurohormonal neurohormonal

neurohormone Nervenhormon *n*, Neurohormon *n*

neurohumor neurohumoraler Wirkstoff *m*

neurohumoral auf neuralem und humoralem Wege wirkend, neurohumoral

neurohypnologist Hypnoseexperte *m*

neurohypnology Lehre *f* von der Hypnose

neurohypophysis Hypophysenhinterlappen *m*

neuroinfection Nervenentzündung *f*

neurokinin Neurokinin *n*

neuroleptic neuroleptisch / Neuroleptikum *n* / **~–induced acute akathisia** neuroleptikainduzierte akute Akathisie *f* / **~–induced acute dystonia** neuroleptikainduzierte akute Dystonie *f* / **~–induced parkinsonism** neuroleptikainduzierter Parkinsonismus *m* / **~–induced supersensitivity psychosis** Supersensitivitätspsychose *f* / **~–induced tardive dyskinesia** neuroleptikainduzierte tardive Dyskinesie *f* / ~ **malignant syndrome** malignes neuroleptisches Syndrom *n* / **basic ~s** Basisneuroleptika *npl* / **broad–spectrum ~s** Breitbandneuroleptika *npl*

neurolinguistic neurolinguistisch

neurolinguistics Neurolinguistik *f*

neurological neurologisch

neurologist Neurologe *m*

neurology Neurologie *f*, Lehre *f* von den Nerven, Nervenheilkunde *f*

neurolymph Zerebrospinalflüssigkeit *f*

neuroma Nerventumor *m*, Neurom *n*

neuromere Nervensegment *n*, Neuromer *n*

neuromodulator Neuromodulator *m*

neuromotor neuromotorisch

neuromuscular neuromuskulär

neuron, neurone Neuron *n*, vollständige Nervenzelle *f*, Neurozyt *m* / ~ **chain** Neuronenkette *f* / ~ **doctrine** Neuronentheorie *f*, Neuronenlehre *f* / **~–theory** Neurontheorie *f* / **adrenergic ~** adrenerges Neuron *n* / **afferent ~** afferentes Neuron *n* / **auditory ~** Hörnervenzelle *f* / **bipolar ~** bipolare Nervenzelle *f* / **centrifugal ~** motorische Nervenzelle *f* / **early–inspiratory ~** frühinspiratorisches Neuron *n* / **efferent ~** efferentes Neuron *n* / **expiratory ~** exspiratorisches Neuron *n* / **integrating ~** integrierendes Neuron *n* / **inter-**

nuncial ~ Schaltneuron *n*, Interneuron *n*, Zwischenneuron *n* / **local** ~ Lokalzelle *f* / **motor** ~ motorisches Neuron *n*, Motoneuron *n* / **multipolar** ~ multipolare Nervenzelle *f* / **noradrenergic** ~ noradrenerges Neuron *n* / **peptidergic** ~ peptiderges Neuron *n* / **peripheral** ~ periphere Nervenzelle *f* / **postganglionic** ~ postganglionäres Neuron *n* / **preganglionic** ~ präganglionäres Neuron *n* / **respiratory** ~ respiratorisches Neuron *n* / **sensory** ~ sensorisches Neuron *n* / **serotoninergic** ~ serotoninerges Neuron *n* / **sympathetic** ~ sympathisches Neuron *n* / **unipolar** ~ unipolares Neuron *n*, unipolare Nervenzelle *f*

neuronal, neuronic neuronal, zu einem Neuron gehörig, ein Neuron betreffend

neuronitis Entzündung *f* von Nervenzellen, Neuritis *f*

neuropath Nervenkranker *m*, Nervenleidender *m*, Neuropath *m*

neuropathia Neuropathie *f*, Nervenschwäche *f*, vegetative Labilität *f*

neuropathic nervenleidend, neuropathisch, für Nervenkrankheiten disponiert

neuropathologist, neuropathist Neuropathologe *m*, Facharzt *m* für Nervenkrankheiten, Neurologe *m*

neuropathology Neuropathologie *f*, Lehre *f* von den Nervenkrankheiten

neuropathy Nervenleiden *n*, Nervenkrankheit *f*, nervöse Veranlagung *f*, Neuropathie *f*

neuropeptide Neuropeptid *n*

neurophrenia hirnorganisch bedingte Verhaltensstörung *f*

neurophysiological neurophysiologisch

neurophysiology Neurophysiologie *f*

neuropil, neuropile, neuropilem Nervenfilz *m*, diffuses Nervennetz *n*, Neuropilem *n*

neuroplasty Nervenplastik *f*

neuroplegic Neuroplegikum *n*, Neuroleptikum *n* / neuroplegisch

neuroplexus Nervengeflecht *n*, Plexus *m*

neuropsychiatric neuropsychiatrisch

neuropsychiatrist Facharzt *m* für Neurologie und Psychiatrie, Facharzt *m* für Nerven und Gemütsleiden, Neuropsychiater *m*, Psychiater *m*

neuropsychiatry Neuropsychiatrie *f*, Nervenheilkunde *f*

neuropsychic neuropsychisch, psychophysiologisch

neuropsychological neuropsychologisch

neuropsychology Neuropsychologie *f*

neuropsychosis organisch bedingte Geistesstörung *f*, Psychose *f*

neurosal neurotisch

neurosciences Neurowissenschaft *f*, Wissenschaft *f* vom Nervensystern

neurosecretion Neurosekretion *f*

neurosensory neurosensorisch, sensorisch

neurosis Neurose *f* / ~ **of abandonment** Verlassenheitsneurose *f* / ~ **due to an accident** Unfallneurose *f*, traumatische Neurose *f* / ~ **of destiny** Schicksalsneurose *f* / **actual** ~ Aktualneurose *f* / **analytic** ~ analytische Neurose *f* / **benign** ~ Neurose *f* mit guter Prognose / **biological** ~ biologisch bedingte Neurose *f* / **cardiac** ~ Herzneurose *f* / **compensating** ~ Begehrensneurose *f*, Rentenneurose *f* / **compulsive** ~ Zwangsneurose *f* / **compulsive–obsessive** ~ Zwangsneurose *f* / **conversional** ~ Konversionsneurose *f* / **cultural** ~ Kulturneurose *f* / **depressive** ~ depressive Neurose *f*, neurotische Depression *f* / **dissociative** ~ Spaltungsneurose *f*, Hysterie *f* / **existential** ~ existenzielle Neurose *f* / **experimental** ~ experimentelle Neurose *f* / **homosexual** ~ homosexuelle Neurose *f* / **hypochondriacal** ~ Organneurose *f*, Hypochondrie *f*, hypochondrische Neurose *f* / **hysterical** ~ Hysterie *f*, Konversionsneurose *f*, hysterische Reaktion *f* / **hysterical ~, dissociative type** hysterische Neurose *f*, dissoziativer Typ *m* / **iatrogenic** ~ iatrogene Neurose *f*, durch ärztliche Einwirkung ausgelöste Neurose *f* / **industrial** ~ Betriebsneurose *f* / **infantile ~** Kindheitsneurose *f* / **intestinal ~** nervöse Darmstörung *f*, Darmneurose *f* / **marginal ~** Randneurose *f* / **mixed ~** Mischneurose *f*, gemischte Neurose *f* / **narcissistic ~** narzistische Neurose *f* / **nuclear ~** Kernneurose *f* / **obsessional ~** Zwangsneurose *f* / **obsessional ~ mechanism** zwangsneurotischer Mechanismus *m* / **obsessive–compulsive ~** Zwangsneurose *f* / **occupational ~** Berufsneurose *f*, Beschäftigungsneurose *f*, Arbeitsneurose *f* / **oral ~** Sprachneurose *f* / **organic ~** Kernneurose *f*, Organneurose *f* / **phobic ~** phobische Neurose *f*, Angstneurose *f* / **posttraumatic ~** posttraumatische Neurose *f* / **professional ~** Berufsneurose *f*, Beschäftigungsneurose *f*, Arbeitsneurose *f* / **reactive ~** reaktive Neurose *f* / **sexual ~** Sexualneurose / **situational ~** reaktive Neurose *f* / **stratifunctional endogenous ~** Schichtneurose *f* / **traumatic ~** Unfallneurose *f*, traumatische Neurose *f*, posttraumatische Neurose *f* / **vasomotor ~** vasomotorische Neurose *f* / **vegetative ~** vegetative Neurose *f* / **visceral ~** Organneurose *f* / **vocational ~** Berufsneurose *f*, Beschäftigungsneurose *f*, Arbeitsneurose *f*

neurosism Neurasthenie *f*

neurosotropic zu Neurosen veranlagt, neurosebereit

neurospasm Neurospasmus *m*, Nervenkrampf *m*

neurosurgeon Neurochirurg *m*

neurosurgery Neurochirurgie *f*, Nervenchirurgie *f*

neurosyphilis Neurosyphilis *f*, Neurolues *f*

neurotensin Neurotensin *n*

neurotherapy, neurotherapeutics Therapie *f* von Nervenleiden, Psychotherapie *f*

neurotic neurotisch / Neurotiker *m*

neuroticism Neurotizismus *m*, neurotische Tendenz *f*, emotionale Labilität *f* / **~ questionnaire** Neurotizismus–Fragebogen *m*

neurotisation Regeneration *f* von durchtrennten Nerven, Nervenregeneration *f*, Neurotisation *f*

neurotomy Nervendurchtrennung *f*, Neurotomie *f*

neurotonia, neurotony Nervendehnung *f*, Neurotonie *f*

neurotoxin Nervengift *n*, Neurotoxin *n*

neurotransmitter Neurotransmitter *m*, Mittlersubstanz *f* an den Synapsen, Überträgerstoff *m* an den Synapsen / **inhibitory ~** synaptischer Hemmstoff *m*

neurotrauma Nervenverletzung *f*, Neurotrauma *n*

neurotropic neurotrop, auf die Nerven wirkend

neurovegetative neurovegetativ

neutral neutral, indifferent

neutralisation Neutralisation *f*

neutraliser Neutralisator *m*, neutralisierend wirkendes Gruppenmitglied *n*

neutrality Neutralität *f* / **psychotherapeutic ~** psychotherapeutische Neutralität *f*

nevus Muttermal *n*, Leberfleck *m*, Naevus *m*

new neu / **~–born** neugeboren / Neugeborenes *n*, neugeborenes Kind *n* / **~–born children** Neugeborene *npl*, neugeborene Kinder *npl*

Newton's law of colour mixture Newton'sches Gesetz *n* der Farbenmischung

next of kin Angehörige *pl*, nächste Verwandte *pl*

nexus Zusammenhang *m*, Verbindung *f*, Verkettung *f*, Verknüpfung *f*, Nexus *m* / **causal ~** Kausalnexus *m*, Kausalzusammenhang *m*

niacin Nikotinsäure *f*, Niazin *n*

niacinamide, nicotinamide Niazinamid *n*, Nikotinsäureamid *n*

nialamide Nialamid *n*

nibble abnagen, kauen

niche Nische *f*

nicotine Nikotin *n* / ~ **dependence** Nikotinabhängigkeit *f*, Nikotinabusus *m* / **~–related** im Zusammenhang mit Nikotin / **~–use disorder** Störung *f* durch Nikotinkonsum / ~ **withdrawal** Nikotinentzug *m*

nickname Spitzname *m*, Kurzname *m*

nictitate blinzeln

nictitating Blinzeln *n* / ~ **membrane** Nickhaut *f* / ~ **reflex** Blinzelreflex *m*, Lidschlussreflex *m*, Kornealreflex *m*

nifedipine Nifedipin *n*

night Nacht *f* / ~ **blind** nachtblind / ~ **blindness** Nachtblindheit *f*, Hemeralopie *f* / **~–cry** Aufschreien *n* im Schlaf, Pavor nocturnus *m* / **~–eating syndrome** Nachtesser–Syndrom *n* / ~ **start** nächtliches Aufschrecken *n* / ~ **terrors** Nachtangst *f*, Pavor nocturnus *m*, Alpdruck *m* / ~ **vision** Nachtsichtigkeit *f*, skotopes Sehen *n*, Dunkelsehen *n* / **~–walker** Nachtwandler *m*, Schlafwandler *m* / **~–walking** Schlafwandeln *n*, Nachtwandeln *n*, Noktambulismus *m*, Somnambulismus *m*

nightmare Alp *m*, Alptraum *m*, Alpdruck *m* / ~ **disorder** Schlafstörung *f* mit Alpträumen

nigrostriatal nigrostriatal

nihilism Nihilismus *m*

nihilistic nihilistisch

niphablepsia Schneeblindheit *f*

nipple Brustwarze *f*, Trinksauger *m* der Säuglingsflasche / ~ **complex** Saugkomplex *m*

nirvana Nirwana *n* / ~ **principle** Nirwanaprinzip *n*, Todestrieb *m*, Thanatostrieb *m*

nirvanism Nirwana–Gefühl *n*

Nissl|'s bodies Nissl–Schollen *fpl* / **~'s granules** Nissl–Schollen *fpl* / **~'s stain** Nissl–Färbung *f* / ~ **substance** basophiles Material *n* der Nissl–Schollen

nisus Anstrengung *f*, Antrieb *m*, Bestreben *n*, eifrige Bemühung *f*

nitrazepam Nitrazepam *n*

nitrogen Stickstoff *m* / ~ **monoxide** Stickoxid *n*, Stickstoffmonoxid *n*

nitroglycerine Nitroglyzerin *n*

N–methyl–D–aspartate N–Methyl–D–Aspartat *n*

noasthenia Geistesschwäche *f*

nociceptive schmerzvermittelnd, nozizeptiv

nociceptor Nozirezeptor *m*, Schmerzrezeptor *m*

noci–influence schädigender Einfluss *m*

nociperception Nozizeption *f*, Schmerzempfindung *f*, Schmerzwahrnehmung *f*, Wahrnehmung *f* schädigender Reize

nocireceptor, nocisensor Nozirezeptor *m*

noctambulant schlafwandelnd, nachtwandelnd

noctambulation, noctambulism Nachtwandeln *n*, Schlafwandeln *n*, Noktambulismus *m*, Somnambulismus *m*

noctambulic nachtwandlerisch

noctambulist Nachtwandler *m*, Schlafwandler *m*

noctiphobia krankhafte Nachtangst *f*, Dunkelangst *f*

nocturnal nächtlich

nocuous schädlich

nodal Knoten–, knotenförmig

no data kein Ergebnis

node Knoten *m* / ~ **of Ranvier** Ranvier'scher Schnürring *m*

nodding spasm Nickkrampf *m*

noegenesis Noogenese *f*, Erkenntnisbildung *f*, gefühlsmäßige Wissensbildung *f*

noegenetic noogen, geistig verursacht, gefühlsmäßig erkennend

noesis Noese *f*, Denkakt *m*, Geistestätigkeit *f*, Verstand *m*

noetic noetisch, verstandesmäßig, logisch

noetics Erkenntnislehre *f*, Noetik *f*

noise Lärm *m*, Geräusch *n*, Rauschen *n*, Störung *f* / ~ **apparatus** Lärmtrommel *f* / ~ **audiogram** Lärmaudiogramm *n* / ~ **box** Lärmapparat *m* / ~ **deafness** Lärmschwerhörigkeit *f* / ~ **effect** Lärmwirkung *f* / ~ **level** Lärmpegel *m*, Geräuschpegel *m* / ~ **pollution** Lärmbelästigung *f* / **ambient** ~ Nebengeräusch *n* / **filtered** ~ gefiltertes Rauschen *n* / **neural** ~ neurales Rauschen *n* / **physiological** ~ physiologisches Geräusch *n* / **random** ~ unregelmäßiger Lärm *m* / **thermal** ~ Wärmerauschen *n* / **visual** ~ visuelles Rauschen *n* / **white** ~ weißes Rauschen *n*

noisiness Lärm *m*, Geräusch *n*

nomadism Nomadentum *n*

nomenclature Nomenklatur *f*, Terminologie *f*

nomifensine Nomifensin *f*

nominal nominal, Nominal–, nominell

nominalism Nominalismus *m*

nomination technique Benennungsmethode *f*

nomogram Nomogramm *n*

nomography Nomographie *f*

nomological nomologisch

nomology Nomologie *f*

nomothetic nomothetisch, Gesetze aufstellend

non nicht, un– / ~**adjustive** unangepasst / ~**coherent** unzusammenhängend, nicht kohärent / ~ **compos mentis** unzurechnungsfähig / ~**contradiction** Vereinbarkeit *f* / ~**ego** Nicht–Ich *n* / ~**erotic** unerotisch / ~**existent** nicht existent, fehlend / ~**excited** nicht erregt / ~**habit forming** keine Gewohnheit bildend, keine Sucht erzeugend / ~**medullated** marklos / ~**observance** Nichtbeobachtung *f* / ~ **profit** nicht auf Gewinn gerichtet, gemeinnützig / ~**response** Nichtbeantwortung *f* / ~**restraint** ohne Zwang / ~**satisfaction** fehlende Befriedigung *f* / ~**sensitive** unempfindlich / ~**sensory** unempfindlich / ~**sequitur** irrige Folgerung *f* / ~**sexual** asexuell, ungeschlechtlich / ~**striated** glatt, nicht gestreift / ~**veneral** außergeschlechtlich

nonacademic nicht–akademisch, ohne Hochschulausbildung, praktisch

nonbeing Nichts *n*, Nichtexistente *n*

noncompliance| with medical treatment Nichtbefolgen *n* der ärztlichen Behandlungsmaßnahmen / ~ **with treatment** Nichtbefolgen *n* von Behandlungsanweisungen

nonconformism Nonkonformismus *m*

nonconformist Nonkonformist *m*, Dissident *m*

nonconformity mangelnde Anpassung *f*, fehlende Übereinstimmung *f*

nonconscious nicht bewusst, unbewusst

noncontingent unabhängig von, ohne Bezug auf

noncontinuity Diskontinuität *f*, Unterbrechung *f* / ~ **theory of learning** Theorie *f* des diskontinuierlichen Lernens

noncorrelated unkorreliert

nondetermination Unbestimmtheit *f*

nondirective nicht–direktiv, non–direktiv, ungelenkt

nondisjunction Non–Disjunktion *f*

noneducable unerziehbar

nonentity Nichtsein *n*, Nichtdasein *n*, Fiktion *f*, unbedeutende Person *f*

nonglandotropic nicht–glandotrop

nonhomogeneous nicht–homogen, inhomogen

nonius Nonius *m*, Gradteiler *m*

nonlanguage test nichtverbaler Test *m*, sprachfreier Test *m*

nonlinear nicht–linear

nonlinearity Nichtlinearität *f*

nonliterate ohne Schriftsprache, primitiv

nonmedullated marklos, markarm

nonmetric nicht–metrisch, nicht–quantifizierbar, nicht–quantifiziert

nonmonotone nicht monoton, nicht eintönig, abwechslungsreich

nonmoral moralfrei, amoralisch, wertungsfrei

nonobjective nicht gegenständlich, gegenstandslos

nonparametric nicht–parametrisch, verteilungsfrei

nonpareil unvergleichlich / unvergleichliche Person *f*, unvergleichliche Sache *f*

nonprescription drug verschreibungsfreies Medikament *n*

nonprofessional personnel Hilfspersonal *n*

nonprofit organisation gemeinnützige Organisation *f*

nonprojective nicht projektiv

nonpropulsive nicht propulsiv

nonpsychiatric nicht psychiatrisch

nonpsychological nicht psychologisch

nonpsychotic nicht psychotisch, ohne psychotische Erscheinungen

nonrandomized nicht nach Zufall ausgewählt

nonrational unrational, irrational

nonreader Nicht–Leser *m*, Analphabet *m*

nonreinforcement Nichtverstärkung *f*

non–REM sleep Non–REM–Schlaf *m*, orthodoxer Schlaf *m*

nonsense Unsinn *m* / **~ cooking** Faseln *n* / **~ correlation** Scheinkorrelation *f* / **~ figure** sinnlose Figur *f* / **~ syllable** sinnlose Silbe *f* / **~ syndrome** Ganser Syndrom *n*, Pseudodemenz *f*, vorgetäuschte Geistesstörung *f*

nonsexual ungeschlechtlich, geschlechtslos, asexuell

nonsocial asozial, unsozial

nonspecific unspezifisch

nonstandard English Umgangsenglisch *n*

nonverbal nichtverbal, sprachfrei

nonviolence Gewaltlosigkeit *f*

nonvoluntary nicht willensmäßig

noopsyche Noopsyche *f*

noradrenaline Noradrenalin *n*

norepinephrine Norepinephrin *n*, Noradrenalin *n* / **~ metabolite** Noradrenalinmetabolit *m*

norm Norm *f*, Standard *m* / **~ line** Normlinie *f* / **~ sending** Anwendung *f* von Normen / **behavioural ~** Verhaltensnorm *f* / **composite ~** zusammengesetzte Norm *f*, kombinierte Norm *f* / **cultural ~** Kulturnorm *f* / **developmental ~** Entwicklungsnorm *f*, Altersnorm *f* / **ideal ~** Idealnorm *f* / **local ~** örtliche Norm *f*, Regionalnorm *f* / **national ~** Volksnorm *f*, nationale Norm *f* / **occupational ~** Berufsnorm *f* / **percentile ~** Perzentilnorm *f*, Prozentrangnorm *f* / **psychic ~** psychische Norm *f* / **social ~** soziale Norm *f*, gesellschaftliche Norm *f* / **statistical ~** statistische Norm *f*

normal normal, Normal–, Standard–

normalisation Normalisierung *f*, Normierung *f*

normalise normalisieren, normieren

normality, normalcy Normalität *f*, Regelmäßigkeit *f*

normative normativ

normosplanchnic normalen Körperbau betreffend

normoventilation Normoventilation *f*

nortriptyline Nortriptylin *n*

nose Nase *f*

nosebrain Riechhirn *n*, Rhinenzephalon *n*

nosoagnosia Nosoagnosie *f*

nosogenesis, nosogeny Krankheitsentwicklung *f*, Nosogenie *f*

nosography Krankheitsbeschreibung *f*, Nosographie *f*

nosological nosologisch

nosologist Nosologe *m*

nosology Krankheitslehre *f*, Nosologie *f*

nosomania Krankheitswahn *m*, Nosomanie *f*, eingebildete Krankheit *f*

nosophilia Krankheitsneigung *f*, Krankheitsbereitschaft *f*, Nosophilie *f*

nosophobe Mensch *m* mit neurotischer Angst, krank zu sein

nosophobia neurotische Angst *f* vor Krankheiten, Nosophobie *f*, Krankheitsfurcht *f*

nostalgia, nostalgy Heimweh *f*, Sehnsucht *f*, sehnsüchtige Erinnerung *f*, Nostalgie *f*

nostalgic heimwehkrank, sehnsuchtsvoll, nostalgisch

nostomania krankhaftes Heimweh *n*

nostril Nasenloch *n*

not otherwise specified nicht näher bezeichnet

notation Bezeichnung *f*, Symbol *n*, Kode *m*, Kodifizierung *f*

note Note *f*, Ton *m*, Klang *m*, Laut *m*, Notiz *f* / beachten, bemerken / **~ blindness** Amusie *f* / **~ taking** Protokollieren *n*, Notizenanfertigung *f*

noteworthy bemerkenswert, beachtenswert

nothingness Nichtsein *n*, Nichts *n*

notice bemerken, beobachten / Nachricht *f*, Beachtung *f*, Notiz *f*

noticeable wahrnehmbar, merklich, bemerkbar / **just ~** eben merklich, gerade wahrnehmbar

notion Begriff *m*, Vorstellung *f* / **~ of force** Kraftbegriff *m* / **intuitive ~** Anschauungsbegriff *m*

notochord Rückenstrang *m*, Chorda dorsalis *f*

noun Substantiv *n*, Hauptwort *n*

nous Intellekt *m*, Geist *m*

novelty Neuheit *f* / **~ seeking** Suche *f* nach neuen Reizen

novice Neuling *m*, Anfänger *m*

novocaine Novocain *n*, Procain *n*

noxa schädigende Ursache *f*, krankheitserzeugende Schädigung *f*, Noxe *f*

noxal schädlich

noxavoidance need Bedürfnis *n* Schäden zu vermeiden

noxious schädlich, verderblich

n–power Machtbedürfnis *n*, Machtmotiv *n*

NREM sleep Non–REM–Schlaf *m*, orthodoxer Schlaf *m*

n–tuple *n*–fach *n*, –faches *n*

nuclear Kern–, nuklear

nucleated kernhaltig

nucleolus Kernkörperchen *n*, Nukleolus *m*

nucleotide Nukleotid *n*

nucleus Kern *m*, Zellkern *m*, Nukleus *m* / **~ caudatus** Nucleus caudatus *m* / **~ cuneatus** Burdach–Strang *m*, Nucleus cuneatus *m* / **~ gracilis** Nucleus gracilis *m*, Goll'scher Kern *m* / **amygdaloid ~** Mandelkern *m* / **basal ~** Basalganglion *n* / **caudate ~** Nucleus caudatus *m*, Schweifkern *m* / **cerebellar ~** Kleinhirnkern *m* / **cuneate ~** Burdach–Strang *m*, Nucleus cuneatus *m* / **dentate ~** Dentatum *n*, Nucleus dentatus *m* / **dorsal–column ~** Hinterstrangkern *m* / **gracile ~** Nucleus gracilis *m*, Gollscher Kern *m* / **haploid ~** Kern *m* mit halber Chromosomenzahl / **lenticular ~** Linsenkern *m*, Nucleus lentiformis *m* / **lentiform ~** Linsenkern *m*, Nucleus lentiformis *m* / **medullary ~** weiße Gehirnsubstanz *f* / **oculomotor ~** Nucleus nervi oculomotorii *m* / **olivary ~** Olivenkern *m* / **red ~** Nucleus ruber *m* / **thalamic ~** Thalamuskern *m* / **trigeminal ~** Trigeminuskern *m*

nudism Nudismus *m*, Nacktkultur *f*, Freikörperkultur *f*

nudity Nacktheit *f*

nudomania Nudomanie *f*

nudophilia Nudophilie *f*

nudophobia Angst *f* vor dem Nackten, Nudophobie *f*

nuisance Schaden *m*, Störung *f*, Ärgernis *n*

null hypothesis Nullhypothese *f* / **~ testing** Testen *n* der Nullhypothese

nulliplex gleicherbig rezessiv

nullity of marriage Nichtigkeit *f* der Ehe

numb benommen, betäubt, empfindungslos, abgestumpft

number Zahl *f*, Anzahl *f*, Ziffer *f*, Nummer *f* / **~ blindness** Zahlenblindheit *f*, Rechenstörung *f*, Akalkulie *f* / **~ combination** Zahlenkombination *f* / **~ completion test** Zahlenergänzungstest *m* / **~ comprehension** Zahlenverständnis *n* / **~ concept** Zahlbegriff *m* / **~ fact** Zahlenkombination *f* / ~ **factor** Rechenfaktor *m*, numerischer Faktor *m* / ~ **form** Zahlendiagramm *n* / ~ **system** Zahlensystem *n* / **binary** ~ binäre Zahl *f* / **discrete** ~ diskrete Zahl *f* / **irrational** ~ irrationale Zahl *f* / **ordinal** ~ Ordinalzahl *f*, Ordnungszahl *f* / **random** ~ Zufallszahl *f* / **rational** ~ rationale Zahl *f*

numbering system Rechensystem *n*, Zahlensystem *n*

numbness Benommenheit *f*, Gefühllosigkeit *f*, Parästhesie *f*, Erstarrung *f*, Betäubung *f*

numerator Zähler *m*

numeric, numerical numerisch, zahlenmäßig

numerology Lehre *f* von der okkulten Bedeutung der Zahlen

numerosity große Zahl *f*, Menge *f* / ~ **perception** Mengenwahrnehmung *f*

numinous numinös, göttlich, geheimnisvoll

nurse Kinderpflegerin *f*, Kindergärtnerin *f*, Krankenschwester *f*, Krankenpfleger *m* / stillen, säugen, pflegen / **~-child** Pflegekind *n* / **psychiatric** ~ Krankenschwester *f* in der Psychiatrie / **registered** ~ examinierte Krankenschwester *f*

nursery Kindertagesstätte *f* / **~-rhyme** Kinderreim *m*, Kinderlied *n* / **~-school** Kindergarten *m* / **~-school student** Kindergartenkind *n*, Vorschulkind *n*

nursing Stillen *n*, Säugen *n*, Pflege *f*, Krankenpflege *f* / ~ **education** Krankenpflegeausbildung *f* / ~ **home** Pflegeheim *n* / **~-mother** Pflegemutter *f* / ~ **student** Krankenpflegeschüler *m*

nurturance Fürsorglichkeit *f*, Pflege- und Schutztendenz *f* / ~ **need** Pflegetrieb *m*

nurture Erziehung *f*, Aufziehen *n*, entwicklungsfördernde Umwelteinflüsse *mpl* / aufziehen, erziehen

nutriance need Nahrungsbedürfnis *n*, Futtertrieb *m*

nutrient Nährstoff *m* / nahrhaft / ~ **content** Nährstoffgehalt *m*

nutriment Nahrung *f*, Lebensmittel *npl*

nutrition Ernährung *f*, Nutrition *f*

nychthemeron, nycthemeron Tag- und Nachtzyklus *m*, ein voller Tag *m* und eine volle Nacht *f*

nyctalgia Nachtschmerz *m*, Nyktalgie *f*

nyctalope Nachtblinder *m*, Tagblinder *m*

nyctalopia Nachtblindheit *f*, Mondblindheit *f*, Tagblindheit *f*, Hemeralopie *f*

nyctalopic nachtblind, tagblind

nyctanopia Nachtblindheit *f*, Mondblindheit *f*, Hemeralopie *f*

nyctaphonia Nyktaphonie *f*

nyctophilia Nyktophilie *f*

nyctophobia Nachtangst *f*, Angst *f* vor der Dunkelheit, Nyktophobie *f*

nympholepsy Liebeswahn *m*

nymphomania Nymphomanie *f*, Mannstollheit *f*, Andromanie *f*, Hysteromanie *f*

nymphomaniac nymphoman, mannstoll, Nymphomanin *f*

nystagmic nystagmisch

nystagmogram Nystagmogramm *n*

nystagmograph Nystagmograph *m*

nystagmus Augenzittern *n*, Nystagmus *m* / ~ **caloric test** Bárány kalorische Prüfung *f* / **caloric** ~ kalorischer Nystagmus *m* / **disjunctive** ~ Einstellungsnystagmus *m* / **galvanic** ~ galvanischer Nystagmus *m* / **kinetic** ~ kinetischer Nystagmus *m* / **lateral** ~ horizontaler Nystagmus *m* / **optokinetic** ~ Eisenbahnnystagmus *m* / **paroxysmal** ~ Nystagmusklonus *m* / **postcaloric** ~ kalorischer Nystagmus *m* / **postrotatory** ~ Drehnystagmus *m*, postrotatorischer Nystagmus *m* / **rotatory** ~ Drehnystagmus *m*, Rotationsnystagmus *m* / **spontaneous** ~ Sponatannystagmus *m* / **undulatory** ~ Pendelnystagmus *m* / **vertical** ~ Vertikalnystagmus *m*

O

obcecation Teilerblindung *f*

obdormition Eingeschlafensein *n* von Gliedern, Taubheit *f* eines Gliedes, Parästhesie *f*

obedience Gehorsam *m*, bedingungsloser Gehorsam *m* / **automatic ~** Befehlsautomatie *f* / **deferred ~** nachträglicher Gehorsam *m*

obese fett, korpulent, dick

obesity Fettleibigkeit *f*, Korpulenz *f*, Übergewicht *n*

object Objekt *n*, Ziel *n*, Zielvorstellung *f*, Absicht *f*, Zweck *m*, Intention *f* / **~ agnosia** Objektagnosie *f* / **~ assembly test** Puzzletest *m*, Legespieltest *m* / **~-assimilation** Assimilation *f*, kognitive Assimilation *f* / **~ attitude** Einstellung *f* zum Versuchsobjekt / **~ blindness** Seelenblindheit *f*, optische Agnosie *f* / **~ cathexis** Objektbesetzung *f* / **~ choice** Objektwahl *f* / **anaclytic ~ choice** anaklitische Objektwahl *f*, Anlehnungstyp *m* der Objektwahl / **~ colour** Objektfarbe *f* / **~ consciousness** Objektbewusstsein *n* / **~ constancy** Dingkonstanz *f*, Wahrnehmungskonstanz *f*, Objektkonstanz *f* / **~ error** Reizirrtum *m* / **~ finding** Objektfindung *f* / **~ of instinct** instinktauslösendes Objekt *n* / **~ libido** Objektlibido *f* / **~ loss** Objektverlust *m*, Liebesverlust *m* / **~ love** Objektliebe *f* / **~ of perception** Wahrnehmungsgegenstand *m* / **~ permanence** Objektpermanenz *f* / **~ recognition** Objekterkennung *f* / **~ relation** Objektbeziehung *f* / **~ relations theory** Objektbeziehungstheorie *f* / **~ relationship** Objektbeziehung *f* / **~ size** Objektgröße *f* / **bad ~** schlechtes Objekt *n* / **good ~** gutes Objekt *n* / **inanimate ~** lebloser Gegenstand *m* / **incestuous ~ choice** inzestuöse Objektwahl *f* / **instinctual ~** instinktauslösendes Objekt *n* / **libidinal ~** Libidoobjekt *n* / **narcissistic ~ choice** narzisstische Objektwahl *f* / **part-~** Teilobjekt *n*, Partialobjekt *n* / **sexual ~** Sexualobjekt *n* / **signified ~** Bezeichnete *n*, bezeichneter Gegenstand *m* / **transitional ~** Übergangsobjekt *n*

objectal Objekt–

objectification Objektivierung *f*, Externalisation *f*, Projektion *f* nach außen

objectify objektivieren, konkretisieren

objection Einwand *m* / **conscientious ~** Kriegsdienstverweigerung *f*

objectivation Objektivierung *f*, Objektivation *f* / **~ of thinking** Objektivierung *f* des Denkens

objective Objektiv *n*, Ziel *n*, Zielvorstellung *f* / objektiv, sachlich, vorurteilslos / **~ of thinking** Denkziel *n* / **basic ~** Grundziel *n*, grundsätzliches Leistungsziel *n* / **behavioural ~** Verhaltensziel *n* / **educational ~** Erziehungsziel *n*, Bildungsziel *n* / **organizational ~** Organisationsziel *n*, Organisationszweck *m*

objectivism Objektivismus *m*

objectivity Objektivität *f*, Sachlichkeit *f*

oblateness, oblativity Abflachung *f*, Abplattung *f* an den Polen

obligate gebunden, verpflichtend, unabdingbar, wichtig

obligation Verpflichtung *f*, Pflicht *f*

obligatory verpflichtend, obligatorisch, verbindlich

oblimax method Oblimax–Methode *f*

oblimin method Oblimin–Methode *f*

oblique schief, schräg, quer, schiefwinklig

obliquity Schrägheit *f*, Schiefheit *f*, Obliquität *f*, Verirrung *f*, Unredlichkeit *f*

obliteration Auslöschung *f*, Löschung *f*, Extinktion *f*, Obliteration *f*

obliviscence Vergesslichkeit *f*

oblongata Medalla oblongata *f*, verlängertes Mark *n*

obmutescence Verlust *m* der Stimme, Stimmlosigkeit *f*, Aphonie *f*

obnubilation Bewusstseinstrübung *f*, Benommenheit *f*, geistige Umnachtung *f*

obscene unzüchtig, obszön

obscenity Unzüchtigkeit *f*, Obszönität *f*, Unanständigkeit *f*

obscurant Bildungsfeind *m* / bildungsfeindlich

obscurantism Verdummung *f*, Bildungshass *m*

observation Beobachtung *f*, Untersuchung *f* / **~ method** Beobachtungsmethode *f* / **concomitant ~** gleichzeitige Beobachtung *f* / **epistemic ~** erkenntnistheoretische Beobachtung *f* / **natural ~** natürliche Beobachtung *f* / **naturalistic ~** natürliche Beobachtung *f* / **random ~** Zufallsbeobachtung *f* / **unobtrusive ~** unauffällige Beobachtung *f*

observational Beobachtungs–

observe beobachten, feststellen, bemerken

observer Beobachter *m* / **matched ~s** gleichwertige Beobachter *mpl* / **participant ~** teilnehmender Beobachter *m*

obsessed besessen, von einer Zwangsvorstellung befallen

obsession Besessenheit *f*, fixe Idee *f*, Zwangsvorstellung *f*, Zwangsgedanke *m*, Obsession *f* / **artificial ~** künstliche Besessenheit *f* / **impulsive ~** Zwangsantrieb *m* / **manifest ~** manifeste Besessenheit *f* / **masked ~** larvierte Zwangsvorstellung *f* / **questioning ~** Fragezwang *m* / **somatic ~** körperliche Besessenheit *f* / **somnambulic ~** somnambule Besessenheit *f*

obsessional Zwangs– / **~–neurotic** zwangsneurotisch

obsessive Zwangs–, zwanghaft / **~–compulsive** zwangsneurotisch, obsessiv–impulsiv

obsolenscence Veralten *n*

obsolescent veraltend

obsolete veraltet, ungebräuchlich, unvollkommen entwickelt

obstacle Hindernis *n* / **~ sense** Hindernissinn *m*

obstetrician Geburtshelfer *m*, Facharzt *m* für Geburtshilfe

obstetrics Geburtshilfe *f*

obstinacy Hartnäckigkeit *f*, Eigensinn *m*

obstinate hartnäckig, eigensinnig, starrköpfig, trotzig

obstipation Verstopfung *f*, Obstipation *f*

obstruction Hindernis *n*, Sperre *f* / **~ box** Hinderniskasten *m* / **~ method** Hindernismethode *f*

obtain erhalten, erreichen

obturator nerve Nervus obturatorius *m*

obtuseness Beschränktheit *f*, Dummheit *f*

obtusion Stumpfwerden *n* / **~ of sensation** Gefühlsabstumpfung *f*

obverse dem Betrachter zugewandt, Vorder–

Occam's razor Sparsamkeitsprinzip *n*, Ökonomie–Prinzip *n*

occasional gelegentlich, Gelegenheits–

occasionalism Okkasionalismus *m*

Occidentalism abendländische Kultur *f*, westliche Zivilisation *f*

occipital Hinterhaupt–, okzipital

occiput Hinterkopf *m*, Okziput *m*

occlude verschließen, separieren

occlusion Schließung *f*, Verschluss *m*, Okklusion *f* / **~ test** Nullversuch *m*

occlusive verschließend, okklusiv

occult verborgen, geheim, magisch, okkult

occultism Okkultismus *m*

occupation Beruf *m*, Beschäftigung *f* / **~ neurosis** Berufsneurose *f*, Beschäftigungsneurose *f*, Arbeitsneurose *f* / **parental ~** Beruf *m* der Eltern

occupational beruflich, Berufs–, Arbeits–, Beschäftigungs–

ocellus Punktauge *n*

ochlophobia Massenangst *f*, Ochlophobie *f*

octave Oktave *f*

octopus Tintenfisch *m*, Oktopus *m*

ocular Augen–, okular

oculist, ocularist Augenarzt *m*

oculocardiac, oculocardial okulokardial, Augen–Herz–

oculogyral, oculogyric Augenbewegungs–, okulogyral

oculomotor, oculomotoric, oculomotive Augenbewegungs–, okulomotorisch, blickmotorisch, Okulomotorius

od Od *n*, angeblich vom Menschen ausstrahlende Kraft *f*

odd ungerade, ungleich, seltsam, sonderbar / **~–even** gerade und ungerade / **~s** Vorteile *mpl*, Chancen *fpl*, Wahrscheinlichkeit *f*

oddity Seltsamkeit *f*, Original *n*, seltsamer Kauz *m*, ungleiche Sache *f* / **~ method** Teilungsmethode *f*

odious verhasst, abscheulich

odontalgia Zahnschmerz *m*

odontogenesis, odontogeny Zahnbildung *f*, Zahnentwicklung *f*, Dentifikation *f*

odoriferous duftend, wohlriechend

odorimetry Odorimetrie *f*, Prüfung *f* des Geruchssinnes, Geruchsmessung *f*

odoriphore Geruchsträger *m*

odorivector Geruchsvektor *m*

odorosity Geruchsintensität *f*

odorous wohlriechend

odour, odor Geruch *m*, Duft *m* / **~ discrimination** Geruchsunterscheidung *f*, Geruchsdiskrimination *f* / **~ prism** Geruchsprisma *n* / **~ stimulus** Geruchsreiz *m* / **~ substance** Duftstoff *m* / **alliaceous ~** lauchartiger Geruch *m* / **ambrosiac ~** würziger Geruch *m*, Amber–Moschusgeruch *m* / **resinous ~** harziger Geruch *m*

odorant Duftstoff *m*

odourless, odorless geruchlos

odynophobia Angst *f* vor Schmerzen

oecological ökologisch

oecology Ökologie *f*, Lehre *f* von den Umweltbeziehungen / **~ of social behaviour** Verhaltenstheorie *f* im sozialen Feld

oedema Ödem *n*, Flüssigkeitsansammlung *f*, Wassersucht *f* / **angioneurotic ~** angioneurotisches Ödem *n*, Quincke–Ödem *n* / **cerebral ~** Hirnödem *n*, Hirnschwellung *f* / **hysterical ~** hysterisches Ödem *n* / **wandering ~** Wanderödem *n*, angioneurotisches Ödem *n*

oedematous ödematös

oedipal ödipal, Ödipus–

Oedipus| complex Ödipuskomplex *m* / **~ situation** Ödipussituation *f* / **complete ~** vollständiger Ödipus *m* / **female ~ complex** weiblicher Ödipuskomplex *m*, Elektrakomplex *m* / **inverted ~ complex** perverser Ödipuskomplex *m*

oenomania Säuferwahnsinn *m*, Oenomanie *f*

oesophagus Speiseröhre *f*, Schlund *m*, Ösophagus *m*

oestrogen Östrogen *n*

oestromania Östromanie *f*, Nymphomanie *f*

oestrum, oestrus Brunst *f*, Brunstzeit *f*, Brunstperiode *f*, Östrus *m*

off–effect Aus–Effekt *m*

offence, offense Angriff *m*, Kränkung *f*, Beleidigung *f*, Straftat *f* / **criminal ~** strafbare Handlung *f* / **sexual ~** Sexualdelikt *n*, Sexualverbrechen *n* / Sexualstraftat *f* / **unnatural ~** widernatürliche Unzucht *f*

offend verstoßen gegen, sich vergehen, verletzen, beleidigen

offender Straftäter *m*, Delinquent *m*, Krimineller *m* / **mentally ill ~** psychisch kranker Straftäter *m* / **sexual ~** Sittlichkeitsverbrecher *m*, Sexualstraftäter *m*

offensive offensiv, Angriffs–, beleidigend

office Funktion *f*, Dienst *m*, Amt *n*, Büro *n* / **~ automation** Büroautomatisierung *f*, Bürorationalisierung *f* / **~ management** Büroorganisation *f*, Büroverwaltung *f*

official offiziell, amtlich, Amts–

officinal offizinell, im Arzneibuch aufgeführt, arzneilich

offshoot Spross *m*, Nachkomme *m*, Seitenlinie *f*, Ableger *m*

offspring Nachkommenschaft *f*, Abkömmling *m*, Kind *n*, Nachwuchs *m*, Brut *f* / **interracial ~** Mischling *m*

ogival Ogiven–, Summenkurven–

ogive Ogive *f*, kumulative Häufigkeitskurve *f*

ohm Ohm *n*

ohmmeter Ohmmeter *n*

Ohm's law Ohm'sches Gesetz *n*

oikomania Raserei *f* gegenüber der eigenen Familie

oikophobia Hausangst *f*, Oikophobie *f*

oikotropic oikotrop, autonom

oinomania Trunksucht *f*, Säuferwahnsinn *m*, Oenomanie *f*

old alt / **~–age** Alter *n*, Greisenalter *n* / Alters– / **~–sighted** alterssichtig, presbyop / **very ~** hochbetagt / Hochbetagte *m,f*

oldsightedness Alterssichtigkeit *f*, Presbyopie *f*

olfactible riechbar, geruchsmäßig wahrnehmbar

olfactie Olfaktie *f*, Riecheinheit *f*

olfaction Geruchssinn *m*, Geruchsvermögen *n*, Riechen *n* / **coloured ~** Farbenriechen *n*

olfactive Riech–, Geruchs–

olfactology Osmologie *f*, Osphresiologie *f*, Lehre *f* vom Geruchssinn

olfactometer Olfaktometer *n*

olfactometry Olfaktometrie *f*, Geruchsprüfung *f*

olfactory Geruchs–, Riech–, olfaktorisch

oligergasia psychische Störung *f*, Geistesstörung *f*, Oligophrenie *f*

oligodendroglia Oligodendroglia *f*, Mikroglia *f* des Zentralnervensystems

oligoencephaly Oligophrenie *f*, Geistesschwäche *f*

oligographia Einsilbigkeit *f* im schriftlichen Ausdruck

oligolalia, oligologia, oligophasia Einsilbigkeit *f*

oligomenorrhea Oligomenorrhoe *f*, zu seltene Menstruationsblutung *f*

oligophrenia Oligophrenie *f*, Geistesschwäche *f*, Schwachsinn *m*, geistige Minderbegabung *f* / **phenylpyruvic ~** Brenztraubensäureschwachsinn *m*, Fölling–Krankheit *f*

oligophrenic geistesschwach, schwachsinnig, geistig minderbegabt, oligophren

oligopsychia psychische Funktionsminderung *f*, Oligophrenie *f*, Schwachsinn *m*

olivary olivenförmig

omen Vorbedeutung *f*, Omen *n*, Vorzeichen *n*

omission Auslassung *f*, Unterlassung *f*, Weglassen *n*, Vergessen *n* / **~ training** Unterlassungstraining *n*

ommatidium Ommatidium *n*, Augenkeil *m* der Facettenaugen

omnibus test Sammeltest *m*, Testserie *f*, Testbatterie *f*

omnipotence Allmacht *f*, Omnipotenz *f* / **~ of the id** Allmacht *f* des Es / **~ of thought** Allmacht *f* der Gedanken, Wunschdenken *n* / **infantile ~** kindliches Wunschdenken *n*

omnipotent allmächtig

onanism Onanie *f*, Masturbation *f*, Selbstbefriedigung *f*, Koitus interruptus *m* / **compulsive ~** zwanghaftes Onanieren *n*, exzessive Onanie *f* / **to practice ~** onanieren, masturbieren

onanist Onanist *m*

onanistic Masturbations–, Onanie–

one–dimensional eindimensional, unidimensional

on–effect Ein–Effekt *m*

oneiric Traum–, traumartig, oneiroid

oneirism Traumzustand *m*

oneiroanalysis Traumdeutung *f*, Traumanalyse *f*

oneirocritic traumdeutend / Traumdeuter *m*

oneirodynia Traumzustand *m*, schwerer Traum *m*, ängstliches Träumen *n*, Oneirodynia *f* / **active ~** Schlafwandeln *n* / **passive ~** Alpdrücken *n*

oneirology Traumlehre *f*, Traumdeutungslehre *f*, Oneirologie *f*

oneiromancy Traumweissagung *f*, Vorahnung *f* aufgrund von Träumen

oneiroscopy Traumdeutung *f*

one–sided einseitig

one–tailed einseitig, gerichtet

one–way Einweg– / **~ mirror** Einweg–Fenster *n* / **~ screen** Einweg–Fenster *n*

oniomania krankhafter Kauftrieb *m*, Kaufsucht *f*, Oniomanie *f*

onirism Traumzustand *m*, Traumgesicht *n*

online| database Online–Datenbank *f* / **~ search** Online–Suche *f*

onliness Tatsache *f* Einzelkind zu sein, Einzelkind–Dasein *n*

onomatology Onomatologie *f*

onomatomania Namenszwang *m*, Wortzwang *m*, Onomatomanie *f*

onomatophobia Wortangst *f*, Namensangst *f*, Onomatophobie *f*

onomatopoeia, onomatopoeisis Onomatopöie *f*, Bildung *f* von Wörtern durch Lautmalerei, Wortmalerei *f*

onomatopoetic, onomatopoeic lautnachahmend, onomatopoetisch

onset Anfang *m*, Beginn *m*, Wirkungseintritt *m*, Anfall *m* / **~ of disorder** Krankheitsbeginn *m* / **with delayed ~** mit verzögertem Beginn / **with ~ during intoxication** mit Beginn während der Intoxikation / **with ~ during withdrawal** mit Beginn während des Entzugs / **with postpartum ~** mit postpartalem Beginn

ontogenesis, ontogeny Ontogenese *f*, Ontogenie *f* / **~ of behaviour** Reifung *f*, Ontogenese *f*

ontogenetic, ontogenic ontogenetisch

ontological ontologisch

ontology Ontologie *f*, Seinslehre *f*

onychophagia, onychophagy Nägelbeißen *n*, Nägelkauen *n*, Onychophagie *f*

onychophagist Nägelbeißer *m*, Nägelkauer *m*

onychotillomania Nagelabdrehen *n*, triebartige Zerstörung *f* der Fingernägel, Onychotillomanie *f*

oogenesis Eientwicklung *f*, Eireifung *f*, Oogenese *f*

oogonium Ureier *npl* im Keimepithel des Ovars, Eimutterzelle *f*, Oogonium *n*

oophoralgia Eierstockschmerz *m*, Ovarialgie *f*

opacity Undurchsichtigkeit *f*, Trübung *f*

opaque undurchsichtig, trüb

open offen / **~–class** gesellschaftlich offen, mobil / **~–cue** mit sichtbaren Lösungshinweisen, mit allen erforderlichen Lösungszeichen / **~–end** offen, mit freier Antwortmöglichkeit, unbegrenzt, ohne vorgegebenes Ende / **~–minded** aufgeschlossen, unvoreingenommen / **~–mindedness** Aufgeschlossenheit *f*, Unvoreingenommenheit *f*, offenes System *n* von Meinungen

openness Offenheit *f*, Aufgeschlossenheit *f*, Offenherzigkeit *f* / **~ to experience** Offenheit *f* für Erfahrungen

operant nicht–reizbedingt, nicht–reizbezogen, operant / Wirkreaktion *f*, Operant *m* / **discriminated ~** nicht–reizbezogene Unterscheidungsreaktion *f*

operate arbeiten, handeln, bewirken, bedienen

operating Operations–, Bedienungs–, Arbeits–

operation Handlung *f*, Operation *f* / **~s research** Operations Research *f*, Entscheidungsforschung *f*, Unternehmensforschung *f* / **concrete ~s** konkrete Handlungen *fpl* / **drive–inducing ~** triebauslösender Vorgang *m* / **empirical ~** empirische Handlung *f* / **formal ~s** formelle Handlungen *fpl* / **infra–logical ~s** prälogische Handlungen *fpl* / **intellectual ~** geistige Handlung *f*, Denkvorgang *m* / **logical ~** logische Operation *f* / **mathematical ~** mathematische Operation *f* / **permissible ~** erlaubte Handlung *f*, korrekte Operation *f* / **sensorimotor ~** sensumotorische Handlung

operational Operations–, Verfahrens–, operational

operationalism, operationism Operationalismus *m*, Operationismus *m*

operative wirksam, in Betrieb befindlich, operativ

operator Operator *m*

operotropism Operotropismus *m*, Orientierung *f* zu einem bestimmten Beruf, Hinwendung *f* zur Arbeit

ophidiophilia krankhaftes Angezogensein *n* von Schlangen

ophidiophobe Mensch *m* der vor Schlangen Angst hat

ophidiophobia, ophidiphobia, ophiophobia krankhafte Furcht *f* vor Schlangen, Schlangenfurcht *f*, Schlangenphobie *f*

ophthalmencephalon Sehlappen *m*, Sehhirn *n*

ophthalmia Augenentzündung *f*

ophthalmic Augen–

ophthalmograph Gerät *n* zur Aufzeichnung von Lesebewegungen der Augen

ophthalmologist Augenarzt *m*, Facharzt *m* für Augenkrankheiten

ophthalmology Augenheilkunde *f*, Ophthalmologie *f*

ophthalmometer Ophthalmometer *n*, Astigmometer *n*, Krümmungsflächenmesser *m*

ophthalmometry Ophthalmometrie *f*

ophthalmopathy Augenleiden *n*, Augenkrankheit *f*

ophthalmoplegia Augenmuskellähmung *f*

ophthalmoscope Augenspiegel *m*, Ophthalmoskop *n*

ophthalmoscopy Augenspiegeln *n*, Ophthalmoskopie *f*

ophthalmostatometer Ophthalmostatometer *n*, Gerät *n* zur Messung der Augenstellung

ophthalmostatometry Ophthalmostatometrie *f*, Messung *f* der Augenstellung

ophthalmotonometer Augendruckmesser *m*, Ophthalmotonometer *n*

ophthalmotonometry Augendruckmessung *f*, Messung *f* des intraokularen Drucks, Ophthalmotonometrie *f*

ophthalmotrope Augenmodell *n*

opiate Opium *n*, Opiat *n*, Schlafmittel *n* / einschläfernd, Beruhigungs– / **~ agonist** Opiatagonist *m* / **~ analgesia** Opiatanalgesie *f* / **~ antagonist** Opiatantagonist *m* / **~ receptor** Opiatrezeptor *m* / **endogenous ~** körpereigenes Opiat *n*

opine meinen

opinion Meinung *f*, Überzeugung *f*, Einstellung *f*, Gutachten *n* / **~ change** Einstellungsänderung *f*, Meinungsänderung *f* / **~ leader** Meinungsführer *m*, Meinungsbildner *m* / **~ poll** Meinungsforschung *f*, Meinungsumfrage *f* / **to ~–poll** nach der Meinung befragen / **~ research** Meinungsforschung *f*, Meinungsumfrage *f* / **~ survey** Meinungsbefragung *f*, Meinungsumfrage *f* / **moderate ~** gemäßigte Einstellung *f* / **psychological ~** psychologisches Gutachten *n* / **public ~** öffentliche Meinung *f*

opinionaire Fragebogen *m* zur Erfassung von Meinungen

opinionated, opinionative eigensinnig, eigenwillig, starrsinnig

opioid Opiat *n*, Opioid *n*, endogenes Opioid *n* / ~ **abuse** Opiatmissbrauch *m* / ~ **addiction** Opiatsucht *f* / ~ **dependence** Opiatabhängigkeit *f* / ~**–induced** opiatinduziert / ~ **intoxication** Opiatintoxikation *f* / ~ **intoxication delirium** Opiatintoxikationsdelir *n* / ~**–related** im Zusammenhang mit Opiaten / ~**–use disorders** Störungen *fpl* durch Opiatkonsum / ~ **withdrawal** Opiatentzug *m*

opiomania Opiumsucht *f*, Morphinismus *m*

opiomaniac opiumsüchtig, morphiumsüchtig / Opiumsüchtiger *m*

opiophile Opiumsüchtiger *m*, Rauschgiftsüchtiger *m*

opisthoporeia unwillkürliches Rückwärtsgehen *n*

opisthotonos Krampf *m* der Rückenmuskulatur, Genickstarrehaltung *f*, Opisthotonus *m*

opium Opium *n* / ~ **addict** Opiumsüchtiger *m* / ~ **alkaloid** Opiumalkaloid *n* / ~ **containing drug** opiumhaltiges Arzneimittel *n* / ~ **derivate** Opiumderivat *n* / ~ **eater** Opiumesser *m* / ~ **habit** Opiumsucht *f*, Morphinismus *m* / ~ **smoker** Opiumraucher *m*

opiumism Opiumsucht *f*

Oppel–Kundt illusion Oppel'sche Täuschung *f*

Oppenheim's reflex Oppenheim–Reflex *m*

oppilation Verstopfung *f*

opponent entgegengesetzt, Gegen– / Antagonist *m* / ~**–colour theory** Gegenfarbentheorie *f* / ~**–process theory** Theorie *f* der antagonistischen Prozesse

opportunism Opportunismus *m*, Anpassungspolitik *f*, Prinzipienlosigkeit *f*

opportunist Opportunist *m*, Anpassungsmensch *m*, Mitläufer *m*

opportunistic opportunistisch

opportunity Gelegenheit *f*, Möglichkeit *f*, Chance *f* / ~ **class** Förderklasse *f*

oppose bekämpfen, sich widersetzen, entgegensetzen, gegenüber stellen

opposite Gegenteil *n* / ~**s test** Test *m* gegensätzlicher Begriffe

opposition Opposition *f*, Gegensatz *m*, Widerstand *m* / ~ **of thumb** Daumenabspreizung *f*

oppress bedrücken, beklemmen, unterdrücken

oppression Bedrückung *f*, Beklemmung *f*, Beklemmungsgefühl *n*, Bedrängnis *f*

oppressive bedrückend, beklemmend

opsin Opsin *n*, Sehstoff *m*, Sehpigment *n*

opsomania Opsomanie *f*

optic, optical optisch, Seh–, Augen–

optician Optiker *m*

optics Optik *f*

optimal optimal

optimism Optimismus *m*, Zuversicht *f*, Lebensbejahung *f* / **oral** ~ oraler Optimismus *m*

Optimist Optimist *m*

optimistic optimistisch, zuversichtlich, hoffnungsvoll

optimize optimieren

optimizing Optimierung *f*

optimum Optimum *n* / optimal

option Wahl *f*, Wahlmöglichkeit *f*, Option *f*

optional Wahl–, freibleibend

optogram Netzhautbild *n*

optokinetic optokinetisch, die Augenbewegungen betreffend

optometer Optometer *n*, Sehweitemesser *m*

optometrical optometrisch

optometrist Optiker *m*

optometry Optometrie *f*, Sehweitebestimmung *f*, Fernpunktbestimmung *f*

optotype Sehprobe *f*, Testtafel *f*, Sehprobentafel *f*

oral oral, mündlich, Mund– / ~**–aggressive** oralaggressiv / ~**–biting** oralsadistisch / ~**–erotic** oral, oralerotisch / ~**–incorporative** durch den Mund einverleibend, oralinkorporativ / ~**–passive** rezeptiv / ~**–sadistic** oralsadistisch

orality Oralität *f*, Oralerotik *f*

orang–outan, orangutan Orang–Utan *m*

orbit Augenhöhle *f*, Orbita *f*

orbital Orbital–, orbital

orbitofrontal orbitofrontal

order Ordnung *f*, Anordnung *f*, Reihenfolge *f*, Befehl *m* / ordnen, anordnen, verordnen, befehlen / **~ of age** Altersstaffel *f* / **~ of birth** Geburtsordnung *f* / **~ of magnitude** Größenordnung *f* / **~ of a matrix** Ordnung *f* einer Matrix / **~ of merit ranking** Bildung *f* einer Rangreihe nach einem bestimmten Merkmal / **~ of merit rating** Vergleichsbeurteilung *f* / **~ need** Ordnungsbedürfnis *n* / **~ of rank** Rangreihe *f*, Rangordnung *f* / **chronological ~** zeitliche Reihenfolge *f* / **cyclic ~** zyklische Reihenfolge *f* / **first–~ factor** Faktor *m* erster Ordnung / **first–~ symptom** Symptom *n* 1. Ranges / **higher–~ conditioning** Konditionierung *f* höherer Ordnung / **higher–~ factor** Faktor *m* höherer Ordnung / **linear ~** lineare Reihe *f* / **moral ~** Sittenordnung *f* / **nth–~ conditioning** Konditionierung *f* *n*–ter Ordnung / **open ~** Wartebefehl *m* / **second–~ conditioning** Konditionierung *f* zweiter Ordnung / **second–~ correlation coefficient** Korrelationskoeffizient *m* zweiter Ordnung / **second–~ factor** Faktor *m* zweiter Ordnung / **second–~ symptom** Symptom *n* 2. Ranges / **serial ~** Reihenfolge *f* / **social ~** Sozialordnung *f*

orderliness Ordentlichkeit *f*, Ordnung *f* / **compulsive ~** zwanghafte Ordentlichkeit *f*, Pedanterie *f*

orderly ordentlich, geregelt

ordinal Ordnungs–, Ordinal–

ordinary ordentlich, gewöhnlich, regelmäßig, üblich

ordinate Ordinate *f*

orectic orektisch, konativ, willensmäßig, gefühlsmäßig, affektiv–antriebhaft

Orestes complex Oresteskomplex *m*, Wunsch *m* des Sohnes, die eigene Mutter zu töten

orexis, orexia Orexie *f*, affektive und konative Aspekte *mpl* einer Handlung, Esslust *f*

organ Organ *n* / **~ donation** Organspende *f* / **~–erotic** organerotisch / **~ eroticism** Organlibido *f* / **~ erotism** Organlibido *f* / **~ inferiority** Organminderwertigkeit *f* / **~ libido** Organlibido *f* / **~ neurosis** Organneurose *f* / **~ of copulation** Begattungsorgan *n*, Penis *m* / **~ of Corti** Corti–Organ *n* / **~ of generation** Fortpflanzungsorgan *n* / **~ of hearing** Gehörorgan *n*, Hörorgan *n* / **~s of reproduction** Fortpflanzungsorgane *npl* / **~ of sight** Sehorgan *n* / **~ of smell** Riechorgan *n* / **~ of speech** Sprechwerkzeug *n* / **~ of taste** Geschmacksorgan *n* / **~ of vision** Sehorgan *n* / **~ pleasure** Organlust *f* / **~ psychosis** Organpsychose *f* / **~ transplantation** Organtransplantation *f* / **acoustic ~** Corti–Organ *n* / **analogous ~** analoges Organ *n* / **copulative ~** Begattungsorgan *n* / **digestive ~s** Verdauungsorgane *npl* / **genital ~** Geschlechtsorgan *n*, Reproduktionsorgan *n* / **gustatory ~** Geschmacksorgan *n* / **homologous ~s** homologe Organe *npl* / **male ~** männliches Glied *n* / **olfactory ~** Geruchsorgan *n* / **perceptive ~s** Wahrnehmungsorgane *npl* / **reproductive ~** Fortpflanzungsorgan *n*, Reproduktionsorgan *n* / **sexual ~** Geschlechtsorgan *n* / **statolithic ~** Makulaorgan *n* / **tactile ~** Tastorgan *n*, Hautsinnesorgan *n* / **vestibular ~** Vestibularapparat *m* / **visual ~** Sehorgan *n* / **vocal ~s** Stimmorgan *n*, Sprechwerkzeuge *npl*

organelle Zellorgan *n*, Organelle *f*

organic organisch, innerlich zusammenhängend, körperlich, somatisch

organicism, organismische Auffasung *f*, Theorie *f* von der organischen Grundlage aller körperlichen und psychischen Störungen, Organizismus *m*

organicity organische Beschaffenheit *f*, organische Grundlage *f*, organische Bedingtheit *f*

organise, organize organisieren, veranstalten

organism Organismus *m* / **cybernetic ~** Regelorganismus *m* / **psychophysiological ~** psychophysiologischer Organismus *m* / **social ~** sozialer Organismus *m* / **unicellular ~** Einzeller *m*, einzelliges Lebewesen *n*

organismic, organismal organismisch

organistic organistisch

organization Organisation *f*, Struktur *f* / **~ centre** Organisator *m*, Organisationszentrum *n* / **~ chart** Organisationsstruktur *f*, Organigramm *n* / **~ development** Organisationsentwicklung *f* / **~ of the ego** Ich–Organisation *f* / **~ of the libido** Organisation *f* der Libido / **autonomous ~** autonome Organisation *f* / **bureaucratic ~** bürokratische Organisation *f* / **centralized ~** zentralisierte Organisation *f* / **foreign ~** Ausländerorganisation *f* / **formal ~** formelle Organisation *f* / **genital ~** Genitalorganisation *f* / **industrial ~** Industrieorganisation *f* / **informal ~** informelle Organisation *f* / **international ~** internationale Organisation *f* / **laryngeal ~** Kehlkopfaufbau *m* / **libidinal~**Organisation *f* der Libido / **logical ~** logische Organisation *f* / **mental ~** geistige Organisation *f* / **non–profit ~** gemeinnützige Organisation *f* / **perceptual ~** Wahrnehmungsorganisation *f* / **professional ~** Berufsverband *m*, Fachverband *m* / **sensory ~** Organisation *f* der Sinneseindrücke / **social ~** soziale Organisation *f*, soziale Struktur *f* / **spatial ~** räumliche Strukturierung *f*, räumliche Organisation *f* / **visceral ~** Struktur *f* der Eingeweide / **visual ~** Organisation *f* des Sehfeldes

organizational Organisations–, organisatorisch

organizator, organizer Organisator *m* / **advance ~** Orientierungszeichen *n*

organogenetic organbildend

organogenic aus einem Organ stammend, aus einem Organ entstanden, somatogen, organogen

organogenesis, organogeny Organbildung *f*, Organogenese *f*

organokinetic Kindesbewegungs–, Glieder bewegend

organoleptic organoleptisch, sinnlich wahrnehmbar

organon wissenschaftliche Methode *f*, Organon *n*, Organ *n*

organophosphate Organophosphat *n*

orgasm Orgasmus *m*, sexueller Höhepunkt *m*, Klimax *m* / **female ~** weiblicher Orgasmus *m* / **male ~** männlicher Orgasmus *m*, Orgasmus *m* des Mannes / **multiple ~** multiple Orgasmen *mpl* / **vaginal ~** Scheidenorgasmus *m*

orgastic orgastisch, Orgasmus betreffend

orgiastic ausschweifend, wild, zügellos

orgone theory Orgon–Theorie *f*

orgy Orgie *f*, Ausschweifung *f*, Orgiasmus *m*

orient, orientate orientieren, informieren, sich orientieren

orientation Orientierung *f*, Ausrichtung *f*, Orientierungssinn *m* / **~ needs** Orientierungsbedürfnisse *npl* / **~ of place** örtliche Orientierung *f* / **~ programme** Einführungsprogramm *n* / **~ reflex** Orientierungsreaktion *f* / **~ response** Orientierungsreaktion *f* / **~ in space** Orientierung *f* im Raum / **~ in time** zeitliche Orientierung *f* / **autopsychic ~** autopsychische Orientierung *f* / **cognitive ~** kognitive Orientierung *f* / **double ~** doppelte Orientierung *f* / **egodystonic sexual ~** egodystone Sexualorientierung *f* / **existential ~** Befindlichkeit *f* / **impaired ~** gestörte Orientierung *f* / **perceptual ~** Orientierung *f* nach der Wahrnehmung, perzeptive Orientierung *f* / **personal ~** persönliche Orientierung *f* / **sexual ~** sexuelle Orientierung *f* / **situational ~** situative Orientierung *f* / **social ~** soziale Orientierung *f* / **spatial ~** räumliche Orientierung *f* / **temporal ~** zeitliche Orientierung *f* / **theoretical ~** theoretische Orientierung *f*

oriented orientiert, informiert

orienting Orientierungs–

origin Ursprung *m*, Nullpunkt *m* / **~ of a nerve** Nervenaustritt *m* / **arbitrary ~** willkürlicher Nullpunkt *m*

original original, ursprünglich, Original–

originality Originalität *f*, Ursprünglichkeit *f*

originate entstehen, herstammen

orphan Waise *f*

orphanage Waisenhaus *n*

orphenadrine Orphenadrin *n*

orthodox orthodox, anerkannt

orthodoxy Orthodoxie *f*, orthodoxe Meinung *f*

orthodromic orthodrom

orthoepy richtige Aussprache *f*

orthogenesis Orthogenese *f*

orthogenetic orthogenetisch

orthogenic heilpädagogisch, korrigierend, gute Entwicklung betreffend

orthogenics Wiedereingliederung *f* emotional gestörter und geistig behinderter Kinder

orthogenital geschlechtlich normal

orthognathism, orthognathy gerade Kieferstellung *f*, Orthognathie *f*

orthognathic, orthognathous mit gerader Kieferstellung, orthognath

orthogonal rechtwinklig, orthogonal

orthogonality Orthogonalität *f*, Rechtwinkligkeit *f*

orthography Rechtschreibung *f*, Orthographie *f*

orthopaedic, orthopedic orthopädisch

orthopaedics, orthopedics, orthopaedy, orthopedy Orthopädie *f*

orthopedagogics Heilpädagogik *f*, Orthopädagogik *f*

orthophoria Ruhelage *f* der Augen, Orthophorie *f*

orthophrenia geistige Gesundheit *f*, Orthophrenie *f*

orthopsychiatry präventive Psychiatrie *f* / **~ for children** vorbeugende Kinderpsychiatrie *f*

orthoptics Augentraining *n*

Orthorater Augentestgerät *n*, Orthorater *m*

orthoscope Orthoskop *n*

orthoscopic normalsichtig

orthoscopy Orthoskopie *f*

orthostatic orthostatisch, aufrecht stehend

orthothymia Orthothymie *f*

os Mund *m*, Knochen *m*

oscillate oszillieren, schwanken, schwingen

oscillation Schwankung *f*, Schwingung *f*, Oszillation *f* / **beating ~** Schwebung *f* / **behavioural ~** Verhaltensschwankung *f*, Schwankung *f* des Reaktionspotenzials / **harmonic ~** harmonische Schwingung *f*, Sinusschwingung *f* / **retinal ~** Netzhautoszillation *f* / **sinoidal ~** Sinusschwingung *f*

oscillator Oszillator *m*, Wellenerzeuger *m*

oscillatory, oscillating oszillierend, schwankend, schwingend

oscillograph Oszillograph *m*

oscillography Oszillographie *f*, Schwingungsmessung *f*

oscillometer Oszillometer *n*, Schwingungsmesser *m*

oscillometry Oszillometrie *f*, Schwingungsmessung *f*

oscilloscope Oszilloskop *n*, Oszillometer *n*

Oseretzky Scale Oseretzky–Test *m*

osmaesthesia, osmesthesia Geruchsempfindlichkeit *f*, Geruchsüberempfindlichkeit *f*

osmatic stark riechend

osmesis Geruchssinn *m*, Geruchsvorgang *m*

osmics Lehre *f* von den Gerüchen

osmoceptor Osmorezeptor *m*

osmology Lehre *f* vom Geruchssinn, Osmologie *f*, Osphresiologie *f*

osmophobia krankhafte Abneigung *f* gegen bestimmte Gerüche, Osmophobie *f*

osmoreceptor, osmoceptor Osmorezeptor *m*, Geruchsrezeptor *m*

osmoregulation Osmoregulation *f*, Regulation *f* des osmotischen Drucks der Zellen

osmosis, osmose Osmose *f*, Konzentrationsausgleich *m* zwischen zwei Flüssigkeiten unterschiedlicher Konzentration über eine semipermeable Membran

osmotaxis Osmotaxis *f*, Bewegungsausrichtung *f* nach den Druckverhältnissen

osmotherapy Osmotherapie *f*, Behandlung *f* durch Einspritzen von Lösungen mit hohem osmotischem Druck

osmotic osmotisch

osphradium Osphradium *n*, Geruchsorgan *n* der im Wasser lebenden Weichtiere

osphresiolagnia geschlechtliche Erregung *f* durch Geruchseinwirkung

osphresiology Lehre *f* vom Geruchssinn, Osphresiologie *f*, Osmologie *f*

osphresiophilia Riechlust *f*, Osphresiophilie *f*

osphresiophiliac Geruchsliebhaber *m*, Duftliebhaber *m*, Riecher *m*

osphresiophobia Angst *f* vor bestimmten Gerüchen

osphresis Geruchssinn *m*

osphretic den Geruchssinn betreffend

osseous knöchern, Knochen–, aus Knochen

ossicle Knöchelchen *n*, Oberknöchelchen *n* / **auditory ~** Gehörknöchelchen *n*

ossification Knochenbildung *f*, Ossifikation *f* / **~ ratio** anatomischer Index *m* / **social ~** Verhaltensrigidität *f*, Inflexibilität *f*

ossify verknöchern, ossifizieren

ostensive anschaulich, scheinbar überzeugend

ostentatious prahlerisch, Prahl–, demonstrativ

osteoacusis, osteoacousia Knochenleitung *f*, Knochenschalleitung *f*

osteoclast Osteoklast *m*

osteoporosis Osteoporose *f*

ostracism gesellschaftliche Ächtung *f*

ostracize gesellschaftlich ächten, aus der Gesehschaft ausschließen

Ostwald colours Ostwald–Farbenkreis *m*, Ostwald–Farbsystem *n*

O technique O–Technik *f*

other sonstige(r), Andere *m,f* / **the ~** der Andere *m*, das Andere *n* / **generalized ~** verallgemeinerter Anderer *m* / **significant ~** bedeutsamer Anderer *m*

otherness Anderssein *n*, Verschiedenheit *f*, Andersgeartetheit *f*

otic Ohr–, Ohren–

otitis Ohrentzündung *f*, Mittelohrentzündung *f* / **~ media** Mittelohrentzündung *f*, Otitis media *f*

otoconia, otoconium Hörstein *m*, Otolith *m*

otocyst Hörbläschen *n*

otolith Hörstein *m*, Otolith *m* / **~ organ** Otolithenmembran *f*

otolithic otolithisch, Hörsteine betreffend

otologist Facharzt *m* für Ohrenkrankheiten, Otologe *m*

otology Ohrenheilkunde *f*, Otologie *f*

otopathy Ohrenleiden *n*

otophone Hörrohr *n*, Hörgerät *n*

otosclerosis Otosklerose *f*

otoscope Ohrspiegel *m*

otospongiosis Otospongiose *f*, Otosklerose *f*

ouija board Alphabettafel *f* für spiritistische Sitzungen

out außen, draußen, hinaus / **~–group** Fremdgruppe *f* / **~–patient** ambulanter Patient *m* / **~–patient department** Poliklinik *f*, Ambulanz *f* / **~–patient treatment** ambulante Behandlung *f*

outbreak Ausbruch *m*, Beginn *m*

outbreeding Paarung *f* außerhalb der eigenen Gruppe, Befruchtung *f* von außen

outburst Ausbruch *m*, Anfall *m* / **~ of temper** Zornesausbruch *m*, Wutanfall *m* / **affective ~** Affektausbruch *m*, Gefühlsausbruch *m*

outcast ausgestoßen, verbannt / Ausgestoßener *m*

outcome Ergebnis *n*, Folge *f* / **psychotherapeutic ~** Ergebnis *n* der Psychotherapie, psychotherapeutischer Erfolg *m*

outer äußerer, externer, Außen– / **~–directed** außen–geleitet

outgoing extravertiert

outgoingness extraversive Haltung *f*, Extraversion *f*

outgrowth Auswuchs *m*

outlet Ausgang *m*, Ausweg *m*, Ausfluss *m*, Absatzmarkt *m*, Absatzmöglichkeit *f*, Verkaufsstelle *f* / **affective ~** affektive Entladung *f*

outline Umriss *m*, Kontur *f* / **facial ~** Gesichtskontur *f*

output Ausstoß *m*, Informationsausgang *m*, Leistung *f*, Output *m*, Ausgang *m*, Ausgangsvariable *f* / **~ data** Ausgabedaten *npl* / **~ equivocation** Empfangsäquivokation *f* / **~ quantity** Ausgangsgröße *f*, Regelgröße *f* / **cardiac ~** Herzminutenvolumen *n*, Herzzeitvolumen *n* / **effective ~** effektive Leistung *f*, tatsächliche Leistung *f*

outreach programme niedrigschwelliges Angebot *n*

outsider Außenseiter *m*, Außenstehender *m*

oval oval

ovaralgia, ovarialgia Eierstockschmerz *m*

O variable organische Variable *f*, organischer Faktor *m*, persönlicher Faktor *m*

ovarian, ovarial ovarial, Eierstock–

ovariectomy, ovariotomy Entfernung *f* des Eierstocks, Ovariektomie *f*

ovariomania Nymphomanie *f*, Mannstollheit *f*

ovary, ovarium Eierstock *m*, Ovarium *n* / **~ disorder** Eierstockerkrankung *f*

over über, vorbei / **~–active** überaktiv / **~–activity** Überfunktion *f*, übermäßige Aktivität *f* / **~–age** über der Altersgrenze liegend, zu alt / **~–anxious** überängstlich / **~–excitability** Übererregbarkeit *f* / **~–excitation** Übererregung *f*, Überreizung *f* / **~–excite** überreizen / **~–exertion** Überanstrengung *f* / **~–fatigue** Übermüdung *f*, Überanstrengung *f* / **~ inclusiveness** Übereinschließung *f* / **~–indulgence** Übermaß *n* / **~–interpretation** Überdeutung *f* / **~–populated** übervölkert / **~ population** Übervölkerung *f* / **~–recruitment** Einstellung *f* einer Personalreserve / **~ talkativeness** Rededrang *m*, Redesucht *f* / **~–the–counter** freiverkäuflich, nicht verschreibungspflichtig

overachievement Mehrleistung *f*, Leistungsüberschuss *m*, über Erwarten gute Schulleistung *f* / **academic ~** über Erwarten gute Schulleistung *f*, Schulleistungsüberschuss *m*

overachiever Mehrleister *m*, über Erwarten guter Schüler *m*, Streber *m*

overall gesamt, Gesamt–

overbearing anmaßend, arrogant, herrisch, autoritär

overcarefulness übermäßige Sorgfalt *f*, peinliche Genauigkeit *f*

overcharge Überbesetzung *f*

overcompensation Überkompensation *f*

overconditioning Überkonditionieren *n*

overconforming unterwürfig, übergehorsam

overcrowding Übervölkerung *f*

overdependent übermäßig abhängig

overdetermination Überdeterminierung *f*, Überdetermination *f*, mehrfache Determination *f*

overdetermined überdeterminiert, mehrfach determiniert, überbestimmt

overeating übermäßiges Essen *n*, Essattacke *f* / **~ associated with other psychological disturbances** Essattacken *fpl* bei sonstigen psychischen Störungen / **compulsive ~** zwanghaftes Überessen *n*, Zwangsessen *n*

overestimation Überbewertung *f*

overexcited überspannt, überreizt

overexclusion zu starke Elimination *f* von (auf einen Reiz) konkurrierenden Reaktionen

overflow Überfluss *m*, Überschwenglichkeit *f* / überfluten, überlaufen

overinclusion zu geringe Elimination *f* von (auf einen Reiz) konkurrierenden Reaktionen

overindividual überindividuell, Gruppen–

overinhibited übermäßig gehemmt, stark gehemmt

overinhibition starke Hemmung *f*

overlap überlagern, überschneiden / Überlagerung *f*, Überschneidung *f*

overlapping Überlagerung *f*, Überschneidung *f* / ~ **element** gemeinsames Element *n* / ~ **factor** gemeinsamer Faktor *m* / ~ **of groups** Gruppenüberschneidung *f* / ~ **of response** Ineinanderlaufen *n* von Aufgaben

overlay Überlagerung *f*

overlearn überlernen

overlearning Überlernen *n*

overload überbelasten, überladen / Überlastung *f*

overmaster überwältigen

overorganization Überorganisation *f*

overpass überstehen, überstreiten / Überführung *f*

overpopulation Übervölkerung *f*

overproduction Überproduktion *f*

overproductivity motorische Unruhe *f*, geistige Unruhe *f*

overprotected übermäßig umsorgt, verwöhnt

overprotection Überbesorgtheit *f*, Verwöhnung *f* / **maternal** ~ übergroße Besorgtheit *f* der Mutter

overprotective überbesorgt, überfürsorglich

overrate überbewerten, überwerten

overreact überreagieren, übermäßig stark reagieren

overreaction Überreaktion *f* / **emotional** ~ übermäßig starke emotionale Reaktion *f*

oversatiation Übersättigung *f*

oversensitive überempfindlich

oversensitivity, oversensitiveness Überempfindlichkeit *f*

oversexed sexbesessen, nymphoman, mit übermäßig starkem Sexualtrieb

overshadow überschatten, in den Schatten stellen

overshoot Umpolarisierung *f*

oversoul Seele *f*, Überseele *f*

overstimulation Überreizung *f*, Reizüberflutung *f*

overstrain Übermüdung *f*, Überanstrengung *f*, Überlastung *f* / überanstrengen, übermüden, überlasten

overstrung überreizt, aufgeregt, enerviert

overt manifest, offen, explizit

overtime Überstunde *f*, Mehrarbeit *f*

overtone Oberton *m* / **harmonic** ~ Oberton *m* / **psychic** ~ Überlagerung *f*

overuse Überbeanspruchung *f*, übermäßiger Gebrauch *m*

overvaluation Überbewertung *f*, Überschätzung *f*

overweight Übergewicht *n*

overwork Arbeitsüberlastung *f*

overwrought überarbeitet, überreizt, erschöpft

oviduct Eileiter *m*, Tube *f*

ovulation Ovulation *f*, Follikelsprung *m* / ~ **inhibitor** Ovulationshemmer *m*

ovule kleines Ei *n*, Ei *n*, Ovulum *n*

ovum Ei *n*, Eizelle *f*, Ovum *n*

own eigene (r, s), persönliche (r, s) / besitzen, zugestehen

ownership Eigentum *n*

oxazepam Oxazepam *n*

oxidase Oxydase *f*

oxidative oxidativ

oxide Oxyd *n* / **nitrous** ~ Lachgas *n*

oximetry Oxymetrie *f*, Sauerstoffbestimmung *f* des arteriellen Blutes

oxyaesthesia, oxyesthesia gesteigerte Gefühlsempfindung *f*

oxycephalous spitzköpfig

oxycephaly Spitzschädel *m*, Oxyzephalie *f*

oxygen Sauerstoff *m* / ~ **capacity** Sauerstoffbindungskapazität *f*, Sauerstoffaufnahmekapazität *f*

oxygenation Verbindung *f* mit Sauerstoff, Oxydation *f*, Sättigung *f* mit Sauerstoff, Oxygenierung *f*

oxygeusia ungewöhnlich scharfer Geschmackssinn *m*, überfeines Geschmacksempfinden *n*

oxyhemoglobin Oxyhämoglobin *n*

oxyopia übernormale Sehschärfe *f*

oxyopter Sehschärfeneinheit *f*

oxyosmia, oxyosphresia überfeiner Geruchssinn *m*

oxyphonia Schrillheit *f* der Stimme, Oxyphonie *f*

oxytocin Oxytozin *n*, Hypophysenhinterlappenhormon *n*

ozostomia übler Mundgeruch *m*

P

pabulum Nahrung *f* / **mental ~** geistige Nahrung *f*

pace Gang *m*, Schritt *m*, Tempo *n* / **~ maker** Schrittmacher *m*, Sinusknoten *m* / **artificial ~ maker** Herzschrittmacher *m* / **~ maker cell** Schrittmacherzelle *f* / **~-maker potential** Schrittmacherpotenzial *n* / **personal ~** Eigentempo *n*

pachymeninx harte Hirnhaut *f*, dura mater *f*, Pachymeninx *f*

pacific friedlich

pacification Beruhigung *f*, Befriedung *f*

pacifism Pazifismus *m*

pacifist Pazifist *m* / pazifistisch

pacing Angleichen *n* des Lernens an die individuellen Gegebenheiten

Pacini's corpuscles Pacini–Körperchen *npl*, Vater–Pacini Körperchen *npl*, Corpuscula lamellosa *npl*

packet switching Datenpaketvermittlung *f*, Methode zur Datenübertragung im Internet

paederast Päderast *m*

paederasty Homosexualität *f* mit Knaben, Unzucht *f* mit Kindern, Päderastie *f*

paederosis Sexualvergehen *n* an Kindern

paedication Homosexualität *f* mit Knaben, Unzucht *f* mit Kindern, Päderastie *f*, Unzucht *f* mit Tieren, Sodomie *f*

paedology Pädologie *f*, Lehre *f* vom Kinde

paedophilia Pädophilie *f*, sexuelle Präferenz *f* für Kinder

paedophobia krankhafte Abscheu *f* vor Kindern

paidicatio Homosexualität *f* mit Knaben, Unzucht *f* mit Kindern, Päderastie *f*, Unzucht *f* mit Tieren, Sodomie *f*

paidology Lehre *f* vom Kinde, Pädologie *f*

paidophilia Liebe *f* zu Kindern, Pädophilie *f*

pain Schmerz *m* / **~ asymbolia** Schmerzasymbolie *f* / **~ centre** Schmerzzentrum *n* / **~-control system** Schmerzkontrollsystem *n* / **~-craving** Freude *f* am Schmerz / **~ disorder** Schmerzstörung *f* / **~ disorder associated with a general medical condition** Schmerzstörung *f* in Verbindung mit medizinischen Krankheitsfaktoren / **~ disorder associated with psychological factors** Schmerzstörung *f* in Verbindung mit psychischen Faktoren / **~ disorder associated with both psychological factors and a general medical factor** Schmerzstörung *f* in Verbindung mit sowohl psychischen Faktoren wie einem medizinischen Krankheitsfaktor / **persistent somatoform ~ disorder** anhaltende somatoforme Schmerzstörung *f* / **psychogenic ~ disorder** psychogenes Schmerzsyndrom *n* / **~ inhibition** Schmerzhemmung *f* / **~ intensity** Schmerzintensität *f* / **~ killer** Analgetikum *n*, Schmerzmittel *n* / **~ management** Schmerzmangement *n* / **~ measurement** Schmerzmessung *f* / **~ perception** Schmerzwahrnehmung *f* / **~ point** Schmerzpunkt *m* / **~ principle** Unlustprinzip *n* / **~ receptor** Schmerzrezeptor *m* / **~-relieving** schmerzstillend / **~ sensation** Schmerzempfindung *f* / **~ sense** Schmerzsinn *m* / **~-sensitive** schmerzempfindlich / **~ spot** Schmerzpunkt *m* / **~ therapy** Schmerztherapie *f* / **~ threshold** Schmerzschwelle *f*, Schmerzgrenze *f* / **~ tolerance** Schmerztoleranz *f* / **~-tolerance threshold** Schmerztoleranzschwelle *f* / **acute ~** akuter Schmerz *m* / **chronic ~** chronischer Schmerz *m* / **deep ~** Tiefenschmerz *m* / **facial ~** Gesichtsschmerz *m* / **functional ~** funktionelle Schmerzen *mpl* / **growing ~s** Wachstumsschmerzen *mpl* / **irradiating ~** Ausstrahlungsschmerz *m* / **myofascial ~** myofaszialer Schmerz *m* / **neuralgic ~** neuralgischer Schmerz *m*, Neuralgie *f* / **primal ~** Urschmerz *m* / **projected ~** projizierter Schmerz *m* / **psychic ~** psychischer Schmerz *m* / **psychogenic ~** psychogener Schmerz *m*, hysterischer Schmerz *m* / **referred ~** Ausstrahlungsschmerz *m*, übertragener Schmerz *m* / **sharp ~** heftiger Schmerz *m* / **somatic ~** somatischer Schmerz *m* / **superficial ~** Oberflächenschmerz *m* / **sympathetic ~** Sympathikusschmerz *m* / **visceral ~** viszeraler Schmerz *m* / **thalamic ~** Thalamusschmerz *m* / **traumatic ~** Wundschmerz *m*

painful schmerzhaft, schmerzend, mühevoll, quälend

painless schmerzlos

painstaking Sorgfalt *f* / sorgfältig, gewissenhaft, arbeitsam

painting Malerei *f*

pair Paar *n* / **~ of opposites** Gegensatzpaar *n* / **matched ~s** Vergleichspaare *npl*

paired Paar–

pairing Paarung *f*, Begattung *f*, Zuordnung *f* / **~ of chromosomes** Chromosomenpaarung *f* / **~–time** Paarungszeit *f*, Balz *f*

palaeoencephalon Urhirn *n*, Althirn *n*, Stammhirn *n*

palaeopallium, paleopallium Palaeokortex *m*, phylogenetisch ältester Teil *m* des Cortex cerebri

palatability Schmackhaftigkeit *f*

palatable schmackhaft

palate Gaumen *m*

pale bleich, blass / erbleichen, blass werden

paleencephalon Paläencephalon *n*, Urhirn *n*, Althirn *n*, Stammhirn *n*

paleoatavistic paläoatavistisch

paleocortex Paläocortex *m*

paleoneurology Paläoneurologie *f*

paleontological paläontologisch

paleontology Paläontologie *f*

paleopathology Paläopathologie *f*

paleopsychic paläopsychisch, primitive Züge des Seelenlebens betreffend

paleopsychology Paläopsychologie *f*

palikinesis, palikinesia Palikinese *f*, unfreiwilliges Wiederholen *n* bestimmter Bewegungen

palilalia stereotypes Wiederholen *n* von Worten und Sätzen, Palilalie *f*

palilexia Palilexie *f*

palingenesis Palingenese *f*, Palingenesis *f*, Wiederholung *f* phylogenetischer Stufen in der Ontogenie, Seelenwanderung *f*

palingenetic palingenetisch

palingraphia Spiegelschrift *f*

palinlexia Rückwärtslesen *n*

palinmnesis Erinnerung *f* vergangener Ereignisse, Wiedererinnerung *f* an vergessene Vorgänge, Palinmnese *f*

palinopsia Palinopsie *f*

palinphrasia, paliphrasia stereotypes Wiederholen *n* von Worten und Sätzen, Palilalie *f*

paliphemia Paliphemie *f*

palipraxia Palipraxie *f*

pallaesthesia, pallesthesia Pallästhesie *f*, Vibrationsempfindung *f*, Vibrationsgefühl *n*, Vibrationssinn *m*

palliative lindernd

pallidum Pallidum *n*

pallium Pallium *n*, Gehirnmantel *m*, Gehirnrinde *f*

pallor große Blässe *f*, blasses Aussehen *n*

palm Handfläche *f*, Handinnenfläche *f*, Handteller *m*

palmaesthesis, palmesthesis, palmaesthesia, palmesthesia Pallästhesie *f*, Vibrationsempfindung *f*, Vibrationsgefühl *n*, Vibrationssinn *m*

palmanaesthesia, palmanesthesia fehlende Vibrationsempfindung *f*

palmar Handflächen–, palmar

palmistry Handlesekunst *f*, Handwahrsagerei *f*, Chiromantik *f*

palmospasm Schüttelkrampf *m*, Zitterkrampf *m*

palp, palpate betasten, befühlen, abtasten

palpable fühlbar, tastbar, greifbar

palpation Betasten *n*, Befühlen *n*, Palpieren *n*

palpebral Augenlid–, palpebral

palpitation Herzklopfen *n*, Palpitation *f* / **nervous ~** unruhiges Herzklopfen *n*, Herzunruhe *f*

palsy Lähmung *f*, Paralyse *f* / **cerebral ~** Gehirnlähmung *f*, zerebrale Lähmung *f*, Zerebralparese *f* / **progressive supranuclear ~** progressive supranukleäre Lähmung *f* / **psychic ~** Seelenlähmung *f* / **shaking ~** Schüttellähmung *f* / **wasting ~** progressive Muskelatrophie *f*

paltry armselig, erbärmlich

pamper verwöhnen

pampered verwöhnt, verzogen

pampering Verwöhnung *f*

panasthenia Neurasthenie *f*

pancreas Pankreas *n*, Bauchspeicheldrüse *f*

pandemonium Reich *n* der bösen Geister, Hölle *f*, Pandämonium *n*

pandiculation Sichräkeln *n*, Bewegung *f* des Sichreckens

Pandy's test Pandy–Probe *f*, Pandy–Reaktion *f*, Pandy–Test *m*

panel Panel *n*, Liste *f* von Versuchspersonen, feste Stichprobe *f* für Befragungen, Testgruppe *f* / **~ design** Plan *m* für eine Paneluntersuchung *f*, Panelversuchsplan *m* / **~ discussion** öffentliche Podiumsdiskussion *f*, Gruppengespräch *n* / **~ meeting** Zusammenkunft *f* gewisser Spezialisten / **~ method** Panelmethode *f*, Paneltechnik *f* / **~ study** Paneluntersuchung *f*, Panelbefragung *f* / **~ technique** Paneltechnik *f*

pang stechender Schmerz. *m*, qualvolle Angst *f* / **~s of conscience** Gewissensbisse *mpl* / **~s of death** Todesangst *f*

pangen Gemmula *f*, Keim *m*

panglossia krankhafte Schwatzsucht *f*

panic Panik *f*, Schrecken *m*, Bestürzung *f* / panisch, wild / in Panik geraten / **~ attack** Panikattacke *f* / **~ disorder** Panikstörung *f*, Paniksyndrom *n* / **~ disorder with (without) agoraphobia** Panikstörung *f* mit (ohne) Agoraphobie / **~–like** panikartig / **~ reaction** Panikreaktion *f* / **homosexual ~** homosexuelle Panik *f*

panophobia, panphobia Furcht *f* vor allen Dingen, Panphobie *f*, Pantophobie *f*

panphagia krankhafte Sucht *f* alles Vorhandene aufzuessen

panpsychism Panpsychismus *m*

pansexualism Pansexualismus *m*

pantalgia Schmerzen *mpl* im ganzen Körper, Panalgie *f*

pantheism Pantheismus *m*

pantheist Pantheist *m*

panting Keuchen *n*, Kurzatmigkeit *f*, Atemnot *f*

pantophobia Furcht *f* vor allen Dingen, Panphobie *f*, Pantophobie *f*

Panum| effect Panum'sches Phänomen *n* / **~ phenomenon** Panum'sches Phänomen *n*

papaverine Papaverin *n*

paper Papier *n*, Abhandlung *f*, Vortrag *m* / **~–and–pencil test** Papier–Bleistift–Test *m*, schriftlicher Test *m*, Paper–Pencil–Test *m* / **sensitive ~** lichtempfindliches Papier *n* / **sensitized ~** lichtempfindliches Papier *n*

papilla Papille *f*, warzenartige Erhebung *f* / **~ of the tongue** Zungenpapille *f* / **acoustic ~** Corti–Organ *n* / **circumvallate ~** Papilla circumvallata *f* der Zunge / **filiform ~** Fadenpapille *f* der Zunge / **foliate ~** Papilla foliata *f*, blätterförmige Zungenpapille *f* / **fungiform ~** pilzförmige Zungenpapille *f* / **gustatory ~** Geschmacksknospe *f* / **lingual ~** Zungenpapille *f* / **nervous ~** Nervenendpapille *f* / **optic ~** Sehnervenpapille *f*, blinder Fleck *m*, Mariotte–Fleck *m* / **vallate ~** Wallpapille *f*

papillary papillenförmig, Papillar–, warzenartig

parabiosis Parabiose *f*, operative Vereinigung *f* zweier Lebewesen, Reizleitungsblock *m*

parabiotic parabiotisch, in Parabiose lebend, durch Leitungsblock gehemmt

parablepsis, parablepsia Sehstörung *f*, falsches Sehen *n*

parabola Parabel *f*

parabulia krankhafte Willensrichtung *f*, Parabulie *f*, Perversion *f* der Willensrichtung

paracentral in der Nähe des Zentrums liegend, zentrumnahe

paracerebellar neben dem Kleinhirn liegend

parachlorophenylalanine Parachlorphenylalanin *n*

parachromatism, parachromatoblepsia gestörtes Farbempfinden *n*, Parachromatismus *m*

parachromatopsia, parachromopsia partielle Farbenblindheit *f*, Dyschromatopsie *f*

paracinesis Koordinationsstörung *f*, Parakinese *f*, verkehrte, unregelmäßige Bewegungen *fpl*

paracrine parakrin

paracusia, paracusis akustische Fehlwahrnehmung *f*, Fehlhören *n*, Parakusis *f*

paradic normal verteilt, entsprechend den Beispielen verteilt

paradigm Paradigma *n*, Muster *n*, Beispiel *n*

paradigmatic paradigmatisch

paradox Widerspruch *m*, Paradox *n*, Paradoxon *n*

paradoxia paradoxer Zustand *m*, Paradoxie *f* / **~ sexualis** Paradoxia sexualis *f*, präpubertäre Geschlechtswünsche *mpl*, sexuelle Begierde *f* im Greisenalter

paradoxial paradox

paraepilepsy leichte Form *f* einer Epilepsie

paraesthesia Hautkribbeln *n*, Sensibilitätsstörung *f*, Parästhesie *f*

paraganglion Paraganglion *n*

paragenital ohne Zeugungsabsicht, paragenital

parageusia, paragetisis Geschmacksstörung *f*, Geschmackshalluzination *f*, Parageusie *f*

parageusic Geschmacksstörung betreffend

paragnosia außersinnliche Wahrnehmung *f*, Hellsehen *n*, Paragnosie *f*

paragrammatism Paragrammatismus *m*, Sprache *f* mit grammatischen oder syntaktischen Störungen

paragrammatize Buchstaben vertauschen

paragraphia Paragraphie *f*, Schreibstörung *f* gekennzeichnet durch Verwendung falscher Wörter oder Buchstaben

parakinesis, parakinesia Koordinationsstörung *f*, Parakinese *f*, verkehrte, unregelmäßige Bewegungen *fpl*

parakinetic parakinetisch, in der Koordination gestört

paralalia Lautverwechslung *f*, Paralalie *f*

paralambdacism Paralambdazismus *m*, Unfähigkeit *f* das „l" auszusprechen

paralanguage Paralinguistik *f*, Wissenschaft *f* von den vokalen Begleitphänomenen der Sprache

paraldehyde Paraldehyd *n*

paralexia Lesestörung *f*, Wortverwechslung *f* beim Lesen, Paralexie *f*, Dyslexie *f*

paralgesia Störung *f* der Schmerzempfindung, schmerzhafte Parästhesie *f*, Paralgesie *f*

paralipophobia Furcht *f* Verantwortlichkeiten zu vernachlässigen, Paralipophobie *f*, Furcht *f* durch das Unterlassen von Handlungen andere Personen in Gefahr zu bringen

parallactic parallaktisch

parallax Parallaxe *f*, parallaktische Verschiebung *f* / ~ **effect** Parallaxeneffekt *m* / ~ **threshold** Parallaxendifferenz *f* / **binocular** ~ binokulare Parallaxe *f*, Konvergenzwinkel *m* / **monocular** ~ monokulare Parallaxe *f*

parallel parallel, Parallel–, entsprechend / Parallele *f*, parallele Linie *f*

parallelism Parallelismus *m*, parallel verlaufende Entwicklung *f* / **cultural** ~ kultureller Parallelismus *m*, parallel verlaufende kulturelle Entwicklung *f* / **psychoneural** ~ psychophysischer Parallelismus *m* / **psychophysical** ~ psychophysischer Parallelismus *m*

parallelogram Parallelogramm *n*

paralog sinnloses zweisilbiges Wort *n*

paralogia Vorbeireden *n*, Paralogie *f* / **thematic** ~ Vorbeireden *n* am Thema

paralogism Fehlschluss *m*, Trugschluss *m*

paralyse, paralyze lähmen, paralysieren

paralysis Lähmung *f*, Paralyse *f* / ~ **agitans** Schüttellähmung *f*, Parkinson–Krankheit *f* / ~ **of the conjugate** Blicklähmung *f* / ~ **of ocular movement** Blicklähmung *f* / **acute sensory** ~ akute Gefühlslähmung *f* / **alcoholic** ~ Alkoholparese *f* / **ambiguo–accessorius–hypoglossal** ~ Jackson–Lähmung *f*, Jackson–Syndrom *n* / **central** ~ zentralbedingte Lähmung *f* / **cerebral** ~ Gehirnlähmung *f* / **complete** ~ vollständige Lähmung *f* / **conjugate** ~ Blicklähmung *f* / **cortical** ~ Rindenlähmung *f* / **facial** ~ Fazialisparese *f*, Gesichtslähmung *f* / **flaccid** ~ schlaffe Lähmung *f* / **functional** ~ hysterische Lähmung *f* / **general** ~ paralytische Demenz *f* / **general** ~ **of the insane** progressive Paralyse *f* / **hysterical** ~ hysterische Lähmung *f*, psychogene Lähmung *f* / **infantile** ~ Kinderlähmung *f* / **juvenile** ~ juvenile Paralyse *f* / **mixed** ~ sensible und motorische Lähmung *f* / **motor** ~ motorische Lähmung *f* / **occupational** ~ Beschäftigungslähmung *f*, berufsbedingte Lähmung *f* / **partial** ~ Teillähmung *f*, partielle Lähmung *f* / **phonetic** ~ Stimmbandlähmung *f* / **progressive** ~ progressive Paralyse *f* / **psychic** ~ Seelenlähmung *f* / **sensomotor** ~ motorische und sensible Lähmung *f* / **sensory** ~ Gefühlsverlust *m* / **spastic** ~ spastische Lähmung *f* / **spastic spinal** ~ spastische Spinalparalyse *f* / **vasomotor** ~ Vasomotorenlähmung *f*

paralytic, paralytical gelähmt, paralytisch / Gelähmter *m*, Paralytiker *m*

parameter Parameter *m*, Kennziffer *f* / ~**s of a distribution** Charakteristika *npl* einer Verteilung / **temporal** ~ Zeitparameter *m*

parametric parametrisch

paramimia Paramimie *f*, Missverhältnis *n* zwischen Gefühlsausdruck und Gefühlslage

paramnesia Erinnerungstäuschung *f*, Pseudoerinnerung *f*, Bekanntheitstäuschung *f*, Paramnesie *f*

paramusia musikalische Aphasie *f*

paraneural nervennah, um den Nerven herumgelegen, paraneural

paranoia Paranoia *f*, Wahn *m*, Wahnvorstellung *f* / ~ **with delusions of jealousy** Eifersuchtswahn *m* / **alcoholic** ~ Alkoholwahn *m* / **climacteric** ~ klimakterische Psychose *f* / **expansive** ~ Expansivparanoia *f* / **involutional** ~ Involutionsparanoia *f* / **litigious** ~ Streitsucht *f*, Prozesssucht *f* / **querulous** ~ Querulantenwahn *m*

paranoiac, paranoic Paranoiker *m* / paranoisch / **litigious** ~ Querulantenwahn *m*, expansive paranoische Reaktion *f*, Kampfparanoia *f*

paranoid paranoisch, paranoid

paranomia Paranomie *f*, Namensaphasie *f*

paranormal paranormal, außerhalb des normal Erklärbaren, okkult

paranosic den primären Krankheitsgewinn betreffend

paranosis primärer Krankheitsgewinn *m*

parapathia, parapathy Parapathie *f*, Sekundärleiden *n*, Neurose *f*

parapathic parapathisch, neurotisch

paraphasia Wortverwechslung *f*, Paraphasie *f*, Paraphrasie *f*, Sprachstörung *f* / **literal ~** Lautverwechslung *f*, literale Paraphasie *f* / **verbal ~** semantische Paraphasie *f*, Wortamnesie *f*, verbale Paraphasie *f*

paraphasic paraphasisch, Wortverwechslungen betreffend

paraphemia Sprachstörung *f*, Paraphrasie *f*, Paraphemie *f*

paraphia Tastsinnanomalie *f*

paraphilia sexuelle Perversion *f*, sexuelle Anomalie *f* / **atypical ~** atypische Paraphilie *f*

paraphiliac sexuell Perverse *m,f* Paraphile *m,f* / parahil

paraphonia Stimmstörung *f*, Überschnappen *n* der Stimme, Paraphonie *f*

paraphora leichte Geistesstörung *f*

paraphrasia Wortverwechslung *f*, Sprachstörung *f*, Paraphrasie *f*, Paraphasie *f*

paraphrenia Paraphrenie *f*, paranoide Entwicklungspsychose *f*

paraphrenic paraphrenisch, Paraphrenie betreffend

paraplectic, paraplegic paraplegisch / Querschnittsgelähmte *m,f*

paraplegia Paraplegie *f*, Querschnittslähmung *f*, doppelseitige Lähmung *f* / **hysterical ~** Pseudoparaplegie *f*

parapraxia, parapraxis Fehlleistung *f*, Fehlhandlung *f*, Parapraxie *f*

parapsychic parapsychisch

parapsychics Parapsychologie *f*, Metapsychik *f*, Metapsychologie *f*

parapsychology Parapsychologie *f*

parapsychosis Denkstörung *f*

pararhotacism Pararhotazismus *m*, Unfähigkeit *f* das „r" korrekt auszusprechen

pararthria Störung *f* der Aussprache, Dysarthrie *f*, Pararthrie *f*

parasagittal parasagittal, neben der Pfeilnaht gelegen

parasexuality sexuelle Perversion *f*, sexuellie Anomalie *f*, Parasexualität *f*

parasigmatism Unfähigkeit *f* Zischlaute richtig auszusprechen, Parasigmatismus *m*

parasite Parasit *m*, Schmarotzer *m*

parasitic parasitär, schmarotzend

parasitism Parasitismus *m*, Schmarotzertum *n*

parasitology Parasitologief, Parasitenkunde *f*

parasitophobia krankhafte Angst *f* vor Parasiten, Parasitophobie *f*

parasympathetic parasympathisch

parasympatholytic parasympatholytisch, den Parasympathikus dämpfend / Parasympatholytikum *n*

parasympathomimetic parasympathomimetisch / Parasympathomimetikum *n*

parasympathicotonia Parasympathikotonie *f*, Parasymphatotonie *f*, Vagotonie *f*

parataxic, paratactic parataxisch

parataxis Parataxie *f*, Verzerrung *f* zwischenmenschlicher Beziehungen

parathormone Nebenschilddrüsenhormon *n*, Parathormon *n*

parathymia Parathymie *f*, Gefühlsstörung *f*, Gefühlsverkehrung *f*

parathyroid Nebenschilddrüse *f*, Epithelkörperchen *n*, Parathyreoidea *f* / neben der Schilddrüse liegend, parathyreoid

paratonia Verspannung *f* willkürlicher Muskeln

paratype Umwelteinflüsse *mpl* während der Entwicklung, Paratypus *m*

paratypic, paratypical atypisch, vom Typ abweichend, Umwelteinflüsse betreffend

parencephalia angeborener Gehirndefekt *m*

parencephalon Kleinhirn *n*

parencephalous hirngeschädigt seit der Geburt

parent Elternteil *m*, Vater *m*, Mutter *f* / **~s** Eltern pl, Vorfahren pl / **~ attitude** Elterneinstellung *f* / **~–child communication** Eltern–Kind–Kommunikation *f* / **~–child relational problem** Eltern–Kind–Problem *n* / **~–child relationship** Eltern–Kind–Beziehung *f* / **~ educational background** Ausbildung *f* der Eltern, Bildungsstand *m* der Eltern / **~ image** Elternbild *n*, Elternimago *f* / **~–run nursery** Kinderladen *m* / **~–school relationship** Eltern–Schule–Beziehung *f* / **~ surrogate** Elternersatz *m* / **~ training** Elterntraining *n* / **~ variance** Herkunftsvarianz *f* / **adoptive ~s** Adoptiveltern pl / **bad ~s** Rabeneltern *pl*, schlechte Eltern *pl* / **combined ~ figure** vereinigte Elternimago *f* / **combined ~s** beide Eltern pl / **expectant ~s** werdende Eltern *pl* / **homosexual ~s** homosexuelle Eltern *pl* / **lesbian ~s** lesbische Eltern *pl*, homosexuelle Eltern *pl* / **single ~** Alleinerzieher *m*

parentage Elternschaft *f*, Vaterschaft *f*, Herkunft *f*, Abstammung *f*

parental elterlich

parentalism übertriebene Dominanz *f* der Eltern über die Kinder, Parentalismus *m*

parenthood Elternschaft *f*, Mutterschaft *f*, Vaterschaft *f* / **~ status** Elternschaft *f*, Elternstatus *m* / **delayed ~** Elternschaft *f* in höherem Lebensalter / **planned ~** Geburtenplanung *f*, Geburtenbeschränkung *f* / **voluntary ~** Geburtenbeschränkung *f*, gewollte Elternschaft *f*

parergasia Parergasie *f*, verkehrte Willenshandlung *f* durch Fehllenkung von Impulsen

parergastic parergastisch, verkehrte Willenshandlungen betreffend

paresis Lähmung *f*, Parese *f* / **~ of the facial nerve** Fazialisparese *f*, Gesichtslähmung *f* / **alcoholic ~** Alkoholparese *f* / **general ~** progressive Paralyse *f* / **juvenile ~** Parese *f* infolge angeborener Syphilis / **occupational ~** Beschäftigungslähmung *f* / **ocular ~** Augenlähmung *f* / **painful ~** schmerzhafte Lähmung *f*

paresthesia Hautkribbeln *n*, Sensibilitätsstörung *f*, Parästhesie *f*

paresthetic parästhetisch

paretic paretisch, gelähmt

pareunia Geschlechtsverkehr *m*, Zeugungsakt *m*, Koitus *m*

parietal parietal, zum Scheitelbein gehörig

parietofrontal Stirnbein und Scheitelbein betreffend, frontoparietal

parieto–occipital Scheitelbein und Hinterhauptbein betreffend, okzipitoparietal

parietotemporal Scheitelbein und Schläfenbein betreffend, temporoparietal

Parinaud|–von Kries theory Parinaud–von–Kries Theorie *f* / **~'s theory** Parinaud–Theorie *f*

parity Gleichheit *f*, Gleichberechtigung *f*, Parität *f* / **~ bit** Paritätsbit *n*, Prüfbit *n*

Parkinson's| disease Parkinson–Krankheit *f*, Paralysis agitans *f*, Schüttellähmung *f* / **~ facies** Maskengesicht *n* / **~ mask** Maskengesicht *n* / **~ syndrome** Parkinson–Syndrom *n*, Parkinsonismus *m*

parkinsonian Parkinson'sche(r, s), Parkinsonismus betreffend / Parkinsonpatient *m*, Parkinsonpatientin *f*

parkinsonism Parkinsonismus *m*, Parkinson–Syndrom *n* / **neuroleptic–induced ~** Pakinsonoid *n*, neuroleptikainduzierter Parkinsonismus *m* / **postencephalitic ~** postenzephalitisches Parkinson–Syndrom *n* / **other drug–induced secondary ~** sonstiger arzneimittelinduzierter sekundärer Parkinsonismus *m* / **secondary ~ due to other external agents** sekundärer Parkinsonismus *m* durch sonstige außere Substanzen

parlance, in common im allgemeinen Sprachgebrauch

parole Bewährung *f*, Bewährungsfrist *f*, bedingte Haftentlassung *f*, Strafaussetzung *f* / **~ officer** Bewährungshelfer *m*

paropsia, paropsis Sehstörung *f*

parorexia krankhaftes Verlangen *n* nach ungewöhnlichen Speisen, anomale Essgelüste *npl*, Parorexie *f*, Pikazismus *m*, Pica–Syndrom *n*

parosmia Geruchstäuschung *f*, Geruchshalluzination *f*, Parosmie *f* Parosphresie *f*

parosmic Geruchstäuschung betreffend

parosphresia, parosphresis Geruchstäuschung *f*, Parosphresie *f*, Parosmie *f*

parotid Ohrspeicheldrüse *f*, Parotis *f*

paroxetine Paroxetin *n*

paroxysm Paroxysmus *m*, krampfartiger Anfall *m*

paroxysmal paroxysmal, krampfartig

parricide Vatermörder *m*, Muttermörder *m*, Elternmörder *m* / Vatermord *m*, Muttermord *m*, Elternmord *m*

parsimony Sparsamkeit *f*

part Teil *m*, Anteil *m* / **~ instinct** Partialtrieb *m*, Triebkomponente *f* / **~ learning** Lernen *n* in Teilen / **~ method of learning** Methode *f* des verteilten Lernens / **~–object** Teilobjekt *n*, Partialobjekt *n* / **~–whole** vom Teil zum Ganzen / **~–whole relation** Beziehung *f* zwischen dem Ganzen und seinen Teilen / **cortical ~** Rindensubstanz *f* / **privy ~s** Geschlechtsteile *npl* / **vital ~** lebenswichtiger Teil *m*

parthenogenesis, parthogenesis Jungfernzeugung *f*, Parthogenese *f*

parthenogenetic parthenogenetisch

parthenophobia krankhafte Angst *f* vor Mädchen, Abneigung *f* gegen junge Mädchen

partial Teil–, teilweise, partial, partiell, Partial– / **lower ~** Fundamentalton *m*, unterer Teilton *m*

partialization Differenzierung *f*

participant Teilnehmer *m* / **~ observation** Beobachtung *f* unter eigener Beteiligung / **~ observer** teilnehmender Beobachter *m*

participation Teilnahme *f*, Beteiligung *f*, Mitwirkung *f*, Mitbestimmung *f*, Partizipation *f* / **~ schedule** Teilnehmer–Beobachtungsliste *f* / **athletic ~** sportliche Aktivität *f* / **mystical ~** Partizipation *f*, „participation mystique“ *f* / **political ~** politische Partizipation *f*

particular besondere(r, s), Sonder–, speziell

particularism Partikularismus *m*

partile Partil *n*, Bereich *m* einer Verteilung

partition Teilung *f*, Zerteilung *f* / **~ measure** Messung *f* eines definierten Teilbereichs

partitive Teil–, Partial–, partitiv

partner Partner *m* / **~ abuse** Partnermisshandlung *f* / **~ choice** Partnerwahl *f* / **~ relational problem** Partnerschaftsproblem *n*

partnership Partnerschaft *f*, Vereinigung *f*

parturition Geburt *f*, Geburtsvorgang *m*, Gebären *n*

party Partei *f* / **political ~** politische Partei *f*

Pascal's triangle Pascal'sches Dreieck *n*

passion Leidenschaft *f*, Sucht *f* / **uncontrolled ~s** unkontrollierte Leidenschaften *fpl*

passive passiv, teilnahmslos

passiveness Passivität *f*, Teilnahmslosigkeit *f*

passivism passive Homosexualität *f*, passive Rolle *f* eines Homosexuellen, Passivismus *m*

passivist passiver Homosexueller *m*

passivity Passivität *f*, Teilnahmslosigkeit *f*, Untätigkeit *f* / **~ need** Entspannungsbedürfnis *n* / **~ phenomena** geistige Automatismen *mpl*, Zwangsbewegungen *fpl*

past vergangen, vorüber / **the ~** die Vergangenheit *f* / **~–pointing** Vorbeizeigen *n*, Dahinterzeigen *n* mit dem Finger

pastoral pastoral, Pastoral–, seelsorgerisch

patella Kniescheibe *f*, Patella *f*

patellar Patellar–, patellar

paternal väterlich, Vater–, väterlicherseits

paternalism Paternalismus *m*, Bevormundung *f* durch Autoritätspersonen

path Bahn *f*, Leitungsbahn *f*, Weg *m*, Pfad *m* / ~ **analysis** Pfadanalyse *f* / ~ **of association** Assoziationsbahn *f* / ~ **of conduction** Leitungsbahn *f* / **afferent** ~ afferente Bahn *f*, sensorische Bahn *f* / **associative** ~ Assoziationsbahn *f* / **auditory** ~ Hörbahn *f* / **conductive** ~ Leitungsbahn *f* / **efferent** ~ efferente Bahn *f*, motorische Bahn *f* / **final common** ~ gemeinsame Endstrecke *f* / **nervous** ~ Nervenbahn *f*

pathernia Gefühlsbetontheit *f*

pathergasia Funktionseinschränkung *f*

pathetic erbärmlich, Mitleid erregend, den Nervus trochlearis betreffend

pathetics pathetische Gefühle *npl*, pathetisches Verhalten *n*, Studium *n* menschlicher Leidenschaften

patheticus Nervus trochlearis *m*, Augenrollnerv *m*

pathic pathisch, leidend, pathologisch

pathogenesis, pathogeny Pathogenese *f*, Entstehungf einer Krankheit

pathogenic, pathogenous, pathogenetic pathogen, krankheitsauslösend

pathognomic, pathognomonic, pathognostic Ausdrucks–, die Ausdruckskunde betreffend, pathognom, pathognomisch, pathognomonisch, für eine Krankheit kennzeichnend

pathognomy Ausdruckskunde *f*, Pathognomik *f*, Symptomenlehre *f*

pathography Krankheitsbeschreibung *f*, Pathographie *f*

pathologic, pathological pathologisch, krankhaft

pathologist Pathologe *m*

pathology Pathologie *f*, Krankheitslehre *f* / ~ **of anxiety** Pathologie *f* der Angst / **constitutional** ~ Konstitutionspathologie *f* / **forensic** ~ gerichtliche Medizin *f* / **functional** ~ Funktionspathologie *f* / **mental** ~ Psychopathologie *f* / **social** ~ Sozialpathologie *f*

pathomimesis, pathomimia, pathomimicry Vortäuschung *f* einer Krankheit, Pathomimie *f*

pathoneurosis krankheitsbegleitende Neurose *f*, Pathoneurose *f*

pathoneurotic pathoneurotisch, krankheitsbegleitende Neurose betreffend

pathophilic pathophil

pathophobia abnorme Furcht *f* vor Krankheiten, Pathophobie *f*

pathopsychology Psychopathologie *f*, Pathopsychologie *f*

pathopsychosis Psychose *f* die auf somatische Funktionen krankheitsauslösend wirkt

pathos Pathos *n*, Leidenschaftlichkeit *f*

pathway Bahn *f*, Nervenbahn *f*, Leitungsbahn *f* / ~**s of associations** Assoziationsbahnen *fpl*, Verbindungsbahnen *fpl* / ~**s of connections** Verbindungsbahnen *fpl*, Assoziationsbahnen *fpl* / **afferent** ~ afferente Nervenbahn *f* / **descending** ~ motorische Bahn *f* / **efferent** ~ efferente Nervenbahn *f* / **motor** ~ motorische Bahn *f* / **neural** ~ Nervenbahn *f* / **optic** ~ Sehbahn *f* / **visual** ~ Sehbahn *f*

patience Geduld *f*, Nachsicht *f*, Ausdauer *f*

patient Kranker *m*, Patient *m* / ~ **abuse** Patientenmissbrauch *m* / ~ **care** Patientenversorgung *f* / ~ **history** Krankengeschichte *f* / ~ **seclusion** Patientenisolierung *f* / ~ **selection** Patientenauswahl *f* / ~**–therapist interaction** Interaktion *f* zwischen Patient und Therapeut / ~**–therapist sexual relations** sexuelle Beziehungen *fpl* zu Patienten / ~ **violence** Patientengewaltätigkeit *f* / **geriatric** ~ geriatrischer Patient *m*, Alterspatient *m* / **hospitalised** ~ Krankenhauspatient *m*, stationärer Patient *m* / **medical** ~ medizinischer Patient *m* / **mental** ~ Geisteskranker *m* / **obsessive** ~ Zwangspsychotiker *m* / **physically ill** ~ körperlich kranker

Patient *m* / **psychiatric ~** psychiatrischer Patient *m* / **surgical ~** chirurgischer Patient *m*, Patient *m* auf einer chirurgischen Station / **terminally ill ~** unheilbar kranker Patient *m*, todkranker Patient *m*

patriarchy, patriarchate Patriarchat *m*, Vaterrecht *n*, Vaterherrschaft *f*

patrilineal vaterrechtlich, patriarchalisch, patrilinear

patriliny Vaterrecht *n*, Patriarchat *n*

patriotism Patriotismus *m*, Vaterlandsliebe *f*

patronage Schutz *m*, Fürsorge *f*, Unterstützung *f*

pattern Muster *n*, Gefüge *n*, Struktur *f*, Anordnung *f*, Konstellation *f*, Konfiguration *f*, Schema *n*, „Pattern" *n*, Gestalt *f* / **~ analysis** multiple Faktorenanalyse *f* / **~ of behaviour** Verhaltensmuster *n*, Verhahensweise *f*, Verhaltensgefüge *n* / **~–case** Musterfall *m* / **~ coherence criterion** strukturelles Kohärenzkriterium *n* / **~ discrimination** Gestaltdiskriminierung *f*, Musterdiskrimination *f* / **~ of leadership** Führungsstil *m* / **~ learning** Lernen *n* von Gestalten / **~ perception** Strukturwahrnehmung *f* / **~ of reinforcement** Verstärkungsplan *m* / **~ similarity** Strukturähnlichkeit *f* / **~ variable** Konfigurationsvariable *f* / **behavioural ~** Verhaltensmuster *n*, Verhaltensgefüge *n*, Verhaltenskonstellation *f* / **constitutional ~** Konstitutionsgefüge *n* / **cultural ~** kulturelles Schema *n* / **dermal ~** Hautstruktur *f* / **dissociative ~** dissoziatves Muster *n* / **eating ~s** Essgewohnheiten *fpl* / **emotional ~** Gefühlsstruktur *f*, emotionelle Struktur *f* / **excitatory ~** Erregungskonstellation *f*, Erregungsmuster *n* / **fixed ~** Erbkoordination *f*, Instinkthandlung *f* / **innate motor ~** angeborene Erbkoordination *f* / **instinctive releasing ~** instinktauslösendes Schema *n* / **motor ~** motorische Gestalt *f* / **neural ~** Nervenstruktur *f*, Nervennetz *n*, Nervengefüge *n* / **perceptual ~** Wahrnehmungskonstellation *f* / **phenomenal ~** erscheinungsmäßige Gegebenheit *f*, Erscheinung *f*, Phänomen *n* / **postural ~** Haltungsstruktur *f* / **psychometric ~** psychometrische Struktur *f* / **sensory ~** Empfindungskonstellation *f* / **total ~** Ganzheitsstruktur *f* / **transgenerational ~** transgenerationales Verhaltensmuster *n*

patternedness Strukturiertheit *f*, Anordnung *f* in Musterform

patterning Strukturieren *n*, Eingruppieren *n*

paucity kleine Zahl *f*, geringe Menge *f*, Mangel *m*

pauper Armer *m*, Unterstützungsempfänger *m*, Sozialhilfeempfänger *m*

pause Pause *f*, Unterbrechung *f* / Pause machen, stoppen, anhalten / **~ group** abgegrenzte Phonemkette *f* / **apnoic ~** apnoische Pause *f*

Pavlovianism Pawlows Theorie *f*

pavor Angst *f* / **~ diurnus** Tagangst *f* / **~ nocturnus** Nachtangst *f*, nächtliches Aufschrecken *n*, Pavor nocturuns *m*

pay–off Belohnung *f* / **~ matrix** Entscheidungsmatrix *f* / **~ schedule** Verstärkerplan *m*

PB| cache besonders schneller Cache–Speicher *m* / **~ words** Liste *f* der phonetisch gleichgewichtigen Wörter

peace Ruhe *f*, Frieden *m* / **~ of mind** psychische Entspannung *f*, seelische Ruhe *f*

peacock blue grünblau

peak Gipfel *m*, Höhepunkt *m*, Spitze *f* / **~ clipping** Auslassen *n* der Sprachteile im hohen Amplitudenbereich / **~ top diagram** Häufigkeitspolygon *n*, Häufigkeitsdiagramm *n*

Pearson| coefficient of correlation Pearson'scher Korrelationskoeffizient *m*, Produkt–Moment–Korrelation *f* / **~'s correlation** Pearson'sche Korrelation *f*, Produkt–Moment–Korrelation *f* / **~ criterion** Pearson–Kriterium *n* / **~ curve** Pearson–Kurve *f*

Pearsonian Pearson–

peccant krankhaft, morbid

peccatophobia krankhafte Furcht *f* zu sündigen

pecking Hacken *n*, Picken *n* / ~ **hierarchy** Hackhierarchie *f* / ~ **order** Hackordnung *f*

peck order Hackordnung *f*

pectoral Brust–, Brustkorb–

peculiarity Eigenheit *f*, Eigentümlichkeit *f*

pedagogic, pedagogical pädagogisch, Erziehungs–, erziehungswissenschaftlich

pedagogue, pedagog Pädagoge *m*, Erzieher *m*, Lehrer *m*, Erziehungswissenschaftler *m*

pedagogy, pedagogics Erziehungswissenschaft *f*, Pädagogik *f* / **curative** ~ Heilpädagogik *f* / **experimental** ~ Schulversuch *m*, experimentelle Pädagogik *f* / **modern**~ moderne Pädagogik *f* / **particular** ~ Sonderpädagogik *f* / **scientific** ~ wissenschaftliche Pädagogik *f* / **therapeutic** ~ Heilpädagogik *f*

pedal Fuß—, die Füße betreffend / Pedal *n*

pedant Pedant *m*, Kleinigkeitskrämer *m*

pedantic pedantisch

pedantry Pedanterie *f*, übersteigerte Ordnungsliebe *f*

pederast Päderast *m*

pederastic päderastisch

pederasty Päderastie *f*, Unzucht *f* mit Knaben

pederosis Päderosis *f*, heterosexuelle Pädophilie *f*, Unzucht *f* mit Kindern des anderen Geschlechts

pedestrian Fußgänger *m* / ~ **accident** Fußgängerunfall *m*

pediatric pädiatrisch, kinderärztlich

pediatrician, pediatrist Kinderarzt *m*, Pädiater *m*

pediatrics, pediatry Kinderheilkunde *f*, Pädiatrie *f*

pedication Homosexualität *f* mit Knaben, Unzucht *f* mit Kindern, Päderastie *f*, Unzucht *f* mit Tieren, Sodomie *f*

pediculophobia krankhafte Furcht *f* vor Läusen, Pedikulophobie *f*

pedigree Stammbaum *m*, Ahnentafel *f* / ~ **studies** genealogische Nachforschungen *fpl*, Familienforschung *f*

pediophobia krankhafte Angst *f* vor Kinder, Pädophobie *f*

pedology Kinderkunde *f*, Pädologie *f*, Paidologie *f*, Lehre *f* vom Kind

pedomorphism Pädomorphismus *m*, Behandlung *f* eines Erwachsenen als Kind, Verhaltensbeschreibung *f* in Kindersprache

pedophilia Pädophilie *f*, sexuelle Liebe *f* zu Kindern

pedophobia krankhafte Angst *f* vor Kinder, Pädophobie *f*

pedopsychiater, pedopsychiatrist Kinderpsychiater *m*

peduncle Stiel *m*, Schenkel *m*, Pedunculus *m* / ~ **of the cerebellum** Kleinhirnstiel *m* / **cerebral** ~ Hirnstiel *m* / **cerebellar** ~ Kleinhirnstiel *m* / **median cerebellar** ~ Brückenschenkel *m*

peduncular stielförmig, den Stiel betreffend, Stiel–

peeper, peeping Tom Voyeur *m* / vorwitzig, neugierig

peer Gefährte *m*, Kollege *m*, Angehöriger *m* der gleichen hierarchischen Stufe, Gleichaltriger *m*, Peer *m* / ~ **counseling** Beratung *f* von Kollegen, Peer–Beratung *f* / ~ **group** Gefährtengruppe *f*, Gruppe *f* Gleichgestellter / ~ **pressure** Bezugsgruppendruck *m* / ~ **rating** Kollegenbeurteilung *f* / ~ **relations** Verhältnis *n* zu Kollegen, Peer–Beziehung *f* / ~ **tutoring** Studienbetreuung *f* durch Studenten, Peer–Unterricht *m*

pegboard Steckbrett *n*

pejorative pejorativ, verschlechternd

pejorism Pessimismus *m*

pellagra Pellagra *f*, Maisesserkrankheit *f*, multiple Avitaminose *f* / ~ **psychosis** Pellagrapsychose *f*

pellet Kügelchen *n*, Pille *f*

pelvis Becken *n*

pemoline Pemolin *n*

penal Straf–, strafbar, strafrechtlich

penalize bestrafen, mit Strafe belegen

penalty Strafe *f*, Geldstrafe *f*

pencil–and–paper test Papier–Bleistift–Test *m*, schriftlicher Test *m*, „Paper–Pencil–Test" *m*

pendulum Pendel *n* / **optical ~** optisches Pendel *n*

penetration Einprägungsgrad *m*, Bekanntheitsgrad *m*, Grad *m* der Benutzung, Eindringung *f*, Durchdringung *f*, Durchbruch *m*

penetrative scharfsinnig, durchdringend

penial, penile Penis–, zum Penis gehörig

peniaphobia Angst *f* vor Armut

penicillin Penicillin *n*

penilingus Genitalkuss *m*, Fellatio *f*

penis Penis *m*, männliches Glied *n* / **~ envy** Penisneid *m*

penitence Reue *f*

penitentiary Straf–, Besserungs– / Strafanstalt *f*, Besserungsanstalt *f*

penological Strafvollzugslehre betreffend

penologist Experte *m* des Strafvollzugs

penology Strafvollzugslehre *f*, Pönologie *f*

pension neurosis Rentenneurose *f*

pentatonic Fünfton–

pentazocine Pentazocin *n*

pentobarbital Pentobarbital *n*

pentose Pentose *f*

pentothal Pentothal *n*, Thiopental *n* / **~ interview** Exploration *f* unter Pentothalgaben

pentylenetetrazol Pentamethylentetrazol *n*

people Volk *n*, Leute *pl*, Menschen *mpl* / **preliterate ~s** Primitivkultur *f*, Kultur *f* ohne Schriftsprache / **sensible ~** vernünftige Leute *pl*, kluge Leute *pl*

peotillomania Pseudomasturbation *f*, kindliches Spiel *n* am Penis, Peotillomanie *f*

pepsin Pepsin *n*

pepsinogen Pepsinogen *n*

peptic Verdauungs–, Magen–, peptisch

peptide Peptid *n* / **~ hormone** Peptidhormon *n* / **gastrointestinal ~** gastrointestinales Peptid *n*

perceive wahrnehmen

percent Prozent *n* / **~ hearing** Hörvermögen *n* in Prozent / **~ hearing loss** Hörverlust *m* in Prozent

percentage Prozentsatz *m* / **~ cumulative distribution** prozentuale Häufigkeitsverteilung *f*, kumulative Prozentverteilung *f* / **~ diagram** Prozentdiagramm *n* / **~ point** Signifikanzniveau *n* ausgedrückt in Prozent / **~ reinforcement** prozentuale Verstärkung, Intervallverstärkung *f* / **~ standard deviation** prozentuale Standardabweichung *f*

percentile Perzentil *n*, Zentil *n*, Hundertstel *n*, Hundertstelwert *m* / **~ band** Perzentilbereich *m* / **~ curve** Perzentilkurve *f*, Prozentrangkurve *f* / **~ graph** Perzentilkurve *f*, Prozentrangkurve *f* / **~ norm** Zentilnorm *f* / **~ range** Zentilrang *m* / **~ rank** Prozentrang *m*, Perzentilwert *m*, Perzentilrang *m* / **~ score** Perzentilwert *m* / **~ scale** Prozentrangskala *f*

percept Wahrnehmung *f*, Wahrnehmungsinhalt *m*

perceptible wahrnehmbar, bemerkbar, merklich

perception Wahrnehmung *f*, Perzeption *f*, Empfindung *f* / **~ of colour** Farbwahrnehmung *f* / **~–consciousness** Wahrnehmungsbewusstsein *n* / **~ deafness** Wahrnehmungstaubheit *f* / **~ of depth** Tiefenwahrnehmung *f*, Tiefenempfindung *f* / **~ disorder** Wahrnehmungsstörung *f* / **~–hallucination** Perzeptionsphantasmen *npl* / **~ illusion** Wahrnehmungstäuschung *f* / **~ of form** Formwahrnehmung *f* / **~ of motion** Bewegungssehen *n* / **~ of movement** Bewegungssehen *n* / **~ set** Wahrnehmungseinstellung *f* / **~ of space** Raumwahrnehmung *f* / **~ of three–dimensional space** plastisches Sehen *n*, dreidimensionale Wahrnehmung *f* / **~**

time Wahrnehmungszeit *f*, Fixationszeit *f* / **auditory ~** Gehörwahrnehmung *f*, auditive Wahrnehmung *f* / **automorphic ~** automorphe Wahrnehmung *f* / **binocular ~** binokulares Sehen *n* / **conscious ~** bewusste Wahrnehmung *f* / **cutaneous ~** Hautempfindung *f* / **delusional ~** schizophrenes Primärerlebnis *n* / **egocentric ~** egozentrische Wahrnehmung *f* / **enriched ~** ausgeschmückte Wahrnehmung *f* / **extrasensory ~** außersinnliche Wahrnehmung *f*, Hellsehen *n*, Telepathie *f* / **gustatory ~** Geschmackswahrnehmung *f* / **haptic ~** Raumwahrnehmung *f* / **impoverished ~** künstlich reizarme Wahrnehmung *f* / **internal ~** innere Wahrnehmung *f* / **interpersonal ~** interpersonale Wahrnehmung *f*, soziale Wahrnehmung *f* / **intersensory ~** Wahrnehmung *f* mit mehreren Sinnesorganen gleichzeitig / **intrapsychic ~** innere Wahrnehmung *f* / **kinaesthetic ~** kinästhetische Wahrnehmung *f* / **literal ~** objektive Wahrnehmung *f*, wahrheitsgetreue Wahrnehmung *f* / **olfactory ~** Geruchswahrnehmung *f* / **physiognomic ~** physiognomische Wahrnehmung *f* / **proprioceptive ~** propriozeptive Wahrnehmung *f* / **reduced ~** reduzierte Wahrnehmung *f* / **selective ~** selektive Wahrnehmung *f* / **sensory ~** Sinnesempfindung *f* / **social ~** soziale Wahrnehmung *f* / **somaesthetic ~** Körperempfinden *n*, somästhetische Wahrnehmung *f* / **spatial ~** Raumwahrnehmung *f*, räumliche Wahrnehmnung *f* / **stereognostic ~** Erkennen *n* von Gegenständen durch Betasten / **stereoscopic ~** Tiefenwahrnehmung *f*, Tiefensehen *n*, räumliche Wahrnehmung *f* / **subconscious ~** unterschwellige Wahrnehmung *f*, unbewusste Wahrnehmung *f* / **subliminal ~** unterschwellige Wahrnehmung *f*, subliminale Wahrnehmung *f* / **tactile ~** taktile Wahrnehmung *f*, Tastwahrnehmung *f* / **tactile–motor ~** taktil–motorische Wahrnehmung *f* / **tactual ~** Tastwahrnehmung *f* / **unconscious ~** unbewusste Wahrnehmung *f* / **visual ~** visuelle Wahrnehmung *f*

perceptional Wahrnehmungs–, Auffassungs–

perceptionism Sensualismus *m*

perceptionist Anhänger *m* des Sensualismus, Sensualist *m*

perceptive wahrnehmend, auffassend, perzeptiv

perceptiveness, perceptivity Wahrnehmungsfähigkeit *f*, Auffassungsvermögen *n*, Einsicht *f*

perceptual Wahrnehmungs–, perzeptiv, wahrnehmend

perceptualization Wahrnehmungsstrukturierung *f*

percipient wahrnehmende Person *f*, Wahrnehmender *m*, Telepath *m*, Empfänger *m*

percussion hammer Perkussionshammer *m*

perfectionism Perfektionismus *m*, Vollkommenheitswahn *m*

perfectionist Perfektionist *m*

performance Ausführung *f*, Verrichtung *f*, Handlung *f*, Leistung *f* / **~ anxiety** Leistungsangst *f*, Angst *f* vor Versagen / **~ appraisal** Leistungsbeurteilung *f*, Leistungsbewertung *f* / **~ box** Versuchskäfig *m* / **~ curve** Leistungskurve *f*, Arbeitskurve *f* / **~ evaluation** Leistungsbeurteilung *f* / **~ scale** Leistungsskala *f* / **~ test** Leistungstest *m*, Geschicklichkeitstest *m* / **~ test of personality** Leistungstest *m* zur Persönlichkeitsmessung / **athletic ~** sportliche Leistung *f* / **long–term ~** Ausdauerleistung *f*, Dauerleistung *f*, Langzeitleistung *f* / **motor ~** motorische Leistung *f*, motorisches Verhalten *n* / **physical ~** physische Leistung *f*, körperliche Leistung *f* / **psychological ~** psychische Leistung *f* / **psychophysical ~** psychophysische Leistung *f* / **sensorimotor ~** sensomotorische Leistung *f*

perfusion Durchblutung *f*, Perfusion *f* / **coronary ~** Koronardurchblutung *f* / **pulmonary ~** Lungenperfusion *f* / **renal ~** Nierendurchblutung *f*

periblepsis Periblepsis *f*

pericardial perikardial, den Herzbeutel betreffend

pericardium Herzbeutel *m*, Perikard *n*

pericaryon, perikaryon der um den Zellkern gelegene Teil *m* der Zelle, Perikaryon *n*

pericerebral um das Gehirn herum gelegen

periganglionic periganglionär, um ein Ganglion herum gelegen

perilymph Labyrinthflüssigkeit *f*, Perilymphe *f*

perimacular um den gelben Fleck herum gelegen

perimeter Gesichtsfeldmesser *m*, Perimeter *n*

perimetry Gesichtsfeldmessung *f*, Perimetrie *f*

perinatal zum Zeitpunkt der Geburt, perinatal

perineural um den Nerv herum gelegen, perineural

perineurium Nervenscheide *f*, Epineurium *n*, Perineurium *n*

period Periode *f*, Zeitabschnitt *m*, Menstruation *f* / ~ **of development** Entwicklungsphase *f* / ~ **of excitement** Erregungsphase *f* / ~ **of puberty** Pubertätszeit *f* / **absolute refractory** ~ absolute Refraktärzeit *f* / **anoestrous** ~ paarungsungünstige Zeit *f* / **childbearing** ~ Fortpflanzungszeit *f* / **climacteric** ~ Wechseljahre *npl*, Klimakterium *n* / **compensatory** ~ kompensatorische Pause *f* / **critical** ~ kritische Phase *f* / **developmental** ~ Entwicklungszeit *f* / **falling–asleep** ~ Einschlafzeit *f* / **hypnagogic** ~ Einschlafzeit *f* / **hypnopompic** ~ Aufwachzeit *f* / **interparoxysmal**~ Zeit *f* zwischen zwei Krampfanfällen / **latent** ~ Latenzzeit *f*, Zeit *f* zwischen Reiz und Reaktion / **monthly** ~ Periode *f*, Menstruation *f* / **natural** ~ natürliche Zeitdauer *f* / **organogenetic** ~ Organbildungszeit *f* / **organokinetic** ~ Periode *f* der Kindsbewegung / **perinatal** ~ Geburtsphase *f*, Geburtsperiode *f* / **postnatal** ~ postnatale Phase *f*, Nachgeburtsperiode *f* / **prenatal** ~ Vorgeburtsperiode *f* / **prodromal** ~ Prodromalstadium *n* / **refractory** ~ Refraktärzeit *f*, Refraktärphase *f*, Refraktärperiode *f*, akoluthe Phase *f* / **sensorimotor** ~ sensumotorisches Stadium *n* / **silent** ~ Ruhezeit *f*, Innervationspause *f*, Innervationsstille *f* / **sleeping** ~ Schlafzeit *f* / **supernormal** ~ über dem Durchschnitt liegende Zeitdauer *f* / **transitional** ~ Übergangszeit *f*

periodic, periodical periodisch

periodicity Periodizität *f* / ~ **analysis** Periodizitätsanalyse *f*

periosteal die Knochenhaut betreffend

peripheral, peripheric peripher, peripher wirkend

peripheralism Peripheralismus *m*, Reflexologie *f*

peripheroceptor sensorischer Nervenendapparat *m*

peripheromittor motorischer Nervenendapparat *m*

peripheroneural zum peripheren Nervensystem gehörig

periphery Peripherie *f* / ~ **of the retina** Netzhautperipherie *f*

periphrastic umschreibend, periphrastisch

peristalsis Peristaltik *f*, Darmtätigkeit *f* / **intestinal** ~ Darmperistaltik *f*

peristaltic peristaltisch / Peristaltik *f*, peristaltische Bewegung *f*

peristasis Milieu *n*, Umgebung *f*, Umwelt *f*

peristatic umweltbedingt, peristatisch

peritoneal Bauchfell–, peritoneal

peritoneum Bauchfell *n*, Peritoneum *n*

permanent dauernd, bleibend, ständig

permeability Durchlässigkeit *f*, Permeabilität *f* / **selective** ~ selektive Permeabilität *f*

permeable durchlässig, permeabel

permeate durchdringen, dringen in, dringen durch

permeation Durchdringung *f*, Penetration *f*

permissible erlaubt, zulässig

permissive nachsichtig, gewährenlassend, tolerant

permissiveness Toleranz *f*, Permissivität *f*, Gewährenlassen *n* / **parental ~** elterliche Nachsicht *f*, elterliche Permissivität *f*

permutation Umstellung *f*, Vertauschung *f*, Permutation *f* / **~ group** Permutationsgruppe *f*

permute, permutate umstellen, vertauschen

pernicious schädlich, verderblich, perniziös

peroxidase Peroxidase *f*

peroxisome Peroxisom *n*, Microbody *m*

perpetrator Täter *m*

perphenazine Perphenazin *n*

perplexed verwirrt, verlegen, bestürzt, unschlüssig

perplexity Verwirrung *f*, Unschlüssigkeit *f*, Ratlosigkeit *f*, Bestürzung *f*

persecuted verfolgt, belästigt

persecution Verfolgung *f* / **~ complex** Verfolgungswahn *m* / **~ mania** Verfolgungswahn *m*

persecutor Verfolger *m*

persecutory Verfolgungs–, verfolgend

perseverance Ausdauer *f*, Beharrlichkeit *f*, Perseveranz *f*

perseverate, persevere perseverieren

perseveration Perseveration *f*, dispositionelle Rigidität *f*, subjektive Wiederholungstendenzen *fpl* / **~ theory** Perseverationstheorie *f*, Konsolidierungstheorie *f*

perseverative perseverativ, ständig wiederkehrend

persist beharren, bestehen auf, beharrlich fortfahren etwas zu tun

persistence Beharren *n*, Beharrlichkeit *f*, Ausdauer *f*, Persistenz *f*, Fortdauer *f* / **~ of vision** Fortdauer *f* von Seheindrücken / **academic ~** schulische Verweildauer *f*

persistency Beharrlichkeit *f*, Ausdauer *f*, Fortdauer *f*

persistent fortdauernd, anhaltend, hartnäckig

person Person *f*, Individuum *n*, Persönlichkeit *f* / **~–environment fit** Person–Umwelt–Kongruenz *f* / **divorced ~** Geschiedene *m,f* / **querulous ~** Querulant *m* / **right–handed ~** Rechtshänder *m* / **single ~** Alleinstehender *m*, Single *m* / **dysthymic ~** Dysthymiker *m* / **unbalanced ~** unausgeglichene Person *f*

persona Persona *f*

personage Persönlichkeit *f*, bedeutende Person *f*, Charakter *m*

personal persönlich, individuell

personalism Personalismus *m*

personalistic personalistisch

personality Persönlichkeit *f*, Charakter *m* / **~ adjustment** Anpassung *f* der Persönlichkeit / **~ and behavioural disorders due to brain disease, damage and dysfunction** Persönlichkeits– und Verhaltensstörungen *fpl* aufgrund einer Krankheit, Schädigung oder Funktionsstörung des Gehirns / **other organic ~ and behavioural disorders due to brain disease, damage and dysfunction** sonstige organische Persönlichkeits– und Verhaltensstörungen *fpl* aufgrund einer Krankheit, Schädigung oder Funktionsstörung des Gehirns / **unspecified organic ~ and behavioural disorders due to brain disease, damage and dysfunction** nicht näher bezeichnete organische Persönlichkeits– und Verhaltensstörungen *fpl* aufgrund einer Krankheit, Schädigung oder Funktionsstörung des Gehirns / **~ assessment** Persönlichkeitsbeurteilung *f* / **~ change** Persönlichkeitsänderung *f*, Charakteränderung *f*, Wesensänderung *f* / **~ change due to a general medical condition** Persönlichkeitsveränderung *f* aufgrund eines medizinischen Krankheitsfaktor / **enduring ~ change after catastrophic experience** andauernde Persönlichkeitsänderung *f* nach Extrembelastung / **enduring ~ change after psychiatric illness** andauernde Persönlichkeitsänderung *f* nach psychischer Erkrankung / **enduring ~ changes, not attributable to**

brain damage and disease andauernde Persönlichkeitsänderungen *fpl*, nicht Folge einer Schädigung oder Krankheit des Gehirns / **troublesome ~ change** störende Persönlichkeitsänderung *f* / **~ characteristic** Persönlichkeitsmerkmal *n* / **~ continuity** Kontinuität *f* der Persönlichkeit / **~ correlate** Persönlichkeitskorrelat *n* / **~ defect** Charaktermangel *m*, Persönlichkeitsstörung *f* / **~ development** Persönlichkeitsentwicklung *f* / **~ deviations** Fehlhaltung *f* der Persönlichkeit / **~ dimension** Persönlichkeitsdimension *f* / **~ disintegration** Persönlichkeitszerfall *m*, Auflösung *f* des Persönlichkeitsgefüges

personality disorder Persönlichkeitsstörung *f* / **~, unspecified** nicht näher bezeichnete Persönlichkeitsstörung *f* / **amoral ~** amoralische Persönlichkeitsstörung *f* / **anankastic ~** anankastische Persönlichkeitsstörung *f* / **antisocial ~** antisoziale Persönlichkeitsstörung *f* / **anxious ~** ängstliche Persönlichkeitsstörung *f* / **asocial ~** asoziale Persönlichkeitsstörung *f* / **atypical ~** atypische Persönlichkeitsstörung *f* / **avoidant ~** vermeidend–selbstunsichere Persönlichkeitsstörung *f* / **dependent ~** abhängige Persönlichkeitsstörung *f*, dependente Persönlichkeitsstörung *f* / **dissocial ~** dissoziale Persönlichkeitsstörung *f* / **emotionally unstable ~** emotional instabile Persönlichkeitsstörung *f* / **histrionic ~** histrionische Persönlichkeitsstörung *f* / **mixed ~** kombinierte Persönlichkeitsstörung *f* / **multiple ~** multiple Persönlichkeitsstörung *f* / **narcissistic ~** narzisstische Persönlichkeitsstörung *f* / **obsessive–compulsive ~** zwanghafte Persönlichkeitsstörung *f* / **organic ~** organische Persönlichkeitsstörung *f* / **paranoid ~** paranoide Persönlichkeitsstörung *f* / **passive–aggressive ~** passiv–aggressive Persönlichkeitsstörung *f* / **posttraumatic ~** traumatische Persönlichkeitsveränderung *f* / **schizoid ~** schizoide Persönlichkeitsstörung *f* / **schizotypal ~** schizotypische Persönlichkeitsstörung *f* / **specific ~** spezifische Persönlichkeitsstörung *f* / **specific ~s, mixed and other ~s, and enduring personality changes** spezifische Persönlichkeitsstörungen *fpl*, kombinierte und sonstige Persönlichkeitsstörungen und anhaltende Persönlichkeitsänderungen

personality| disorganization Persönlichkeitsabbau *m* / **sociopathic ~ disturbance** Soziopathie *f* / **~ dynamics** Persönlichkeitsdynamik *f* / **~ factor** Persönlichkeitsfaktor *m* / **~ formation** Persönlichkeitsbildung *f*, Charakterbildung *f* / **~ function** Persönlichkeitsfunktion *f* / **~ hierarchy** hierarchische Struktur *f* der Persönlichkeit / **~ identity** Identität *f* der Persönlichkeit / **~ integration** Persönlichkeitsorganisation *f* / **~ inventory** Persönlichkeitsfragebogen *m* / **~ measure** Persönlichkeitsmessung *f*, Persönlichkeitstest *m* / **nonprojective ~ measure** nichtprojektiver Persönlichkeitstest *m* / **projective ~ measure** projektiver Persönlichkeitstest *m* / **~ organization** Persönlichkeitsorganisation *f* / **~ panels** Persönlichkeitsstruktur *f* / **~ pattern disturbance** Störung *f* der Persönlichkeitsstruktur / **~ problem** Persönlichkeitsproblem *n* / **~ process** Persönlichkeitsprozess *m*, intrapersonaler Persönlichkeitsprozess *m* / **~ profile** Persönlichkeitsprofil *n* / **~ questionnaire** Persönlichkeitsfragebogen *m* / **~ reorganization** Umorientierung *f* der Persönlichkeit / **~ research** Persönlichkeitsforschung *f* / **~ scale** Persönlichkeitsfragebogen *m* / **~ sphere** Persönlichkeitssphäre *f* / **~ split** Doppel–Ich *n* / **~ structure** Persönlichkeitsstruktur *f* / **~ study** Persönlichkeitsforschung *f* / **~ survey** Persönlichkeitsuntersuchung *f* / **~ syndrome** Persönlichkeitssyndrom *n* / **~ test** Persönlichkeitstest *m* / **~ theory** Persönlichkeitstheorie *f* / **~ trait** Charaktereigenschaft *f*, Persönlichkeitsmerkmal *n* / **~ trait disturbance** Charakterstörung *f* / **~ trend** Charakterrichtung *f* / **~ type** Persönlichkeitstyp *m* / **~ variable** Persönlichkeitsvariable *f* / **~ as a whole** Gesamtpersönlichkeit *f* / **aggressive ~** aggressive Persönlichkeit *f* / **alternating ~** gespaltene Persönlichkeit *f* / **anal ~** analer Charakter *m* / **antisocial ~** Psychopath *m*, dissoziale Persönlichkeit *f*, antisoziale Persönlichkeit *f* / **"as if" ~** „als–ob"–Persönlichkeit *f* / **asocial ~** asoziale Persönlichkeit *f* / **asthenic ~** asthenische Persönlichkeit *f*, Astheniker *m* / **authoritarian ~** autoritäre Persönlichkeit *f* / **avoidant ~** hypersensitive Persönlichkeit *f* / **basic ~ structure** grundlegende Persönlichkeitsstruktur *f* / **common ~** vorherrschende Charakterzüge *mpl* / **compulsive ~** Zwangscharakter *m*, Zwangsneurotiker *m* / **conforming ~** konformistische Persönlichkeit *f* / **cycloid ~** zykloide Persönlichkeit *f* / **cyclophrenic ~** zyklophrene Persönlichkeit *f* / **cyclothymic ~** zyklothymer Typ *m* / **decompensated ~** unausgeglichene Persönlichkeit *f* / **dependent ~** dependente Persönlichkeit *f* / **describing ~ test** beschreibender Persönlichkeitstest *m* / **disordered ~** gestörte Persönlichkeit *f* / dissociated gespaltene Persönlichkeit *f* / **double ~** Spaltung *f* der Persönlichkeit, Doppel–Ich *n* / **dual ~** Spaltung *f* der Persönlichkeit, Doppel–Ich *n*, doppelte Persönlichkeit *f* / **emotionally unstable ~** labile Persönlichkeit *f* / **epileptoid ~** epileptoider Typ *m* / **ethnocentric ~** ethnozentrische Persönlichkeit *f* / **expanded ~** expansiver Typus *m* / **explosive ~** aufbrausende Persönlichkeit *f* / **hostile ~** aggressive Persönlichkeit *f* / **hysterical ~** hysterische Persönlichkeit *f* / **immature ~** unreife Persönlichkeit *f* / **implicit ~ theory** implizite Persönlichkeitstheorie *f* / **inadequate ~** unangepasste Persönlichkeit *f* / **inferior ~** fehlangepasste Persönlichkeit *f* / **integrated ~** integrierte Persönlichkeit *f*, in–sich–geschlossene Persönlichkeit *f* / **maladjusted ~** unangepasste Persönlichkeit *f* / **masochistic ~** masochistische Persönlichkeit *f* / **mentally defective ~** schwachsinnige Person *f* / **modal ~** Modalpersönlichkeit *f* / **momentary ~** im Augenblick vorherrschende Persönlichkeitsstruktur *f* / **multiple ~** multiple Persönlichkeit *f* / **narcissistic ~** narzisstische Persönlichkeit *f* / **neurotic ~** neurotische Persönlichkeit *f* / **obsessive–compulsive ~** zwanghafte Persönlichkeit *f* / **oral ~** orale Persönlichkeit *f* / **organic ~ syndrome** organisch bedingtes Persönlichkeitssyndrom *n* / **paranoid ~** paranoide Persönlichkeit *f*, paranoider Typ *m* / **passive–aggressive ~** passiv–aggressive Persönlichkeit *f* / **pathological ~** pathologische Persönlichkeit *f*, krankhafte Persönlichkeit *f* / **perverse ~** perverse Persönlichkeit *f* / **primary ~** Ausgangspersönlichkeit *f* / **psychoanalytic ~ factors** psychoanalytische Persönlichkeitsfaktoren *mpl* / **psychopathic ~** psychopathische Persönlichkeit *f*, abnorme Persönlichkeit *f* / **psychotic ~** psychotische Persönlichkeit *f* / **sadistic ~** sadistische Persönlichkeit *f* / **sadomasochistic ~** sadomasochistische Persönlichkeit *f* / **schizoid ~** schizoide Persönlichkeit *f* / **schizotypal ~** schizotypische Persönlichkeit *f* / **secondary ~** krankhaft veränderte Persönlichkeit *f* / **sociopathic ~** sozial abartige Persönlichkeit *f* / **split ~** gespaltene Persönlichkeit *f* / **split ~ delusion** Doppelgängerwahn *m* / **submissive ~** unterwürfige Persönlichkeit *f* / **total ~** Gesamtpersönlichkeit *f* / **weak ~** schwache Persönlichkeit *f*

personalize personifizieren, verkörpern

personification, personalisation, personation Personifizierung *f*, Verkörperung *f*, Personifikation *f*

personify verkörpern, personifizieren

personnel Personal *n*, Belegschaft *f* / **~ counselor** Personalberater *m* / **~ development** Personalentwicklung *f* / **~ director** Personalleiter *m*, Personaldirektor *m* / **~ evaluation** Personalbeurteilung *f* / **~ management** Personalleitung *f*, Personalführung *f*, Personal–Management *n*, Personalwesen *n*, Menschenführung *f* / **~ manager** Personalleiter *m*, Personalchef *m* / **~ placement** Personaleinsatz *m*, Personalvermittlung *f* / **~ policy** Personalpolitik *f*, Personalrichtlinie *f* / **~ promotion** personelle Beförderung *f* / **~ psy-**

chology angewandte Psychologie *f* im Rahmen der Personalführung, Psychologie *f* im Personalwesen / ~ **recruitment** Personaleinstellung *f*, Personalbeschaffung *f* / ~ **rotation** Personalwechsel *m*, Personalversetzung *f* / ~ **selection** Personalauslese *f*, Personalauswahl *f* / ~ **supply** Personalersatz *m*, Personalangebot *n* / ~ **termination** Beendigung *f* von Arbeitsverhältnissen, Personalentlassung *f* / ~ **training** Weiterbildung *f* des Personals, Personalschulung *f* / **clerical** ~ Bürokräfte *fpl*, Büropersonal *n* / **disabled** ~ behindertes Personal *n* / **educational** ~ Lehrkörper *m* / **industrial** ~ Industriebeschäftigte *pl*, Angestellte *pl* in der Industrie / **medical** ~ medizinisches Personal *n* / **nonprofessional** ~ Laien *mpl*, Hilfspersonal *n* / **paramedical** ~ medizinisches Hilfspersonal *n* / **paraprofessional** ~ nichtakademisches Fachpersonal *n* / **professional** ~ Fachkräfte *fpl*, Fachpersonal *n* / **secretarial** ~ Schreibkräfte *fpl*, Sekretärinnen *fpl* / **subprofessional** ~ gehobene Sachbearbeiter *mpl*, Assistenten *mpl* / **technical** ~ technisches Personal *n*

personology Personologie *f*

perspective Perspektive *f* / ~ **size** perspektivische Größe *f* / **aerial** ~ Luftperspektive *f*, atmosphärische Perspektive *f* / **alternating** ~ wechselnde Perspektive *f* / **ambiguous** ~ mehrdeutige Perspektive *f* / **angular** ~ Winkelperspektive *f* / **atmospheric** ~ Luftperspektive *f*, atmosphärische Perspektive *f* / **binocular** ~ binokulare Perspektive *f*, Querdisparation *f* / **future** ~ Zukunftsperspektive *f* / **linear** ~ lineare Perspektive *f* / **reversible** ~ wechselnde Perspektive *f*, Umkehrperspektive *f* / **temporal** ~ Zeitperspektive *f*

perspicacity geistiger Scharfblick *m*

perspicuity Klugheit *f*, Scharfsinn *m*

perspiration Schweiß *m*, Schwitzen *n*, Transpirieren *n*

perspire schwitzen, transpirieren

perstimulatory Dauerreizung betreffend, aufgrund andauernder Reizung

persuade überreden, überzeugen, verleiten

persuasibility Beeinflussbarkeit *f*, Überredbarkeit *f*, Persuabilität *f*

persuasion Überredung *f*, Überzeugung *f*, Beeinflussung *f*, Persuasion *f* / ~ **therapy** Persuasionstherapie *f*

persuasive überredend, überzeugend

pertinence, pertinency Angemessenheit *f*, Eignung *f*

perturbation Störung *f*

pervasive tiefgreifend, durchdringend

perverse pervers, widernatürlich, geschlechtlich abnorm

perverseness, perversity Perversion *f*, Widernatürlichkeit *f*, Perversität *f*

perversion Perversion *f*, widernatürliche Abweichung *f* / **infantile polymorphous** ~ infantil–polymorphe Perversion *f* / **osphresiophilic** ~ Geruchsperversion *f* / **sexual** ~ sexuelle Perversion *f*, krankhafte geschlechtliche Abweichung *f*

pervert verführen, sittlich verderben / Perverser *m*, sexuell abartig veranlagter Mensch *m*

perverted pervers, widernatürlich, geschlechtlich abnorm

pervertedness Pervertiertheit *f*, Widernatürlichkeit *f*, sexuelle Abnormität *f*

pervigilium Schlaflosigkeit *f*, Pervigilium *n*

pessimism Pessimismus *m* / **oral** ~ oraler Pessimismus *m*

pessimist Pessimist *m*

pessimistic pessimistisch

pet Haustier *n* / ~ **therapy** Haustier unterstützte Therapie *f*

Peter principle Peter–Prinzip *n*, Beförderung *f* zur Inkompetenz

petit mal kleiner epileptischer Anfall *m*, Petit mal *n* / ~ **epilepsy** Petit–mal–Epilepsie *f* / ~ **with head retropulsion** Petit mal retropulsif

petrifaction Versteinerung *f*, Petrifizierung *f*

petrol sniffing Benzinismus *m*, Benzinsucht *f*, Benzinomanie *f*

petting Petting *n*, Liebkosung *f*

peyote Peyoti *f*, Peyote *f*, meskalinhaltiges Kakteengift *n* / **~ cult** Peyote–Kult *m* / **~ dance** ekstatischer Fruchtbarkeitstanz *m* mit Einnahme von Meskalinkörnern, Peyote Tanz *m*

peyotism Peyotismus *m*, indianische Religion *f* die Peyote bei der Gottesverehrung einsetzt

p factor P–Faktor *m*, Perseverationsfaktor *m*

pfropfhebephrenia Pfropfhebephrenie *f*

pfropfschizophrenia Pfropfschizophrenie *f*

phacoscope, phakoscope Phakoskop *n*, Linsenmessgerät *n*

phacoscopy, phakoscopy Linsenmessung Phakoskopie *f*

phagocyte Phagozyt *m*, Fresszelle *f*

phagocytosis Phagozytose *f*

phagomania Phagomanie *f*, Fresssucht *f*

phagophobia Furcht *f* vor dem Schlucken, Phagophobie *f*

phagotherapy Mastkur *f*

phallic phallisch, Penis–

phallicism, phallism Phalluskult *m*, Phallusverehrung *f*

phallus Phallus *m*, Penis *m*, männliches Glied *n* / **~ worship** Phalluskult *m*, Phallusverehrung *f*

phantasm Wahngebilde *n*, Trugbild *n*, Sinnestäuschung *f*, Erscheinung *f*

phantasmagorial unwirklich, eingebildet, traumhaft

phantasmal, phantasmic eingebildet, unwirklich, halluzinatorisch

phantasmatology Lehre *f* vom Okkultismus, Lehre *f* von den Geistererscheinungen

phantasmoscopia Halluzination *f*

phantasy Phantasie *f*, Einbildung *f*, Einbildungskraft *f* / **~ of destruction** Destruktionsphantasie *f*, Zerstörungsphantasie *f* / **conscious ~** bewusste Einbildung *f* / **primal ~** Urphantasie *f* / **unconscious ~** unbewusste Phantasie *f*

phantom Phantom *n*, Trugbild *n*, Illusion *f*, Sinnestäuschung *f* / **~ extremity** Phantomglied *n* / **~ image** Phantomklang *m* / **~ limb** Phantomglied *n* / **~ sensation** Phantomschmerz *m* / **~ sound** Phantomklang *m*

pharmacist Apotheker *m*

pharmacological pharmakologisch

pharmacology Arzneimittelkunde *f*, Pharmakologie *f*

pharmacomania Arzneimittelsucht *f*, Pharmakomanie *f*

pharmacon Droge *f*, Pharmakon *n*

pharmacophilia leichte Arzneimittelsucht *f*

pharmacophobia krankhafte Angst *f* vor Drogeneinnahme, Furcht *f* vor Arzneimitteleinnahme

pharmacopsychiatric pharmakopsychiatrisch

pharmacopsychiatry Pharmakopsychiatrie *f*

pharmacopsychology Pharmakopsychologie *f*, Psychopharmakologie *f*

pharmacopsychopathology Pharmakopsychopathologie *f*

pharmacopsychosis durch Arzneimittel ausgelöste Psychose *f*, Pharmakopsychose *f*

pharmacotherapy Behandlung *f* mit Arzneimitteln, Pharmakotherapie *f*

pharyngal, pharyngeal Rachen–, Pharynx–, pharyngeal

pharynx Pharynx *m*, Rachen *m*, Schlund *m*

phase Phase *f*, Stadium *n*, Entwicklungsstufe *f* / **~ angle** Phasenwinkel *m* / **~ change beat** Phasenänderungsschlag *m* / **~ change effect** Phasenänderungseffekt *m* / **~ s of development** Entwicklungsphasen *fpl*, Entwicklungsstufen *fpl* / **~ difference** Phasendifferenz *f* / **~ displacement** Phasenverschiebung *f* / **~ of equalization** Ausgleichsphase *f* / **~ of involution** Rückbildungsphase *f* / **~ of life**

problem Problem *n* einer Lebensphase / **~ of sleep** Schlafstadium *n*, Schlafphase *f* / **~ rule** Phasenregel *f*, Phasengesetz *n* / **~ sequence** Phasenfolge *f* / **~ sequence theory** Theorie *f* der Phasenfolgen / **~ space** Phasenraum *m* / **~ structure grammar** Phasenstruktur–Grammatik *f* / **active ~** floride Phase *f* / **anal ~** anale Phase *f* / **anal–sadistic ~** analsadistische Phase *f* / **associative ~** Assoziationsphase *f* / **cannibalic ~** kannibalische Phase *f* / **developmental ~** Entwicklungsphase *f* / **developmental ~ of apperception** Apperzeptionsstadium *n* / **depressive ~** depressive Phase *f* / **effective ~** Wirkungsphase *f* / **endogenous–cyclothymic ~** endogen–zyklothyme Phase *f* / **genital ~** genitale Phase *f* / **libidinal ~** Libidostufe *f* / **negative ~** negative Phase *f* / **neonatal ~** Neugeborenenphase *f* / **oral–biting ~** oral–sadistische Phase *f* / **oral–incorporative ~** oral–inkorporative Phase *f* / **out–of ~** phasenverschoben / **paradoxal ~** paradoxe Phase *f* / **persecutory ~** Verfolgungsphase *f* / **phallic ~** phallische Phase *f*, phallisches Stadium *n* / **pregenital ~** prägenitale Phase *f* / **preoedipal ~** Präödipusphase *f* / **prodromal ~** Prodromalstadium *n* / **refractory ~** Refraktärphase *f*, Refraktärstadium *n* / **transitional ~** Übergangsphase *f*, Durchgangsphase *f* / **ultraparadoxal ~** ultraparadoxe Phase *f* / **urethral ~** Urethralstadium *n*

phasic phasisch, Phasen–

phenacetin Phenazetin *n*

phenaglycodol Phenaglykodol *n*

phenakistoscope Phenakistoskop *n*, Drehscheibe *f* zur Erzeugung bewegter Bilder

phencyclidine Phencyclidin *n* / **~ abuse** Phencyclidinmissbrauch *m* / **~ dependence** Phencyclidinabhängigkeit *f* / **~–induced** phencyclidininduziert / **~ intoxication** Phencyclidinintoxikation *f* / **~ intoxication delirium** Phencyclidinintoxikationsdelir *n* / **~–related disorders** Störungen *fpl* im Zusammenhang mit Phencyclidin / **~–like related disorders** Störungen *fpl* im Zusammenhang mit phencyclidinähnlichen Substanzen

phenelzine Phenelzin *n*

phenethylamine Phenäthylamin *n*

pheniprazine Pheniprazin *n*

phenmetrazine Phenmetrazin *n*

phenobarbital, phenobarbitone Phenobarbital *n*

phenomenal phänomenal, Erscheinungs–

phenomenalism Phänomenalismus *m*, Phänomenologie *f*

phenomenalistic phänomenalistisch

phenomenism Phänomenismus *m*, prälogische Deutungsweise *f*, Ursache–Wirkung–Umkehr *f* in der Deutung von Phänomenen

phenomenistic phänomenistisch, prälogisch

phenomenological phänomenologisch

phenomenology Phänomenologie *f* / **integral ~** integrale Phänomenologie *f*, Gesamtschau *f*

phenomenon Phänomen *n*, Erscheinung *f*, Symptom *n* / **anticipatory ~** antizipatorisches Phänomen *n* / **autokinetic–~** autokinetisches Phänomen *n* / **bioelectric ~** bioelektrische Erscheinung *f* / **compulsive ~** Zwangserscheinung *f* / **covariant ~** Kovarianzphänomen *n* / **déjà–vu ~** Déjà–vu–Phänomen *n* / **dissociative ~** dissoziatives Phänomen *n* / **entoptic ~** entoptische Erscheinung *f* / **functional ~** funktionales Phänomen *n* / **idiophonic ~** Eigenklangphänomen *n* / **iterative ~** Iterativphänomen *n* / **obsessional ~** Zwangserscheinung *f* / **parapsychological ~** parapsychologisches Phänomen *n* / **senile ~** Alterserscheinung *f* / **social ~** soziales Phanomen *n* / **stepwise ~** Stufenphänomen *n*

phenomotive Phäno–Motiv *n*

phenothiazine Phenothiazin *n* / **~ derivative** Phenothiazinderivat *n*

phenotype Phänotypus *m*, äußeres Erscheinungsbild *n*

phenotypical, phenotypic phänotypisch

phenoxybenzamine Phenoxybenzamin *n*

phenyl Phenyl *n*

phenylalanine Phenylalanin *n*

phenylethylamine Phenyläthylamin *n*

phenylketonuria Phenylketonurie *f*, Phenylbrenztraubensäure–Schwachsinn *m*, Fölling–Krankheit *f*

phenylketonuric phenylbrenztraubensauer, phenylketonurisch

phenylpyruvic Phenylbrenztraubensäure–, phenylbrenztraubensauer

phenytoin Phenytoin *n*, Diphenylhydantoin *n*

pheromones Pheromone *npl*, Sexuallockstoffe *mpl*

phi Phi *n* / **~ coefficient** Phi–Koeffizient *m* / **~–gamma function** Phi–Gamma–Funktion *f*, psychometrische Funktion *f* / **~–gamma hypothesis** Phi–Gamma–Hypothese *f* / **~–phenomenon** Phi–Phänomen *n*

philander hofieren, umwerben, umschmeicheln

philanthrope, philanthropist Menschenfreund *m*, Philanthrop *m*

philanthropic menschenfreundlich, philanthropisch

philanthropy Philanthropie *f*, Menschenliebe *f*

philocratic machtliebend, philokratisch

philogenesis, philogenics, philogeny Stammesgeschichte *f*, Entwicklungsgeschichte *f*, Phylogenese *f*, Phylogenie *f*

philology Philologie *f*, Sprachwissenschaft *f*

philomimesia unwiderstehlicher Drang *m* nachzuahmen

philoneism Neuigkeitssucht *f*, Neophilismus *m*

philosophical philosophisch

philosophy Philosophie *f* / **~ of life** Lebensphilosophie *f* / **"as if" ~** Philosophie *f* des „als ob" / **mental ~** geisteswissenschaftliche Psychologie *f*, verstehende Psychologie *f* / **natural ~** Naturphilosophie *f*

philtre, philter Liebestrank *m*, Aphrodisiakum *n*

phlegm Phlegma *n*, Trägheit *f*

phlegmatic phlegmatisch, gleichgültig, träge

phobia Phobie *f*, krankhafte Angst *f*, Furcht *f* / **cardiac ~** Herzangstsyndrom *n*, Herzphobie *f* / **simple ~** einfache Phobie *f* / **social ~** soziale Phobie *f* / **specific (isolated) ~** spezifische (isolierte) Phobie *f*

phobiac Phobiker *m*, Phobikerin *f*

phobic phobisch, angstbedingt

phobophobia Angst *f* vor Angstzuständen, Phobophobie *f*, Angsterwartung *f*

phobotaxis Phobotaxis *f*, ungerichtete Schreckreaktion *f*

phon Phon *n* / **~ scale** Phonskala *f*

phonasthenia Stimmschwäche *f*, Phonasthenie *f*

phonation Lautbildung *f*, Stimmbildung *f*, Phonation *f*

phonautograph Lautaufzeichnungsgerät *n*, Phonautograph *m*

phone Laut *m*, Phonem *n*

phoneidoscope Phoneidoskop *n*, Gerät *n* zur Sichtbarmachung von Schallwellen

phonelescope Phoneleskop *n*, Gerät *n* zur Messung und photographischen Aufzeichnung von Schallwellen

phoneme Phonem *n*, akustische Sinnestäuschung *f*, Hörhalluzination *f*, Stimmenhören *n*

phonemics, phonematics Lautlehre *f*, Phonemik *f*, Phonematik *f*, Phonologie *f*

phonendoscope Phonendoskop *n*, Hörrohr *n* mit Lautverstärker, Membranstethoskop *n*

phonetic phonetisch

phonetician Phonetiker *m*, Lautforscher *m*

phonetics Phonetik *f*, Lautlehre *f*

phoniatrics, phoniatry Stimmheilkunde *f*, Phoniatrie *f*

phonic lautlich, akustisch, Laut–, phonisch

phonics Akustik *f*

phonism Phonismus *m*, akustische Synästhesie *f*

phonodeik Gerät *n* zur photographischen Aufzeichnung von Schallwellen, Phonedeik *m*

phonogram Lautaufzeichnung *f*, Phonogramm *n*

phonology Lautlehre *f*, Phonologie *f*, Phonemik *f*, Phonematik *f*

phonomania Mordsucht *f*, Phonomanie *f*

phonometer Lautstärkemesser *m*, Phonometer *n*

phonometry Lautstärkemessung *f*, Phonometrie *f*

phonopathy Stimmleiden *n*, Stimmerkrankung *f*, Stimmstörung *f*

phonophobia Angst *f* vor dem Sprechen, Angst *f* vor Geräuschen, Phonophobie *f*

phonoprojectoscope Gerät *n* zur Sichtbarmachung von Schallschwingungen

phonopsy, phonopsia Phonopsie *f*, visuelle Synästhesie *f*

phonoscope Phonoskop *n*, Mikrophonstethoskop *n*

phoria Abweichen *n* der Sehachse

phorometer Gerät *n* zur Messung der Sehachsenabweichung, Phorometer *n*

phorometry Messung *f* der Sehachsenabweichung, Phorometrie *f*

phose subjektive Lichtempfindung *f*

phosphate Phosphat *n*

phosphatase Phosphatase *f*

phosphatide Phosphatid *n*

phosphene Lichterscheinung *f* im Auge ohne normal–visuelle Reizung, Phosphen *n*

phosphodiesterase Phosphodiesterase *f*

phosphoinositol Phosphoinositol *n*

phospholipid Phospholipid *n*

phosphorus Phosphor *m*

phosphorylase Phosphorylase *f*

phosphorylation Phosphorylierung *f*

phot Phot *n*

photaesthesia, photesthesia Lichtempfindlichkeit *f*, Lichtscheu *f*

photerythrous rotempfindlich

photic photisch, Licht betreffend

photism Photismus *m*, optische Synästhesie *f*, durch Farben hervorgerufene Tonempfindungen *fpl*

photistic Licht–

photoaesthesimeter, photoesthesimeter Photoästhesimeter *n*, Gerät *n* zur Messung der Lichtempfindlichkeit

photochemical photochemisch

photochemistry Photochemie *f*, Lichtchemie *f*

photochromatic photochromatisch

photocopy Fotokopie *f* / **~ machine** Fotokopiermaschine *f*, Fotokopierautomat *m*

photoelectric photoelektrisch

photogenesis Lichtentstehung *f*, Lichtproduktion *f*

photogenic, photogenous lichterzeugend, lichtausstrahlend, leuchtend

photokinesis Photokinese *f*, Bewegung *f* durch Lichtenergie

photokinetic photokinetisch, durch Lichtenergie bewegt

photokymograph Photokymograph *m*, Lichtkurvenschreiber *m*

photolysis Zersetzung *f* durch Licht, Photolyse *f*

photoma Photom *n*, entoptische Helligkeitsempfindung *f*

photomania Photomanie *f*, krankhaftes Verlangen *n* nach Licht und Sonne

photometer Lichtstärkemesser *m*, Photometer *n* / **integrating ~** Photometer *n*

photometric photometrisch

photometry Lichtmessung *f*, Photometrie *f* / **heterochromatic ~** heterochromatische Photometrie *f*, Messung *f* der Intensität verschiedenfarbigen Lichts / **visual ~** Messung *f* der Lichtintensität in den Sehrezeptoren

photon Photon *n*, Lichtquant *n*

photopathy Phototrauma *n*, Lichtschädigung *f*

photoperceptive lichtempfindlich, auf Lichtstrahlen reagierend

photophobia Lichtscheu *f*, Photophobie *f*, Heliophobie *f*

photophobic lichtscheu, photophob

photopia Helladaptation *f*

photopic Helligkeits–, photopisch

photopsia, photopsy subjektive Lichterscheinungen *fpl*, subjektive Lichteindrücke *mpl*, Photopsie *f*

photoptic photoptisch, subjektive Lichteindrücke betreffend

photoptometer Lichtstärkemesser *m*

photoptometry Messung *f* der Lichtstärkeempfindung

photoreception Lichtempfindung *f*

photoreceptive lichtempfindlich

photoreceptor Photorezeptor *m*, lichtwahrnehmende Nervenendzelle *f*, lichtempfindlicher Nerv *m*

photosensitisation Photosensibilisierung *f*, Empfindlichwerden *n* gegen Licht

photosensitive lichtempfindlich

photosensitivity Lichtempfindlichkeit *f*

phototaxis Phototaxis *f*, Phototropismus *m*

phototherapy Lichttherapie *f*, Lichtbehandlung *f*, Phototherapie *f*

phototropism Phototropismus *m*, Phototaxis *f*

phrase Satzteil *m*, idiomatischer Ausdruck *m*, Phrase *f* / **~ marker** Formationsmarker *m*, P–Marker *m* / **~ structure grammar** Phrasenstrukturgrammatik *f*, Konstituentengrammatik *f*, IC–Grammatik *f* / **phonemic ~** abgegrenzte Phonemkette *f* / **phonological ~** ausgedehnte Intonationsstruktur *f*

phrenasthenia Geistesschwäche *f*, geistiger Defekt *m*, Debilität *f*, Schwachsinn *m*

phrenasthenic geistesschwach, debil, schwachsinnig

phrenesis Wahnsinn *m*, Raserei *f*, Tobsucht *f*

phrenetic wahnsinnig, rasend, tobend

phrenic Zwerchfell–

phrenitis Gehirnentzündung *f*, Phrenitis *f*

phrenolepsia Zwangsvorstellung *f*

phrenological phrenologisch

phrenologist Phrenologe *m*, Anhänger *m* der Gall'schen Schädellehre

phrenology Phrenologie *f*, Lehre *f* von der Charakterdeutung aus der Schädelform

phrenopathy Geisteskrankheit *f*

phthiriophobia krankhafte Angst *f* vor Läusen

phthisiomania Phthisiomanie *f*, krankhafte Überzeugung *f* an Tuberkulose zu leiden

phthisiophobia Phthisiophobie *f*, irrationale Furcht *f* vor Tuberkulose

phyletic phylogenetisch / Stammesphyloanalyse *f*, Phyloanalyse *f*

phylobiology Phylobiologie *f*, Stammesbiologie *f*

phylogenesis, phylogeny Phylogenese *f*, Phylogenie *f*, Stammesgeschichte *f*, Entwicklungsgeschichte *f*

phylogenetic, phylogenic entwicklungsgeschichtlich, phylogenetisch, stammesgeschichtlich

phylum Klasse *f*, Abteilung *f* des Tier– oder Pflanzenreichs

physical physikalisch, körperlich, physisch

physicalism Physikalismus *m*

physicalistic physikalistisch

physician Arzt *m*

physicist Physiker *m*

physicochemical physikalisch–chemisch

physics Physik *f*

physiochemical biochemisch

physiochemistry Biochemie *f*

physiogenesis Embryologie *f*

physiognomic, physiognomical physiognomisch, Gesichtsausdrucks

physiognomy Gesichtsausdruck *m*, Physiognomie *f*, Physiognomik *f*

physiologic, physiological physiologisch

physiologist Physiologe *m*

physiology Physiologie *f*

physioneurosis echte Neurose *f*

physiopathic echte Neurosen betreffend

physiopathology pathologische Physiologie *f*, Physiopathologie *f*

physiopsychic leibseelisch, Leibseele–

physiotherapy Krankengymnastik *f*, Physiotherapie *f*

physique Körperbau *m*

physostigmine Physostigmin *n*, Eserin *n* / **~ salicylate** Physostigmin *n*, Eserin *n*

piano theory Resonanztheorie *f* / **~ of hearing** Resonanztheorie *f*

pial die weiche Hirnhaut betreffend

pia mater weiche Hirnhaut *f*, Piamater *f*

pica Pica *f*, absonderlicher Appetit *m*, perverser Geschmack *m*, Pikazismus *m*, Pica–Syndrom *n* / **~ of infancy and childhood** Pica *f* im frühen Kindesalter

picketing Aufstellen *n* von Streikposten

Pick's| atrophy of the frontal lobe Stirnhirn–Pick *m* / **~ disease** Pick–Hirnatrophie *f*, Pick–Krankheit *f* / **~ disease, temporal lobe form** Schläfenlappen–Pick *m*

pickwickian syndrom Pickwick–Syndrom *n*, Pickwickier–Syndrom *n*

picrogeusia bitterer Geschmack *m*, Pikrogeusie *f*

picrotoxin Pikrotoxin *n*

pictograph, pictogram Bildzeichen *n*, Bildsymbol *n*, graphische Darstellung *f*

pictorial Bild–

picture Bild *n* / **~ arrangement** Bilderordnen *n* / **~ arrangement test** Bilderordnungstest *m* / **~ of character** Charakterbild *n* / **~ completion test** Bildergänzungstest *m* / **~ of the fantasy** Phantasievorstellung *f* / **~ frustration test** Frustrationstest *m* / **~ interpretation** Bildbetrachtung *f*, Bildbeschreibung *f* / **clinical ~** Erscheinungsbild *n*, Zustandsbild *n*, Krankheitsbild *n*, Syndrom *n* / **imaginary ~** Vorstellungsbild *n*, Phantasiebild *n* / **incomplete ~ test** Bildergänzungstest *m* / **retinal ~** Netzhautbild *n*

Piderit drawings Piderit–Zeichnungen *fpl*

pie graph, pie chart graphische Darstellung *f* durch Kreissektoren

piece Stück *n* / **~ rate wages** Akkordlohn *m* / **~ work** Akkordarbeit *f*

piecemeal stückweise, einzeln, zerstückelt

piesaesthesia, piesesthesia Drucksinn *m*

piesimeter, piesometer Hautdruckmesser *m*

pigment Pigment *n*, Farbstoff *m* / **~ cell** Pigmentzelle *f* / **visual ~** Sehfarbstoff *m*

pigmentary Pigment–

pigmentation Pigmentierung *f*, Färbung *f*, Pigmentablagerung *f*

pilar, pilary das Haar betreffend, pilar

pill Pille *f*

pillars of Corti Corti–Pfeilerzellen *fpl*

pilocarpine Pilokarpin *n*

piloerection Piloerektion *f*, Aufrichten *n* der Haare

pilomotor haaraufrichtend, Gänsehaut hervorrufend, pilomotorisch

pilot study, pilot survey, pilot experiment Pilotstudie *f*, Leitstudie *f*, Voruntersuchung *f*, Erkundungsexperiment *n*

pilose behaart, haarig

Piltdown man Piltdown–Mensch *m*, Sussex–Mensch *m*

pimozide Pimozid *n*

pincer technique Greiftechnik *f*, Umklammerungstechnik *f*

pineal pineal, Zirbeldrüsen–

pinealectomy Zirbeldrüsenresektion *f*, Epiphysenektomie *f*

pinna Ohrmuschel *f*, äußeres Ohr *n* / ~ **reflex** Ohrmuschelreflex *m*

pins and needles Ameisenlaufen *n*, Kribbeln *n*, eingeschlafene Glieder *npl*, Parästhesie *f*

piperazine Piperazin *n*

Piper's law Piper'sches Gesetz *n*

pipradol Pipradol *n*

piracetam Piracetam *n*

pitch Tonhöhe *f* / ~ **brightness** Tonhelligkeit *f*, Klanghelligkeit *f* / ~ **discrimination** Tonhöhenunterscheidung *f*, Tonhöhendiskrimination *f* / ~ **fork** Stimmgabel *f* / ~ **limit** Hörschwelle *f*, Hörgrenze *f* / ~ **perception** Tonhöhenwahrnehmung *f* / ~ **pipe** Orgelpfeifen *fpl* / ~ **residue** Hörrest *m* / ~ **scale** Tonskala *f* / **absolute** ~ absolutes Gehör *n* / **equal** ~ **contour** Linie *f* gleicher Tonhöhe / **lower** ~ **limit** untere Hörschwelle *f* / **relative** ~ relatives Gehör *n* / **standard** ~ Normalton *m* / **upper** ~ obere Hörschwelle *f*

Pithecanthropus Pithekanthropus *m*, Javamensch *m*

pithecoid affenartig, zu den Menschenaffen gehörig, pithekoid

pithiatic, pithiatric suggerierbar, beeinflussbar, suggestiv

pithiatism Suggestionstherapie *f*

pithiatry Suggestionsbehandlung *f*

pituitary hypophysär, Hypophysen– / Hypophyse *f*, Hirnanhangdrüse *f*

pixel Pixel *n*, Bildpunkt *m* im Bildschirm

pity Mitleid *n*, Bedauern *n*

place Ort *m*, Platz *m*, Stelle *f* / ~ **conditioning** Konditionieren *n* der Ortspräferenz / ~ **disorientation** örtliche Desorientiertheit *f*, Desorientiertheit *f* nach Raum / ~ **learning** Ortslernen *n* / ~ **principle of hearing** Resonanztheorie *f* / ~ **theory** Resonanztheorie *f*

place under guardianship entmündigen

placebo Placebo *n*, Plazebo *n*, Scheinmedikament *n*, Leerpräparat *n* / ~ **effect** Placeboeffekt *m* / ~ **response** Placeboeffekt *m* / ~ **therapy** Plazebotherapie *f* / ~ **test** Plazeboversuch *m*

placement Platzierung *f*, Einsatz *m*, Personaleinsatz *m* / ~ **office** Arbeitsamt *n*, Stellenvermittlungsbüro *n* / ~ **test** Auswahlverfahren *n*, Klassifikationstest *m* / **educational** ~ schulische Einstufung *f*, Schullaufbahnentscheidung *f*

placenta Plazenta *f*, Mutterkuchen *m*, Nachgeburt *f*

placidity Gelassenheit *f*, Gemütsruhe *f*

Placido's disk Keratoskop *n*, Placido–Scheibe *f*

plan Plan *m*, Methode *f*, Verfahren *n*, System *n* / **objective** ~ objektiver Plan *m* / **subjective** ~ subjektiver Plan *m*

planchette herzförmiges Brett *n* mit Rollen und Schreibvorrichtung (für automatische Aufzeichnungen bei spiritistischen Sitzungen), Planchette *f*

plane Ebene *f*, Fläche *f* / eben, flach / **focal** ~ Brennfläche *f*, Brennlinie *f* / **medial** ~ Medianebene *f* / **median** ~ Medianebene *f* / **principal** ~ Hauptebene *f* / **sagittal** ~ Sagittalebene *f* / **separating** ~ Trennfläche *f*

planimeter Flächenmesser *m*, Planimeter *n*

planimetry Planimetrie *f*

planning Planung *f* / ~ **department** Planungsabteilung *f*, Abteilung *f* für Arbeitsvorbereitung / **urban** ~ Stadtplanung *f* / **vocational** ~ berufliche Planung *f*

planomania pathologischer Wandertrieb *m*, krankhafter Trieb *m* von Zuhause auszubrechen und die gesellschaftlichen Fesseln abzuwerfen

planophrasia Ideenflucht *f*

plantar Fußsohlen–, plantar

plantigrade Sohlengänger *m* / auf die ganze Sohle auftretend

plasma Plasma *n* / ~ **cell** Plasmazelle *f* / ~ **membrane** Plasmahaut *f*, Zellmembran *f*

plastic plastisch

plasticity Plastizität *f*, Formbarkeit *f* / **~ of the libido** Plastizität *f* der Libido / **neural ~** neurale Plastizität *f*

plate Platte *f*, Tafel *f* / **basal ~** Basalplatte *f* / **coloured ~ s** farbige Tafeln *fpl* / **dorsal ~** Dorsalplatte *f* / **inverted ~** umgekehrte Tafel *f* / **medullary ~** Neuralplatte *f* / **metallic ~** Metallplatte *f* / **motor ~** motorische Endplatte *f* / **neural ~** Neuralplatte *f*, Nervenplatte *f* / **pseudoisochromatic ~s** pseudoisochromatische Tafeln *fpl*, Ishihara–Tafeln *fpl* / **sensitive ~** lichtempfindliche Platte *f* / **sensitized ~** lichtempfindliche Platte *f* / **terminal ~** Nervenendplatte *f*

plateau Plateau *n* / **~ formation** Plateaubildung *f* / **~ phase** Plateauphase *f* / **~ test** Plateautest *m*

platform, orgasmic orgastische Manschette *f*

Platonic platonisch

platonisation Idealisierung *f*, Sublimation *f*, Platonisierung *f*

platonist Platoniker *m*

platycephalia, platycephalism, platycephaly Flachköpfigkeit *f*, Plattköpfigkeit *f*, Platyzephalie *f*

platycephalic, platycephalous flachköpfig, plattköpfig, platyzephal

platycephalus Flachkopf *m*, Plattkopf *m*, Platyzephalus *m*

platykurtic flachgipflig, abgeflacht, platykurtisch

plausibility Wahrscheinlichkeit *f*, Plausibilität *f*, Glaubwürdigkeit *f*

play Spiel *n* / spielen / **~ analysis** Spielanalyse *f* / **~–down** herabspielen / **~ group** Spielgruppe *f* / **~ instinct** Spieltrieb *m* / **~ need** Spielbedürfnis *n* / **~–pen** Laufgitter *n* für Kinder / **~ projection** Spielprojektion *f* / **~–room** Spielzimmer *n*, Spielraum *n* / **~ technique** Spieltherapie *f*, Spieltechnik *f* / **~ therapy** Spieltherapie *f* / **fair ~** ehrliches Verhalten *n*, Fair play *n* / **free ~** freies Spiel *n* / **organized ~** geregeltes Spiel *n*, geleitetes Spiel *n* / **parallel ~** paralleles Spiel *n* / **projective ~** projektives spielerisches Gestaltungsverfahren *n* / **symbolic ~** symbolisches Spiel *n*

playback Wiedergabe *f*

playful spielend, scherzhaft, ausgelassen

playfulness Spielerei *f*, Ausgelassenheit *f*

playground Spielplatz *m*, Schulhof *m*

pleasant erfreulich, angenehm, liebenswürdig / **~–unpleasant** angenehm–unangenehm

pleasantness Heiterkeit *f*, Freundlichkeit *f*

pleasurable Lust–, lustvoll, hedonisch

pleasure Lust *f*, Freude *f*, Vergnügen *n* / **~ within anxiety** Angstlust *f* / **~–appetite** Esslust *f* / **~ centre** Lustzentrum *n* / **~ in eating** Esslust *f* / **~–ego** Lust–Ich *n* / **~ in evacuating** Entleerungslust *f*, Exkretionslust *f* / **~ from gratification** Befriedigungslust *f* / **~ in hating** Hasslust *f* / **~ in movement** Bewegungslust *f* / **~ object** Lustobjekt *n* / **~–pain principle** Lust–Unlust–Prinzip *n* / **~ in pain** Schmerzlust *f* / **~ principle** Lustprinzip *n* / **~–seeking** vergnügungssüchtig / **functional ~** Funktionslust *f* / **sensual ~** sinnliche Lust *f* / **solitary ~** Masturbation *f*, Onanie *f*

pleiotropia, pleiotropism Pleiotropie *f*, Polyphänie *f*

pleomorphic, pleomorphous vielgestaltig, in mehreren Formen vorkommend, polymorph, pleomorph

pleomorphism Vielgestaltigkeit *f*, Polymorphismus *m*, Pleomorphismus *m*

pleonexia Geiz *m*, Habsucht *f*, heftiges Verlangen *n*

plesiomorphic, plesiomorphous von nahezu gleicher Gestalt

plesiomorphism nahezu gleiche Gestalt

plethoric vollblütig

plethysmogram Volumenpulskurve *f*, Plethysmogramm *n*

plethysmograph Plethysmograph *m*, Volumenpulskurvenschreiber *m*

plethysmographic plethysmographisch

plethysmography Aufzeichnung *f* von Volumenpulskurven, Plethysmographie *f*

plethysmometry Plethysmometrie *f*, Volumenmessung *f*

plexus Geflecht *n*, Nervengeflecht *n*, Plexus *m* / **brachial ~** Brachialplexus *m* / **cervical ~** Halsnervengeflecht *n* / **coeliac ~** Sonnengeflecht *n* / **hypogastric ~** autonomes Nervengeflecht *n* / **lumbosacral ~** Beingeflecht *n* / **myenteric ~** Auerbach–Plexus *m*, Plexus myentericus *m* / **solar ~** Sonnengeflecht *n*, Solarplexus *m* / **submucous ~** Meißner–Plexus *m*, Plexus submucosus *m*

pliability, pliancy Anpassungsfähigkeit *f*, Flexibilität *f*, Nachgiebigkeit *f*, Beeinflussbarkeit *f*

pliable anpassungsfähig, flexibel, nachgiebig, beeinflussbar

plosive Verschlusslaut *m* / Verschluss *m*

plot aufzeichnen, graphisch darstellen

plotting of curves Kurvenaufzeichnung *f*, Kurvenauswertung *f*

plunger Taucher *m*

pluralism Pluralismus *m* / **~ of feelings** Pluralismus *m* der Gefühle

pluralistic pluralistisch

plurality Vielzahl *f*, Mehrheit *f*

plurel Klasse *f*, Kategorie *f*, Gruppe *f*

plus plus, extra, Mehr–

plutomania Sucht *f* nach Reichtum, Plutomanie *f*

pneograph Atemkurvenschreiber *m*

pneometer Spirometer *n*

pneoscope Pneumograph *m*

pneuma Lebenshauch *m*, Seele *f*, Pneuma *n*

pneumatic pneumatisch, luftgefüllt, Luft–

pneumatogram Atmungskurve *f*, Pneumatogramm *n*

pneumatograph Pneumatograph *m*, Gerät *n* zur Aufzeichnung von Atemkurven

pneumatography Atemkurvenaufzeichnung *f*, Pneumatographie *f* / **cerebral ~** Pneumenzephalographie *f*

pneumatology Atmungslehre *f*, Pneumologie *f*

pneumatometer Atemluftmesser *m*, Pneumatometer *n*, Spirometer *n*

pneumatotherapy Luftbehandlung *f*, Pneumatotherapie *f*

pneumencephalography Luftenzephalographie *f*, Pneumenzephalographie *f*

pneumocardiograph Luftkardiograph *m*, Pneumokardiograph *m*

pneumoencephalogram Pneumenzephalogramm *n*, Luftenzephalogramm *n*

pneumoencephalography Pneumenzephalographie *f*, Luftenzephalographie *f*

pneumogastric pneumogastrisch, Magen und Lunge betreffend

pneumogram Pneumatogramm *n*, Atmungskurve *f*

pneumograph Pneumatograph *m*, Gerät *n* zur Aufzeichnung von Atemkurven

pneumography Atemkurvenaufzeichnung *f*, Pneumatographie *f*

pneumometer Pneumatometer *n*, Spirometer *n*

pneumonia Lungenentzündung *f*, Pneumonie *f*

pneumothorax Pneumothorax *m*

poetry Dichtung *f*, Dichtkunst *f*, Poesie *f* / **~ therapy** Poesietherapie *f*

Poetzl phenomenon Poetzl–Phänomen *n*

Poggendorff illusion Poggendorf'sche Täuschung *f*

poikilotherm wechselwarmes Tier *n*

poikilothermal, poikilothermic wechselwarm, poikilotherm

point Punkt *m*, Spitze *f* / hinweisen, zeigen, punktieren / **~ binomial** Binomialverteilung *f* / **~ biserial correlation** punktbiseriale Korrelation *f* / **~ of convergence**

Konvergenzpunkt *m* / ~ **density** Punktedichte *f* / ~ **of departure** Ausgangspunkt *m* / ~ **estimation** Punktschätzung *f* / ~ **of fixation** Fixationspunkt *m* / ~**-hour ratio** Durchschnitt *m* der erzielten Klassennoten / ~ **of initiation** Ausgangspunkt *m* / ~**-to-point correspondence** Punkt-für Punkt-Entsprechung *f* / ~**-to-point projection** Punkt-für-Punkt-Projektion *f* / ~ **of reference** Bezugspunkt *m* / ~ **of regard** Fixationspunkt *m*, Blickpunkt *m* / ~ **sampling** punktuelle Stichprobenerhebung *f* / ~ **scale** Punkteskala *f* / ~ **score** Punktwert *m*, Rohwert *m* / ~ **score system** Punktebewertungssystem *n* / ~ **source** punktförmige Lichtquelle *f* / ~ **of subjective equality** Punkt *m* subjektiver Gleichheit, Äquivalenzpunkt *m* / ~ **of symmetry** Symmetriepunkt *m*, Äquivalenzpunkt *m* / ~ **system** Punktesystem *n* / **affective nodal** ~**s** affektive Knotenpunkte *mpl* / **anchoring** ~ Bezugspunkt *m* / **cardinal** ~ Hauptpunkt *m* / **cold** ~ Kältepunkt *m* / **congruent** ~ **s** kongruente Punkte *mpl* / **corresponding retinal** ~**s** korrespondierende Netzhautpunkte *mpl* / **critical** ~ kritischer Punkt *m* / **cut-off** ~ Entscheidungspunkt *m*, Grenzwert *m* / **disparate retinal** ~**s** disparate Netzhautpunkte *mpl* / **excitatory** ~ Erregungspunkt *m* / **far** ~ Fernpunkt *m* / **focal** ~ Brennpunkt *m* / **hot** ~ Wärmepunkt *m* / **identical** ~**s** identische Netzhautpunkte *mpl* / **indifferent** ~ Indifferenzpunkt *m* / **motor** ~ elektrischer Reizpunkt *m* / **near** ~ Nahpunkt *m* / **neutral** ~ Indifferenzpunkt *m* / **principal** ~ Augenpunkt *m*, Gesichtspunkt *m* / **retinal** ~ Netzhautpunkt *m* / **visual** ~ Blickpunkt *m* / **vital** ~ lebenswichtiger Punkt *m*

pointillism, pointillisme, pointillage Punktmalerei *f*

poise Gleichgewicht *n*, innere Ausgeglichenheit *f*, Gelassenheit *f* / **sanguine** ~ zuversichtliches Gleichgewicht *n* / **tough** ~ festes Gleichgewicht *n*

poised schwebend, ruhend

poison Gift *n* / vergiften / ~ **dependence** Gifthunger *m* / ~**-pen psychotherapy** Schreiben *n* zorniger Briefe zu kathartischen Zwecken (jedoch ohne Absendung)

poisoning Vergiftung *f*, Intoxikation *f* / **occupational** ~ beruflich bedingte Vergiftung *f*

poisonous giftig, toxisch

Poisson| distribution Poisson-Verteilung *f* / ~**'s distribution** Poisson-Verteilung *f* / ~ **index of dispersion** Poisson Streuungsindex *m* / ~ **series** Poisson-Reihe *f*

polar polar, entgegengesetzt

polarimeter Polarimeter *n*

polarimetry Polarimetrie *f*

polarisation Polarisation *f*, optische Drehung *f* / ~ **brushes** Polarisationsbündel *npl*

polariscope Polarimeter *n*

polarised polarisiert

polarity Polarität *f* / ~ **of nervous conduction** Polarität *f* der Nervenleitung

pole Pol *m*

policlinic Stadtkrankenhaus *n*, Poliklinik *f*

policy Grundsatz *m*, Richtlinie *f*, Politik *f* / ~ **making** Betreiben *n* von Politik, Politisieren *n*, Treffen *n* politischer Entscheidungen / **foreign** ~ Außenpolitik *f* / **social** ~ Sozialpolitik *f*

polio spinale Kinderlähmung *f*, Poliomyelitis *f*

poliomyelitis spinale Kinderlähmung *f*, Poliomyelitis *f* / **acute anterior** ~ Heine-Medin-Krankheit *f* / **cerebral** ~ zerebrale Kinderlähmung *f*

politeness Höflichkeit *f*

political politisch

politician Politiker *m*

politics Politik *f*

poll Meinungsumfrage *f*, Umfrage *f*, Befragung *f*, Abstimmung *f*, Stimmenzählung *f*, Kopf *m* / ~ **question** Interviewfrage *f*

pollakisuria, pollakiuria häufiges Harnlassen *n*, Pollakisurie *f*

polling Wahl *f*, Stimmabgabe *f*, Wahlbeteiligung *f*

pollinosis Heuschnupfen *m*, Heufieber *n*

pollster Meinungsforscher *m*, Meinungsforscherin *f*, Interviewer *m*, Interviewerin *f*

pollution Pollution *f*, Samenerguss *m* / Umweltverschmutzung *f* / **nocturnal ~** nächtlicher Samenerguß *m*, Spermaentleerung *f* im Schlaf

Pollyanna blinder Optimist *m*

polyaesthesia, polyesthesia mehrfaches Fühlen *n* eines Berührungsreizes

polyandrous polyandrisch

polyandry Polyandrie *f*, Vielmännerei *f*

polychromasia Polychromasie *f*, Polychromatophilie *f*

polychromatic polychromatisch, mehrfarbig

polychromatophilia Polychromatophilie *f*

polychromic mehrfarbig, vielfarbig

polyclinic stationäre Klinik *f* für alle Krankheiten

polycythemia Polycythämie *f*, Polyzythämie *f*

polydactyl mit überzähligen Fingern versehen

polydactylia, polydactylism, polydactyly Vorhandensein *n* überzähliger Finger, Polydaktylie *f*

polydipsia krankhafter Durst *m*, Polydipsie *f*

polydiurnal mehrmals täglich

polydrug abuse Polytoxikomanie *f*

polygamist Polygamist *m*, Anhänger *m* der Polygamie

polygamous polygam, polygamisch

polygamy Polygamie *f*

polygenes Polygene *npl*

polyglot mehrsprachig, vielsprachig / Polyglotte *m,f*

polygon Polygon *n*, Vieleck *n*

polygonal polygonal, mehrwinklig

polygraph Lügendetektor *m*, Polygraph *m*

polygynous polygyn, mit mehreren Frauen verheiratet

polygyny Vielweiberei *f*, Polygynie *f*

polyideism Polyideismus *m*, Fülle *f* der Gedanken, Gesamtheit *f* psychischer Tätigkeit

polylogia Polyphrasie *f*, Logomanie *f*, Logorrhoe *f*, Redefluss *m*, Schwatzsucht *f*

polymorphic, polymorphous polymorph, vielgestaltig / **~ perverse** polymorph–pervers

polymorphism Vielgestaltigkeit *f*, Polymorphie *f*

polyneural polyneural, mehrere Nerven betreffend

polyneuritic polyneuritisch

polyneuritis Polyneuritis *f* / **alcoholic ~** Alkoholpolyneuritis *f*

polyneuropathy Erkrankung *f* mehrerer Nerven

polyopia, polyopsia, polyopy Mehrfachsehen *n*, Polyopie *f*, Polyopsie *f*

polypathia Multimorbidität *f*

polypeptide Polypeptid *n*

polyphaenia Polyphänie *f*

polyphagia Gefräßigkeit *f*, Bulimie *f*, Polyphagie *f*

polyphobia multiple Angst *f*

polyphony Vielstimmigkeit *f*, Polyphonie *f*

polyphrasia Polyphrasie *f*, Logorrhoe *f*, Logomanie *f*

polypnoea, polypnea schnelles Atmen *n*, Polypnoe *f*

polypragmasy Vielgeschäftigkeit *f*, Polypragmasie *f*

polyradiculoneuritis Polyradikuloneuritis *f*, Guillain–Barré–Syndrom *n*

polysaccharide Polysaccharid *n*

polysubstance dependence Polytoxikomanie *f* / **~–related disorder** Störung *f* im Zusammenhang mit multiplen Substanzen

polysynaptic polysynaptisch, mehrere Synapsen betreffend

polytheism Polytheismus *m*, Vielgötterei *f*

polytrophia Überfütterung *f*

polyuria krankhafte Vermehrung *f* der Harnmenge, Polyurie *f*

polyvalence Polyvalenz *f*, Vielwertigkeit *f*

polyvalent polyvalent, vielwertig

ponderable wägbar, abwägbar

ponderal Gewichts–

ponophobia krankhafte Angst *f* vor Schmerz

pons Brücke *f*, Pons *f* / ~ **Varolii** Varolsbrücke *f* Pons Varoli *f*

pool of pain, primal Urschmerzfundus *m*

pooling Zusammenlegung *f*, Zusammenfassung *f*, Pooling *n*

popular populär, beliebt, weitverbreitet, gängig

popularity Popularität *f*, Beliebtheit *f*

population Bevölkerung *f*, Population *f*, Grundgesamtheit *f* / ~ **characteristics** Bevölkerungsmerkmale *npl* / ~ **control** Geburtenkontrolle *f* / ~ **genetics** Bevölkerungsgenetik *f* / ~ **group** Bevölkerungsgruppe *f* / **infinite** ~ unbestimmte Population *f*

porencephaly Porenzephalie *f*

poriomania Poriomanie *f*, krankhafter Wandertrieb *m*

pornographer Verfasser *m* pornographischer Literatur

pornographic pornographisch, obszön

pornographomania Sucht *f* obszöne Dinge zu verfassen, Pornographomanie *f*

pornography Pornographie *f*, obszöne Darstellungen *fpl*

porphyria Porphyrie *f*, Entgleisung *f* des Porphyrinstoffwechsels

porropsia Porropsie *f*, Wahrnehmungsanomalie *f* mit Verkleinerung der Objekte

port Datenkanal *m*, Anschlussstelle *f* für Peripheriegeräte an einen Rechner

Porter's law Porters Gesetz *n*

Porteus| maze test Porteus–Labyrinth–Test *m* / ~ **test** Porteus–Test *m*

portrait Bild *n* / ~ **of character** Charakterbild *n*

pose Haltung *f*, Pose / hinstellen, in Positur stellen

posiomania periodische Trunksucht *f*, Quartalsäufertum *n*, Dipsomanie *f*

posit voraussetzen, postulieren

position Lage *f*, Stellung *f*, Position *f* / ~ **of checkmate** Mattstellung *f* / ~ **factor** Positionseffekt *m*, Bevorzugung *f* aufgrund der Lage / ~ **in the family** Geburtsordnung *f* / ~ **habit** Gewohnheit *f* zum gleichen Ort zurückzukehren / ~ **preference** Bevorzugung *f* aufgrund der Position, Positionseffekt *m* / ~ **response** Lageantwort *f* / ~ **therapy** Positionstherapie *f* / **a fronte** ~ Koitus *m* von vorn / **a tergo** ~ Koitus *m* von hinten / **depressive** ~ depressive Position *f* / **focal** ~ thematische Position *f* / **ordinal** ~ Position *f* in einer Ordinalskala / **paranoid** ~ paranoide Position *f* / **paranoid–schizoid** ~ paranoid–schizoide Position *f* / **primary** ~ normale Augenstellung *f* / **serial** ~ Stellung *f* in einer Reihe, Rangfolge *f* / **serial** ~ **effect** Reihen–Stellen–Phänomen *n*, Positionseffekt *m* / **social** ~ soziale Position *f*, sozialer Stand *m* / **socio–economic** ~ soziale Position *f*, sozialer Stand *m*

positional positionell, Positions–

positive positiv / ~**–negative** zwischen Annäherungs– und Vermeidungstendenz / ~**–negative ambivalent** positiv zu negativ ambivalent / ~**–positive** zwischen zwei Annäherungstendenzen

positivism Positivismus *m* / **logical** ~ logischer Positivismus *m*, wissenschaftlicher Empirismus *m*

positron emission tomography Positronenemissionstomographie *f*, PET

possessed besessen

possession Besitz *m*, Besessenheit *f* / ~ **disorder** Bessessenheitszustand *m* / **demoniacal** ~ Dämonismus *m*

possessive nach Besitz strebend

possessiveness, possessivity Besitzstreben *n*, Tendenz *f* zum Festhalten

possibility Möglichkeit *f*

possible möglich, denkbar

postactivation potential Postaktivationspotenzial *n*

postambivalent nachambivalent

postcentral hinter einem Hirnzentrum gelegen

postcerebral hinter einem Hirnzentrum gelegen

postcoital nach dem Koitus auftretend

postcornu Hinterhorn *n*

postcure Nachbehandlung *f*

postencephalitic postenzephalitisch

postepileptic nach dem epileptischen Anfall

posterior hintere(r, s), Hinter–

postexperimental nach dem Experiment liegend

postganglionic postganglionär, hinter einem Ganglion liegend

postgraduate postgraduiert, nach der Graduierung, nach dem Diplom, postuniversitär

posthypnotic posthypnotisch

postinfectuous nach einer Infektion auftretend

posting Verschicken *n* von Artikeln in eine Newsgroup

postmature überreif

postmodernism Postmoderne *f*

postnatal nach der Geburt, postnatal

postoperative postoperativ

postpartum nach der Geburt

postpituitary den Hypophysenhinterlappen betreffend

postpuberal, postpubertal nach der Pubertät auftretend

postremity Postremität *f*, Verstärkung *f* des zuletzt aufgetretenen Reizes vor einer Reaktion

postsynaptic postsynaptisch, hinter einer Synapse gelegen

posttesting Nachtesten *n*, Durchführen *n* eines Kontrolltests

posttetanic posttetanisch

posttraumatic posttraumatisch

posttreatment Nachbehandlungf / **~ follow–up** Katamnese *f*

postulate Postulat *n*, Annahme *f* / voraussetzen, annehmen

postulational auf Postulaten basierend, hypothetisch–deduktiv

postural Lage–, Haltungs–

posture Positur *f*, Stellung *f*, Körperhaltung *f* / **~ reflex** Stellreflex *m*

potamophobia krankhafte Angst *f* vor Flüssen

potassium Kalium *n* / **~ chloride** Kaliumchlorid *n* / **~ flux** Kaliumstrom *m* / **~ ion** Kaliumion *n* / **~ pump** Kaliumpumpe *f*

potator Trinker *m*

potence, potency Potenz *f* ,Vermögen *n*, Macht *f*, Wirkung *f* / **impaired ~** Potenzstörung *f*, Impotenz *f* / **magic ~** magische Gewalt *f* / **orgastic ~** orgastische Potenz *f* / **sexual ~** Potenz *f*, geschlechtliche Potenz *f*, Zeugungsfähigkeit *f*

potent mächtig, stark, gewaltig, potent

potential Potenzial *n*, Spannung *f* / potenziell, möglich / **human ~ movement** Bewegung *f* für Selbstverwirklichung / **~ of cerebral cortex** Hirnrindenpotenzial *n* / **~ of hydrogen value** pH–Wert *m* / **auditory evoked ~** auditiv evoziertes Potenzial *n* / **bio–electrical ~** bioelektrisches Potenzial *n* / **cochlear ~s** Mikrophonpotenziale *npl* / **corneoretinal ~** Korneoretinalpotenzial *n*, korneoretinales Bestandspotenzial *n* / **cortical ~** Rindenpotenzial *n* / **cortical evoked ~** evoziertes Rindenpotenzial *n*, kortikal evoziertes Potenzial *n* / **dendritic ~** Dendritenpotenzial *n* / **effective excitatory ~** effektives Reaktionspotenzial *n* / **evoked ~** Reizpotenzial *n*, Reaktionspotenzial *n*, evoziertes Potenzial *n* / **excitatory ~** Erregungspotenzial *n*, Reaktionspotenzial *n* / **excitatory postsynaptic ~** postsynaptisches Erregungspotenzial *n* / **inhibitory ~** Hemmungspotenzial *n* / **inhibitory postsynaptic ~** postsynaptisches Hemmungspotenzial *n*, inhibitorisch–postsynaptisches Potenzial *n* / **local excitatory ~** lokales Erregungspotenzial *n* / **maintained ~** Bestandspotenzial *n*, Ruhepotenzial *n* / **microphonic ~s** Mikrophonpotenziale *npl* / **olfactory evoked ~** durch Gerüche evoziertes Reaktionspotenzial *n*, olfaktorisch evoziertes Potenzial *n* / **paroxysmal ~** Spitzenpotenzial *n* / **postsynaptic ~** postsynaptisches Potenzial *n* / **resting ~** Ruhepotenzial *n*, Bestandspotenzial *n* / **reversal ~** Umkehrpotenzial *n* / **slow ~** langsames Potenzial *n* / **somatosensory evoked ~** somatosensorisch evoziertes Potenzial *n* / **spinal ~** Rückenmarkspotenzial *n* / **suicidal ~** Suizidalität *f* / **synaptic ~** synaptisches Potenzial *n*, Synapsenpotenzial *n* / **vital ~** Vitalpotenzial *n* / **visual evoked ~** visuell evoziertes Potenzial *n*

potentiality Möglichkeit *f*, latente Kraft *f*

potentiation Potenzierung *f* / **tetanic ~** tetanische Potenzierung *f*

potlach Geschenk *n*, Indianerwettkampf *m* mit Zerstörung von Besitztümern

potomania Trunksucht *f*, Potomanie *f*

poverty Armut *f*, Mangel *m* / **~ area** Elendsviertel *n*, Elendsquartier *n*, Armenviertel *n* / **~ of speech** Sprachverarmung *f* / **dire ~** schreckliche Armut *f*

power Kraft *f*, Stärke *f*, Vermögen *n*, Fähigkeit *f*, Macht *f*, Einfluss *m* / **~ of absorption** Saugkraft *f* / **~ of apprehension** Auffassungsfähigkeit *f* / **~ complex** Machtkomplex *m* / **~ of comprehension** Begriffsfähigkeit *f* / **~ of concentration** Konzentrationsvermögen *n*, Konzentrationsfähigkeit *f* / **~ of configuration** Gestaltungskraft *f* / **~ curve** Leistungskurve *f* / **~ drive** Machttrieb *m*, Machtstreben *n* / **~ factor** Energiefaktor *m* / **~ fields** Kraftfelder *npl* / **~ figure** Autoritätsperson *f* / **~ function** Leistungsfähigkeit *f* eines statistischen Tests, Potenzfunktion *f* / **~ of imagination** Vorstellungskraft *f* / **~ instinct** Machttrieb *m* / **~ of intuition** Anschauungsvermögen *n* / **~ law** Potenzgesetz *n* / **~ of a statistical test** Leistungsfähigkeit *f* eines statistischen Tests / **~ of suggestion** Suggestionskraft *f* / **~ test** Niveautest *m*, Power–Test *m* / **~ of vision** Sehkraft *f* / **~ want** Machtstreben *n*, Machtbedürfnis *n* / **attractive ~** Anziehungskraft *f* / **coercive ~** brachiale Gewalt *f* / **configurative ~** Gestaltungskraft *f* / **creative ~** schöpferische Kraft *f* / **discriminating ~** Unterscheidungsempfindlichkeit *f* / **discriminatory ~** Unterscheidungsempfindlichkeit *f* / **discursive ~** schlussfolgerndes Denken *n* / **estimative ~** Schätzfähigkeit *f* / **executive ~** Vollzugsgewalt *f*, Macht *f* / **generative ~** Zeugungsfähigkeit *f* / **instrumental ~** instrumentelle Macht *f* / **mental ~** Geisteskraft *f* / **reasoning ~** Denkvermögen *n*, Intelligenz *f* / **refractive ~** Brechungsvermögen *n* / **resolving ~** Auflösungsvermögen *n* / **social ~** gesellschaftliche Macht *f*, sozialer Einfluss *m* / **statistical ~** statistische Teststärke *f* / **visual ~** Sehkraft *f*

powerful mächtig, kräftig, einflussreich

powerless machtlos, kraftlos, unfähig

practical praktisch, angewandt

practicalness Geschicktheit *f*

practice Übung *f*, Praxis *f* / üben / **~ curve** Übungskurve *f* / **~ effect** Übungseffekt *m*, Übungswirkung *f* / **~ limit** Übungsgrenze *f* / **~ material** Übungsmaterial *n* / **~ period** Übungszeitraum *m* / **~ phase** Übungsphase *f* / **~ theory** Übungstheorie *f* / **distributed ~** verteilte Übung *f*, Wiederholung *f* in Abständen / **massed ~** massierte Übung *f*, gedrängtes Lernen *n* / **medical ~** ärztliche Praxis *f* / **negative ~** negative Übung *f* / **private ~** Privatpraxis *f* / **religious ~s** religiöse Riten *mpl*, religiöse Bräuche *mpl* / **spaced ~** verteilte Übung *f*, verteiltes Lernen *n* / **supervi-**

sory ~s test Test *m* des Vorgesetztenverhaltens / **unspaced ~** gedrängtes Lernen *n*, gedrängte Übung *f*

practician Praktiker *m*

practitioner, general Allgemeinmediziner *m*, praktischer Arzt *m*

practicum studienbegleitendes Praktikum *n* / **~ supervision** Praktikumsbetreuung *f*

practise üben

practising Üben *n*, Übung *f*

praecox vorzeitig, frühreif, praecox

Prader–Willi syndrome Prader–Willi–Syndrom *n*

pragmatagnosia Nichterkennen *n* von Gegenständen, Pragmatagnosie *f*

pragmatamnesia Verlust *m* des Erinnerungsvermögens für Gegenstände, Pragmatamnesie *f*

pragmatic, pragmatical pragmatisch, sachlich

pragmatics Pragmatik *f*

pragmatism Pragmatismus *m*

praise loben / Lob *n*

praxernia praktisches gewissenhaftes Verhalten *n*, konventioneller Sinn *m* für das Praktische, Praxernie *f*

praxia Praxie *f*, Handlungsgestalt *f*

praxinoscope Praxinoskop *n*

praxiology Neobehaviorismus *m*

praxis Praxis *f*, Handlung *f*

prayer Gebet *n*, Beter *m*, Beterin *f*

preadolescence Vorreifezeit *f*

preadolescent Präadoleszente *m,f*

preadult jugendlich, vor dem Erwachsenenalter liegend

preambivalent vorambivalent

precausality vorkausales Denken *n*, Präkausalität *f*, Vorkausalität *f*

precentral vor dem Zentrum gelegen

precentre, precenter Vorzentrum *n*, vorläufiger Mittelpunkt *m*

precipitate übereilt, überstürzt, plötzlich

precipitation Übereilung *f*, Überstürzung *f*, Hast *f*

précis Zusammenenfassung *f*, Inhaltsangabe *f*, Resümee *n*

precise genau, bestimmt, präzis, richtig

preciseness Genauigkeit *f*, Pedanterie *f*

precision Genauigkeit *f*, Präzision *f* / **~ alternative** „Oder"–Antwort *f* / **~ law** Prägnanzgesetz *n* / **relative ~** relative Genauigkeit *f*

preclude ausschließen

precocious frühreif

precocity, precociousness Frühreife *f* / **sexual ~** sexuelle Frühreife *f*, vorzeitige Geschlechtsreife *f*

precodingVorkodierung *f*, vorherige Klasseneinteilung *f*

precognition Hellsehen *n*, Präkognition *f*, Prophetie *f*

preconceived vorgefasst, vorher ausgedacht

preconception Vorurteil *n*, vorgefasste Meinung *f*, Vorbegriff *m*

preconceptual vorbegrifflich

precondition Vorbedingung *f* / **~ of anxiety** Angstbedingung *f*

preconditioning Vorbedingen *n*, Vorkonditionieren *n*, Präkonditionierung *f* / **sensory ~** sensorisches Vorkonditionieren *n*

preconscious Vorbewusstes *n* / vorbewusst

preconsciousness Vorbewusstsein *n*

precornu Vorderhorn *n*

precox vorzeitig, frühreif, praecox

precuneus Vorkeil *m*

predelay Verzögerung *f*, Vorverzögerung *f*

predelinquent potenzieller Straftäter *m*

predelirium Prädelirium tremens *n*

predetermine vorherbestimmen, im Voraus bestimmen

predicament Kategorie *f*, Klasse *f*

predicate behaupten, aussagen / Prädikat *n*, Aussage *f*

predication Behauptung *f*, Aussage *f*, Predigt *f*

predicative prädikativ

predict vorhersagen

predictability Vorhersagbarkeit *f*, Prognostizierbarkeit *f*, Vorhersage *f*, Voraussage *f*, Prognose *f*

prediction Vorhersage *f*, Voraussage *f*, Prognose *f* / **~ error** Vorhersagefehler *m* / **clinical ~** klinische Prognose *f* / **differential ~** differenzielle Vorhersage *f* / **statistical ~** statistische Vorhersage *f*

predictive Vorhersage–

predictor Vorhersageinstrument *n*, Vorhersagevariable *f*, Prädiktor *m*

predilection Vorliebe *f*

predispose prädisponieren, empfänglich machen

predisposed empfänglich, veranlagt, prädisponiert

predisposing predisponierend

predisposition Disposition *f*, Veranlagung *f*, Prädisposition *f*, Anlage *f* / **genetic ~** erbliche Veranlagung *f*, genetische Anlage *f* / **hereditary ~** erbliche Veranlagung *f*, erbliche Disposition *f*

prednisolone Prednisolon *n*

predominance Vorherrschen *n*, Übergewicht *n*, Vorwiegen *n* / **~ of the unconscious** Vorherrschaft *f* des Unbewussten

predominant dominierend, vorherrschend

predominantly vorwiegend, in erster Linie

predormitium, predormition Einschlafstadium *n* / **~ thoughts** Einschlafdenken *n*

predyslexic im Vorfeld einer Lesestörung

preemptive Prioritäts–, Ausschließlichkeits–

preepileptic präepileptisch

preexperimental vor dem Experiment liegend

prefer vorziehen

preference Bevorzugung *f*, Vorliebe *f*, Vorzug *m*, Präferenz *f* / **~ inventory** Interessenfragebogen *m* / **~ measure** Maß *n* der Bevorzugung, Präferenzmessverfahren *n* / **~ method** Wahlmethode *f*, Vorzugsmethode *f* / **~ procedure** Wahlverfahren *n*, Vorzugsmethode *f* / **~ scale** Bevorzugungsskala *f* / **~ test** Bevorzugungstest *m*, Interessentest *m* / **aesthetic ~** künstlerische Bevorzugung *f*, ästhetische Präferenz *f* / **occupational ~** berufliche Präferenz *f*, Berufsneigung *f* / **occupational ~ inventory** Berufsinteressentest *m* / **vocational ~** Berufsneigung *f*

preferential Vorzugs–, bevorzugt

prefiguration vorherige Darstellung *f*, Vorbild *n*

preformation Präformation *f*, Vorausbildung *f* / **~ theory** Präformationstheorie *f*

preformed vorgebildet, angelegt, präformiert

preformism Präformationstheorie *f*

prefrontal präfrontal

preganglionic präganglionär, vor einem Ganglion liegend

pregeniculum body äußerer Kniehöcker *m*

pregenital prägenital, vorgenital

pregenitality prägenitale Phase *f*

pregnance Prägnanz *f* / **~ theory** Prägnanztheorie *f*

pregnancy Schwangerschaft *f*, Gravidität *f* / **~ phobia** Schwangerschaftsphobie *f* / **~ psychosis** Schwangerschaftspsychose *f* / **~ test** Schwangerschaftstest *m* / **adolescent ~** Schwangerschaft *f* im Jugendalter / **false ~** Pseudogravidität *f*, Scheinschwangerschaft *f* / **hysteric ~** eingebildete Schwangerschaft *f* / **hysterical ~** eingebildete Schwangerschaft *f* / **nervous ~** psychogene Schwangerschaft *f* / **spurious ~** Scheinschwangerschaft *f* / **teenage ~** Schwangerschaft *f* bei einer Minderjährigen

pregnant gravid, schwanger

prehensile greiffähig, Greif–

prehension Greifen *n*, Greifvorgang *m*, geistiges Erfassen *n* / **~ test** Greiftest *m*

prehypophysis Hypophysenvorderlappen *m*

prejudgement, prejudgment Vorurteil *n*

prejudice Vorurteil *n*, Voreingenommenheit *f* / **racial ~** rassisches Vorurteil *n* / **religious ~** religiöses Vorurteil *n* / **social ~** soziales Vorurteil *n*

prelinguistic, prelingual vorsprachlich

preliterate ohne Schriftsprache, primitiv

prelogical prälogisch, vorlogisch

Premack's principle Premack–Prinzip *n*

premaniacal vormanisch, unmittelbar vor einem manischen Anfall liegend

premanifestation Vorgestalt *f*

premarital vorehelich

premature frühreif

prematurity Frühreife *f*, Unreife *f*

premedication Vorbehandlung *f*

premeditation Vorbedacht *m*

premenstrual prämenstruell

premise, premiss Voraussetzung *f*, Prämisse *f* / voraussetzen, vorausschicken

premonition Warnung *f*, Vorahnung *f*, Vorgefühl *n*

premonitory warnend, prämonitorisch

premorbid kränklich, krankhaft, prämorbid

premorbidity Prämorbidität *f*, vor Beginn einer Krankheit auftretende Anomalie *f*

premotor prämotorisch

prenatal pränatal, vorgeburtlich

preneurotic präneurotisch, im Vorfeld einer Neurose befindlich

prenubile noch nicht heiratsfähig

prenuptial vorehelich

preoccupation Voreingenommenheit *f*, Versunkensein *n*, Vertieftsein *n*

preoccupied in Anspruch genommen, zerstreut, geistesabwesend

preoedipal, pre–Oedipal präödipal

preovulatory präovulatorisch

preparalytic präparalytisch

preparation Vorbereitung *f*, Präparation *f*

preparatory vorbereitend, Vorbereitungs–

preparedness Bereitschaft *f*

preperceive eine Erwartungshaltung besitzen, eine Wahrnehmungseinstellung bilden

prepercept Inhalt *m* einer Erwartungshaltung

preperception Erwartungshaltung *f*, Wahrnehmungseinstellung *f*

preperceptual Wahrnehmungseinstellungs–, antizipatorisch wahrnehmend

preponderance Überwiegen *n*, Übergewicht *n* / **~ of responses to colour** Farbreaktion *f* / **directional ~** Überwiegen *n* einer Blickrichtung

prepossession Voreingenommenheit *f*, Vorurteil *n*

prepotence Vorherrschen *n*

prepotency Vorherrschaft *f*, Vormacht *f*, stärkere Vererbungskraft *f*

prepotent vorherrschend, dominant

prepsychopathic präpsychopathisch

prepsychotic präpsychotisch

prepuberal, prepubertal Vorpubertäts–, vor der Pubertät liegend

prepuberty Vorpubertät *f*, Präpubertät *f*

prepulse inhibition Schreckreflexhemmung *f*

presbyacusia, presbyacusis Altersschwerhörigkeit *f*, Presbyakusis *f*

presbyatrics, presbyatry Geriatrie *f*, Wissenschaft *f* von den Alterskrankheiten

presbyophrenia Altersdemenz *f*, Presbyophrenie *f*

presbyopia Alterssichtigkeit *f*, Presbyopie *f*

presbyopic alterssichtig

preschizophrenia beginnende Schizophrenie *f*, Vorfeld *n* einer manifesten Schizophrenie

preschool Vorschul–

prescription drugs verschreibungspflichtige Medikamente *npl*

presence Vorhandensein *n*, Anwesenheit *f* / **~ of mind** Geistesgegenwart *f* / **psychic ~** geistige Präsenz *f*, Geistesgegenwart *f*

presenile präsenil

presenility vorzeitige Alterung *f*, Präsenilität *f*

present gegenwärtig, vorhanden / Gegenwart *f*, Präsenz *f* / vorführen, darbieten, präsentieren, überreichen / **psychological ~** psychische Präsenzzeit *f* / **sensory ~** psychische Präsenzzeit *f* / **specious ~** scheinbare Gegenwart *f*, psychische Präsenz *f*

presentable vorzeigbar, präsentierbar

presentation Darbietung *f*, Vorstellung *f* / **~ method** Darbietungsmethode *f* / **~ mode** Darbietungsweise *f* / **graphic ~** graphische Darstellung *f* / **stereoscopic ~** stereoskopische Darbietung *f*, räumliche Darbietung *f* / **tachistoscopic ~** tachistoskopische Darbietung *f*

presentiment Vorahnung *f*, Vorgefühl *n*

preservation Erhaltung *f* / **~ of self** Selbsterhaltung *f* / **~ of the species** Arterhaltung *f*

preservative erhaltend, Schutz– / Schutzmittel *n*, Präservativ *n*

preside den Vorsitz führen, präsidieren, herrschen

press Umwelteinfluss *m*, Umwelteffekt *m*, „press" *n* / **~–need** Thema *n*

pressor blutdruckerhöhend / blutdruckerhöhendes Mittel *n*

pressoreceptive auf Druckreiz reagierend, pressorezeptiv

pressoreceptor Druckrezeptor *m*, Pressorezeptor *m*

pressure Druck *m*, Drang *m* / **~ balance** Druckwaage *f* / **~ block** Druckblock *m* / **~ blower** Gebläse *n* / **~ on the brain** Hirndruck *m* / **~ gradient** Druckgradient *m* / **~ group** Lobby *f*, Interessengruppe *f* / **~ level** Druckpegel *m*, Druckniveau *n* / **~ point** Druckpunkt *m*, Gefäßdruckpunkt *m* / **~ sensation** Druckempfindung *f* / **~ sense** Drucksinn *m* / **~ sensibility** Druckempfindlichkeit *f*, Drucksensibilität *f* / **~ spot** Druckpunkt *m* / **~ stimulus** Druckreiz *m* / **~ of thought** Gedankendrängen *n*, Gedankenjagen *n* / **~ toward uniformity** Druck *m* zu gleichförmigem sozialen Verhalten / **acoustic ~ level** Schalldruckpegel *m* / **barometric ~** Luftdruck *m* / **cerebral ~** Hirndruck *m* / **diastolic ~** diastolischer Blutdruck *m* / **intracranial ~** Schädelinnendruck *m* / **minimal audible ~** eben hörbarer Schalldruck *m* / **osmotic ~** osmotischer Druck *m* / **precordial ~** Präkordialangst *f* / **social ~** sozialer Druck *m* / **static ~** statischer Druck *m* / **systolic ~** systolischer Blutdruck *m*

prestige Prestige *n* / **~ bias** Verfälschung *f* durch Prestigeeinflüsse / **~ motive** Prestigebedürfnis *n* / **~ suggestion** Prestigesuggestion *f*

prestretching Vordehnung *f*

prestriate vor dem Corpus striatum liegend

presumption Annahme *f*, Vermutung *f*, Anmaßung *f*

presumptive mutmaßlich, präsumptiv

presumptuous eingebildet, anmaßend, vermessen

presuppose voraussetzen, postulieren

presupposition Voraussetzung *f*, Postulat *n*

presymbolic vorsymbolisch

presynaptic präsynaptisch, vor einer Synapse gelegen

pretence, pretense Anspruch *m*, Anmaßung *f*, Vorspiegelung *f*

pretend vorgeben, vortäuschen

pretest Vortest *m*, Probebefragung *f*

pretesting Vortesten *n*, Vortest *m*

prevalence Prävalenz *f*

prevalent vorherrschend, weit verbreitet, häufig

prevenception Empfängnisverhütung *f*

prevention Prävention *f*, Verhütung *f*, Verhinderung *f*, Prophylaxe *f* / **~ of accidents** Unfallverhütung *f* / **~ of conception** Empfängnisverhütung *f* / **primary ~** primäre Prävention *f* / **secondary ~** sekundäre Prävention *f* / **tertiary ~** tertiäre Prävention *f*

preventive vorbeugend, präventiv

preverbal präverbal, vorsprachlich

previous vorhergehend, früher

prevision Vorhersehen *n*, Voraussicht *f*, Ahnung *f*

Preyer's pinna reflex Preyer–Ohrmuschelreflex *m*

priapism Priapismus *m*, Dauererektion *f* des Penis

prick stechen, punktieren, mit Punkten versehen / **~ test** Prick–Test *m*

prickings of conscience Gewissensbisse *mpl*

pride Stolz *m*, Hochmut *m* / **~ system** System *n* des neurotischen Stolzes / **neurotic ~** neurotischer Stolz *m*

primacy Primat *m*, Vorrang *m*, Priorität *f* / **~ effect** Primat–Effekt *m* / **~ of the genitals** Genitalprimat *m* / **~–recency effect** Primat–Rezenz–Effekt *m* / **~ zone** Primatzone *f* / **genital ~** Genitalprimat *m* / **motor ~ theory** Theorie *f* des Bewegungsprimats / **oral ~** oraler Primat *m* / **phallic ~** Genitalprimat *m*

prima facie dem ersten Anschein nach, auf den ersten Eindruck

primal erster, frühester, Ur– / Urerlebnis *n*

primary ursprünglich, primär, Ur– / Grundfarbe *f* / **psychological ~** psychologische Grundfarbe *f*

primates Menschenaffen *mpl*, Primaten pl

prime erster, frühester, Haupt–, Grund–, wichtigster

primidone Primidon *n*

priming assoziative Aktivierung *f*, Priming *n* / **semantic ~** semantisches Priming *n*

primipara Erstgebärende *f*

primiparity erstmaliges Gebären *n*

primiparous erstgebärend

primitivation, primitivisation Regression *f*, Rückschritt *m*, Primitivierung *f*

primitive ursprünglich, primitiv, Grund–

primitiveness Primitivität *f*, Ursprünglichkeit *f*

primitivism Primitivismus *m*, Glaube *m* an das Primitive

primordial ursprünglich, primär, primitiv

primordium Anlage *f*

principal Haupt–, führend, hervorragend / Rektor *m*, Direktor *m*, Vorgesetzter *m*, Hauptperson *f*

principle Prinzip *n*, Grundsatz *m* / **~ of advantage** Gesetz *n* des Vorteils / **~ of analogy** Analogieprinzip *n* / **~ of associative shifting** Prinzip *n* der assoziativen Verschiebung / **~ of belongingness** Zugehörigkeitsgesetz *n* / **~ of concurrency** Übereinstimmungsprinzip *n* / **~ of configuration** Gestaltungsprinzip *n* / **~ of constance** Konstanzprinzip *n* / **~ of constancy** Konstanzprinzip *n* / **~ of contemporaneity** Gleichzeitigkeitspostulat *n* / **~ of continuity** Kontinuitätsprinzip *n* / **~ of contradiction** Gesetz *n* des Widerspruchs / **~ of correspondence** Korrespondenzprinzip *n* / **~ of creative resultants** Prinzip *n* der schöpferischen Synthese / **~ of disuse** Entwöhnungsprinzip *n* / **~ of duality** Dualitätsprinzip *n* / **~ of dynamogenesis** dynamogenetisches Prinzip / **~** / **~ of economy** Sparsamkeitsprinzip *n*, Ökonomieprinzip *n* / **~ of Gestalt** Gestaltprinzip *n*, Gestaltgesetz *n* / **~ of impressiveness** Prinzip *n* der Beeindruckbarkeit / **~ of inertia** Trägheitsprinzip *n* / **~ of intimacy** Prinzip *n* der Vertrautheit / **~ of isomorphism** Isomorphieprinzip *n* / **~ of maturation** Reifeprinzip *n* / **~ of multiple control** Prinzip *n* der Mehrfachsicherung / **~ of multiple functions** Prinzip *n* der Mehrfachfunktion / **~ of multiple reaction** Prinzip *n* der Mehrfachreaktion / **~ of multiple response** Prinzip *n* der Mehrfachantwort / **~ of neuronic inertia** Prinzip *n* der Neuronenträgheit, Trägheitsprinzip *n* / **~ of parsimony** Sparsamkeitsprinzip *n*, Ökonomieprinzip *n*, Morgans Kanon *m* / **~ of pleasure** Lustprinzip *n* / **~ of proximity** Gesetz *n* der Nähe / **~ of reality** Realitätsprinzip *n* / **~ of relativity** Relativitätsprinzip *n* / **~ of stability** Stabilitätsprinzip *n* / **~ of suf-**

ficient reason Prinzip *n* des hinreichenden Grundes / **~ of varied reaction** Prinzip *n* der Mehrfachreaktion / **all–or–nothing ~** Alles–oder–Nichts–Gesetz *n* / **descriptive ~** Prinzip *n* der Beschreibung / **economic ~** ökonomisches Prinzip *n* / **fundamental ~** Grundprinzip *n* / **indicating ~** Leitsatz *m* / **phylogenetic ~** phylogenetisches Prinzip *n*, biogenetisches Grundgesetz *n* / **subtractive ~** subtraktives Prinzip *n*

print drucken / Druck *m*, Abdruck *m*

printing Drucken *n*, Druckschrift *f*, Druckbuchstaben *mpl*

prior vorhergehend, früher

priority Priorität *f*, Vorrang *m*

prism Prisma *n* / **~ diopter** prismatische Standardabweichung *f*

prismatic prismatisch

prison Gefängnis *n*, Haftanstalt *f* / **~ depression** Haftdepression *f* / **~ inmate** Häftling *m*, Strafgefangener *m* / **~ personnel** Gefängnispersonal *n* / **~ psychosis** Haftpsychose *f*

prisoner Häftling *m*, Strafgefangene *m,f* / **~ dilemma game** Häftlingsdilemmaspiel *n* / **~'s psychosis** Ganser'sches Syndrom *n*, simulierte Geistesstörung *f* / **~ of war** Kriegsgefangene *m,f*

privacy Privatleben *n*, Privatsphäre *f*

private privat, Privat–, persönlich, vertraulich

privation Entbehrung *f*, Entziehung *f*

privilege Privileg *n*, Vorrecht *n*

proactive proaktiv

probabilism Probabilismus *m*

probabilistic probabilistisch

probability Wahrscheinlichkeit *f* / **~ chart** Wahrscheinlichkeitstafel *f* / **~ of correlation** Korrelationswahrscheinlichkeit *f* / **~ curve** Wahrscheinlichkeitskurve *f* / **~ density function** Wahrscheinlichkeitsdichtefunktion *f* / **~ distribution** Wahrscheinlichkeitsverteilung *f* / **~ element** Wahrscheinlichkeitselement *n* / **~ function** Wahrscheinlichkeitsfunktion *f* / **~ integral** Wahrscheinlichkeitsintegral *n* / **~ judgment** Wahrscheinlichkeitsschluss *m*, Wahrscheinlichkeitsurteil *n* / **~ learning** Wahrscheinlichkeitslernen *n* / **~ matching** Wahrscheinlichkeitsangleichung *f* / **~ measure** Wahrscheinlichkeitsmaß *n* / **~ ratio** Wahrscheinlichkeit *f*, Grad *m* der Wahrscheinlichkeit / **~ of response** Verhaltenswahrscheinlichkeit *f* / **~ sample** Wahrscheinlichkeitsstichprobe *f* / **~ space** Wahrscheinlichkeitsraum *m* / **~ table** Wahrscheinlichkeitstafel *f* / **~ theory** Wahrscheinlichkeitstheorie *f* / **a posteriori ~** empirische Wahrscheinlichkeit *f* / **complementary ~** Komplementärwahrscheinlichkeit *f* / **compound ~** gemeinsame Wahrscheinlichkeit *f* / **conditional ~** bedingte Wahrscheinlichkeit *f* / **contingent ~** bedingte Wahrscheinlichkeit *f* / **differential–~ hypothesis** Premack–Prinzip *n*, Hypothese *f* der differenziellen Auftretenswahrscheinlichkeit / **discriminating ~ of a test** Unterscheidungswahrscheinlichkeit *f* eines Tests / **empirical ~** empirische Wahrscheinlichkeit *f* / **joint ~** gemeinsame Wahrscheinlichkeit *f* / **normal ~** normale Wahrscheinlichkeit *f* / **random ~** Zufallswahrscheinlichkeit *f* / **statistical ~** statistische Wahrscheinlichkeit *f*, statistische Sicherheit *f* / **subjective ~** subjektive Wahrscheinlichkeit *f*

probable wahrscheinlich

probation Prüfung *f*, Probe *f*, Bewährung *f* / **~ officer** Bewährungshelfer *m*

probationer Kandidat *m*, auf Bewährung freigelassener Sträfling *m*

probe Untersuchung *f*, Prüfung *f* / untersuchen, prüfen

probenecid Probenecid *n*

problem Problem *n*, schwierige Aufgabe *f* / **~ area** Problembereich *m* / **~ behaviour** abnormes Verhalten *n*, Problemverhalten *n* / **~ box** Problemkäfig w / **~ check list** Problemfragebogen *m* / **~ child** Problemkind *n*, schwererziehbares Kind *n* / **~ drinking** Problemtrinken *n* / **~ method**

Problemverfahren *n* / ~ **personality** schwierige Persönlichkeit *f* / ~ **situation** Problemsituation *f* / ~ **solving** Problemlösung *n* / ~**–solving behaviour** Problemlöseverhalten *n* / **academic** ~ Schwierigkeiten *fpl* in Schule oder Studium / **marital** ~ Eheproblem *n* / **occupational** ~ Berufsproblem *n* / **psychosocial and environmental** ~**s** psychosoziale und umweltbedingte Probleme *npl* / **rational** ~ **solving** rationale Problemlösung *f* / **relational** ~ zwischenmenschliches Problem *n* / **religious or spiritual** ~ religiöses oder spirituelles Problem *n*

problematic, problematical problematisch, schwierig, fraglich

procaine Procain *n*

procedure Verfahren *n*, Methode *f* / ~ **of average error** Methode *f* des mittleren Fehlers, Herstellungsmethode *f* / ~ **of exhaustion** Anpassungsverfahren *n* / ~ **of mean error** Methode *f* des mittleren Fehlers / ~ **of reproduction** Herstellungsmethode *f* / **clinical** ~ Behandlungsmethode *f* / **counterbalanced** ~ Ausgleichsmethode *f* / **flooding** ~**s** Überflutungstherapie *f* / **implosive** ~ Implosionstherapie *f*, Überflutungstherapie *f* / **psychoanalytic** ~ psychoanalytische Methode *f* / **selective** ~ Auswahlverfahren *n*

proceed vorgehen, verfahren

proceeding Vorgehen *n*, Verfahren *n*, Handlung *f*

procephalic Vorderhaupts–

process Verfahren *n*, Prozess *m*, Vorgang *m*, Fortsatz *m* / ~ **of adaptation** Anpassungsvorgang *m* / ~ **of association** Assoziationsvorgang *m* / ~ **attitude** Bewusstseinshaltung *f* / ~ **of consciousness** Bewusstseinsvorgang *m* / ~ **of development** Entwicklungsprozess *m* / ~ **of disintegration** Auflösungsvorgang *m* / ~ **of displacement** Verschiebungsprozess *m* / ~ **of equilibration** Äquilibrationsprozess *m* / ~ **error** Verfahrensfehler *m*, Prozessfehler *m* / ~ **of gratification** Belohnungsprozess *m*, Befriedigungsablauf *m* / ~ **of growth** Wachstumsvorgang *m* / ~ **of individualisation** Individualisierung *f*, Individualisierungsprozess *m* / ~ **of the mind** Denkvorgang *m* / ~ **psychosis** chronische Psychose *f*, Prozesspsychose *f* / ~ **schizophrenia** chronische Schizophrenie *f*, Prozessschizophrenie *f* / ~ **of thought** Denkprozess *m*, Denkvorgang *m* / **associative** ~ Assoziationsvorgang *m*, assoziativer Prozess *m* / **autonomic** ~ Ablauf *m* im autonomen Nervensystem / **central** ~ Vorgang *m* im ZNS, zentraler Prozess *m* / **ciliary** ~ Ziliarfortsatz *m* / **cognitive** ~ kognitiver Prozess *m*, Denkvorgang *m* / **developmental** ~ Entwicklungsprozess *m* / **discriminal** ~ Unterscheidungsprozess *m* / **dual–**~ **theory** Zweifaktorentheorie *f* / **educational** ~ Erziehungsprozess *m* / **excitatory** ~ Erregungsablauf *m* / **formal** ~ **test** Test *m* der formellen Vorgehensweise / **founding** ~ grundlegender Vorgang *m* / **higher mental** ~**es** höhere geistige Prozesse *mpl* / **hypothetical** ~ hypothetischer Vorgang *m* / **hypothetical** ~ **variable** hypothetische Prozessvariable *f*, intervenierende Prozessvariable *f* / **intersensory** ~ intersensorischer Prozess *m*, zwischen Sinnesorganen ablaufender Prozess *m* / **latent** ~ latenter Prozess *m* / **legal** ~ Rechtsverfahren *n*, Prozess *m* / **legislative** ~ Gesetzgebungsverfahren *n* / **maturing** ~ Reifevorgang *m* / **mediating** ~ vermittelnder Prozess *m* / **mental** ~ geistiger Prozess *m*, Denkvorgang *m* / **motor** ~ Bewegungsablauf *m*, Bewegungsvorgang *m*, motorischer Prozess *m* / **neural** ~ Nervenfortsatz *m* / **neurotic** ~ neurotischer Vorgang *m* / **orectic** ~ orektischer Vorgang *m* / **organizational** ~ Organisationsprozess *m* / **paranoid** ~ paranoider Prozess *m* / **perceptual** ~ Wahrnehmungsvorgang *m*, Wahrnehmungsprozess *m* / **perceptual motor** ~ sensumotorischer Prozess *m* / **physiological** ~ physiologischer Prozess *m* / **political** ~ politischer Prozess *m*, politischer Vorgang *m* / **primal** ~ Primärprozess *m*, Primärvorgang *m* / **primary** ~ Primärprozess *m*, Primärvorgang *m* / **psychomotor** ~ psychomotorische Koordination *f* / **psychotherapeutic ~** psychotherapeutischer Prozess *m*, psychotherapeutische Interaktion *f* / **regulatory ~** Regelungsvorgang *m* / **secondary ~** sekundäärer Prozess *m*, Sekundärvorgang *m* / **selective ~** Selektionsvorgang *m* / **sensory ~** Wahrnehmungsprozess *m*, Wahrnehmungsvorgang *m* / **sensory motor ~** sensumotorische Koordination *f* / **social ~** soziale Prozess *m*, soziale Interaktion *f*, sozialer Vorgang *m* / **symbolic ~** symbolischer Prozess *m* / **therapeutic ~** therapeutischer Prozess *m*, Therapieverlauf *m* / **transverse ~** Querfortsatz *m* / **unconscious ~** unbewusster Prozess *m* / **visual ~** Sehvorgang *m* / **vital ~** Lebensablauf *m*

processing Verfahrens–, Verarbeitungs– / Verarbeitung *f*, Bearbeitung *f* / **cognitive ~ speed** kognitive Verarbeitungsgeschwindigkeit *f* / **random ~** Zufallsverfahren *n* / **sequential ~** sequenzielle Strategie *f*, sequenzielle Vorgehensweise *f*

processomania Streitsucht *f*, Prozesswütigkeit *f*

processor Datenverarbeitungsmaschine *f*, Zentraleinheit *f* / **~ storage** Hauptspeicher *m*

prochlorperazine Prochlorperazin *n*

proclivity Hang *m*, Neigung *f*

procoverant eine im Stillen über sich selbst hergesagte positive Feststellung *f*

procrastination Verzögerung *f*, Aufschieben *n*, Verschleppung *f*

procreation Fortpflanzung *f*, Zeugung *f*, Reproduktion *f*

procreative Zeugungs–, zeugungsfähig

procreator Erzeuger *m*, Vater *m*

proctalgia, proctagra Afterschmerz *m*

procure beschaffen, erlangen, Kuppelei treiben

procurer Kuppler *m*, Zuhälter *m*

prodigality Verschwendung *f*

prodigy Wunder *n* / **~ infant** Wunderkind *n*

prodromal vorausgehend, prodromal, prämonitorisch

prodrome Prodrom *n*, Prodomalerscheinung *f*, Vorzeichen *n*, Frühsymptom *n*

product Produkt *n* / **~ design** Produktgestaltung *f* / **~ group manager** Produktgruppenleiter *m* / **~ image** Produktbild *n*, Produkt–Image *n* / **~ manager** Produkt–Manager *m* / **~ matrix** Produktmatrix *f* / **~ moment** Produktmoment *n* / **~ moment coefficient of correlation** Produkt–Moment–Korrelationskoeffizient *m* / **~ moment correlation** Produkt–Moment–Korrelation *f*, Pearson–Korrelation *f* / **~ of the fantasy** Phantasieprodukt *n* / **~ scale** Vergleichsskala *f*, Ergebnisskala *f*

production Produktion *f*, Herstellung *f* / **~ curve** Produktionskurve *f* / **~ method** Herstellungsverfahren *n* / **~ procedure** Herstellungsverfahren *n* / **~ process** Produktionsvorgang *m* / **~ theory** Produktionstheorie *f* / **intentional ~ or feigning of symptoms or disabilities, either physical or psychological (factitious disorder)** artifizielle Störung *f* (absichtliches Erzeugen oder Vortäuschen von körperlichen oder psychischen Symptomen oder Behinderungen) / **restricted ~ curve** eingeschränkte Produktionskurve *f*

productive produktiv, schöpferisch

productivity, productiveness Produktivität *f*, schöpferische Leistung *f*, Kreativität *f* / **~ incentive system** Anreizsystem *n* zur Produktivitätssteigerung / **imaginal ~ test** Test *m* der schöpferischen Phantasie

profanity Vulgärsprache *f*

profession Beruf *m*, Stand *m*

professional beruflich, Berufs– / Fachmann *m*

professionalism Berufsausübung *f*, Berufsausbildung *f*, Professionalismus *m*

proficiency Fertigkeit *f*, Tüchtigkeit *f*, Leistung *f*, Meisterschaft *f* / **~ test** Begabungstest *m*, Fertigkeitstest *m*

profile Profil *n* / ~ **analysis** Profilanalyse *f* / ~ **chart** Profil *n*, Profildarstellung *f* / ~ **test** Profiltest *m*, Profilverfahren *n* / **educational** ~ Schulleistungsprofil *n* / **mental** ~ Charakterdiagramm *n*, Persönlichkeitsprofil *n* / **psychic** ~ Persönlichkeitsprofil *n*, Charakterdiagramm *n* / **psychological** ~ Testprofil *n*, psychologisches Profil *n*

profound schwerste(r), tief, tiefreichend, nachhaltig

progeny Nachkommenschaft *f*, Kinder *npl*

progeria Progerie *f*, Hutchinson–Guilford–Krankheit *f*, Vergreisung *f* im Kindesalter

progestational prämenstruell, vor der Monatsblutung

progesterone Progesteron *n*, Gelbkörperhormon *n*

progestin Gestagen *n*

prognathism, prognathy vorstehender Kiefer *m*, Prognathie *f*

prognathous mit vorstehendem Kinn, prognath

prognose, prognosticate prognostizieren, vorhersagen, Prognose stellen

prognosis Prognose *f*, Voraussage *f*, Vorhersage *f* / **bad** ~ ungünstige Prognose *f* / **long–term** ~ Langzeitprognose *f*

prognostic prognostisch / Anzeichen *n*, Vorzeichen *n*

programmatic programmatisch, schematisch

programme, program Programm *n*, Plan *m* / programmieren, ein Programm erstellen / ~ **control** Folgeregelung *f* / ~ **development** Programmentwicklung *f* / ~ **evaluation** Programmbeurteilung *f*, Programmevaluation *f* / ~ **flow chart** Programmablaufplan *m* / ~ **instruction** Programmunterweisung *f* / **branched** ~ verzweigtes Programm *n* / **educational** ~ Bildungsprogramm *n* / **executive** ~ Steuerprogramm *n*, Organisationsprogramm *n* / **independent living** ~ Behindertenselbsthilfeprogramm *n* / **linear** ~ Einwegprogramm *n*, lineares Programm *n* / **stored–**~ **machine** speicherprogrammierte Rechenanlage *f* / **social** ~ sozialpolitisches Programm *n*

programmed programmiert

programmer Programmierer *m*

programming, programing Programmierung *f* / ~ **language** Programmiersprache *f* / **extrinsic** ~ externe Programmsteuerung *f* / **intrinsic** ~ immanente Programmsteuerung *f* / **neurolinguistic** ~ neurolinguistisches Programmieren *n*

progress Fortschritt *m* / Fortschritte machen / **social** ~ sozialer Fortschritt *m*

Progression Fortschritt *m*, Progression *f*, Reihe *f* / **arithmetical** ~ arithmetische Reihe *f* / **backward** ~ Retropulsion *f* / **geometrical** ~ geometrische Reihe *f*

progressive zunehmend, fortschreitend, progressiv

prohibition Verbot *n* / ~ **against incest** Inzestverbot *n*

project projizieren / Projekt *n*, Entwurf *m*, Plan *m* / ~ **evaluation** Projektevaluierung *f*, Wirkungsanalyse *f* bei Projekten / ~ **follow–through** Durchführung *f* eines Projekts, Projektablauf *m* / ~ **method** Projektmethode *f*

projection Projektion *f*, Projizierung *f* / ~ **of affect** Affektprojektion *f* / ~ **area** Projektionsfeld *n*, sensorisches Rindenfeld *n* / ~ **centre** Projektionszentrum *n*, Projektionsfeld *n*, sensorisches Rindenfeld *n* / ~ **fiber** Projektionsfaser *f* / ~ **neuron** Projektionsneuron *n* / ~ **system** Projektionssystem *n* / ~ **test** projektiver Test *m*, projektives Verfahren *n* / ~ **tract** Projektionsbahn *f* / **assimilative** ~ Projektion *f*, Hinausverlagerung *f* / **auditory** ~ **area** Hörzentrum *n* / **disowning** ~ Projektion *f* verleugneter Triebwünsche / **excentric** ~ exzentrische Projektion *f* / **mental** ~ Projektion *f* / **optical** ~ Bildprojektion *f* / **visual** ~ Sehprojektion *f*

projective projektiv

projectivity projektives Verhalten *n*

projectoscope Projektionsapparat *m*, Epidiaskop *n*

projicient projizierend

prolactin Prolaktin *n*, Laktationshormon *n* / **~ inhibiting hormone** Prolaktin–Inhibiting–Hormon *n*, PIH, Prolaktin–Inhibiting–Faktor *m*, PIF / **~ releasing hormone** Prolaktin–Releasing–Hormon *n*, PRH, Prolaktin–Releasing–Faktor *m*, PRF

prolan Prolan *n* / **~ A** follikelstimulierendes Hormon *n* / **~ B** interstitielle–Zellen–stimulierendes Hormon *n*

prolegomenon Einleitung *f*, Vorbemerkung *f*

prolepsis vorzeitiges Eintreten *n* eines Anfalls, Prolepsis *f*, vorwegnehmende Antwort *f*

proliferation Wucherung *f*, Proliferation *f*

prolific fruchtbar, produktiv

prolificacy, prolificity Fruchtbarkeit *f*, Produktivität *f*

proline Prolin *n*

prolixity Weitschweifigkeit *f*

prolonged verlängert, protrahiert

promazine Promazin *n*

promethazine Promethazin *n*

prominence Vorsprung *m*, Erhöhung *f*

promiscuity Promiskuität *f*, häufig wechselnder Geschlechtsverkehr *m*

promiscuous gemischt, gemeinschaftlich

promotion Förderung *f*, Beförderung *f*

prompt Wink *m*, Denkanstoß *m*, Eingabeaufforderung *f* / **formal ~** formaler Denkanstoß *m* / **thematic ~** inhaltlicher Denkanstoß *m*

prompting Lernhilfe *f*, Prompting *n*, Anbieten *n* von Lernhilfen, Abrufreiz *m*, Souffliermethode *f*, Sicherungsverfahren *n* / **connotative ~** Anbieten *n* von Bezugspunkten / **denotative ~** Anbieten *n* von andeutungsweisen Lernhilfen

pronation Pronation *f*, Einwärtsdrehung *f*

prone geneigt, neigend, veranlagt

proneness Neigung *f*, Veranlagung *f*, Hang *m*

pronoun Pronomen *n*, Fürwort *n*

pronouncedness Klarheit *f*, Deutlichkeit *f*

pronunciation Aussprache *f*

proof Beweis *m*, Nachweis *m*, Probe *f*, Prüfung *f* / **material ~** konkreter Beweis *m* / **substantial ~** wesentlicher Beweis *m*, schlüssiger Beweis *m*

proof|reader's illusion Korrektorentäuschung *f* / **~ reading** Korrekturlesen *n*

propaedeutic, propaedeutical, propedeutic, propedeutical propädeutisch, einführend, Einführungs–

propaedeutics Propädeutik *f*, Einführungskurs *m*, Vorbereitungsübung *f*

propaganda Propaganda *f*, Werbung *f*, Reklame *f* / **~ analysis** Propagandaanalyse *f* / **~ medium** Werbeträger *m*, Werbemedium *n*

propagandize propagieren, Propaganda treiben

propagate fortpflanzen, ausbreiten, verbreiten, propagieren, Propaganda machen

propagation Fortpflanzung *f*, Zeugung *f*, Ausbreitung *f*, Verbreitung *f* / **~ of the species** Arterhaltung *f*

propanolol Propanolol *n*

propensity, propension Trieb *m*, Antrieb *m*, Triebkraft *f* natürliche Neigung *f* / **innate ~** Instinkt *m*

property Eigenschaft *f*, Eigentümlichkeit *f*, Attribut *n*, Grundeigenschaft *f* / Eigentum *n* / **derived ~** abgeleitete Eigenschaft *f* / **dynamic ~** dynamische Eigenschaft *f*

prophecy Vorhersage *f*, Prophezeiung *f* / **~ formula** Vorhersageformel *f* / **self–defeating ~** Vorhersage *f* die durch unterlassenes Handeln nicht erfüllt wird / **self–fulfilling ~** selbsterfüllende Prophezeihung *f*, Rosenthal–Effekt *m*, Pygmalion–Effekt *m*

prophylactic vorbeugend, prophylaktisch / Vorbeugungsmittel *n*, Verhütungsmittel *n*, Prophylaktikum *n*, Präventivmittel *n*

prophylaxis, prophylaxy Vorbeugung *f*, Prophylaxe *f*

propinquity Nähe *f*, nahe Verwandtschaft *f*

proportion Proportion *f*, Größenverhältnis *n*

proportional proportional, verhältnismäßig, in richtigem Verhältnis

proportionality Proportionalität *f*, Verhältnismäßigkeit *f*, Verhältnis *n*

proportionate proportioniert, in richtigem Verhältnis stehend, angemessen, ausgeglichen

propose vorschlagen

proposition Behauptung *f*, Feststellung *f*, Lehrsatz *m*, Vorschlag *m* / **identical ~** identische Feststellung *f*

propositional Satz–

propriate selbstverwirklichend, Selbstverwirklichungs–

propriety Angemessenheit *f*, Richtigkeit *f*, Anstand *m* / **~ of conduct** anständiges Betragen *n*

proprioception Eigenwahrnehmung *f*, Muskelsinn *m*, Propriozeption *f*

proprioceptive propriozeptiv

proprioceptor Propriozeptor *m*

propriospinal propriospinal

proprium Proprium *n*, Selbst *n*, Ich *n*

propulsion Antrieb *m*, unwillkürliches Nachvornelaufen *n*, Propulsion *f*

propulsive nach vorne treibend, propulsiv

prose Prosa *f*, Prosatext *m*

prosencephalon Vorhirn *n*, Prosenzephalon *n*

prosody Prosodie *f*, Satzrhythmus *m*, Sprechrhythmus *m*

prosopagnosia Prosopagnosie *f*, physiognomische Agnosie *f*, Unvermögen *n* ein bestimmtes Gesicht als solches zu erkennen

prosopalgia Trigeminusneuralgie *f*, Gesichtsschmerz *m*, Prosopalgie *f*, Gesichtsneuralgie *f*

prosoponeuralgia Gesichtsneuralgie *f*

prosopospasm Gesichtskrampf *m*, Gesichtszuckung *f*, Tic *m*, Prosopospasmus *m*, Fazialiskrampf *m*

prospect Aussicht *f*, Ausblick *m*, Erwartung *f*, voraussichtlicher Kunde *m*, Interessent *m*

prospective voraussichtlich

prospermia vorzeitige Ejakulation *f*, Prospermie *f*

prostaglandin Prostaglandin *n*

prostate Prostata *f*, Vorsteherdrüse *f*

prosthesis Prothese *f*, Kunstglied *n*

prosthetic prothetisch

prostigmin, prostigmine Prostigmin *n*

prostitute Prostituierte *f*, Dirne *f* / gewerbsmäßige Unzucht betreiben, prostituieren, anschaffen gehen

prostitution Prostitution *f* / **~ complex** Prostitutionskomplex *m*

prostration Erschöpfungszustand *m*, Kraftlosigkeit *f*, Prostration *f* / **nervous ~** Nervenschwäche *f*, Neurasthenie *f*, nervöse Erschöpfung *f*

protagonist Hauptfigur *f*, Hauptperson *f*

protan, protanomal Protanomale *m,f*

protanomalous rotschwach

protanomaly Rotschwäche *f*

protanope Rotblinder *m*

protanopia Rotblindheit *f*, Protanopie *f*, Anerythropsie *f*

protanopic rotblind, protanop

protease Protease *f*

protection Schutz *m* / **~ complex** Schutzkomplex *m* / **~ against external stimuli** äußerer Reizschutz *m* / **~ against internal stimuli** innerer Reizschutz *m* / **~ against stimuli** Reizschutz *m*

protective schützend, Schutz–

protector Beschützer *m*, Schutzmittel *n*, Schutz *m*

protein Eiweiß *n*, Eiweißkörper *m*, Protein *n* / **~ biosynthesis** Proteinbiosynthese *f* / **~ deficiency disorder** Proteinmangelerscheinung *f*, Eiweißmangelkrankheit *f* /

~ hormone Proteinhormon *n* / **~ kinase** Proteinkinase *f* / **~ metabolism** Proteinstoffwechsel *m*, Eiweißstoffwechsel *m* / **~ sensitisation** Einweißsensibilisierung *f* / **~ shock therapy** Eiweißschockbehandlung *f* / **~ synthesis** Eiweißsynthese *f*, Proteinsynthese *f* / **~ therapy** Eiweißkörpertherapie *f*, Umstimmungstherapie *f* / **vegetable ~** pflanzliches Eiweiß *n*

proteinase Proteinase *f*

protension Ausdehnung *f*, Dauer *f*

protensity Dauer *f*, Zeitausdehnung *f*, subjektive Zeitdauer *f*

protest Protest *m*, Einspruch *m* / protestieren, Protest einlegen / **~ child** schwieriges Kind *n* / **masculine ~** männlicher Protest *m*

protestation Beteuerung *f*, Einspruch *m*, Protesterklärung *f*

prothesis Prothese *f*, Kunstglied *n*

prothetic prothetisch

prothrombin Prothrombin *n*

protocol Protokoll *n* / **~ sentences** Protokoll–Sätze *mpl*

proton Proton *n*

protopathic protopathisch, idiopathisch

protopathy Protopathie *f*

protoplasm Protoplasma *n*, Zytoplasma *n*

protoplasmatic, protoplasmic Protoplasma–, protoplasmatisch

prototaxic prototaktisch

prototype Prototyp *m*, Urbild *n*, Muster *n*, Vorbild *n*

protovertebra Ursegment *n*, Muskelursegment *n*, Metamer *n*, Somit *n*

protozoology Lehre *f* von den Protozoen, Protozoenkunde *f*, Protozoologie *f*

protozoon Urtierchen *n*, Protozoon *n*

protracted protrahiert, verzögert, verlängert

proud stolz

proverbs test Sprichwort–Test *m*

provertebra Urwirbel *m*, Ursegment *n*

provider Provider *m*, Online–Dienst *m*

provisional vorläufig, provisorisch

provocation Provokation *f*, Reizung *f* / **~ of an attack** Anfallsauslösung *f* / **~ by cardiazol** Cardiazolprovokation *f*

proximal körpernah, proximal / **~–distal** proximal–distal

proximity Nähe *f*, Proximität *f*

proximodistal proximodistal

proxy server spezieller Server *m* von Internet–Providern, Proxy–Server *m*, lokaler Zwischenspeicher *m*

Pr scale Skala *f* zur Messung von Rassenvorurteilen

prude Spröde *m,f*, Prüde *m,f*

prudery, prudishness Prüderie *f*, Sprödigkeit *f*

prudish prüde, spröde

pruriginous juckend, pruriginös

pruritus Hautjucken *n*, Pruritus *m*

pselaphesia Tastsinn *m*

psellism Stottern *n*, Stammeln *n*, Psellismus *m*

P sensor P–Sensor *m*, Proportionalsensor *m*

pseudaesthesia, pseudesthesia eingebildete Empfindung *f*, Phantomschmerz *m*, Pseudoästhesie *f*

pseudoanaemia, pseudoanemia Scheinanämie *f*, Pseudoanämie *f*

pseudoangina pectoris Pseudoangina pectoris *f*

pseudoataxia Pseudoataxie *f*, ataxieähnlicher Zustand *m*

pseudoathetosis Pseudoathetose *f*

pseudoblepsia, pseudoblepsis Pseudoblepsie *f*, visuelle Halluzination *f*

pseudochromaesthesia, pseudochromesthesia Farbenhören *n*, Phonopsie *f*, Schallphotismus *m*

pseudoclonus Pseudoklonus *m*

pseudocommunication falsche Kommunikation *f*, Pseudokommunikation *f*

pseudoconditioning Pseudokonditionierung *f*

pseudoconfusion psychogener Dämmerzustand *m*

pseudocrisis falsche Krise *f*, Pseudokrise *f*

pseudocyesis eingebildete Schwangerschaft *f*, Scheinschwangerschaft *f*

pseudodebility Pseudodebilität *f*

pseudodementia Pseudodemenz *f*

pseudoemotion eingebildete Emotion *f*, Pseudoemotion *f*

pseudofovea Pseudofovea *f*

pseudofrigidity Pseudofrigidität *f*, eingebildete Frigidität *f*

pseudogeuesthesia Pseudogeuästhesie *f*

pseudogeusia Pseudogeusie *f*, Geruchsillusion *f*

pseudohallucination Pseudohalluzination *f*, subjektiv unwahre Trugwahrnehmung *f*, Phantasmie *f*

pseudohermaphrodite Pseudohermaphrodit *m*, Scheinzwitter *m*

pseudohermaphroditic pseudohermaphroditisch, scheinzwitterig

pseudohermaphroditism Pseudohermaphroditismus *m*, Scheinzwittertum *n*, scheinbarer Hermaphroditismus *m*

pseudoimpotence Pseudoimpotenz *f*, eingebildete Impotenz *f*

pseudoisochromatic pseudoisochromatisch

pseudolalia Scheinsprache *f*, Pseudosprache *f*

pseudolanguage Scheinsprache *f*, Pseudosprache *f*

pseudologia, pseudology Lügensucht *f* / **~ fantastica** krankhafte Lügensucht *f*, Pseudologia phantastica *f*

pseudomania krankhaftes Lügen *n*, Pseudomanie *f*

pseudomasturbation spielerische Onanie *f*, Peniszupfen *n*

pseudomembrane falsche Membran *f*, Pseudomembran *f*

pseudomemory Pseudoerinnerung *f*, Bekanntheitstäuschung *f*, Erinnerungstäuschung *f*, Pseudomnesie *f*

pseudomnesia Erinnerungstäuschung *f*, Erinnerungsillusion *f*, Pseudomnesie *f*

pseudomyopia Scheinmyopie *f*, Pseudomyopie *f*

pseudoneurosis Scheinneurose *f*, Pseudoneurose *f* / **somatogenic ~** somatogene Pseudoneurose *f*

pseudonystagmus Pseudonystagmus *m*

pseudoparalysis Scheinlähmung *f*, Pseudoparalyse *f*

pseudoperception Scheinwahrnehmung *f*, Pseudowahrnehmung *f*

pseudophone Pseudophon *n*

pseudoplegia hysterische Lähmung *f*

pseudopodium, pseudopod Pseudopodium *n*, Scheinfüßchen *n*

pseudopregnancy Scheinschwangerschaft *f*, hysterische Schwangerschaft *f*, eingebildete Schwangerschaft *f*

pseudopresentiment falsche Vorahnung *f*, scheinbare Ahnung *f*

pseudopsia Illusion *f*, visuelle Halluzination *f*, illusionäres Sehen *n*

pseudopsychology Scheinpsychologie *f*

pseudoreaction Pseudoreaktion *f*

pseudoreflex Pseudoreflex *m*, unterscheidende Wirkreaktion *f*, nicht–reizbezogene Unterscheidungsreaktion *f*

pseudoreliability Pseudoreliabilität *f*, Scheinreliabilität *f*

pseudoremininscence Erinnerungstäuschung *f*, Erinnerungsillusion *f*, Konfabulation *f*

pseudoscope Pseudoskop *n*

pseudoscopy Pseudoskopie *f*

pseudosmia Geruchshalluzination *f*

pseudostupor Pseudostupor *m*

pseudoword Pseudowort *n*

psi Psi *n*, Bezeichnung *f* für „Psychisches“, Bezeichnung *f* für „Parapsychisches“ / **~ process** Psi–Funktion *f* / **~ system** Psi–System *n*

psilocybin Psilocybin *n*

psittacism Psittazismus *m*, automatische Lautfolge *f* die an Vogelzwitschern erinnert

psopholalia Lallen *n*

psychaesthesia, psychesthesia Psychästhesie *f*, seelische Empfindsamkeit *f*

psychaesthetic, psychesthetic psychisch empfindsam, psychisch empfindlich, psychästhetisch

psychagogue Psychagoge *m*

psychagogy, psychagogia Psychagogik *f*

psychalgia psychisch bedingter Schmerz *m*, Psychalgie *f*

psychanalysis Psychoanalyse *f*

psychanopsia Seelenblindheit *f*

psychasthenia Psychasthenie *f*

psychasthenic psychasthenisch

psyche Psyche *f*, Geist *m*, Seele *f*

psychedelic psychedelisch, bewusstseinserweiternd / Psychedelikum *n*

psycheism Mesmerismus *m*, Hypnotismus *m*

psychergograph Psychergograph *m*

psychergometer Psychergograph *m*

psychesthesia Psychästhesie *f*, seelische Empfindsamkeit *f*

psychesthetic psychästhetisch, psychisch empfindlich

psychiater Psychiater *m*

psychiatric psychiatrisch

psychiatrics Psychiatrie *f*, Lehre *f* von den Geistesstörungen und Geisteskrankheiten

psychiatrist Psychiater *m* / **industrial ~** Betriebspsychiater *m*

psychiatrize psychiatrisch deuten

psychiatry Psychiatrie *f*, Lehre *f* von den Geistesstörungen und Geisteskrankheiten / **administrative ~** administrative Psychiatrie *f* / **adolescent ~** Jugendpsychiatrie *f* / **biological ~** biologische Psychiatrie *f* / **criminal ~** Kriminalpsychopathologie *f* / **cross–cultural ~** transkulturelle Psychiatrie *f* / **cultural ~** Kulturpsychiatrie *f* / **descriptive ~** beschreibende Psychiatrie *f* / **dynamic ~** dynamische Psychiatrie *f* / **existential ~** existenzielle Psychiatrie *f* / **experimental ~** experimentelle Psychiatrie *f* / **forensic ~** forensische Psychiatrie *f*, Gerichtspsychiatrie *f* / **geriatric ~** geriatrische Psychiatrie *f* / **legal ~** Gerichtspsychiatrie *f*, gerichtliche Psychiatrie *f* / **military ~** Wehrpsychiatrie *f* / **orthomolecular ~** Orthomolekularpsychiatrie *f* / **pastoral ~** seelsorgerische Psychiatrie *f* / **prophylactic ~** präventive Psychiatrie *f* / **psychoanalytic ~** psychoanalytische Psychiatrie / **social ~** soziale Psychiatrie *f*, Sozialpsychiatrie *f* / **transcultural ~** kulturunabhängige Psychiatrie *f*, transkulturelle Psychiatrie *f*

psychic Medium *n*, zum Spiritismus neigender Mensch *m*

psychic, psychical psychisch, seelisch, psychologisch, geistig

psychics Psychologie *f*, Seelenkunde *f*

psychism Psychismus *m*, Parapsychologie *f*

psychoacoustics Psychoakustik *f*

psychoanaleptic psychoanaleptisch / Psychoanaleptikum *n*

psychoanalyse psychoanalysieren, analysieren, psychoanalytisch behandeln

psychoanalysis Pschychoanalyse *f*, psychoanalytische Therapie *f* / **classical ~** klassische Psychoanalyse *f* / **didactic ~** Lehranalyse *f* / **existential ~** existenzielle Psychoanalyse *f* / **transactional ~** Transaktionsanalyse *f* / **wild ~** wilde Psychoanalyse *f*, Amateur–Psychoanalyse *f*

psychoanalyst, psychoanalyzer Psychoanalytiker *m*

psychoanalytic psychoanalytisch

psychoasthenia Psychasthenie *f*

psychoasthenics Lehre *f* von den psychischen Störungen

psychobiochemist Psychobiochemiker *m*

psychobiochemistry Psychobiochemie *f*

psychobiogram Psychobiogramm *n*

psychobiography psychologische Lebensbeschreibung *f*, psychologische Biographie *f*

psychobiological psychobiologisch

psychobiologist Psychobiologe *m*

psychobiology Psychobiologie *f*

psychocatharsis Katharsis *f*, Psychokatharsis *f*, seelische Läuterung *f*

psychoceramic sonderbarer Kauz *m*, Verrückter *m*

psychochemical psychochemisch / Psychopharmakon *n*

psychochemistry Psychochemie *f*

psychochromaesthesia, psychochromesthesia Farbenhören *n*, Phonopsie *f*, Schallphotismus *m*, Psychochromästhesie *f*

psychochronometry Reaktionszeitmessung *f*

psychodelic Psychedelikum *n*, psychedelisch, psychodelisch, bewusstseinserweiternd

psychodiagnosis Psychodiagnose *f*

psychodiagnostic psychodiagnostisch

psychodiagnostics Psychodiagnostik *f*

psychodometer Psychodometer *n*, Reaktionszeitmesser *m*

psychodometry Psychodometrie *f*, Reaktionszeitmessung *f*

psychodrama Psychodrama *n*

psychodynamic psychodynamisch

psychodynamics Psychodynamik *f*, Lehre *f* von den psychischen Funktionen

psychodysleptic psychodysleptisch, halluzinatorisch / Psychodysleptikum *n*, Halluzinogen *n*

psychoeducation psychoedukativer Ansatz *m*

psychoendocrinology Psychoendokrinologie *f*

psychoenergizer Psychoenergetikum *n*, Psychostimulantium *n*

psychoepilepsy idiopathische Epilepsie *f*

psychogalvanic psychogalvanisch

psychogalvanometer Psychogalvanometer *n*

psychogenesis, psychogeny Psychogenese *f*, Entwicklung *f* des Psychischen, Entwicklung *f* des Seelischen

psychogenetics Lehre *f* von der Entwicklung des Psychischen, Entwicklungspsychologie *f*

psychogenia Psychogenie *f*, Verursachung *f* von Krankheiten aufgrund psychischer Ereignisse

psychogenic, psychogenetic, psychogenous psychogen, seelisch bedingt, psychogenetisch

psychogeriatrics Psychogeriatrie *f*

psychogerontology psychologische Altersforschung *f*

psychognosis, psychognostics, psychognosy Psychognostik *f*, psychologisch–wissenschaftlich fundierte Menschenkenntnis *f*, Studium *n* der Seelenvorgänge

psychognostic psychognostisch

psychogram, psychograph Psychogramm *n* / **individual ~** individuelles Psychogramm *n*

psychographer, psychographist Verfasser *m* eines Psychogramms, Verfasser *m* einer psychologischen Biographie

psychography, psychographics Psychographie *f*

psychohistorian Psychohistoriker *m*, Historiker *m* mit psychologischer Orientierung, Psychologe *m* der historische Motivationsstrukturen studiert

psychohistorical psychohistorisch

psychohistory psychologisch interpretierte Geschichte *f*, psychologisch gedeutete Biographie *f*, Wissenschaft *f* von der psychologischen Geschichtsdeutung, Psychohistorie *f*

psychoid psychoid, seelenartig / Psychoid *n*, vorseelische Ganzheit *f*

psychokinesis Psychokinese *f*

psychokym Psychokym *n*, Gesamtheit *f* der psychischen Energie

psycholagny Psycholagnie *f*, geistige Masturbation *f*, durch Phantasievorstellungen erzeugte geschlechtliche Erregung *f*

psycholepsy Psycholepsie *f*

psycholeptic psycholeptisch / Psycholeptikum *n*

psycholinguistics Psycholinguistik *f*

psychologic, psychological psychologisch, psychisch, seelisch

psychologism Psychologismus *m*

psychologist Psychologe *m* / **~ attitude** Psychologeneinstellung *f* / **~'s fallacy** Psychologen–Trugschluss *m*, psychologischer Trugschluss *m* / **analytical ~** analytischer Psychologe *m* / **clinical ~** klinischer Psychologe *m* / **consulting ~** beratender Psychologe *m*, in der Beratung tätiger Psychologe *m* / **educational ~** Schulpsychologe *m*, pädagogischer Psychologe *m* / **experimental ~** Experimentalpsychologe *m* / **industrial ~** Arbeitspsychologe *m*, Betriebspsychologe *m* / **military ~** Militärpsychologe *m* / **social ~** Sozialpsychologe *m*

psychologize psychologisch erklären, psychologisieren

psychologue Psychologe *m*

psychology Psychologie *f* / **~ education** Psychologieausbildung *f* / **~ of adolescence** Jugendpsychologie *f* / **~ of aging** Alterspsychologie *f*, Gerontopsychologie *f* / **~ of apperception** Appperzeptionspsychologie *f* / **~ of art** Kunstpsychologie *f* / **~ of behaviour** Verhaltenspsychologie *f* / **~ of conduct** Verhaltenspsychologie *f* / **~ of culture** Kulturpsychologie *f* / **~ of depths** Tiefenpsychologie *f* / **~ of expression** Ausdruckspsychologie *f* / **~ of individuality** Persönlichkeitspsychologie *f* / **~ of learning** Lernpsychologie *f* / **~ of perception** Wahrnehmungspsychologie *f*, Psychologie *f* der Wahrnehmung / **~ of religion** Religionspsychologie *f* / **~ of sport** Sportpsychologie *f* / **~ of the ego** Ich–Psychologie *f* / **~ of thinking** Denkpsychologie *f* / **~ of understanding** philosophische Psychologie *f* / **abnormal ~** Psychopathologie *f* / **academic ~** philosophische Psychologie *f* / **Adlerian ~** Adler'sche Psychologie *f* / **adolescent ~** Jugendpsychologie *f*, Psychologie *f* des Jugendalters / **aeronautical ~** Luftfahrtpsychologie *f* / **aesthetic ~** ästhetische Psychologie *f* / **analytic ~** analytische Psychologie *f* / **applied ~** angewandte Psychologie *f* / **architectural ~** Architekturpsychologie *f* / **atomistic ~** atomistische Psychologie *f*, Elementenpsychologie *f* / **behavioristic ~** behavioristische Psychologie *f*, Behaviorismus *m* / **biological ~** biologische Psychologie *f*, physiologische Psychologie *f* / **clinical ~** klinische Psychologie *f* / **clinical ~ internship** klinisch–psychologisches Assistentenjahr *n* / **cognitive ~** kognitive Psychologie *f* / **collective ~** Kollektivpsychologie *f*, Massenpsychologie *f*, Gruppenpsychologie *f* / **comparative ~** vergleichende Psychologie *f* / **complex ~** komplexe Psychologie *f* / **constitutional ~** Konstitutionspsychologie *f* / **criminal ~** Kriminalpsychologie *f* / **critical ~** kritische Psychologie *f* / **cross cultural ~** kulturvergleichende Psychologie *f* / **cultural ~** Kulturpsychologie *f* / **descriptive ~** deskriptive Psychologie *f*, beschreibende Psychologie *f* / **developmental ~** Entwicklungspsychologie *f* / **differential ~** differenzielle Psychologie *f* / **dynamic ~** dynamische Psychologie *f* / **eclectic ~** eklektische Psychologie *f* / **ecological ~** ökologische Psychologie *f*, Ökopsychologie *f* / **economic ~** Wirtschaftspsychologie *f* / **educational ~** pädagogische Psychologie *f*, Erziehungspsychologie *f* / **empirical ~** empirische Psychologie *f* / **environmental ~** Umweltpsychologie *f*, ökologische Psychologie *f*, Ökopsychologie *f* / **esthetic ~** ästhetische Psychologie *f* / **existential ~** Existenzpsychologie *f* / **experimental ~** experimentelle Psychologie *f*, Experimentalpsychologie *f* / **forensic ~** forensische Psychologie *f*, Gerichtspsychologie *f* / **Freudian ~** Freud'sche Psychologie *f* / **functional ~** Funktionalismus *m* / **general ~** allgemeine Psychologie *f* / **genetic ~** Erbpsychologie *f*, psychologische Genetik *f*, Entwicklungspsychologie *f*, genetische Psychologie *f* / **geriatric ~** Psychologie *f* des Alterns / **Herbartian ~** Herbart'sche Psychologie *f* / **hodological ~** Hodologie *f* / **holistic ~** organismische Psychologie *f*, Ganzheitspsychologie *f* / **hormic ~** hormische Psychologie *f* / **humanistic ~** humanistische Psychologie *f* / **idiographic ~** beschreibende Psychologie *f* / **individual ~** Individualpsychologie *f* / **industrial ~** Industriepsychologie *f*, Arbeitspsychologie *f*, Betriebspsychologie *f* / **intentional ~** teleologische Psychologie *f*, hormische Psychologie *f* / **interbehavioural ~** Interaktionspsychologie *f* / **introspective ~** introspektive Psychologie *f* / **Jungian ~** Jung'sche Psychologie *f* / **legal ~** Rechtspsychologie *f* / **literary ~** Literaturpsychologie *f* / **mathematical ~** mathematische Psychologie *f* / **medical ~** medizinische Psychologie *f* / **military ~** Wehrpsychologie *f*, Militärpsychologie *f* / **molar ~** molare Psychologie *f* / **molecular ~** molekulare Psychologie *f* / **morbid ~** Psychopathologie *f* / **neo–Freudian ~** Neo–Freud'sche Psychologie *f* / **new ~** moderne Psychologie *f* / **nomothetic ~** wissenschaftliche Psychologie *f*, nomothetische Psychologie *f* / **objective ~** objektive Psychologie *f* / **occupational ~** Berufspsychologie *f* / **ontogenetic ~** ontogenetische Psychologie *f* / **organismic ~** organismische Psychologie *f* / **organistic ~** organismische Psychologie *f* / **organizational ~** Organisationspsychologie *f* / **pastoral ~** Pastoralpsychologie *f* / **pathological ~** Pathopsychologie *f*, Psychopathologie *f* / **perceptual ~** Wahrnehmungspsychologie *f* / **personalistic ~** Personalismus *m*, personalistische Psychologie *f* / **phenomenological ~** phänomenologische Psychologie *f* / **philosophical ~** philosophische Psychologie *f*, verstehende Psychologie *f* / **physiological ~** physiologische Psychologie *f* / **political ~** politische Psychologie *f* / **popular ~** Populärpsychologie *f* / **practical ~** praktische Psychologie *f*, angewandte Psychologie *f* / **probabilistic ~** probabilistische Psychologie *f* / **purposive ~** hormische Psychologie *f*, teleologische Psychologie *f* / **racial ~** Rassenpsychologie *f* / **rational ~** verstehende Psychologie *f* / **recreational ~** Freizeitpsychologie *f* / **scientific ~** naturwissenschaftliche Psychologie *f* / **social ~** Sozialpsychologie *f* / **statistical ~** statistische Psychologie *f* / **structural ~** strukturelle Psychologie *f*, Strukturalismus *m* / **subjective ~** subjektivierende Psychologie *f* / **systematic ~** systematische Psychologie *f* / **topological ~** topologische Psychologie *f*, Vektorpsychologie *f* / **transpersonal ~** transpersonale Psychologie *f* / **variational ~** differenzielle Psychologie *f* / **vocational ~** Berufspsychologie *f*, Psychologie *f* der Berufswahl

psycholysis Psycholyse *f*

psycholytic psycholytisch, psychodysleptisch, halluzinatorisch / Psycholytikum *n*, Halluzinogen *n*

psychomathematics mathematische Psychologie *f*

psychometer Wahrsager *m*, psychometrisches Messinstrument *n*

psychometric psychometrisch

psychometrician, psychometrist Psychometriker *m*, Testpsychologe *m*

psychometrics Psychometrie *f*, Messung *f* psychischer Erscheinungen

psychometrizing (parapsychologische) Psychometrie *f*

psychometry Psychometrie *f*

psychomobility psychische Mobilität *f*

psychomorphism Psychomorphismus *m*, Zuerkennung *f* psychischer Vorgänge an Tiere und unbelebte Objekte

psychomotility Psychomotilität *f*, Psychomotorik *f*

psychomotor psychomotorisch

psychoneural leibseelisch, psychophysisch, neuropsychisch

psychoneuroimmunology Psychoneuroimmunologie *f*

psychoneurosis Psychoneurose *f*

psychoneurotic psychoneurotisch / Psychoneurotiker *m*

psychonomic psychonom, physischer Gesetzmäßigkeit unterliegend

psychonomics, psychonomy psychische Gesetzmäßigkeit *f*

psychonosis Geisteskrankheit *f*

psychonosology Lehre *f* von den psychischen Krankheiten, Klassifikation *f* psychischer Störungen

psycho–organic psychoorganisch

psychopaedagogics, psychopaedagogy Psychopädagogik *f*

psychoparesis Geistesschwäche *f*

psychopath Psychopath *m*

psychopathic psychopathisch

psychopathist Psychiater *m*

psychopathological psychopathologisch

psychopathologist Psychopathologe *m*

psychopathology Psychopathologie *f*, Pathopsychologie *f* / **~ of child** Psychopathologie *f* des Kindes / **sexual ~** Sexualpsychopathologie *f*

psychopathy, psychopathia Psychopathie *f* / **~ sexualis** Psychopathia sexualis *f*, Perversion *f*

psychopedagogics, psychopedagogy Psychopädagogik *f*

psychopedics Psychopädie *f*, klinische Kinderpsychologie *f*, Kinder– und Jugendpsychiatrie *f*

psychopharmacological pharmakopsychologisch, psychopharmakologisch

psychopharmacology Psychopharmakologie *f*

psychophobia Abneigung *f* gegen psychologische Betrachtungen

psychophylaxis Psychohygiene *f*

psychophysical psychophysisch, leibseelisch, Leib–Seele–

psychophysicist Psychophysiker *m*, Anhänger *m* der Psychophysik

psychophysics Psychophysik *f*, Leib–Seele–Lehre *f*, Wissenschaft *f* von den Beziehungen zwischen physischen Reizen und den entsprechenden psychischen Erlebnissen / **outer ~** äußere Psychophysik *f*

psychophysiological psychophysiologisch

psychophysiologist Psychophysiologe *m*

psychophysiology physiologische Psychologie *f*, Psychophysiologie *f*

psychoplasticity psychische Formbarkeit *f*, Plastizität *f* der Psyche

psychoplegic Psychoplegikum *n*, Neuroleptikum *n*

psychoprophylactic psychoprophylaktisch

psychoprophylaxis Psychoprophylaxe *f*, Psychohygiene *f*

psychoreactive psychoreaktiv

psychoreflexology Psychoreflexologie *f*

psychosensorial, psychosensory psychosensorisch

psychosexual psychosexuell

psychosexuality psychische Aspekte *mpl* der Sexualität

psychosis Psychose *f*, Geisteskrankheit *f*, Irresein *n* / **~ due to alcoholism** Alkoholpsychose *f* / **~ of association** Begleitpsychose *f* / **~ of depersonalization** Entfremdungspsychose *f* / **~ of reference** Beziehungspsychose *f* / **acute ~** akute Psychose *f* / **affective ~** affektive Psychose *f*, Affektpsychose *f* / **alcoholic ~** Alkoholpsychose *f*, Säuferpsychose *f* / **alternating ~** zirkuläre Psychose *f*, alternierende Psychose *f*, zirkuläres Irresein *n* / **arteriosclerotic ~** arteriosklerotische Psychose *f* / **associated ~** Begleitpsychose *f* / **atypical ~** atypische Psychose *f* / **benign ~** gutartig verlaufende Psychose *f* / **brief reactive ~** kurze reaktive Psychose *f* / **chronic ~** chronische Psychose *f* / **circular ~** zirkulare Psychose *f*, zirkuläres Irresein *n*, zyklische Psychose *f* / **climacteric ~** Involutionspsychose *f*, klimakterische Psychose *f*, Psychose *f* der Wechseljahre / **constitutional ~** Konstitutionspsychose *f*, Organpsychose *f* / **collective ~** Massenpsychose *f*, Gemeinschaftspsychose *f* / **cyclic ~** zirkuläres Irresein *n*, zyklische Psychose *f*, zirkuläre Psychose *f* / **degenerative ~** Degenerationspsychose *f*, Defektpsychose *f* / **depressive ~** Depression *f* / **deteriorative ~** Entartungspsychose *f* / **diabetic ~** Diabetespsychose *f* / **dysthymic ~** dysthymische Psychose *f* / **eclamptic ~** eklamptische Psychose *f* / **emotional ~** Affektpsychose *f* / **endogenous ~** endogene Psychose *f* / **epileptic ~** Epilepsiepsychose *f* / **exogenous ~** exogene Psychose *f* / **experimental ~** experimentelle Psychose *f* / **functional ~** funktionelle Psychose *f* / **gestational ~** Schwangerschaftpsychose *f*, Gestationspsychose *f*, Generationspsychose *f* / **hallucinatory ~** halluzinatorische Psychose *f* / **heriditary ~** Erbpsychose *f* / **iatrogenic ~** iatrogene Psychose *f* / **idiophrenic ~** organische Schwangerschaftspsychose *f* / **infantile ~** Kinderpsychose *f*, infantile Psychose *f*, kindliche Psychose *f* / **intermittent ~** intermittierende Psychose *f* / **involutional ~** Involutionspsychose *f*, klimakterische Psychose *f* / **involutional paranoid ~** paranoide Involutionspsychose *f* / **juvenile ~** juvenile Psychose *f* / **litigious ~** Prozesspsychose *f* / **manic ~** Manie *f* / **manic–depressive ~** manisch–depressive Erkrankung *f*, manisch–depressive Psychose *f* / **marginal ~** Randpsychose *f* / **menstrual ~** Menstruationspsychose *f* / **oneiroid ~** oneiroide Psychose *f* / **organic ~** organische Psychose *f* / **paranoid ~** Paranoia *f*, paranoide Psychose *f* / **periodic ~** periodisches Irresein *n*, zirkuläres Irresein *n*, zyklische Psychose *f* / **polyneuritic ~** Korsakow–Psychose *f*, Korsakow–Syndrom *n*, polyneuritische Psychose *f* / **postinfectious ~** postinfektiöse Psychose *f* / **postoperative ~** postoperative Psychose *f* / **post partum ~** Wochenbettpsychose *f* / **presenile ~** präsenile Psychose *f* / **pubertal ~** Pubertätspsychose *f* / **puerperal ~** Puerperalpsychose *f*, Wochenbettpsychose *f* / **reactive ~** reaktive Psychose *f*, abnorme Erlebnisreaktion *f* / **recurrent ~** rezidivierende Psychose *f*, wiederkehrende Psychose *f* / **schizoaffective ~** schizoaffektive Psychose *f*, schizoaffektive Störung *f* / **senile ~** Alterspsychose *f* / **situational ~** Situationspsychose *f* / **symbiotic ~** symbiotische Psychose *f* / **symbiotic infantile ~** symbiotische infantile Psychose *f* / **symptomatic ~** symptomatische Psychose *f* / **terminal ~** Endpsychose *f* / **toxic ~** Intoxikationspsychose *f* / **transitory ~** transitorisches Irresein *n* / **traumatic ~** Unfallpsychose *f*, traumatische Psychose *f* / **tropical ~** Tropenkoller *m* / **unspecified nonorganic ~** nicht näher bezeichnete nichtorganische Psychose *f* / **windigo ~** Windigo–Psychose *f*, Psychose *f* mit Kannibalismus

psychosocial psychosozial

psychosociology Psychosoziologie *f*, Sozialpsychologie *f*

psychosoma, psychosome Psychosoma *f*, Leib–Seele–Einheit *f*

psychosomatic psychosomatisch

psychosomatics Psychosomatik *f*

psychosophy philosophische Psychologie *f*

psychostatics psychische Struktur *f*, Psychostruktur

psychostatistics psychologische Statistik *f*

psychosurgery Psychochirurgie *f*

psychosyndrome Psychosyndrom *n*

psychosynthesis Psychosynthese *f*

psychotaxis unbewusste gedankliche Anpassung *f*, Psychotaxis *f*

psychotechnical psychotechnisch

psychotechnician Psychotechniker *m*

psychotechnics Psychotechnik *f*

psychotechnologist praktischer Psychologe *m*, Psychotechniker *m*, Fachpsychologe *m* im Bereich der angewandten Psychologie

psychotechnology angewandte Psychologie *f*, Psychotechnologie *f*

psychotherapeutic, psychotherapeutical psychotherapeutisch

psychotherapeutics Psychotherapie *f*

psychotherapic psychotherapeutisch

psychotherapist, psychotherapeutist Psychotherapeut *m* / **~ attitudes** Psychotherapeuteneinstellungen *fpl* / **~ trainee** Psychotherapeut *m* in Ausbildung

psychotherapy Psychotherapie *f* / **~ training** Psychotherapieausbildung *f* / **Adlerian ~** individualpsychologische Therapie *f* / **adolescent ~** Jugendlichenpsychotherapie *f* / **ambulatory ~** ambulante Psychotherapie *f* / **analytic ~** analytische Psychotherapie *f* / **bionomic ~** bionome Psychotherapie *f* / **brief ~** Kurzpsychotherapie *f* / **client–centered ~** klientbezogene Psychotherapie *f*, nicht–direktive Psychotherapie *f* / **collective ~** kollektive Psychotherapie *f* / **eclectic ~** eklektische Psychotherapie *f* / **existential ~** existenzielle Psychotherapie *f* / **experiential ~** Erfahrungspsychotherapie *f* / **expressive ~** Ausdruckspsychotherapie *f*, expressive Psychotherapie *f* / **forensic ~** forensische Psychotherapie *f* / **geriatric ~** geriatrische Psychiatrie *f*, Alterspsychotherapie *f* / **individual ~** Einzelpsychotherapie *f* / **interpersonal ~** interpersonelle Psychotherapie *f* / **non–directive ~** nicht–direktive Psychotherapie *f* / **persuasive ~** Persuasionstherapie *f* / **psychoanalytically oriented ~** tiefenpsychologisch fundierte Psychotherapie *f* / **rational–emotive ~** rational–emotive Therapie *f*, rationale Psychotherapie *f* / **reconstructive ~** aufbauende Psychotherapie *f* / **supportive ~** stützende Psychotherapie *f*, unterstützende Psychotherapie *f* / **uncovering ~** aufdeckende Psychotherapie *f*

psychotic psychotisch / Psychotiker *m*

psychoticism Psychotizismus *m*

psychotogenic psychotogen, psychodysleptisch

psychotomimetic psychotomimetisch, psychosomimetisch

psychotonic psychotonisch

psychotoxic psychotoxisch / Psychotoxikon *n*, Psychosomimetikum *n*, Halluzinogen *n*

psychotropic psychotrop, auf die Psyche wirkend

psychotropy Psychotropie *f*

psychovegetative psychovegetativ

psychovitalism Psychovitalismus *m*

psychroaesthesia, psychroesthesia Psychroästhesie *f*, subjektives Kältegefühl *n*

psychroalgia Kälteschmerz *m*, Psychroalgie *f*

psychrophobia Kälteangst *f*, krankhafte Furcht *f* vor Kälte, Psychrophobie *f*

psywar psychologische Kriegführung *f*

P technique P–Technik *f*

pterophagia Essen *n* von Federn

ptosis Ptosis *f*, Oberlidlähmung *f*

puberal, pubertal Pubertäts–, pubertär

puberty Pubertät *f* / **~ rites** Pubertätsriten *mpl*, Mannbarkeitsriten *mpl* / **late ~** Spätpubertät *f* / **precocious ~** frühzeitige Pubertät *f*, Frühreife *f*

pubes Schamhaare *npl*, Schamgegend *f*

pubescence Pubertätseintritt *m*, Pubeszenz *f*

pubescent pubertierend, in der Pubertät befindlich, pubeszent

pubic Scham

pubis Schambein *n*

public öffentlich / Öffentlichkeit *f*, Publikum *n*, Hörerschaft *f*, Auditorium *n* / **~ relations** Öffentlichkeitsarbeit *f*, Public Relations *fpl*

publication Veröffentlichung *f*, Publikation *f*, Werk *n*

publicity Werbung *f*, Propaganda *f*, Öffentlichkeitsarbeit *f*, Reklame *f* / **~ medium** Werbeträger *m*, Werbemedium *n* / **free ~** Gratiswerbung *f*, kostenlose Reklame *f*

pudenda Schamteile *npl*, Schamgegend *f*, Scham *f*

puerile kindisch, knabenhaft, unreif

puerilism, puerility Puerilismus *m*, kindisches Verhalten *n*

puerilistic läppisch

puerperal Kindbett–, puerperal

pugnacious streitsüchtig, kampflustig

pugnacity Kampflust *f*, Streitsucht *f* / **~ erg** Aggressionsmotiv *n*

Pulfrich| effect Pulfrich–Effekt *m* / **~ phenomenon** Pulfrich–Phänomen *n*

pull Anziehungskraft *f*, Zug *m*

pulmonary Lungen–, pulmonal

pulsatile, pulsating pulsierend, rhythmisch, schlagend

pulsation Pulsation *f*, Pulsschlag *m*, rhythmisches Schlagen *n*

pulse Puls *m*, Pulsschlag *m* / **~ quality** Pulsqualität *f* / **~ rate** Pulsfrequenz *f* / **~ wave** Pulswelle *f* / **~ wave velocity** Pulswellengeschwindigkeit *f* / **anacrotic ~** anakroter Puls *m* / **arterial ~** arterieller Puls *m*, Arterienpuls *m* / **dicrotic ~** dikroter Puls *m*, doppelschlägiger Puls *m*

pulvinar Pulvinar *n*, hinteres Ende *n* des Thalamus im Gehirn

punch card, punched card Lochkarte *f* / **~ method** Lochkartenmethode *f* / **~ technique** Lochkartentechnik *f*

punch–drunk syndrome Boxerenzephalopathie *f*, Boxer–Syndrom *n*

punctate punktiert

punctiform punktförmig

punctuality Pünktlichkeit *f*

punctuate punktieren, betonen, unterstreichen

punctuation Punktierung *f*

puncture Punktion *f*, Einstich *m* / **lumbar ~** Lumbalpunktion *f*

punisher Strafreiz *m*

punishment Strafe *f*, Bestrafung *f* / **~ dream** Straftraum *m* / **~ fantasy** Straftraum *m*, Strafphantasie *f* / **capital ~** Todesstrafe *f* / **contingent ~** bedingte Strafe *f* / **corporal ~** körperliche Strafe *f*, körperliche Züchtigung *f* / **natural ~** natürliche Strafe *f* / **negative ~** negative Bestrafung *f*

punitive Straf–, strafend, punitiv

pupa Puppe *f*, Larve *f*

pupal das Puppenstadium betreffend

pupate sich verpuppen

pupil Schüler *m* / **weak ~** schwacher Schüler *m*

pupil Pupille *f* / **~ dilating drug** pupillenerweiterndes Mittel *n* / **~ dilation** Pupillenerweiterung *f* / **~ of the eye** Pupille *f* / **~ reflex** Pupillenreflex *m* / **~ size** Pupillengröße *f* / **artificial ~** künstliches Sehloch *n* / **contracted ~** enge Pupille *f* / **dilated ~** erweiterte Pupille *f*

pupillary Pupillen–

pupillometer Pupillometer *n*, Pupillenmesser *m*

pupillometry, pupillometrics Pupillenmessung *f*

pupilloscope Skiaskop *n*

pupilloscopy Skiaskopie *f*

purchase pattern Käuferverhalten *n*, Einkaufsverhalten *n* des Konsumenten

pure rein

purgation Katharsis *f*, Abreagieren *n*, Läuterung *f*

purification compulsion Reinigungszwang *m*

purity Reinheit *f* / **colorimetric ~** kolorimetrische Reinheit *f*

Purkinje| afterimage zweites Nachbild *n*, Purkinje–Nachbild *n* / **~ cell** Purkinje–Zelle *f* / **~ corpuscle** Purkinje–Zelle *f* / **~ effect** Purkinje–Phänomen *n*, Purkinje–Effekt *m* / **~ figures** Purkinje–Aderfigur *f* / **~ phenomenon** Purkinje–Phänomen *n* / **~–Sanson images** Purkinje–Sanson–Spiegelbilder *npl*, Reflexbilder *npl*

puromycin Puromycin *n*

purple Purpur *n* / purpurfarben / ~ **ring** Purpurring *m* / **retinal** ~ Sehpurpur *n* / **visual** ~ Sehpurpur *n*, Rhodopsin *n*, Erythropsin *n*

purport Bedeutung *f*, Sinn *m*, Inhalt *m*

purpose Absicht *f*, Ziel *n*, Zweck *m*, Vorsatz *m*, Intention *f* / ~ **psychosis** Zweckpsychose *f*

purposeful beabsichtigt, zielbewusst, zweckmäßig

purposefulness Zielbewusstheit *f*, Entschlossenheit *f*

purposive zielgerichtet, zielbewusst, zweckgerichtet

purposiveness Zielgerichtetheit *f*, Zielstrebigkeit *f*

purposivism Intentionalismus *m*, Lehre *f* von der Zielstrebigkeit

pursuit Folgen *n*, Verfolgen *n* / ~ **pendulum** Schwingpendel *n* / ~ **reaction** visuellmotorische Reaktion *f* / ~ **rotor** „pursuit rotor" *m*, Gerät *n* zur Prüfung der visuellmotorischen Reaktion, Ziel– und Markenverfolgungsapparat *m* / ~ **test** Prüfung *f* der visuell–motorischen Reaktion / **ocular** ~ visuelles Nachfolgen *n* / **rotary** ~ Verfolgen *n* von bewegten Objekten

pursuitmeter Gerät *n* zur Messung der visuell–motorischen Koordination, Pursuitmeter *n* / **rotary** ~ Gerät *n* zur Messung der visuell–motorischen Koordination bei Drehbewegungen

putrefaction Fäulnis *f*

putrefactive fäulniserregend

putrid faul, faulig, putrid

putting through automatisch–mechanisches Gliedertraining *n* / ~ **puzzle** Problem *n*, Rätsel *n* / ~ **box** Problemkäfig *m*, Problemkasten *m* / ~ **test** Puzzle–Test *m*, Legespiel–Test *m*

pygmalionism Pygmalionismus *m*, sexuelle Erregung *f* beim Beschauen oder Betasten von Standbildern

pyknic, pycnic pyknisch

pyknolepsy, pycnoepilepsy, pyknoepilepsy Pyknolepsie *f*, epileptiforme Anfälle *mpl*

pyknomorph, pyknomorphic pyknomorph

pyknomorphy Pyknomorphie *f*

pyloric Magenausgangs–, Pylorus–

pylorus Magenausgang *m*, Pförtner *m*, Pylorus *m*

pyramid Pyramide *f*

pyramidal pyramidenförmig, pyramidal

pyramidotomy Durchtrennung *f* der Pyramidenbahn, Pyramidotomie *f*

pyretogenetic, pyretogenic, pyretogenous fiebererzeugend, pyrogen

pyrexia, pyrexy Fieberanfall *m*, Fieberzustand *m*, Pyrexie *f*

pyriform birnenförmig

pyrogenetic, pyrogenic, pyrogenous fiebererzeugend, pyrogen

pyrolagnia, pyrolagny Pyrolagnie *f*, sexuelle Erregung *f* durch Brandstiftung

pyromancy Feuerkult *m*

pyromania Pyromanie *f*, pathologische Brandstiftung *f*, Brandstiftungstrieb *m* / **erotic** ~ Pyrolagnie *f*, sexuelle Erregung *f* durch Brandstiftung

pyromaniac Pyromaner *m*, dranghafter Brandstifter *m* / pyroman, triebhaft Brände legend

pyrophobia krankhafte Angst *f* vor Feuer, Pyrophobie *f*

pyrosis Sodbrennen *n*, Pyrosis *f*

Q

Q data Q–Daten *npl*

Q fever psychosis Q–Fieber–Psychose *f*

Q method Fragebogenmethode *f*

Q score Q–Wert *m*

Q sort Q–Sortierung *f* / **~ testing technique** Q–Sort–Verfahren *n*

Q technique Q–Technik *f*

quack Quacksalber *m*, Kurpfuscher *m* / **~ remedy** Schwindelmedikament *n*

quackery Quacksalberei *f*, Scharlatanerie *f*

quadrangle Viereck *n*

quadrangular viereckig

quadrant Quadrant *m*, Viertelkreis *m*

quadrantal Quadranten

quadrantanopsia Verlust *m* des Sehvermögens in einem Sehfeldquadranten

quadratic quadratisch

quadrature Quadratur *f*

quadrigemina Vierhügelgegend *f*

quadrigeminal Vierhügel–

quadrilateral vierseitig

quadriplegia Lähmung *f* aller vier Extremitäten, Quadriplegie *f*, Tetraplegie *f*

quadrisyllabic viersilbig

quadrumane Vierhänder *m*

quadrumanous, quadrumanal vierhändig

quadruped Vierfüßer *m*, Vierfüßler *m*

quadrupedal vierfüßig

quadruplet Vierling *m*

quaint wunderlich, malerisch, urig

quaintness malerischer Anblick *m*, Kuriosität *f*

quale abstrakte Erfahrungseinheit *f*, beziehungslose Sinnesempfindung *f*

qualification Qualifikation *f*, Eignung *f*, Befähigung *f*, Tauglichkeit *f*, Fähigkeit *f* / **with ~** unter Vorbehalt, mit Einschränkungen

qualifier Merkmal *n*, Unterscheidungskriterium *n*

qualitative qualitativ

quality Qualität *f*, Eigenschaft *f*, Beschaffenheit *f*, Eigenart *f* / **~ assurance** Qualitätssicherung *f* / **~ circle** Qualitätszirkel *m* / **~ complex** Begriffszerfall *m* / **~ control** Qualitätskontrolle *f* / **~ management** Qualitätssicherung *f*, Qualitätsmanagement *n* / **~ of care** Versorgungsqualität *f*, Betreuungsqualität *f* / **~ of education** Bildungsqualität *f* / **~ of form** Formqualität *f*, Gestaltqualität *f* / **~ of form theory** Theorie *f* der Gestaltqualität / **~ of Gestalt** Gestaltqualität *f*, Formqualität *f* / **~ of life** Lebensqualität *f* / **~ of performance** Qualität *f* der Leistung / **~ of services** Qualität *f* der Dienstleistungen / **~ of work life** Arbeitsplatzqualität *f* / **~ scale** qualitative Skala *f* / **educational ~** Bildungsqualität *f* / **palaeoatavistic ~** paläoatavistische Qualität *f* / **primary ~** Urqualität *f*, Primäreigenschaft *f* / **secondary ~** sekundäre Qualität *f* / **sensory ~** Sinnesqualität *f*

qualm Gewissensbiss *m*, Zweifel *m*

qualmish unwohl, niedergeschlagen

quandary verzwickte Lage *f*, Verlegenheit *f*

quanta Quanten *npl* / **~ theory** Quantentheorie *f*

quantal diskontinuierlich

quantification Quantifikation *f*, Quantifizierung *f*

quantify quantifizieren

quantitative quantitativ

quantity Quantität *f*, Menge *f* / **imaginary ~** imaginäre Zahl *f*, imaginäre Menge *f*

quantum Menge *f*, Größe *f*, Quantum *n* / **~ theory** Quantentheorie *f* / **sensory ~** Wahrnehmungsgröße *f*, sensorische Größe *f*

quarrel Streit *m*, Zank *m* / sich zanken, sich streiten

quarreller, quarreler Streitsüchtiger *m*, Zankhahn *m*

quarrelsome streitsüchtig, zänkisch

quarrelsomeness Streitsucht *f*

quart Viertel *n*, Quart *f*

quartile Quartil *n* / **~ deviation** Quartilabweichung *f* / **~ interval** Quartilintervall *n* / **~ range** Quartilbereich *m*, Quartilintervall *n* / **~ score** Quartilwert *m*

quartimax rotation Quartimax–Rotation *f*, Quartimax–Methode *f*

quasi Quasi– / **~ experiment** Quasi–Experiment *n* / **~ measurement** Quasi–Messung *f*, Messung *f* in relativen Werten / **~ need** Quasi–Bedürfnis *n* / **~ scale** Quasi–Skala *f*

queasiness übertriebene Gewissenskrupel *mpl*, Überempfindlichkeit *f*, Übelkeit *f*

queer komisch, sonderbar, homosexuell / Homosexueller *m*

querulance Querulantentum *n*, Querulantenwahn *m*

querulent Querulant *m* / querulierend, nörgelnd

querulous querulierend, nörgelnd

querulousness Querulantentum *n*, Nörgelsucht *f*

query Frage *f*, Zweifel *m* / fragen, in Zweifel ziehen

quest for significance Geltungsstreben *n*, Geltungsdrang *m*

question Frage *f*, Problem *n*, Fragen *n* / fragen, befragen / **closed ~** gebundene Frage *f*, geschlossene Frage *f* / **fixed–alternative ~** Frage *f* mit gebundener Aufgabenbeantwortung / **leading ~** Suggestivfrage *f* / **open ~** offene Frage *f*, ungebundene Frage *f* / **open–end ~** offene Frage *f* / **restricted ~** gebundene Frage *f* / **unrestricted ~** offene Frage *f*, ungebundene Frage *f*

questionary, questionnaire Fragebogen *m*, Frageliste *f* / **~ data** Q–Daten *npl* / **~ method** Fragebogenmethode *f*

questioning Befragung *f*, Vernehmung *f* / fragend, kritisch

quick schnell, lebhaft

quiddity eigentliches Wesen *n*, Spitzfindigkeit *f*

quiescence Ruhe *f*

quiet ruhig, still, gelassen / Ruhe *f*

Quincke's| oedema Quincke–Ödem *n* / **~ tube** Quincke–Röhre *f*

quinidine Chinidin *n* / **~ sulfate** Chinidinsulfat *n*

quinine Chinin *n* / **~ sulfate** Chininsulfat *n*

quinpirole Quinpirol *n*

quint Quinte *f*

quintal Zentner *m*

quintessence Quintessenz *f*, Kern *m*, Inbegriff *m*

quintile Quintil *n*, fünfter Teil *m* einer Verteilung

quiver Zittern *n*, Beben *n*

quiz mündliche Prüfung *f*, Examen *n*, Quiz *n*, Frage– und Antwortspiel *n*

quota Quote *f*, Anteil *m* / **~ of affect** Affektbetrag *m* / **~ control** Quotensystem *n*, Stichprobenauswahl *f* nach Quoten / **~ sample** Quotenstichprobe *f* / **~ sampling** Quotenmethode *f*, Stichprobenauswahl *f* nach Quoten

quotidian täglich

quotient Quotient *m* / **~ of achievement** Leistungsquotient *m* / **~ of instruction** Erziehungsquotient *m* / **~ of intelligence** Intelligenzquotient *m*, IQ *m* / **conceptual ~** Begriffsquotient *m* / **developmental ~** Entwicklungsquotient *m* / **educational ~** Erziehungsquotient *m* / **respiratory ~** respiratorischer Quotient *m* / **social ~** Sozialquotient *m*

R

rabble Mob *m*, Pöbel *m*, lärmender Haufen *m* / **~–rouser** Agitator *m*, Demagoge *m*, Aufwiegler *m*, Aufrührer *m*

rabdomancy, rhabdomancy Wünschelrutengehen *n*, Aufsuchen *n* von Wasser mit Hilfe von Wünschelruten

rabid wütend, tollwütig

rabidness Wut *f*, Tollheit *f*, Verrücktheit *f*

rabies Tollwut *f* Rabies *f*

race Rasse *f* / **~ and ethnic discrimination** ethnische und nationale Diskriminierung *f* / **~ consciousness** Rassenbewusstsein *n*, Rassenideologie *f* / **~ difference** Rassenunterschied *m* / **~ discrimination** Rassendiskriminierung *f* / **~ hatred** Rassenhass *m* / **~ mixture** Rassenkreuzung *f* / **~ prejudice** rassisches Vorurteil *n* / **~ psychology** Rassenpsychologie *f* / **~ relations** Rassenbeziehungen *fpl*

racial rassisch, Rassen–

racialism, racism Rassismus *m*, Rassenfanatismus *m*, Rassenhass *m*, Rassenpolitik *f*, Rassentheorie *f*, Rassenlehre *f*

radial radial, strahlenförmig

radian Radian *m*

radiance, radiancy Leuchtdichte *f*, Strahlungsintensität *f*

radiant strahlend, Strahlungs–

radiate strahlenförmig, Strahlen– / strahlen, ausstrahlen

radiation Strahlung *f*, Ausstrahlung *f* / **~ therapy** Strahlentherapie *f* / **auditory ~** Hörstrahlung *f* / **electromagnetic ~** elektromagnetische Strahlung *f* / **optic ~** Sehstrahlung *f* / **thalamic ~** Thalamusstil *m*

radical gründlich, fundamental, radikal / Wurzel *f*, Radikal *n* / **free ~** freies Radikal *n*

radicalism Radikalismus *m*, Gründlichkeit *f* / **political ~** politischer Radikalismus *m*

radiculitis Wurzelentzündung *f*, Radikulitis *f*

radio Rundfunk *m*, Radio *n*

radiogram Röntgenaufnahme *f*, Röntgenbild *n*

radiograph Röntgenaufnahme *f*

radiologist Radiologe *m*, Röntgenologe *m*, Röntgenfacharzt *m*

radiology Strahlenkunde *f*, Radiologie *f*, Röntgenologie *f*

radiometer Strahlungsmesser *m*, Radiometer *n*

radiometry Strahlenmessung *f*, Radiometrie *f*

radiosensitiveness, radiosensitivity Strahlenempfindlichkeit *f*, Strahlensensibilität *f*

radiotherapy Strahlentherapie *f*, Radiotherapie *f*

radius Radius *m*, Halbmesser *m*

radix Wurzel *f*

rage Wut *f*, Raserei *f*, Zorn *m* / rasen, toben / **nonadjustive ~** unangepasste Wut *f* / **sham ~** Scheinwut *f*

railway phobia Eisenbahnphobie *f*

ramble unzusammenhängend reden, vom Thema abschweifen

rambling gedankliche Abschweifung *f*, Gedankenflucht *f* / unzusammenhängend, weitschweifig, gedankenflüchtig

ramification Verzweigung *f*, Verästelung *f*, Auswirkung *f*, Ramifikation *f* / **nervous ~** Nervenverästelung *f* / **terminal ~** Endverzweigung *f*

ramous verzweigt, verastelt

ramp rasen, toben, wüten

rampageous wild, wütend, tobend, ausgelassen

Ramsey Hunt syndrome Ramsey Hunt–Syndrom *n*

ramus Ast *m*, Zweig *m*, Ramus *m* / **~ communicans albus** weißer Verbindungsast *m*, Ramus communicans albus *m* / **~ of nerve** Nervenast *m* / **white ~** weißer Nervenast *m*

rancour, rancor Groll *m*, Erbitterung *f*, Hass *m*

random zufällig, Zufalls–, wahllos, stochastisch / **at ~** aufs Geratewohl, zufällig

randomization zufällige Aufteilung *f*, Zufallsauswahl *f*, Randomisierung *f*

randomize zufällig auswählen, auslosen

randomizer Zufallsgenerator *m*, Gerät *n* zur Herstellung von Zufallszahlen

randomness Zufälligkeit *f*

range Bereich *m*, Variationsbreite *f*, Streuung *f*, Streubreite *f* / **~ of accomodation** Akkomodationsbreite *f* / **~ of action** Wirkungsbereich *m* / **~ of adaptation** Adaptationsbreite *f* / **~ of attention** Aufmerksamkeitsumfang *m* / **~ of audibility** Hörbereich *m*, Hörfeld *n* / **~ of colours** Farbspektrum *n*, Farbpalette *f* / **~–finding** Telemetrie *f*, Entfernungsmessung *f* / **~ of hearing** Hörbereich *m*, Hörweite *f* / **~ scale** Skalenbreite *f* / **~ of scatter** Streubereich *m* / **~ of thoughts** Ideenkreis *m* / **~ of vision** Gesichtsfeld *n* / **discriminating ~** Trennbereich *m* / **interquartile ~** Quartilabstand *m* / **neutral ~** Indifferenzbereich *m* / **normal ~** Normalbereich *m* / **out–of–~ judges** Urteile *npl* außerhalb des angebotenen Beurteilungsbereiches / **operating ~** Arbeitsbereich *m* / **semi–interquartile ~** Quartilabweichung *f*, mittlere Quartilabweichung *f* / **short–~ impact** kurzfristige Wirkung *f* / **visual ~** Sehweite *f*

rank Rang *m*, Rangplatz *m* in eine Rangreihe bringen, einreihen, klassifizieren / **~ correlation** Rangkorrelation *f* / **~–difference correlation** Rangkorrelation *f* / **~–order** Rangordnung *f*, Rangreihe *f* / **~–order correlation** Rangkorrelation *f* / **~–order method** Rangreihenbildung *f*, Rangreihenmethode *f* / **relative ~** relativer Rangplatz *m*, relative Position *f* / **social ~** sozialer Stand *m*, sozialer Status *m*

ranking Rangfolge *f*, Rangreihe *f*, Rangordnung *f*, Rangreihenbilden *n* / **~ list** Rangreihe *f*, Rangliste *f* / **~ order** Rangordnung *f*, Rangreihe *f* / **~ method** Rangreihenmethode *f*, Rangreihenbildung *f* / **~ principle** Rangordnungsprinzip *n* / **high ~** hohe Einstufung *f*, hohe Platzierung *f*

Ranschburg| inhibition Ranschburg'sche Hemmung *f* / **~ phenomenon** Ranschburg'sches Phänomen *n*

Ranvier|'s constrictions Ranvier–Schnürringe *mpl* / **nodes of ~** Ranvier–Schnürringe *mpl*

rap leichter Schlag *m*, Klaps *m*, Rüffel *m*, Verweis *m*

rape vergewaltigen / Vergewaltigung *f*, Notzucht *f* / **~ and murder** Lustmord *m* / **~ trauma syndrome** Vergewaltigungssyndrom *n* / **anal ~** anale Vergewaltigung *f*

raphe Raphe *f*

rapidity Schnelligkeit *f* / **~ of movements** Bewegungsschnelligkeit *f*

rapport Rapport *m*, innere Übereinstimmung *f* / **affective ~** affektiver Rapport *m*, emotionale Beziehung *f*, affektiver Kontakt *m* / **emotional ~** affektiver Rapport *m*, emotionale Beziehung *f*

rapture Entzücken *n*, Verzückung *f*, Ekstase *f* / **~ of the deep** Tiefenrausch *m*

raptus Raptus *m*, anfallsartige, aggressive Handlung *f*, Wutanfall *m*

rarefaction Verflüchtigung *f*, Minderung *f*, Verfeinerung *f*

rash Kurzschlussreaktion *f*, Unbesonnenheit *f*, Ausschlag *m* / rasch, voreilig

rat Ratte *f* / **~ learning** Lernverhalten *n* der Ratten, Lernen *n* bei Ratten / **white ~** weiße Ratte *f*, Albino Ratte *f*

ratchet mechanism Verschlussmechanismus *m*

rate Verhältnis *n*, Anteil *m*, Quote *f*, Häufigkeit *f* / bewerten, beurteilen, schätzen / **~ of absenteeism** Abwesenheitsquote *f*, Fehlzeitquote *f* / **~ buster** Akkordbrecher *m*, Stachanow–Arbeiter *m*, Norm–Überfüller *m* / **~ of change** prozentuale Veränderung *f* / **~ of forgetting** Schnelligkeit *f* des Vergessens / **~ of growth** Wachstumsrate *f* / **~ of learning** Lerntempo *n* / **~ of responding** Reaktionsrate *f* / **~ of response** Reaktionsrate *f* / **~ revision** Akkordüberprüfung *f*, Änderung *f* der Arbeitsnormen / **~ of scanning** Abtastgeschwindigkeit *f* / **~ score** Verhältniswert *m* / **~ of speech** Sprechtempo *n* / **~ of success** Erfolgsziffer *f* / **~ test** Schnelligkeitstest *m* / **~ of wages** Lohnniveau *n*, Lohnsatz *m* / **~ of work** Arbeitsleistung *f*, Produktivität *f* / **basal metabolic ~** Grundumsatz *m* / **cardiac ~** Herzfrequenz. *f*, Pulszahl *f* / **compensatory ~** Kompensationsgrad *m* / **differential ~ reinforcement** differenzielle Verstärkung *f* unterschiedlicher Häufigkeit / **metabolic ~** Grundumsatz *m*, Stoffwechselumsatz *m* / **overall ~** Gesamthäufigkeit *f*, Gesamtfrequenz *f* / **terminal ~** Endhäufigkeit *f*

ratee Beurteilter *m*, beurteilte Person *f*

rater Beurteiler *m*, Schätzer *m*

rating Beurteilung *f*, Bewertung *f*, Einstufung *f*, Schätzung *f*, Rating *n* / **~–scale** Rating–Skala *f*, Schätzskala *f*, Bewertungsskala *f*, Beurteilungsskala *f* / **~ scale method** Methode *f* der Schätzskala / **graphic ~ scale** graphisches Einstufungssystem *n* / **sociometric ~** soziometrische Einschätzung *f*

ratio Verhältnis *n*, Kennziffer *f*, Häufigkeit *f* / **~–delay studies** Multimomentverfahren *n* / **~ estimation** Verhältnisschätzung *f* / **~ reinforcement** Verhältnisverstärkung *f* / **~ scale** Verhältnisskala *f* / **affective ~** Farbenindex *m* / **binaural ~** Schalldruckdifferenz *f* / **diathetic ~** diathetische Proportion *f* / **fixed–~ schedule** feste Verhältnisfolge *f* / **fixed–~ reinforcement** Verstärkung *f* in festgelegtem Verhältnis, fester Quotenverstärkungsplan *m*, feste Verhältnisfolge *f* / **Mendelian ~** Mendel'sches Zahlenverhältnis *n* / **therapeutic ~** therapeutische Breite *f* / **variable ~** variables Verhältnis *n*, variable Quote *f* / **variable–~ reinforcement** variable Quotenverstärkung *f* / **variable–~ schedule** veränderliche Verhältnisfolge *f*, variabler Quotenverstärkungsplan *m*

ratiocination Folgerung *f*, Schlussfolgerung *f*

rational rational, vernunftsgemäß, vernünftig, mit Vernunft begabt

rationale logische Grundlage *f*, Grund *m*, Rechtfertigung *f*, Prinzip *n*

rationalisation Rationalisierung *f*, Rationalisation *f*

rationalise rationalisieren

rationalism Rationalismus *m*

rationalist Rationalist *m*, Vernunftsmensch *m*

rationality Rationalität *f*, Vernünftigkeit *f*, klarer Verstand *m*

Rauwolfia Rauwolfia *f*

ravage Verheerung *f*, Verwüstung *f*

rave fantasieren, delirieren, irre reden, toben

ravenous gierig, heißhungrig, gefräßig

raving Delirium *n*, Gefasel *n*, unsinniges Gerede *n*, Fieberwahn *m*

ravish fortreißen, entzücken, entführen, schänden

raw roh, Roh–, unverarbeitet

ray Strahl *m* / **~ of direction** Richtungsstrahl *m* / **~ of light** Lichtstrahl *m* / **biotic ~s** Lebensstrahlen *mpl* / **caloric ~s** Wärmestrahlen *mpl* / **infrared ~s** Infrarotstrahlen *mpl* / **luminous ~s** Spektralstrahlen *mpl* / **ultraviolet ~s** Ultraviolettstrahlen *mpl*

Rayleigh equation Rayleigh–Gleichung *f*

Raynaud's disease Raynaud–Krankheit *f*, Raynaud–Syndrom *n*

reabsorb rückresorbieren, wiederaufnehmen

reabsorption Reabsorption *f*, Rückresorption *f*, Wiederaufnahme *f* / ~ **rate** Reabsorptionsrate *f*

reaccustom wieder gewöhnen an

react reagieren

reactance Reaktanz *f*, Blindwiderstand *m* / **psychological** ~ psychologische Reaktanz *f*

reactiometer Reaktionsprüfgerät *n*

reaction Reaktion *f*, Reizantwort *f* / ~ **of adaptation** Anpassungsreaktion *f* / ~ **arc** Reflexbogen *m* / ~ **chain** Reaktionskette *f*, Verhaltensfolge *f* / ~ **to crisis** Krisenreaktion *f*, Stressreaktion *f* / ~ **curve** Reaktionskurve *f* / ~ **of exhaustion** Erschöpfungsreaktion *f* / **~–evocation potentiality** Reaktionspotential *n* / ~ **of flight** Fluchtreaktion *f* / ~ **formation** Reaktionsbildung *f* / ~ **generalisation** Reaktionsgeneralisierung *f* / ~ **key** Reaktionstaste *f* / ~ **latency** Reaktionslatenz *f* / ~ **level** Reaktionsniveau *n*, Reaktionsebene *f* / ~ **of the surrounding medium** Reaktion *f* auf die Umwelt / ~ **pattern** Reaktionsmuster *n*, Reaktionsnorm *f* / ~ **period** Reaktionszeit *f* / ~ **potential** Reaktionspotential *n* / ~ **psychology** Reaktionspsychologie *f* / ~ **psychosis** Reaktionspsychose *f*, reaktive Psychose *f* / ~ **summation** Reaktionssummation *f* / ~ **system** Aktionssystem *n* / ~ **threshold** Reaktionsschwelle *f* / **~–time** Reaktionszeit *f* / **~–time method** Reaktionsmethode *f* / ~ **to a trauma** Traumareaktion *f*, Erlebnisreaktion *f* / ~ **to restraint** Verbotsreaktion *f* / ~ **to severe stress, and adjustment disorders** Reaktionen *fpl* auf schwere Belastungen und Anpassungsstörungen / ~ **type** Reaktionstyp *m* / ~ **variable** Reaktionsvariable *f* / **adjustive** ~ Anpassungsreaktion *f* / **affective** ~ Affektreaktion *f*, Affekthandlung *f* / **alerting** ~ Alarmreaktion *f* / **all–or–none** ~ Alles–oder–Nichts–Reaktion *f* / **anergastic** ~ psychoorganisches Syndrom *n* / **antedating** ~ antizipatorische Reaktion *f* / **anticipatory** ~ antizipatorische Reaktion *f* / **antisocial** ~ asoziales Verhalten *n* / **assaultive** ~ Angriffsreaktion *f*, Angriffsverhalten *n* / **associative** ~ Assoziationsreaktion *f* / **asthenic** ~ Schwächereaktion *f* / **autonomic** ~ autonome Reaktion *f* / **avoiding** ~ Vermeidungsreaktion *f* / **catastrophic** ~ Katastrophenreaktion *f* / **catathymic** ~ katathyme Reaktion *f* / **circular** ~ Kreisreaktion *f* / **compensatory** ~ Kompensationsreaktion *f*, kompensatorische Reaktion *f* / **compulsive** ~ Zwangsreaktion *f* / **conditioned** ~ bedingte Reaktion *f*, konditionierte Reaktion *f* / **confirming** ~ Betätigungsreaktion *f* / **deferred** ~ verzögerte Reaktion *f*, aufgeschobene Reaktion *f* / **delayed** ~ verzögerte Reaktion *f*, Spätreaktion *f*, aufgeschobene Reaktion *f* / **demonstrative** ~ demonstrative Reaktion *f* / **depressive** ~ depressive Reaktion *f* / **destructive** ~ destruktive Reaktion *f* / **differential** ~ differenzierte Reaktion *f* / **discriminatory** ~ unterscheidende Reaktion *f* / **disergastic** ~ disergastische Reaktion *f* / **disjunctive** ~ disjunktive Reaktion *f* / **dissociative** ~ Abspaltung *f*, Dissoziation *f* / **dysergastic** ~ abnorme Reaktion *f* / **dyssocial** ~ strafbares Verhalten *n* / **emotional** ~ Affektreaktion *f*, Gefühlsreaktion *f* / **false** ~ Fehlreaktion *f* / **following** ~ Folgeverhalten *n* / **galvanic** ~ galvanische Hautreaktion *f* / **gastrointestinal** ~ Magendarmreaktion *f* / **hyperergastic** ~ manische Reaktion *f* / **hyperintensive** ~ Überreaktion *f* / **hypoergastic** ~ depressive Reaktion *f* / **hypochondric** ~ hypochondrische Reaktion *f* / **hypothymergastic** ~ körperliche Reaktion *f* bei Niedergeschlagenheit / **hysterical** ~ hysterische Reaktion *f* / **incompatible** ~ inkompatibles Verhalten *n* / **induced** ~ induzierte Reaktion *f* / **intentional** ~ willkürliche Reaktion *f* / **investigatory** ~ Untersuchungsreaktion *f*, Orientierungsreaktion *f* / **learned** ~ erlernte Reaktion *f* / **local galvanic** ~ lokale galvanische Hautreaktion *f* / **muscular** ~ Muskelreaktion *f* / **negative therapeutic** ~ negative therapeutische Reaktion *f* / **neurotic** ~ neurotische Reaktion *f* / **neurotic–depressive ~** reaktive neurotische Depression *f*, neurotisch–depressive Reaktion *f* / **obsessive ~** Zwangsreaktion *f* / **obsessive–compulsive ~** zwangsneurotische Reaktion *f*, obsessiv–kompulsive Reaktion *f* / **operant ~** Wirkreaktion *f*, Operant *m* / **optokinetic ~** optokinetische Reaktion *f* / **orienting ~** Orientierungsreaktion *f*, Orientierungsreflex *m* / **orthostatic ~** Aufstehreaktion *f* / **paranoid ~** paranoide Reaktion *f* / **parergastic ~** psychotische Falschreaktion *f* / **passive–aggressive ~** passiv–aggressives Verhalten *n* / **phobic ~** phobische Reaktion *f*, Angstreaktion *f* / **photophobic ~** Lichtscheu *f*, Photophobie *f* / **positive supporting ~** Unterstützungsreaktion *f* / **protective ~** Schutzreaktion *f* / **psychasthenic ~** psychasthenische Reaktion *f*, Psychasthenie *f* / **psychical ~** psychische Reaktion *f* / **psychoneurotic ~** Psychoneurose *f* / **psychotic depressive ~** psychotische depressive Reaktion *f* / **rebellious ~** Widerstandsreaktion *f* / **retarded conditioned ~** verzögerte konditionierte Reaktion *f* / **schizophrenic ~** schizophrene Reaktion *f* / **selected ~** Wahlreaktion *f* / **serial ~** Kettenreaktion *f*, Serienhandlung *f* / **sexual ~** sexueller Reflex *m* / **situational ~** situative Reaktion *f* / **tertiary circular ~** tertiäre Kreisreaktion *f* / **thymergastic ~** thymergastische Reaktion *f*, pathologisch–affektives Verhalten *n* / **unconditioned ~** unkonditionierte Reaktion *f* / **voluntary ~** willkürliche Reaktion *f* / **what–is–that ~** Orientierungsreaktion *f*

reactivate reaktivieren

reactivation Reaktivierung *f*

reactive reaktiv

reactivist psychology Reaktivismus *m*, reaktivistische Psychologie *f*

reactivity Reaktionsfähigkeit *f*, Reagibilität *f*, Reaktivität *f* / **~ effect** reaktiver Effekt *m* / **cardiovascular ~** kadiovaskuläre Reaktivität *f*

reactology Verhaltenswissenschaft *f*, Lehre *f* vom menschlichen Verhalten

reactor reagierende Person *f*

Read's| delivery method Read Entbindungsverfahren *n* / **~ preparation for labor** Read Entbindungsverfahren *n*

read lesen, studieren

readability Lesbarkeit *f*, Textverständlichkeit *f*

readable lesbar

readaptation Wiedereingewöhnung *f*

reader interest research Leserforschung *f*, Leseranalyse *f*

readiness Bereitschaft *f*, Bereitwilligkeit *f*, Vorbereitung *f* / **~ grouping** Eingruppierung *f* nach Fähigkeitsniveaus / **~ potential** Bereitschaftspotential *n* / **~ of speech** Sprachgewandtheit *f*, Sprachfertigkeit *f* / **maturational ~** Reife *f*, Reifevoraussetzung *f*

reading Lesen *n* / **~ ability** Lesefertigkeit *f*, Lesefähigkeit *f* / **~ achievement** Leseleistung *f* / **~ age** Lesealter *n* / **~ aloud** Lautlesen *n* / **~ aptitude** Lesefertigkeit *f* / **~–book** Lesebuch *n* / **~ centre** Lesezentrum *n* / **~ chart** Leseprobentafel *f* / **~ comprehension** Leseverständnis *n* / **~ development** Leseentwicklung *f* / **~ device** Lesehilfe *f*, Lesegerät *n* / **~ disability** Leseunvermögen *n*, Lese–Rechtschreibeschwäche *f*, Leseschwäche *f* / **~ disorder** Lesestörung *f* / **developmental ~ disorder** entwicklungsbezogene Lesestörung *f* / **specific ~ disorder** umschriebene Lesestörung *f* / **~ education** Leseunterricht *m* / **~ habit** Lesegewohnheit *f* / **~ ladder** nach Schwierigkeitsgrad abgestuftes Lesematerial *n* / **~ material** Lesematerial *n* / **~ measure** Messen *n* der Leseleistung, Lesetest *m* / **~ quotient** Lesequotient *m* / **~ readiness** Lesereife *f*, Lesebereitschaft *f* / **~ skill** Lesefertigkeit *f* / **~ span** Lesbarkeitsgrenze *f*, Gedächtnisspanne *f* / **~ speed** Lesegeschwindigkeit *f* / **~ test** Lesetest *m* / **backward ~** Rückwärtslesen *n* / **oral ~** Lautlesen *n* / **oral ~ habit** Gewohnheit *f* beim Lesen die Lippen mitzubewegen / **remedial ~** heilpädagogisches Lesetraining *n*, Leseförderunterricht *m* / **selected ~s** ausgewählte Literatur *f* / **silent ~** lautloses Lesen *n*, stilles Lesen *n*

readjustment Wiedereingewöhnung *f*, Wiedereingliederung *f*, Wiederherstellung *f* / **psychosocial ~** psychosoziale Wiedereingliederung *f*, psychosoziale Wiederanpassung *f*

readmission erneute Einlieferung *f*, Wiedereinlieferung *f*

reafference Reafferenz *f* / **~ principle** Reafferenzprinzip *n*

reagent Reagens *n*

real real, wirklich, echt

realisation Verwirklichung *f* / **symbolic ~** symbolische Wunscherfüllung *f*

realism Realismus *m* / **fortuitous ~** Zufallsrealismus *m* / **moral ~** moralischer Realismus *m* / **psychological ~** psychologischer Realismus *m*

realistic realistisch, sachlich

reality Realität *f*, Wirklichkeit *f* / **~ adaptation** Realitätsanpassung *f*, Anpassung *f* an die Wirklichkeit / **~ awareness** Realitätsbewusstsein *n* / **~ ego** Real–Ich *n* / **~ feeling** Wirklichkeitsgefühl *n* / **~ principle** Realitätsprinzip *n* / **~ sense** Realitätssinn *m*, Wirklichkeitssinn *m* / **~ situation** objektive Situation *f*, Realität *f* / **~ testing** Realitätsprüfung *f* / **~ therapy** Realitätstherapie *f* / **objective ~ level** objektives Realitätsniveau *n* / **psychic ~** psychische Realität *f* / **psychological ~** psychische Realität *f* / **social ~** soziale Wirklichkeit *f* / **virtual ~** virtuelle Realität *f*

rearing Erziehung *f*, Aufzucht *f*

rearrangement Neuordnung *f*, Umordnung *f*, Umwandlung *f* / **~ test** Ordnungstest *m*

reason Grund *m*, Beweggrund *m*, Motiv *n*, Vernunft *f* / denken, schließen, urteilen

reasonable vernünftig, verständig, angemessen

reasoning logisches Denken *n*, schlussfolgerndes Denken *n*, Urteilen *n* / **~ test** Test *m* des logischen Denkens / **abstract ~** logisches Denken *n*, abstraktes Denken *n* / **affective ~** affektives Denken *n*, Affektivlogik *f* / **arithmetical ~** rechnerisches Denken *n* / **deductive ~** deduktives Denken *n* / **false ~** Denkfehler *m* / **inductive–deductive ~** schlussfolgerndes Denken *n*, konvergentes Denken *n*, induktiv–deduktiv logisches Denken *n* / **logical ~** logisches Denken *n* / **shrewd ~** scharfsinniges Schlussfolgern *n* / **syllogistic ~** syllogistisches Denken *n*, schlussfolgerndes Denken *n*

reassurance Beruhigung *f*, Rückversicherung *f*, Bestätigung *f*, Zusicherung *f*

rebel Rebell *m*, Aufrührer *m* / rebellisch, aufrührerisch / rebellieren, sich auflehnen

rebellion Rebellion *f*, Revolte *f*, Auflehnung *f*, Aufruhr *f* / **adolescent ~** Auflehnung *f* der Jugend, Jugendrevolte *f*

rebelliousness Widerspenstigkeit *f* / **neurotic ~** neurotischer Widerstand *m*

rebirth fantasy Wiedergeburtsphantasie *f*

rebound phenomenon Rückstoßeffekt *m*, Rebound–Phänomen *n*

rebuke tadeln, zurechtweisen / Tadel *m*, Vorwurf *m*

rebus writing Malen *n* von Bilderrätseln

rebuttal Widerlegung *f*

recalcitrant widerspenstig / Widerspenstiger *m*

recall Erinnerung *f*, Reproduzieren *n*, Wachrufen *n*, Abruf *m* / erinnern, ins Gedächtnis zurückrufen / **~ method** Gedächtnismethode *f*, Reproduktionsverfahren *n*, Wiedererkennungsverfahren *n* / **~ procedure** Reproduktionsverfahren *n*, Wiedererkennungsverfahren *n* / **~ score method** Methode *f* der behaltenen Glieder / **~ test** Gedächtnistest *m* / **aided ~** Gedächtnisstütze *f*, Erinnerungshilfe *f* / **cued ~** hinweisgeleitetes Reproduzieren *n* / **free ~** freies Reproduzieren *n*, freie Erinnerung *f* / **ideational ~** Erinnerungsvorstellung *f* /

serial ~ serielles Reproduzieren *n* / **unaided ~** Erinnerung *f* ohne Gedächtnishilfe

recapitulate rekapitulieren, kurz wiederholen

recapitulation Rekapitulation *f*, kurze Wiederholung *f* / **~ principle** Wiederholungsprinzip *n*, biogenetisches Grundgesetz *n* / **~ theory** Rekapitulationstheorie *f*, biogenetisches Grundgesetz *n*

receive empfangen, erhalten

receiver Empfänger *m* / **~ operating characteristic** Leistungsfunktion *f* des Empfängers, Empfänger–Verhaltenscharakteristik *f*

recency Neuheit *f* / **~ effect** Rezenz–Effekt *m*, Recency–Effekt *m* / **~ principle** Neuheitsprinzip *n*

recent neulich, kürzlich, rezent, jüngst

recenter umstrukturieren

recentring, recentering Umzentrierung *f*, Umstrukturierung *f*

recept eingeprägte Vorstellung *f*, Standard–Vorstellungsbild *n*

reception Empfang *m*, Aufnahme *f* / **cold ~** kühle Aufnahme *f*

receptive empfänglich, aufnahmefähig, rezeptiv

receptiveness Aufnahmefähigkeit *f*, Rezeptivität *f*, Empfänglichkeit *f*, Empfindlichkeit *f*

receptivity Aufnahmefähigkeit *f*, Rezeptivität *f* / **sexual ~** sexuelle Rezeptivität *f*

receptor Rezeptor *m*, Sensor *m*, Aufnahmeorgan *n* / **~ adaptation** Rezeptoradaptation *f* / **~ binding** Rezeptorbindung *f* / **~ blockade** Rezeptorblock *m*, Rezeptorblockade *f* / **~–cell potential** Sinneszellenpotential *n* / **~ field** rezeptorisches Feld *n* / **~ potential** Rezeptorpotential *n* / **~ unit** Rezeptoreinheit *f* / **alpha–adrenergic ~** alpha–adrenerger Rezeptor *m* / **beta–adrenergic ~** beta–adrenerger Rezeptor *m* / **chemical ~** Chemorezeptor *m* / **cholinergic ~** cholinerger Rezeptor *m* / **cold ~** Kälterezeptor *m* / **cutaneous ~** Hautrezeptor *m* / **kinaesthetic ~** Propriozeptor *m* / **mechanosensitive ~** Mechanosensor *m*, mechanosensitiver Rezeptor *m* / **muscarinic ~** muskarinartiger Rezeptor *m* / **neural ~** Rezeptor *m*, Sinnesorgan *n* / **nicotinic ~** nikotinerger Rezeptor *m* / **on ~** An–Rezeptor *m* / **on–off ~** An–Aus Rezeptor *m* / **secondary ~ cell** sekundäre Sinneszelle *f* / **sensory ~** sensorischer Rezeptor *m*, Sensor *m*

recess Pause *f*, Unterbrechung *f*, Ferien *f*

recessive rezessiv

recessiveness Rezessivität *f* / **genetic ~** rezessive Vererbung *f*, genetische Rezessivität *f*

recidivation, recidivism Rückfall *m*, Rückfälligkeit *f*

recidivist rückfälliger Verbrecher *m*, Rückfälliger *m*

recidivous rückfällig

recipathy gegenseitige Sympathie *f*

recipient Empfänger *m*

reciprocal reziprok

reciprocate gegenseitig beeinflussen, erwidern, sich erkenntlich zeigen

reciprocity Gegenseitigkeit *f*, Wechselseitigkeit *f*, Wechselwirkung *f* / **~ law** Gesetz *n* der Wechselwirkung, Block'sches Gesetz *n* / **~ principle** Gegenseitigkeitsprinzip *n*, Bunsen–Roscoe–Gesetz *n*

recitation Vortragen *n*, Rezitieren *n*, Hersagen *n*, Rezitation *f* / **~ procedure** Rezitationsmethode *f* / **socialized ~** Rede–und Antwort–Spiel *n* in einer Lerngruppe

recitative Rezitativ *n*, dramatischer Sprechgesang *m*

recite rezitieren, vortragen, hersagen

reckless unbesonnen, unbekümmert, leichtsinnig

recklessness Unbesonnenheit *f*, Unbekümmertheit *f*, Leichtsinn *m*

reclusion Einsamkeit *f*, Zurückgezogenheit *f*, Einzelhaft *f*

recoding erneute Codierung *f*, Umkodierung *f*

recognition Erkennen *n*, Wiedererkennen *n*, Erkenntnis *f*, Anerkennung *f* / **~ method** Wiedererkennungsmethode *f* / **~ need** Bedürfnis *n* nach Anerkennung / **~ procedure** Wiedererkennungsmethode *f* / **~ span** Gedächtnisspanne *f* / **~ test** Erkennungstest *m*, Erinnerungstest *m* / **~ vocabulary** passives Vokabular *n* / **audio–visual ~** audiovisuelles Erkennen *n* / **false ~** Erinnerungstäuschung *f*, Bekanntheitstäuschung *f* / **social ~** soziale Anerkennung *f*

recognitive erkennbar, erkenntlich

recognizable erkennbar, wiedererkennbar

recognize erkennen, wiedererkennen

recollect sich erinnern

recollection Erinnerung *f*, Gedächtnis *n*

recombination Rekombination *f* / **homologous ~** homologe Rekombination *f*, legitime Rekombination *f* / **illegitimate ~** illegitime Rekombination *f*, nichthomologe Rekombination *f*

recommendation Empfehlung *f*

recondition rekonditionieren

reconditioning Rekonditionieren *n*

reconsider nochmals überdenken, von neuem erwägen, überprüfen

reconsideration nochmalige Überlegung *f*, nochmalige Erwägung *f*

reconstruction Wiederherstellung *f*, Rekonstruktion *f* / **~ method** Rekonstruktionsmethode *f* / **~ procedure** Rekonstruktionsmethode *f*

record aufzeichnen, aufnehmen, registrieren, protokollieren / Protokoll *n*, Niederschrift *f*, Aufzeichnung *f* / **academic ~s** schulische Leistungsnachweise *mpl* / **anecdotal ~** unsystematische Aufzeichnung *f* / **cumulative ~** additive Aufzeichnung *f*, kumulative Aufzeichnung *f*, kumulierter Durchschnitt *m* der erzielten Klassennoten seit der Aufnahmeprüfung / **medical ~** Krankenblatt *n*, ärztliche Befundkarte *f*, medizinische Falldokumentation *f*

recorder Protokollführer *m*, Aufnahmegerät *n*

recording Aufzeichnung *f*, Aufnahme *f*, Protokoll *n*, Ableitung *f* / **~ condition** Ableitbedingung *f* / **~ electrode** Ableitelektrode *f* / **~ on paper–tape** Aufzeichnung *f* auf Lochstreifen / **~ of punched–card data** Aufzeichnung *f* von Lochkartendaten / **~ system** Aufzeichnungssystem *n* / **bipolar ~** bipolare Ableitung *f* / **extracellular ~** extrazelluläre Ableitung *f* / **intracellular ~** intrazelluläre Ableitung *f* / **isotonic ~** isotonische Registrierung *f* / **monopolar ~** monopolare Ableitung *f*

recovery Erholung *f*, Wiederherstellung *f*, Genesung *f* / **~ phase** *f* Erregungsrückbildungsphase *f* / **~ pulse sum** Erholungspulssumme *f* / **complete ~** völlige Wiederherstellung *f* / **partial ~** Teilgenesung *f*, Defektheilung *f* / **spontaneous ~** spontane Erholung *f*, spontanes Wiederauftreten *n*

recreation Erholung *f*, Freizeitgestaltung *f* / **~ area** Erholungsgebiet *n* / **~ therapy** Übungstherapie *f*, Entspannungstherapie *f*, kreative Therapieform *f*

recruit anwerben, rekrutieren, ergänzen

recruitment Anwerbung *f*, Rekrutierung *f*, Recruitment *n* / **~ of loudness** Rekrutierung *f* durch Lautstärke, Hörregression *f* / **excitatory ~** Erregungsausbreitung *f* / **inhibitory ~** Hemmungsausbreitung *f*

rectangular rechteckig, rechtwinklig

rectification Berichtigung *f*, Verbesserung *f*, Umwandlung *f* von Wechselstrom in Gleichstrom, Gleichrichtung *f* / **delayed ~** verzögerte Gleichrichtung *f*

rectifier Gleichrichter *m*

rectify korrigieren, verbessern, berichtigen, gleichrichten

rectilinear, rectilineal geradlinig, linear

rectilinearity Geradlinigkeit *f*, Linearität *f*, Rectus externus *m*

rectum Enddarm *m*

rectitude Aufrichtigkeit *f*, charakterliche Geradlinigkeit *f*, Redlichkeit *f*

rectus Musculus rectus *m* / ~ **tendon** Augenbewegungsmuskel *m* / **external ~** Seitenwender *m*, Musculus rectus lateralis *m* / **internal ~** Senker *m*, Musculus rectus inferior *m*

recuperate sich erholen, genesen

recuperation Erholung *f*, Genesung *f*, Rekonvaleszenz *f*

recur sich wiederholen, wiederauftreten, rezidivieren, wiederkehren

recurrence Wiederauftreten *n*, Rückfall *n*

recurrent periodisch, sich wiederholend, wiederkehrend, wiederauftretend, rekurrent, regressiv, rückläufig

recursive rekursiv

red Rot *n* / rot / ~ **blindness** Rotblindheit *f*, Anerythropsie *f* / **~-green blindness** Rot–Grünblindheit *f* / **~-sighted** rotsichtig / ~ **vision** Rotsehen *n*, Erythropsie *f* / **visual ~** Sehrot *n*

redintegration Erneuerung *f*, Wiederherstellung *f*, Reintegration *f*

redirection Umleitung *f*, Umadressierung *f* / ~ **activity** Ersatzhandlung *f*

reduce reduzieren, vermindern

reduced reduziert

reduction Reduktion *f*, Rückführung *f*, Verminderung *f*, Verringerung *f*, Rückbildung *f* / ~ **ad absurdum** Beweis *m* des Widersinns / ~ **division** Reduktionsteilung *f* / ~ **screen** Reduktionsschirm *m*, Lochschirm *m* / ~ **of stimuli** Reizverminderung *f*

reductionism Reduktionismus *m*

reductive reduktiv

redundancy, redundance Redundanz *f*, Weitschweifigkeit *f* / ~ **check** Redundanzkontrolle *f* / ~ **learning** Redundanz *f* beim Lernen / ~ **theory of learning** Redundanztheorie *f* des Lernens

redundant redundant, überflüssig, weitschweifig

reduplication Verdoppelung *f*, Wiederholung *f*, Reduplikation *f*

reeducate umerziehen, umschulen

reeducation Umerziehung *f*, Umschulung *f*

reefer Rauschgiftzigarette *f*, Marihuanazigarette *f*

reemployment Rückkehr *f* ins Berufsleben

reenactment Wiederholung *f* / **emotional ~** emotionales Abreagieren *n*

reenforcement Verstärkung *f*

reentry student Wiedereinsteiger *m* ins Bildungssystem

reevaluation nochmalige Auswertung *f*, Wiederholung *f* der Auswertung

reexamination Nachprüfung *f*, Nachuntersuchung *f*, Wiederholungsprüfung *f*

reexamine nachprüfen, nachuntersuchen, erneut prüfen

refer sich beziehen, verweisen

reference Bezug *m*, Referenz *f* / ~ **axis** Bezugsachse *f* / ~ **electrode** indifferente Elektrode *f* / ~ **frame** Bezugsrahmen *m*, Bezugssystem *n* / ~ **frequency** Normalfrequenz *f*, Normalton *m* / ~ **group** Bezugsgruppe *f* / ~ **input** Führungsgröße *f* / ~ **intensity** Bezugslautstärke *f* / ~ **signal** Sollwert *m* / ~ **sound** Normalton *m* / ~ **sound pressure** Normalschalldruck *m* / ~ **stimulus** Ankerreiz *m*, Bezugsreiz *m* / ~ **system** Bezugssystem *n* / ~ **vector** Bezugsvektor *m* / **acoustic ~ pressure** Normalschalldruck *m* / **objective ~** objektiver Bezug *m* / **religious ~ group** religiöse Bezugsgruppe *f*

referent Bezugsobjekt *n*, Bezugspunkt *m* / ~ **power** persönliche Macht *f*

referral Überweisung *f*, Überwiesener *m* / **professional ~** Überweisung *f* zu einem Fachmann, Überweisung *f* zur Fachbehandlung

refined verfeinert, verbessert

refixation erneute Fixation *f*

reflect reflektieren, nachdenken, widerspiegeln, zurückstrahlen

reflected reflektiert

reflecting, reflective reflektierend / Reflektieren *n*, Reflexion *f* / ~ **of light** Lichtreflexion *f*

reflection Reflexion *f*, Nachdenken *n*, Introspektion *f*, Spiegelung *f*, Rückstrahlung *f* / **~ of feeling** Widerspiegelung *f* von Gefühlen / **~ response** Spiegeldeutung *f* / **corneal ~** Hornhautspiegelung *f* / **specular ~** Spiegelung *f*

reflectiveness Besinnung *f*, Reflexivität *f*

reflector Reflektor *m*, Scheinwerfer *m*

reflex Reflex *m* / reflektorisch, Reflex– / **~ action** Reflexhandlung *f*, Reflexbewegung *f* / **~ arc** Reflexbogen *m* / **~ automatism** Reflexautomatik *f* / **~ bladder** Reflexblase *f* / **~ centre** Reflexzentrum *n* / **~ chain** Reflexkette *f*, Verhaltenskette *f* / **~ circle** Reflexkreis *m* / **~ circuit** Reflexbogen *m* / **~ conduction** Reflexleitung *f* / **~ after discharge** Reflex *m* nach Entladung / **~ doctrine** Reflexlehre *f* / **~ epilepsy** Reflexepilepsie *f* / **~ excitability** Reflexerregbarkeit *f* / **~ facilitation** Reflexbahnung *f* / **~ fatigue** Reflexermüdung *f* / **~ inhibition** Reflexhemmung *f* / **~ integration** Reflexintegration *f* / **~ irradiation** Reflexausbreitung *f*, Reflexirradiation *f* / **~ latency** Reflexverzögerung *f*, Reflexlatenz *f*, Reflexzeit *f* / **~ movement** Reflexbewegung *f* / **~ neurosis** reaktive Neurose *f*, Reflexneurose *f* / **~ path** Reflexbahn *f* / **~ reserve** Reflexreserve *f*, Reaktionsreserve *f* / **~ of self–defence** Abwehrreflex *m*, Schutzreflex *m* / **~ sensitization** Reflexsensibilisierung *f* / **~ spasm** Reflexkrampf *m* / **~ strength** Reflexstärke *f* / **~ summation** Reflexsummation *f*, Reflexsummierung *f* / **~ therapy** Reflextherapie *f* / **~ time** Reflexzeit *f* / **~ tonus** Reflextonus *m* / **~ tract** Reflexbahn *f* / **abdominal ~** Bauchdeckenreflex *m*, Abdominalreflex *m* / **abnormal ~** Reflexanomalie *f* / **absent ~** fehlender Reflex *m* / **acoustic ~** Hörreflex *m* / **acquired ~** erworbener Reflex *m* / **adversive ~** Adversionsreflex *m*, Zuwendungsreflex *m* / **affective ~** Affektreflex *m* / **alimentary ~** Nahrungsreflex *m* / **allied ~es** Reflexsynergie *f* / **antagonistic ~** antagonistischer Reflex *m* / **attitudinal ~** Stellungsreflex *m*, Haltungsreflex *m* / **audito–oculogyric ~** akustisch bedingter Sehbewegungsreflex *m* / **autogenic ~** Eigenreflex *m* / **autonomic ~** autonomer Reflex *m*, vegetativer Reflex *m*, selbständiger Reflex *m* / **brisk ~** lebhafter Reflex *m* / **cleaning ~** Wischreflex *m* / **closing ~** Schließreflex *m* / **compensatory ~** Ausgleichsreflex *m* / **compound ~** komplexer Reflex *m* / **conditional ~** bedingter Reflex *m*, konditionierter Reflex *m* / **conditioned ~** bedingter Reflex *m*, konditionierter Reflex *m* / **conditioned ~ mechanism** bedingter Reflexbogen *m* / **conjunctival ~** Blinzelreflex *m* / **contralateral ~** kontralateraler Reflex *m*, gekreuzter Reflex *m* / **corneal ~** Hornhautreflex *m*, Kornealreflex *m*, Lidschlussreflex *m*, Lidschlagreflex *m* / **cranial ~** Hirnnervenreflex *m* / **cremasteric ~** Kremasterreflex *m* / **crossed ~** gekreuzter Reflex *m* / **cutaneous ~** Hautreflex *m* / **cutaneous secretory ~** Hautsekretionsreflex *m* / **deep ~** Tiefenreflex *m* / **defensive ~** Abwehrreflex *m*, Schutzreflex *m* / **delayed ~** verzögerter Reflex *m*, Spätreflex *m* / **delayed conditional ~** verzögerter bedingter Reflex *m* / **direct ~** direkter Reflex *m* / **disynaptic ~** disynaptischer Reflex *m* / **embrace ~** Umklammerungsreflex *m* / **enteroceptive ~** enterozeptiver Reflex *m* / **exteroceptive ~** exterozeptiver Reflex *m* / **feeble ~** verminderter Reflex *m* / **galvanic ~** psychogalvanische Reaktion *f* / **genital ~** Genitalreflex *m* / **grasping ~** Greifreflex *m* / **heteronymous ~** heteronymer Reflex *m* / **homolateral ~** homolateraler Reflex *m*, direkter Reflex *m* / **homonymous ~** homonymer Reflex *m* / **hyperactive ~** gesteigerter Reflex *m* / **ideomotor ~** ideomotorischer Reflex *m*, Haab–Reflex *m* / **inborn ~** angeborener Reflex *m* / **increased ~** gesteigerter Reflex *m* / **incremental ~** ansteigender Reflex *m* / **inhibitory ~** Hemmreflex *m* / **initial ~** Initialreflex *m* / **investigatory ~** Untersuchungsreaktion *f*, Orientierungsreaktion *f* / **intrinsic ~** Eigenreflex *m* / **laryngeal ~** Kehlkopfreflex *m* / **learned ~** erlernter

Reflex *m* / **lumbar ~** Lumbalreflex *m* / **mandibular ~** Unterkieferreflex *m* / **medullar ~** Medullarreflex *m* / **monosynaptic ~** monosynaptischer Reflex *m* / **motor ~** motorischer Reflex *m* / **multisynaptic ~** polysynaptischer Reflex *m* / **muscular ~** Muskelreflex *m* / **myotatic ~** Streckreflex *m* / **nasal ~** Niesreflex *m* / **nociceptive ~** Schmerzreflex *m* / **oculocardiac ~** Bulbusdruckreflex *m* / **orienting ~** Orientierungsreaktion *f*, Orientierungsreflex *m*, Untersuchungsreaktion *f* / **palatal ~** Gaumenreflex *m* / **palmar ~** Palmarreflex *m*, Volarreflex *m* / **patellar ~** Patellarreflex *m*, Kniesehnenreflex *m* / **pharyngeal ~** Rachenreflex *m* / **photomotor ~** photomotorischer Reflex *m* / **pilomotor ~** pilomotorischer Reflex *m*, Gänsehautreflex *m* / **plantar ~** Plantarreflex *m*, Fußsohlenreflex *m* / **polysynaptic ~** polysynaptischer Reflex *m* / **positive supporting ~** Unterstützungsreaktion *f* / **postural ~** Stellreflex *m*, Lagereflex *m* / **preconditioned ~** vorbedingter Reflex *m* / **prepotent ~** dominanter Reflex *m*, vitaler Reflex *m* / **primary ~** Grundreflex *m* / **proprioceptive ~** propriozeptiver Reflex *m*, Eigenreflex *m* / **protective ~** Schutzreflex *m*, Abwehrreflex *m* / **psychic ~** Psychoreflex *m* / **psychogalvanic ~** psychogalvanische Reaktion *f*, galvanische Hautreaktion *f* / **psychomotor ~** psychomotorischer Reflex *m*, Aufmerksamkeitsreflex *m* / **pupillary ~** Pupillenreflex *m*, Lichtreflex *m* / **radial ~** Radialreflex *m* / **rectal ~** Analreflex *m* / **red ~** Rot–Reflexion *f* / **regional ~** segmentaler Reflex *m* / **reinforced ~** verstärkter Reflex *m*, gebahnter Reflex *m*, intensivierter Reflex *m* / **renorenal ~** renorenaler Reflex *m*, Schmerz *m* in der gesunden Niere / **retarded conditioned ~** verzögerter bedingter Reflex *m*, verspäteter bedingter Reflex *m* / **righting ~** Stellreflex *m* / **sacral ~** sakraler Reflex *m* / **salivary ~** Speichelreflex *m* / **secondary conditioned ~** sekundärer bedingter Reflex *m* / **secretory ~** sekretorischer Reflex *m* / **segmental ~** segmentaler Reflex *m* / **senile ~** Altersreflex *m* / **sexual ~** Sexualreflex *m* / **simple ~** unkonditionierter Reflex *m* / **skeletal ~** Skelettreflex *m* / **sluggish ~** träger Reflex *m* / **spinal ~** spinaler Reflex *m*, Rückenmarksreflex *m* / **stapedial ~** Stapediusreflex *m* / **static ~** Gleichgewichtsreflex *m* / **statotonic ~** Haltungsreflex *m* / **sucking ~** Saugreflex *m* / **superficial ~** Oberflächenreflex *m* / **suprapubic ~** Reflex *m* der unteren Bauchdecke / **swallowing ~** Schluckreflex *m* / **tonic ~** tonischer Reflex *m* / **unconditional ~** unbedingter Reflex *m*, unkonditionierter Reflex *m* / **unconditioned ~** unbedingter Reflex *m*, unkonditionierter Reflex *m* / **unequal ~** ungleicher Reflex *m* / **vasomotor ~** vasomotorischer Reflex *m* / **vesical ~** Blasenreflex *m* / **visceromotor ~** viszeromotorischer Reflex *m* / **vomiting ~** Brechreflex *m* / **weak ~** schwacher Reflex *m* / **winking ~** Lidreflex *m*, Lidschlagreflex *m*

reflexion Reflexion *f*, Nachdenken *n*, Spiegelung *f* / **diffuse ~** diffuse Reflexion *f* / **direct ~** direkte Reflexion *f* / **matt ~** Mattreflexion *f*

reflexivity Reflexivität *f*

reflexogenic, reflexogenous reflexauslösend, reflexogen

reflexograph Reflexograph *m*, Reflexschreiber *m*

reflexology Reflexologie *f*, Psychoreflexologie *f*, Reflexlehre *f*

reflexometer Reflexometer *n*

reflexometry Reflexmessung *f*

reflexotherapy Reflextherapie *f*

reflux Rückfluss *m*

reform reformieren, umgestalten, verbessern / Reform *f*, Umgestaltung *f* / **educational ~** Schulreform *f*, Bildungsreform *f*, Reform *f* des Ausbildungswesens / **social ~** Sozialreform *f*

reformation Umgestaltung *f*, Verbesserung *f*, Reformierung *f*

reformatory Besserungsanstalt *f*, Jugendstrafanstalt *f* / Reform–, Besserungs–

reformism Reformismus *m*

reformist Reformer *m*, Reformist *m*

refract brechen

refracting brechend, Brechungs–

refraction Brechung *f*, Lichtbrechung *f*, Strahlenbrechung *f* / ~ **of colour** Farbenbrechung *f* / ~ **error** Brechungsfehler *m* / ~ **of light** Lichtbrechung *f* / ~ **of sound** Schallbrechung *f* / **double** ~ Doppelbrechung *f* / **single** ~ Einfachbrechung *f*

refractive Brechungs–

refractivity Brechungsvermögen *n*, Brechungskraft *f*, Lichtbrechungsvermögen *n*

refractometer Refraktometer *n*, Brechungsmesser *m*

refractometry Refraktometrie *f*, Messung *f* des Brechungsvermögens

refractory refraktär, widerspenstig

refrangibility Brechbarkeit *f*

refrangible brechbar

refresher course Auffrischungskurs *m*, Wiederholungskurs *m*, Übungskurs *m*

refrigeration Abkühlung *f*, Abkühlen *n*, Temperaturverminderung *f* des Körpers

refringence Brechungsvermögen *n*, Lichtbrechungsvermögen *n*

refringent brechend

refugee Flüchtling *m*

refusal Verweigerung *f*, Weigerung *f*

refutable widerlegbar

refutation Widerlegung *f*

refute widerlegen

regain wiedergewinnen, wiedererlangen

regard ansehen, betrachten, beachten, achten / Blick *m* / **unconditional positive** ~ unbedingte positive Zuwendung *f*

regenerate erneuern, regenerieren, sich neu bilden / regeneriert

regenerating regenerierend, sich neu bildend

regeneration Wiederherstellung *f*, Neubildung *f*

regimen Kur *f*, gesundheitsgemäße Lebensweise *f*

regiminal eine gesundheitsgemäße Lebensweise betreffend

region Region *f*, Gebiet *n*, Gegend *f*, Zone *f*, Bereich *m* / ~ **of development** Entwicklungsgebiet *n*, Entfaltungszone *f* / ~**s of personality** Persönlichkeitsregionen *fpl* / **anal** ~ Analgegend *f*, Analbereich *m* / **cardiac** ~ Herzgegend *f* / **connected** ~ verbundene Region *f* / **cranial** ~ Schädelregion *f* / **critical** ~ kritischer Bereich *m* / **frontal** ~ Stirngegend *f* / **gustatory** ~ Geschmackszentrum *n* / **incident** ~ zugehörige Region *f* / **lumbosacral** ~ Lendenkreuzbeingegend *f* / **motoric** ~ motorische Region *f* / **motor–perceptual** ~ motorisch perzeptive Region *f* / **neighbouring** ~ Nachbarregion *f* / **neutral** ~ neutrale Region *f* / **olfactory** ~ Riechzentrum *n*, Riechlappen *m* / **oral** ~ Mundgegend *f* / **parietal** ~ Scheitelgegend *f* / **psychological** ~ psychologische Region *f* / **pubic** ~ Schamgegend *f* / **synaptic** ~ Synapsengegend *f* / **temporal** ~ Schläfengegend *f* / **vertebral** ~ Wirbelsäulengegend *f*

regional regional, örtlich

register registrieren, aufzeichnen, einschreiben / Stimmumfang *m*, Tonlage *f* / **vocal** ~ Stimmumfang *m*, Stimmbereich *m*

registered eingetragen, gesetzlich geschützt, diplomiert, staatlich zugelassen

registrar Registrator *m*, Archivar *m*

registration Einschreibung *f*, Registrierung *f*, Anmeldung *f*

regnancy Herrschaft *f*, dominante Erfahrungsgestalt *f*

regnant herrschend, dominierend, vorherrschend

regress sich zurückbilden, regredieren, auf eine tiefere Stufe zurückfallen

regression Regression *f*, Rückschritt *m*, Rückfall *m*, Rückbildung *f* / ~ **analysis** Regressionsanalyse *f* / ~ **coefficient** Regressionskoeffizient *m* / ~ **curve** Regressionskurve *f* / ~ **equation** Regressionsgleichung *f* / ~ **estimate** Regressionsschätzung *f* / ~ **of libido** Regression *f* der Libido / ~ **line** Regressionslinie *f* / ~ **neurosis** Regressionsneurose *f*, Regression *f* / ~ **surface** Regressionskurve *f*, Regressionsfläche *f* / ~ **time** Regressionszeit *f* / ~ **weight** Regressionskoeffizient *m* / **auditory** ~ Hörverlust *m* / **curvilinear** ~ **line** kurvilineare Regressionslinie *f* / **ergic** ~ Triebregression *f* / **filial** ~ Regression *f* der Nachkommen, Regression *f* / **libidinal** ~ Regression *f* der Libido / **linear** ~ lineare Regression *f* / **multiple** ~ multiple Regression *f* / **multiple** ~ **equation** multiple Regressionsgleichung *f* / **nonlinear** ~ nicht–lineare Regression *f* / **oral** ~ Regression *f* auf die orale Stufe / **partial** ~ Triebregression *f* / **partial–**~ **equation** partielle Regressionsgleichung *f* / **phenomenal** ~ Wahrnehmungsregression *f*, phänomenale Regression *f* / **rectilinear** ~ lineare Regression *f* / **skew** ~ nicht–lineare Regressionslinie *f* / **spontaneous** ~ spontane Rückbildung *f* / **statistical** ~ statistische Regression *f* / **temporal** ~ temporäre Regression *f*

regressive regressiv

regret bedauern, bereuen / Bedauern *n*, Reue *f*

regroup umgruppieren, neu einteilen, neu einstufen

regrowth neues Wachstum *n*

regular normal, regulär, gleichmäßig

regularity Gleichmäßigkeit *f*, Regelmäßigkeit *f*, Richtigkeit *f*

regularize regeln, genau festlegen

regulate regeln, regulieren, ordnen

regulation Regelung *f*, Regulierung *f*, Vorschrift *f* / ~ **of birth** Geburtenregelung *f* / **metabolic** ~ Stoffwechselregulation *f*

regulator Ordner *m*, Regler *m*, Reguliervorrichtung *f*

regulatory regulierend, regelnd, ordnend

regurgitation Regurgitation *f*, Würgebewegung *f*, Würgen *n*, Rückstauung *f*

rehabilitation Rehabilitation *f*, Umschulung *f*, Wiedereingliederung *f* / ~ **centre** Rehabilitationszentrum *n* / ~ **counseling** Rehabilitationsberatung *f* / ~ **counselor** Rehabilitationsberater *m* / ~ **education** Rehabilitationsausbildung *f* / **active** ~ aktive Umgewöhnung *f* / **cognitive** ~ kognitive Rehabilitation *f* / **motor** ~ motorische Rehabilitation *f* / **neuropsychological** ~ neuropsychologische Rehabilitation *f* / **psychosocial** ~ psychosoziale Rehabilitation *f* / **vocational** ~ berufliche Rehabilitation *f*

rehearsal Probe *f*, Wiederholung *f*, inneres Hersagen *n*, Übung *f* / **behavioural** ~ Verhaltensübung *f* / **cognitive** ~ kognitive Übung *f*

reification Verdinglichung *f*, Konkretisierung *f*

reify verdinglichen

reincarnation Wiedergeburt *f*, Reinkarnation *f*

reinfection neue Infektion *f*, Wiederansteckung *f*, Reinfektion *f*

reinforce verstärken, bekräftigen, festigen

reinforced verstärkt, gefestigt

reinforcement Verstärkung *f*, Wiederverstärkung *f*, Festigung *f*, Bekräftigung *f* / ~ **agent** Verstärkungsmittel *n*, Verstärker *m* / ~ **amount** Verstärkungsbetrag *m* / ~ **delay** Verstärkungsaufschub *m* / ~ **gradient** Verstärkungsgradient *m* / ~ **hypothesis** Verstärkungshypothese *f* / ~ **retroaction paradox** Paradox *n* der retroaktiven Verstärkung / ~ **schedule** Verstärkerplan *m* / **concurrent** ~ **schedule** gleichzeitiger Verstärkerplan *m* / ~ **value** Verstärkungswert *m* / **accidental** ~ zufällige Verstärkung *f* / **alternative** ~ alternierende Verstärkung *f* / **aperiodic** ~ aperiodische Verstärkung *f* / **autogenic** ~ autogene Verstärkung *f* / **chained** ~ Verstärkungsfolge *f* / **concurrent** ~ Simultanverstärkung *f* / **conditioned** ~ bedingte Verstärkung *f*, konditionierte Verstärkung *f* / **conditioned negative** ~ bedingte negative Verstärkung *f* / **continuous** ~

Immerverstärkung *f*, kontinuierliche Verstärkung *f* / **covert ~** verdeckte Verstärkung *f* / **delayed ~** verzögerte Verstärkung *f* / **differential ~** unterschiedliche Verstärkung *f*, differenzielle Verstärkung *f* / **differential ~ of high rates** differenzielle Verstärkung *f* großer Häufigkeit / **differential ~ of low rates** differenzielle Verstärkung *f* geringer Häufigkeit / **differential ~ of other behaviour** differenzielle Verstärkung *f* anderen Verhaltens / **discriminative ~** diskriminierende Verstärkung *f* / **episodic ~** episodische Verstärkung *f*, gelegentliche Verstärkung *f* / **external ~** äußere Verstärkung *f* / **extrinsic ~** äußere Verstärkung *f* / **free ~** nicht-kontingente Verstärkung *f* / **heterogeneous ~** heterogene Verstärkung *f* / **homogeneous ~** homogene Verstärkung *f* / **immediate ~** unmittelbare Verstärkung *f*, direkte Verstärkung *f* / **inadvertent ~** unbeabsichtigte, versehentliche Verstärkung *f* / **incidental ~** zufällige Verstärkung *f* / **intermittent ~** partielle Verstärkung *f*, gelegentliche Verstärkung *f*, intermittierende Verstärkung *f* / **internal ~** innere Verstärkung *f* / **interpolated ~** interpolierte Verstärkung *f* / **intrinsic ~** innere Verstärkung *f* / **irrelevant ~** irrelevante Verstärkung *f* / **multiple ~** Mehrfachverstärkung *f* / **negative ~** negative Verstärkung *f* / **neural ~** neurale Verstärkung *f* / **noncontingent ~** nicht kontingente Verstärkung *f* / **nonverbal ~** nonverbale Verstärkung *f* / **operant ~ schedule** nicht reizbezogener Verstärkungsplan *m* / **partial ~** partielle Verstärkung *f*, gelegentliche Verstärkung *f*, intermittierende Verstärkung *f* / **partial ~ effect** Partialverstärkungseffekt *m* / **periodic ~** periodische Verstärkung *f* / **positive ~** positive Verstärkung *f* / **pre delay ~** Verstärkung *f* mit Zwischenverzögerung / **primary ~** primäre Verstärkung *f* / **random ~** Verstärkung *f* in zufälligen Intervallen / **reactive ~** Reaktionsverstärkung *f* / **reciprocal ~** reziproke Verstärkung *f* / **reproductive ~** reproduktive Verstärkung *f* / **secondary ~** sekundäre Verstärkung *f* / **sequential ~** sequenzielle Verstärkung *f* / **serial ~** Serienverstärkung *f* / **social ~** soziale Verstärkung *f* / **terminal ~** Endverstärkung *f* / **verbal ~** verbale Verstärkung *f* / **vicarious ~** stellvertretende Verstärkung *f*

reinforcer Verstärker *m*, Verstärkungsmittel *n* / **back–up ~** Eintauschverstärker *m* / **conditioned ~** bedingter Verstärker *m* / **generalized ~** generalisierter Verstärker *m* / **intrinsic ~** innerer Verstärker *m* / **negative ~** negativer Verstärker *m* / **positive ~** positiver Verstärker *m* / **primary ~** primärer Verstärker *m* / **secondary ~** sekundärer Verstärker *m* / **social ~** sozialer Verstärker *m*

reinforcing verstärkend

reinstatement Wiedereinsetzung *f*, Wiedereinstellung *f*, Wiederherstellung *f*

reintegration Erneuerung *f*, Wiederherstellung *f*, Reintegration *f*

Reissner's| fibre Reissner–Faden *m* / **~ membrane** Reissner–Membran *f*

reject ablehnen, abweisen, verstoßen, verwerfen

rejected abgelehnt, zurückgewiesen, ausgestoßen

rejection Ablehnung *f*, Zurückweisung *f*, Abweisung *f*, Abstoßungsreaktion *f* / **~ error** Fehler *m* erster Art, Typ I–Fehler *m* / **~ line** Rejektionslinie *f* / **~ need** Ablehnungsbedürfnis *n* / **~ reaction** Abstoßungsreaktion *f* / **~ region** Rejektionsbereich *m* / **~ response** Abstoßungsreaktion *f* / **maternal ~** Ablehnung *f* durch die Mutter / **opinionated ~** Ablehnung *f* aufgrund eines Vorurteils / **parental ~** Ablehnung *f* durch die Eltern / **paternal ~** Ablehnung *f* durch den Vater

rejuvenate verjüngen, sich verjüngen

rejuvenation Verjüngung *f*

relapse Rückfall *m*, Rezidiv *n* / rezidivieren, einen Rückfall erleiden / **~ prevention** Rückfallprävention *f*

relapsing rezidivierend, Rückfall–

relata Bezugsgegenstände *mpl*, Bezugsobjekte *npl*

related to im Zusammenhang mit

relatedness Verwandtschaft *f*, verwandtschaftliches Verhältnis *n*

relation Beziehung *f*, Verhältnis *n*, Rapport *m*, Relation *f* / **~ learning** Lernen *n* von Beziehungen / **~ of dependence** Abhängigkeitsbeziehung *f* / **allelomorphic ~** allelomorphe Beziehung *f* / **all–or–nothing ~** Alles–oder–Nichts–Gesetz *n* / **causal ~** Kausalzusammenhang *m* / **functional ~** funktionelle Beziehung *f* / **human ~s** zwischenmenschliche Beziehungen *fpl*, „human relations" *pl* / **human ~s training** Kontakttraining *n*, gruppendynamisches Training *n* / **industrial ~s** Beziehungen *fpl* zwischen Arbeitgeber und Arbeitnehmern, Beziehungen *fpl* zwischen den Sozialpartnern / **intergenerational ~s** Generationenbeziehungen *fpl* / **intergroup ~s** Beziehungen *fpl* zwischen Gruppen / **international ~s** internationale Beziehungen *fpl* / **interpersonal ~** zwischenmenschliche Beziehung *f* / **male–female ~s** Geschlechterbeziehungen *fpl* / **marital ~s** eheliche Beziehungen *fpl*, Partnerbeziehungen *fpl* / **mechanical ~s test** Test *m* zur Erfassung mechanischer Beziehungen / **public ~s** Öffentlichkeitsarbeit *f*, Public Relations *fpl* / **racial and ethnic ~s** ethnische und nationale Beziehungen *fpl* / **sexual ~** Geschlechtsbeziehung *f*, sexuelle Beziehung *f* / **social ~** Sozialbeziehung *f*, soziale Interaktion *f* / **spatial ~s** Raumbeziehungen *fpl*

relational Beziehungs–, Relations–, relational

relationship Beziehung *f* Verhältnis *n*, Verbindung *f*, Verwandtschaft *f* / **~ system** Verwandtschaftssystem *n* / **~ termination** Beendigung *f* einer Beziehung / **~ therapy** therapeutischer Aufbau *m* von Bindungen, Paartherapie *f* / **causal ~** Kausalzusammenhang *m* / **curvilinear ~** kurvilineare Beziehung *f* / **heterosexual ~** heterosexuelle Beziehung *f* / **inverse ~** Umkehrbeziehung *f*, negative Korrelation *f* / **isomorphic ~** Isomorphie–Beziehung *f* / **objectal ~** Objektbeziehung *f* / **positional ~** Lagebeziehung *f* / **social ~** Sozialbeziehung *f*, soziale Interaktion *f* / **sexual ~ disorder** sexuelle Beziehungsstörung *f*

relative relativ, verhältnismäßig / Verwandte *m,f*

relativism Relativismus *m* / **cultural ~** Kulturrelativismus *m*

relativity Relativität *f* / **~ attitude** relativistische Einstellung *f* / **~ law** Relativitätssatz *m*

relax sich entspannen, erschlaffen, ausruhen

relaxation Entspannung *f*, Lockerung *f*, Relaxation *f*, Erholung *f* / **~ feeling** Gefühl *n* der Entspannung / **~ techniques** Entspannungstechniken *fpl* / **~ therapy** Entspannungstherapie *f*, Relaxationstherapie *f* / **progressive ~** progressive Entspannung *f*

relaxed entspannt, gelockert, spannungslos

relaxing entspannend, mild

relearning Wiederlernen *n*

release freilassen, loslassen, freigeben, entbinden / Befreiung *f*, Erlösung *f*, Auslösung *f*, Ausschüttung *f* / **~ mechanism** Auslösemechanismus *m* / **~ phenomenon** Auslösephänomen *n* / **~ therapy** kathartische Psychotherapie *f*, befreiende Psychotherapie *f* / **emotional ~** Affektauslösung *f* / **innate ~ mechanism** angeborener Auslösemechanismus *m* / **institutional ~** Anstaltsentlassung *f*

releaser Auslöser *m* / **~ mechanism** Auslösemechanismus *m* / **behavioural ~** Auslöser *m* / **vocal ~** stimmlicher Auslöser *m*, Stimme *f* als Auslöser

releasing auslösend, Auslöse– / **~ hormone** Releasinghormon *n*

relevance, relevancy Relevanz *f*, Erheblichkeit *f*, Bedeutung *f* / **~ therapy** Relevanztherapie *f*

reliability Reliabilität *f*, Zuverlassigkeit *f* / **~ coefficient** Reliabilitätskoeffizient *m* / **~ test** Reliabilitätsprüfung *f* / **~ of a test** Testzuverlässigkeit *f*, Testreliabilität *f* / **interrater ~** Interrater–Reliabilität *f* / **inter–scorer ~** Auswerteobjektivität *f* / **random halves ~** Halbierungsreliabilität *f* / **sampling ~** Stichprobenreliabilität *f* / **split–half ~** Halbierungsreliabilität *f* / **statistical ~** statistische Zuverlässigkeit *f*, statistische Reliabilität *f*

reliable zuverlässig, vertrauenswürdig, verlässlich

relief Erleichterung *f*, Entlastung *f*, Befreiung *f*, Linderung *f*

relieve befreien, entlasten, lindern, beseitigen

religion Religion *f*

religiosity Religiosität *f*

religious religiös, fromm

relinquishment of aggressivity Aggressionsverzicht *m*

REM dream REM–Traum *m* / **~ dream deprivation** Traumentzug *m* wahrend der REM–Phase / **~ sleep** REM–Schlaf *m*, paradoxer Schlaf *m*

Remak's| band Achsenzylinder *m* / **~ fibres** marklose Nervenfasern *fpl*

remarriage Wiederverheiratung *f*

remedial heilend, kurativ, Heilungs–, Heil–

remedy Heilmittel *n*, Arznei *f*, Abhilfe *f* / heilen, abhelfen, abstellen / **~ of choice** Mittel *n* der Wahl / **chemical ~** Chemotherapeutikum *n* / **specific ~** spezifisches Heilmittel *n*

remember sich erinnern, erinnern

remembering Erinnern *n*, Erinnerungsvorgang *m* / **selective ~** selektives Erinnern *n*

remembrance Erinnerung *f*, Gedächtnis *n* / **~ hallucination** Erinnerungshalluzination *f* / **deceptive ~** Erinnerungsfälschung *f* / **delusive ~** Erinnerungstäuschung *f* / **visual ~** optisches Erinnerungsbild *n*

reminiscence Erinnerung *f*, Reminiszenz *f*, Wiedererinnerung *f*

remission Remission *f*, Remissionsgrad *m*, Nachlassen *n*, Abnahme *f*, Besserung *f* / **~ specifier** Zusatzkodierung *f* für Remissionsgrad / **in full ~** vollremittiert / **in partial ~** teilremittiert / **spontaneous ~** Spontanremission *f*

remit nachlassen, weichen, zurückgehen

remittent nachlassend, remittierend

remonstrance Protest *m*, Einspruch *m*

remorse Gewissensbisse *npl*, Reue *f*

remorseless unbarmherzig, erbarmungslos, unerbittlich

remote entfernt, unbedeutend, schwach

removal Entfernung *f*, Beseitigung *f*, Abtransport *m* / **~ depression** Umzugsdepression *f*

remove entfernen, beseitigen, herausnehmen

remuneration Belohnung *f*, Vergütung *f*, Remuneration *f*

renal renal, Nieren–

renew erneuern, wiederherstellen, wieder beginnen

renewal Erneuerung *f*

renifleur Renifleur *m*

renin Renin *n* / **~–angiotensin–aldosterone system** Renin–Angiotensin–Aldosteron–System *n*

renorenal renorenal

renounce verzichten, versagen, aufgeben

Renshaw| cell Renshaw–Zelle *f* / **~ inhibition** Renshaw–Hemmung *f*

renunciation Verzicht *f*, Entsagung *f*, Selbstverleugnung *f* / **~ of an instinct** Triebverzicht *m* / **instinctual ~** Triebverzicht *m*

reorganisation Reorganisation *f*, Neugestaltung *f*, Umstrukturierung *f*, Reparation *f* im ZNS / **~ principle** Reorganisationsprinzip *n* / **~ theory** Umstrukturierungstheorie *f*

reorganise reorganisieren, neu einteilen, neu aufbauen

reorientation Neuorientierung *f*

reparation Wiedergutmachung *f*

repeat wiederholen

repeatability Wiederholbarkeit *f*

repercussion Rückwirkung *f*, Nachwirkung *f*, Auswirkung *f*, Widerhall *m*

repercussive rückwirkend, nachwirkend, widerhallend

repertory, repertoire Repertoire *n*, Verzeichnis *n* / **behavioural ~** Verhaltensrepertoire *n*

repetition Wiederholung *f* / **~ compulsion** Wiederholungszwang *m* / **compulsive ~** Wiederholungszwang *m* / **distributed ~** Wiederholung *f* in Abständen, verteilte Wiederholung *f* / **spaced ~** verteilte Wiederholung *f*, Wiederholung *f* in Abständen / **unspaced ~** massierte Wiederholung *f*

repetitive, repetitious sich wiederholend

replacement Ersatz *m* / **~ therapy** Substitutionstherapie *f*

replica Kopie *f*, Nachbildung *f*

replicate wiederholen, kopieren, nachahmen

replication Wiederholung *f*, Bildung *f* von Substraten mit identischen Parametern / **~ therapy** Replikationstherapie *f*, Wiederholung *f* problematischer Lebenssituationen bei der klinischen Therapie / **experimental ~** Versuchswiederholung *f*, experimentelle Replikation *f*

repolarisation Wiederherstellung *f* des Membranpotenzials, Erregungsrückbildung *f*, Repolarisation *f* / **~ phase** Repolarisationsphase *f*

report berichten, darstellen, beschreiben / Bericht *m*, Protokoll *n* / **annual ~** Jahresbericht *m* / **educational ~** Erziehungsbefund *m* / **psychological ~** psychologisches Gutachten *n*

represent vorstellen, darstehen, repräsentieren

representation Vorstellung *f*, Vorstellungsbild *n*, Bild *n*, Darstellung *f*, Repräsentation *f* / **central ~** zentrale Repräsentation *f* / **collective ~** Kollektivvorstellung *f* / **double ~** doppeltes Vorstellungsbild *n* / **graphical ~** graphische Darstellung *f* / **spatial ~** Raumvorstellung *f*

representative repräsentativ, typisch, Durchschnitts–, stellvertretend / Repräsentant *m*, Beauftragter *m*, Vertreter *m* / **~ of an instinct** Triebrepräsentant *m* / **ideational ~** Vorstellungsrepräsentanz *f*, Vorstellungsrepräsentant *m* / **instinctual ~** Triebrepräsentant *m* / **psychical ~** psychische Repräsentanz *f*

representativity, representativeness Repräsentativität *f*

repress verdrängen, unterdrücken

repressed verdrängt, unterdrückt / Verdrängtes *n*

repression Verdrängung *f*, Repression *f*, Informationsverdrängung *f* / **~ of instincts** Triebverdrängung *f* / **~ process** Verdrängungsvorgang *m* / **~ resistance** Verdrängungswiderstand *m* / **~ sensitisation** Sensibilisierung *f* gegen Verdrängungen / **attempted ~** Verdrängungsversuch *m* / **miscarried ~** missglückte Verdrängung *f* / **organic ~** organische Verdrängung *f*, anterograde Amnesie *f* / **primal ~** Primärverdrängung *f* / **primary ~** Primärverdrängung *f* / **secondary ~** Sekundärverdrängung *f* / **successful ~** erfolgreiche Verdrängung *f* / **unsuccessful ~** missglückte Verdrängung *f*

repressive verdrängend, repressiv

repressor Repressor *m*

reprobation Missbilligung *f*

reproduce wiedergeben, reproduzieren, sich fortpflanzen, sich vermehren

reproducibility Reproduzierbarkeit *f*, Reproduktionsfähigkeit *f* / **~ coefficient** Koeffizient *m* der Wiederholbarkeit

reproduction Reproduktion *f*, originalgetreue Kopie *f*, Faksimile *n*, Wiederhervorbringen *n*, Fortpflanzung *f* / **~ method**

Reproduktionsmethode *f* / ~ **procedure** Reproduktionsverfahren *n* / **asexual** ~ ungeschlechtliche Fortpflanzung *f*, Parthenogenese *f* / **imperfect** ~ unvollständige Erinnerung *f* / **sexual** ~ geschlechtliche Fortpflanzung *f* / **successive** ~ sukzessive Reproduktion *f* / **unisexual** ~ Jungfernzeugung *f*, Parthenogenese *f*

reproductive reproduktiv, Fortpflanzungs–

reproductiveness Reproduzierbarkeit *f*, Zeugungsfähigkeit *f*

reproof Verweis *m*, Tadel *m*

repudiation Ablehnung *f*, Verwerfung *f*, Zurückweisung *f*

repugnance Abneigung *f*, Aversion *f*, Antipathie *f*, Widerwille *m* / ~ **to faeces** Koprophobie *f* / ~ **to feces** Koprophobie *f*

repulsion Abneigung *f*, Widerwille *m*, Ekel *m*

repulsive abstoßend, widerlich, ekelhaft

reputation Ruf *m*, Ansehen *n* / ~ **rating** Einstufung *f* nach Ansehen / ~ **test** Imagetest *m*

request Anfrage *f*, Nachfrage *f*, Ersuchen *n* / bitten, ersuchen

required erforderlich, notwendig

requiredness Erfordertheit *f*, Gefordertheit *f*

requirement Erfordernis *n*, Bedürfnis *n*, Bedingung *f*

requisite erforderlich, notwendig / Erfordernis *n*, notwendige Bedingung *f*

rereading erneutes Lesen *n* / ~ **method** Methode *f* des Wiederlesens / ~ **procedure** Methode *f* des Wiederlesens

research Forschung *f*, Untersuchung *f* / forschen, untersuchen, Forschung treiben / ~ **design** Untersuchungsplan *m* / ~ **and development** Forschung *f* und Entwicklung *f* / ~ **diagnostic criteria** diagnostische Forschungskriterien *npl* / ~ **hypothesis** Forschungshypothese *f* / ~ **laboratory** Forschungslabor *n* / ~ **method** Forschungsmethode *f* / ~ **scientist** Forscher *m*, Wissenschaftler *m* / ~ **system** Forschungssystem *n* / ~ **work** Forschungsarbeit *f* / **applied** ~ angewandte Forschung *f* / **basic** ~ Grundlagenforschung *f* / **cross–sectional** ~ Querschnittsuntersuchung *f* / **empirical** ~ empirische Forschung *f* / **experimental** ~ experimentelle Untersuchung *f* / **fundamental** ~ Grundlagenforschung *f* / **genetic** ~ Vererbungsforschung *f* / **interdisciplinary** ~ interdisziplinäre Forschung *f* / **longitudinal** ~ Längsschnittuntersuchung *f* / **operational** ~ Operations Research *n* / **psychical** ~ parapsychologische Untersuchung *f* / **scientific** ~ wissenschaftliche Untersuchung *f*

researcher Forscher *m*, Marktforscher *m*, Meinungsforscher *m*

resemblance Ähnlichkeit *f* / **marital** ~ Ähnlichkeit *f* zwischen Eheleuten / **protective** ~ Schutzfärbung *f*

resemble ähneln, ähnlich sein

resentful ärgerlich, grollend, nachtragend

resentment Entrüstung *f*, Ärger *m*, Groll *m*, Ressentiment *n*

reserpine Reserpin *n*

reserve, reservation Zurückhaltung *f*, Verschlossenheit *f*, Reserve *f* / ~ **volume** Restvolumen *n*, Residualvolumen *n* / **operant** ~ Reflexreserve *f*

reserved reserviert, zurückhaltend

residency Facharztausbildung *f* / **medical** ~ Facharztausbildung *f*

resident innewohnend, fest ansässig / Bewohner *m*

residual residual, Rest–

residue, residuum Rest *m*, Rückstand *m*, Residuum *n* / ~**s method** Residualmethode *f* / **archaic** ~ archaischer Rest *m*

resign aufgeben, verzichten auf, entsagen

resignation Resignation *f*, Entsagung *f*, Verzicht *m* / **dynamic** ~ dynamischer Verzicht *m*, dynamische Resignation *f* / **neurotic** ~ neurotischer Verzicht *m*, neurotische Resignation *f* / **religious** ~ Entsagung *f*, religiös bedingter Verzicht *m*

resigned ergeben, entsagungsvoll, resigniert

resilience Elastizität *f*, Spannkraft *f*, Widerstandsfähigkeit *f*, Belastbarkeit *f*

resinous harzig

resistance Widerstand *m*, Resistenz *f*, Resistance *f* / **~ in dream interpretation** Widerstand *m* bei der Traumdeutung / **~ by the ego/of the ego** Ich–Widerstand *m* / **~ to extinction** Löschungsresistenz *f* / **~ by the id/of the id** Es–Widerstand *m* / **~ phase** Widerstandsphase *f* / **~ sensation** Widerstandsgefühl *n* / **~ to stress** Belastungsfähigkeit *f* / **~ by the superego/of the superego** Überich–Widerstand *m* / **~ to therapy** Therapieresistenz *f* / **~ due to transference** Übertragungswiderstand *m* / **~ by the unconscious/of the unconscious** Widerstand *m* des Unbewussten / **conscious ~** bewusster Widerstand *m* / **cutaneous ~** Hautwiderstand *m* / **expiratory ~** exspiratorische Resistance *f* / **internal ~** innerer Widerstand *m* / **passive ~** passiver Widerstand *m* / **psychotherapeutic ~** psychotherapeutischer Widerstand *m* / **synaptic ~** Synapsenwiderstand *m* / **unconscious ~** unbewusster Widerstand *m*

resistant widerstandsfähig, resistent / **~ to environmental influences** widerstandsfähig gegenüber Milieueinflüssen / **~ to treatment** therapieresistent

resistivity Widerstandsfähigkeit *f*

resocialisation Resozialisierung *f* / **psychosocial ~** gesellschaftliche Wiedereingliederung *f* Resozialisierung *f*

resoluteness Entschlossenheit *f*, Festigkeit *f*

resolution Entschluss *m*, Entschlossenheit *f*, Mut *m*, Auflösung *f*, Zerlegung *f*

resolve lösen, bestimmen, entscheiden, beschließen

resonance Resonanz *f*, Mitklingen *n*, Widerhall *m* / **~ box** Resonanzkasten *m* / **~–place theory** Resonanztheorie *f* / **~ theory** Resonanztheorie *f* / **~–volley theory** Wellendispersionstheorie *f* / **magnetic ~ imaging** Magnetresonanztomographie *f* / **nuclear magnetic ~** Kernspinresonanz *f* / **nuclear magnetic ~ imaging** Kernspinresonanztomographie *f* / **tympanic ~** tympanitischer Schall *m*, Tympanie *f*

resonant nachhallend, widerhallend, mitschwingend

resonate widerhallen, erklingen, ertönen

resonator Resonator *m*, Resonanzkörper *m*

resorption Resorption *f*, Aufsaugung *f*

resort Zuflucht nehmen, Gebrauch machen von / **~ to violence** Gewalt anwenden

resound widerhallen, ertönen, erschallen

resource Mittel *n*, Hilfsmittel *n*, Hilfsquelle *f* / **~ allocation** Ressourcenzuweisung *f* / **~ teacher** Aushilfslehrer *m*, Hilfslehrer *m* / **uniform ~ locator (URL)** Internetadresse *f*, URL / **human ~s** Personalwesen *n*

resourceful wendig, findig, geistig beweglich

respect Achtung *f*, Ehrerbietung *f*, Respekt *m* / schätzen, achten, Rücksicht nehmen

respectability Achtbarkeit *f*, Anständigkeit *f*, Schicklichkeit *f*

respiration Atmung *f*, Respiration *f* / **~ stimulating drug** Atemstimulans *n*, atmungsanregende Substanz *f* / **artificial ~** künstliche Beatmung *f*

respiratory Atem–, Atmungs–, respiratorisch

respire atmen

respirometry Messung *f* der Atembewegungen, Atemmessung *f*

respite care Pflege *f* durch Angehörige

respondent reagierend, antwortend / reagierende Person *f*

response Reaktion *f*, Reizantwort *f*, Antwort *f*, Reflex *m* / **~ adequacy** Angemessenheit *f* der Reaktion / **~ amplitude** Reaktionsamplitude *f*, Reaktionsstärke *f* / **~ attitude** Reaktionseinstellung *f* / **~ bias** Reaktionsverzerrung *f*, konstanter Reaktionsfehler *m* / **~ circuit** Reflexbogen *m* /

~ class Reaktionsklasse *f* / **~ contingent test** adaptiv–antwortabhängiger Test *m* / **~ cost** Verstärkerentzug *m* / **~ to demand** Leistungsanspruch *m* / **~ differentiation** Reaktionsdifferenzierung *f* / **~ dispersion** Reaktionszerfall *m* / **~ duration** Reaktionsdauer *f* / **~ equivalence** Reaktionsäquivalenz *f* / **~ frequency** Reaktionshäufigkeit *f* / **~ function** Funktion *f* einer Reaktion / **~ generalisation** Reaktionsgeneralisierung *f* / **~ hierarchy** Antworthierarchie *f*, Reaktionshierarchie *f* / **~ instance** Reaktion *f*, Einzelreaktion *f* / **~ intensity** Reaktionsstärke *f*, Reaktionsintensität *f* / **~ key** Reaktionstaste *f* / **~ lag** Reaktionsverzögerung *f* / **~ latency** Reaktionszeit *f*, Latenzzeit *f*, Latenz *f* / **~ learning** Reaktionslernen *n* / **~ magnitude** Reaktionsstärke *f* / **~ measurement** Reaktionsmessung *f* / **~ occurrence** Eintritt *m* einer Reaktion / **~–oriented psychologies** Verhaltenspsychologien *fpl* / **~ parameter** Reaktionsparameter *m* / **~ pattern** Reaktionsmuster *n* / **~ prevention** Reaktionsverhinderung *f* / **~ probability** Reaktionswahrscheinlichkeit *f* / **~–produced stimulus** reaktionsbedingter Reiz *m* / **~ psychology** Verhaltenspsychologie *f* / **~ rate** Reaktionsrate *f* / **~–reference** Reaktionsbezug *m* / **~ schema** Reaktionsschema *n*, Reaktionsmuster *n* / **~ set** Antworttendenz *f*, Reaktionstendenz *f*, Response–Set *m* / **~ speed** Reaktionsgeschwindigkeit *f* / **~ to a stimulus** Reizbeantwortung *f* / **~ strength** Antwortstärke *f*, Reaktionsstärke *f* / **~ system** Reaktionssystem *n* / **~ threshold** Reaktionsschwelle *f* / **~ time** Reaktionszeit *f* / **~ type** Reaktionstyp *m* / **~ variable** Reaktionsvariable *f* / **~ variability** Reaktionsvariabilität *f*, Reaktionsstreuung *f* / **abient ~** Vermeidungsreaktion *f* / **achromatic ~** Farbdeutung *f* zu schwarz und weiß / **acquired ~** erlernte Reaktion *f* / **adaptive ~** Anpassungsreaktion *f* / **adrenergic ~ state** adrenergischer Reaktionszustand *m* / **all–or–none ~** Alles–oder–Nichts–Reaktion *f* / **alternate–~ test** Alternativantworttest *m* / **alternating ~** wechselnde Reaktion *f* / **antagonistic ~** antagonistische Reaktion *f*, Gegenreaktion *f* / **antedating ~** antizipatorische Reaktion *f* / **anticipatory ~** antizipatorische Reaktion *f* / **arbitrary ~** Willkürreaktion *f* / **assertive ~** Durchsetzungsreaktion *f* / **chained ~s** Verhaltenskette *f* / **cochlear ~** Cochlea–Reflex *m*, Cochlea–Mikrophonpotential *n* / **conditioned ~** bedingte Reaktion *f*, konditionierte Reaktion *f*, bedingter Reflex *m* / **conditioned emotional ~** konditionierte emotionale Reaktion *f* / **constructed ~** selbstproduzierte Antwort *f* / **consummatory ~** Vollzugshandlung *f*, Zielhandlung *f* / **covert ~** verdeckte Reaktion *f*, verdecktes Verhalten *n*, gedankliche Antwort *f* / **cutaneous pupillary ~** Haut–Pupillen–Reflex *m* / **defensive ~** Schutzreflex *m* / **delayed ~** verzögerte Reaktion *f* / **delayed ~ set** verzögerte Reaktionstendenz *f* / **delayed conditioned ~** verzögerter bedingter Reflex *m* / **deviant ~ tendency** abweichende Reaktionstendenz *f* / **differential ~** selektive Reaktion *f* / **distal ~** distale Reaktion *f* / **electrodermal ~** psychogalvanische Reaktion *f*, galvanische Hautreaktion *f* / **elicited ~** ausgelöste Reaktion *f*, provozierte Reaktion *f* / **emotional ~** Gefühlsreaktion *f*, emotionale Reaktion *f* / **explicit ~** offene Reaktion *f*, offen gezeigte Reaktion *f* / **extrinsic motor ~** Fremdreflex *m* / **following ~** geprägte Reaktion *f* / **free–~** mit offener Antwort, mit ungebundener Aufgabenbeantwortung / **free–~ method** Methode *f* mit ungebundener Aufgabenbeantwortung / **glandular ~** Drüsenreaktion *f* / **humorous ~** humorvolle Deutung *f* / **ideomotor ~** ideomotorische Reaktion *f* / **implicit ~** implizite Reaktion *f*, verdeckte Reaktion *f* / **incompatible ~** unvereinbare Reaktion *f* / **individual ~** Individualantwort *f* / **inflammatory ~** Entzündungsreaktion *f* / **intentional ~** willkürliche Reaktion *f* / **investigatory ~** Orientierungsreaktion *f*, Untersuchungsreaktion *f* / **kinaesthetic ~** Bewegungsantwort *f* / **mediated ~** vermittelte Reaktion *f* / **med-**

iating ~ vermittelnde Reaktion *f* / **mimetic** ~ Nachahmungsreaktion *f*, nachahmendes Verhalten *n* / **multiple** ~ **test** Test *m* mit mehreren richtigen Antwortmöglichkeiten / **negative** ~ Vermeidungsreaktion *f* / **oculomotor** ~ reaktive Augenbewegung *f* / **operant** ~ operante Reaktion *f*, nichtreizgebundene Reaktion *f* / **optomotor** ~ optomotorische Reaktion *f* / **orienting** ~ Orientierungsreaktion *f*, Untersuchungsreaktion *f* / **original** ~ Originalantwort *f* / **overt** ~ offene Reaktion *f*, offen gezeigte Reaktion *f*, ausdrückliche Antwort *f* / **perceptual** ~ **disposition** perzeptionelle Reaktionsdisposition *f* / **pilomotor** ~ pilomotorische Reaktion *f*, Gänsehaut *f* / **popular** ~ Vulgärantwort *f* / **preparatory** ~ Vorbereitungsreaktion *f* / **prepotent** ~ dominante Reaktion *f* / **protective** ~ Schutzreaktion *f*, Schutzantwort *f*, Schutzbehauptung *f* / **proximal** ~ proximale Reaktion *f* / **psychogalvanic** ~ psychogalvanische Reaktion *f*, galvanische Hautreaktion *f* / **pupillary** ~ Pupillenreaktion *f* / **selected** ~ Auswahlantwort *f* / **selective** ~ selektive Reaktion *f* / **serial** ~ Serienreaktion *f*, Reaktionsfolge *f* / **species–specific** ~ artspezifische Reaktion *f* / **starting** ~ Umklammerungsreaktion *f* / **static** ~ Gleichgewichtsreflex *m* / **statokinetic** ~ statokinetischer Reflex *m*, Gleichgewichtsreflex *m* bei Bewegungen / **stereotyped** ~ stereotype Reaktion *f* / **Thorndikian** ~ Thorndike–Reaktion *f* / **total** ~**s** Anzahl *f* der Deutungen / **unconditioned** ~ unbedingte Reaktion *f*, unkonditionierte Reaktion *f*, unbedingter Reflex *m* / **vasomotor** ~ vasomotorischer Reflex *m* / **voluntary motor** ~ Willkürmotorik *f* / **vulgar** ~ Vulgärantwort *f* / **whole** ~ Ganzantwort *f* / **withdrawing** ~ Rückzugsreaktion *f*

responsibility Verantwortung *f*, Verantwortlichkeit *f*, Verpflichtung *f*, Zuständigkeit *f*, Aufgabe *f* / **civil** ~ Zurechnungsfähigkeit *f* / **criminal** ~ Schuldfähigkeit *f*, strafrechtliche Verantwortlichkeit *f* / **diminished criminal** ~ verminderte Schuldfähigkeit *f* / **moral** ~ moralische Verantwortung *f*

responsible verantwortlich, verantwortungsvoll

responsive reaktionsfähig, reagierend

responsiveness Reaktionsfähigkeit *f*, Reagibilität *f*, Antwortbereitschaft *f*, Ansprechbarkeit *f* / **whole–hearted** ~ Verständnis *n*

rest Ruhe *f*, Ausruhen *n*, Entspannung *f*, Rest *m* / ruhen, ausruhen, schlafen, übrigbleiben, bleiben / ~ **cure** Ruhekur *f* / ~ **pause** Ruhepause *f*, Pause *f* / ~ **period** Ruhepause *f* / ~ **tremor** Ruhetremor *m* / **mnemic** ~ Erinnerungsspur *f*

resting Ruhe–, ruhend

restitution Wiederherstellung *f*, Abheilung *f*, Restitution *f*

restless unruhig, ruhelos

restlessness Ruhelosigkeit *f*, Unruhe *f*, Schlaflosigkeit *f*, psychomotorische Unruhe *f* / **unstable** ~ innere Getriebenheit *f*, flatterhafte Unstetigkeit *f*

restoration Wiederherstellung *f*, Erholung *f* / ~ **of working capacity** Wiederherstellung *f* der Arbeitsfähigkeit / **spontaneous** ~ Spontanerholung *f*

restrain hindern, hemmen, einschränken

restraint Einschränkung *f*, Beschränkung *f*, Hinderung *f*, Freiheitsbeschränkung *f*, Zwangsmaßnahmen *fpl* / **chemical** ~ Zwangsberuhigung *f* von Geisteskranken mit Medikamenten / **dietary** ~ gezügeltes Essverhalten *n* / **emotional** ~ emotionale Kontrolle *f* / **mechanical** ~ Festschnallen *n* von Geisteskranken / **moral** ~ Enthaltsamkeit *f* / **physical** ~ körperliche Zwangsmaßnahmen *fpl*

restriction Einschränkung *f*, Beschränkung *f*, Restriktion *f* / ~ **of the ego** Ich–Einschränkung *f* / **genetically determined** ~**s** erbbedingte Beschränkungen *fpl*

restrictive einschränkend, beschränkend, restriktiv

restructure umstrukturieren

restructuring Umstrukturierung *f* / **cognitive ~** kognitive Umstrukturierung *f* / **perceptual ~** Wahrnehmungsumstrukturierung *f*

restructurisation Umstrukturierung *f*

result sich ergeben, folgen, führen zu / Ergebnis *n*, Folge *f*, Wirkung *f*, Resultat *n*, Konsequenz *f* / **~ of examination** Untersuchungsergebnis *n* / **~ of stimulation** Reizerfolg *m* / **~ of treatment** Behandlungsergebnis *n* / **early ~s** vorläufige Befunde *mpl* / **positive ~** positives Ergebnis *n*

resultant Resultante *f* / resultierend

resumption Wiederaufnahme *f*, Wiederbeginn *m* / **~ of interrupted actions** Wiederaufnahme *f* von unterbrochenen Handlungen

resuscitation Wiederbelebung *f*, Reanimation *f* / **~ limit** Strukturerhaltungszeit *f*, Wiederbelebungszeit *f*

resynthesis Wiedervereinigung *f*, neue Synthese *f*

retain behalten

retaliation Vergeltung *f*

retardate Zurückgebliebene *m,f*, Spätentwickler *m*, Retardierte *m,f*

retardation Verlangsamung *f*, Verzögerung *f*, Retardation *f*, Retardierung *f* / **~ in maturation** Reifungsverzögerung *f* / **~ of stimulation** Reizhemmung *f* / **cultural familial mental ~** psychosoziale Retardierung *f* / **educational ~** Schulversagen *n*, schulisches Zurückbleiben *n* / **familial ~** erblich bedingte Debilität *f* / **mental ~** geistige Behinderung *f*, Intelligenzminderung *f*, Retardierung *f*, Hypophrenie *f*, Minderbegabung *f* / **mental ~, severity unspecified** geistige Behinderung *f* mit unspezifischem Schweregrad / **mild mental ~** leichte geistige Behinderung *f* / **moderate mental ~** mittelschwere geistige Behinderung *f* / **profound mental ~** schwerste geistige Behinderung *f* / **psychic ~** psychische Retardierung *f* / **psychosocial mental ~** psychosoziale Retardierung *f*, geistige Behinderung *f* psychosozialen Ursprungs / **secondary mental ~** erworbene Debilität *f* / **severe mental ~** schwere geistige Behinderung *f*

retarded zurückgeblieben, behindert, retardiert, unterentwickelt / **educable mentally ~** geistig behinderte Person *f* die erziehbar ist, geistig Behinderte *m,f* mit Bildungsfähigkeiten / **institutionalised mentally ~** geistig behindertes Heimkind *n*, geistig Behinderter *m* in institutioneller Pflege / **mentally ~** geistig behindert / geistig Behinderte *m,f* / **profoundly mentally ~** geistig schwer Behinderte *m,f* / **severely mentally ~** imbezill, geistig stark behindert / **trainable mentally ~** geistig behinderte Person *f* die ausbildbar ist

retention Behalten *n*, Zurückhaltung *f*, Retention *f*, Retentionsfähigkeit *f* / **~ curve** Behaltenskurve *f*, Vergessenskurve *f* / **~ defect** Behaltensstörung *f*, Gedächtnisstörung *f* / **~ of faeces** Obstipation *f*, Verstopfung *f* / **~ hysteria** Retentionshysterie *f* / **~ measure** Gedächtnistest *m* / **~ need** Retentionsbedürfnis *n* / **~ of urine** Harnverhaltung *f* / **immediate ~** unmittelbares Behalten *n* / **selective ~** selektives Behalten *n* / **visual ~ test** Test *m* des visuellen Behaltens

retentive behaltend, zurückhaltend, verhaltend

retentiveness, retentivity Merkfähigkeit *f*, Fähigkeit *f* gut zu behalten / **~ of memory** Merkfähigkeit *f* / **extreme ~** abnorm gutes Gedächtnis *n*, Hypermnesie *f*

retest Testwiederholung *f*, Retest *m* / erneut testen, wiedertesten / **~ consistency** Testwiederholungsreliabilität *f*, Retest–Konsistenz *f*

reticence Zurückhaltung *f*, Verschwiegenheit *f*

reticent zurückhaltend, verschwiegen

reticular retikulär, netzartig

reticulate netzartig, retikulär / netzförmig anlegen

reticulum Retikulum *n*, Netzwerk *n* / **endoplasmic ~** endoplasmatisches Retikulum *n*

retina Retina *f*, Netzhaut *f* / **detached ~** abgelöste Netzhaut *f*

retinal Netzhaut–, Retina–

retinene Retinin *n*

retinitis Netzhautentzündung *f*, Retinitis *f* / **~ pigmentosa** Retinitis pigmentosa *f*, Pigmententartung *f* der Netzhaut

retinopathy Netzhauterkrankung *f*, Retinopathie *f*

retinoscope Augenspiegel *m*, Skiaskop *n*

retinoscopy Retinoskopie *f*, Skiaskopie *f*

retinotopic retinotop

retire zurückziehen, pensionieren, abtreten, in den Ruhestand treten

retirement Pensionierung *f*, Ruhestand *m*, Rücktritt *m* / **~ community** Altenwohnsitze *mpl* / **early ~** vorzeitige Pensionierung *f*

retraction Zurückziehen *n*, Sich–Zurückziehen *n*, Retraktion *f* / **~ of publication** Publikationsrücknahme *f*

retraining Umschulung *f* / **occupational ~** berufliche Umschulung *f*

retreat Rückzug *m* / nachgeben, sich zurückziehen / **~ to immaturity** Regression *f* / **~ from reality** Realitätsflucht *f* / **erotic ~** erotischer Rückzug *m*

retrieval Abruf *m* aus dem Gedächtnis / **cued ~** spezifisch signalisierter Abruf *m* / **noncued ~** unspezifisch signalisierter Abruf *m*

retrieving Abrufen *n* aus dem Gedächtnis

retroact zurückwirken, reagieren

retroaction Rückwirkung *f* / **negative ~** retroaktive Hemmung *f*, rückwirkende Hemmung *f*

retroactive retroaktiv, rückwirkend

retrobulbar retrobulbär, hinter dem Augapfel liegend

retrocede zurückgehen, rückübertragen

retrocognition unmittelbare Wahrnehmung *f* vergangener Ereignisse

retrocopulation Koitus *m* von hinten, Coitus a tergo *m*

retroflexed nach hinten gebeugt, zurückgelehnt

retroflexion Retroflexion *f*, Rückwärtsbeugung *f*

retrograde retrograd, rückläufig / rückwärts gehen, zurückgehen

retrography Spiegelschrift *f*

retrogress zurückgehen, rückentwickeln, degenerieren

retrogression Rückschritt *m*, Rückentwicklung *f*, Degeneration *f*

retrogressive rückschreitend, zurückgehend

retrospect Rückblick *m*, Rückschau *f* / zurückblicken

retrospection Rückblick *m*, Rückschau *f*

retrospective retrospektiv, zurückblickend, rückschauend

retroversion Rückwärtsbeugung *f*

retrovirus Retrovirus *n*

Rett's disorder Rett–Störung *f* / **~ syndrome** Rett–Syndrom *n*

return zurückkehren, wiederkehren, erwidern / Rückkehr *f*, Wiederkehr *f* / **~ of the repressed** Wiederkehr *f* des Verdrängten, Rückkehr *f* des Verdrängten / **~ sweep** Augenbewegung *f* beim Zeilenlesen / **diminishing ~** fallender Aufwandsertrag *m*

revaluation Aufwertung *f*

revalue aufwerten

reveal enthüllen, offenbaren, zeigen

revendication neurosis Prozessneurose *f*, Rentenneurose *f*

revenge rächen / Rache *f*, Revanche *f*

revengefulness Rachgier *f*, Rachsucht *f*

reverberate widerhallen, erschallen, ertönen

reverberation Widerhall *m*, Echo *n*

reverence Verehrung *f*, Reverenz *f*

reversal Umkehr *f*, Umkehrung *f* / ~ **design** Umkehrmethode *f*, Reversionsexperiment *n* / ~ **effect** Umkehreffekt *m* / ~ **formation** Reaktionsbildung *f*, Gefühlsverkehrung *f*, Umkehrbildung *f* / ~ **learning** Umkehrlernen *n* / ~ **into the opposite** Umkehrung *f* ins Gegenteil / ~ **of affect** Affektverkehrung *f* / ~ **shift** innerdimensionales Umlernen *n* / **non~ shift** außerdimensionales Umlernen *n*

reverse umgekehrt / Gegenteil *m*

reversed umgekehrt

reversibility Reversibilität *f*, Umkehrbarkeit *f* / ~ **by negation** Umkehr *f* durch Negation / ~ **by reciprocity** Umkehr *f* durch Umdrehung

reversible reversibel, umkehrbar, Umkehr–

reversion Rückschlag *m*, Umkehr *f*, Reversion *f* / ~ **figure** Reversionsfigur *f*, Kippfigur *f*, Vexierfigur *f*, Umschlagfigur *f* / ~ **picture** Umspringbild *n*, Umschlagfigur *f*

revert zurückfallen, in einen früheren Zustand zurückkehren

revery, reverie Träumerei *f* / **directed ~ therapy** gelenkte Traumtherapie *f*

review Überprüfung *f*, Inspektion *f*, Rezension *f* / überprüfen, nochmal durchdenken, kritisieren / ~ **passage** Wiederholungsstrecke *f*

revision Revision *f*, nochmalige Durchsicht *f* / **secondary ~** sekundäre Bearbeitung *f*

revival Wiederaufleben *n*, Reproduktion *f*, Erinnerung *f*

revivification Wiederaufleben *n*

revolution Revolution *f*, Umsturz *m* / **political ~** politischer Umsturz *m*

reward Belohnung *f* / belohnen / ~ **allocation** Belohnungszuteilung *f* / ~ **expectancy** Belohnungserwartung *f*, Antizipation *f* der Belohnung / ~ **learning** Lernen *n* durch Belohnung / ~ **schedule** Verstärkungsplan *m*, Belohnungsplan *m* / ~ **situation** Belohnungssituation *f* / **conditioned ~** konditionierte Belohnung *f* / **delayed ~** verzögerte Belohnung *f* / **external ~** externale Belohnung *f* / **extraneous ~** externe Belohnung *f* / **extrinsic ~** externe Belohnung *f* / **internal ~** internale Belohnung *f*, in der Handlung liegende Belohnung *f* / **intrinsic ~** in der Handlung liegende Belohnung *f* / **monetary ~** Entlohnung *f*, finanzielle Belohnung *f* / **negative ~** negative Belohnung *f*, Strafe *f* / **positive ~** Belohnung *f*, positive Belohnung *f* / **preferred ~** bevorzugte Belohnung *f* / **primary ~** primäre Verstärkung *f* / **secondary ~** sekundäre Verstärkung *f* / **sedative ~** abschließende Belohnung *f* / **stimulating ~** stimulierende Belohnung *f*

rewriting rule Satzerzeugungsregel *f*, Ersetzungsregel *f*

RF center RF–Zentrum *n*

Rh incompatibility Rhesusfaktor–Unverträglichkeit *f*

rhabdomancy Weissagung *f* mittels Zauberstäben

rhabdophobia Angst *f* vor Stöcken, Rhabdophobie *f*

rhathymia Rhathymie *f*, Sorglosigkeit *f*, Unbesorgtheit *f*, Unbekümmertheit *f*

rheobase, rheobasis Rheobase *f*, galvanische Reizschwelle *f*, Reizschwelle *f* bei elektrischer Gleichstromreizung

rheoencephalography Schädelrheographie *f*, Rheoenzephalographie *f*

rheometer Galvanometer *n*, Blutstromschnelligkeitsmesser *m*

rheoscope Galvanoskop *n*

rheoscopic galvanoskopisch

rheostat Rheostat *m*, Vorschaltwiderstand *m*

rheotaxis Rheotaxis *f*, Bewegungsrichtung *f* von Organismen

rheotrope Stromwender *m*, Gleichrichter *m*

rheotropism Rheotropismus *m*, Rheotaxis *f*, Bewegungsrichtung *f* von Organismen

rhesus monkey, rhesus, rhesus macaque Rhesusaffe *m*

rhesus system Rhesus–System *n*

rhetoric Rhetorik *f*, Redekunst *f*

rhinaesthesia, rhinesthesia Geruchssinn *m*

rhinencephalic Riechhirn–

rhinencephalon Riechhirn *n*, Rhinenzephalon *n*

rhinism Näseln *n*, Rhinolalie *f*

rhinolalia Näseln *n*, Rhinolalie *f*

rhinology Nasenheilkunde *f*, Rhinologie *f*

rhinophonia Näseln *n*, Rhinophonie *f*, Rhinolalie *f*

rhinoscope Nasenspiegel *m*, Rhinoskop *n*

rhinoscopic rhinoskopisch

rhinoscopy Untersuchung *f* mittels Nasenspiegel, Rhinoskopie *f*

rhizopod Wurzelfüßler *m*, Rhizopod *m*

rhodopsin Sehpurpur *m*, Rhodopsin *n*, Erythropsin *n*

rhombencephalon Rautenhirn *n*, Rhombenzephalon *n*

rhotacism fehlerhafte Aussprache *f* des Buchstaben „r", Rhotazismus *m*, Stammeln *n*

rhypophagy Schmutzessen *n*, Dreckessen *n*, Kotessen *n*

rhypophobia Schmutzangst *f*, Rhypophobie *f*, Mysophobie *f*

rhythm Rhythmus *m* / **~ method** Knaus–Ogino–Methode *f*, Methode *f* der zeitlichen Enthaltsamkeit / **alpha ~** Alpha–Rhythmus *m* / **autogenic ~** Eigenrhythmus *m* / **beta ~** Beta–Rhythmus *m* / **biological ~** biologischer Rhythmus *m*, Lebensrhythmus *m* / **bright ~** Belichtungsrhythmus *m* / **circadian ~** Schlaf–Wach–Rhythmus *m*, Tagesrhythmus *m*, zirkadianer Rhythmus *m* / **cortical ~** Großhirnrhythmus *m* / **daily ~** Tagesrhythmus *m* / **delta ~** Delta–Rhythmus *m* / **diurnal ~** tagesperiodischer Rhythmus *m* / **human biological ~** biologischer Rhythmus *m* beim Menschen / **mating ~** Begattungsrhythmus *m* / **own ~** Eigenrhythmus *m* / **respiratory ~** Atemrhythmus *m* / **sleeping–waking ~** Schlaf–Wach–Rhythmus *m* / **spontaneous ~** Spontanrhythmus *m* / **subjective ~** subjektiver Rhythmus *m* / **working ~** Arbeitsrhythmus *m*

rhythmic, rhythmical rhythmisch

rib Rippe *f*

ribonuclease Ribonuklease *f*

ribose Ribose *f*

ribosome Ribosom *n*

rickets Rachitis *f*, englische Krankheit *f*

rickety rachitisch

riddance reflex Befreiungsreflex *m*, Abschüttelreflex *m*

Ridgway colours Ridgway–Farben *fpl*

right rechts, richtig, angemessen, recht / Recht *n* / **~–angled** rechtwinklig / **~–handed** rechtshändig / **~–handedness** Rechtshändigkeit *f* / **~–hander** Rechtshänder *m* / **~s of men** Menschenrechte *npl* / **~–preponderance** Überwiegen *n* der rechten Seite / **~ to treatment** Recht *n* auf Behandlung / **civil ~s** Bürgerrechte *npl*, Menschenrechte *npl* / **civil ~s movement** Bürgerrechtsbewegung *f* / **deprived of civil ~s** entmündigt / **human ~s** Menschenrechte *npl*

righteousness Rechtschaffenheit *f*

righting Aufrichten *n* / **~ reaction** Aufrichtungsreaktion *f* / **~ reflex** Aufrichtungsreflex *m* / **~ response** Aufrichtungsreaktion *f* / **visual ~ reflexes** Sehstellreflexe *mpl*

rightness Richtigkeit *f*, Korrektheit *f*

rigid rigide, starr, steif

rigidity Rigidität *f*, Starrheit *f*, Inflexibilität *f*, Unbeweglichkeit *f*, Starre *f*, Bewegungssperre *f* / **affective ~** Affektsteifigkeit *f*, Affektlahmheit *f* / **cataleptic ~** kataleptische Bewegungsunfähigkeit *f* / **cataleptiform ~** kataleptiforme Starre *f* / **decerebrate ~** Enthirnungsstarre *f*, Dezerebrierungsstarre *f* / **hypnotic ~** hypnotische Starre *f* / **mental ~** geistige Inflexibilität *f*, geistige Rigidität *f* / **muscular ~** Muskelstarre *f* / **psychic ~** psychische Rigidität *f*, psychische Inflexibilität *f*

rigor Rigor *m*, Muskelstarre *f* / **~ mortis** Totenstarre *f*

Riley–Day syndrome Riley–Day–Syndrom *n*

ringing in the ears Ohrenklingen *n*, Tinnitus *m*

riot Aufruhr *m*, Aufstand *m*, Unruhen *fpl*, Ausschweifung *f* / **racial ~s** Rassenunruhen *fpl*

rioter, riotist Aufrührer *m*, Randalierer *m*

ripen reifen, sich entwickeln

ripeness Reife *f*

risibility Lachlust *f*

risible Lach–, lächerlich

risk Risiko *n*, Gefährdung *f* / **~ analysis** Risikoanalyse *f* / **~ factor** Risikofaktor *m* / **~ level** Konfidenzbereich *m*, Risikobereich *m*, Signifikanzniveau *n* / **~ management** Risiko–Management *n* / **~ perception** Risikowahrnehmung *f* / **~–taking** Risikobereitschaft *f*, Risikoverhalten *n* / **~–taking behaviour** Risikoverhalten *n* / **at–~ population** Risikogruppe / **occupational ~** Berufsgefährdung *f*

risperidone Risperidon *n*

ritanserin Ritanserin *n*

rite Ritus *m*, Ritual *n*, Zeremonie *f*, Brauch *m* / **~s of passage** Übergangsriten *mpl*, Initiationsriten *mpl*

ritual Ritual *n* / rituell / **obsessional ~** Zwangsritual *n*

ritualisation Ritualisierung *f*

ritualistic rituell, ritualistisch, zeremoniell

rivalry Rivalität *f*, Konkurrenz *f*, Nebenbuhlerschaft *f*, Wetteifer *m*, Wettstreit *m* / **binocular ~** Rivalitat *f* der Sehfelder / **envious ~** neidischer Wettstreit *m* / **fraternal ~** Bruderzwist *m* / **jealous ~** Nebenbuhlerschaft *f*, eifersüchtige Rivalität *f* / **neural ~** Wettstreit *m* von Nervenimpulsen / **religious ~** religiöser Zwist *m* / **retinal ~** Wettstreit *m* der Sehfelder / **sibling ~** Geschwisterrivalität *f*

robbery Diebstahl *m*, Raub *m*

roborant stärkend, roborierend / Stärkungsmittel *n*, Roborans *n*

robot Roboter *m*, menschliche Maschine *f*

robotism Mechanisierung *f*

R occurence Reaktionshäufigkeit *f*, Auftreten *n* einer Reaktion

rock music Rock–Musik *f*

rocking Schaukeln *n*, Wiegen *n* / Schaukel–

rod Stäbchen *n* / **~ cell** Stäbchenzelle *f* / **~ and cone vision** Stäbchen–und–Zapfen–Sehen *n* / **~s and cones** Stäbchen– und Zapfenschicht *f* / **~s of Corti** Corti–Pfeilerzellen *fpl* / **~ vision** Dämmerungssehen *n* / **divining ~** Wünschelrute *f* / **retinal ~** Netzhautstäbchen *n*, Stäbchen *n*

roentgeno|graphy Röntgenverfahren *n*, Röntgenfotografie *f* / **~phoby** Röntgenophobie *f*, krankhafte Angst *f* vor Röntgenstrahlen

Rolandic fissure Rolando–Furche *f*, Zentralfurche *f*

Rolando's sulcus Rolando–Furche *f*, Zentralfurche *f*

role Rolle *f* / **~ behaviour** Rollenverhalten *n*, rollenkonformes Verhalten *n* / **~ conflict** Rollenkonflikt *m* / **~ expectation** Rollenerwartung *f* / **~ incompatibility** Unverträglichkeit *f* von Rollen / **~ model** Rollenmodell *n* / **~ perception** Rollenwahrnehmung *f* / **~–playing** Rollenspiel *n* / **~–playing method** Methode *f* des Rollenspiels / **~ satisfaction** Rollenzufriedenheit *f* / **~ strain** Rollenzwang *m*, Rollendruck *m* / **~ taking** Rollenübernahme *f* / **~ theory** Rollentheorie *f* / **~ trait** Rollenmerkmal *n* / **achieved ~** erreichte Rolle *f* / **imposed ~** auferlegte Rolle *f* / **parental ~** Elternrolle *f* / **personal ~–definition** persönliche Rollenauffassung *f* / **prescribed ~** vorgeschriebene Rolle *f* / **social ~** soziale Rolle *f*

romance Liebesbeziehung *f*

romancing Fabulieren *n*, Aufschneiden *n*

romanticism romantischer Charakter *m*, romantische Einstellung *f*, Romantizismus *m*

Romberg's| sign Romberg–Zeichen *n* / **~ symptom** Romberg–Zeichen *n* / **~ test** Romberg–Versuch *m*

room Raum *m*, Zimmer *n* / **~ mate** Zimmergenosse *m* / **anechoic ~** schalltoter Raum *m* / **distorted ~** verzerrter Raum *m*, Ames'scher Raum *m* / **sound–proof ~** schalldichter Raum *m*

root Wurzel *f* / **~ conflict** Kernproblem *n*, Kernkonflikt *m* / **~–mean–square** mittlere Quadratwurzel *f* / **anterior ~ of spinal nerves** Vorderwurzel *f* der Spinalnerven / **dorsal ~** hintere Wurzel *f*, Dorsalwurzel *f* / **efferent ~** vordere Wurzel *f* / **motor ~** motorische Wurzel *f* / **posterior ~** hintere Wurzel *f* / **sensory ~** sensible Wurzel *f* / **spinal ~** Rückenmarkwurzel *f* / **square ~** Quadratwurzel *f* / **ventral ~** vordere Wurzel *f*, ventrale Wurzel *f*

Rorschach| category Rorschach Einteilung *f* / **~ Inkblots test** Rorschach–Formdeuteversuch *m* / **~ method** Rorschach–Verfahren *n* / **~ ranking test** Rorschach Rangreihentest *m* / **~ test** Rorschachtest *m* / **~ test card** Rorschachtafel *f*

Rossolimo| profile Rossolimo–Profil *n* / **~'s sign** Zehenreflex *m*, Rossolimo–Reflex *m* / **~'s reflex** Rossolimo–Reflex *m*, Zehenreflex in

rostral rostral, zum Kopfende hin gelegen

rotary, rotatory rotierend, kreisend

rotate rotieren, drehen, sich drehen

rotating rotierend, kreisend

rotation Rotation *f*, Achsendrehung *f*, Drehung *f* / **~ chair** Drehstuhl *m* / **~ disk** Kreiselscheibe *f* / **~ of factor axes** Rotation *f* der Faktorenachsen / **~ method** Rotationsmethode *f* / **~ nystagmus** Drehnystagmus m / **~ perception** Rotationswahrnehmung *f* / **~ sense** Drehsinn *m* / **~ table** Drehtisch *m*, Rotationstisch *m* / **~ test** Rotationstest in, Drehversuch in / **coloured ~ disk** Farbenkreisel *m*, Farbscheibe *f* / **mental ~** mentale Rotation *f* / **oblique ~** schiefwinkelige Rotation *f*, oblique Rotation *f* / **orthogonal ~** orthogonale Rotation *f* / **statistical ~** statistische Rotation *f*

rotator Drehmuskel *m*, Rotator *m*

rotatory rotierend, durch Rotation bedingt, Rotations–, sich drehend

rote rein mechanisch, durch bloße Übung, auswendig

rough rauh, uneben, grob

roughness Rauheit *f*, Rauhigkeit *f*, Grobheit *f*

rounded abgerundet, aufgerundet, ungefähr, Näherungs–

rounding Abrundung *f*, Aufrundung *f* / **~ of data** Aufrundung *f* oder Abrundung *f* von Daten

router Router *m*, Computersystem *n* zur Verbindung von zwei Netzwerken

routine Routine / **executive ~** ausführendes Programm *n*, Organisationsprogramm *n* / **narrow ~** Eingleisigkeit *f* / **supervisory ~** Führungserfahrung *f*

routing Leitweg *m*

row Reihe *f*

R–R law R–R–Gesetz *n*

R technique R–Technik *f*

rubella Röteln *fpl* / **~ deaf** taub aufgrund von Röteln

Rubin's| figure Rubin–Figur *f* / **~ goblet–profile figure** Rubins Kelch–Profil–Figur *f* / **~ test** Rubin–Methode *f*

rubric Überschrift *f*, Rubrik *f*

ructation Aufstoßen *n*

rude barsch

rudiment Rudiment *n*, erster Ansatz *m*

rudimentary rudimentär, nicht voll entwickelt

Ruffini| body Ruffini–Körperchen *n* / **~ cylinder** Ruffini–Körperchen *n* / **~ corpuscle** Ruffini–Körperchen *n* / **~ papillary endings** Ruffini–Nervenendpapillen *fpl* / **~ plumes** Ruffini–Nervenendpapillen *fpl*

rule Regel *f* / ~ **of conduct** Verhaltensnorm *f* / ~**–example method** Regel–Beispiel–Methode *f* / ~ **of a single variable** Regel *f* einer einzigen unabhängigen Variable *n* / **analytic** ~ analytische Grundregel *f* / **fundamental** ~ Grundregel *f*

Rulon test Rulon–Konsistenzkoeffizient in

rumination Nachsinnen *n*, Überdenken *n*, Rumination *f*, psychische Rumination *f* / ~ **disorder** Störung *f* mit Rumination, Ruminationsstörung *f* / ~ **disorder of infancy** Rumination *f* im Kleinkindalter / **obsessive** ~ zwanghaftes Grübeln *n*

rumor Gerücht *n*

run Lauf *m*, Durchlauf in / laufen, durchlaufen / ~ **test** Zeitreihentest in

runaway Ausreißer *m* / durchgegangen, fortgelaufen / ~ **behaviour** Weglaufen *n*, Ausreissen *n*, Fluchtverhalten *n*

running Laufen *n* / **long–distance** ~ Langstreckenlauf *m*

runway Laufsteg *m*, Gehweg *m*

rupophobia Schmutzangst *f*, Rhypophobie *f*, Mysophobie *f*

rupture Riss *m*, Ruptur *f*, Bruch *m*

rural ländlich, bäuerlich, Land–

rut Brunst *f*, Brunstzeit *f*, Brunft *f* / ~**–formation** Bildung *f* von Zwangsideen

rutting Brunst *f*, Brunft *f* / brünstig, Brunst–, Brunft– / ~ **season** Brunstzeit *f* / ~ **time** Brunstzeit *f*

R variable Reaktionsvariable *f*

S

sabotage Sabotage *f* / **masochistic ~** masochistische Sabotage *f*

saccade Sakkade *f*

saccadic ruckartig, sakkadisch, saccadiert

saccharin Saccharin *n*, Süßstoff *m*

saccule, sacculus Säckchen *n*, Sacculus *m*

Sachs' disease Sachs–Krankheit *f*, amaurotische Idiotie *f*

sacral sakral, Kreuzbein–

sacralisation Sakralisation *f*, angeborene Lendenwirbelsäulenanomalie *f*

sacred heilig, geheiligt, geistlich

sacrum Kreuzbein *n*, Sakrum *n*

sad traurig

sadism Sadismus *m* / **anal ~** Analsadismus *m* / **inverted ~** invertierter Sadismus *m* / **oral ~** oraler Sadismus *m* / **primal ~** primärer Sadismus *m* / **sexual ~** sexueller Sadismus *m*

sadist Sadist *m*

sadistic sadistisch / **~–masochistic** sadistisch–masochistisch, sadomasochistisch

sadness Traurigkeit *f* / **vital ~** vitale Traurigkeit *f*

sado–masochism Sadomasochismus *m* / **sexual ~** Sadomasochismus *m*

sado–masochistic sadomasochistisch

safeguard schützen, bewahren / Schutz *m*, Sicherung *f*

safety Sicherheit *f* / **~ belt** Sicherheitsgurt *m* / **~ device** Schutzmechanismus *m*, Sicherheitsvorrichtung *f* / **~ factor** Sicherheitsfaktor *m* / **~ hazard** Unfallgefahr *f*, Sicherheitsrisiko *n* / **~ limit** Sicherheitsgrenze *f* / **~ margin** Sicherheitsmarge *f* / **~ measures** Unfallverhütungsmaßnahmen *fpl* / **~ need** Sicherheitsbedürfnis *n* / **industrial ~** Sicherheit *f* am Arbeitsplatz, Sicherheit *f* in der Industrie / **occupational ~** Sicherheit *f* am Arbeitsplatz

sagacious klug, scharfsinnig

sagaciousness, sagacity Klugheit *f*, Scharfsinn *m*

sage klug, weise

sagittal sagittal, pfeilartig

Saint Vitus' dance Veitstanz *m*, Chorea minor *f*

Salaam| convulsion Salaamkrampf *m*, Nickkrampf *m*, Blitzkrampf *m* / **~ spasm** Salaamkrampf *m*, Nickkrampf *m*

sales Verkauf *m* / **~ aptitude** Eignung *f* für den Verkauf / **~ aptitude test** Test *m* zur Prüfung der Verkaufseignung / **~ comprehension test** Test *m* zur Prüfung des Verkaufswissens / **~ management** Verkaufsleitung *f* / **~ motivation inventory** Fragebogen *m* zur Erfassung der Verkaufsmotivation / **~ personnel** Verkaufspersonal *n* / **~ promotor** Verkaufsförderer *m* / **~ promotion** Verkaufsförderung *f*

salesmanship Verkaufsgewandtheit *f*, Verkaufstüchtigkeit *f*

salience, saliency Bedeutsamkeit *f*, Abhebung *f*

salient hervortretend, hervorspringend

saline salzig

saliva Speichel *m*

salivant speicheltreibend

salivary Speichel–, speichelig

salivation Speichelabsonderung *f*

salivomania Spucksucht *f*, Salivomanie *f*

Salpêtrière school Salpêtrière–Schule *f*

salpingectomy Eileiterentfernung *f*, Tubenresektion *f*, Salpingektomie *f*

salpinx Eileiter *m*, Tube *f*, Salpinx *f*, Ohrtrompete *f*, Eustach'sche Röhre *f*

saltation Veitstanz *m*, Mutation *f* / saltatorische Erregungsleitung *f*

saltatory springend, Mutations–

saltiness Salzigkeit *f*, Salzgeschmack *m*

salty salzig

salvarsan Salvarsan *n*

sameness Gleichheit *f*

sample Stichprobe *f* / Stichproben erheben / **~ bias** Stichprobenfehler *m* / **~ census** Stichprobenerhebung *f* / **~ design** Planung *f* einer Stichprobenerhebung / **~ estimate** Stichprobenschätzung *f* / **~ group** Stichprobe *f* / **~ interview** Stichprobeninterview *n* / **~ mean** Stichprobenmittel *n* / **~ overlap** Stichprobenüberlappung *f* / **~ parameter** Stichprobenparameter *m* / **~ size** Stichprobengrösse *f* / **~ space** Stichprobenbereich *m* / **~ survey** Umfrage *f* bei einer Stichprobe / **adequate ~** hinreichend große Stichprobe *f* / **controlled ~** kontrollierte Stichprobe *f* / **dependent ~** abhängige Stichprobe *f* / **independent ~** unabhängige Stichprobe *f* / **matched ~** Parallelstichprobe *f*, zugeordnete Stichprobe *f* / **random ~** unausgelesene Stichprobe *f*, Zufallsstichprobe *f* / **representative ~** repräsentative Stichprobe *f* / **selected ~** ausgewählte Stichprobe *f*, ausgewählte Gruppe *f* / **small ~ theory** Theorie *f* der kleinen Stichproben / **statistical ~** repräsentative Stichprobe *f*, statistische Stichprobe *f* / **statistical ~ parameter** statistischer Stichprobenparameter *m* / **stratified ~** geschichtete Stichprobe *f*, stratifizierte Stichprobe *f* / **systematic ~** systematische Stichprobe *f* / **unbiased ~** unverzerrte Stichprobe *f*, erwartungstreue Stichprobe *f*

sampling Stichprobenerhebung *f*, Stichprobenauswahl *f*, Stichprobenzusammenstellung *f* / **~ design** Planung *f* von Stichprobenerbebungen, Anlage *f* von Stichprobenerhebungen / **~ error** Stichprobenfehler *m* / **~ fluctuation** Stichprobenschwankung *f* / **~ method** Stichprobenverfahren *n*, Stichprobenmethode *f* / **~ population** Population *f* für eine Stichprobenauswahl, Grundgesamtheit *f* für eine Stichprobenauswahl / **~ without replacement** Stichprobenauswahl *f* ohne Ersatz / **~ servo** Korrekturregulativ *n* bei einer Stichprobenerhebung / **~ stability** Stichprobenstabilität *f*, Stichprobenbeständigkeit *f* / **~ technique** Stichprobenverfahren *n* / **~ theory** Theorie *f* der Stichprobenauswahl / **~ validity** Stichprobenvalidität *f* / **~ variability** Stichprobenschwankungen *fpl* / **accidental ~** zufällige Stichprobenauswahl *f* / **biased ~** systematischer Stichprobenfehler *m*, fehlerhafte Stichprobenzusammenstellung *f* / **controlled ~** kontrollierte Stichprobenauswahl *f* / **direct ~** kontrollierte Stichprobenauswahl *f* / **disproportional ~** disproportionale Stichprobenerhebung *f* / **domal ~** Stichprobenerhebung *f* nach Wohneinheiten / **double ~** doppelte Stichprobenerhebung *f* / **extensive ~** breitgefächerte Stichprobe *f* / **haphazard ~** zufällige Stichprobenauswahl *f* / **horizontal ~** horizontale Stichprobenauswahl *f* / **intensive ~** intensive Stichprobe *f* / **matched ~** Parallelisieren *n* / **proportional ~** proportionale Stichprobenerhebung *f* / **purposive ~** kontrollierte Stichprobe *f* / **random ~** Zufallsauswahl *f*, Erhebung *f* einer unausgelesenen Stichprobe, Zufallsstichprobenzusammenstellung *f* / **representative ~** repräsentative Stichprobe *f* / **situational ~** Erhebung *f* einer Situationsstichprobe / **stratified ~** Erhebung *f* einer stratifizierten Stichprobe, Erhebung *f* einer geschichteten Stichprobe / **vertical ~** vertikale Stichprobenauswahl *f*

sanative heilend, heilsam

sanatorium Sanatorium *n*, Heilstätte *f*, Genesungsheim *n*

sanction Sanktion *f*, Genehmigung *f*, Strafmaßnahme *f* / **social ~** soziale Sanktion *f*

Sandström's| bodies Epithelkörperchen *npl*, Sandström–Körperchen *npl*, Nebenschilddrüsen *fpl* / **~ glands** Nebenschilddrüsen *fpl*, Sandström–Körperchen *npl*

sane geistig gesund

sanguine, sanguineous sanguinisch, leichtblütig, optimistisch, zuversichtlich

sanguineness Zuversichtlichkeit *f*, zuversichtliches Gleichgewicht *n*, heiteres Temperament *n*

sanguinic Sanguiniker *m*

sanitation Hygiene *f*, Gesundheitswesen *n*

sanity, saneness geistige Gesundheit *f*, normale Geistesverfassung *f* / **mental ~** geistige Gesundheit *f*

Sanson images Purkinje–Sanson–Spiegelbilder *npl*, Reflexbilder *npl*

santonin Santonin *n*

saphead Tölpel *m*, Hohlkopf *m*

sapid schmackhaft

sapidity Schmackhaftigkeit *f*

sapphic lesbisch

sapphism Sapphismus *m*, weibliche Homosexualität *f*, lesbische Liebe *f*, Tribadismus *m*

sarcasm Sarkasmus *m*, bitterer Spott *m*

sarcastic sarkastisch

sarco|de tierisches Protoplasma *n* / **~lemma** Sarkolemm *n*, Plasmalemm *n* der Muskelfaser / **~ma** Sarkom *n*, bösartige Gewebsgeschwulst *f* / **~mere** Sarkomer *n* / **~plasm** Sarkoplasma *n* / **~plasmic** sarkoplasmatisch

satanophobia krankhafte Angst *f* vor dem Teufel

sate, satiate sättigen, übersättigen

sated, satiated übersättigt

satiating sättigend

satiation Sättigung *f* / **~ effect** psychische Sättigung *f*, Sättigungseffekt *m* / **~ hypothesis** Sättigungshypothese *f* / **~ point** Sättigungspunkt *m* / **cortical ~** kortikale Sättigung *f*

satiety Sattheit *f*, Übersättigung *f*, Überdruss *m*

satisfaction Befriedigung *f* / **~ of instinct** Triebbefriedigung *f* / **instinctual ~** Triebbefriedigung *f* / **marital ~** partnerschaftliche Zufriedenheit *f* / **sexual ~** sexuelle Zufriedenheit *f* / **substitute ~** Ersatzbefriedigung *f*

satisfier Mittel *n* zur Befriedigung

satisfy befriedigen, zufriedenstellen

saturate sättigen

saturated gesättigt

saturation Sättigung *f*, Faktorenladung *f* / **~ point** Sättigungspunkt *m* / **~ scale** Sättigungsskala *f* / **~ therapy** Übersättigungstherapie *f* / **~ voltage** Sättigungsspannung *f*

satyriasis, satyromania, satyrism Satyriasis *f*, Satyromanie *f*, krankhafte Steigerung *f* des männlichen Sexualbegehrens

satyromaniac Satyromaner *m*, an übersteigerter Sexualität leidender Mann *m*

Savart wheel Savart–Scheibe *f*

saving Ersparnis *f* / **~ method** Ersparnismethode *f* / **~ procedure** Ersparnismethode *f*

savour Geschmack *m*

scala Treppe *f* / **~ media** mittlere Treppe *f* / **~ tympani** Paukentreppe *f* / **~ vestibuli** Vorhoftreppe *f*

scalability Skalierbarkeit *f*

scalable skalierbar

scale Skala *f*, Stufenleiter *f*, Maßstab *m*, Tonleiter *f*, Test *m* / **~ analysis** Skalenanalyse *f* / **~ caption** Skalenbeschreibung *f* / **~ of colours** Farbenskala *f* / **~ interval** Skalenintervall *n* / **~ level** Skalenniveau *n* / **~ of measurement** Messskala *f* / **~ points** Skalenpunkte *mpl* / **~ of psychomotor development** Stufenleiter *f* der psychomotorischen Entwicklung / **~ of reproducibility** Skalenreproduzierbarkeit *f* / **~ of salaries** Gehaltsstufen *fpl* / **~ of tones** Tonskala *f* / **~ value** Skalenwert *m* / **absolute ~** Absolutskala *f*, Verhältnisskala *f* / **additive ~** Intervallskala *f* / **analytical ~** diagnostischer Test *m* / **a priori ~** vorher definierte Skala *f* / **A–S ~** Antisemitismus–Skala *f* / **auditory ~** Gehörempfindlichkeitsskala *f* / **chromatic ~** chromatische Tonleiter *f* / **classificatory ~** Nominalskala *f* / **continuous ~** kontinuierliche Skala *f* / **cumulative ~** Häufigkeitsskala *f*, kumulative Skala *f*, Guttman–Skala *f* / **derived ~** abgeleitete Skala *f* / **designatory ~** Nominalskala *f* / **developmental ~** Entwicklungstest *m* / **diatonic ~** diatonische Tonleiter *f* / **discontinuous ~** diskontinuierliche Skala *f* / **discrete ~** diskreter Maßstab *m* / **equal–tempered ~** gleichmäßige Skala *f* / **fundamental ~** Grundskala *f* / **graphic ~** graphische Beurteilungsskala *f* / **ipsative ~** ipsative Messskala *f* / **isochron ~** Isochronskala *f* / **joint ~** kombinierte Skala *f* / **logarithmic ~** logarithmische Skala *f* / **major ~** Dur–Tonleiter *f* / **mental ~** psychologische Skala *f* / **minor ~** Moll–Tonleiter *f* / **nominal ~** Nominalskala *f* / **ordered metric ~** Ordinalskala *f* / **ordinal ~** Ordinalskala *f* / **pentatonic ~** Fünftonskala *f* / **percentile ~** Prozentrangskala *f*, Perzentilskala *f* / **psychological ~** psychologische Skala *f* / **sensory ~** Empfindungsskala *f* / **social ~** soziale Stufenleiter *f* / **spectral ~** Spektralskala *f* / **spectral chromatic ~** Spektralfarbenband *n* / **subjective ~** subjektive Skala *f* / **tempered ~** temperierte Stimmung *f* / **tonal ~** Tonskala *f* / **unidimensional ~** eindimensionale Skala *f* / **verbal ~** sprachlicher Test *m*, verbaler Test *m*

scaling Skalierung *f* / **ipsative ~** ipsative Messung *f* / **multidimensional ~** mehrdimensionale Skalierung *f*

scallop bogenförmiger Ausschnitt *m*

scalogram Skalogramm *n*, Häufigkeitsskala *f*, Guttman–Skala *f*, kumulative Skala *f* / **~ analysis** Skalogrammanalyse *f* / **~ board** Skalogramm–Formular *n*

scalp Kopfhaut *f*

scan abtasten, kritisch prüfen, zerlegen

scanning Abtasten *n*, Beobachten *n*, Szintigraphie *f* / skandierend / **~ machine** Analysegerät *n* / **~ strategy** Strategie *f* des langsamen Abtastens / **biased ~** gerichtetes Beobachten *n*

scansion Skandieren *n*, Skandierung *f*

scapegoat Sündenbock *m*

scaphocephalic, scaphocephalous kahnschädelig

scaphocephalus Kahnschädel *m*

scaphocephaly Kahnschädeligkeit *f*

scapula Schulterblatt *n*, Skapula *f*

scatological, scatologic Kot–, obszön, pornographisch

scatology Untersuchung *f* von Exkrementen, Kotforschung *f*

scatophagous kotessend, koprophag

scatophagy Kotessen *n*, Koprophagie *f*

scatter Streuung *f* / streuen / **~ analysis** Streuungsanalyse *f* / **~ diagram** Streudiagramm *n* / **~ phenomenon** Dispersionsphänomen *n*

scattered zerstreut liegend, verstreut, zerfahren

scattergram Streudiagramm *n*

scattering Streuung *f*, Dispersion *f*

scatterplot Streudiagramm *n*

scedastic skedastisch, die Streuung der Variablen in einer bivariaten Verteilung betreffend

scedasticity Skedastizität *f*, Streuung *f* der Variablen in einer bivariaten Matrix

scene Szene *f* / **~ of seduction** Verführungsszene *f* / **primal ~** Urszene *f* / **traumatic ~** traumatische Erfahrung *f*

scent Duft *m*, Geruch *m*

scentless geruchlos

sceptic Skeptiker *m*, Zweifler *m*

sceptical skeptisch, misstrauisch

scepticism Skeptizismus *m*

Schaffer's collaterals Schaffer–Kollateralen *fpl*

schedule Plan *m*, Schema *n*, Folge *f* / **~ of reinforcement** Verstärkungsplan *m* / **chained ~ of reinforcement** Kettenverstärkung *f* / **concurrent ~ of reinforcement** Parallelverstärkungsplan *m* / Verstärkungsplan *m* / **alternative ~** Vorzugsfolge *f*, Alternativplan *m* / **chained ~** Kettenfolge *f*, Verkettungsplan *m* / **concurrent ~** Simultanfolge *f* / **conjunctive ~** Doppelfolge *f*, Konjunktivplan *m* / **developmental ~** Entwicklungsstufen *fpl* / **fixed–interval ~** gleiche Zeitspannenfolge *f* / **fixed–ratio ~** gleiche Verhältnisfolge *f* / **interlocked ~** Verschachtelungsplan *m* / **intermittent ~** gelegentliche Folge *f*, gelegentliche Verstärkung *f* / **interpolated ~** Einsatzfolge *f* / **mixed ~** Mischfolge *f* / **multiple ~** Mischfolge *f* mit Kontrollreiz

schema Schema *n*, Ordnungsmuster *n*, Diagramm *n* / **cognitive ~** kognitives Schema *n* / **perceptual ~** Wahrnehmungsschema *n*, Wahrnehmungssystem *n* / **sensorimotor ~** sensumotorisches Schema *n*

schematic schematisch

schematism, schematisation Schematisierung *f*, Schematismus *m*

schematize schematisch darstellen, bildlich darstellen

scheme Plan *m*, Projekt *n*, Schema *n*, Programm *n* / entwerfen, planen / **~ of colour** Farbzusammenstellung *f*

schemograph Gerät *n* zur Bestimmung der Gesichtsfeldgrenzen

schism Schisma *n*, Spaltung *f*, Trennung *f*

schismatic schismatisch, abtrünnig

schismogenesis Entstehung *f* von Abspaltungen

schizoaffective schizoaffektiv

schizobulia Willensspaltung *f*, Schizobulie *f*

schizogonic, schizogenic, schizogenous sich durch Spaltung vermehrend

schizogony, schizogenesis Vermehrung *f* durch Spaltung, Schizogonie *f*

schizoid schizoid / Schizoider *m*

schizoidia, schizoidism Schizoidie *f*, Persönlichkeitsspaltung *f* leichteren Grades, Schizoidismus *m*

schizophasia, schizophrasia Schizophasie *f*, unverständliche Sprache *f*

schizophrenia Schizophrenie *f*, Spaltungsirresein *n* / **~–like** schizophreniform / **~, unspecified** nicht näher bezeichnete Schizophrenie *f* / **acute ~** akute Schizophrenie *f* / **ambulatory ~** ambulatorische Schizophrenie *f* / **autistic ~** autistische Schizophrenie *f* / **catatonic ~** katatone Schizophrenie *f*, Katatonie *f*, kataton–schizophrenes Syndrom *n* / **cenesthetic ~** zönästhetische Schizophrenie *f* / **constitutional ~** konstitutionelle Schizophrenie *f* / **hebephrenic ~** hebephrene Schizophrenie *f*, Hebephrenie *f*, Jugendirresein *n* / **latent ~** Borderline–Schizophrenie *f* / **mixed ~** gemischte Schizophrenie *f* / **other ~** sonstige Schizophrenie *f* / **paranoid ~** paranoide Schizophrenie *f*, Paranoia *f* / **periodic ~** periodische Schizophrenie *f* / **prepsychotic ~** Borderline–Schizophrenie *f* / **pseudoneurotic ~** pseudoneurotische Schizophrenie *f* / **pseudopsychopathic ~** pseudopsychopathische Schizophrenie *f* / **psychoneurotic ~** psychoneurotische Schizophrenie *f* / **reactive ~** reaktive Schizophrenie *f*, Reaktionspsychose *f* / **residual ~** schizophrenes Residuum *n* / **simple ~** einfache Schizophrenie *f*, Schizophrenia simplex *f* / **undifferentiated ~** undifferenzierte Schizophrenie *f*

schizophreniac, schizophrene Schizophrener *m*, an Schizophrenie Leidender *m*

schizophrenic schizophren, Schizophrenie– / Schizophrene *m,f*

schizophreniform schizophreniform

schizophrenogenic schizophrenieerzeugend, schizophrenogen

schizophrenosis schizophrene Erkrankung *f*

schizothyme Schizothymer *m*, schizothymer Typus *m*

schizothymia Schizothymie *f*

schizothymic, schizothymous schizothym

schizotypal schizotyp

scholaptitude Schuleignung *f*, schulische Begabung *f*

scholar Schüler *m*, Stipendiat *m*, Gelehrter *m*

scholarship Gelehrsamkeit *f*, Stipendium *n*

scholastic schulisch, scholastisch

Scholasticism Scholastik *f*

school Schule *f* / ~ **achievement** Schulleistung *f* / ~ **adjustment** schulische Anpassung *f* / ~ **age** Schulalter *n* / ~ **age child** Schulkind *n*, Kind *n* im Schulalter, schulpflichtiges Kind *n* / ~ **attendance** Schulbesuch *m* / ~ **backwardness** Rückstand *m* in der Schule / ~**–boy** Schüler *m* / ~ **counseling** Schulberatung *f* / ~ **counselor** Schuljugendberater *m* / ~ **difficulty** Schulschwierigkeit *f*, Schulproblem *n* / ~ **dropout** Schulversager *m*, Schulabbrecher *m* / ~ **enrollment** Einschulung *f*, Schulanmeldung *f* / ~ **environment** Schulmilieu *n*, Umfeld *n* der Schule / ~ **expulsion** Entfernung *f* von der Schule, Verweisung *f* / ~ **facilities** schulische Einrichtungen *fpl* / ~ **failure** Schulversagen *n* / ~ **federal aid** Ausbildungsförderung *f* / ~ **financial assistance** finanzielle Ausbildungsförderung *f* / ~ **graduation** Schulabschluss *m* / ~ **inadaptation** mangelnde Anpassung *f* in der Schule / ~ **integration** schulische Integration *f* / ~ **learning** schulisches Lernen *n* / ~ **leaver** Schulabgänger *m* / ~**–leaving age** Schulentlassungsalter *n* / ~ **library** Schulbücherei *f* / ~ **motivation analysis** Analyse *f* der Schulmotivation / ~ **neurosis** Schulneurose *f* / ~ **phobia** Schulangst *f* / ~ **principal** Schulleiter *m*, Direktor *m* der Schule / ~ **psychologist** Schulpsychologe *m* / ~ **psychology** Schulpsychologie *f* / ~ **readiness** Schulreife *f* / ~ **refusal** Schulverweigerung *f* / ~ **retention** Schulverbleib *m* / ~ **selection** Schulauswahl *f* / **elementary** ~ **student** Grundschüler *m* / ~ **superintendent** Schulrat *m* / ~ **suspension** Schulverweis *f* auf Zeit / **elementary** ~ **teacher** Grundschullehrer *m* / ~**–to–work transition** Übergang *m* Schule–Beruf / ~ **transition** Schul- bzw. Klassenübergang *m* / ~ **truancy** Schulschwänzen *n* / **Austrian** ~ Österreichische Schule *f*, Grazer Schule *f* / **elementary** ~ Grundschule *f* / **Freudian** ~ Freud'sche Schule *f* / **Freudian psychoanalytic** ~ Freud'sche psychoanalytische Schule *f* / **grammar** ~ Hauptschule *f* [in USA], höhere Schule *f* [in Großbritannien] / **high** ~ höhere Schule *f*, Schule *f* der Sekundarstufe / **high** ~ **graduate** Abiturient *m* / **high** ~ **student** Schüler *m* der Sekundarstufe / **institutional** ~ Anstaltsschule *f* / **intermediate** ~ Mittelschule *f* / **junior high** ~ Mittelstufe *f* des Gymnasiums / **neo–Freudian** ~ Neopsychoanalytische Schule *f* / **neopsychoanalytic** ~ Neopsychoanalytische Schule *f* / **non-graded** ~ klassenlose Schule *f*, Schule *f* ohne Klassenaufteilung, Schule *f* ohne Altersklassen / **primary** ~ Grundschule *f*, Volksschule *f* / **primary** ~ **student** Grundschüler *m*, Volksschüler *m* / **private** ~ **education** Privatschulausbildung *f* / **psychoanalytic** ~ psychoanalytische Schule *f* / **public** ~ staatliche Schule *f* [*in USA*], Privatschule *f* [*in Großbritannien*] / **rural** ~ Landschule *f* / **special** ~ Sonderschule *f*, Hilfsschule *f* / **technical** ~ Gewerbeschule *f*, gewerbliche Berufsschule *f*, technische Schule *f* / **vocational** ~ Berufsschule *f* / **vocational** ~ **student** Berufsschüler *m*

schooling Unterricht *m*, Schulerziehung *f*, Schulbesuch *m*

Schultz's disease Agranulozytose *f*

Schwann| cell Schwann–Zelle *f* / ~**'s membrane** Schwann–Scheide *f*, Neurilemm *n* / ~**'s sheath** Schwann–Scheide *f*, Neurilemm *n* / ~**'s white substance** Schwann'sche weiße Substanz *f*

sciascope Skiaskop *n*

sciatalgia Ischiasschmerz *m*

sciatica Ischias *n,m*

science Wissenschaft *f*, Naturwissenschaft *f*, Wissen *n* / **~ achievement** naturwissenschaftliche Leistung *f* / **~ education** naturwissenschaftlicher Unterricht *m*, naturwissenschaftliche Ausbildung *f* / **~ of human behaviour** Wissenschaft *f* vom menschlichen Verhalten / **~ of mind** Geisteswissenschaft *f* / **basic ~** Grundwissenschaft *f* / **behavioural ~s** Verhaltenswissenschaften *fpl* / **cultural ~** Geisteswissenschaft *f*, Kulturwissenschaft *f* / **educational ~** Erziehungswissenschaft *f*, Pädagogik *f* / **empirical ~** Erfahrungswissenschaft *f*, empirische Wissenschaft *f* / **medical ~** Medizin *f* / **mental ~** Geisteswissenschaft *f* / **moral ~** Sittenlehre *f*, Ethik *f* / **natural ~** Naturwissenschaft *f* / **nomothetic ~** nomothetische Wissenschaft *f* / **normative ~** normative Wissenschaft *f* / **paramedical ~** medizinische Hilfswissenschaft *f* / **political ~** politische Wissenschaft *f*, Politologie *f* / **social ~** Sozialwissenschaft *f* / **social ~ psychology** geisteswissenschaftliche Psychologie *f*

scientific wissenschaftlich, systematisch

scientist Wissenschaftler *m*, Naturwissenschaftler *m*

scintillate funkeln, flimmern

scintillation Funkensehen *n*, Skotom *n*

sciosophist Pseudowissenschaftler *m*

sciosophy Pseudowissenschaft *f*

sclera Sklera *f*, Lederhaut *f* des Auges / **~ layer** Skleraschicht *f*

scleroderma, sclerodermia Sklerodermie *f*

sclerosis Sklerose *f* / **arterial ~** Arteriosklerose *f* / **cerebral ~** Hirnsklerose *f*, Zerebralsklerose *f* / **cerebrospinal ~** multiple Sklerose *f* / **coronary ~** Koronarsklerose *f* / **disseminated ~** multiple Sklerose *f* / **focal ~** Herdsklerose *f* / **insular ~** multiple Sklerose *f*, Polysklerose *f* / **multiple ~** multiple Sklerose *f*

sclerotic sklerotisch

scoliosis Skoliose *f*, seitliche Rückgratverkrümmung *f*

scope Bereich *m*, Rahmen *m*

scopic Sicht–, Ables–

scopolamine Skopolamin *n*, Hyoszin *n* / **~ hydrobromide** Skopolamin *n*, Hyoszin *n*

scopophilia Schautrieb *m*, Voyeurtum *n*, Skopophilie *f*

scopophiliac Voyeur *m*

scopophobia Skopophobie *f*, zwanghafte Angst *f* dem Anblick Anderer ausgesetzt zu sein

scorching brenzlig

score Punktwert *m*, Punktzahl *f*, Messwert *m*, Punkt *m* / Punkte erreichen, nach Punkten auswerten / **~ equation** Testwertangleichung *f* / **~ of scatter** Streuwert *m* / **additonal ~** Zusatzwert *m* / **composite ~** Gesamtwert *m* / **critical ~** kritischer Wert *m* / **crude ~** Rohwert *m*, Annäherungswert *m* / **cut–off ~** Cut–Off–Wert *m*, Schwellenwert *m* / **cutting ~** kritischer Wert *m*, Grenzwert *m*, Trennpunkt *m* / **derived ~** abgeleiteter Messwert *m* / **global ~** Gesamtwert *m* / **graphic ~** graphisch dargestellter Messwert *m* / **gross ~** Rohwert *m* / **interactive ~** Interaktionswert *m* / **normalized ~** normalisierter Punktwert *m* / **objective ~** objektiver Punktwert *m* / **obtained ~** Rohwert *m*, erzielter Punktwert *m* / **operant ~** Ergebnis *n*, Aktionswert *m* / **original ~** Rohwert *m* / **percentile ~** Prozentwert *m* / **raw ~** Rohwert *m* / **reduced ~** reduzierter Punktwert *m* / **representative ~** repräsentativer Wert *m* / **rough ~** Rohwert *m* / **sigma ~** Standardmesswert *m* / **sociometric ~** soziometrischer Wert *m* / **standard ~** Standardwert *m* / **standard gross ~** Standardrohwert *m* / **total ~** Gesamtwert *m*, Summe *f* / **total weighted ~** gewichteter Gesamtwert *m* / **transmuted ~** transponierter Punktwert *m*, umgewandelter Punktwert *m* / **true ~** wahre Punktzahl *f*, wahrer Wert *m* / **ungrouped ~s** ungruppierte Punktwerte *mpl* / **weighted ~** gewogener Punktwert *m*, gewichtetes Maß *n* / **z ~** Standardmesswert *m*, z–Wert *m*

scorer „Punktemacher" *m* / **top ~** Proband *m* mit Spitzenpunktwerten

scoring Bewertung *f*, Auswertung *f*, Punktebewertung *f*, Testwertvergabe *f* / **~ sheet** Auswertungsbogen *m*, Auswertungsformular *n*, Auswertungstabelle *f* / **automated ~** maschinelle Testauswertung *f* / **differential ~** Mehrfachauswertung *f*, differenzielle Testauswertung *f* / **multiple ~** Mehrfachauswertung *f* / **objective ~** objektive Auswertung *f* / **subjective ~** subjektive Auswertung *f*

scoterythrous rotblind, protanop

scotoma Gesichtsfeldausfall *m*, Skotom *n* / **central ~** Zentralskotom *n* / **scintillating ~** Flimmerskotom *n*

scotometer Skotometer *n*

scotometry Skotometrie *f*, Gesichtsfeldausfallmessung *f*

scotomisation Skotomisation *f*, Realitätsleugnung *f*

scotomize die Realität verleugnen, verleugnen

scotophilia Drang *m* zur Dunkelheit, Skotophilie *f*

scotophobia Angst *f* vor Dunkelheit, Skotophobie *f*, Dunkelangst *f*, Nyktophobie *f*

scotophobic, scotophobical skotophobisch, Angst vor der Dunkelheit betreffend

scotopia Dämmerungssehen *n*

scotopic skotopisch, Dunkelsehen betreffend

scotoscopy Skiaskopie *f*, Schattenprobe *f*

scratch reflex Kratzreflex *m*

scratching Kratzen *n*

scream Schrei *m* / **primal ~** Urschrei *m* / **primal ~ therapy** Urschreitherapie *f*

screen Schirm *m*, Bildschirm *m*, Scheibe *f*, Abschirmung *f* / untersuchen, überprüfen / **~ memory** Deckerinnerung *f* / **~ resolution** Bildschirmauflösung *f* / **~ test** Selektionstest *m*, Siebtest *m* / **one–way ~** einseitig durchsichtige Scheibe *f*, Einweg–Scheibe *f*

screening grobe Auslese *f*, Vorauswahl *f*, Screening *n* / **~ efficiency** Effizienz *f* der Vorauswahl / **~ test** Siebtest *m*, Screening–Test *m* / **psychological ~ inventory** psychologisches Vorauswahlverfahren *n*

scribble Gekritzel *n*, Kritzelei *f*

scribomania Kritzelsucht *f*, Schreibsucht *f*

script Manuskript *n*, Originaltext *m*

scriveners' palsy Schreibkrampf *m*

scruple Skrupel *m*, Bedenken *n* / Bedenken haben, zweifeln

scrupulosity, scrupulousness peinliche Genauigkeit *f*, Überängstlichkeit *f*, Gewissenhaftigkeit *f*, Bedenken *n*

scrupulous überbedenklich, ängstlich, übergenau

scrutinize genau prüfen, untersuchen

scrutiny Überprüfung *f*, Untersuchung *f*

scrying Kristallvision *f*

sculpturing Bildhauerei *f*, Schnitzen *n*, Plastizieren *n*, Formen *n*

S–curve S–Kurve *f*

séance spiritistische Sitzung *f*, Séance *f*

search Suche *f*, Forschen *n*, Streben *n* / **~ for glory** Ruhmsucht *f*, Geltungssucht *f* / **~ model** Forschungsvorhaben *n*, Forschungshypothese *f* / **visual ~** visueller Suchprozess *m*

seasickness Seekrankheit *f*

seat Sitz *m* / **~ of consciousness** Sitz *m* des Bewusstseins / **~ of mind** Sitz *m* der Seele

sebaccous Talg–

sebastomania religiöser Wahnsinn *m*

seclude sich absondern, abgesondert leben, abschließen

seclusion Absonderung *f*, Zurückgezogenheit *f*, Isolation *f* / **~ need** Bedürfnis *n* nach Privatsphäre

seclusive verschlossen, abgesondert

seclusiveness Isolation *f*, Absonderung *f*

secobarbital Secobarbital *n*

second zweite (r, s), nächste (r, s) / Zweiter *m*, Nächster *m*, Sekunde *f* / beistehen, unterstützen, helfen

secondary sekundär, untergeordnet, Neben–, Folge–, erworben

secrecy Verschwiegenheit *f*, Schweigepflicht *f*, Amtsverschwiegenheit *f*, Geheimhaltung *f*

secreta Ausscheidungen *fpl*

secrete absondern, ausscheiden

secretin Sekretin *n*

secretion Sekretion *f*, Absonderung *f*, Sekret *n* / **~ of saliva** Speichelsekretion *f* / **~ of sweat** Schweißabsonderung *f* / **internal ~** innere Sekretion *f* / **internal–~ gland** Drüse *f* mit innererer Sekretion, endokrine Drüse *f* / **pancreatic ~** Pankreassekretion *f* / **psychic ~** psychisch bedingte Sekretion *f* / **salivary ~** Speichelsekretion *f*

secretive verschlossen, verschwiegen

secretiveness Verschwiegenheit *f*

secretory Sekret–, sekretorisch

sect Sekte *f*

sectarian sektiererisch / Sektenanhänger *m*, Sektierer *m*

section Schnitt *m* / **cross–~** Querschnitt *m* / **golden ~** goldener Schnitt *m* / **longitudinal ~** Längsschnitt *m* / **transverse ~** Querschnitt *m*

sectioning Aufteilung *f*, Eingruppierung *f*

sector Sektor *m*, Abschnitt *m* / **~s of research** Forschungsgebiete *npl* / **positional ~** Positionssegment *n*, Positionssektor *m* / **private ~** privater Sektor *m* / **public ~** öffentlicher Sektor *m*

secular jahrhundertlang, jahrhundertalt, säkular, weltlich

securing Schutz–, Sicherheits–

security Sicherheit *f*, Schutz *m* / **maximum ~ facilities** Sicherungsverwahrung *f* / **~ measure** Sicherheitsmaßnahme *f* / **~ motive** Sicherheitsmotiv *n* / **emotional ~** emotionale Sicherheit *f* / **social ~** Sozialversicherung *f*, Rentenversicherung *f*, soziale Sicherung *f* / **social ~ benefit** Sozialleistung *f*

sedation Beruhigung *f*, Sedierung *f* / **~ threshold** Sedierungsschwelle *f*

sedative beruhigend, sedierend / Beruhigungsmittel *n*, Sedativum *n* / **nervous ~** Nervenmittel *n*, Sedativum *n*

seduce verführen

seducer Verführer *m*

seduction Verführung *f*

seductive verführerisch

sedulous fleißig, emsig

sedulousness Fleiß *m*

see sehen, beobachten, wahrnehmen, verstehen

seed Samen *m*

seeing Sehen *n*, Sehvermögen *n*

segment Segment *n*, Abschnitt *m* / **~ illusion** Segmenttäuschung *f* / **cranial ~** Schädelsegment *n* / **distal ~** distales Segment *n* / **neural ~** Medullarsegment *n*, Neuromer *n* / **primitive ~** Ursegment *n*, Metamer *n* / **spinal ~** Rückenmarkssegment *n* / **vertebral ~** Wirbelabschnitt *m*

segmental segmentär, Segment–

segregation Trennung *f*, Segregation *f*, Bevölkerungstrennung *f*, Aufspaltung *f* von Genpaaren / **~ law** Vererbungsgesetz *n* / **perceptual ~** Trennung *f* von Wahrnehmungsfeldern

seismaesthesia, seismesthesia Vibrationsempfindung *f*

seizure Anfall *m*, Attacke *f*, Ictus *m* / **~ discharge** Anfallsentladung / **apoplectic ~** Schlaganfall *m*, Apoplexie *f* / **audiogenic ~** audiogener Anfall *m*, audiogener Krampfanfall *m* / **convulsive ~** Krampfanfall *m* / **epileptic ~** epileptischer Anfall *m* / **epileptiform ~** epilepsieähnlicher Anfall *m* / **focal ~s** Herdanfall *m* / **generalized tonic–clonic ~s** Grand–mal–Status *m* / **hysteriform ~** hysterieähnlicher Anfall *m* / **jackknife ~** Blitzkrampf *m*,

Petit mal propulsif *n* / **pychomotor ~** psychomotorischer Anfall *m* / **retropulsive ~** Retropulsiv–Petit–mal *n*

sejunction Sejunktion *f*, Auflösung *f* von Assoziationen

select auswählen

selected ausgewählt

selection Auswahl *f*, Auslese *f*, Selektion *f* / **~ and placement** Personalauslese *f* und Personaleinsatz *m* / **~ characteristics** Auswahlkriterien *npl*, Selektionsmerkmale *npl* / **~ device** Ausleseinstrument *n* / **~ index** Selektionsindex *m* / **~ method** Ausleseverfahren *n* / **~ process** Auswahlverfahren *n*, Auswahlprozess *m* / **~ ratio** Ausleseverhältnis *n* / **~ test** Auslesetest *m*, Auswahlantworttest *m* / **artificial ~** künstliche Zuchtwahl *f* / **educational ~** schulische Auslese *f* / **functional ~** funktionelle Auslese *f*, natürliche Auslese *f* / **individual ~** Einzelauswahl *f* / **natural ~** natürliche Auslese *f*, natürliche Selektion *f*, biologische Auslese *f*, natürliche Zuchtwahl *f* / **occupational ~** Eignungsauslese *f*, Berufsauslese *f* / **proportional ~** Auswahl *f* in entsprechendem Verhältnis / **random ~** Zufallsauswahl *f* / **reproductive ~** genetische Auslese *f* / **social ~** Partnerwahl *f*, soziale Auslese *f* / **vocational ~** Eignungsauslese *f*, Berufsauslese *f*

selective auswählend

selectivity Trennschärfe *f*, Selektivität *f*

selenoplegia, selenogamia Mondsüchtigkeit *f*, Somnambulismus *m*, Schlafwandeln *n*

self Selbst *n* / **~–abasement** Selbsterniedrigung *f* / **~–abnegation** Selbstverleugnung *f* / **~–absorbed** in sich versunken, in sich gekehrt / **~–absorption** Selbstversunkenheit *f* / **~–abuse** Onanie *f*, Masturbation *f* / **~–acceptance** Selbstbejahung *f* / **~–accusation** Selbstbeschuldigung *f* / **~–activity** Eigenaktivität *f* / **~–actualisation** Selbstverwirklichung *f*, Selbstrealisierung *f*, Selbstaktualisierung *f* / **~–actualisation need** Bedürfnis *n* der Selbstverwirklichung / **~–adjustive** selbstdirektiv / **~–administering** selbst durchzuführend / **~–admiration** Selbstbewunderung *f*, Einbildung *f* / **~–aggrandizement** Selbsterhöhung *f*, Selbstverherrlichung *f* / **~–alienation** Selbstentfremdung *f* / **~–analysis** Selbstanalyse *f* / **~–apparent** offensichtlich, augenscheinlich / **~–appraisal** Selbstbeurteilung *f*, Selbsteinschätzung *f* / **~–approval** Selbstgefälligkeit *f* / **~–assertion** Selbstbehauptung *f* / **~–assertive** rechthaberisch, autoritär / **~–assertiveness** Selbstbehauptung *f* / **~–assessment** Selbsteinschätzung *f*, Selbstbeurteilung *f* / **~–assumed** selbsteingenommen, eingebildet / **~–assumption** Einbildung *f*, Eigendünkel *m* / **~–assurance** Selbstvertrauen *n* / **~–assured** selbstsicher, selbstbewusst / **~–attitude** Selbstbewertung *f* / **~–awareness** Selbstbewusstsein *n*, Ich–Bewusstsein *n*, Selbstverständnis *n* / **~–care skill** Selbsthilfefertigkeit *f*, Selbsthilfevermögen *n* / **~–centred** ichbezogen, egozentrisch / **~–centredness** Ich–Bezogenheit *f*, Egozentrismus *m*, Selbstsucht *f* / **~–coloured** einfarbig, naturfarben / **~–command** Selbstbeherrschung *f*, Selbstkontrolle *f* / **~–complacency** Selbstgefälligkeit *f* / **~–complacent** selbstgefällig / **~–comprehension** Selbstverständnis *n*, Selbstbewusstsein *n* / **~–conceit** Eigendünkel *m*, Einbildung *f* / **~–conceited** eingebildet / **~–concept** Selbstbild *n*, Selbstkonzept *n* / **academic ~–concept** Selbstkonzept *n* der schulischen Begabung / **~–confidence** Selbstvertrauen *n*, Selbstsicherheit *f* / **~–confident** selbstbewusst, selbstsicher / **~–confinement** Selbstbefangenheit *f* / **audiovisual ~–confrontation** audiovisuelle Selbstkonfrontation *f* / **~–congruence** Selbstkonguenz *f*, Übereinstimmung *f* mit sich selbst / **~–conscious** befangen, verlegen, bewusst / **~–consciousness** Befangenheit *f*, Verlegenheit *f*, Selbstbewusstsein *n* / **~–consideration** Nachdenken *n* über sich selbst / **~–consistency** Beständigkeit *f*, Selbstkonsistenz *f* / **~–contained** in sich abgeschlossen, unabhängig / **~–containment** Unabhängigkeit *f* / **~–contempt** Selbstverachtung *f* / **~–contradictory** sich selbst widersprechend / **~–control** Selbstbeherrschung *f*, Selbstkontrolle *f* / **~–controlled** selbstbeherrscht / **~–correlation** Autokorrelation *f* / **~–criticism** Selbstkritik *f* / **~–cure** Selbstheilung *f* / **~–defeating behaviour** selbstblockierendes Verhalten *n* / **~–defeating prophecy** Vorhersage *f* die durch unterlassenes Handeln nicht erfüllt wird / **~–deceit** Selbsttäuschung *f*, Selbstbetrug *m* / **~–deception** Selbstbetrug *m*, Selbsttäuschung *f* / **~–defence** Selbstverteidigung *f* / **~–defense** Selbstverteidigung *f* / **~–delusion** Selbsttäuschung *f* / **~–demand schedule** Fütterung *f* entsprechend dem Bedürfnis des Säuglings / **~–denial** Selbstverleugnung *f* / **~–dependence** Selbständigkeit *f*, Unabhängigkeit *f* / **~–depreciation** Selbstherabsetzung *f* / **~–destruction** Selbstzerstörung *f*, Selbstmord *m* / **~–destructive behaviour** selbstzerstörerisches Verhalten *n* / **~–detachment** Selbstdistanzierung *f* / **~–determination** Selbstbestimmung *f* / **~–determined** selbstbestimmt / **~–development** persönliche Entwicklung *f*, eigene Weiterbildung *f*, Selbstverwirklichung *f* / **~–direction** Selbstbestimmung *f* / **~–directional** selbstbestimmt / **~–discipline** Selbstdisziplin *f*, Selbstkontrolle *f* / **~–disclosure** Selbsteinbringung *f* / **~–disparagement** Selbsterniedrigung *f* / **~–display** Angeberei *f*, Prahlerei *f* / **~–distribution** Selbstgliederung *f* / **~–distrust** mangelndes Selbstvertrauen *n*, Schüchternheit *f* / **~–dynamism** Selbstdynamik *f* / **~–educated** autodidaktisch / **~–effacement** bescheidene Zurückhaltung *f* / **~–effacing** bescheiden, zurückhaltend / **~–efficacy** Selbstwirkung *f* / **~–employed** selbstandig erwerbstätig / **~–employment** Selbständigkeit *f* / **~–esteem** Selbstachtung *f*, Selbstwertgefühl *n* / **~–evaluation** Selbsteinschätzung *f*, Selbstbewertung *f* / **~–evident** selbstverständlich / **~–exaltation** Großtuerei *f*, Prahlerei *f* / **~–examination** Gewissensprüfung *f*, Selbstuntersuchung *f* / **medical ~–examination** medizinische Selbstuntersuchung *f* / **~–excitation** Selbsterregung *f* / **~–exhibition** Angeberei *f*, Prahlerei *f* / **~–explanatory** keiner Erklärung bedürfend / **~–expression** Ausdruck *m* der eigenen Persönlichkeit / **~–extinction** neurotische Selbstentfremdung *f* / **~–feeding** automatische Fütterung *f* / **~–feeling** Selbstgefühl *n* / **~–fertilisation** Selbstbefruchtung *f* / **~–forgetfulness** Selbstvergessenheit *f*, Selbstlosigkeit *f* / **~–fulfilling prophecy** selbsterfüllende Prophezeiung *f* / **~–fulfillment** Selbsterfüllung *f*, Selbstverwirklichung *f* / **~–glorification** Selbstverherrlichung *f* / **~–government** Autonomie *f*, Selbstverwaltung *f* / **~–gratification** Befriedigung *f* der Selbstwertgefühle / **~–handicapping strategy** Selbstbehinderungsstrategie *f* / **~–hatred** Selbsthass *m* / **~–help** Selbsthilfe *f*, eigene Anstrengung *f* / **~–help group** Selbsthilfegruppe *f* / **~–help technique** Selbsthilfetechnik *f* / **~–humiliation** Selbsterniedrigung *f* / **~–hypnosis** Selbsthypnose *f*, Autohypnose *f* / **~–ideal** Selbstideal *n* / **~–identification** Identifikation *f* des Selbst / **~–image** Selbstbild *n* / **~–immolation** Selbstaufopferung *f* / **~–importance** Selbstüberhebung *f*, Wichtigtuerei *f* / **~–important** überheblich, wichtigtuerisch / **~–improvement** selbständige Weiterbildung *f* / **~–induction** Eigenerregung *f* / **~–indulgence** Genusssucht *f*, rücksichtslose Befriedigung *f* eigener Bedürfnisse / **~–inflicted** selbstzugefügt / **~–inflicted wound** Selbstverletzung *f* / **~–injury** Selbstverstümmelung *f* / **~–instructional training** Selbstinstruktionstraining *n* / **~–interest** Eigeninteresse *n* / **~–inventory** Selbsterkennungsfragebogen *m* / **~–involved** persönlich beteiligt / **~–justification** Selbstrechtfertigung *f* / **~–knowledge** Selbsterkenntnis / **~–love** Eigenliebe *f* / **~–made** aus eigener Kraft emporgekommen / **~–maintenance** Selbstbehauptung *f* / **~–management** Selbstkontrolltechniken *fpl*, Selbst–Management *n* / **~–marking** selbstauswertend / **~–mastery** Selbstbeherrschung *f*, Selbstkontrolle *f* / **~–maximation** Selbsterhöhung *f* / **~–medication** Selbstmedikation *f* / **~–monitoring** Selbstüberwachung *f*, Selbstbeobachtung *f* / **~–motion** Selbstbewegung *f* / **~–murder** Selbstmord *m* / **~–mutilation** Selbstverstümmelung *f* / **~–observation** Selbstbeobachtung *f*, Introspektion *f* / **~–opinion** Dünkel *m*, Einbildung *f* / **~–opinionated** eigensinnig, dickköpfig / **~–orientation** Selbstfindung *f*, Selbsterfahrung *f* / **~–oriented** persönlich, ich–zentriert / **~–other system** Selbstauffassung *f* und das Bild *n* vom Anderen / **~–pacing** Selbstbestimmen *n* des Lerntempos / **~–percept** wahrgenommenes Selbst *n*, Selbstbild *n* / **~–perception** Selbstwahrnehmung *f* / **~–pity** Selbstmitleid *n* / **~–pollution** Onanie *f*, Masturbation *f*, Selbstbefleckung *f* / **~–possessed** selbstbeherrscht / **~–possession** Selbstbeherrschung *f* / **~–preservation** Selbsterhaltung *f* / **~–psychology** Ich–Psychologie *f*, Selbst–Psychologie *f* / **~–punishment** Selbstbestrafung *f* / **~–punishment mechanism** Selbstbestrafungsmechanismus *m* / **~–rating** Selbstbeurteilung *f*, Selbstbewertung *f* / **~–realisation** Selbstverwirklichung *f*, Selbstrealisierung *f*, Selbstaktualisierung / **~–recitation** Aufsagen *n*, wiederholtes Vorsagen *n* / **~–reference** Selbstbezug *m* / **~–referral** Eigeninitiative *f* zur Behandlung / **~–regard** Selbstgefühl *n* / **~–regulating** selbststeuernd / **~–regulation** Selbststeuerung *f*, Selbstregelung *f* / **~–reinforcement** Selbstverstärkung *f* / **~–rejection** Selbstablehnung *f* / **~–reliance** Selbstvertrauen *n* / **~–reliant** selbstvertrauend / **~–renunciation** Selbstverleugnung *f* / **~–report** Selbstbericht *m* / **~–report inventory** Selbsterkennungsfragebogen *m* / **~–repression** Verdrängung *f* eigener Triebe / **~–reproach** Selbstbeschuldigung *f*, Selbstvorwurf *m* / **~–respect** Selbstachtung *f* / **~–restraint** Selbstbeschränkung *f*, Selbstbeherrschung *f* / **~–revelation** Selbstenthüllung *f* / **~–reward** Selbstbelohnung *f* / **~–righteous** selbstgerecht / **~–righteousness** Selbstgerechtigkeit *f* / **~–sacrifice** Selbstaufopferung *f* / **~–salience** strukturelles Hervortreten *m* des Selbst / **~–same** selbstidentisch / **~–satisfaction** Selbstzufriedenheit *f* / **~–satisfied** selbstzufrieden / **~–scoring** Selbstauswertung *f*, automatisch auswertend / **~–searching** Selbstprüfung *f* / **~–seeking** selbstsüchtig, egoistisch / **~–selection** Selbstbedienung *f* / **~–sentiment** Selbstgefühl *n*, Selbstwertgefühl *n* / **~–starter** Person *f* mit Initiative / **~–stimulation** Autostimulation *f*, Selbstreizung *f* / **~–study** Selbstbeobachtung *f*, Introspektion *f* / **~–submission** Selbstunterwerfung *f* / **~–sufficiency** Selbstgenügsamkeit *f*, Autarkie *f* / **~–sufficient** selbstgenügsam / **~–suggestion** Selbstsuggestion *f*, Autosuggestion *f* / **~–supporting** Selbstversorger– / **~–sure** selbstsicher / **~–sureness** Selbstsicherheit *f* / **~–surrender** Selbstaufgabe *f* / **~–system** Selbstsystem *n*, Selbstwertsystem *n* / **~–talk** Selbstgespräch *n* / **~–taught** autodidaktisch / **~ theory** Selbsttheorie *f* / **~–tranquilisation** Selbstruhigstellung *f* / **~–treatment** Selbstbehandlung *f* / **~–trust** Selbstvertrauen *n* / **~–will** Sturheit *f*, Eigensinn *m* / **~–willed** eigenwillig, eigensinnig / **~–worth** Selbstwert *m* / **actual ~** aktuelles Selbst *n* / **central ~** zentrales Selbst *n* / **conscious ~** bewusstes Selbst *n* / **divided ~** gespaltenes Selbst *n* / **ethical ~** ethisches Selbst *n* / **glorified ~** idealisiertes Selbst *n* / **ideal ~** ideales Selbst *n* / **idealised ~** idealisiertes Selbst *n* / **looking–glass ~** Spiegelselbst *n* / **narcistic ~** narzisstisches Selbst *n* / **narcistic ~–sentiment** narzisstisches Selbstgefühl *n* / **negative ~–feeling** negatives Selbstgefühl *n*, Minderwertigkeitsgefühl *n* / **other ~** anderes Ich *n*, „alter ego" *n* / **perceived ~** wahrgenommenes Selbst *n* / **phenomenal ~** phänomenales Selbst *n*, wahrgenommenes Selbst *n* / **positive ~–feeling** positives Selbstgefühl *n* / **primitive ~** primitives Selbst *n* / **real ~** reales

Selbst *n* / **social ~** soziales Selbst *n* / **subliminal ~** unterschwelliges Selbst *n* / **tribal ~** Stammesselbst *n*

selfhood personales Selbst *n*, eigentliches Selbst *n*, Proprium *n*

selfish eigennützig, selbstsüchtig, egoistisch

selfishness Selbstsucht *f*, Egoismus *m*

sella turcica Türkensattel *m*, Sella turcica *f*

semantic semantisch

semantics Semantik *f*, Wortbedeutungslehre *f*, Semiologie *f* / **applied ~** angewandte Semantik *f*, Semantik *f* / **general ~** allgemeine Semantik *f* / **generative ~** generative Semantik *f*

semantisation Semantisierung *f*, Ritualisierung *f*

semantogenic durch Bedeutungsfehlinterpretation verursacht

semasiology historische Semantik *f*, Bedeutungslehre *f*, Lehre *f* von den Änderungen der Wortbedeutungen, Semasiologie *f*

semblance äußere Gestalt *f*, Form *f*, Erscheinung *f*

semeiology, semeiotics Semiologie *f*, Lehre *f* von den Zeichen, Semiotik *f*, Symptomatologie *f*

semen Samen *m*, Sperma *n*

semicircular halbkreisförmig / **~s** Bogengänge *mpl*

semiconscious bei teilweisem Bewusstsein, somnolent, halbbewusst

semiconsciousness Dämmerzustand *m*

semidelirium Halbdelirium *n*

semilogarithmic semilogarithmisch, halblogarithmisch

seminal Samen–, Sperma–

semiology Semiologie *f*, Lehre *f* von den Zeichen, Semiotik *f*, Symptomatologie *f*

semiopathic abnormen Zeichengebrauch betreffend

semiotic semiologisch, semiotisch

semiotics Semiotik *f*, allgemeine Zeichenlehre *f*, Semiologie *f*

semiprogrammed halbprogrammiert

semipublic halböffentlich

semitone Halbton *m*

semitrance oberflächlicher Trancezustand *m*

semiunconscious bei halbem Bewusstsein, im Dämmerzustand

semiunconsciousness Dämmerzustand *m*, Halbbewusstsein *n*

semivowel Halbvokal *m*

senescence Altern *n*, Altwerden *n*, Seneszenz *f*, Vergreisung *f*

senescent alternd, altwerdend

senile senil, altersschwach

senilism vorzeitiges Altern *n*, Senilismus *m*

senility Senilität *f*, Altersschwäche *f* / **premature ~** vorzeitiges Altern *n*, Senilismus *m*

seniority höheres Alter *n*, höheres Dienstalter *n*, Seniorität *f*, Vorrang *m*

senium Greisenalter *n*, Senium *n* / **~ praecox** vorzeitiges Altern *n*

sensa Sinnesempfindungen *fpl*, Sinneseindrücke *mpl*

sensation Sinnesempfindung *f*, Sinneseindruck *m*, Empfindung *f*, Sensation *f* / **~ of colour** Farbempfindung *f* / **~ difference** Empfindungsunterschied *m* / **~ of discomfort** Unbehaglichkeitsgefühl *n* / **~ of dizziness** Schwindelgefühl *n* / **~ of fatigue** Ermüdungsempfindung *f* / **~ of floating** Schwebegefühl *n* / **~ of hearing** Hörempfindung *f* / **~ increment** Anwachsen *n* der Empfindungsstärke / **~ level** Tonhöhe *f*, Empfindungsniveau *n* / **~ modality** Empfindungsmodalität *f* / **~ quality** Empfindungsqualität *f* / **~ seeking** Reizsuche *f*, Sensationslust *f* / **~ of taste** Geschmacksempfinden *n* / **~ of thirst** Durstgefühl *n*, Durstempfindung *f* / **~ threshold** Empfindungsschwelle *f* / **~ of touch** Tastempfindung *f* / **~ type** Empfindungstypus *m* / **~ unit** Empfindungseinheit *f* / **auditory ~** Gehörempfindung *f* / **auditory ~ level** Hörschwelle *f* / **cold ~** Kälteempfindung *f* / **common ~** Gemeingefühl *n*, Organempfindung *f* / **concomi-**

tant ~ Begleitgefühl *n*, Nebenempfindung *f* / **cutaneous** ~ Hautsinn *m*, Hautempfindung *f* / **dermal** ~ Hautsinn *m*, Hautempfindung *f* / **double** ~ Doppelempfindung *f* / **general** ~ Allgemeingefühl *n*, Allgemeinempfindung *f* / **genital** ~ Geschlechtsempfindung *f*, Sexualempfindung *f* / **gustatory** ~ Geschmacksempfindung *f* / **liminal** ~ Mindestempfindung *f* / **maximal** ~ Maximalempfindung *f* / **motor** ~ Bewegungsempfindung *f* / **muscular** ~ Muskelempfindung *f* / **negative** ~ unterschwellige Empfindung *f* / **olfactory** ~ Geruchsempfindung *f* / **organic** ~ Organempfindung *f* / **phrictopathetic** ~ Gänsehautempfindung *f* / **pleasurable** ~ Lustgefühl *n* / **premonitory** ~ Vorgefühl *n*, Aura *f* / **proprioceptive** ~ Tiefensensibilität *f*, propriozeptive Empfindung *f* / **referred** ~ Trugempfindung *f*, Empfindung *f* an reizentfernter Stelle / **sexual** ~ sexuelle Empfindung *f*, Geschlechtsempfindung *f* / **subjective** ~ subjektive Empfindung *f* / **tactile** ~ Tastempfindung *f* / **tactual** ~ Tastempfindung *f* / **tendinous** ~ Sehnenempfindung *f* / **tonal** ~ Tonempfindung *f* / **transferred** ~ Empfindung *f* an reizentfernter Stelle / **vascular** ~ Gefäßempfindung *f* / **vibratory** ~ Vibrationsempfindung *f*, Vibrationsgefühl *n* / **visual** ~ Gesichtsempfindung *f* / **warm** ~ Wärmeempfindung *f*

sensational sinnlich, Empfindungs–, sensationell

sensationalism Sensualismus *m*, Effekthascherei *f*

sense Sinn *m*, Sinnesfunktion *f*, Gefühl *n*, Bedeutung *f* / empfinden, sinnlich wahrnehmen, fühlen / ~ **appetite** fühlbares Verlangen *n* / ~ **of autonomy** Gefühl *n* der Selbständigkeit / ~ **of balance** Gleichgewichtssinn *m* / ~ **of belonging** Zugehörigkeitsgefühl *n* / ~ **of cold** Kaltsinn *m* / ~ **of colour** Farbensinn *m* / ~ **of community** Gemeinschaftsgefühl *n* / ~ **datum** Sinnesempfindung *f*, Sinneseindruck *m*, Sinnesdatum *n* / ~ **of direction** Richtungssinn *m* / ~ **discrimination** sensorisches Unterscheidungsvermögen *n* / ~ **distance** Empfindungsunterschied *m* / ~ **of duty** Pflichtgefühl *n* / ~ **of equilibrium** Gleichgewichtssinn *n*, praktischer Sinn *m* / ~ **experience** sensorische Erfahrung *f* / ~ **feeling** ambivalente Sinnesempfindung *f* / ~ **for form,** / ~ **of form** Formensinn *m* / ~ **of guilt** Schuldgefühl *n*, Schuldbewusstsein *n* / ~ **of hearing** Gehör *n*, Gehörsinn *m* / ~ **of humour** Sinn *m* für Humor / ~ **illusion** Sinnestäuschung *f* / ~ **impression** Sinneseindruck *m* / ~ **of inferiority** Minderwertigkeitsgefühl *n* / ~ **intuition** sinnliche Erfassung *f* / ~ **limen** Empfindungsschwelle *f* / ~ **modality** Sinnesmodalität *f*, Modalität *f* / ~ **of order** Ordnungssinn *m* / ~ **organ** Sinnesorgan *n* / ~ **perception** Sinneswahrnehmung *f* / ~ **of posture** Stellungssinn *m* / ~ **power** Sinneskraft *f* / ~ **of pressure** Drucksinn *m* / ~ **process** sensorischer Prozess *m* / ~ **of proportion** Maßbegriff *m*, Sinn *m* für die Wirklichkeit / ~ **quality** Empfindungsqualität *f* / ~ **ratios method** Verhältnisherstellungsmetbode *f* / ~ **of reality** Wirklichkeitssinn *m*, Realitätssinn *m* / ~ **of sight** Gesichtssinn *m*, Sehvermögen *n*, Sehen *n* / ~ **of smell** Geruchssinn *m*, Geruchsvermögen *n* / ~ **of space** Raumsinn *m*, Raumgefühl *n* / ~ **of taste** Geschmackssinn *m* / ~ **threshold** Empfindungsschwelle *f* / ~ **of touch** Tastsinn *m*, Tastgefühl *n* / ~ **unit** Sinneseinheit *f* / ~ **of vision** Gesichtssinn *m*, Sehen *n* / **antithetical** ~ **of primal words** Gegensinn *m* der Urworte / **chemical** ~ chemischer Sinn *m* / **common** ~ gesunder Menschenverstand *m* / **contrary** ~ **of primal words** Gegensinn *m* der Urworte / **corporate** ~ Zusammengehörigkeitsgefühl *n*, Verbundenheitsgefühl *n* / **cutaneous** ~ Hautsinn *m* / **dermal** ~ Hautsinn *m* / **distant** ~ Fernsinn *m* / **equal** ~ **differences method** Methode *f* der gleicherscheinenden Intervalle / **external** ~ Exterozeptor *m* / **genesic** ~ Geschlechtsinstinkt *m* / **higher** ~**s** höhere Sinne *mpl* / **internal** ~**s** viszerale Sinne *mpl*, Interozeptoren *mpl* / **joint** ~ Muskelsinn *m*, Kinästhesie *f* / **kinaesthetic ~** Muskelsinn *m*, Kinästhesie *f* / **labyrinthine ~** Gleichgewichtssinn *m* / **moral ~** Sittlichkeitsgefühl *n* / **motor ~** Bewegungssinn *m* / **muscular ~** Muskelsinn *m* / **olfactory ~** Geruchssinn *m*, Riechvermögen *n* / **postural ~** Lagesinn *m*, Lageempfindung *f* / **proprioceptive ~** Propriozeptor *m* / **reproductive ~** Fortpflanzungstrieb *m* / **sexual ~** Geschlechtssinn *m* / **sixth ~** sechster Sinn *m* / **somaesthetic ~** Somasthesie *f* / **spatial cutaneous ~** Raumsinn *m* der Haut / **special ~** spezieller Sinn *m* / **static ~** Gleichgewichtssinn *m* / **stereognostic ~** Formensinn *m* / **systemic ~** Interozeptor *m*, Viszerozeptor *m* / **tactile ~** Tastsinn *m* / **tactual ~** Tastsinn *m* / **vestibular ~** Gleichgewichtssinn *m* / **vital ~** Vitalgefühl *n*, Lebensgefühl *n* / **vomeronasal ~** vomeronasaler Sinn *m*

senseless sinnlos, bewusstlos

sensibilia wahrnehmbare Dinge *npl*

sensibility Sensibilität *f*, Empfindlichkeit *f*, Empfindungsfähigkeit *f*, Empfindungsvermögen *n*, Feinfühligkeit *f* / **common ~** Gemeingefühl *n*, Gemeinempfindung *f* / **cutaneous ~** Hautempfindlichkeit *f*, Hautsensibilität *f* / **deep ~** Tiefensensibilität *f* / **differential ~** Unterschiedsempfindlichkeit *f* / **diminished ~** Sensibilitätsverminderung *f* / **epicritic ~** epikritische Sensibilität *f* / **kinaesthetic ~** Bewegungsempfindlichkeit *f* / **labyrinthine ~** Gleichgewichtsempfindung *f* / **luminous ~** Lichtempfindlichkeit *f* / **pallaesthetic ~** Vibrationsempfinden *n* / **perceptual ~** Wahrnehmungsempfindlichkeit / **proprioceptive ~** Lagesinn *m* / **protopathic ~** protopathische Sensibilität *f* / **subcutaneous ~** Tiefensensibilität *f* / **superficial ~** Oberflächensensibilität *f* / **vibratory ~** Vibrationsempfinden *n*

sensible wahrnehmbar, fühlbar, bemerkbar, empfindlich, vernünftig, verständig

sensibleness Wahrnehmbarkeit *f*, Empfindlichkeit *f*, Vernünftigkeit *f*, Klugheit *f*

sensing Empfinden *n*, Fühlen *n*

sensitisation Sensibilisierung *f*, Sensitivierung *f*, Informationsempfänglichkeit *f* / **~ period** Sensibilisierungszeit *f*, Belichtungszeit *f* / **~ repression** Sensibilisierung *f* gegen Verdrängungen / **~ time** Sensibilisierungszeit *f*, Belichtungszeit *f* / **covert ~** verdeckte Sensibilisierung *f*

sensitive empfindsam, empfindlich, empfindend, sensitiv / **~ to cold** kälteempfindlich / **~ to colours** farbempfindlich / **~ to noise** lärmempfindlich / **~ to touch** berührungsempfindlich / **abnormally ~** überempfindlich / **highly ~** hochempfindlich

sensitiveness Empfindlichkeit *f*, Empfindungsfähigkeit *f*, Empfindungsvermögen *n*, Sensibilität *f*, Sensitivität *f* / **~ to cold** Kälteempfindlichkeit *f* / **~ to pressure** Druckempfindlichkeit *f* / **~ to touch** Berührungsempfindlichkeit *f* / **chromatic ~** Farbempfindlichkeit *f* / **differential ~** Unterschiedsempfindlichkeit *f* / **excessive ~** Überempfindlichkeit *f*

sensitivity Empfindlichkeit *f*, Empfindungsfähigkeit *f*, Empfindungsvermögen *n*, Sensibilität *f*, Sensitivität *f* / **~ to cold** Kälteempfindlichkeit *f* / **~ group** Selbsterfahrungsgruppe *f* / **~ to interference** Interferenzneigung *f*, Konfliktbereitschaft *f* / **~ to light** Lichtempfindlichkeit *f* / **~ to pain** Schmerzempfindlichkeit *f* / **~ to pressure** Druckempfindlichkeit *f* / **~ to stimuli** Reizempfindlichkeit *f* / **~ training** Training *n* von Selbst– und Fremdwahrnehmung, Sensitivitätstraining *n* / **absolute ~** absolute Empfindungsschwelle *f* / **cultural ~** kulturelle Sensitivität *f* / **dermal ~** Hautempfindlichkeit *f* / **dermatoptic ~** Lichtempfindlichkeit *f* der Haut / **differential ~** Unterschiedsempfindlichkeit *f* / **epicritic ~** Empfindlichkeit *f* für Hautreize / **liminal ~** Schwellenempfindlichkeit *f* / **partially disturbed ~** Empfindungsdissoziation *f* / **social ~** soziales Gespür *n* / **spectral ~** spektrale Unterschiedsempfindlichkeit *f* / **spectral visual ~** spektrale Hellempfindlichkeitskurve *f* / **terminal ~** maximale Empfindlichkeit *f* / **thermal ~** Temperaturempfindlichkeit *f*, Wärmeempfindlichkeit *f* / **visceral ~** Körpergefühl *n*, Körperempfinden *n* / **visual ~** Sehempfindlichkeit *f*

sensitize sensibilisieren, empfindlich machen, gefühlsempfindlich machen

sensitizer sensibilisierender Reiz *m*, Sensibilisator *m*

sensitizing Sensibilisieren *n*

sensomotor sensomotorisch, sensumotorisch

sensor Sensor *m*, Rezeptor *m*, Messfühler *m* / **~ potential** Sensorpotenzial *n* / **D ~** Differenzialsensor *m* / **differential ~** Differenzialsensor *m* / **osmoreceptive ~** Geruchsrezeptor *m* / **P ~** Proportionalsensor *m*, P–Sensor *m* / **PD ~** Proportional–Differenzialsensor *m*, PD–Sensor *m* / **proportional–differential ~** Proportional–Differenzialsensor *m*, PD–Sensor *m*

sensorial sensorisch, Sinnes–, Empfindungs–

sensorimotor sensomotorisch, sensumotorisch

sensorimuscular Muskelempfindung betreffend

sensorium Sinnesapparat *m*, Sinneszentren *npl*, Sensorium *n*, Bewusstsein *n*

sensory Sinnes–, Empfindungs–, sensorisch, sensibel

sensual sinnlich, erotisch, wollüstig

sensualise sinnlich machen, geschlechtlich erregen

sensualism Sensualismus *m*, sinnliche Veranlagung *f*

sensualist Sensualist *m*, Sinnenmensch *m*

sensuality Sinnlichkeit *f* / **~ erg** narzisstisches Motiv *n*

sensum Sinnesempfindung *f*, Sinneseindruck *m*

sensuous sinnlich, lebensbejahend

sensus communis gesunder Menschenverstand *m*

sentence Satz *m* / **~–completion test** Satzergänzungstest *m* / **~ comprehension** Satzverständnis *n* / **~–repetition test** Satzwiederholungstest *m* / **~ structure** Satzstruktur *f* / **ambiguous ~** mehrdeutiger Satz *m* / **disarranged–~ test** Satzordnungstest *m* / **dissected–~ test** Satzordnungstest *m* / **incomplete–~ test** Satzergänzungstest *m* / **negative ~** Satzverneinung *f*

sentience Empfindung *f*, Gefühl *n* / **~ need** Bedürfnis *n* nach Gefühlsempfindungen

sentiendum Empfindung *f*

sentient empfindend, fühlend

sentiment Sentiment *n*, Gefühl *n*, Gesinnung *f*, Motivziel *n*

sentimentality Sentimentalität *f*, Empfindsamkeit *f*, Schwärmerei *f*

separate trennen / getrennt

separation Trennung *f* / **~ anxiety** Trennungsangst *f* / **~ anxiety disorder** Störung *f* mit Trennungsangst, Angstsyndrom *n* mit Trennungsangst / **~ anxiety disorder of childhood** emotionale Störung *f* mit Trennungsangst des Kindesalters / **~ device** Trenngerät *n*, Weiche *f* / **~ reaction** Trennungsreaktion *f* / **marital ~** Trennung *f* der Ehepartner, Trennung *f* von Tisch und Bett, Partnertrennung *f*

septal Septum–, Scheidewand–

septum Scheidewand *f*, Septum *n* / **~ pellucidum** Septum pellucidum *n*, Scheidewand *f* zwischen den Vorderhörnern der Seitenventrikel des Gehirns / **internasal ~** Nasenscheidewand *f*

sequela Folgezustand *m*, Folgeerkrankung *f*

sequence Reihenfolge *f*, Reihe *f*, Folge *f* / **~ of observations** Beobachtungsreihe *f* / **~ preference** sequenzielle Präferenz *f* / **developmental ~** Entwicklungsphasen *fpl* / **numerical ~ of data** numerische Datenfolge *f*

sequential sequenziell, schrittweise erfolgend

serendipity zufälliges Finden *n*, zufällige Entdeckung *f*

serial Serien–, Reihen–, in Serien / periodische Zeitschrift *f*

seriatim der Reihe nach

seriation Anordnung *f* in Reihen, Reihenfolge *f*

series Serie *f*, Reihe *f* / **~ effect** serieller Effekt *m*, Reiheneffekt *m* / **~ of experiments** Versuchsreihe *f* / **~ of observations** Beobachtungsreihe / **~ of reactions** Reaktionskette *f* / **~ of responses** Reaktionskette *f* / **~ resistance** Vorschaltwiderstand *m*, Rheostat *m* / **~ of stimuli** Reizserie *f* / **ascending–descending ~** aufsteigendes–absteigendes Verfahren *n* / **complementary ~** Ergänzungsreihe *f* / **experimental ~** Versuchsreihe *f*, Versuchsserie *f* / **identical ~** gleiche Reihe *f* / **statistical ~** statistische Reihe *f*

serious schwer, ernst, gefährlich

seriousness Ernsthaftigkeit *f*, Ernst *m*

serotonergic serotonerg

serotonin Serotonin *n*, Enteramin *n* / **~ agonist** Serotoninagonist *m* / **~ antagonist** Serotoninantagonist *m* / **~ metabolite** Serotoninmetabolit *m* / **~ precursor** Serotoninvorläufer *m* / **~–reuptake inhibitor** Serotonin–Wiederaufnahmehemmer *m*

sertraline Sertralin *n*

serum albumin Serumalbumin *n*

servant Diener *m*, Beamte *m*, Beamtin *f* / **civil ~** Staatsbeamter *m*

server Server *m*

service Dienst *m*, Dienstleistung *f*, Service *m* / **~ personnel** Dienstleistungsberufe *mpl* / **advisory ~** Beratungsdienst *m* / **integrated ~s** Verbundsystem *n* psychosozialer Betreuung *n* / **protective ~** Schutzdienst *m* / **social ~s** Sozialeinrichtungen *fpl*, soziale Dienste *mpl*, soziale Dienstleistungen *fpl*

serviceable nützlich, brauchbar, dauerhaft

servile untertänig, unterwürfig, servil

servility Unterwürfigkeit *f*, Servilität *f*

servitude sklavische Abhängigkeit *f* / **penal ~** Zwangsarbeit *f*, Zuchthausstrafe *f*

servo, servomechanism Servomechanismus *m*, Regelmechanismus *m*

servomotor Servomotor *m*

sessile sitzend

session Sitzung *f* / **experimental ~** experimentelle Sitzung *f*, Versuch *m*

set Einstellung *f*, Haltung *f*, Ausgerichtetsein *n*, Tendenz *f*, Gruppe *f*, Serie *f* / setzen, stellen, legen / **~–back** Rückschlag *m*, Rückfall *m* / **~ point** Sollwert *m* / **~ point adjustment** Sollwertverstellung *f* / **~ theory** Einstellungstheorie *f* / **~–up** Anordnung *f* / aufstellen, konfigurieren, vorbereiten / **~ of values** Wertausrichtung *f* / **abstract ~** abstrakte Ausrichtung *f*, abstrakte Wahrnehmungstendenz *f* / **cognitive ~** kognitives Schema *n* / **determining ~** determinierende Tendenz / **experimental ~–up** Versuchsanordnung *f* / **hypnotic ~** posthypnotischer Auftrag *m* / **mental ~** mentale Einstellung *f*, geistig–seelische Einstellung *f* / **motor ~** motorische Reaktionsbereitschaft *f* / **neural ~** Bahnung *f*, Reaktionsbereitschaft *f* / **objective ~** objektive Einstellung *f*, objektive Erwartungshaltung *f* / **organic ~** körperliche Einstellung / **perceptual ~** Wahrnehmungseinstellung *f*, Wahrnehmungstendenz *f* / **perseverative ~** Perseverationstendenz *f* / **postural ~** gespannte Haltung *f* / **preparatory ~** angespannte Reaktionsbereitschaft *f* / **situational ~** Reizaufnahmebereitschaft *f* / **unconscious ~** unbewusste Tendenz *f*, unbewusste Einstellung *f*

setting Anordnung *f*, Arrangement *n*, Einrichten *n*, fachspezifische Differenzierung *f* / **experimental ~** Versuchsanordnung *f*

severe schwer, ernst, heftig

severing Durchtrennung *f* / **~ of a nerve** Nervdurchtrennung *f*

severity Schwere *f*, Strenge *f*, Härte *f*, Schweregrad *m*

sex Geschlecht *n* / Geschlechts–, Sexual– / **~ act** Geschlechtsakt *m* / **~ aim** geschlechtlicher Zweck *m* / **~ anomaly** Anomalie *f* der Geschlechtsorgane, geschlechtliche Abweichung *f*, sexuelle Deviation *f* / **~ appeal** sexuelle Anziehungskraft *f*, Sex appeal *m* / **~ cell** Geschlechtszelle *f* / **~ change** Geschlechtsumwandlung *f* / **~ character** Geschlechtsmerkmal *n* / **~ chromosome** Geschlechtschromosom *n* / **~ crime** Sexualverbrechen *n* / **~ cycle** Geschlechtszyklus *m* / **~ delinquency** Sexualverbrechen *n* / **~ determination** Geschlechtsbestimmung *f* / **~ differences** Geschlechtsunterschiede *mpl* / **~ differentiation** Geschlechtsdifferenzierung *f* / **~ discrimination** Diskrimination *f* aufgrund des Geschlechts / **~ distribution** Geschlechtsverhältnis *n* in der Bevölkerung / **~ drive** Geschlechtstrieb *m* / **~ education** Sexualkunde *f*, sexuelle Aufklärung *f*, Sexualerziehung *f* / **~ erg** Sex–Erg *n* / **~ feeling** erotisches Gefühl *n* / **~ flush** Hautrötung *f* bei sexueller Stimulation / **~ game** sexuelles Vorspiel *n* / **~ gland** Geschlechtsdrüse *f* / **~ hormone** Geschlechtshormon *n*, Sexualhormon *n* / **~ hygiene** Sexualhygiene *f* / **~ identity** geschlechtliche Identität *f* / **~ infantilism** sexueller Infantilismus *m* / **~–influenced character** geschlechtsabhängiges Merkmal *n* / **~ intergrade** Hermaphrodit *m*, Intersexualität *f* / **~ latency** sexuelle Latenzphase / **~–limited character** geschlechtsbezogenes Merkmal *n* / **~–linked** geschlechtsgebunden / **~–linked character** geschlechtsspezifisches Merkmal *n* / **~–linked developmental difference** geschlechtsgebundener Entwicklungsunterschied *m* / **~–linked hereditary disorder** geschlechtsgebundene Erbkrankheit *f* / **~ need** geschlechtliches Bedürfnis *n*, sexuelles Bedürfnis *n* / **~ object** sexuelles Triebziel *n*, Sexualobjekt *n* / **~ offense** Sexualverbrechen *n*, Sittlichkeitsdelikt *n* / **~ organs** Geschlechtsorgane *npl* / **~ perversion** sexuelle Perversion *f*, sexuelle Deviation *f* / **~ ratio** Geschlechtsverhältnis *n* in der Bevölkerung / **~ recognition** Geschlechtserkennung *f* / **~ reversal** Geschlechtsumwandlung *f* / **~ rivalry** geschlechtliche Rivalität *f* / **~ role** geschlechtsspezifische Rolle *f*, Geschlechtsrolle *f* / **~ sensation** Geschlechtsempfindung *f*, sexuelle Empfindung *f* / **~ therapy** Sexualtherapie *f* / **~ want** sexuelles Bedürfnis *n*, sexueller Wunsch *m* / **anatomic ~** anatomisches Geschlecht *n* / **female ~** weibliches Geschlecht *n* / **male ~** männliches Geschlecht *n* / **primary ~ character** primäres Geschlechtsmerkmal *n* / **repressed ~** verdrängte Sexualität / **secondary ~ character** sekundäres Geschlechtsmerkmal *n*

sexed mit starker Libido ausgestattet

sexiness sexuelle Attraktivität *f*, erotischer Reiz *m*

sexism Sexismus *m*

sexless geschlechtslos, ungeschlechtlich, asexuell, agamisch

sexological sexologisch, Sexualwissenschaft betreffend

sexologist Sexualwissenschaftler *m*

sexology Sexualwissenschaft *f*, Sexologie *f*

sextile Sechstel *n*

sexual geschlechtlich, sexuell, Sexual–, Geschlechts–

sexualisation Sexualisierung *f*

sexualise sexualisieren

sexuality Sexualität *f*, Geschlechtlichkeit *f* / **dual ~** dualer Liebesmodus *m* / **female ~** weibliche Sexualität *f* / **infantile ~** infantile Sexualität *f*, frühkindliche Sexualität *f* / **pregenital ~** prägenitale Sexualität *f*

sexually attracted to sexuell orientiert auf

sexy sexy, scharf, sexuell aufregend

s factor s–Faktor *m*, spezifischer Faktor *m*

shade Schatten *m*, Schattierung *f*, Farbnuance *f*

shading Schattierung *f* / **~ response** Schattierungsdeutung *f* / **~ shock** Dunkelschock *m*

shadow Schatten *m* / **~ test** Skiaskopie *f* / **acoustic ~** Schallschatten *m* / **coloured ~** Farbschatten *m*, farbiger Schatten *m* / **coloured ~ experiment** Experiment *n* mit farbigen Schatten

shadowing verschwommene mystische Darstellung *f*

shake schütteln / Schütteln *n*, Zittern *n* / **~s** Schüttelfrost *m*

shallow oberflächlich

sham vortäuschen, simulieren, sich verstellen / Nachahmung *f*, Täuschung *f*, Simulation *f* / nachgemacht, falsch, Schein– / **~ feeding** Scheinfütterung *f* / **~ rage** unechte Wut *f*, Scheinwut *f*

shaman Schamane *m*, Heilkundiger *m*

shamanism Schamanismus *m*

shame Scham *f*, Schande *f*

shamming Täuschung *f*, Verstellung *f*, Simulation *f*

shape Form *f*, Gestalt *f*, Struktur *f*, Anordnung *f*, Konfiguration *f*, Gefüge *n* / formen, gestalten / **~ constancy** Formkonstanz *f*, Gestaltkonstanz *f*, Dingkonstanz *f* / **~ of curve** Kurvengestalt *f*, Kurvenform *f* / **~ perception** Gestaltwahrnehmung *f*, Formwahrnehmung *f* / **good ~** gute Form *f*

shapeless formlos, gestaltlos, ungestaltet

shapelessness Formlosigkeit *f*, Gestaltlosigkeit *f*

shaping Annäherungskonditionierung *f*, Verhaltensformung *f* / **~ of behaviour** Verbaltensformung *f*

shared gemeinsam, zusammen teilhabend

shareware Shareware *f*

sharing Teilen *n*, Abgeben *n*

sharp scharf, spitz, scharfsinnig, intelligent, um einen halben Ton erhöht / **~–looking** intelligent aussehend

sharpening Überspitzung *f*, starke Akzentuierung *f*

sharpness Schärfe *f* / **~ of sight** Sehschärfe *f*

sheath Scheide *f*, Hülle *f* / **~ of Schwarm** Schwarm–Scheide *f* / **medullary ~** Markscheide *f*, Myelinscheide *f* / **neural ~** Nervenscheide *f*, Schwann–Scheide *f* / **nucleated ~** Neurilemm *n* / **primitive ~** Neurilemm *n*

Sheldon types Sheldon–Typen *mpl*

shell Schild *n*, Granate *f* / **~ shock** Kriegsneurose *f* / **~ shock neurosis** Kriegsneurose *f*, Kommotionsneurose *f* / **~ shock psychosis** Kommotionspsychose *f*

shelter Schutzhaus *n* / beschützen

shibboleth Erkennungswort *n*, Losungswort *n*, Stichwort *n*

shield Schild *n*, Schutz *m*, Abschirmung *f* / **protective ~** Reizschutz *m*, Schutzschild *n*

shift Wechsel *m*, Veränderung *f*, Schicht *f* / **~ work** Schichtarbeit *f* / **binaural ~** Differenzschwebung *f* links–rechts / **fixed ~** feste Schicht *f* / **nonreversal ~ learning** Lernen *n* mit Dimensionswechsel, Umlernen *n* / **risky ~ effect** Risikoschubeffekt *m* / **rotating ~s** Wechselschicht. *f*

shifting Verschiebung *f*, Wechsel *m* eines Gedankens

shiftless träge, unfähig, hilflos

shock Schock *m* / schocken / **~ absorber** Pufferreiz *m*, Eisbrecherfrage *f* / **~ effect** Schockwirkung *f* / **~ reaction** Schockreaktion *f* / **~ therapy** Schocktherapie *f*, Schockbehandlung *f* / **~ treatment** Schockbehandlung *f* / **anaphylactic ~** anaphylaktischer Schock *m* / **cardiovascular ~** Kreislaufschock *m* / **cerebral ~** Hirnschock *m* / **circulatory ~** Kreislaufschock *m* / **commotional ~** Kommotionsschock *m* / **convulsive ~ therapy** Krampfbehandlung *f* / **delayed ~** Spätschock *m*, verzögerter Schock *m* / **electric ~** Elektroschock *m* / **electric ~ treatment** Elektroschockbehandlung *f* / **electroconvulsive ~** Elektroschock *m* / **electroconvulsive ~ therapy** Elektrokrampfbehandlung *f*, Elektroschocktherapie *f* / **emotional ~** seelischer Schock *m* / **hematogenic ~** Volumenmangelschock *m* / **hypoglycaemic ~** hypoglykämischer Schock *m*, Insulinschock *m* / **hypovolemic ~** Volumenmangelschock *m* / **mental ~** psychischer Schock *m* / **nervous ~** Nervenschock *m* / **neurogenic ~** Nervenschock *m* / **psychic ~** psychischer Schock *m*, seelischer Schock *m* / **sexual ~** sexuelles Trauma *n* / **spinal ~** spinaler Schock *m* / **therapeutic ~** therapeutischer Schock *m* / **traumatic ~** traumatischer Schock *m*, Unfallschock *m*

shocked erschüttert, fassungslos, außer Fassung, geschockt

shoplifting Ladendiebstahl *m*

short kurz, knapp / **~–circuit** Kurzschluss *m* / **~–circuit theory** Kurzschlusstheorie *f* / **~–circuiting** Kurzschließen *n* / **~–circuiting law** Kurzschlussgesetz *n* / **~–circuiting theory** Kurzschlusstheorie *f* / **~–headed** kurzköpfig / **~–range** kurzfristig / **~–sighted** kurzsichtig, myop / **~–sightedness** Kurzsichtigkeit *f*, Myopie *f* / **~–tempered** reizbar / **~–term** kurzfristig, unmittelbar

shortage Mangel *m*, Knappheit *f*

shortening Abkürzung *f* Verkürzung *f*

shortness Kürze *f*, Mangel *m* / **~ of breath** Kurzatmigkeit *f*, Atemnot *f*, Dyspnoe *f* / **~ of memory** Gedächtnisschwäche *f*

"shoulds" ideale Sollvorgaben *fpl*

showmanship Fähigkeit *f* sich selbst in gutes Licht zu rücken, geschickte Zurschaustellung *f*

shrewd klug, scharfsinnig

shrewedness Scharfsinn *m*, Klugheit *f*

shrink schrumpfen, zusammenschrumpfen, eingehen

shrinkage Schwund *m*, Abnahme *f*

shunt Nebenschluss *m* / aufschieben, parallel schalten

shut schließen, verschließen / **~ away** sich absondern / **~ in** einschließen / **~–in personality** verschlossene Persönlichkeit *f*, Introvertierter *m* / **~ off** abschließen, verschließen / **~ out** ausschließen, sperren, blockieren

shutting off reality, shutting out reality Realitätsleugnung *f*

shuttle box Doppelkäfig *m* mit Pendeltür, „Shuttle–Box“ *f* / **~ grid** Gitterrost *m* einer „Shuttle–Box“ / **~ hurdle** Hürde *f* in einer „Shuttle–Box“

shy scheu, schüchtern, zurückhaltend, verlegen

shyness Scheu *f*, Schüchternheit *f*, Verlegenheit *f*

sib Blutsverwandter *m*, Blutsverwandtschaft *f* / blutsverwandt

sibling Bruder *m*, Schwester *f* / **~s** Geschwister pl / **~ incest** Bruder–Schwester–Inzest *m* / **~ relation** Geschwisterbeziehung *f* / **~ relational problem** Problem *n* zwischen Geschwistern / **~ rivalry** Geschwisterrivalität *f* / **~ rivalry disorder** emotionale Störung *f* mit Geschwisterrivalität *f*

sickle–cell disease Sichelzellenerkrankung *f*

sickness Krankheit *f* / **induced ~** Induktionskrankheit *f* / **sleeping ~** Schlafkrankheit *f*, Encephalomyelitis equina *f* / **sleepy ~** Schlafkrankheit *f*, Encephalitis lethargica *f*

sick–rate Krankenstand *m*, Erkrankungsziffer *f*

sidedness Seitenbevorzugung *f*, Seitendominanz *f*, Lateralität *f*

side–effect Nebenwirkung *f*

siderodromophobia Eisenbahnphobie *f*, Siderodromophobie *f*

sidetone Nebenton *m*, Nebengeräusch *n*

Sidman avoidance Sidman–Vermeidung *f*, kontinuierliche Vermeidung *f*

sigh seufzen / Seufzer *m*

sight Sehen *n*, Aussehen *n*, Anblick *m*, Sehvermögen *n*, Visus *m* / **~ angle** Sehwinkel *m* / **~ conservation class** Klasse *f* für Sehbehinderte / **~ line** Sehachse *f*, Visierlinie *f* / ~ **method** Seh–Lese–Methode *f* / ~**–reading** Vom–Blatt–Lesen *n* / ~**–saving class** Schulklasse *f* für Sehbehinderte / ~**–testing** Sehprüfung *f* / ~ **vocabulary** bildhaft erlernte Wörter *npl* / **far** ~ Weitsichtigkeit *f*, Hypermetropie *f* / **long** ~ Weitsichtigkeit *f*, Hypermetropie *f* / **near** ~ Kurzsichtigkeit *f* / **old** ~ Alterssichtigkeit *f*, Presbyopie *f* / **partial** ~ Teilerblindung *f* / **second** ~ zweites Gesicht *n* / **short** ~ Kurzsichtigkeit *f*, Myopie *f* / **unequal** ~ Anisometropie *f* / **weak** ~ Schwachsichtigkeit *f*, Asthenopie *f*

sighted sehend, –sichtig / **far–**~ weitsichtig, hypermetrop / **long–**~ weitsichtig, hypermetrop / **partially** ~ partiell Sehgeschädigte *m,f* / **short–**~ kurzsichtig

sighting Sichten *n*, Visieren *n* / ~ **line** Visierlinie *f*, Sehachse *f* / ~ **test** Prüfung *f* der Augendominanz

sigma Standardabweichung *f*, Millisekunde *f* / ~ **measure** Standardwert *m* / ~ **score** Standardwert *m* / ~ **value** Standardwert *m* / **partial** ~ Standardschätzfehler *m*

sigmatism Lispeln *n*, Sigmatismus *m*

sigmoid S–förmig

sign Zeichen *n*, Anzeichen *n*, Symptom *n* / ~ **of affect** Affektsignal *n* / ~ **of depersonalisation** Depersonalisationserscheinung *f* / ~ **of depression** Depressionserscheinung *f* / ~ **gestalt** Zeichen–Gestalt *f* / ~ **gestalt theory** Zeichen–Gestalt–Theorie *f* / ~ **language** Zeichensprache *f*, Gebärdensprache *f* / ~ **learning** Zeichenlernen *n* / ~ **object** Zeichen–Gestalt *f* / ~**s of senility** Alterserscheinungen *fpl* / ~**–significance relation** Beziehung *f* zwischen Zeichen und Bedeutung, Erwartung *f* / ~ **stimulus** Signalreiz *m* / ~ **test** Zeichentest *m*, Vorzeichentest *m* / **electrical** ~ **of excitation** elektrisches Anzeichen *n* der Erregung / **local** ~ Lokalzeichen *n* / **pathognomic** ~**s** pathognomische Zeichen *npl* / **pathological** ~ pathologisches Zeichen *n* / **prodromal** ~ Vorzeichen *n* / **supernormal** ~ **stimulus** Über das Normale hinausgehender Signalreiz *m* / **temporal** ~ Zeitzeichen *n* / **with predominantly psychological (physical)** ~**s and symptoms** mit vorwiegend psychischen (körperlichen) Zeichen *npl* und Symptomen *npl*

signal Signal *n*, Zeichen *n*, Anzeichen *n* / ~ **of affect** Affektsignal *n* / ~ **amplification** Signalverstärkung *f* / ~ **of anxiety** Angstsignal *n* / ~ **detection theory** Signalentdeckungstheorie *f*, Signaldetektionstheorie *f* / ~ **intensity** Signalstärke *f* / ~ / ~ **noise ratio** Signal–Störspannungsverhältnis *n* / ~ **system** Signalsystem *n* / ~ **transformation** Signalumwandlung *f* / **controlling** ~ Stellgröße *f* / **warning** ~ Warnsignal *n*, Warnzeichen *n*

signalisation Signalisation *f*, Signalfunktion *f*, Signaltätigkeit *f*

signalling system Signalsystem *n* / **verbal** ~ verbales Signalsystem *n*

signature Unterschrift *f*, Lokalzeichen *n*, digitale Unterschrift *f* unter einer E–Mail / **local** ~ Lokalzeichen *n*

significance Bedeutung *f*, Sinn *m*, Signifikanz *f* / ~ **level** Signifikanzniveau *n* / **statistical** ~ statistische Signifikanz *f*

significant bedeutsam, signifikant / ~ **one** Person *f*, die einem etwas bedeutet / ~ **other** Bezugsperson *f*

significate Bezeichnetes *n*

signification Bedeutung *f*, Sinn *m*

signify bezeichnen, bedeuten

sildenafil Sildenafil *n*

silent schweigend, still

silliness Dummheit *f*, Torheit *f*, Albernheit *f*

silly dumm, einfältig, unklug, töricht

similar ähnlich, gleich

similarities test Gemeinsamkeitentest *m*

similarity Ähnlichkeit *f*, Gleichartigkeit *f* / ~ **paradox** Skaggs–Robinson–Hypothese *f*, Hypothese *f* über die Auswirkung der Ähnlichkeit von Lerninhalten auf das Behalten

Simmonds' disease Simmonds Krankheit *f*, Hypophysenvorderlappeninsuffizienz *f*

simple einfach, klar / **~–hearted** arglos / **~–minded** arglos, leichtgläubig

simplex einfach / Simplex *n*

simplicity Einfachheit *f*, Unkompliziertheit *f* / **~ canon** Sparsamkeitsprinzip *n*, Ökonomieprinzip *n*

simplification Vereinfachung *f*

simulate simulieren, sich verstellen, vortäuschen

simulation Simulation *f*, Verstellung *f*, Vortäuschung *f* / **~ game** Simulationsspiel *n*, Simulation *f*

simulator Simulator *m*, Ausbildungsgerät *n*, Übungsgerät *n*, Simulant *m*

simultaneity, simultaneousness Gleichzeitigkeit *f*, Synchronizität *f*

simultaneous gleichzeitig, simultan

sin Sünde *f*, Vergehen *n* / sündigen, eine Sünde begehen, verstoßen gegen

sincerity, sincereness Offenheit *f*, Aufrichtigkeit *f*, Ehrlichkeit *f*

sine Sinus *m* / **~ wave** Sinuswelle *f*

sinful sündig, unmoralisch

singing Singen *n*

single einfach, allein, alleinstehend, ledig, einzig, ehrlich, aufrichtig / Alleinstehende *m,f*, Single *m* / **~–hearted** aufrichtig, treu / **~–minded** zielbewusst, zielstrebig / **~–mindedness** Aufrichtigkeit *f*, Zielstrebigkeit *f*

singleness Einsamkeit *f*, Alleinsein *n*, Singledasein *n* / **~ of heart** Aufrichtigkeit *f* / **~ of purpose** Zielstrebigkeit *f*

singleton Einzelgeburt *f*, Einzelwesen *n*

singularism Monismus *m*

sinister links, linksliegend, linkshändig, unheilvoll, unheimlich, böse

sinistrad linksgerichtet, linkstendierend, nach links hin

sinistral linksseitig / Linkshänder *m*

sinistrality Linksdominanz *f*, Linkshändigkeit *f*

sinistrocerebral zur linken Hemisphäre gehörig

sinistromanual linkshändig

sinistrosis traumatische Neurose *f*, Unfallneurose *f*

sinking Beklommenheit *f*

sinus Sinus *m* / **cerebral ~** Hirnsinus *m* Hirnhohlraum *m* / **cranial ~** Schädelhohlraum *m* / **frontal ~** Stirnhöhle *f* / **occipital ~** Sinus occipitalis *m* / **paranasal ~** Nasennebenhöhle *f*

sinusitis Nebenhöhlenentzündung *f*, Sinusitis *f*

sinusoid Sinusschwingung *f*

sinusoidal sinusförmig

siren Sirene *f*, Verführerin *f*, Signalgerät *n*

sister Schwester *f*

sitomania Fresssucht *f*, Sitomanie *f*

sitophobia krankhafte Angst *f* vor dem Essen, Sitophobie *f*

sitting Sitzung *f*

situation Situation *f*, Lage *f*, Zustand *m* / **~ analysis** Situationsanalyse *f* / **~ neurosis** reaktive Neurose *f*, Situationsneurose *f* / **~–process** Situationsverlauf *m* / **~ psychosis** Situationspsychose *f* / **~ under stress** Stresssituation *f*, belastende Situation *f* / **~ therapy** Milieutherapie *f* / **~ test** Situationstest *m* / **analytic ~** analytische Situation *f* / **difficult ~** schwierige Lage *f*, Zwangslage *f* / **environmental ~** Milieusituation *f* / **experimental ~** Versuchssituation *f* / **hidden–cue ~** Lernvorgang *m* mit verstecktem Auslösereiz / **overlapping ~** Überschneidungssituation *f* / **social ~** soziale Struktur *f* einer Situation, soziales Feld *n* / **total ~** psychologisches Feld *n*, Lebensraum *m*, Verhaltensfeld *n*

situational Situations–, Lage–

situationalism, situationism Situationalismus *m*

sixth sechste(r, s) / Sechstel *n*

size Größe *f* / **~–age confusion** Altersfehleinschätzung *f* aufgrund der Größe / **~ of the brain** Gehirnvolumen *n* / **~ constancy** Größenkonstanz *f*, Dingkonstanz *f*

/ ~ **discrimination** Größenunterscheidung *f*, Größendiskrimination *f* / **~–weight illusion** Größen–Gewichts–Täuschung *f*, Charpentier–Koseleff–Täuschung *f*, optische Gewichtstäuschung *f* / **apparent ~** scheinbare Größe / **pupillary ~** Pupillengröße *f*, Öffnungsgröße *f* der Pupille

Sjögren–Larssen syndrome Sjögren–Larssen–Syndrom *n*

Skaggs–Robinson| hypothesis Skaggs–Robinson–Hypothese *f*, Hypothese *f* über die Auswirkung der Ähnlichkeit von Lerninhalten auf das Behalten / ~ **phenomenon** Skaggs–Robinson–Hypothese *f*

skeletal Skelett–

skeleton Skelett *n*, Knochengerüst *n*, Gerippe *n* / ~ **form** Skelettform *f*

staff Stammbelegschaft *f*

skeptic Skeptiker *m*, Zweifler *m*

skeptical skeptisch, misstrauisch, zweifelnd

skepticism Skeptizismus *m*, Skepsis *f*, Zweifel *m*

skew schief, schräg / schief werden, knicken / **~–eyed** schielend

skewed schief, asymmetrisch

skewness Schiefe *f*, Asymmetrie *f* / ~ **of distribution** Asymmetrie *f* einer Verteilung, schiefe Verteilung *f*

skiascope Skiaskop *n*, Augenspiegel *m*

skiascopy Skiaskopie *f*, Schattenprobe *f*

skilful, skillful geschickt, gewandt

skill Fertigkeit *f*, Geschicklichkeit *f*, Gewandtheit *f* / ~ **learning** Erlernen *n* von Fertigkeiten / ~ **sequence** optimale Handlungsfolge *f* / **academic ~s disorder** Schulleistungsstörung *f* / **basic ~** Grundfertigkeit *f* / **fine motor ~** feinmotorische Geschicklichkeit *f* / **fine motor ~ learning** Lernen *n* feinmotorischer Fertigkeiten / **fundamental ~** Grundfertigkeit *f* / **gross motor ~** grobmotorische Geschicklichkeit *f* / **gross motor ~ learning** Lernen *n* grobmotorischer Fertigkeiten / **manual ~** Handfertigkeit *f* / **motor ~** motorische Geschicklichkeit *f*, motorische Fertigkeit *f* / **motor ~s disorders** Störung *f* der motorischen Fertigkeiten / **parenting ~s** Elternfertigkeiten *fpl* / **perceptual–motor ~** sensumotorische Geschicklichkeit *f* / **secretarial ~** Sekretariatstechnik *f* / **social ~** soziale Fertigkeit *f* / **social ~s training** Training *n* sozialer Fertigkeiten / **technical ~** technische Geschicklichkeit *f*

skilled geschickt, gewandt, erfahren

skim rasch durchlesen, überfliegen

skimming rasches Durchlesen *n*, Überfliegen *n*

skin Haut / ~ **conduction** Hautleitung *f* / ~ **disease** Hautkrankheit *f*, Dermatose *f* / ~ **disorder** Hautkrankheit *f*, Hautleiden *n* / **allergic ~ disorder** allergische Hautkrankheit *f* / ~ **electrical properties** hautelektrische Eigenschaften *fpl*, Hautleitfähigkeit *f* / ~ **eroticism** Hauterotik *f* / ~ **erotism** Hauterotik *f* / ~ **neurosis** Hautneurose *f*, Dermatoneurose *f* / ~ **potential** Hautpotenzial *n* / ~ **reflex** Hautreflex *m*, Hautreaktion *f* / ~ **resistance** Hautwiderstand *m* / **basal ~ resistance** basaler Hautwiderstand *m* / ~ **sensation** Hautempfindung *f* / ~ **sense** Hautsinn *m* / ~ **temperature** Hauttemperatur *f* / **anserine ~** Gänsehaut *f* / **electric ~ response** psychogalvanische Reaktion *f* / **galvanic ~ reflex** psychogalvanische Reaktion *f* / **galvanic ~ response** psychogalvanische Reaktion *f*, galvanische Hautreaktion *f* / **psychogalvanic ~ reflex** psychogalvanische Reaktion *f*, galvanische Hautreaktion *f* / **smooth ~** weiche Haut *f*, glatte Haut *f*

Skinner| box Skinner'scher Kasten *m*, Skinner–Box *f* / **~'s operant conditioning** operantes Konditionieren *n* nach Skinner

skip springen, überspringen, auslassen / Sprung *m*, Auslassen *n*

skipping Überspringen *n* von Klassen, Auslassen *n*

skull Schädel *m*

slang Berufsjargon *m*, Fachsprache *f*, Slang *m*, saloppe Umgangssprache

slant schiefe Lage *f*, Neigung *f*, Neigungswinkel *m*

slanted geneigt

slanting schief, schräg

slate–writing Schreiben *n* auf Schiefertafel

slave Sklave *m* / ~ **system** Servomechanismus *m*

slavery Sklaverei *f*, sklavische Abhängigkeit *f*

sleep Schlaf *m* / ~ **apnea syndrome** Schlaf–Apnoe–Syndrom *n* / ~ **center** Schlafzentrum *n* / ~ **curve** Schlafkurve *f* / ~ **deprivation** Schlafentzug *m*, Schlafdeprivation *f* / **post–ictal** ~ Terminalschlaf *m*

sleep disorder Schlafstörung *f* / ~ **due to a general medical condition** Schlafstörung *f* aufgrund eines medizinischen Krankheitsfaktors / **circadian rhythm** ~ Schlafstörung *f* mit Störung des zirkadianen Rhythmus / **alcohol–induced** ~ alkoholinduzierte Schlafstörung *f* / **amphetamine–induced** ~ amphetamininduzierte Schlafstörung *f* / **breathing–related** ~ atmungsgebundene Schlafstörung *f* / **nonorganic** ~ nichtorganische Schlafstörung *f* / **primary** ~ primäre Schlafstörung *f* / **substance–induced** ~ substanzinduzierte Schlafstörung *f*

sleep| disturbance Schlafstörung *f* / ~ **drunkenness** Schlaftrunkenheit *f* / ~ **epilepsy** Schlafepilepsie *f* / ~ **inducing drug** Schlafmittel *n* / ~ **onset** Schlafeintritt *m*, Somnolenz *f* / ~ **paralysis** Wachanfall *m* / ~ **rituals** Einschlafzeremoniell *n* / ~ **spindle** Schlafspindel *f* / ~ **talking** Sprechen *n* im Schlaf / ~ **terrors** Pavor nocturnus *m* / ~ **treatment** Schlafkur *f*, Schlaftherapie *f* / **~–wake cycle** Schlaf–Wach–Zyklus *m* / **~–walker** Schlafwandler *m*, Nachtwandler *m*, Somnambuler *m* / ~ **walking** Schlafwandeln *n*, Nachtwandeln *n*, Somnambulismus *m* / **~–walking disorder** Schlafstörung *f* mit Schlafwandeln / **broken** ~ Schlafunterbrechung *f* / **continuous** ~ Dauerschlaf *m* / **deep** ~ Tiefschlaf *m* / **disturbed** ~ Schlafstörung *f* / **dreaming** ~ Traumschlaf *m* / **fast** ~ fester Schlaf *m*, tiefer Schlaf *m* / **healing** ~ Heilschlaf *m* / **hypnotic** ~ Hypnose *f* / **induced** ~ künstlich erzeugter Schlaf *m* / **light** ~ leichter Schlaf *m* / **natural** ~ natürlicher Schlaf *m* / **non–REM** ~ Non–REM–Schlaf *m*, orthodoxer Schlaf *m*, traumloser Schlaf *m* / **orthodox** ~ orthodoxer Schlaf *m*, traumloser Schlaf *m*, synchronisierter Schlaf *m* / **paradoxical** ~ paradoxer Schlaf *m* / **paroxysmal** ~ Schlafanfall *m* / **REM** ~ paradoxer Schlaf *m*, Traumschlaf *m* / **sound** ~ fester Schlaf *m*, tiefer Schlaf *m* / **synchronized** ~ synchronisierter Schlaf *m*, orthodoxer Schlaf *m* / **therapeutical** ~ Heilschlaf *m*, Schlaftherapie *f* / **troubled** ~ Schlafstörung *f*

sleeper effect „sleeper"–Effekt *m*, Inkubationseffekt *m*

sleepiness Schläfrigkeit *f*, Somnolenz *f* / **morbid** ~ Bettsucht *f*

sleepless schlaflos

sleeplessness Schlaflosigkeit *f*, Insomnie *f*

sleepy schläfrig, müde

sliding–filament theory Gleitfilamenttheorie *f*

slim schlank, dünn

slip Lapsus *m*, Fehler *m*, Versehen *n* / ~ **comparison** gleitender Vergleich *m* / ~ **of the pen** Verschreiben *n*, Schreibfehler *m* / ~ **of speech** Versprecher *m*, Lapsus linguae *m* / ~ **of the tongue** Versprecher *m*, Lapsus linguae *m* / **Freudian** ~ Freud'sche Fehlleistung *f*, Freud'scher Versprecher *m*

slope Neigung *f*, Schräge *f* / ~ **of a curve** Neigungswinkel *m* einer Kurve / **minimal** ~ minimaler Gradient *m*

slow langsam, schwer von Begriff, schwerfällig / **~–learning** langsam auffassend

slowing down Verlangsamung *f*, Hemmung *f*

slowness Trägheit *f* / ~ **of reaction** Reaktionsträgheit *f*

sluggish träge, faul, verzögert, schwerfällig, lustlos

sluggishness Trägheit / ~ **of the mind** geistige Trägheit *f*, verzögerter Gedankenablauf *m*

slum Elendsviertel *n*, Slum *m*

slychology Psychologie *f* zum Zwecke der Verführung, ausbeutende Psychologie *f*

small klein, gering, unbedeutend

smartness Lebhaftigkeit *f*, Geschicklichkeit *f*, Gewandtheit *f*, Eleganz *f* / **hypomanic** ~ Lebhaftigkeit *f* / **manic** ~ Lebhaftigkeit *f*

smell Geruchssinn *m*, Geruch *m*, Duft *m* / riechen, duften / ~ **blindness** Geruchsblindheit *f*, Anosmie *f* / ~**–brain** Riechhirn *n*, Rhinenzephalon *n* / ~ **centre** Riechzentrum *n*, Geruchszentrum *n* / ~ **compensation** Geruchsneutralisation *f* / ~ **perception** Geruchswahrnehmung *f* / ~ **prism** Geruchsprisma *n* / ~ **quality** Geruchsqualität *f*

smeller Riecher *m*

smelliness übler Geruch *m*, Gestank *m*

smelling Riechen *n* / **coloured** ~ Synästhesie *f*, Riechen *n* bei gleichzeitiger Farbwahrnehmung

smelly übelriechend, stinkend

smile Lächeln *n* / lächeln

smoking Rauchen *n* / ~ **cessation** Raucherentwöhnung *f*

smooth glatt, weich

smoothing Glätten *n*, Ausgleichen *n*, Nivellierung *f*, Ausgleich *m*

smoothness Glätte *f*, Weichheit *f*

smut Zote *f*, Schlüpfrigkeit *f*

snake phobia Schlangenfurcht *f*, krankhafte Furcht *f* vor Schlangen

sneezing reflex Niesreflex *m*

Snellen's| chart Snellen'sche Tafel *f* / ~ **letters** Snellen'sche Tafel *f* / ~ **test** Snellen'sche Sehprobe *f*

sniffing Schnüffeln *n*

snore Schnarchen *n*

snorer Schnarcher *m*, Schnarcherin *f*

snow Schnee *m*, Kokain *n* / ~**–blind** schneeblind / ~**–blindness** Schneeblindheit *f*

snowbird Kokainsüchtiger *m*

snuffle Schnüffeln *n*, Näseln *n* / schnüffeln, näseln, durch die Nase sprechen

snuffling näselnd / geschlossenes Näseln *n*

sob schluchzen

sobbing schluchzend

sober nüchtern, besonnen, gemäßigt, vernünftig / ~**–minded** besonnen, ruhig / ~**–mindedness** Besonnenheit *f*, Ruhe *f*

soberness, sobriety Nüchternheit *f*, Alkoholabstinenz *f* / Besonnenheit *f*, Ruhe *f*

sociability Soziabilität *f*, Geselligkeit *f* / ~ **rating** Beurteilung *f* der Soziabilität

sociable gesellig, umgänglich

social sozial, gesellschaftlich, Sozial– / ~**–minded** gesellschaftlich ausgerichtet, sozial orientiert

socialisation Sozialisation *f*, Sozialisierung *f*, Vergesellschaftung *f* / **political** ~ politische Sozialisation *f*

socialise sozialisieren, gesellig machen, vergesellschaften

socialism Sozialismus *m*

sociality Geselligkeit *f*, Geselligkeitstrieb *m*, Gesellschaftstrieb *m*

sociatry Soziatrie *f*

societal die Gesellschaft betreffend, gesellschaftliche Gruppen betreffend, Gesellschafts–

society Gesellschaft *f* / **nonliterate** ~ schriftlose Kultur *f*, schriftlose Gesellschaft *f* / **permissive** ~ Gesellschaft *f* die alles erlaubt, permissive Gesellschaft *f*

sociobiology Soziobiologie *f*

sociocentre zentrale Figur *f*, sozialer Mittelpunkt *m*, Beliebtheitsführer *m*

sociocentrism Gruppenegoismus *m*, Soziozentrismus *m*

sociodrama Soziodrama *n*, Soziogenesis *f*

socioeconomic sozioökonomisch, sozial und wirtschaftlich

sociogenesis Soziogenese *f*, Entstehen *n* sozialen Verhaltens

sociogenetic soziogenetisch

sociogerontology soziologische Altersforschung *f*

sociogram Soziogramm *n*

sociography Soziographie *f*, graphische Darstellung *f* sozialen Verhaltens

sociolinguistics Soziolinguistik *f*

sociological soziologisch

sociologist Soziologe *m*

sociology Soziologie / **~ of work** Industriesoziologie *f* / **industrial ~** Industriesoziologie *f* / **psychological ~** psychologische Soziologie *f*

sociometric soziometrisch

sociometry, sociometrics Soziometrie *f*

socionomics Sozionomie *f*, Lehre *f* vom Einfluss nicht–sozialer Faktoren auf soziale Gebilde

sociopath gesellschaftsfeindliche Person *f*, Soziopath *m*, gesellschaftlich abartige Person *f*

sociopathic soziopathisch, im sozialen Verhalten abartig

sociopathology Soziopathologie *f*, Sozialpathologie *f*

sociopathy Soziopathie *f*

sociophilia Soziophilie *f*

sociophobia Soziophobie *f*

sociopsychiatry Sozialpsychiatrie *f*, soziale Psychiatrie *f*

sociopsychological sozialpsychologisch

sociotherapy Sozialtherapie *f*, Soziotherapie *f*

sociotype sozialer Typus *m*

socius soziales Wesen *n*, Sozius *m*, Mitglied *n* der Gesellschaft

sodium Natrium *n* / **~ amytal** Amobarbitalnatrium *n* / **~ bromide** Natriumbromid *n* / **~ chloride** Natriumchlorid *n*, Salz *n* / **~ ions** Natriumionen *npl* / **~ pentobarbital** Pentobarbitalnatrium *n* / **~ pentothal** Pentothalnatrium *n* / **~–potassium adenosine triphosphatase** Natrium–Kalium–ATPase *f* / **~–potassium pump** Natrium–Kalium–Pumpe *f*

sodomist, sodomite Sodomit *m*, Sodomitin *f*

sodomy Sodomie *f*, Sexualverkehr *m* mit Tieren

soft weich, mild, leise

softening Erweichung *f*, Malazie *f* / **~ of the brain** Gehirnerweichung *f*, Enzephalomalazie *f* / **cerebral ~** Gehirnerweichung *f*, Enzephalomalazie *f*

softness Weichheit *f*, Milde *f*, Nachgiebigkeit *f*

software Software *f*, EDV–Programme *npl*

sole reflex Fußsohlenreflex *m*, Plantarreflex *m*

solidarity Solidarität *f*, Zusammengehörigkeitsgefühl *n*

solidity Festigkeit *f*, Solidität *f*, Zuverlässigkeit *f*

soliloquize mit sich selbst reden

soliloquy Selbstgespräch *n*

solipsism Solipsismus *m*

solipsistic solipsistisch, egozentrisch

solitary einsam, allein, alleinlebend

solo Solo *n*

solubility Löslichkeit *f*

soluble löslich, lösbar

solution Lösung *f* / **~ learning** Erlernen *n* von Lösungen / **auxiliary ~** Ersatzlösung *f*, Hilfslösung *f* / **comprehensive ~** Gesamtlösung *f*, umfassende Lösung *f* eines Konfliktes / **hypertonic ~** hypertone Lösung / **hypotonic ~** hypotone Lösung *f* / **neurotic ~** neurotische Konfliktlösung *f* / **oblique ~** oblique Faktorenstruktur *f* / **optimal ~** beste Lösung *f* / **orthogonal ~** orthogonale Faktorenstruktur *f*

solvable lösbar

solve auflösen, lösen

solvent Lösungsmittel *n* / **~ abuse** Lösungsmittelmissbrauch *m*, Schnüffelsucht *f* / **volatile ~** flüchtiges Lösungsmittel *n*

solving of problems Lösung *f* von Problemen, Problemlösung *f*

soma Soma *n*, Körper *m*

somaesthesia, somaesthesis, somataesthesia, somatesthesia Körpergefühl *n*, körperliches Empfinden *n*, Somästhesie *f*

somaesthetic Körpergefühl betreffend

somagenic, somatogenic somatogen, körperlich verursacht

somatalgia somatischer Schmerz *m*, Somatalgie *f*, Körperschmerz *m*

somatic somatisch, körperlich, physisch, Körper–

somaticovisceral somatoviszeral

somatization Somatisierung *f*, Konversion *f*, Somatisierungssyndrom *n* / **~ disorder** Somatisierungsstörung *f*

somatist Somatiker *m*

somatagnosia Verlust *m* des Körpergefühls, Somatoagnosie *f*

somatoform somatoform

somatogenesis Somatogenese *f*

somatogenic somatogen, in den Körperzellen entstehend

somatological somatologisch

somatology Somatologie *f*, Lehre *f* vom Körper

somatomedin Somatomedin *n*

somatomegaly Riesenwuchs *m*

somatoneurosis Somatoneurose *f*

somatophrenia Krankheitseinbildung *f*, Somatophrenie *f*

somatoplasm Somatoplasma *n*, Körperzellenplasma *n*

somatopsyche Somatopsyche *f*, Leibseele *f*

somatopsychic somatopsychisch, psychosomatisch

somatopsychosis Somatopsychose *f*, seelisch bedingtes Körperleiden *n*

somatosensory somatosensorisch, Körperempfindungs–

somatosexuality körperliche Sexualität *f*

somatostatin Somatostatin *n*

somatotherapy körperliche Behandlung *f*

somatotonia Somatotonie *f*

somatotonic somatotonisch

somatotopy Somatotopie *f*

somatotropin Somatotropin *n*

somatotype Somatotyp *m*, Körperbautyp *m*

somatotypology Somatotypologie *f*, Typologie *f* nach Körperbau und Konstitution

somatropin, somatotropin Wachstumshormon *n*, Somatotropin *n*

somatovisceral somatoviszeral

somesthesia, somesthesis Körpergefühl *n*, körperliches Empfinden *n*, Somästhesie *f*

somesthetic Körpergefühl betreffend

somite Somit *m*, Ursegment *n*, Metamer *n*

somnambulate nachtwandeln, schlafwandeln

somnambulism, somnambulance, somnambulation Schlafwandeln *n*, Nachtwandeln *n*, Somnambulismus *m*

somnambulist, somnambulator Schlafwandler *m*, Somnambuler *m*, Nachtwandler *m*

somnambulistic schlafwandlerisch, nachtwandlerisch, somnambul

somniferous schlafbringend, schlaferzeugend

somniloquence, somniloquism, somniloquy Sprechen *n* im Schlaf, Sprechen *n* in hypnotischem Zustand

somniloquist im Schlaf Sprechender *m*, unter Hypnose Sprechender *m*

somnipathy Schlafstörung *f*, hypnotischer Schlafzustand *m*

somnolence Somnolenz *f*, Schlafsucht *f*, Schläfrigkeit *f*

somnolent somnolent, schlafsüchtig

somnolism Hypnose *f*, Trance *f*

sonance, sonancy Stimmhaftigkeit *f*

sonant stimmhafter Laut *m* / stimmhaft

sone Sone *n*, Maß *n* der Lautstärkeempfindung

sonic Schall–, akustisch, den Schall betreffend

sonometer Sonometer *n*, Gerät *n* zur Bestimmung der Hörschärfe

sonority, sonorousness Klang *m*, Klangfülle *f*

sonorous tönend, klingend, klangvoll

sophism Sophismus *m*, Trugschluss *m*, Spitzfindigkeit *f*

sophist Sophist *m*

sophistic sophistisch, spitzfindig

sophisticated hochentwickelt, intellektuell, überkultiviert

sophistication Sophisterei *f*, Trugschluss *m*, Fälschung *f*, Intellektualismus *m*

sophistry Sophistik *f*, Spitzfindigkeit *f*

sophomania Sophomanie *f*

sophrologia Sophrologie *f*

sopor Sopor *m*, Bewusstseinseinschränkung *f* mittleren Grades, soporöser Zustand *m*, Schlafsucht *f*

soporific, soporiferous schlaferzeugend, einschläfernd

sorcery Zauberei *f*, Magie *f*

soreness Schmerzhaftigkeit *f*, Empfindlichkeit *f*

sorority Studentinnenverbindung *f* / ~ **membership** Mitgliedschaft *f* in einer Studentinnenverbindung

sorrow Leid *n*, Kummer *m*

sorter Sortiermaschine *f*, Sortierer *m* / **circular** ~ Rundsortierer *m*

sorting Sortieren *n* / ~ **method** Sortiermethode *f* / ~ **of punched card data** Sortieren *n* von Lochkartendaten / ~ **system** Sortiersystem *n* / ~ **test** Sortiertest *m*

Sotos' syndrome Sotos–Syndrom *n*

souffle blasendes Geräusch *n*

soul Seele *f* / ~ **blindness** Seelenblindheit *f*, optische Agnosie *f* / ~**–image** Seelenbildnis *n* / ~ **pain** Psychalgie *f*, Seelenschmerz *m* / ~ **theory** Seelentheorie *f*

sound Ton *m*, Schall *m*, Klang *m*, Geräusch *n* / tönen, klingen, schallen / gesund, normal, intakt / ~ **amplification** Lautverstärkung *f* / ~ **auditory localisation** Schallokalisation *f* / ~ **barrier** Schallmauer *f*, Schallgrenze *f* / ~ **board** Resonanzboden *m* / ~ **box** Klangkörper *m* / ~ **cage** Raum *m* zur Schallokalisation / ~**–conducting** schalleitend / ~ **conduction** Schalleitung *f* / ~ **density** Schalldichte *f* / ~ **energy density** Schallenergiedichte *f* / ~ **energy flux** Schallenergiefluss *m*, Schalleitung *f* / ~ **field** Schallfeld *n* / ~ **flutter** auditives Flimmern *n* / ~ **frequency** Schallfrequenz *f* / ~ **Gestalt** Klanggestalt *f*, Tongestalt *f* / ~ **image** Schallbild *n*, Tonbild *n* / ~ **intensity** Schallintensität *f*, Schallstärke *f* / ~ **interference** Schallinterferenz *f* / ~ **key** Schallschlüssel *m* / ~ **level** Schallpegel *m* / ~**–level control** Lärmbekämpfung *f* / ~ **localisation** Schallokalisation *f*, Schallokalisierung *f* / ~ **of mind** geistig gesund / ~ **mixture** Schallmischung *f* / ~ **pendulum** Schallpendel *n* / ~**–perceiving** schallempfindend, Schallempfindungs– / ~ **perception** Tonwahrnehmung *f*, Schallempfindung *f* / ~ **perimeter** Tonperimeter *m*, Tonumfang *m* / ~ **perimetry** Tonperimetrie *f* / ~ **pressure** Schalldruck *m* / ~ **pressure level** Schalldruckniveau *n*, Schalldruckpegel *m* / ~**–proof** schalldicht / ~ **protection** Schallschutz *m*, Lärmschutz *m* / ~**–ranging** Schallmessung *f*, Schalllokalisierung *f* / ~ **reference intensity** Normalschallstärke *f* / ~ **reflection** Schallreflektion *f* / ~ **sensation level** Niveau *n* der Schallempfindung / ~ **shadow** Tonschatten *m* / ~ **source** Schallquelle *f* / ~ **spectrogram** Schallspektrogramm *n* / ~ **spectrograph** Schallspektrograph *m* / ~ **substitution** Schallersatz *m* / ~ **symbolism** Lautsymbolik *f* / ~ **track** Tonspur *f* / ~ **unit** Lautstärkeeinheit *f* / ~ **wave**

Schallwelle *f* / **aperiodic ~** unregelmäßiger Ton *m* / **clear ~** heller Laut *m* / **compound ~** Klang *m*, Tongemisch *n* / **dull ~** dumpfer Schall *m* / **entotic ~** im Ohr selbst entstehendes Geräusch *n*, entotisches Geräusch *n* / **full ~** voller Schall *m*, voller Klang *m* / **infra–audible ~** Infraschall *m* / **instantaneous ~ pressure** unmittelbarer Schalldruck *m* / **maximum ~ pressure** Scheitelwert *m* des Schalldrukkes / **mean ~ intensity** mittlere Lautstärke *f* / **reflected ~** Echo *n*, reflektierter Schall *m* / **subjective ~** Stimmenhören *n* / **ultra–audible ~** Ultraschall *m*

sounding schallend, tönend / **~–board** Schallbrett *n*, Resonanzboden *m*

soundness of mind Zurechnungsfähigkeit *f*

Souque's phenomenon Souque–Phänomen *n*

sour sauer

source Quelle *f*, Ursprung *m* / **~ of error** Fehlerquelle *f* / **~ of infection** Infektionsquelle *f* / **~ of the instinct** Triebquelle *f* / **~ of message** Nachrichtenquelle *f* / **~ of sound** Schallquelle *f* / **~ of stimulation** Reizquelle *f* / **~ trait** Wurzeleigenschaft *f*, Grundeigenschaft *f*, Grundwesenszug *m* / **constitutional ~ trait** konstitutionelle Wurzeleigenschaft *f* / **electric ~** Spannungsquelle *f* / **extended ~** vergrößerte Lichtquelle *f* / **primary ~** Primärquelle *f* / **secondary ~** Sekundärquelle *f*

sourness saurer Geschmack *m*, Säuerlichkeit *f*, Verdrießlichkeit *f*, Verbitterung *f*

space Raum *m*, Zeitraum *m*, Zwischenraum *m* / verteilen, einteilen / **~ blindness** Raumblindheit *f* / **~ craft** Raumfahrzeug *n* / **~ error** Raumfehler *m*, Positionsirrtum *m* / **~ factor** Faktor *m* der räumlichen Vorstellung / **~ feeling** Raumempfinden *n* / **~ flight** Raumfahrt *f* / **~ illusion** Raumtäuschung *f* / **~ image** Raumbild *n* / **~ interval** Raumintervall *m*, Zwischenraum *m*, Abstand *m* / **~ limitation** Raumbegrenzung *f* / **~ of free movement** frei zugänglicher Raum *m* / **~ orientation** Raumorientierung *f*, Orientierung *f* im Raum / **~ perception** Raumwahrnehmung *f* / **~ relations** Raumbezeichungen *fpl* / **~–time sense** Raum–Zeitgefühl *n* / **anatomical dead ~** anatomischer Totraum *m* / **auditory ~** Hörraum *m* / **communal ~** Gemeinschaftsraum *m* / **conceptual ~** begrifflicher Raum *m* / **extracellular ~** Extrazellularraum *m* / **Euclidean ~** euklidischer Raum *m* / **functional dead ~** funktioneller Totraum *m* / **hodological ~** hodologischer Raurn *m* / **intermediate ~** Zwischenraum *m* / **intracellular ~** Intrazellularraum *m* / **medullary ~** Markraum *m* / **personal ~** persönlicher Raum *m* / **physiological dead ~** physiologischer Totraum *m* / **pleural ~** Pleuralspalt *m* / **psychological ~** psychologischer Raum *m*, Lebensraum *m* / **subdural ~** Subduralraum *m* / **visual ~** Sehraum *m* / **white ~ response** Zwischenfigur–Deutung *f* / **working ~** Arbeitsraum *m*, Arbeitsumfeld *n*

spaced verteilt, auseinanderliegend

spacing Verteilen *n*, Aufteilen *n*, Auseinanderziehen *n*

span Spanne *f*, Spannweite *f*, Umfang *m* / **~ of apprehension** Auffassungsumfang *m*, Erfassungsspannweite *f* / **~ of attention** Aufmerksamkeitsumfang *m* / **~ of consciousness** Bewusstseinsumfang *m*, Bewusstseinsenge *f* / **~ of memory** Gedächtnisspanne *f* / **~ of movement** Bewegungsausdehnung *f* / **~ of perception** Wahrnehmungsumfang *m* / **auditory ~** auditive Gedächtnisspanne *f*

spank den Hintern versohlen

spare sparsam, kärglich, überflüssig / sparen, verschonen

sparetime Freizeit *f* / **~ planning** Freizeitgestaltung *f*

spark Funke *m*, Funken *m* / **~ chronoscope** Funkenchronoskop *n* / **~ method** Funkenmethode *f*

sparkling Glitzern *n*, Funkeln *n*

spasm Krampf *m*, Verkrampfung *f*, Spasmus *m* / **~ centre** Krampfzentrum *n* / **cerebral ~** hirnbedingter Krampf *m* / **clonic**

~ klonischer Krampf *m*, Klonus *m* / **dancing ~** Bamberger'sche Krankheit *f* / **emotional ~** Affektkrampf *m* / **epileptic ~** epileptischer Krampf *m* / **facial ~** Gesichtszuckung *f*, Fazialiskrampf *m* / **functional ~** Überanstrengungskrampf *m* / **mimic ~** Gesichtskrampf *m* / **nictitating ~** Blinzelkrampf *m*, Spasmus nictitans *m* / **nodding ~** Nickkrampf *m*, Salaamkrampf *m*, Blitzkrampf *m* / **occupational ~** Beschäftigungskrampf *m*, Überanstrengungskrampf *m* / **phonic ~** Stimmkrampf *m* / **professional ~** Berufsneurose *f* / **saltatory ~** Bamberger'sche Krankheit *f*, saltatorischer Reflexkrampf *m* / **shaking ~** Schüttelkrampf *m*, Zitterkrampf *m* / **tonic ~** tonischer Krampf *m* / **tonoclonic ~** tonisch–klonischer Krampf *m* / **vaginal ~** Scheidenkrampf *m* / **visual ~** Blickkrampf *m* / **winking ~** Blinzelkrampf *m*, Spasmus nictitans *m*

spasmoarthria krampfhaftes Sprechen *n*

spasmodic krampfartig, krampfhaft, spasmodisch

spasmodyspnoea krampfbedingte Dyspnoe *f*, krampfbedingte Atemnot *f*

spasmology Krampflehre *f*, Spasmologie *f*

spasmolysis Krampflösung *f*, Spasmolyse *f*

spasmolytic krampflösend, spasmolytisch / Spasmolytikum *n*, krampflösendes Mittel *n*

spasmophemia Stottern *n*

spasmophilia Krampfneigung *f*, Krampfbereitschaft *f*, Spasmophilie *f*

spasmophilic, spasmophile krampfgeneigt, krampfbereit, spasmophil

spasmus Krampf *m*, Spasmus *m* / **~ nutans** Nickkrampf *m*, Salaamkrampf *m*, Spasmus nutans *m*

spastic spastisch, krampfartig, krampfhaft, Krampf–

spasticity Krampfneigung *f*, spastischer Zustand *m*, Spastik *f*, Spastizität *f*

spatial räumlich, Raum–

spatiality räumlicher Charakter *m*

spatiotemporal raumzeitlich

spay die Eierstöcke entfernen, sterilisieren

spaying weibliche Kastration *f*

speaker Sprecher *m*, Redner *m* / **native ~** Muttersprachler *m*

speaking Sprechen *n* / **automatic ~** automatisches Sprechen *n* / **public ~** Sprechen *n* vor Publikum

Spearman|–Brown formula Spearman–Brown–Formel *f* / **~–Brown prophecy formula** Spearman–Brown–Formel *f* / **~ footrule** Spearman–Rangkorrelation *f* / **~ rank correlation** Spearman Rangkorrelation *f*

special besondere(r, s), spezielle(r, s), Spezial–, Sonder–

specialisation Spezialisierung *f*, fachliche Vertiefung *f* / **academic ~** Vertiefung *f* in einem Schulleistungsfach, schulische Spezialisierung *f* / **professional ~** berufliche Spezialisierung *f*

specialist Fachmann *m*, Spezialist *m* / **~ leader** Führer *m* aufgrund fachlicher Qualifikation / **mental ~** Psychiater *m*

speciality Besonderheit *f*, charakteristisches Merkmal *n*

specialized spezialisiert

species Art *f*, Spezies *f* / **~ difference** Artenmerkmal *n* / **~ heredity** artspezifische Vererbung *f*, Genotypus *m* / **~ recognition** Arterkennung *f* / **~ reflex** Artreflex *m* / **~–specific** artspezifisch / **~ specifity** Artspezifität *f*

specific spezifisch, speziell, arteigen / **~ to the species** artspezifisch

specification Spezifikation *f*, genaue Beschreibung *f* / **~ equation** Spezifikationsgleichung *f*

specificity spezifische Charakteristik *f*, spezifische Eigenart *f*, Spezifizität *f*, spezifische Varianz *f*

specifier Zusatzcodierung *f* / **rapid–cycling ~** Zusatzcodierung *f* „mit rapid cycling" / **seasonal pattern ~** Zusatzcodierung *f* „mit saisonalem Muster"

specify spezifizieren, genau beschreiben

specimen Muster *n*, Probe *f*, Exemplar *n*

specious trügerisch, Schein–, blendend, fadenscheinig

speciousness trügerischer Schein *m*

spectator Zuschauer *m*

spectral spektral, Spektral–

spectre Erscheinung *f*, Phantom *n*, Hirngespinst *n*

spectrocolorimeter Gerät *n* zum Nachweis der Farbenblindheit

spectrocolorimetry Messung *f* der Farbenschwäche

spectrograph Spektrograph *m*

spectrometer Spektrometer *n*

spectrometry Spektrometrie *f*

spectrophobia Spiegelfurcht *f*, Eisoptrophobia *f*

spectrophotometer Spektrophotometer *n*

spectrophotometric spektrophotometrisch

spectrophotometry Spektrophotometrie *f*

spectroscope Spektroskop *n*

spectroscopic spektroskopisch

spectroscopy Spektroskopie *f*

spectrum Spektrum *n*, Farbenbild *n* / **~ colours** Spektralfarben *fpl* / **~ line** Spektrallinie *f* / **~ locus** Spektralbereich *m* / **acoustic ~** akustisches Spektrum *n* / **auditory ~** Bereich *m* der hörbaren Frequenzen / **broad ~** breites Spektrum *n* / **electromagnetic ~** elektromagnetisches Spektrum *n* / **ocular ~** Nachbild *n* / **prismatic ~** Prismenspektrum *n* / **visible ~** sichtbares Spektrum *n*

specular Spiegel–, spiegelnd

speculation Spekulation *f*, Vermutung *f*, unbewiesene Theorie *f* / **obsessive ~** zwanghafte Spekulation *f*

speech Sprache *f*, Sprechen *n*, Rede *f* / **~ abnormality** Sprachstörung *f* / **~ anxiety** Sprechangst *f* / **~ audiometry** Sprachaudiometrie *f* / **~ block** Sprechhemmung *f* / **~ centre** Sprachzentrum *n* / **~ characteristic** Sprachcharakteristik *f* / **~ deafness** Sprachtaubheit *f*, Worttaubheit *f* / **~ defect** Sprachfehler *m*, Sprachstörung *f* / **~ development** Sprachentwicklung *f* / **retarded ~ development** Sprachentwicklungsstörung *f* / **~ difficulty** Sprachschwierigkeit *f* / **~ disabled** sprachbehindert, Sprachbehinderte *m,f* / **~ discrimination** Sprachwahrnehmung *f*, Sprachunterscheidung *f* / **~ disorder** Sprachstörung *f* / **~ function** Sprechfunktion *f* / **~ handicapped** sprachbehindert / **~ impediment** Sprachfehler *m* / **~ measures** Sprachtest *m* / **~ pause** Sprechpause *f* / **~ perception** Sprachwahrnehmung *f* / **~ pitch** Sprechhöhe *f*, Sprechstimmlage *f* / **~ processing** Sprachverarbeitung *f*, Sprechvorgang *m* / **~ rate** Sprechtempo *n* / **~ reading** Lippenlesen *n* / **~ rhythm** Sprechrhythmus *m* / **~ synthesizer** Apparat *m* zur künstlichen Sprachproduktion / **~ therapeutist** Sprachtherapeut *m*, Logopäde *m* / **~ therapist** Sprachtherapeut *m*, Logopäde *m* / **~ therapy** Sprachtherapie *f*, Logopädie *f* / **~ training** Sprachtraining *n* / **accelerated ~** schnelle Sprache *f* / **articulate ~** artikulierte Sprache *f* / **ataxic ~** ataktische Sprache *f* / **auditory ~ area** auditives Sprachzentrum *n* / **auditory ~ centre** auditives Sprachzentrum *n* / **automated ~ recognition** automatische Spracherkennung *f* / **automatic ~** automatisches Hersagen *n* / **clipped ~** verkürzte Sprechweise *f* / **compressed ~** gepresste Sprache *f*, komprimierte Sprache *f* / **cortical ~ area** Sprachzentrum *n* / **covert ~** innere Sprache *f* / **defective ~** Sprechanomalie *f*, Sprachstörung *f* / **delayed ~** verzögertes Sprechen *n* / **delusional ~** wahnhafte Sprache *f* / **disorganized ~** desorganisierte Sprache *f* / **egocentric ~** egozentrische Redeweise *f* / **filtered ~** gefilterte Sprache *f* / **implicit ~** innere Sprache *f* / **incoherent ~** unzusammenhängende Sprache *f*, verwirrte Sprache *f* / **infantile ~** Babysprache *f*, Kindersprache *f* / **inner ~** inneres Sprechen *n* / **internal ~** inneres Sprechen *n* / **motor ~ area** motorisches Sprachzentrum *n*, Broca'sches Sprachzentrum *n* /

motor ~ centre motorisches Sprachzentrum *n*, Broca'sches Sprachzentrum *n* / **pantomimic ~** Pantomimensprache *f* / **scanning ~** skandierende Sprache *f* / **scattered ~** Sprachzerfall *m* / **sensory ~ centre** sensorisches Sprachzentrum *n*, Wernicke'sches Sprachzentrum *n* / **slow ~** Bradylalie *f* / **spastic ~** spastische Sprache *f* / **specific ~ articulation disorder** Artikulationsstörung *f* / **subvocal ~** inneres Sprechen *n*, subvokales Sprechen *n* / **synthetic ~** synthetische Sprache *f*, Maschinensprache *f* / **tangential ~** sprunghafte Sprache *f* / **telegraphic ~** Sprache *f* im Telegrammstil / **visible ~** sichtbare Sprache *f* / **visual ~ centre** optisches Sprachzentrum *n*, Lesezentrum *n*

speed Geschwindigkeit *f* / Speed *n* / **~ of apperception** Apperzeptionsgeschwindigkeit *f* / **~ of data–processing** Geschwindigkeit *f* der Datenverarbeitung / **~ factor** Faktor *m* „Geschwindigkeit" / **~ of forgetting** Schnelligkeit *f* des Vergessens / **~ limit** Höchstgeschwindigkeit *f*, Tempolimit *n* / **~ of perception** Wahrnehmungsgeschwindigkeit *f* / **~ of performance** Leistungsgeschwindigkeit *f* / **~ score** Rohwert *m* eines Schnelligkeitstests / **~ test** Schnelligkeitstest *m* / **~–up** Beschleunigung *f* / beschleunigen, anspornen / **clerical ~** Schnelligkeit *f* bei Büroarbeiten, Arbeitsschnelligkeit *f* / **individual ~** persönliches Tempo *n* / **perceptual ~** Auffassungsgeschwindigkeit *f* / **reading ~** Lesegeschwindigkeit *f* / **saccadic ~** ruckartiger Bewegungsablauf *m*

speeding–up Beschleunigung *f*, Vergrößerung *f*, Leistungserhöhung *f*

speedometer Geschwindigkeitsmesser *m*, Tachometer *n*

speedy geschwind, schnell, unverzüglich

spell kurze Zeitdauer *f*, bestimmte Arbeitsleistung *f*, Talisman *m*, Anfall *m* / buchstabieren, richtig schreiben / **~s of dizziness** kurze Schwindelanfälle *mpl* / **breath–holding ~** respiratorische Affektanfälle *mpl*, Schreikrämpfe *mpl*, Wutkrämpfe *mpl* / **dizzy ~s** kurze Schwindelanfälle *mpl*

spelling Buchstabieren *n*, Rechtschreibung *f*, Orthographie *f* / **~ demon** Fehlerteufel *m* / **specific ~ disorder** isolierte Rechtschreibstörung *f*

sperm Sperma *n*, Samen *m* / **~ cell** Samenzelle *f*

spermatic Sperma–, Samen–, samenführend

spermatophobia Spermatophobie *f*

spermatozoal Spermatozoen–

spermatozoon, spermatozoid Spermatozoon *n*, Samenzelle *f*

sphagiasm, sphagiasmus Petit mal *n*, Epilepsia minor *f*

spheral, spherical sphärisch, rund

sphere Sphäre *f*, Bereich *m* / **~ of feelings** Gefühlssphäre *f* / **deep ~** Tiefenschicht *f* / **instinctual ~** Triebsphäre *f* / **psychosomatic ~** psychosomatischer Bereich *m* / **volitional ~** Willenssphäre *f*

spheric, spherical sphärisch

spherometer Krümmungsmesser *m*

sphincter Schließmuskel *m*, Sphinkter *m* / **~ control** Sphinkterbeherrschung *f* / **~ education** Reinlichkeitserziehung *f*, Sauberkeitsgewöhnung *f* / **~ morality** anales Verhalten *n*

sphygmogram Pulskurve *f*, Sphygmogramm *n*

sphygmograph Sphygmograph *m*, Pulsschreiber *m*

sphygmographic sphygmographisch, Pulsaufzeichnung betreffend

sphygmography Sphygmographie *f*, Pulsschreibung *f*

sphygmomanometer Sphygmomanometer *n*, Blutdruckmesser *m*

sphygmomanometry Blutdruckmessung *f*

sphygmophone Gerät *n* das den Puls hörbar macht

spicy würzig

spider phobia Spinnenphobie *f*

Spielmeyer–Vogt disease Stock–Spielmeyer–Vogt Syndrom *n*, Batten–Mayou Syndrom *n*

spike Spitzenpotential *n*, Spike *m* / **~s** Krampfspitzen *fpl* im EEG / **~ discharge** Spitzenentladung *f* / **~ sand waves** Krampfspitzen *fpl* / **initial ~** Initialzacke *f*

spina Dorn *m*, Wirbelfortsatz *m*, Spina *f* / **~ bifida** Spina bifida *f*, Wirbelspalt *m*

spinal spinal, Rückenmarks–

spindle Spindel *f* / **~ tendon** Sehnenspindel *f* / **muscular ~** Muskelspindel *f* / **neuromuscular ~** Muskelspindel *f* / **neurotendinous ~** Sehnenspindel *f*

spine Rückgrat *n*, Wirbelsäule *f*, Spina *f* / **neural ~** Rückgrat *n*, Rückenmark *n*

spinocerebellar Rückenmark und Kleinhirn betreffend

spinose, spinous dornig, spinös

spiral spiralförmig

spirit Geist *m*, Seele *f*, Spiritus *m* / **~ of solidarity** Geist *m* der Solidarität / **~ possession** Besessenheit *f* / **~–rapping** Geisterklopfen *n* / **high ~s** gehobene Stimmung *f* / **low ~s** gedrückte Stimmung *f*

spirited geistvoll, lebendig, feurig

spiritism Spiritismus *m*, Geisterglaube *m*

spiritual geistig, seelisch, spirituell, intellektuell

spiritualism Spiritualismus *m*, Spiritismus *m*, Geisterglaube *m*

spiritualist Spiritualist *m*, Spiritist *m*

spirituality geistige Eigenschaft *f*, Geistigkeit *f*, Spiritualität *f*

spirituous alkoholisch, alkoholhaltig, Alkohol–

spirogram Aufzeichnung *f* der Atembewegungen, Spirogramm *n*

spirograph Spirograph *m*

spirometer Spirometer *n*

spirometric spirometrisch

spirometry Messung *f* der Atmung, Spirometrie *f*

spite Groll *m*, Ressentiment *m* / ärgern, kränken

splanchnic Eingeweide–, viszeral

spleen Tick *m*, schlechte Laune *f*, Hypochondrie *f* / Milz *f*

splenetic schlecht gelaunt, mürrisch / Hypochonder *m*

split Spaltung *f*, Halbierung *f* / gespalten / **~–ballot technique** Parallelfragemethode *f* / **~–brain** split brain, gespaltenes Gehirn *n* / **~–half correlation** Korrelation *f* nach der Halbierungsmethode / **~–half method** Halbierungsmethode *f*, Testhalbierungsmethode *f* / **~–off** abgespalten

splitter Haarspalter *m*, überpedantischer Systematiker *m*

splitting Spaltung *f* / **~ of consciousness** Bewusstseinsspaltung *f* / **~ of the ego** Spaltung *f* des Ichs, Ich–Spaltung *f* / **~ of the object** Objektspaltung *f* / **~–off** Abspaltung *f*, Dissoziation *f* / **~ of the personality** Persönlichkeitsspaltung *f*

spoiled verwöhnt, verzogen, Stör–

spongioblast Spongioblast *m*, Neurogliamutterzelle *f*

spontaneity Spontanität *f*, unmittelbare Handlungsauslösung *f* / **~ test** Test *m* der Spontanität / **~ therapy** Soziodrama *n*, Spontanitätstherapie *f* / **~ training** Spontanitätsübung *f*

spontaneous spontan, unwillkürlich, aus innerem Antrieb, Spontan–

sport Sport *m*, Spiel *n*, Kurzweil *f* / **~ performance** sportliche Leistung *f* / **~ psychology** Sportpsychologie *f* / **~s spectator** Sportzuschauer *m* / **~ training** Sporttraining *n* / **competitive ~** Leistungssport *m* / **high–performance ~s** Leistungssport *m*

spot Fleck *m*, kurze Werbesendung *f*, Punkt *m* / **~–pattern test** Test *m* mit gruppierten Punkten / **bright–~ experiment** Lichtfleckexperiment *n* / **blind ~** blinder Fleck *m*, Mariottescher Fleck *m*, Sehnerveneintritt *m*, Papille *f* / **cold ~** Kältepunkt *m* / **hot ~** Wärmepunkt *m* / **identical ~s of the retina** deckungsgleiche Punkte *mpl* / **sensory ~** Sinnespunkt *m*, Rezeptor *m* / **warm ~** Wärmepunkt *m* / **yellow ~** gelber Fleck *m*, Macula lutea *f*

spouse Ehepartner(in) *m,f*, Ehegatte *m*, Ehegattin *f* / **~ abuse** Misshandlung *f* des Ehepartners

spread Ausdehnung *f*, Ausbreitung *f* / **~ of effect** Effektausbreitung *f*, Effektbereich *m* / **~ of excitation** Erregungsausbreitung *f* / **~ phenomenon** Streuungsphänomen *n*, Dispersionsphänomen *n* / **associative ~** zufälliges Lernen *n* / **electrotonic ~** elektrotonische Ausbreitung *f* / **passive ~** passive Ausbreitung *f*

spreading Ausdehnung *f*, Ausbreitung *f* / **~ depression** ausgedehnte Depression *f*, „spreading depression" *f* / **~ effect** Breitenwirkung *f* / **~ of effect** Wirkungsbereich *m*, Wirkungsausbreitung *f*

spring grip Reaktionstaste *f*

spurious falsch, unecht, Pseudo–, unehelich

spuriousness Unechtheit *f*, Falschheit *f*, Unehelichkeit *f*

spurt Spurt *m*, kurzzeitige hohe Anstrengung *f* / **beginning ~** Initialspurt *m* / **initial ~** Initialspurt *m*

square Quadrat *n*, Viereck *n* / quadratisch, viereckig / quadrieren / **~ contingency** Chi–Quadrat *n* / **~ lattice** quadratisches Gitter *n* / **~ matrix** quadratische Matrix *f* / **~ measure** Quadratmaß *n* / **~–root** Quadratwurzel *f* / **~ wave** quadratische Welle *f* / **inverse ~ law** Gesetz *n* der Umkehrung des Quadrates / **Latin ~** lateinisches Quadrat *n* / **least–~s method** Methode *f* der kleinsten Quadrate / **mean ~** mittleres Quadrat *n* / **mean ~ deviation** mittlere Quadratabweichung *f*

squareness das Viereckige *n*, Ehrlichkeit *f*

squeal grell schreien, kreischen / Schrei *m*, lautes Kreischen *n*

squealer Petzer *m*

squeamish übergewissenhaft, skrupulös, leicht Ekel empfindend

squint Schielen *n*, Strabismus *m* / **convergent ~** Einwärtsschielen *n* / **divergent ~** Auswärtsschielen *n* / **downward ~** Abwärtsschielen *n* / **external ~** Auswärtsschielen *n* / **latent ~** latentes Schielen *n*, Heterophorie *f* / **upward ~** Aufwärtsschielen *n* / **vertical ~** Aufwärtsschielen *n*, Höhenschielen *n*

S–R, stimulus–response Reiz *m* — Reaktion *f* / **~ association** Reiz–Reaktionsverbindung *f* / **~ law** Reiz–Reaktionsgesetz *n* / **~ theory** Reiz–Reaktionstheorie *f*

S–S, stimulus,stimulus Reiz *m* — Reiz *m* / **~ association** Reiz Reizverbindung *f* / **~ learning** Orientierungslernen *n* / **~ theory** Reiz–Reiztheorie *f*

stabilimeter Stabilimeter *n*, Gerät *n* zur Registrierung von Körperbewegungen

stability Stabilität *f*, Zuverlässigkeit *f*, Retest–Reliabilität *f* / **~ coefficient** Zuverlässigkeitskoeffizient *m* / **emotional ~** emotionale Stabilität *f* / **functional ~** Funktionsstabilität *f* / **occupational ~** berufliche Stabilität *f* / **statistical ~** statistische Signifikanz *f*, statistische Stabilität *f*

stable stabil, fest, beständig

staccato abgehackt, skandiert, staccato

staff Personal *n*, Belegschaft *f*, Angestellten *pl*, Mitarbeiter *mpl*, Stabspersonal *n* / **~ function** Stabsfunktion *f*

stage Stadium *n*, Phase *f*, Periode *f*, Stufe *f*, Bühne *f* / **~ of developing apperception** Apperzeptionsstadium *n*, Apperzeptionskategorie *f* / **~ of development** Entwicklungsstufe *f* / **~ fright** Lampenfieber *n* / **~ of latency** Latenzperiode *f*, Latenzphase *f* / **~ of libidinal organisation** Libidostufe *f* / **~ of mechanization** Stadium *n* der Mechanisierung / **~ of object love** Objektstufe *f* / **~ play** Bühnenspiel *n*, Theaterspiel *n* / **~ by stage combination therapy** sukzessive Kombinationstherapie *f* / **anal ~** anale Phase *f* / **anal–expulsive ~** anal–expulsive Phase *f*, anale Ausstoßungsphase *f* / **anal–retentive ~** anal–retentive Phase *f*, anale Retentionsphase *f* / **anal–sadistic ~** analsadistische Phase *f* / **cannibalistic ~** oral–aggressive Phase *f* / **developmental ~** Entwicklungsstufe *f*, Entwicklungsphase *f* / **ejective ~** Projektionsphase *f* / **experimental ~** Versuchsstadium *n* / **genital ~** genital Phase *f*, genitale Stufe *f* / **libidinal ~** Libidostufe *f* / **oedipal ~** Ödipusphase *f* / **oral ~** orale Phase *f*, orale Stufe *f* / **oral–biting ~** orale Beißphase *f* / **oral–erotic ~** oralerotische Phase *f* / **oral–sadistic ~** oralsadistische Phase *f* / **pastoral ~** pastorale Phase *f* / **phallic ~** phallische Phase *f* / **pregenital ~** prägenitale Phase *f* / **prelingual ~** vorsprachliche Phase *f* / **prenatal developmental ~s** pränatale Entwicklungsstufen *fpl* / **prepsychopathic ~** Präpsychopathie *f* / **primary ~** Primärstadium *n* / **prodromal ~** Prodromalstadium *n* / **projective ~** projektive Phase *f* / **psychosexual ~** psychosexuelle Phase *f* / **psychosocial ~** psychosoziale Phase *f* / **realistic ~** realistisches Stadium *n* / **resting ~** Ruhephase *f*, Ruheperiode *f* / **scribbling ~** Kitzelstadium *n* / **static ~** Dauerzustand *m* / **three–~** dreistufig, dreiphasisch / **transitional ~** Übergangsphase *f*

staircase Treppe *f* / **~ illusion** Treppentäuschung *f* / **~ phenomenon** Treppenphänomen *n*

stamina Kraft *f*, Ausdauer *f*, Widerstandskraft *f*

stammer Stammeln *n*, Stottern *n* / stammeln, stottern

stammering Stammeln *n*, Stottern *n* / **idiopathic ~** Stottern *n*, Stammeln *n*

stamping–in effect Prägungseffekt *m*

stance reflex Haltungsreflex *m*

standard Standard *m*, Norm *f*, Durchschnitt *m* / normal, Normal–, Standard– / **~ behaviour event** typisches Verhalten *n* / **~ deviation** Standardabweichung *f* / **~ difference** Standardunterschied *m* / **~ Einthoven's triangle** Standardableitung *f* nach Einthoven / **~ error** Standardfehler *m* / **~ error of estimate** Standardschätzfehler *m* / **~ error of mean** Standardfehler *m* / **~ error of measurement** Standardmessfehler *m* / **~ error of sampling** Standardstichprobenfehler *m* / **~ group** Normgruppe *f*, Standardgruppe *f* / **~ interpersonal behaviour event** typisches Sozialverhalten *n* / **~ of living** Lebensstandard *m* / **~ measure** Standardwert *m* / **~ observer** Normalbeobachter *m* / **~ of performance** Leistungsmaßstab *m* / **~ pitch** Normalfrequenz *f*, Normalton *m* / **~ psychiatric nomenclature** Psychiatrische Standard–Nomenklatur *f* / **~ score** Standardwert *m* / **~ stimulus** Standardreiz *m*, Normalreiz *m* / **~ test** standardisierter Test *m* / **~ weight** Normalgewicht *n* / **deviate ~** abweichende Norm *f* / **professional ~** beruflicher Standard *m* / **social ~** soziale Norm *f* / **tonal ~** Vergleichston *m*, Normalton *m*

standardisation Standardisierung *f*, Normierung *f*, Normung *f* / **~ group** Eichgruppe *f*, Normgruppe *f* / **~ requirement** Anforderung *f* an eine Standardisierung / **~ of tests** Teststandardisierung *f*, Testeichung *f*, Testnormierung *f* / **~ sample** Standardisierungsstichprobe *f*

standardize standardisieren, normieren

Stanford| achievement test Stanford–Leistungstest *m* / **~–Binet scale** Stanford–Binet–Test *m* / **~–Binet test** Stanford–Binet–Test *m*

stanine Stanine *n* / **~ scale** Stanine–Skala *f* / **~ score** Stanine–Wert *m*

stapedius Steigbügelmuskel *m* / **~ reflex** Stapediusreflex

stapes Steigbügel *m*, Stapes *m*

star Star *m*, hervorragender Mensch *m*

starfish Seestern *m*

starting beginnend, Anfangs–

startle aufschrecken, erschrecken / Erschrecken *n*, Überraschung *f* / **~ pattern** Schreckreaktion *f* / **~ reaction** Schreckreaktion *f*, Zusammenschrecken *n* / **~ reflex** Schreckreaktion *f*, Schreckreflex *m* / **~ response** Schreckreaktion *f*

startling erschreckend, überraschend, alarmierend, Schreck–

starvation Hungern *n*, Verhungern *n*

stasibasiphobia Angst *f* zu gehen und zu stehen, Stasobasophobie *f*

stasiphobia Angst *f* zu stehen, Stasophobie *f*

stasis Stehen *n*, Stauung *f*, Stockung *f* / **~ edema, oedema** Stauungsödem *n*

state Zustand *m*, Lage *f* / **~ anxiety** Situationsangst *f* / **~–dependent learning** zustandabhängiges Lernen *n* / **~ factor** Zustandsfaktor *m* / **~–forming insects** staatenbildende Insekten *npl* / **~ of agitation** Erregungszustand *m* / **~ of anxiety** Angstzustand *m* / **~ of consciousness** Bewusstseinszustand *m* / **altered ~s of consciousness** veränderte Bewusstseinszustände *mpl* / **~ of depression** Depressionszustand *m* / **~ of development** Entwicklungszustand *m* / **~ of disorientation** Verwirrtheit *f* / **~ of excitation** Erregungszustand *m* / **~ of exhaustion** Ermüdungszustand *m*, Erschöpfungszustand *m* / **~ of health** Gesundheitszustand *m*, Befinden *n* / **~ of inhibition** Hemmungszustand *m* / **~ of mind** Geisteszustand *m* / **~ of tension** Spannungszustand *m* / **~ of training** Trainingszustand *m* / **~ of transition** Übergangszustand *m* / **affective ~** Erregungszustand *m* / **amnesic ~** Amnesie *f* / **cataleptoid ~** kataleptischer Zustand *m* / **central inhibitory ~** Zustand *m* langandauernder Hemmung im ZNS / **confusional ~** Verwirrtheitszustand *m* / **conscious ~** Bewusstseinszustand *m* / **crepuscular ~** Dämmerungszustand *m* / **cyclothymic ~** zyklothymer Zustand *m* / **dangerous ~** gefährlicher Zustand *m* / **delirious ~** deliranter Zustand *m* / **depressive ~** Depression *f* / **dreamlike ~** oneiroide Erlebnisform *f*, oneiroider Zustand *m* / **dreamy ~** traumhafte Bewusstseinsstörung *f* / **emotional ~** Gemütszustand *m*, emotionaler Zustand *m*, Befinden *n* / **epileptic ~** Status epilepticus *m* / **euphoric ~** euphorischer Zustand *m* / **excitatory ~** Erregungszustand *m* / **finite ~** vollständige Bestimmung *f* / **finite ~ grammar** vollständig bestimmte Grammatik *f* / **finite ~ language** vollständig bestimmte Sprache *f* / **hypnagogic ~** Einschlafzustand *m*, hypnagoger Zustand *m* / **hypnoid ~** hypnoider Zustand *m*, leichte Hypnose *f* / **hypnopompic ~** Zustand *m* des Aufwachens, hypnopomper Zustand / **hypothetical ~ variable** hypothetische Zustandsvariable *f* / **lacunar ~** lakunäres Syndrom *n* / **mental ~** Geisteszustand *m*, psychischer Befund *m* / **neurotic ~** neurotischer Zustand *m* / **new German ~** neues Bundesland *n* / **obsessional ~** zwanghafte Lage *f* / **obsessive ~** Zwang *m* / **physiological ~** physiologischer Zustand *m* / **psychomotor ~** psychomotorischer Status *m* / **refractory ~** Refraktärstadium *n*, Refraktärzeit *f*, Refraktärphase *f* / **satisfying ~ of affairs** befriedigender Zustand *m* / **stationary ~** stationärer Zustand *m* / **syntonic ~** ausgeglichene, einheitliche Stimmung *f*, Syntonie *f* / **thymic ~** Status thymicolymphaticus *m*

statement Behauptung *f*, Feststellung *f*, Äußerung *f*

static statisch, bewegungslos, ruhend, fest

station Stellung *f*, Stand *m*, Position *f*

stationary stationär, in Ruhe befindlich, feststehend

statistical statistisch

statistics Statistik *f* / **Bayesian ~** Bayes–Statistik *f* / **deductive ~** Inferenzstatistik *f* / **descriptive ~** deskriptive Statistik *f*, beschreibende Statistik *f* / **inferential ~** Inferenzstatistik *f* / **multivariate ~** multivariate Statistik *f* / **nonparametric ~** verteilungsfreies Verfahren *n*, nichtparametrische Statistik *f* / **parametric ~** parametrisches Verfahren *n*, parametrische Statistik *f* / **psychological ~** Psychometrie *f* / **vital ~** Biostatistik *f*, Bevölkerungsstatistik *f*

statocyst Statozyste *f*

statokinetic statokinetisch

statolith Statolith *m*, Gehörsteinchen *n*

statometer Statometer *n*, Vorrichtung *f* zur Ermüdungsmessung

stature Statur *f*, Gestalt *f*, Figur *f*, Wuchs *m*

status Status *m*, soziale Stellung *f* / **~–centered leadership** direktive Führung *f* / **~ discrepancy** Statusdiskrepanz *f* / **~ epilepticus** Status epilepticus *m* / **~ gradient** Statusgradient *m* / **~ grouping** Gliederung *f* nach Status / **~ leader** Führer *m* aufgrund seines Status / **~ mark** Statuszeichen *n*, Statussymbol *n* / **~ need** Statusstreben *n* / **~ seeker** Person *f* mit starkem Statusstreben / **~ striving** Statusstreben *n* / **~ symbol** Statussymbol *n* / **~ value** Statuswert *m* / **achieved ~** erreichter Status *m*, erreichte Stellung *f*, erworbene Position *f* / **ascribed ~** zugeschriebene Position *f* / **emotional ~** Gefühlslage *f*, Stimmung *f* / **marital ~** Familienstand *m* / **mental ~** Geisteszustand *m*, psychischer Befund *m* / **occupational ~** beruflicher Status *m* / **social ~** sozialer Status *m* / **socioeconomic ~** sozioökonomischer Status *m*

statuvolence Selbsthypnose *f*, Autosuggestion *f*

statuvolent selbsthypnotisch

steadiness Beständigkeit *f*, Gleichmäßigkeit *f*, Stetigkeit *f*, Bewegungsruhe *f* / **~ apparatus** Tremometer *n*, Gerät *n* zur Messung der Zitterbewegungen / **~ tester** Tremometer *m*, Gerät *n* zur Messung der Zitterbewegungen / **wary, controlled ~** Behutsamkeit *f*

steady state Fließgleichgewicht *n*, dynamisches Gleichgewicht *n*, Steady state *n*

stealing Stehlen *n*, Diebstahl *m* / **pathological ~** pathologisches Stehlen *n*, Kleptomanie *f*

S technique S–Technik *f*

Stein–Leventhal syndrome Stein–Leventhal–Syndrom *n*, polyzystisches Ovarium *n*

Stellwag's sign Stellwag–Zeichen *n*

stem Stamm *m* / **~ length** Stammlänge *f*, Körperlänge *f* ohne Extremitäten

sten scale Standardskala *f* mit 10 Unterteilungen, Sten–Werte–Skala *f*

stencil Schablone *f*

stenocephalous schmalköpfig

stenocephaly, stenocephalia Schmalköpfigkeit *f*

stenosis Stenose *f*

stenothermal stenotherm

stentor Stentor *m*, übergroße Lautstärke *f*

step Schritt *m*, Stufe *f*, Lerneinheit *f* / **~ by step** Schritt für Schritt, schrittweise / **~ interval** Klassenintervall *n*, Klassengröße *f*, Klassenbreite *f* / **equal ~s** gleiche Abstände *mpl* / **twelve–~ programme** Zwölfstufenprogramm *n*

stepchild Stiefkind *n*

stepfamily Stieffamilie *f*

stepfather Stiefvater *m*

stepmother Stiefmutter *f*

stepparents Stiefeltern *pl*

stepping reflex Schreitreflex *m*

steradian räumlicher Winkel *m*

stereoacuity stereoskopische Schärfe *f*, Tiefenschärfe *f*

stereoagnosis Tastlähmung *f*, Stereoagnosie *f*, Tastblindheit *f*

stereoanaesthesia, stereoanesthesia Tastblindheit *f*, Unempfindlichkeit *f*, Stereoanästhesie *f*

stereocilium Stereozilie *f*

stereognosis Fähigkeit *f* Gegenstände durch Betasten zu erkennen, Tasterkennen *n*, Stereognostik *f*

stereognostic stereognostisch

stereogram Raummessbild *n*, Stereogramm *n*

stereokinesis Stereokinese *f*

stereophonic stereophonisch

stereophony Stereophonie *f*

stereopsis stereoskopisches Sehen *n*, dreidimensionales Sehen *n*, Tiefensehen *n*

stereoscope Stereoskop *n*

stereoscopic stereoskopisch

stereoscopy stereoskopisches Sehen *n*, Stereoskopie *f*

stereotaxic, stereotactic stereotaktisch

stereotaxis Stereotaxis *f*, Stereotropismus *m*, Kontakttropismus *m*

stereotropism Stereotropismus *m*, Stereotaxis *f*

stereotype stereotyp / Stereotyp *n*

stereotyped stereotyp

stereotypy Stereotypie *f* / ~ **of language** Sprachstereotypie *f*

sterile unfruchtbar, steril

sterilisation Sterilisation *f*, Unfruchtbarmachung *f*, Kastration *f*

sterilise sterilisieren, unfruchtbar machen

sterility Sterilität *f*, Unfruchtbarkeit *f*, Unfruchtbarmachung *f*

Stern variator Stern'scher Tonvariator *m*

steroid Steroid *n*, Kortikosteroid *n*, Steroidhormon *n* / ~ **hormone** Steroidhormon *n*

stethograph Stethograph *m*, Pneumatograph *m*

stethography Stethographie *f*, Pneumatographie *f*

stethoscope Stethoskop *n*, Hörrohr *n*

Stevens' power function Stevens–Potenzfunktion *f*

sthenia Stärke *f* Kraft *f*, Körperkraft *f*, Sthenie *f*

sthenic stark, kräftig, sthenisch

sticktest Stick–Test *m*, Goldstein–Test *m*

stiff steif, rigide, starr

stiffening Steifen *n*, Versteifung *f*, Erstarrung *f*

stiffness Steifheit *f*, Starre *f*, Starrheit *f*, Rigidität *f*

stigma Stigma *n*, Kennzeichen *n*, Mal *n* / ~**ta of degeneration** Degenerationszeichen *npl*

stigmatisation Stigmatisation *f*, Auftreten *n* der Wundmale Christi

stigmatise stigmatisieren, brandmarken

stilb Stilb *n*, Einheit *f* der Leuchtdichte

Stiles–Crawford effect Stiles–Crawford–Effekt *m*

stillbirth Totgeburt *f*

Stilling|'s colour tables Stilling–Tafeln *fpl* / ~ **test** Sehprobe *f* mit Stilling–Tafeln

stimulant Stimulans *n*, Anregungsmittel *n* / stimulierend, anregend / **cerebral** ~ Weckmittel *n*, Weckamin *n* / **genital** ~ Aphrodisiakum *n* / **nervous** ~ Nervenreizmittel *n*

stimulate stimulieren, anregen, erregen, reizen, motivieren

stimulating anregend, stimulierend, reizend, motivierend

stimulation Stimulation *f*, Reizung *f*, Anregung *f*, Stimulierung *f* / ~ **seeking** Reizsuche *f* / **adrenergic** ~ adrenergische Reizung *f* / **afferent** ~ afferente Reizung *f*, afferente Stimulation *f* / **auditory** ~ akustische Reizung *f*, auditive Stimulation *f* / **aversive** ~ aversive Reizung *f*, aversive Stimulation *f* / **bipolar** ~ bipolare Reizung *f* / **central** ~ Reizung *f* des Zentralnervensystems / **cerebral** ~ Hirnreizung *f* / **dichoptic** ~ dichoptische Stimulation *f* / **dichotic** ~ dichotische Reizung *f*, dichotische Stimulation *f* / **diencephalic** ~ Zwischenhirnreizung *f* / **electrical** ~ elektrische Reizung *f*, elektrische Stimulation *f* / **environmental** ~ Anregung *f* durch die Umwelt / **excessive** ~ Reizüberflutung *f* / **extracellular** ~ extrazelluläre Reizung *f* / **galvanic** ~ galvanische Reizung *f* / **genital** ~ Reizung *f* der Geschlechtsorgane, Stimulation *f* der Genitalien / **mechanical** ~ mechanische Reizung *f* / **olfactory** ~ Geruchsstimulation *f*, Reizung *f* des Geruchssinns / **optimal** ~ Reizoptimum *n* / **perceptual** ~ perzeptive Stimulation *f* / **photopic** ~ photopische Reizung *f*, photische Stimulation *f* / **prismatic** ~ Prismenstimulation *f*, prismatische Reizung *f* / **reduced** ~ Reizverminderung *f* / **scotopic** ~ skotopische Reizung *f*, skotopische Stimulation *f* / **selective ~** selektive Reizung *f* / **sensory ~** Sinnesreizung *f* / **sexual ~** sexuelle Stimulation *f* / **somaesthetic ~** somästhetische Stimulation *f* / **subliminal ~** unterschwellige Reizdarbietung *f* / **subthreshold ~** unterschwellige Reizung *f* / **tactual ~** taktile Stimulation *f*, taktile Reizung *f* / **tetanic ~** tetanische Reizung *f* / **thermal ~** thermische Reizung *f* / **vestibular ~** Vestibulum–Reizung *f* / **visual ~** visuelle Reizung *f*, visuelle Stimulation *f*

stimulator Stimulator *m*, Stimulationsapparatur *f*, Reizelektrode *f*

stimulogenous reizbedingt, durch Erregung verursacht

stimulus Reiz *m*, Stimulus *m* / **~ ambiguity** Stimulusambiguität *f*, Mehrdeutigkeit *f* eines Reizes / **~ artefact** Reizeinbruch *m*, Reizartefakt *n* / **~ attenuation** Stimulusabschwächung *f*, Reizdämpfung *f* / **~ attitude** Reizobjekteinstellung *f* / **~–bound** reizgebunden / **~ change** Stimulusveränderung *f*, Reizwechsel *m* / **~ complexity** Stimuluskomplexität *f*, Reizkomplexität *f* / **~ compound** Reizkomplex *m* / **~–conducting** reizleitend / **~ conduction** Reizleitung *f*, Reizfortpflanzung *f* / **~ continuum** Reizkontinuum *n*, Reizserie *f* / **~ control** Stimuluskontrolle *f*, Reizkontrolle *f*, Reizsteuerung *f* / **~ deprivation** Reizentzug *m*, Stimulusdeprivation *f* / **~ differentiation** Reizdifferenzierung *f*, Reizunterscheidung *f* / **~ discharge** Reizentladung *f*, Reizabfuhr *f* / **~ discrimination** Stimulusdiskrimination *f*, Reizdiskriminierung *f* / **~ duration** Stimulusdauer *f*, Reizdauer *f* / **~ equivalence** Reizäquivalent *n*, Reizentsprechung *f* / **~ error** Reizirrtum *m*, Reizfehler *m*, Reizquellenaufmerksamkeitsfehler *m* / **~ exposure time** Reizdauer *f*, Dauer *f* der Reizwirkung / **~ field** Reizfeld *n* / **~ figure** Reizfigur *f* / **~ frequency** Stimulusfrequenz *f*, Reizhäufigkeit *f* / **~ function** Reizfunktion *f* / **~ generalisation** Reizgeneralisierung *f*, Stimulusgeneralisation *f* / **~ hallucination** Reizhalluzination *f* / **~–induced** reizbedingt, durch Reize ausgelöst / **~ intensity** Stimulusintensität *f* / **~–intensity dynamism** Reizintensitätsdynamik *f* / **~ interval** Stimulusintervall *n*, reizfreies Intervall *n* / **~ item** festgelegter Denkanstoß *m* / **~ limen** Reizschwelle *f*, Reizlimen *n* / **~ method** Reizmethode *f* / **~ modality** Reizmodalität *f* / **~ novelty** Stimulusneuheit *f*, Neuartigkeit *f* eines Reizes / **~ object** Reizobjekt *n* / **~ offset** Stimulusende *n* / **~ onset** Stimulusbeginn *m* / **~ organisation** Reizorganisation *f* / **~ parameter** Stimulusparameter *m*, Reizgrößen *fpl*, Reizparameter *m* / **~ pattern** Reizmuster *n* / **~ population** Reizmenge *f* / **~ presentation** Reizdarbietung *f* / **~ presentation method** Stimulusdarbietungsmethode *f* / **~ quality** Reizqualitat *f* / **~ range** Reizbereich *m* / **~–response** Reiz–Reaktion *f* / **~–response correlation** Reiz–Reaktionskorrelation *f* / **~–response device** Reiz–Reaktionsgerät *n* / **~–response psychology** Reiz–Reaktionspsychologie *f* / **~–response theory** Reiz–Reaktionstheorie *f*, Stimulus–Response–Theorie *f* / **~ salience** Stimulusaugenfälligkeit *f*, Anreizhervorhebung *f* / **~–sampling theory** Reiz–Stichprobentheorie *f* / **~ scale** Reizskala *f*, Reizintensitätsskala *f* / **~ sensation** Reizempfindung *f* / **~ set** Reizeinstellung *f* / **~ similarity** Stimulusähnlichkeit *f*, Reizähnlichkeit *f* / **~ situation** Reizsituation *f* / **~ structure** Reizstruktur *f* / **~ substitution** Reizsubstitution *f* / **~ summation** Reizsummation *f* / **~ threshold** Reizschwelle *f*, Reizlimen *n*, Empfindungsschwelle *f*, Schwellenwert *m* / **~ trace** Reizspur *f* / **~ value** Reizwert *m* / **~ variability** Stimulusvariabilität *f*, Reizänderung *f*, Reizschwankung *f* / **~ variable** Reizvariable *f* / **~ word** Reizwort *n* / **acoustic ~** akustischer Reiz *m* / **adequate ~** adäquater Reiz *m* / **afferent ~ interaction** Interaktion *f* afferenter Reize / **ambiguous ~** ambivalenter Reiz *m*, zweideutiger Reiz *m* / **anomalous ~** unangepasster Reiz *m* / **auditory ~** Gehörreiz *m* / **aversive ~** aversiver Reiz *m* /

brief–~ therapy Schocktherapie *f*, Behandlung *f* mit milden Schocks / **cold ~** Kältereiz *m* / **conditional ~** bedingter Reiz *m* / **conditioned ~** bedingter Reiz *m*, konditionierter Reiz *m* / **conditioning ~** konditionierender Reiz *m* / **constant ~** konstanter Reiz *m* / **constant ~ method** Methode *f* der konstanten Reize / **consummatory ~** Zielreiz *m*, konsumatorischer Reiz *m* / **differentiating ~** Differenzierungsreiz *m* / **directing ~** Lenkreiz *m* / **discrete ~** einzelner Reiz *m*, diskontinuierlicher Reiz *m* / **discriminative ~** Unterscheidungsreiz *m*, diskriminativer Reiz *m*, Wahlreiz *m*, differenzierender Reiz *m* / **distal ~** distaler Reiz *m* / **effective ~** wirksamer Reiz *m*, funktionaler Reiz *m* / **electric ~** elektrischer Reiz *m* / **endogenous ~** endogener Reiz *m* / **excitatory ~** Reiz *m*, Erregungsauslöser *m* / **exogenous ~** exogener Reiz *m* / **external ~** Außenreiz *m* / **extra ~** Zusatzreiz *m* / **gustatory ~** Geschmacksreiz *m* / **inadequate ~** inadäquater Reiz *m*, unangepasster Reiz *m* / **incidental ~** zufälliger Reiz *m* / **ineffective ~** unwirksamer Reiz *m* / **inhibitory ~** Hemmreiz *m* / **instinctive ~** Triebreiz *m* / **instinctual ~** Triebreiz *m* / **liminal ~** Schwellenreiz *m* / **maintaining ~** Erhaltungsreiz *m* / **maximal ~** maximaler Reiz *m* / **mediated ~ generalization** vermittelte Reizgeneralisierung *f* / **molar ~ trace** molare Reizspur *f* / **motor ~** Bewegungsreiz *m* / **neutral ~** neutraler Reiz *m* / **normal ~** Normalreiz *m* / **novel ~** neuartiger Reiz *m* / **perseverative ~ trace** perseverierende Reizspur *f*, Nacherregung *f* / **physical ~** körperlicher Reiz *m*, Reiz *m* / **pictorial ~** Bild–Stimulus *m* / **prepotent ~** dominanter Reiz *m* / **primary ~** Primärreiz *m*, Ankerreiz *m* / **primary ~ generalization** primäre Reizgeneralisierung *f* / **private ~** persönlicher Reiz *m* / **proprioceptive ~** propriozeptiver Reiz *m* / **proximal ~** proximaler Reiz *m*, körpernaher Reiz *m* / **punctiform ~** punktförmiger Reiz *m* / **pure–~ act** reine Reizhandlung *f* / **reinforcing ~** verstärkender Reiz *m*, Verstärker *m* / **releasing ~** Auslöser *m* / **sensory ~** Sinnesreiz *m* / **signalling ~** Signalreiz *m* / **social ~** sozialer Reiz *m* / **structured ~** strukturierter Reiz *m* / **subliminal ~** unterschwelliger Reiz *m* / **supraliminal ~** überschwelliger Reiz *m* / **terminal ~** Reizmaximum *n* / **thermal ~** Wärmereiz *m* / **unconditioned ~** unbedingter Reiz *m*, unkonditionierter Reiz *m*, unkonditionierter Stimulus *m* / **unitary ~** Einheitsreiz *m*, Bezugsreiz *m*, Ankerreiz *m* / **utilized ~** Nutzreiz *m* / **variable ~** variabler Reiz *m* / **verbal ~** verbaler Stimulus *m* / **warning ~** Warnreiz *m*

stirps, stirpes Erbanlage *f*, Erbmerkmale *npl*, Stamm *m*, Geschlecht *n*, Familienzweig *m*

stirrup Steigbügel *m*

stochastic stochastisch, wahrscheinlichkeitsstatistisch

stock Stamm *m*, Herkunft *f*, Abstammung *f* / **~–breeder** Züchter *m* / **~–breeding** Aufzucht *f*

stocky untersetzt, kurz

stoic stoisch, gelassen / Stoiker *m*

stoicism Stoizismus *m*, Gelassenheit *f*, Gleichmut *m*

stolidness Gleichmut *m*, Schwerfälligkeit *f*, Stumpfheit *f*

stolparsomnia Schläfrigkeit *f*

stomach Magen *m* / **~ breathing** Bauchatmung *f* / **~ emptying** Magenentleerung *f* / **~ rumbles** Magenknurren *n* / **~ wall** Magenwand *f* / **nervous ~** nervöser Magen *m* / **sensitive ~** empfindlicher Magen *m*

stone Stein *m* / **~ age** Steinzeit *f* / **~–deaf** stocktaub / **biliary ~** Gallenstein *m*

stooge Vertrauter *m* des Versuchsleiters, kooperierende Versuchsperson *f*

stoppage Anhalten *n*, Unterbrechen *n*

stopwatch Stoppuhr *f*, Chronometer *n*

storage Speicher *m*, Speicherung *f* / **~ capacity** Speicherkapazität *f* / **~ cell** Speicherzelle *f*, Speicherelement *n* / **~ device**

Speicher *m*, Speichervorrichtung *f* / ~ **period** Speicherzeitraum *m* / ~ **time** Speicherungszeit *f* / **digital** ~ digitaler Speicher *m* / **long–term** ~ Langzeitspeicher *m* / **short–term** ~ Kurzzeitspeicher *m*

storing Speichern *n*, Speicherung *f* / ~ **of data** Datenspeicherung *f*

storm Sturm *m* / toben, wüten / **~–and–stress period** Sturm–und–Drangzeit *f*

story recall test Nacherzähltest *m*

storytelling Erzählen *n* / ~ **technique** Erzählmethode *f* / **mutual** ~ Methode *f* des gegenseitigen Erzählens

stoutness Stärke *f*, Festigkeit *f*, Mut *m*, Ausdauer *f*, Beleibtheit *f*

strabismal Schiel–

strabismometer, strabometer Strabometer *n*, Gerät *n* zur Messung des Schielwinkels

strabismus, strabism Schielen *n*, Strabismus *m* / **convergent** ~ Einwärtsschielen *n* / **divergent** ~ Auswärtsschielen *n* / **external** ~ Auswärtsschielen *n* / **internal** ~ Einwärtsschielen *n* / **paralytic** ~ Lähmungsschielen *n* / **vertical** ~ Aufwärtsschielen *n*, Abwärtsschielen *n*

strabometry Strabometrie *f*, Schielwinkelmessung *f*

straight gerade, direkt, geradlinig

straight–edge experiment Rechteckexperiment *n*

strain Anstrengung *f*, Anspannung *f*, Beanspruchung *f*, Belastung *f*, Überanstrengung *f* / beanspruchen, überbeanspruchen / **emotional** ~ emotionale Belastung *f* / **nervous** ~ nervliche Überbelastung *f* / **physical** ~ physische Belastung *f*

strained überbelastet, gespannt

stranger reaction Reaktion *f* gegenüber Fremden

strangulate strangulieren, erdrosseln

strangulated eingeklemmt

strangulation Erwürgen *n*, Erdrosseln *n*, Strangulation *f*

strangury, stranguria Harnzwang *m*, Blasendrang *m*, Strangurie *f*

strategy Strategie *f*, geplante Vorgehensweise *f* / **coping** ~ Verarbeitungsstrategie *f*

stratification Schichtung *f* / ~ **of personality** Schichtenaufbau *m* der Persönlichkeit / ~ **theory** schichtentheoretisches Modell *n* / **social** ~ soziale Schichtung *f*

stratified geschichtet, stratifiziert

stratify schichten, stratifizieren

Stratton's experiment Stratton'scher Versuch *m*

stratum Stratum *n*, Lage *f*, Schicht *f*

straw poll Probeabstimmung *f*

stream Strom *m*, Fluss *m*, Lauf *m* / ~ **of consciousness** Bewusstseinsstrom *m* / ~ **of thinking** Gedankenfluss *m* / ~ **of thought** Gedankenstrom *m*, Gedankenfluss *m*

streaming Einordnung *f* von Schülern in die adäquate Klasse, fächerübergreifende Differenzierung *f*, Einrichtung *f* von Leistungsklassen

strength Stärke *f*, Kraft *f*, Muskelkraft *f* / ~ **of a colour** Farbintensität *f* / **~–duration curve** Reiz–Zeit–Spannungskurve *f* / ~ **of the ego** Ich–Stärke *f* / ~ **of a habit** Gewohnheitsstärke *f* / ~ **of mind** Charakterstärke *f* / ~ **of response** Reaktionsstärke *f*, Stärke *f* eines Verhaltens / ~ **of will** Willensstärke *f*, Entschlossenheit *f* / **associative** ~ Assoziationsstärke *f* / **emotional** ~ Gefühlsstärke *f* / **physical** ~ körperliche Stärke *f*, physische Stärke *f* / **reproductive** ~ Reaktionsstärke *f*

strephosymbolia Strephosymbolie *f*, seitenverkehrte Wahrnehmung *f* von Gedrucktem

stress Stress *m*, Belastung *f*, Beanspruchung *f*, Druck *m*, Spannung *f* / betonen, den Akzent legen auf / ~ **damage** Stressschaden *m* / ~ **interview** Stressinterview *n* / ~ **management** Stressverarbeitung *f* / ~ **reaction** Stressreaktion *f*, Stressauswirkung *f* / **~–related physiological response**

körperliche Stressreaktion *f* / ~ **relaxation** Stressrelaxation *f* / ~ **situation** Stresssituation *f*, Drucksituation *f* / ~ **syndrome** Stresssyndrom *n* / ~ **test** Stresstest *m* / ~ **tolerance** Stresstoleranz *f* / **acute ~ disorder** akute Belastungsstörung *f* / **acute ~ reaction** akute Belastungsreaktion *f* / **emotional ~** seelische Belastung *f* / **environmental ~** Umweltstress *m* / **occupational ~** beruflicher Stress *m*, berufliche Belastung *f* / **physiological ~** physiologischer Stress *m* / **posttraumatic ~ disorder** posttraumatische Belastungsstörung *f*, posttraumatische Stressreaktion *f*, akute Belastungsreaktion *f* / **psychic ~** psychischer Stress *f* / **psychological ~** psychische Belastung *f*, psychischer Stress *m* / **severe ~** schwere Belastung *f* / **situational ~ test** Stresstest *m*, Stresssituationstest *m* / **social ~** sozialer Stress *m* / **systemic ~** allgemeiner, korperlicher Stress *m*

stressor Stressauslöser *m*, Stressfaktor *m*, stressauslösender Reiz *m*

stretch Spannung *f*, Anspannung *f*, Streckung *f* / ~ **break** Entspannungspause *f* / ~ **reflex** Streckreflex *m*, Dehnungsreflex *m* / ~ **receptor** Dehnungsrezeptor *m*

striate, striated gestreift

striatum Corpus striatum *n*

stricture Stenose *f*

stridor dentium Zähneknirschen *n*

strike Streik *m*, Schlag *m*

string galvanometer Band–Galvanometer *n*

striosome Striosom *n*

strip Streifen *m* / ~ **key** Testauswertungsschlüssel *m* / ~ **record** alphabetische Aktenablage *f* / **metal ~** Metallamelle *f*

striped gestreift

strith Merkmalsklasse *f* einer Population

strive streben, sich bemühen

striving Strebung *f*, Drang *m* / ~ **for admiration** Geltungsstreben *n*, Geltungsdrang *m* / ~ **for esteem** Geltungsstreben *n*, Geltungsdrang *m*

stroboscope Stroboskop *n*

stroboscopic stroboskopisch

stroboscopy Stroboskopie *f*

stroke Anfall *m*, Schlaganfall *m*, Ictus *m* / ~ **volume** Schlagvolumen *n* / **apoplectic ~** Apoplexie *f*, Schlaganfall *m* / **cerebral ~** Hirnschlag *m*, Schlaganfall *m*

strong stark, charakterstark, fest

structural strukturell, Struktur–

structuralisation Strukturierung *f*

structuralism Strukturalismus *m*

structuralist Strukturalist *m*, Anhänger *m* des Strukturalismus

structuration, structuralisation Strukturierung *f* / **hierarchic ~ of character** Charakteraufbau *m*, Tektonik *f* des Charakters

structure Struktur *f*, Aufbau *m*, Gefüge *n*, Gliederung *f*, Anordnung *f*, Gestalt *f* / strukturieren, gliedern / ~ **of the body** Körperbau *m* / ~ **of the dream** Traumstruktur *f* / **~–function reaction** umfassende Reaktion *f*, Globalreaktion *f* / ~ **of intelligence** Intelligenzstruktur *f* / ~ **psychology** Strukturpsychologie *f* / ~ **of a region** Struktur *f* einer Region / ~ **of a stimulus** Reizstruktur *f* / ~ **word** Funktionswort *n* / **associative ~** assoziative Struktur *f* / **biological ~** biologische Struktur *f*, Organstruktur *f* / **cognitive ~** kognitive Struktur *f* / **factorial ~** Faktorenstruktur *f* / **latent ~ analysis** Analyse *f* latenter Strukturen / **mental ~** geistige Struktur *f*, psychische Struktur *f* / **motivational ~** Motivationsstruktur *f* / **organizational ~** Organisationsstruktur *f* / **perceptual ~** Wahrnehmungsstruktur *f* / **phenomenological ~** Erscheinungsfeld *n* / **psychic ~** psychische Struktur *f* / **psychological ~** psychische Struktur *f* / **simple ~** einfache Struktur *f*, Einfachstruktur *f* / **social ~** soziale Struktur *f*, Sozialstruktur *f* / **syntactic ~** Syntax *f* / **vestigial ~** rudimentäre Struktur *f*

structured strukturiert, gegliedert

structureless strukturlos, amorph

structuring Strukturierung *f*, Gliederung *f*

structuronomic nach strukturellen Gesetzmäßigkeiten, strukturgesetzlich

struggle kämpfen / Kampf *m* / **~ for existence** Existenzkampf *m* / **~ for life** Existenzkampf *m*, Kampf *m* ums Überleben / **~ reflex** Kampfreflex *m* / **mental ~** geistig–seelischer Kampf *m*

struma Kropf *m*

strychnine Strychnin *n*

strychninism Strychninvergiftung *f*, Strychninismus *m*

strychninomania Strychninpsychose *f*

stubborn eigensinnig, hartnäckig, dickköpfig, trotzig

stubbornness Eigensinn *m*, Hartnäckigkeit *f*

Student's| distribution Student–Verteilung *f* / **~ test** Student–Test *m*

student Student *m*, Studierender *m*, Schüler *m* / **~ activism** studentischer Aktivismus *m* / **~ admission criteria** Hochschulzulassungskriterien *npl* / **~ attitudes** Einstellung *f* der Studenten / **~ attrition** Studentenschwund *m* / **~ characteristics** Studentenmerkmale *npl* / **~ personnel work** studentische Persönlichkeitsbildung *f* / **~ protest** studentischer Protest *m* / **~ record** studentischer Leistungsnachweis *m*, Zeugnis *n* / **~ teacher** Lehramtsreferendar *m*, studentische Lehrkraft *f* / **~ teaching** Lehrprobe *f*, Lehramtspraktikum *n* / **foreign ~** ausländischer Student *m* / **medical ~** Medizinstudent *m* / **postgraduate ~** Doktorand *m* / **preschool ~** Kindergartenkind *n*

studious eifrig, fleißig

study studieren, untersuchen, erforschen / Studium *n*, Studie *f*, Untersuchung *f*, Erforschung *f* / **~ of fatigue** Ermüdungsforschung *f* / **~ group** Arbeitskreis *m*, Arbeitsgemeinschaft *f*, Studiengruppe *f* / **~ habit** Lerngewohnheit *f*, Studiergewohnheit *f* / **~ of local conditions** Milieustudie *f* / **~ skill** Lernmethode *f*, Lernverfahren *n* / **~ of values** Untersuchung *f* der Wertvorstellungen, Erfassung *f* der Interessen / **cross–cultural ~** kulturvergleichende Untersuchung *f* / **cross–sectional~** Querschnittuntersuchung *f* / **double–blind ~** Doppelblindversuch *m* / **experimental ~ design** Versuchsplan *m* / **follow–up ~** Nachuntersuchung *f* / **foreign ~** Auslandsstudium *n* / **longitudinal ~** Längsschnittuntersuchung *f* / **preliminary ~** Voruntersuchung *f* / **prospective ~** prospektive Studie *f* / **psychological ~** psychologische Untersuchung *f* / **repeat–~** Wiederholung *f*, Wiederholungsuntersuchung *f* / **retrospective ~** retrospektive Studie *f* / **social ~** soziales Fach *n*, Sozialkunde *f*, Gemeinschaftskunde *f* / **social studies education** sozialwissenschaftliche Ausbildung *f*, Sozialkunde *f*

stump Stumpf *m*, Amputationsstumpf *m* / **~ hallucination** Amputationstäuschung *f*

stupemania manischer Stupor *m*

stupid dumm, albern, töricht, stumpfsinnig, stupide

stupidity Stupidität *f*, Stumpfsinn *m*, Dummheit *f*, Albernheit *f*

stupor Stupor *m*, Erstarrung *f*, Bewegungssperre *f*, Benommenheit *f*, Stumpfsinn *m* / **benign ~** gutartiger Stupor *m* / **catatonic ~** katatoner Stupor *m* / **depressive ~** depressiver Stupor *m* / **dissociative ~** dissoziativer Stupor *m* / **emotional ~** Emotionsstupor *m*, Affektstupor *m*, Affektleere *f* / **epileptic ~** epileptische Starre *f* / **hypoglycaemic ~** hypoglykämische Benommenheit *f* / **postepileptic ~** postepileptischer Stupor *m* / **schizophrenic ~** schizophrener Stupor *m*

stutter stottern, stammeln / Stottern *n*, Stammeln *n*

stutterer Stotterer *m*

stuttering Stottern *n*, Stammeln *n*, Balbuties *f*

style Stil *m*, Ausdrucksweise *f* / **~ of life** Lebensstil *m*, Lebensplan *m* / **cognitive ~** kognitiver Stil *m* / **new–~ examination** Test *m* mit gebundener Aufgabenbeantwortung / **old–~ examination** Essay–

Test *m*, Test *m* mit freier Aufgabenbeantwortung / **perceptual ~** Wahrnehmungsstil *m*

stylistic stilistisch, Stil–

stylistics Stilistik *f*, Stil *m*

stylus Stift *m*, Griffel *m*, Taststift *m* / **~ maze** Stiftlabyrinth *n*

subacute subakut, weniger heftig verlaufend

subception unterschwellige Wahrnehmung *f*

subconscious unterbewusst / Unterbewusste *n*

subconsciousness Unterbewusstsein *n*

subcortex Subkortex *m*, Teile *mpl* unterhalb der Großhirnrinde

subcortical subkortikal, unterhalb der Gehirnrinde liegend

subculture Subkultur *f*, Teil *m* einer Kultur

subcutaneous subkutan, unter der Haut gelegen

subdelirium leichtes Delirium *n*

subdrepressive subdepressiv

subdivision Unterteilung *f*, Unterabteilung *f*

subdue unterwerfen, unterjochen

subduedness Unterwürfigkeit *f*

subgoal Nebenziel *n*, Teilziel *n*

subgroup Untergruppe *f*

subharmonic Unterton *m*, Unterschwingung *f*

subhuman annähernd menschlich

subject Subjekt *n*, Person *f*, Versuchsperson *f*, Proband *m*, Thema *n*, Betreff *m*, Fach *n* / unterwerfen, sich aussetzen / **~–matter** Gegenstand *m*, Stoff *m* / **compulsory ~** Pflichtfach *n* / **experimental ~** Versuchsperson *f* / **main ~** Hauptfach *n* / **major ~** Hauptfach *n* / **minor ~** Nebenfach *n* / **optional ~** Wahlfach *n* / **pyknic ~** Pykniker *m* / **required ~** Pflichtfach *n*

subjectify subjektivieren

subjection Unterwerfung *f*, Abhängigkeit *f*

subjective subjektiv

subjectivism Subjektivismus *m*

subjectivity Subjektivität *f*

subjugate unterwerfen

subjugation Unterwerfung *f*

sublimate sublimieren / sublimiert

sublimation Sublimierung *f*, Sublimation *f*

sublime erhaben, hoch, sublim

subliminal unterschwellig, subliminal

sublimity Erhabenheit *f*, Höhepunkt *m*, höchster Grad *m*

sublingual sublingual, unter der Zunge liegend

submarginal unter einer Grenze gelegen

submental unter dem Kinn gelegen

submerge untertauchen, unterdrücken / **the ~d tenth** die Entrechteten *mpl*

submission Unterwerfung *f*

submissive unterwürfig

submissiveness Ergebenheit *f*, Unterwürfigkeit *f*

submit unterbreiten, einreichen

subnormal unternormal, subnormal / **educationally ~** schwer erziehbar

subnormality Subnormalität *f* / **mental ~** Debilität *f*, Geistesschwäche *f*

subordinate untergeordnet / Untergebener *m*

subordination Unterordnung *f*

subprofessional Assistenten–, fachlich nicht voll ausgebildet

subroutine Unterprogramm *n*

subsample Teilstichprobe *f*

subsampling Teilstichprobenerhebung *f*

subservience Unterwürfigkeit *f*

subservient unterwürfig

subshock therapy Therapie *f* mit leichten Schocks

subsidence Abnahme *f*, Nachlassen *n*, Sinken

subsidiation Mittel–Zweck–Relation *f*, Unterordnung *f* / **dynamic ~** dynamische Unterordnung *f*

substance Substanz *f*, Stoff *m* / **~ abuse** Substanzmissbrauch *m* / **~ dependence** Substanzabhängigkeit *f*, Abhängigkeit *f* von psychotropen Substanzen / **~–induced anxiety disorder** substanzinduzierte Angststörung *f* / **~–induced delirium** substanzinduziertes Delir *n* / **~–induced mood disorder** substanzinduzierte affektive Störung *f* / **~–induced persisting amnestic disorder** persistierende substanzinduzierte amnestische Störung *f* / **~–induced persisting dementia** persistierende substanzinduzierte Demenz *f* / **~–induced psychotic disorder** substanzinduzierte psychotische Störung *f* / **~–induced sleep disorder** substanzinduzierte Schlafstörung *f* / **~ intoxication** Substanzintoxikation *f* / **~ intoxication delirium** Substanzintoxikationsdelir *n* / **~ learning** Bedeutungslernen *n* / **~ memorisation** Bedeutungslernen *n* / **~–related disorder** Störung *f* im Zusammenhang mit psychotropen Substanzen / **other ~–related disorders** Störungen *fpl* im Zusammenhang mit anderen Substanzen / **unknown ~–related disorders** Störungen *fpl* im Zusammenhang mit unbekannten Substanzen / **~ use disorders** Störungen *fpl* durch psychotrope Substanzen, Störungen *fpl* durch Substanzkonsum, substanzinduzierte organisch bedingte psychische Störungen *fpl* / **~ withdrawal** Substanzentzug *m* / **~ withdrawal delirium** Substanzentzugsdelir *n* / **blocking ~** Blocker *m* / **dotted ~** Nervenfilz *m*, diffuses Nervennetz *n* / **excitatory ~** Erregungsstoff *m* / **gray ~** graue Hirnsubstanz *f* / **inhibitory ~** Hemmsubstanz *f* / **medullary ~** Marksubstanz *f* / **mental ~** seelische Substanz *f* / **molecular ~** Nervenfilz *m*, diffuses Nervennetz *n* / **neurohumoral ~** neurohumorale Substanz *f* / **photosensitive ~** lichtempfindliche Substanz *f* / **psychic ~** seelische Substanz *f* / **stimulating ~** Reizstoff *m* / **visual ~** Sehstoff *m* / **white ~** weiße Hirnsubstanz *f*

substantia Substanz *f*, Stoff *m* / **~ alba** weiße Hirnsubstanz *f* / **~ grisea** graue Hirnsubstanz *f* / **~ nigra** Nucleus niger *m*

substantial wesentlich, materiell, substanziell

substantiation Substantiation *f*, Verwirklichung *f*, Bestätigung *f*

substantive wirklich, real, wesentlich / Substantiv *n*, Hauptwort *n*

substitute ersetzen, austauschen / Ersatz *m*, Stellvertreter *m* / stellvertretend, Ersatz– / **~ activity** Ersatzhandlung *f*, Übersprungshandlung *f* / **~ formation** Ersatzbildung *f* / **~ for masturbation** Onanieersatz *m*, Masturbationsersatz *m* / **~ for a symptom** Symptomersatz *m* / **regressive ~** Ersatz *m* durch Regression

substitution Ersatz *m*, Substitution *f* / **~ method** Substitutionsmethode *f* / **~ neurosis** Substitutionsneurose *f* / **~ test** Substitutionstest *m* / **~ therapy** Substitutionstherapie *f*

substitutive Ersatz–, substituierend

substrate, substratum Substratum *n*, Teil *n* einer Schicht, Unterschicht *f*

subsume subsumieren, zusammenfassen unter, einbegreifen

subsynaptic subsynaptisch

subsystem Teilsystem *n*, Teilanlage *f*

subtest Untertest *m*, Subtest *m*

subthalamus Subthalamas *m*, unterer Teil *m* des Thalamus

subtheory Teiltheorie *f*

subthreshold unterschwellig, subliminal

subtraction Subtraktion *f*, Abzug *m* / **~ method** Subtraktionsmethode *f*

subtractive abziehend, Abzugs–, Subtraktions–

subversion Subversion *f*, Unterwanderung *f*, Umsturz *m*

subversive subversiv, untergrabend, umstürzlerisch

subvocal lautlos, subvokal

subvocalisation subvokales Sprechen *n*, lautloses Sprechen *n*, subvokale Sprachbildung *f*

sub–whole Teilganzes *n*

success Erfolg *m* / **~ of therapy** Behandlungserfolg *m* / **occupational ~** Berufserfolg *m*, beruflicher Erfolg *m* / **occupational ~ prediction** Vorhersage *f* des Berufserfolgs, Berufserfolgsprognose *f*

successful erfolgreich, gelungen

succession Folge *f*, Nachfolge *f*

successive aufeinanderfolgend, sukzessiv

succinylcholine Succinylcholin *n*, Suxamethoniumchlorid *n*, Bernsteinsäure–bischolinester *m*

succorance Unterstützung *f*, Unterstützungstendenz *f* / **~ need** Unterstützungsbedürfnis *n* / **repressed ~** verdrängtes Unterstützungsbedürfnis *n*

succubus Succubus *m*, weiblicher Dämon *m* der mit Männern geschlechtlich verkehrt

suck saugen

sucking Saugen *n* / saugend, Saug– / **~ reflex** Saugreflex *m* / **~ of thumb** Daumenlutschen *n* / **nonnutritive ~** Saugen *n* ohne Nahrungsaufnahme

suckling Säugling *m*, Säugen *n*, Saugvorgang *m*

suction Saugen *n*, Saugakt *m*

sudation Schweißabsonderung *f*, Schweißsekretion *f*

sudden plötzlich, unvorhergesehen, unerwartet

sudomotor, sudoriferous, sudorific, sudoriparous schweißtreibend, schweißproduzierend

suffer leiden, erleiden, ertragen

suffering leidend, krank / Leiden *n* / **mental ~** seelisches Leiden *n* / **physical ~** körperliches Leiden *n*

sufficient genügend, ausreichend, hinreichend

suffocate ersticken

suffocation Ersticken *n*, Asphyxie *f*

suggest suggerieren, vorschlagen, anregen

suggestibility Suggestibilität *f*, Beeinflussbarkeit *f*

suggestible suggestibel, beeinflussbar

suggestion Suggestion *f*, Vorschlag *m* / **~ therapy** Suggestionstherapie *f* / **hypnotic ~** hypnotischer Befehl *m* / **negative ~** negative Suggestion *f* / **posthypnotic ~** posthypnotische Suggestion *f*, posthypnotischer Befehl *m* / **self–~** Autosuggestion *f* / **therapeutic ~** therapeutische Suggestion *f* / **verbal ~** Verbalsuggestion *f*

suggestive suggestiv

suggestiveness Gedankenanregung *f*, Anspielung *f*, Zweideutigkeit *f*

sui generis einzigartig

suicidal suizidal, selbstmörderisch, Selbstmord–

suicide Selbstmord *m*, Suizid *m*, Freitod *m*, Selbsttötung *f*, Selbstmörder *m*, Suizidant *m* / **~ prevention** Selbstmordverhütung *f*, Suizidprophylaxe *f*, Suizidprävention *f* / **~ prevention centre** Zentrum *n* zur Suizid–Prävention / **assisted ~** unterstützter Suizid *m* / **attempted ~** Selbstmordversuch *m*, Suizidversuch *m* / **collective ~** gemeinsamer Suizid *m* / **double ~** Doppelselbstmord *m*, Doppelsuizid *m* / **to commit ~** Selbstmord begehen / **a potential ~** Lebensmüde *m,f*

suicidology Suizidologie *f*

suigenderism nicht–geschlechtlicher Umgang *m* mit Personen des eigenen Geschlechts, Kameradschaft *f*

sulcal, sulcate gefurcht

sulcus Sulcus *m*, Furche *f* / **~ centralis** Zentralfurche *f*, Sulcus centralis *m* / **calcarine ~** Sulcus calcarinus *m* / **central ~** Zentralfurche *f*, Sulcus centralis *m* / **cerebellar ~** Kleinhirnfurche *f* / **cerebral ~** Rindenfurche *f*

sulkiness schlechte Laune *f*, Schmollen *n*

sulpiride Sulpirid *n*

sum Summe *f* / **~ of excitation** Erregungssumme *f* / **~ score** Summenwert *m* / **~ total** Gesamtsumme *f* / **algebraic ~** algebraische Summe *f*

summarize zusammenfassen, resümieren

summarizing Zusammenfassung *f*, Resümee *n*, Übersicht *f*

summary zusammenfassend, summarisch / Übersicht *f*, Abriss *m*, Zusammenfassung *f*

summating Summations–

summation Summation *f* Summierung *f* / **~ curve** Summenkurve *f*, kumulative Häufigkeitskurve *f*, Ogive *f*, Summenfrequenzpolygon *n* / **~ effect** Summationseffekt *m* / **~ method** Summationsmethode *f* / **~ potential** Summationspotential *n* / **~ of stimuli** Reizsummierung *f*, Summation *f* der Reize / **~ time** Summationszeit *f* / **~ tone** Summationston *m* / **sensory ~** Reizsummation *f*, Reizsummierung *f* / **sensory ~ effect** Reizsummierungseffekt *m* / **spatial ~** räumliche Summation *f* / **temporal ~** zeitliche Summation *f*

superactivity Überfunktion *f*, motorische Unruhe *f*

superadd hinzufügen

superconscious das Bewusstsein überschreitend

superconstancy Überkonstanz *f*

superego Über–Ich *n* / **~ conflict** Über–Ich–Konflikt *m* / **~ integration** Über–Ich–Integration *f* / **~ motivation** Über–Ich–Motivation *f* / **~ resistance** Über–Ich–Widerstand *m*

superexcitation Übererregung *f*, Überreizung *f*

superexcite übererregen, überreizen

superficial oberflächlich, an der Oberfläche befindlich

superfluous überflüssig

superhuman übermenschlich / Übermensch *m*

superimpose auflegen, hinzufügen, überlagern

superior höher, überlegen / Vorgesetzter *m*

superiority Überlegenheit *f* / **~ complex** Superioritätskomplex *m*, Überlegenheitskomplex *m* / **~ feeling** Überlegenheitsgefühl *n* / **~ need** Bedürfnis *n* nach Überlegenheit / **emotional ~** emotionale Überlegenheit *f*

superman Übermensch *m*

supernatural übernatürlich

supernaturalism Wunderglaube *m*, Supernaturalismus *m*

supernormal über das Normale hinausgehend, übernormal

superordination Überordnung *f*, Höhergruppierung *f*

superoxide dismutase Superoxiddismutase *f*

supersaturate übersättigen

supersensitive überempfindlich

supersensitivity Überempfindlichkeit *f* / **~ to stimuli** Reizüberempfindlichkeit *f*

supersonic sehr hochfrequent, überschallschnell, Ultraschall–, Überschall–

superstition Aberglaube *m*

superstitious abergläubisch

superstructure Oberbau *m*, Überbau *m* / **mental ~** seelischer Überbau *m* / **psychic ~** psychischer Überbau *m* / **psychological ~** psychischer Überbau *m*

supervalent qualitative Steigerung *f* / **social ~** sozial bedingte Qualitätssteigerung *f*

supervision Supervision *f*, Überwachung *f*, Aufsicht *f*, Leitung *f*, Kontrolle *f* / **~ of conduct** Führungsaufsicht *f* / **democratic ~** demokratische Führung *f* / **lower ~** unterste Führungsebene *f* / **professional ~** Supervision *f*

supervisor Vorgesetzter *m*, untere Führungskraft *f* / **~–employee interaction** Vorgesetzten–Untergebenen–Interaktion *f*

/ ~ **training** Vorgesetztenschulung *f* / **first–line** ~ Meister *m*, Vorarbeiter *m*, Werkführer *m*

supervisory Aufsichts–, geführt, kontrolliert

supination Auswärtsdrehung *f*, Supination *f*

supine auf dem Rücken liegend

supple anpassungsfähig, geschmeidig

supplement Ergänzung *f*, Nachtrag *m*, Supplement *n*

supplemental ergänzend, Ergänzungs–

suppleness Anpassungsfähigkeit *f*, Flexibilität *f*, Umstellbarkeit *f*

support ertragen, dulden, unterstützen, helfen, fördern / Unterstützung *f*, Hilfe *f*, Erhaltung *f* / ~ **for a theory** Untermauerung *f* einer Theorie / ~ **group** unterstützende Gruppe *f* / **social** ~ **network** soziales Unterstützungsnetzwerk *n*

supportive unterstützend, helfend, Unterstützungs–

supposition Voraussetzung *f*, Annahme *f*, Postulat *n*

suppress unterdrücken, hemmen, dämpfen

suppressant Hemmer *m*, Blocker *m* / **autonomic** ~ Ganglienblocker *m*

suppressed gehemmt, verhalten, unterdrückt

suppressibility Zurückhaltung *f*

suppression Unterdrückung *f*, Hemmung *f*, Verdrängung *f* / ~ **areas** Hemmungsfelder *npl* / **conditioned** ~ konditionierte Hemmung *f* / **monocular** ~ Unterdrückung *f* der Wahrnehmungsreize eines Auges / **social** ~ gesellschaftliche Unterdrückung *f*

suppressive unterdrückend, hemmend

suppressor Hemmer *m*, Suppressor *m* / ~ **areas** Suppressor–Felder *npl*, Hemmbereiche *mpl*, Hemmzentren *npl* / ~ **variable** Suppressorvariable *f*

supraliminal über einem Schwellenwert liegend, überschwellig

supraordinate übergeordnet

suprapubic über dem Schambein liegend

suprarenal Nebennieren–

suprarenin, suprarenalin Adrenalin *n*, Suprarenin *n*, Epinephrin *n*

suprasegmental segmentübergreifend

surdimute, surdomute taubstumm / Taubstumme *m,f*

surdimutism Taubstummheit *f*

surdity Taubheit *f*

surface Oberfläche *f* / ~ **anaesthesia** Oberflächenanästhesie *f* / ~ **colour** Oberflächenfarbe *f* / ~ **electrode** Oberflächenelektrode *f* / ~ **of consciousness** Bewusstseinsoberfläche *f* / ~ **structure** Oberflächenstruktur *f* / ~ **therapy** zudeckende Psychotherapie *f* / ~ **trait** Oberflächenmerkmal *n*, Oberflächeneigenschaft *f*, Oberflächenwesenszug *m* / **olfactory** ~ Riechfläche *f* / **reflecting** ~ spiegelnde Oberfläche *f*, reflektierende Oberfläche *f* / **refracting** ~ brechende Fläche *f* / **transparent** ~ **colour** transparente Oberflächenfarbe *f*

surgence, surgency Aufgeschlossenheit *f*, unbekümmertes, sorgloses Verhalten *n*

surgent aufgeschlossen

surgeon Chirurg *m*

surgery Chirurgie *f* / **cerebral** ~ Gehirnchirurgie *f* / **dental** ~ Zahnchirurgie *f*, Kieferchirurgie *f* / **neuro**~ Nervenchirurgie *f*, Neurochirurgie *f* / **plastic** ~ plastische Chirurgie *f*

surgical chirurgisch, operativ

surprise Überraschung *f*, Verwunderung *f*, Erstaunen *n*

surrender Aufgabe *f*, Kapitulation *f* / aufgeben, verzichten / **altruistic** ~ altruistischer Verzicht *m* / **psychotic** ~ psychotischer Zerfall *m*, Versandung *f*

surreptitious durch Betrug erlangt, betrügerisch, erschlichen, heimlich, verstohlen

surrogate Ersatz *m*, Stellvertreter *m*, Surrogat *n* / ~ **parents** Ersatzeltern *pl*, Vormund *m*

surround Lebensbedingungen *fpl*, unmittelbare Umgebung *f* / ~ **inhibition** Hemmung *f* durch die Umgebung

surroundings Umgebung *f*, Umwelt *f*, Milieu *n*

sursumduction Bewegung *f* nach oben

sursumvergence Aufwärtsbewegung *f* nur eines Auges

surveillance Überwachung *f*, Aufsicht *f*, Kontrolle *f*

survey Untersuchung *f*, Überprüfung *f*, Befragung *f*, Umfrage *f* / ~ **method** Befragungsmethode *f* Erhebungsmethode *f* / ~ **research** Erkundungsuntersuchung *f* / ~ **test** Befragungstest *m* / **interpretative ~** Motivumfrage *f*, Ursachenuntersuchung *f* / **normative ~** Normenfeststellung *f*, Normierung *f*

survival Überleben *n* / ~ **instinct** Überlebenstrieb *m*, Selbsterhaltungstrieb *m* / ~ **of the fittest** Überleben *n* der Tüchtigsten, positive Auswahl *f* / ~ **value** Überlebenswert *m*, arterhaltender Wert *m*

survivor Überlebender *m*, Hinterbliebener *m* / ~ **syndrome** Überlebendensyndrom *n*

susceptibility Anfälligkeit *f*, Empfänglichkeit *f*, Empfindlichkeit *f*, Rezeptivität *f* / **hypnotic ~** Hypnotisierbarkeit *f*, Hypnoseempfänglichkeit *f*

susceptible empfänglich, empfindlich, sensibel, zugänglich, besetzbar

suspect beargwöhnen, Misstrauen hegen, verdächtigen

suspense Aussetzung *f*, Aufschub *m*, Ungewissheit *f* / **in ~** in der Schwebe

suspension Suspension *f*, Enthebung *f*, Suspendierung *f*

suspicion Verdacht *m* / Misstrauen *n*, Argwohn *m*

suspicious verdächtig, argwöhnisch, misstrauisch

sustained andauernd, anhaltend, ununterbrochen, gleichmäßig

suture Naht *f*, Nahtstelle *f*

S variable S–Variable *f*, Reizvariable *f*

swaddle in Windeln legen, wickeln

swarm schwärmen, wimmeln, sich drängeln / Schwarm *m*, Menschenschwarm *m*, Bienenschwarm *m*

sweat Schweiß *m* / schwitzen, transpirieren / ~ **gland** Schweißdrüse *f*

sweating Transpiration *f*, Schwitzen *n*, Schweißabsonderung *f*, Schweißsekretion *f*

sweet süß

sweetness Süße *f*

swallowing Schlucken *n*

swelling Schwellung *f*, Anschwellung *f*

swim bladder Schwimmblase *f*

swimming Schwimmen *n*

swindle beschwindeln, betrügen / Schwindel *m*, Betrug *m*

Swindle's ghost verlängerte positive Nachempfindung *f*

swindling betrügerisch, Schwindel

swing Schaukel *f* / **haunted ~** Geisterschaukel *f* / **haunted ~ illusion** Schaukelillusion *f*

switchboard Schalttafel *f*, Schaltbrett *n* / ~ **learning** Schaltbrettlernen *n*

switch resistance Vorschaltwiderstand *m*

swoon Ohnmacht *f*, Ohnmachtsanfall *m* / ohnmächtig werden

sycophancy Kriecherei *f*

sycophant Kriecher *m*, Schmeichler *m*

sycophantic, sycophantish kriecherisch

Sydenham's chorea Veitstanz *m*, Chorea / ~ **minor** *f* Sydenham–Chorea *f*

syllabism Silbenschrift *f*, skandierende Sprechweise *f*

syllable Silbe *f* / **~–span test** Test *m* des unmittelbaren Behaltens von Silben / **senseless ~** sinnlose Silbe *f*

syllogism Syllogismus *m*, Vernunftschluss *m*

Sylvius| aqueduct Aquaeductus cerebri *n* / **~ fissure** Silvius–Furche *f*, Sulcus lateralis *m* / **~ sulcus** Sulcus lateralis *m*, Silvius–Furche *f*

symbiosis Symbiose *f*, Zusammenleben *n* zum beiderseitigen Nutzen / **biological ~** Symbiose *f*, biologische Symbiose *f*

symbiotic symbiotisch, in Symbiose lebend, partnerschaftlich

symbol Symbol *n*, Zeichen *n*, Sinnbild *n* / **~ cathexis** Symbolbesetzung *f* / **~ of a construct** Konstruktsymbol *n* / **~–digit test** Zahlensymboltest *m* / **~ erotism** Symbolerotik *f* / **~–substitution test** Symboltest *m*, Zeichensymboltest *m* / **anticipatory ~** Zeichen *n*, antizipatorisches Symbol *n* / **expressive ~** Ausdruckssymbol *n* / **mnemic ~** Erinnerungssymbol *n* / **phallic ~** Phallussymbol *n* / **propositional ~** Satzzeichen *n* / **sexual ~** Sexualsymbol *n*, sexuelles Symbol *n* / **universal ~** universelles Symbol *n*

symbolic symbolisch / Symbolische *n*

symbolisation Symbolisation *f*, Symbolisierung *f*, Versinnbildlichung *f*

symbolism Symbolismus *m*, Symbolik *f* / **phonetic ~** phonetischer Symbolismus *m*, Lautsymbolik *f*

symbolize symbolisieren, sinnbildlich darstellen

symbolophobia Symbolophobie *f*, Zwangsvorstellung *f* dass ein Ereignis symbolhaften Charakter habe und Unglück anzeige

symmetrical symmetrisch

symmetry Symmetrie *f*

sympathectomy Sympathikusdurchtrennung *f*, Entfernung *f* sympathischer Ganglien

sympathetic sympathisch, verständnisvoll, mitfühlend, Sympathikus–, das sympathische Nervensystem betreffend

sympathicoadrenal sympathikoadrenal

sympatheticotonia, sympathicotonia Sympathikotonie *f*, gesteigerte Erregbarkeit *f* des Sympathikus

sympatheticotonic, sympathicotonic sympathikoton

sympathicus Sympathikus *m*, Nervus sympathicus *m*

sympathin Sympathin *n* / **exhibitory ~** Noradrenalin *n* / **inhibitory ~** Adrenalin *n*

sympathism Neigung *f* zu Suggestionseinflüssen

sympathist suggestibler Mensch *m*

sympathize sympathisieren, mitfühlen

sympatholytic, sympathicolytic sympathikolytisch / Sympathikolytikum *n*

sympathomimetic, sympathicomimetic sympathikomimetisch / Sympathikomimetikum *n*

sympathy Sympathie *f*, Verständnis *n*, Mitgefühl *n*, Mitleid *n*, Anteilnahme *f*

symposium Symposion *n*, wissenschaftliche Tagung *f*

symptom Symptom *n*, Anzeichen *n* / **~ analysis** Symptomanalyse *f* / **~ checklist** Symptomliste *f* / **~ choice** Symptomwahl *f* / **~ cluster** Syndrom *n*, Symptomenkomplex *m* / **~ complex** Syndrom *n*, Symptomenkomplex *m* / **~ displacement** Symptomverschiebung *f* / **~ formation** Symptombildung *f* / **~ neurosis** symptomatische Neurose *f* / **~ of depersonalisation** Depersonalisationserscheinung *f* / **~ of depression** Depressionserscheinung *f* / **~ of withdrawal** Entzugssymptom *n* / **~ provocation** Symptomprovokation *f* / **~ remission** Abklingen *n* der Symptome, Symptomremission *f* / **~ removal** Symptombeseitigung *f* / **~ substitute** Symptomersatz *m* / **~ substitution** Symptomverschiebung *f* / **~ value** Symptomwert *m* / **accompanying ~** Begleitsymptom *n* / **autoplastic ~** autoplastisches Krankheitsbild *n* / **axial ~** Achsensymptom *n* / **basic ~s** Grundsymptome *npl* / **concomitant ~** Begleitsymptom *n* / **dissociative ~** dissoziatives Symptom *n* / **entoptic ~** entoptische Erscheinung *f* / **entotic ~** entotische Erscheinung *f* / **extrapyra-**

midal ~ extrapyramidales Symptom *n* / **focal** ~ Herdsymptom *n* / **focal cerebral** ~ zerebrales Herdsymptom *n* / **negative** ~ negatives Symptom *n* / **neurological** ~ neurologisches Symptom *n* / **neurotic** ~**s** neurotische Symptome *npl* / **positive** ~ positives Symptom *n* / **positive and negative** ~**s** Positiv– und Negativsymptomatik *f* / **premonitory** ~ Prodrom *n*, Frühsymptom *n* / **primary** ~**s** Grundsymptome *npl* / **prodromal** ~ Prodrom *n*, Vorzeichen *n* / **psychiatric** ~ psychiatrisches Symptom *n* / **subjective** ~ subjektives Symptom *n*

symptomatic symptomatisch, charakteristisch, bezeichnend

symptomatology Symptomatologie *f*, Semiotik *f*, Semiologie *f* / **clinical** ~ Lehre *f* von den Krankheitsbildern

synaesthesia Mitempfindung *f*, Synästhesie *f*

synapse Synapse *f*, Nervenverbindungsstelle *f*, Umschaltstelle *f* / ~ **time** synaptische Überleitungszeit *f* / **axoaxonic** ~ axoaxonische Synapse *f* / **axodentritic** ~ axodendritische Synapse *f* / **axosomatic** ~ axosomatische Synapse *f* / **chemical** ~ chemische Synapse *f* / **dendrodentric** ~ dendrodendritische Synapse *f* / **electrical** ~ elektrische Synapse *f* / **electrically transmitting** ~ elektrische Synapse / **excitatory** ~ exzitatorische Synapse *f* / **inhibitory** ~ hemmende Synapse *f* / **myoneural** ~ myoneuronale Synapse *f* / **neuromuscular** ~ neuromuskuläre Synapse *f* / **neuro–neuronal** ~ neuro–neuronale Synapse *f* / **somato–somatic** ~ somato–somatische Synapse *f*

synapsis Synapse *f*

synaptic synaptisch

synaptology Synaptologie *f*, Lehre *f* von den Synapsen

synchronicity Gleichzeitigkeit *f*, Synchronizität *f*

synchronisation Synchronisation *f*

synchronism, synchronia, synchrony Synchronismus *m*, Gleichzeitigkeit *f*

synchronizer Synchronisator *m*

synchronizing Synchronisierung *f*, Synkretismus *m*

synchronous gleichzeitig, synchron

syncope Ohnmacht *f*, Bewusstlosigkeit *f*, Synkope *f* / **laryngeal** ~ Kehlkopfschlag *m*

syncretic, syncretistic synkretisch

syncretism Synkretismus *m*, Verschmelzung *f* verschiedener heidnischer Kulte

syncytium Synzytium *n*, Zellverband *m* / **functional** ~ funktionelles Synzytium *n*

syndactylism, syndactylia, syndactyly Syndaktylie *f*, zusammengewachsene Finger *mpl*

syndactylous mit zusammengewachsenen Fingern

syndrome Syndrom *n*, Symptomenkomplex *m*, Krankheitsbild *n* / ~ **of approximate answers** Ganser'sches Syndrom *n*, Syndrom *n* einer vorgetäuschten Geistesstörung / ~ **of de Sanctis and Cacchione** de Sanctis–Cacchione Syndrom *n* / ~ **of general neurosis** Syndrom *n* einer Allgemeinneurose / ~ **of reference** Beziehungssyndrom *n* / **adiposogenital** ~ Fröhlich Syndrom *n* / **affective** ~ Affektsyndrom *n* / **amnesic** ~ amnestisches Syndrom *n* / **amnestic** ~ amnestisches Syndrom *n* / **apallic** ~ apallisches Syndrom *n* / **behavioural** ~**s associated with physiological disturbances and physical factors** Verhaltensauffälligkeiten *fpl* in Verbindung mit körperlichen Störungen und Faktoren / **cavernous** ~ Foix–Syndrom *n* / **choreic–athetotic** ~ choreatisch–athetotisches Syndrom *n* / **culture–specific** ~ kulturspezifisches Syndrom *f* / **delusional** ~ Wahnkomplex *m* / **depressive** ~ depressives Syndrom *n*, depressiv–zyklothymes Syndrom *n* / **dysglandular** ~**s** dysglandulare Syndrome *npl* / **dysmnesic** ~ dysmnestisches Syndrom *n* / **expansive** ~ expansives

Syndrom *n* / **extrapyramidal ~** striopallidärer Symptomenkomplex *m* / **frontal ~** Stirnhirnsyndrom *n* Syndrom *n* des Frontallappens / **hepatocerebral ~** hepatozerebrales Syndrom *n* / **hyperkinetic ~** hyperkinetisches Syndrom *n* / **neuroleptic malignant ~** malignes neuroleptisches Syndrom *n* / **nuclear ~** Kernsyndrom *n* / **occipital ~** Hinterhauptsyndrom *n* / **organic amnesic ~, not induced by alcohol and other psychoactive substances** organisches amnestisches Syndrom *n*, nicht durch Alkohol oder sonstige psychotrope Substanzen bedingt / **organic delusional ~** organisch bedingtes Wahnsyndrom *n* / **organic mental ~** organisch bedingtes psychisches Syndrom *n* / **paranoic ~** paranoides Syndrom *n* / **polyneuritic ~** Korsakow–Syndrom *n* / **postconcussional ~** organisches Psychosyndrom *n* nach Schädelhirntrauma, postkommotionelles Syndrom *n* / **postencephalitic ~** postenzephalitisches Syndrom *n* / **presuicidal ~** präsuizidales Syndrom *n* / **psycho–organic ~** psychoorganisches Syndrom *n* / **thalamic ~** Thalamussyndrom *n*, Déjérine–Roussy–Syndrom *n* / **transitional ~** Durchgangssyndrom *n* / **unspecified behavioural ~s associated with physiological disturbances and physical factors** nicht näher bezeichnete Verhaltensauffälligkeiten *fpl* bei körperlichen Störungen und Faktoren

syndromic Syndrom–, Symptomenkomplex betreffend

syndromogenetic syndromogenetisch

synecology Lehre *f* von den Beziehungen zwischen Lebensgemeinschaften und ihrer Umwelt

synectics Synektik *n*

synergia, synergy, synergism Synergie *f*, Zusammenwirken *n*, Koordination *f*, Synergismus *m* / **effective ~** wirksame Koordination *f*

synergic, synergetic, synergistic synergistisch, zusammenwirkend

synergist Synergist *m*, mitwirkender Muskel *m*

synergize zusammenarbeiten, zusammenwirken

synesthesia, synesthesis Mitempfindung *f*, Synästhesie *f*

syngamy geschlechtliche Fortpflanzung *f*

synkinesia, synkinesis begleitende Bewegung *f*, Assoziationsbewegung *f*, Synkinese *f*

synkinetic sich miteinander bewegend

synonym Synonym *n*

synonym–antonym test Test *m* gleicher und gegensätzlicher Begriffe

synonymy Synonymie *f*, Lehre *f* von der Ähnlichkeit der Begriffsbedeutungen

synopsia, synopsy Farbenhören *n*, Phonopsie *f*, Synopsie *f*, Pseudochromästhesie *f*, Synopsis *f*

synopsis vergleichende Übersicht *f*, Zusammenschau *f*, Synopse *f*

synoptic nebeneinandergereiht, übersichtlich, synoptisch, Farbenhören betreffend

syntactic syntaktisch

syntactics Syntax *f*

syntality Syntalität *f*, Charakter *m* einer Gruppe

syntax Satzlehre *f*, Syntax *f*

syntaxic syntaktisch, erfahrungsmäßig übereinstimmend

synthesis Synthese *f*, Zusammenfügen *n*, Verbindung *f* / **creative ~** schöpferische Synthese *f* / **morphological ~** morphologische Synthese *f*, Gestaltsynthese *f* / **selective ~** selektive Verbindung *f*

synthetic synthetisch, künstlich hergestellt

syntoid, syntone, syntonic ausgeglichen, synton

syntony, syntonia Syntonie *f*, Ausgeglichenheit *f*

syntropic gleichgerichtet

syphilis Syphilis *f*, Lues *f*

syphilophobia, syphilomania Angst *f* vor Syphiliserkrankung, Syphilophobie *f*

syphilophobic syphilophob

syphilopsychosis durch Syphilis hervorgerufene Psychose *f*, Syphilopsychose *f*

syringomyelia Syringomyelie *f*

syringomyelitis Syringomyelitis *f*

system System *n* / **~s analysis** Systemanalyse *f* / **~s analyst** Systemanalytiker *m* / **~ equation** Systemgleichung *f* / **~ of education** Erziehungssystem *n* / **~ performance** Systemleistung *f* / **~s research** Systemforschung *f* / **~ segregation** Systemtrennung *f* / **~ specifications** Systemspezifizierungen *fpl* / **general ~s theory** allgemeine Systemtheorie *f* / **acoustic ~** Gehörsystem *n* / **adrenergic nervous ~** adrenergisches Nervensystem *n* / **afferent nervous ~** sensorisches Nervensystem *n* / **anatomical ~** anatomisches System *n* / **ascending reticular activating ~** aufsteigendes retikuläres Aktivierungssystem *n* / **autonomic nervous ~** antonomes Nervensystem *n*, vegetatives Nervensystem *n* / **binary ~** Binärsystem *n* / **biospheric ~** Biosphärensystem *n* / **cardiovascular ~** Herz–Kreislauf–System *n*, kardiovaskuläres System *n* / **causal ~** Kausalsystem *n* / **central nervous ~** Zentralnervensystem *n* / **centrencephalic ~** zentrales Gehirnsystem *n* / **cerebrospinal ~** Zerebrospinalsystem *n* / **closed ~** geschlossenes System *n* / **collateral ~** Kollateralsystem *n* / **compulsive ~** Zwangssystem *n* / **conceptual nervous ~** begriffliches Nervensystem *n* / **conducting ~** Reizleitungssystem *n* / **cultural ~** Kultursystem *n* / **digestive ~** Verdauungssystem *n* / **digestive ~ disorder** Erkrankung *f* des Verdauungssystems / **dynamic ~** dynamisches System *n* / **educational ~** Erziehungssystem *n* / **endocrine ~** endokrines System *n* / **enteric nervous ~** Darmnervensystem *n* / **extrapyramidal ~** extrapyramidales System *n* / **gastrointestinal ~** Magen–Darm–System *n*, Verdauungssystem *n* / **general ~s theory** Systemtheorie *f* / **glandular ~** Drüsensystem *n* / **hierarchical ~** Hierarchie *f*, hierarchisches System *n* / **higher motor ~** höhere Motorik *f* / **higher nervous ~ activity** höhere Nerventätigkeit *f* / **hormonic ~** Hormonsystem *n* / **hypothalamo–hypophyseal ~** Hypothalamus–Hypophysen–System *n* / **hypothalamo–pituitary–adrenal ~** Hypothalamus–Hypophysen–Nebennierensystem *n* / **interoceptive ~** Eingeweidenervensystem *n* / **involuntary nervous ~** vegetatives Nervensystem *n* / **labyrinthine ~** Gleichgewichtsorgan *n*, Ohrlabyrinth *n* / **lemniscal ~** Lemniskussystem *n*, Hinterstrangsystem *n* / **limbic ~** limbisches System *n* / **linear ~** lineares System *n* / **lymphatic ~** lymphatisches System *n* / **manual ~** manuelles System *n* / **mechanical ~** mechanisches System *n* / **metric ~** metrisches System *n* / **mnemonic ~** mnemonisches System *n* / **monochromatic ~** monochromatisches System *n* / **motor ~** motorisches System *n*, Motorik *f* / **muscular ~** Muskulatur *f* / **musculoskeletal ~** Skelettmuskelsystem *n* / **nervous ~** Nervensystem *n* / **nervous ~ disorder** Störung *f* des Nervensystems, Erkrankung *f* des Nervensystems / **neurohumoral ~** neurohumorales System *n* / **neuroleptic malignant ~** malignes neuroleptisches Syndrom *n* / **neurovegetative ~** neurovegetatives System *n* / **nocifensor ~** autonomes System *n* der schmerzleitenden Hautfasern / **oikotropic ~** Ökosystem *n*, autonomes System *n* / **on/off ~** Ein–Aus–System *n* / **open ~** offenes System *n* / **optical ~** optisches System *n* / **orthosympathetic nervous ~** sympathisches Nervensystem *n* / **parasympathetic ~** parasympathisches System *n*, Parasympathikus *m* / **parasympathetic nervous ~** parasympathisches Nervensystem *n*, Parasympathikus *m* / **peripheral nervous ~** peripheres Nervensystem *n* / **photopic ~** photopisches System *n*, Tagessehsystem *n* / **pituitary–adrenocortical ~** Hypophysen–Nebennierenrinden–System *n* / **political economic ~** politisch–ökonomisches System *n* / **postural motor ~** Stützmotorik *f* / **projective ~** Projektionssystem *n* / **pyramidal ~** Pyramidenbahnsystem *n* /

refracting optical ~ System *n* der Lichtbrechung / **reproductive ~** Genitalapparat *m* / **respiratory ~** Atmungsorgane *npl*, Atemsystem *n* / **reticular activating ~** retikuläres Aktivierungssystem *n* / **scotopic ~** Dämmerungsapparat *m* / **second signalling ~** zweites Signalsystem *n* / **sensory ~** Sinnesnervensystem *n* / **social ~** Sozialsystem *n* / **somatic nervous ~** animales Nervensystem *n*, somatisches Nervensystem *n* / **somatosensory ~** Somatosensorik *f* / **specific ~** funktionsspezifisches System *n* / **spinal motor ~** Spinalmotorik *f* / **statistical ~** statistisches System *n* / **sudomotor ~** Sudomotorsystem *n* / **sympathetic ~** Sympathikussystem *n* / **sympathetic nervous ~** sympathisches Nervensystem *n*, Sympathikussystem *n* / **thalamic reticular ~** retikuläres System *n* des Thalamus / **transverse ~** T–System *n*, transversales Röhrensystem *n* / **urogenital ~** Urogenitalsystem *n* / **vegetative nervous ~** vegetatives Nervensystem *n*, autonomes Nervensystem *n* / **vestibular ~** Gleichgewichtsapparat *m*, Vestibularsystem *n* / **visceral ~** Viszeralnervensystem *n* / **voluntary muscular ~** Willkürmuskulatur *f*

systematic systematisch, methodisch geordnet, planvoll

systematisation Systematisierung *f*

systematize systematisieren, in ein System bringen

systemic Allgemein–, generalisiert, den Körper betreffend

systole Systole *f*

systolic systolisch

Szondi| table Szondi–Bilderserie *f* / **~ test** Szondi–Test *m*

T

tabacism, tabagism Nikotinvergiftung *f*

tabes Schwindsucht *f*, Rückenmarksschwindsucht *f* / ~ **dorsalis** Rückenmarksschwindsucht *f*, Tabes *f*, lokomotorische Ataxie *f*

table Tabelle *f*, Verzeichnis *n*, Tisch *m* / ~ **of contents** Inhaltsverzeichnis *n* / ~**–lifting** Tischrücken *n* / ~ **of logarithms** Logarithmentafel *f* / ~**–rapping** Tischrücken *n* / ~**–turning** Tischklopfen *n* / **chronological** ~ Zeittafel *f* / **fourfold** ~ Vierfelder–Tafel *f* / **hierarchical** ~ hierarchische Tafel *f*, Baumdiagramm *n* / **logarithmic** ~ Logarithmentafel *f* / **mental–age–grade** ~ Tabelle *f* der Intelligenzaltersstufen / **net** ~ Kurvendiagramm *n* / **pseudo–isochromatic** ~**s** pseudoisochromatische Tafeln *fpl* / **statistical** ~ statistische Tabelle *f* / **two–way** ~ Streudiagramm *n*

taboo, tabu Tabu *n*, Verbot *n* / tabu, unberührbar, verboten / **social** ~ soziales Tabu *n*

taboparesis Taboparalyse *f*

tabula rasa völlige Leere *f*, Tabula rasa *f*

tabulate in eine Tabelle aufnehmen, auszählen

tabulation Auszählung *f*, Tabellierung *f*

tachistoscope Tachistoskop *n*

tachogram Geschwindigkeitskurve *f*

tachometer Geschwindigkeitsmesser *m*

tachycardia Tachykardie *f*, Pulsbeschleunigung *f*

tachycardiac an Tachykardie leidend, mit zu hoher Pulsfrequenz

tachykinin Tachykinin *n*

tachylalia Tachylalie *f*, überhastetes Sprechtempo *n*, Tachyphrasie *f*

tachylogia übermäßig schnelles Sprechen *n*, Tachylogie *f*

tachymeter Geschwindigkeitsmesser *m*

tachyphagia übermäßig schnelles Essen *n*, Schlingen *n*, Tachyphagie *f*

tachyphasia übermäßig schnelle Sprache *f*, Tachyphasie *f*

tachyphemia pathologisches Versiegen *n* der Artikulation, Tachyphemie *f*

tachyphrasia überhastetes Sprechtempo *n*, Tachyphrasie *f*, Tachylalie *f*

tachyphrenia krankhaft gesteigerte Geistestätigkeit *f*

tachypnoea, tachypnea hohe Atemfrequenz *f*, schnelles Atmen *n*, Tachypnoe *f*

tacit still, stillschweigend

taciturn schweigsam, verschlossen

tact Takt *m*, Feingefühl *n*, Taktgefühl *n* / ~ **function** Taktfunktion *f*

tactic taktisch, planvoll, klug

tactile tastbar, greifbar, taktil

tactism Taxis *f*, Raumorientierung *f*, Tropismus *m*

tactlessness Taktlosigkeit *f*

tactometer Taktometer *m*, Tastempfindungsmesser *m*, Tastgefühlsprüfer *m*

tactor Tastkörperchen *n*

tactual tastbar, Berührungs–, Tast–

tactus Tastsinn *m*

taedium vitae Lebensmüdigkeit *f*, Lebensüberdruss *m*

taenia Taenia *f*

taeniophobia krankhafte Angst *f* vor Bandwürmern

tail äußerer Teil *m* einer Verteilung / **~ assumption** Annahme *f* über die Seiten einer Verteilung

taint Fleck *m*, Makel *n* / **hereditary ~** erbliche Belastung *f*

tainted belastet, erblich belastet

Talbot|'s law Talbot'sches Gesetz *n*, Talbot–Plateau'sches Gesetz *n* / **~–Plateau law** Talbot–Plateau'sches Gesetz *n*, Talbot'sches Gesetz *n*

tale, fairy Märchen *n*

talent Talent *n*, Begabung *f*, Hochbegabung *f* / **musical ~s test** Musik–Begabungstest *m*

talented begabt, talentiert / **very ~** hochbegabt

talion Vergeltung *f* / **~ dread** Furcht *f* vor Vergeltung / **~ principle** Vergeltungsprinzip *n*

talipes Klumpfuß *m*

talisman Talisman *m*, Amulett *n*

talk reden, sprechen, sich unterhalten / Gespräch *n*, Rede *f*, Vortrag *m* / **~ insanely** irrereden, phantasieren

talkative gesprächig, geschwätzig, redselig

talkativeness Geschwätzigkeit *f*, Gesprächigkeit *f*, Redseligkeit *f*

talking Unterhaltung *f*, Sprechen *n* / **~ cure** Redekur *f* / **~ out** Aussprechen *n*, Aussprache *f* / **subvocal ~** lautloses Sprechen *n*

tally registrieren, eine Strichliste machen

tambour Trommel *f*, Registriertrommel *f*

tame zahm / zähmen, bändigen

taming Zähmung *f*, Bändigung *f*

tandem Tandem *n* / **~ reinforcement** Tandemverstärkung *f*, Doppelverstärkung *f* / **~ schedule** Tandemplan *m*, Tandemfolge *f*

tangential tangential

tangoreceptor Tastkörperchen *n*, Tastsinnesorgan *n*, Tangorezeptor *m*

tantrum Wutanfall *m*, Temperamentsausbruch *m*

tanyphonia dünne, metallische Stimme *f*

tap klopfen, leicht schlagen, punktieren / Klopfen *n*, leichter Schlag *m* / **spinal ~** Lumbalpunktion *f*

tape Band *n* / **~–to–card converter** Magnetband–Karten–Wandler *m* / **~–recorder** Tonbandgerät *m*, Magnetophon *n* / **magnetic ~** Magnetband *n*

taphophilia, taphephilia krankhafte Vorliebe *f* für Gräber und Friedhöfe, Taphophilie *f*

taphophobia, taphephobia krankhafte Angst *f* vor Gräbern, Furcht *f* lebendig begraben zu werden

tapping Klopfen *n* / **~ board** Klopfbrett *n* / **~ speed** Klopfgeschwindigkeit *f* / **~ test** Klopftest *m*, Tapping–Test *m*

tarantism Tanzwut *f*

taraxein Taraxein *n*

Tarchanoff phenomenon Tarchanoff–Effekt *m*, psychogalvanische Reaktion *f*

target Zielscheibe *f*, Ziel *n* / **~ area** Ziel *n*, Zielbereich *m* / **~ behaviour** Zielverhalten *n* / **~ group** Zielgruppe *f* / **~ population** Zielpopulation *f*, Zielgruppe *f* / **~ symptom** Zielsymptom *n* / **~ test** Zieltest *m*, Genauigkeitstest *m*

Tartini's tone Differenzton *m*

tasikinesia motorische Unruhe *f*, Tasikinesie *f*

task Aufgabe *f* / **~ analysis** Arbeitsanalyse *f*, Arbeitsplatzanalyse *f*, Aufgabenanalyse *f* / **~ characteristic** Aufgabenmerkmal *n* / **~ complexity** Aufgabenkomplexität *f* / **~ demand** Aufgabenanforderung *f* / **~ difficulty** Aufgabenschwierigkeit *f*, Aufgabenkomplexität *f* / **~ energy** Energie *f* zur Erledigung von Aufgaben / **~ force** Arbeitsgruppe *f*, Arbeitsgemeinschaft *f*, Projektgruppe *f* / **~ group** Arbeitsgemeinschaft *f*, Arbeitskreis *m*, Projektgruppe *f*, Arbeitsgruppe *f* / **~–irrelevant** nicht–aufgabenbezogen / **~–oriented** aufgabenbezogen / **~–orientation** Ausrichtung *f* auf eine Aufgabe, Aufgabenzentrierung *f* / **~–set** Reaktionshaltung *f* /

closed ~ abgeschlossene Aufgabe *f* / **interrupted ~** unterbrochene Handlung *f* / **manual ~** manuelle Aufgabe *f* / **propaedeutic ~** vorbereitende Aufgabe *f*, Einführungsaufgabe *f* / **technical ~** technische Aufgabe *f* / **unfinished ~** unerledigte Handlung *f*

taste Geschmack *m*, Geschmackssinn *m* / schmecken, versuchen, prüfen / **~ acuity** Geschmacksschärfe *f* / **~ blindness** Geschmacksblindheit *f* / **~ bud** Geschmacksknospe *f*, Schmeckbecher *m*, Geschmacksbecher *m* / **~ bulb** Geschmacksknospe *f*, Schmeckbecher *m* / **~ cell** Geschmackszelle *f*, Schmeckzelle *f* / **~ centre** Geschmackszentrum *n* / **~ discrimination** Geschmacksunterscheidung *f* / **~ disorder** Geschmacksstörung *f* / **~ perception** Geschmackswahrnehmung *f* / **~ stimulation** Geschmacksreizung *f*, gustatorische Stimulation *f* / **~ stimulus** Schmeckreiz *m* / **~ tetrahedon** Geschmackstetraeder *n* / **excessively sensitive ~** Hypergeusie *f* / **telaesthetic ~** außersinnliche Geschmackswahrnehmung *f*

tasteful geschmackvoll

tasteless geschmacklos

taster Schmecker *m*, Koster *m*

tasting Verkostung *f*, Geschmacksprobe *f*

tattoo tätowieren / Tätowierung *f*

tau Tau *n* / **~ coefficient of correlation** Kendall'scher Korrelationskoeffizient τ *m* / **~ effect** Tau–Phänomen *n*, Gelb'sches–Phänomen *n*

taurine Taurin *n*

tautological dasselbe besagend, tautologisch

tautology Tautologie *f*, Wiedergabe *f* des gleichen Sachverhalts durch zwei Synonyme

tautophone Tautophon *n*, Gerät *n* zur Wiedergabe undeutlicher Laute

tautophony Wiederholung *f* des gleichen Lautes, Tautophonie *f*

taxis Taxis *f*, Tropismus *m*, Raumorientierung *f*

taxonomic, taxonomical klassifizierend, Klassifizierungs–

taxonomist klassifizierender Systematiker *m*

taxonomy, taxology Klassifizierung *f*, Systematik *f*, Taxonomie *f* / **numerical ~** numerische Taxonomie *f*

Tay–Sachs disease Tay–Sachs–Idiotie *f* / **~ syndrome** Tay–Sachs–Syndrom *n*

Taylor–Russel tables Taylor–Russel–Tabellen *fpl*

Taylor system Taylor–System *n*, Taylorismus *m*

Taylorism Taylorismus *m*

T data Testdaten *npl*, T–Daten *npl*

t distribution t–Verteilung *f*

teach lehren, unterrichten / **~–in** agitative Umfunktionierung *f* einer Lehrveranstaltung

teachable lehrbar, gelehrig

teacher Lehrer(in) *m,f*, Lehrkraft *f*, Lehrperson *f* / **~ aide** Hilfslehrer *m* / **~ attitude** Lehrereinstellung *f* / **~ characteristics** Lehrermerkmale *npl*, Charakteristika *npl* eines Lehrers / **~ education** Lehrerausbildung *f* / **~ effectiveness** Lehrereffizienz *f* / **~ effectiveness evaluation** Beurteilung *f* des Lehrererfolges / **~ expectation** Lehrererwartung *f* / **~–made test** von einem Lehrer entwickelter Test *m* / **~ personality** Lehrerpersönlichkeit *f* / **~ recruitment** Lehrerrekrutierung *f*, Auswahl *f* und Einstellung *f* von Lehrern, Lehrerstellenbesetzung *f* / **~–student interaction** Lehrer–Schüler–Interaktion *f* / **~ supply** Lehrernachwuchs *m*, Lehrerersatz *m* / **~ tenure** Lehrerplanstelle *f* / **~ training** Lehrerausbildung *f* / **cooperating ~** kooperierender Lehrer *m*, Mentor *m* / **in-service ~ education** Lehrerweiterbildung *f*, Lehrerfortbildung *f* / **preschool ~** Kindergartenerzieher *m* / **preservice ~** angehender Lehrer *m*

teaching Unterricht *m*, Schulerziehung *f*, Lehren *n* / Lehr–, Unterrichts–, lehrend / **~ aids** Unterrichtshilfsmittel *npl*, Lehrhilfsmittel *npl* / ~ **by discovery** Lehren *n* durch Entdecken, Lehren *n* durch Selbstfindenlassen / ~ **effectiveness** Unterrichtserfolg *m*, Wirkung *f* des Unterrichts / ~ **engineer** Lehringenieur *m* / ~ **internship** Zeit *f* als Lehramtsanwärter / ~ **machine** Lehrautomat *m*, Lehrmaschine *f*, Lernmaschine *f* / ~ **method** Lehrmethode *f* / ~ **staff** Lehrkörper *m*, Lehrerschaft *f*, Dozentenschaft *f* / **general** ~ allgemeine Unterweisung *f* / **initial** ~ **alphabet** Unterrichtsalphabet *n* für Anfänger / **primary** ~ Erstunterweisung *f*, Grundschulunterricht *m* / **private** ~ Privatunterricht *m* / **programmed** ~ programmierte Unterweisung *f*, programmierter Unterricht *m* / **public** ~ staatliches Schulwesen *n* / **technic** ~ Fachunterricht *m*, technischer Unterricht *m*

team Arbeitsgruppe *f*, Mannschaft *f*, Gruppe *f* / ~ **leader** Gruppenführer *m*, Leiter *m* einer Gruppe, Teamleiter *m* / **~–spirit** Mannschaftsgeist *m*, Teamgeist *m* / **~–teaching** Gruppenunterricht *m*, Teamunterricht *m* / **~–work** Zusammenarbeit *f*, Gruppenarbeit *f*, Teamarbeit *f*

tear Träne *f*

tearfulness Weinen *n* / **episode of** ~ Weinkrampf *m*

tease aufreizen, necken, reizen

teasing Neckerei *f*, Stichelei *f*

technic Technik *f*, Methode *f*, Verfahren *n*

technical technisch, fachmännisch, Fach–

technics Technik *f*, Technologie *f*

technique Technik *f*, Methode *f*, Verfahren *n* / **active** ~ aktive Technik *f* / **cognitive** ~ kognitive Technik *f* / **correlational** ~ Korrelationsmethode *f* / **disguised** ~ larviertes Verfahren *n* / **graphomotor** ~ schreibmotorisches Verfahren *n* / **memorizing** ~ Technik *f* des Behaltens, Mnemotechnik *f*, Lerntechnik *f* / **multiple–discriminant** ~ multiple Unterscheidungstechnik *f* / **non–analytical ~s** nicht–analytische Psychotherapie *f* / **odd–even** ~ Halbierungsmethode *f* nach Geraden und Ungeraden / **operating** ~ Bedienungsverfahren *n*, Arbeitsmethode *f* / **paradoxical** ~ paradoxe Technik *f* / **precoital** ~ Vorspiel *n* / **projective** ~ projektives Verfahren *n*, projektiver Test *m* / **psychoanalytic** ~ psychoanalytische Methode *f* / **psychotherapeutic** ~ psychotherapeutisches Verfahren *n*, psychotherapeutische Technik *f* / **social** ~ gesellschaftliche Methode *f*, soziale Technik *f* / **sociometric** ~ soziometrisches Verfahren *n* / **stereotaxic** ~ stereotaktisches Operationsverfahren *n*, stereotaktische Technik *f* / **therapeutic** ~ Heilverfahren *n*, Heilmethode *f*, Therapieverfahren *n*

technological technologisch

technologist Technologe *m*

technology Technologie *f* / **educational** ~ Methodik *f*, Erziehungstechnologie *f* / **instructional** ~ Unterrichtsmethodik *f* / **reproductive** ~ Reproduktionstechnologie *f*

technopsychology Psychotechnik *f*, Technopsychologie *f*

tectology Strukturlehre *f*, Lehre *f* vom organischen Aufbau

tectonics Tektonik *f*, Aufbau *m*, Struktur *f*

tectorial bedeckend, Deck–

tedious langweilig, weitschweifig, ermüdend

teenager Minderjährige *m,f*, Teenager *m*

teeny–bopper junger Teenager *m*

teeth Zähne *mpl* / **nocturnal** ~ **grinding** nächtliches Zähneknirschen *n*

teething Zahnen *n*

teetotal abstinent, enthaltsam

teetotalism Abstinenz *f*, Enthaltsamkeit *f*

teetotaller Abstinenzler *m*, Antialkoholiker *m*, Nichttrinker *m*

tegmentum Tegmentum *n*, Dach *n*, Haube *f*

teichopsia Flimmerskotom *n*, Teichopsie *f*

telaesthesia Hellsehen *n*, Telästhesie *f*, Fernwahrnehmung *f*

telebinocular Gerät *n* zur stereoskopen Augenuntersuchung

teleceptor Telerezeptor *m*, sensible Nervenendzelle *f* die aus der Entfernung gereizt wird

telecommand fernsteuern

telecommunication Telekommunikation *f*, Fernmeldetechnik *f* / ~ **media** Telekommunikationsmedien *npl*

teleconferencing Telekonferenz *f*

telegnosis Hellsehen *n*, Telepathie *f*, außersinnliche Wahrnehmung *f*

telegnostic telepathisch, hellsehend

telegony Fernzeugung *f*, Telegonie *f*

telekinesis, telecinesis Telekinese *f*, Bewegen *n* von Gegenständen durch okkulte Kräfte

telekinetic telekinetisch

telemetry Telemetrie *f*, Entfernungsmessung *f*

telencephalic telenzephal, Endhirn–

telencephalon Endhirn *n*, Telenzephalon *n*

teleneurite Endbäumchen *n*, Telodendron *n*

teleoceptor, teleoreceptor Telerezeptor *n*, sensible Nervenendzelle *f* die aus der Entfernung gereizt wird

teleological zweckbestimmt, teleologisch

teleology Teleologie *f*, Lehre *f* von der Zweckbestimmtheit

teleonomic teleonomisch, zielgesetzlich

telepathic telepathisch

telepathise durch Telepathie beeinflussen

telepathist Telepath *m*

telepathy Telepathie *f*, Gedankenübertragung *f*

telephone Telefon *n* / ~ **hot lines** Notrufdienste *mpl* / ~ **survey** telefonische Umfrage *f* / ~ **system** Telefonsystem *n* / ~ **theory** Frequenztheorie *f*, Telefontheorie *f* / ~ **theory of hearing** Frequenztheorie *f* / ~ **support service** Telefonseelsorge *f*

telephonophobia Telefonangst *f*

teleplasma Teleplasma *n*

telergy Gedankenübertragung *f*, Befehlsübertragung *f* durch lautlose Anordnung

telesis Vollendung *f*, Erfüllung *f*

telestereoscope, teleostereoscope Telestereoskop *n*

telesthesia Hellsehen *n*, Telästhesie *f*, Fernwahrnehmung *f*

telesthetic hellseherisch, telästhetisch

teletactor Teletaktor *m*, Gerät *n* zur Übertragung von Schallwellen auf die Haut

teletherapeutics, teletherapy Fernbehandlung *f*, Suggestionsbehandlung *f*

teletype Fernschreiber *m* / ~ **writer** Fernschreiber *m*

television Fernsehen *n* / ~ **advertising** Fernsehwerbung *f* / ~ **disease** Fernsehkrankheit *f* / ~ **viewer** Fernsehzuschauer *m* / ~ **viewing** Fernsehverhalten *n* / **educational** ~ Schulfernsehen *n*, Telekolleg *n*, Bildungsfernsehen *n*

telic zielstrebig, zielorientiert, zweckvoll, final

telodendrion, telodendron Nervenendbäumchen *n*, Telodendrion *n*

telotaxis Telotaxis *f*, Raumorientierung *f* in Richtung auf eine (von mehreren) Reizquelle(*n*)

telotism vollständiger Funktionsablauf *m*, vollständige Erektion *f* des Penis

temerity Verwegenheit *f*, Tollkühnheit *f*, Unbesonnenheit *f*

temper Charakteranlage *f*, Charaktereigenschaft *f*, Temperament *n*, Wut *f* / ~ **tantrum** Wutanfall *m*

temperament Temperament *n*, Gemütsart *f* / ~ **scale** typologische Skala *f* / ~ **traits** Temperamentsdimensionen *fpl* / **atrabilious** ~ Melancholie *f* / **choleric** ~ cholerische Veranlagung *f* / **lymphatic** ~ phlegmatische Veranlagung *f* / **melancholic** ~ melancholische Veranlagung *f* / **nervous** ~ nervöse Veranlagung *f* / **phlegmatic** ~ phlegmatische Veranlagung *f* / **sanguine** ~ sanguinische Veranlagung *f*

temperamental launisch, launenhaft, unstet, temperamentvoll

temperance Enthaltsamkeit *f*, Mäßigkeit *f*, Temperenz *f* / ~ **movement** Mäßigkeitsbewegung *f*, Temperenzbewegung *f* / ~ **society** Temperenzgesellschaft *f*

temperate mäßig, enthaltsam

temperature Temperatur *f* / ~ **curve** Temperaturkurve *f* / ~ **effect** Temperaturwirkung *f* / ~ **illusion** Temperaturtäuschung *f* / ~ **perception** Temperaturwahrnehmung *f* / ~ **sensation** Temperaturempfinden *n* / ~ **sense** Temperatursinn *m*, Wärmesinn *m* / ~ **sensitivity** Temperaturempfindlichkeit *f*, Wärmesensibilität *f* / ~ **spot** Temperaturpunkt *m* / **comfortable** ~ Behaglichkeitstemperatur *f*

template, templet Schablone *f*, Formatvorlage *f* / ~ **matching** Auflegen *n* einer Schablone

tempo Tempo *n*, Geschwindigkeit *f* / **conceptual** ~ konzeptuelles Tempo *n* / **personal** ~ persönliches Tempo *n*

temporal zeitlich, temporal, zur Schläfe gehörig, Schläfen–

temporality Zeitlichkeit *f*, Dauer *f*

temporary vorübergehend, zeitweilig, temporär

tempt verführen, verlocken, auf die Probe stellen

temptation Versuchung *f*, Verlockung *f*, Verführung *f*

tenacity Hartnäckigkeit *f*, Zähigkeit *f*, Tenazität *f*

tendency Tendenz *f*, Neigung *f*, Disposition *f*, Anlage *f*, Hang *m*, Bereitschaft *f* / ~ **to attacks** Anfallsbereitschaft *f* / ~ **to convulsions** Krampfneigung *f* / ~ **of extension** Streckungstendenz *f* / ~ **in situations** Situationstendenz *f* / **acquired** ~ erworbene Tendenz *f*, Gewohnheit *f* / **behavioural** ~ Verhaltenstendenz *f* / **central** ~ zentrale Tendenz *f* / **central** ~ **error** Fehler *m* der zentralen Tendenz / **constitutional** ~ Veranlagung *f* / **determining** ~ determinierende Tendenz *f* / **directive** ~ determinierende Tendenz *f* / **final** ~ finale Tendenz *f* / **inherited** ~ angeborene Tendenz *f* / **instinctive** ~ Triebtendenz *f* / **masochistic–passive** ~ masochistisch–passive Neigung *f* / **native** ~ angeborene Tendenz *f* / **neurotic** ~ neurotische Tendenz *f*, Neurotizismus *m* / **perseverative** ~ Perseverationstendenz *f* / **psychotic** ~ psychotische Tendenz *f* / **suicidal** ~ Selbstmordneigung *f*, Suizidalität *f*

tendential, tendentious, tendencious tendenziell, tendenziös, zweckbestimmt, Tendenz–

tender zart, empfindlich, schmerzhaft / ~–**hearted** weichherzig / ~–**minded** introvertiert / Introvertierter *m*

tenderness Zartheit *f*, Empfindlichkeit, Zärtlichkeit *f*, Schmerzhaftigkeit *f*

tendinous sehnig, Sehnen–

tendon Sehne *f* / ~ **jerk** Sehnenreflex *m* / ~ **organ** Sehnenspindel *f* / ~ **reflex** Sehnenreflex *m* / ~ **sensation** Sehnenempfindung *f* / ~ **spindle** Sehnenspindel *f* / **patellar** ~ Kniesehne *f*, Patellarsehne *f* / **patellar** ~ **reflex** Patellarreflex *m*, Kniesehnenreflex *m*

tenesmus Drang *m*, Tenesmus *m*, Darmzwang *m* / **rectal** ~ Stuhldrang *m* / **vesical** ~ Harndrang *m*, Blasenzwang *m*, Strangurie *f*

tenet Grundsatz *m*, Lehre *f*, Meinung *f*

tenia Taenia *f*

teniophobia krankhafte Angst *f* vor Bandwürmern

tenotic sehnig, Sehnen–

tense gespannt, straff

tenseness Spannung *f*, Straffheit *f*

tensinflexia angespannte Starrheit *f*

tension Spannung *f*, Gespanntheit *f*, Tension *f* / ~ **headache** Spannungskopfschmerz *m* / ~ **law** Spannungsgesetz *n* / ~ **movement** Bewegung *f* gespannter Muskeln / ~ **of muscle** Muskelspannung *f*, Muskelanspannung *f* / ~ **reduction** Spannungslösung *f*, Spannungsverminderung *f* / ~–**relaxation dimension** Dimension *f* der Spannung–Entspannung / ~ **release**

Spannungslösung *f* / ~ **state** Spannungszustand *m* / ~ **system** Spannungssystem *n* / **affective** ~ emotionale Spannung *f* / **conflictual** ~**s** Konfliktspannungen *fpl* / **emotional** ~ emotionale Spannung *f* / **ergic** ~ nicht abgeführte Triebspannung *f* / **muscular** ~ Muskelspannung *f* / **nervous** ~ nervöse Erregbarkeit *f* / **premenstrual** ~ prämenstruelles Syndrom *n* / **psychic** ~ psychische Spannung *f* / **sexual** ~ sexuelle Spannung *f* / **social** ~ soziale Spannung *f*

tensional Spannungs–

tensive Spannung verursachend

tensor Spannmuskel *m*, Tensor *m* / ~ **tympani** Spannmuskel *m* des Trommelfells

tentacle Fühler *m*, Greifarm *m*

tentative versuchsweise, Versuchs–, Probe–

tentiginous krankhaft wollüstig

tentigo krankhaft gesteigerter Geschlechtstrieb *m*

tentum Penis *m*

tenuity Dünnheit *f*, Schlankheit *f*, Zartheit *f*

tenuous dünn, schlank, zart, anfällig

tenure feste Anstellung *f*, Daueranstellung *f* / **occupational** ~ feste berufliche Anstellung *f*

teratism Missbildung *f*, Deformität *f*

teratogen Teratogen *n*

teratogenic Missbildungen verursachend

teratology Lehre *f* von den Missgeburten, Teratologie *f*

teratophobia krankhafte Angst *f* vor einer Missgeburt, Teratophobie *f*

term Ausdruck *m*, Fachausdruck *m*, Begriff *m*, Bezeichnung *f*, Glied *n*, Frist *f*, bestimmte Zeitdauer *f*, zeitliche Grenze *f* / **long–**~ langfristig / **long–**~ **features** Längsschnitt–Einheit *f* / **objective** ~ objektiver Begriff *m* / **short–**~ kurzfristig / **short–**~ **features** Querschnitt–Einheit *f* / **technical** ~ Fachausdruck *m*

terminal terminal, End– / **synaptic** ~ synaptische Nervenendigung *f*

termination Beendigung *f*, Ende *n* / ~ **of analysis** Beendigung *f* einer Analyse / ~ **of pregnancy** Schwangerschaftsabbruch *m*

terminative enden, beenden

terminological terminologisch

terminology Fachsprache *f*, Terminologie *f*, Nomenklatur *f* / **psychological** ~ psychologische Fachsprache *f*, psychologische Terminologie *f* / **traditional** ~ traditionelle Nomenklatur *f*, veraltete Terminologie *f*

ternary ternär, aus drei Elementen bestehend

terrible schrecklich, furchtbar, entsetzlich

territoriality Territorialverhalten *n*

territory Gebiet *n*, Bereich *m*

terror Schrecken *m*, schreckliche Furcht *f*

terrorism Terrorismus *m*, Schreckensherrschaft *f*

tertiary an dritter Stelle stehend, drittgradig, tertiär

tesselated mosaikartig

test Test *m*, Prüfung *f*, Probe *f*, Versuch *m* / testen, prüfen, erproben, untersuchen / ~ **of ability** Eignungstest *m*, Fähigkeitstest *m* / ~ **administration** Testdurchführung *f*, Testdarbietung *f* / ~ **age** Testalter *n* / ~ **analysis** Testanalyse *f* / ~ **anxiety** Prüfungsangst *f*, Testangst *f* / ~ **for aphasia** Aphasieprüfung *f* / ~ **of auditory acuity** Hörschärfeprobe *f* / ~ **battery** Testbatterie *f*, Testreihe *f* / ~ **bias** Testbias *m* / ~ **blank** Testblatt *n*, Testformular *n* / ~ **campaign** Testkampagne *f* / ~ **card** Testtafel *f*, Sehprobentafel *f* / ~ **chart** Testtafel *f*, Sehprobentafel *f* / ~ **coaching** Testtraining *n* / ~ **for colour blindness** Test *m* zur Prüfung der Farbenblindheit, Sehprüfung *f* mit pseudoisochromatischen Tafeln / ~ **construction** Testkonstruktion *f* / ~ **for creativity** Kreativitätstest *m* / ~ **data** T–Daten *npl* / ~ **of diffused attention** Test *m* der Aufmerksamkeitsstreuung / ~ **form** Test *m*, Testform *f* / ~ **of independence** Homogenitätsindex *m*, Prüfung *f* der Unabhängigkeit / **~ of intercorrelation** Intertestkorrelation *f* / **~ interpretation** Testinterpretation *f* / **~ item** Testaufgabe *f*, Testitem *n* / **~ market** Testmarkt *m* / **~ of maximum performance** Höchstleistungstest *m* / **~ of mental maturity** Prüfung *f* der geistigen Reife / **~ norm** Testnorm *f* / **~ normalisation** Testeichung *f*, Teststandardisierung *f* / **~ panel** Untersuchungsgruppe *f*, Testgruppe *f* / **~ performance** Testleistung *f* / **~ of personality** Persönlichkeitstest *m* / **~ of the plates** Plattentest *m* / **~ procedure** Testverfahren *n* / **~ profile** Testprofil *n* / **~ reliability** Testreliabilität *f*, Reliabilität *f*, Zuverlässigkeit *f* / **~ representativeness** Repräsentativität *f* des Tests / **~–retest coefficient** Retest–Reliabilitätskoeffizient *m* / **~–retest method** Methode *f* der Testwiederholung / **~–retest reliability** Retest–Reliabilität *f* / **~–retest technique** Methode *f* der Testwiederholung / **~ of sales aptitude** Eignungstest *m* für Verkäufer / **~ scale** Testskala *f* / **~ scaling** Testskalierung *f* / **~ score** Testwert *m*, Testpunktwert *m* / **~ of significance** Signifikanztest *m* / **~ standardization** Testeichung *f*, Teststandardisierung *f*, Testnormierung *f* / **~ taking** Testverhalten *m* / **~ theory** Testtheorie *f* / **~ tone** Testton *m* / **~ validation** Testvalidierung *f* / **~ validity** Testvalidität *f*, Testgültigkeit *f* / **~ value** Testwert *m* / **~ vector** Vektor *m*, Testvektor *m* / **~ for visual acuity** Sehschärfetest *m* / **~–wise** testerfahren / **~–wiseness** Testerfahrung *f*, Testerfahrenheit *f* / **~ of work stability** Prüfung *f* der Arbeitsbeständigkeit / **analytic ~** analytischer Test *m* / **assymmetric ~** einseitiger Test *m* / **audiometric ~** Hörschärfeprüfung *f* / **auditory ~** Hörtest *m* / **automated ~ interpretation** maschinelle Interpretation *f* von Testdaten / **blind ~** Blindversuch *m* / **class–free ~** Test *m* der frei von sozioökonomischen Faktoren ist / **clerical ~** Eignungstest *m* für Büroarbeiten, Bürofertigkeitstest *m* / **comparative ~** Vergleichsuntersuchung *f*, Paralleluntersuchung *f* / **composite ~** zusammengesetzter Test *m*, Testbatterie *f* / **cultural ~ bias** kulturelle Testverzerrung *f* / **culture–free ~** kulturunabhängiger Test *m* / **developmental ~** Entwicklungstest *m* / **diagnostic ~** diagnostischer Test *m* / **double–blind ~** Doppelblindversuch *m* / **educational ~** Schultest *m* / **empirical ~** empirischer Test *m* / **individual ~** Einzeltest *m* / **informal ~** informeller Test *m* / **instructional ~** Test *m* zur Prüfung von Lernfortschritten / **matching ~** Zuordnungstest *m* / **mental ~** Intelligenztest *m*, Fähigkeitstest *m* / **motor ~** motorischer Test *m* / **multiple–choice ~** Test *m* mit Mehrfachwahlantworten / **multivariate ~** multivariates Prüfverfahren *n* / **music ~** Musik–Begabungstest *m* / **nonparametric ~** nichtparametrisches Prüfverfahren *n* / **nonparametric statistical ~** nichtparametrischer statistischer Test *m* / **nonverbal ~** sprachfreier Test *m*, nichtverbaler Test *m* / **objective ~** objektiver Test *m* / **occupational ~** Berufstest *m* / **omnibus ~** Sammeltest *m*, Testserie *f* / **one–sided ~** einseitiger Test *m* / **one–tailed ~** einseitiger Test *m*, gerichteter Test *m* / **one–tailed ~ of significance** einseitiger Signifikanztest *m* / **oral ~** mündliche Prüfung *f* / **ordering ~** Ordnungstest *m* / **parallel ~** Kontrollversuch *m*, Paralleltest *m* / **parametric ~** parametrisches Prüfverfahren *n* / **parametric statistical ~** parametrischer statistischer Test *m* / **pointing ~** Zeigeversuch *m* / **postural ~** Haltungstest *m* / **prognostic ~** prognostischer Test *m*, Vorhersagetest *m* / **projective ~** projektiver Test *m*, Projektionstest *m* / **psychological ~** psychologischer Test *m* / **psychometric ~** psychometrischer Test *m* / **psychomotor ~** psychomotorischer Test *m* / **psychophysiological ~** psychophysiologischer Test *m* / **right–and–wrong ~** Test *m* mit Antwortvorgabe „richtig–falsch" / **same–opposite ~** Test *m* mit Antwortvorgabe „gleich–entgegengesetzt" / **scaled ~** skalierter Test *m*, geeichter Test *m*, normierter Test *m* / **scholastic ~** Schultest *m*, Schulleistungstest *m* / **self–administering**

~ Test *m* zur Selbstdurchführung / **self–marking ~** Test *m* mit automatischer Selbstauswertung / **sequential ~** sequenzieller Test *m* / **serial ~** Reihenuntersuchung *f* / **situational ~** Situationstest *m* / **smelling ~** Geruchsprobe *f* / **socioeconomie–free ~** Test *m* der frei von sozioökonomischen Faktoren ist / **sociometric ~** soziometrischer Test *m* / **spiral ~** Spiraltest *m*, Test *m* mit zunehmend schwieriger werdenden Aufgaben der gleichen Aufgabenart / **standardized ~** standardisierter Test *m* / **statistical ~** statistischer Test *m*, Signifikanztest *m*, Signifikanzprüfung *f* / **stylistic ~** Stiltest *m*, stilistischer Test *m* / **subjective ~** subjektiver Test *m* / **timed ~** Test *m* mit Zeitbegrenzung, zeitlich limitierter Test *m* / **true–false ~** Test *m* mit Wahlantworten „richtig–falsch" / **two–sided ~** zweiseitiger Test *m* / **two–tailed ~** zweiseitiger Test *m* / **two–tailed ~ of significance** zweiseitiger Signifikanztest *m* / **unspeeded ~** Test *m* ohne Zeitbegrenzung / **verbal ~** verbaler Test *m*, sprachlicher Test *m*

testability Prüfbarkeit *f*, Untersuchbarkeit *f*

testable prüfbar, untersuchbar

testee Testperson *f*, Prüfling *m*, Proband *m*

tester Prüfer *m*, Versuchsleiter *m*, Testleiter *m*

testes Hoden *m*, Testes *mpl*, Testikel *mpl* / **~ disorder** Hodenerkrankung *f*

testicle Hoden *m*, Testikel *mpl*

testify bezeugen

testimony Zeugnis *n*, Beweis *m*, Aussage *f* / **legal ~** Zeugenaussage *f* vor Gericht

testiness Empfindlichkeit *f*, Gereiztheit *f*, Verdrießlichkeit *f*

testing Testen *n*, Probe *f*, Testabnahme *f* / **~ chamber** Testraum *m* / **~ for reality** Realitätsprüfung *f* / **~ method** Testmethode *f*, Testverfahren *n*, Prüfverfahren *n* / **probabilistic ~ model** probabilistisches Testmodell *n* / **projective ~ technique** projektive Testmethode *f* / **~ the limits** Ausreizen *n* der letzten Möglichkeiten, Testen *n* des Grenzbereichs, komplettierende Nachuntersuchung *f* / **~ of vision** Sehprüfung *f*, Sehprobe *f* / **~ with regard to reality** Realitätsprüfung *f* / **adaptive ~** adaptives Testen *n* / **animal ~** tierexperimentelle Untersuchung *f* / **individual ~** Einzeltestung *f* / **preschool ~** Testen *n* von Vorschulkindern / **sequential ~** Anwendung *f* sequenzieller Tests, sukzessives Testen *n*

testis Hoden *m*

testosterone Testosteron *n*

testwiseness Testerfahrenheit *f*

tetanal, tetanic tetanisch, tetanusbedingt

tetanise tetanisieren, Starrkrampf hervorrufen

tetanism Übererregbarkeit *f* der Muskulatur

tetanoid tetanoid, starrkrampf ähnlich

tetanophobia krankhafte Angst *f* vor Tetanie, Tetanophobie *f*

tetanus Tetanus *m*, Wundstarrkrampf *m* / **~ toxin** Tetanustoxin *n*

tetany Tetanie *f*, Erkrankung *f* durch neuromuskuläre Übererregbarkeit

tetartanopia, tetartanopsia Tetratanopie *f*, Blau–Gelbblindheit *f*

tetrabenazine Tetrabenazin *n*

tetracaine Tetracain *n*

tetraceptor theory Vier–Rezeptoren–Theorie *f*

tetrachoric tetrachorisch, Vierfelder–

tetrachromatic vierfarbig

tetrachromatism Vier–Farben–Theorie *f*

tetrad Tetrade *f* / **~ criterion** Tetradenkriterium *n* / **~ difference** Tetradendifferenz *f* / **~ difference criterion** Kriterium *n* der Tetradendifferenz / **~ equation** Tetradengleichung *f*

tetraethyl|ammonium Tetraäthylammonium *n* / **~ thiuram disulfide** Tetraäthylthiuramdisulfid *n*, Disulfiram *n*

tetrahedron Tetraeder *n*

tetrahydrocannabinol Tetrahydrocannabinol *n*, THC

tetraiodothyronine Tetrajodthyronin *n*

tetraplegia Tetraplegie *f*, Lähmung *f* aller vier Extremitäten

tetrodotoxin Tetrodotoxin *n*

text Text *m*, Wortlaut *m* / **~–blindness** Wortblindheit *f*, Alexie *f* / **~ error** Textfehler *m* / **~ structure** Textstruktur *f*

textbook Lehrbuch *n* / **programmed ~** Lehrprogrammtext *m*, programmiertes Lehrbuch *n*, algorithmisches Lehrbuch *n*

textual textlich, Text–, wortgetreu, wörtlich

textural strukturartig, Struktur–

texture Struktur *f*, Gefüge *n*, Gewebe *n* / **~ gradient** Strukturgradient *m* / **~ perception** Wahrnehmung *f* der Oberflächenstruktur / **~ response** Strukturdeutung *f* / **causal ~** Interdependenz *f* von Umweltvorgängen, Wirkungsgefüge *n*

t function t–Funktion *f*, t–Verteilung *f*

T group Trainingsgruppe *f*, Selbsterfahrungsgruppe *f*

thalamencephalon Thalamenzephalon *n*, Teil *m* des Zwischenhirns

thalamic Sehhügel–, Thalamus–, thalamisch

thalamotomy Thalamotomie *f*, Thalamusoperation *f*

thalamus Thalamus *m*, Sehhügel *m* / **extrinsic ~** extrinsischer Thalamus *m* / **intrinsic ~** intrinsischer Thalamus *m* / **optic ~** Sehhügel *m*

thalassophobia krankhafte Angst *f* vor dem Meer, Thalassophobie *f*

thalidomide Thalidomid *n*, *N*–Phthalylglutaminsäureimid *n*, Contergan *n*

thanatology Lehre *f* vom Tod, Thanatologie *f*

thanatomania ständig wiederkehrende Selbstmordabsicht *f*

thanatophobia krankhafte Angst *f* vor dem Tode, Thanatophobie *f*

Thanatos Thanatos *m*, Tod *m* / **~ instinct** Todestrieb *m*, Thanatostrieb *m*

thanatosis Totstellreflex *m*, Thanatose *f*

thaumatrope Stroboskop *n*, Wunderscheibe *f*, Thaumatrop *n*

thaumatropy Prüfung *f* mittels Thaumatrop

theatrotherapy Therapie *f* mittels Theaterspiel

Theelin Theelin *n*, Östron *n*, Follikelhormon *n*

theft Diebstahl *m*

theism Theismus *m*, Glaube *m* an einen Gott

T helper cell T–Helfer–Zelle *f*

thema Thema *n*

thematic thematisch

theme Thema *n*, Leitmotiv *n*, Motiv *n* / **~–centered interaction** themenzentrierte Interaktion *f*

theocracy Theokratie *f*, Gottesherrschaft *f*

theomancy Weissagung *f* aus göttlicher Eingebung, Theomantie *f*

theomania religiöser Wahnsinn *m*, Theomanie *f*

theomaniac an religiösem Wahnsinn Leidender *m*

theopathy Gotteserfahrung *f*, göttliche Erleuchtung *f*

theophobia krankhafte Gottesfurcht *f*, Theophobie *f*

theophylline Theophyllin *n*

theorem Lehrsatz *m*, Theorem *n* / **~ of escape** Dissonanztheorem *n* / **Bayesian ~** Bayes–Theorem *n*, Bayes–Gesetz *n*, Bayes–Statistik *f*

theoretical theoretisch, rein gedanklich, spekulativ

theoretician, theorist Theoretiker *m*

theory Theorie *f*, Lehre *f* / **~ of association** Assoziationstheorie *f* / **~ of audition** Hörtheorie *f* / **~–begging** fehlerhafte Verquickung *f* von Theorie und Empirie / **~ of cognitive dissonance** Theorie *f* der kognitiven Dissonanz / **~ of colours** Farbtheorie *f*, Farbenlehre *f* / **~ of colour vision** Theorie *f* des Farbensehens / **~ of combinations** Kombinatorik *f* / **~ of**

control Regeltheorie *f* / ~ **of development** Entwicklungstheorie *f* / ~ **of disuse** Entwöhnungstheorie *f* / ~ **of dreams** Traumlehre *f*, Traumtheorie *f* / ~ **of education** Erziehungstheorie *f*, pädagogische Theorie *f* / ~ **of the emotions** Gefühlstheorie *f* / ~ **of evolution** Evolutionstheorie *f* / ~ **of excitation** Theorie *f* der Erregung, Erregungsgesetze *npl* / ~ **of expression** Ausdruckstheorie *f* / ~ **of facilitation** Bahnungstheorie *f*, Ausschleifungstheorie *f* / ~ **of forgetting** Theorie *f* des Vergessens / ~ **formulation** Theorienbildung *f* / ~ **of games** Spieltheorie *f* / ~ **of hearing** Hörtheorie *f* / ~ **of the instincts** Triebtheorie *f*, Trieblehre *f*, Instinkttheorie *f* / ~ **of intelligence** Intelligenztheorie *f* / ~ **of interference** Interferenztheorie *f*, Überlagerungstheorie *f* / ~ **of knowledge** Erkenntnistheorie *f* / ~ **of learning** Lerntheorie *f* / ~ **of memory** Gedächtnistheorie *f* / ~ **of neurosis** Neurosenlehre *f*, Neurosentheorie *f* / ~ **of objects** Gegenstandstheorie *f* / ~ **of perception** Wahrnehmungstheorie *f* / **constitutional** ~ **of personality** Konstitutionslehre *f* / ~ **of probability** Wahrscheinlichkeitstheorie *f* / ~ **of seduction** Verführungstheorie *f* / ~ **of sex** Sexualtheorie *f* / ~ **of signal detectability** Signalentdekkungstheorie *f*, Signaldetektionstheorie *f* / ~ **of vision** Sehtheorie *f* / ~ **verification** Überprüfung *f* einer Theorie, Verifikation *f* einer Theorie / ~ **X** X–Theorie *f*, pessimistische Theorie *f* des Verhaltens in Organisationen / ~ **Y** Y–Theorie *f*, optimistische Theorie *f* des Verhaltens in Organisationen / **analytic** ~ psychoanalytische Theorie *f* / **bifactorial** ~ **of conditioning** Zweifaktorentheorie *f* des Konditionierens / **biosocial** ~ Biosoziologie *f* / **causal** ~ Kausaltheorie *f* / **central** ~ **of thinking** periphere Denktheorie *f* / **cloacal** ~ Kloakentheorie *f* / **cognitive** ~ **of learning** kognitive Lerntheorie *f* / **complementary** ~ Komplementärtheorie *f* / **cybernetic** ~ Kybernetik *f* / **Darwinian** ~ Abstammungslehre *f*, Darwinismus *m* / **developmental** ~ Entwicklungstheorie *f* / **ding–dong** ~ onomatopoetische Theorie *f*, Theorie *f* von der Entstehung der Worte durch Lautmalerei / **dynamic** ~ dynamische Theorie *f* / **economic** ~ **of libido** ökonomische Theorie *f* der Libido / **egoistic** ~ **of dreams** egoistische Traumtheorie *f* / **genetic** ~ genetische Theorie *f* / **holistic** ~ Holismus *m*, Ganzheitstheorie *f* / **hormic** ~ hormische Psychologie *f* / **humoral** ~ Humorallehre *f* / **ideomotor** ~ ideomotorische Theorie *f* / **instinctual** ~ Trieblehre *f*, Triebtheorie *f*, Instinkttheorie *f* / **intellectualist** ~ intellektualistische Theorie *f* / **interjectional** ~ Interjektionstheorie *f* / **lamarckian** ~ Lamarckismus *m* / **mathematical** ~ **of learning** mathematische Lerntheorie *f* / **mechanistic** ~ mechanistische Theorie *f*, Mechanismus *m* / **Mendelian** ~ Mendel'sche Vererbungstheorie *f* / **motor** ~ motorische Theorie *f*, motorische Prozesstheorie *f* / **motor** ~ **of consciousness** motorische Bewusstseinstheorie *f* / **multimodal** ~ **of intelligence** multifaktorielle Intelligenztheorie *f*, multimodale Intelligenztheorie *f* / **nativistic** ~ nativistische Theorie *f* / **new–look** ~ Theorie *f* der neuen Aufmachung / **onomatopoeic** ~ onomatopoetische Theorie *f*, Theorie *f* von der Entstehung der Worte durch Lautmalerei / **onomatopoetic** ~ onomatopoetische Theorie *f*, Theorie *f* von der Entstehung der Worte durch Lautmalerei / **organismic** ~ organismische Theorie *f* / **photochemical** ~ photochemische Theorie *f* / **photoelectric** ~ photoelektrische Theorie *f* / **physiological** ~ physiologische Theorie *f*, James–Lange'sche Theorie *f* / **psychoanalytic** ~ psychoanalytische Theorie *f* / **psychodynamic** ~ psychodynamische Theorie *f* / **segmental** ~ Segmenttheorie *f* / **social** ~ Sozialtheorie *f*, Gesellschaftstheorie *f* / **subjective** ~ subjektive Theorie *f* / **thalamic** ~ **of emotion** Thalamus–Gefühlstheorie *f* / **trichromatic** ~ Drei–Farben–Theorie *f*, Young–Helmholtz'sche Dreikomponententheorie *f* / **tridimensional** ~ **of feeling** dreidimensionale Gefühlstheorie *f*, alghedonische Gefühlstheorie *f* / **vascular ~ of thermal sensitivity** Gefäßtheorie *f* der Wärmeempfindung / **vertebral ~ of the skull** vertebrale Schädeltheorie *f*

theotherapy Gesundbeten *n*

therapeutic therapeutisch, Behandlungs–

therapeutics Therapeutik *f*, Lehre *f* von der Behandlung der Krankheiten, Therapie *f* / **empirical ~** Erfahrungsheilkunde *f* / **mental ~** Psychotherapie *f* / **rational ~** rationale Psychotherapie *f* / **suggestive ~** Suggestionsbehandlung *f*

therapist, therapeutist Therapeut *m* / **~ attitude** Therapeuteneinstellung *f* / **~ characteristics** Therapeutenmerkmale *fpl* / **~ effectiveness** Therapeutenerfolg *m* / **~ experience** Therapeutenerfahrung *f* / **~–patient interaction** Interaktion *f* zwischen Therapeut und Patient / **~–patient sexual relations** sexuelle Beziehungen *fpl* zu Patienten / **~ personality** Persönlichkeit *f* des Therapeuten / **~ role** Rolle *f* des Therapeuten / **~ selection** Therapeutenwahl *f* / **~ trainee** Therapeut *m* in Ausbildung / **multiple ~** Mehrfachtherapeut *m* / **occupational ~** Beschäftigungstherapeut *m* / **physical ~** Heilgymnast *m*, Physiotherapeut *m*

therapy Therapie *f*, Behandlung *f* / **active ~** aktive Psychotherapie *f* / **adjuvant ~** Unterstützungstherapie *f* / **analytic ~** tiefenpsychologische Therapie *f* / **aversive ~** Aversionstherapie *f* / **behavioural ~** Verhaltenstherapie *f* / **biological ~** biologische Heilweise *f* / **cathartic ~** kathartische Therapie *f*, kathartische Methode *f* / **client–centered ~** Patienten zentrierte Therapie *f*, nicht–direktive Psychotherapie *f* / **cognitive ~** kognitive Therapie *f*, kognitive Verhaltenstherapie *f*, Erkenntnistherapie *f* / **conjoint ~** Mitbehandlung *f*, Ko–Therapie *f*, gemeinsame Therapie *f* / **convulsive ~** Krampftherapie *f* / **directed reverie ~** katathymes Bilderleben *n* / **directive ~** gelenkte Therapie *f*, direktive Psychotherapie *f* / **dynamic ~** dynamische Psychotherapie *f* / **electroconvulsive ~** Elektroschockbehandlung *f* / **existential ~** existenzielle Therapie *f*, Existenzialtherapie *f* / **expressive ~** Ausdruckstherapie *f* / **flooding ~** Überflutungstherapie *f* / **gymnastic ~** Heilgymnastik *f* / **hypoglycaemic ~** Insulinschocktherapie *f* / **implosive ~** Überflutungstherapie *f*, Implosionstherapie *f* / **individual ~** Einzelpsychotherapie *f* / **integrative ~ approach** integrativer Therapieansatz *m* / **interpretative ~** Interpretationstherapie *f*, direktive Therapie *f* / **marital ~** Partnertherapie *f*, Ehetherapie *f* / **medical ~** ärztliche Behandlung *f* / **mental ~** Psychotherapie *f* / **nondirective ~** nicht–direktive Psychotherapie *f*, Klienten–zentrierte Therapie *f* / **occupational ~** Arbeitstherapie *f*, Beschäftigungstherapie *f* / **on agonist ~** bei agonistischer Therapie / **organic ~** Organtherapie *f* / **out–patient ~** ambulante Therapie *f* / **persuasive ~** Persuasionstherapie *f*, Überredungstherapie *f* / **physical ~** Physiotherapie *f*, Krankengymnastik *f* / **primal ~** Primärtherapie *f*, Urschreitherapie *f* / **psychedelic ~** psychedelische Behandlung *f* / **psychoanalytic~** Psychoanalyse *f*, psychoanalytische Therapie *f* / **rational–emotive ~** rationale Psychotherapie *f*, rational–emotive Therapie *f* / **recreational ~** Kurerholung *f* / **semantic ~** Bedeutungstherapie *f* / **situational ~** Milieutherapie *f* / **social ~** Sozialtherapie *f*, Soziotherapie *f* / **special ~** spezielles therapeutisches Verfahren *n* / **supportive ~** unterstützende Therapie *f* / **symptomatic ~** symptomatische Therapie *f* / **vocational ~** Arbeitstherapie *f*

therblig Therblig *m*

theriomimikry, theriomimicry Tarnung *f* der Tiere

theriomorphic tiersymbolisch, tiergestaltig, theriomorph

theriomorphism Tiersymbolik *f*, tiersymbolische Darstellung *f*

thermae Thermalquellen *fpl*

thermaesthesia, thermesthesia Wärmeempfindlichkeit *f*, Wärmesinn *m*, Thermorezeption *f*

thermaesthesiometer Wärmeempfindlichkeitsmesser *m*

thermal thermal, Wärme–

thermalgesia übermäßige Wärmeempfindlichkeit *f*, Thermästhesie *f*

thermalgia brennender Schmerz *m*, Thermalgie *f*

thermic thermisch, Wärme–

thermistor Thermistor *m*

thermoaesthesial, thermoesthesia Wärmesinn *m*, Wärmeempfindlichkeit *f*

thermoaesthesiometer, thermoesthesiometer Wärmeempfindlichkeitsmesser *m*

thermoanaesthesia Verlust *m* des Wärmesinns

thermoanalgesia Unempfindlichkeit *f* gegen Wärme

thermocouple Fernthermometer *n*

thermogenesis Thermogenese *f*, Wärmebildung *f*

thermohypaesthesia, thermohypesthesia geringe Empfindlichkeit *f* gegen Wärme

thermohyperaesthesia, thermohyperesthesia Überempfindlichkeit *f* gegen Wärme

thermohyperalgesia Wärmeüberempfindlichkeit *f*

thermoperception Thermoperzeption *f*

thermophobia krankhafte Angst *f* vor Hitze

thermoreceptor Thermorezeptor *m*, temperaturempfindendes Nervenendorgan *n*

thermoregulation Wärmeregulation *f*, Thermoregulation *f*

thermoregulator Temperaturregler *m*, Thermostat *m*

thermosensor Thermosensor *m*

thermostat Thermostat *m*

thermotactic, thermotaxic thermotaktisch, thermotrop

thermotaxis Thermotaxis *f*, Thermotropismus *m*, durch Wärme bedingte Bewegung *f*

thermothesiometer Wärmeempfindlichkeitsmesser *m*

thermotropism Thermotaxis *f*, Thermotropismus *m*, durch Wärme bedingte Bewegung *f*

thesaurus Wortschatz *m*, Lexikon *n*, Thesaurus *m*

thesis wissenschaftliche Arbeit *f*, Diplomarbeit *f*, These *f*

theta| rhythm Theta–Rhythmus *m* / **~ wave** Theta–Welle *f*

they–group Fremdgruppe *f*

thigh Schenkel *m*

thiamine, thiamin Thiamin *n*, Aneurin *n*, Vitamin B *n*

thigmaesthesia, thigmesthesia Tastempfindung *f*, Tastsinn *m*

thigmotaxis Berührungsreiz *m*, Reizung *f* durch Berührung, Thigmotaxis *f*, Kontakttropismus *m*

thigmotropic thigmotrop

thigmotropism Kontakttropismus *m*, Reizung *f* durch Berührung

thing Ding *n*, Sache *f*, Gegenstand *m* / **~ image** Sachvorstellung *f*, Dingvorstellung *f* / **~ by itself** Ding–an–Sich *n* / **~ language** gegenständliche Sprache *f* / **~ presentation** Sachvorstellung *f*, Dingvorstellung *f*

thinking Denken *n* / **~ aloud** lautes Denken *n* / **~ type** Denktypus *m* / **abstract ~** abstraktes Denken *n* / **archaic ~** archaisches Denken *n* / **associative ~** assoziatives Denken *n* / **atavistic ~** atavistisches Denken *n*, archaisches Denken *n* / **autistic ~** autistisches Denken *n*, Autismus *m*, Wunscherfüllungsdenken *n* / **convulsive ~** Zwangsdenken *n* / **conceptual ~** begriffliches Denken *n*, konzeptionelles Denken *n* / **concrete ~** anschauliches Denken *n* / **constructive ~** konstruktives Denken *n* / **convergent ~** konvergentes Denken *n* / **creative ~** kreatives Denken *n*, Kreativität *f* / **dereistic ~** dereistisches

Denken *n*, Autismus *m* / **diffuse ~** weitschweifiges Denken *n* / **directed ~** gesteuertes Denken *n* / **disordered ~** gestörtes Denken *n* / **divergent ~** divergentes Denken *n* / **dreamlike ~** traumartiges Denken *n* / **epistemic ~** intellektuelles Denken *n* / **forced ~** Gedankeneingebung *f* / **goal–directed ~** zielgerichtetes Denken *n* / **imageless ~** unanschauliches Denken *n*, abstraktes Denken *n* / **intuitive ~** intuitives Denken *n*, sprunghaftes Denken *n* / **logical ~** logisches Denken *n* / **magic ~** magisches Denken *n*, Wunscherfüllungsdenken *n* / **obsessional ~** Zwangsdenken *n* / **obsessive ~** Zwangsdenken *n* / **operative ~** operatives Denken *n* / **overinclusive ~** Übereinschließung *f* / **preconscious ~** vorbewusstes Denken *n* / **prelingual ~** vorsprachliches Denken *n* / **prelogical ~** vorlogisches Denken *n* / **primitive ~** archaisches Denken *n* / **rational ~** rationales Denken *n*, logisches Denken *n* / **recursive ~** rekursives Denken *n*, Denken *n* in Verschachtelungen / **scattered ~** konfuses Denken *n* / **selective ~** selektives Denken *n* / **subjective ~** subjektives Denken *n* / **substitutive ~** Ersatzdenken *n* / **wishful ~** Wunschdenken *n*

thiopental Thiopental *n*

thioridazine Thioridazin

thiotixene Thiotixen *n*

thiouracil Thiourazil *n*

thirst Durst *m*, Durstempfindung *f* / **~–quenching** durststillend / **~ threshold** Durstschwelle *f* / **excessive ~** Polydipsie *f*, krankhafter Durst *m* / **diminished ~** verminderter Durst *m* / **hypovolemic ~** hypovolämischer Durst *m* / **insensible ~** verminderter Durst *m* / **osmotic ~** osmotischer Durst *m* / **subliminal ~** verminderter Durst *m*

thirstiness Durstempfindung *f*, Durstgefühl *n*

thobbing emotional beeinflusstes Denken *n*, vorurteilsbehaftetes Denken *n*

thoracic, thoracal thorakal, Brust–, Brustkorb–

thoracolumbar thorakolumbal, Brust und Lendengegend betreffend

thorax Brustkorb *m*, Brust *f*, Thorax *m*

Thorndike| handwriting scale Thorndikes Handschriftenskala *f* / **~'s trial–and–error learning** Thorndikes Versuch–und–Irrtum–Lernen *n*

thoroughness Gründlichkeit *f* / **slow ~** Passivität *f*

thought Gedanke *m* / **~–blocking** Denkhemmung *f*, Gedankenabreißen *n*, Gedankenblockade *f* / **~ cathexis** Denkbesetzung *f* / **~ content** Denkinhalt *m* / **~ deprivation** *f* Gedankenentzug *m* / **~ disorder** Denkstörung *f* / **~ disturbance** Denkstörung *f* / **~ echoing** Gedankenhören *n* / **~ element** gedankliches Element *n* / **~ experiment** Denkexperiment *n* / **~ hearing** Gedankenhören *n* / **~ identity** Denkidentität *f* / **~ impulses** Denkimpulse *mpl*, Denkantriebe *mpl* / **~ insertion** Gedankeneingebung *f* / **~ process** Denkvorgang *m*, Denkprozess *m* / **~ psychology** Denkpsychologie *f* / **~ questions** Denkfragen *fpl* / **~ reading** Gedankenlesen *n* / **~ stopping** Gedankenstopp *m* / **~ transference** Gedankenübertragung *f*, Telepathie *f* / **~ withdrawal** Gedankenentzug *m* / **~ work** Denkarbeit *f* / **creative ~** schöpferisches Denken *n* / **dereistic ~** dereistisches Denken *n*, autistisches Denken *n* / **discursive ~** abschweifendes Denken *n* / **disordered ~s** verworrenes Denken *n* / **formal ~** formales Denken *n* / **imageless ~** unanschaulisches Denken *n*, abstraktes Denken *n* / **intuitive ~** Intuition *f*, intuitives Denken *n* / **mixed obsessional ~s and acts** Zwangsgedanken *mpl* und –handlungen *fpl*, gemischt / **obsessional ~** Zwangsgedanke *m* / **obsessive ~** Zwangsgedanke *m* / **predominantly obsessional ~s or ruminations** vorwiegend Zwangsgedanken *mpl* oder Grübelzwang *m* / **preconceptual ~** vorbegriffliches Denken *n* / **suicidal ~s**

Selbstmordgedanken *mpl* / **supervalent ~** überwertiger Gedanke *m*, Zwangsgedanke *m* / **symbolic ~** symbolisches Denken *n*

threat Drohung *f* / **~ behaviour** Drohgebärde *f*, drohendes Verhalten *n* / **~ posture** Drohhaltung *f*, Drohgebärde *f* / **homeostatic ~** Bedrohung *f* einer Homeostase

threcia Ängstlichkeit *f*, Schüchternheit *f*, Zaghaftigkeit *f*

three drei / **~–colour theory** Dreifarbentheorie *f*, Young–Helmholtz'sche Theorie *f*, Dreikomponententheorie *f* / **~–component theory** Dreikomponententheorie *f*, Dreifarbentheorie *f*, Young–Helmholtz'sche Theorie *f* / **~ dimensional** dreidimensional / **epileptic ~–phase crisis** epileptische Dreiphasenkrise *f*

threshold Schwelle *f*, Wahrnehmungsschwelle *f* / **~ audiometry** Schwellenaudiometrie *f* / **~ determination** Reizschwellenbestimmung *f*, Wahrnehmungsschwellenbestimmung *f* / **~ difference** Schwellenunterschied *m*, eben wahrnehmbarer Unterschied *m* / **~ excitation** Schwellenreiz *m* / **~ for bodily motion** Grenze *f* der körperlichen Bewegung / **~ of audibility** Hörschwelle *f* / **~ of consciousness** Bewusstseinsschwelle *f* / **~ of contrast** Kontrastschwelle *f* / **~ of discomfort** Schmerzschwelle *f* / **~ of distinction** Unterschiedsschwelle *f*, Grenzreiz *m* / **~ of disturbance** Störungsschwelle *f* / **~ of feeling** Empfindungsschwelle *f* / **~ of pain** Schmerzgrenze *f* / **~ of rotation** Rotationsgrenze *f* / **~ of sensation** Empfindungsschwelle *f*, Reizschwelle *f*, Sinnesreizschwelle *f*, Schwellenwert *m* / **~ of successiveness** Hörfolgeschwelle *f* / **~ of tonality** Tonschwelle *f* / **~ stimulus** Schwellenreiz *m* / **absolute ~** unterste Reizschwelle *f*, absolute Schwelle *f* / **absolute auditory ~** absolute Hörschwelle *f* / **auditory ~** Hörschwelle *f* / **differential ~** Unterschiedsschwelle *f* / **lower ~** untere Reizschwelle *f* / **lowered ~** Schwellensenkung *f* / **momentary ~** augenblickliche Schwelle *f* / **olfactory ~** Geruchsschwelle *f* / **relative differential ~** relative Unterschiedsschwelle *f* / **sensory ~** Reizschwelle *f*, Empfindungsschwelle *f*, Schwellenwert *m* / **simultaneous ~** Simultanschwelle *f* / **spatial ~** Raumschwelle *f* / **successive ~** Sukzessionsschwelle *f* / **terminal ~** maximale Reizgrenze *f* / **upper ~** obere Reizschwelle *f* / **vibrotactile ~** Schwelle *f* der Vibrationsempfindung, vibrotaktile Schwelle *f* / **visual ~** Sehschwelle *f*

thrill plötzliche seelische Erregung *f*, Entzücken *n*, Erzittern *n*, Vibrieren *n* / **~ of joy** freudige Erregung *f* / **~ of horror** Schauer *m*, Erschaudern *n*

throat clearing tic Räuspertic *m*

thrombin Thrombin *n*

thrombocyte Thrombozyt *m*, Blutplättchen *n*

thrombokinase, thromboplastin Thrombokinase *f*, Thromboplastin *n*

thrombosis Thrombose *f* / **cerebral ~** Gehirnthrombose *f* / **coronary ~** Koronarthrombose *f*, Herzinfarkt *m* / **deep–vein ~** tiefe Venenthrombose *f*

thrombotic thrombotisch

thumb Daumen *m* / **~ reflex** Daumenreflex *m* / **~ sucking** Daumenlutschen *n*

Thurstone| scale Thurstone–Skala *f* / **~'s theory of primary mental abilities** Thurstones Theorie *f* der Primärfaktoren der Intelligenz

thwart vereiteln, frustrieren

thymectomy Thymusentfernung *f*, Thymektomie *f*

thymergastic thymergastisch, pathologisch affektiv

thymia affektiver Zustand *m*

thymic Thymus–

thymine Thymin *n*

thymogenic thymogen, durch Emotionen ausgelöst

thymoleptics Thymoleptika *npl*

thymopsyche Thymopsyche *f*, Gemütsanteil *m* im Seelenleben

thymus Thymus *m*, Thymusdrüse *f* / ~ **gland** Thymusdrüse *f*

thyrasthenia durch Schilddrüsenunterfunktion bedingte Neurasthenie *f*

thyrogenic, thyrogenous thyrogen, von der Schilddrüse verursacht

thyroglobulin Thyreoglobulin *n*

thyroid Schilddrüse *f*, Thyreoidea *f*, Schilddrüsen–, thyroid / ~ **disorders** Schilddrüsenstörungen *fpl* / ~ **extract** Schilddrüsenextrakt / ~ **gland** Schilddrüse *f* / ~ **hormone** Schilddrüsenhormon *n* / ~ **stimulating hormone** Thyreotropin *n*, thyreotropes Hormon *n* / **accessory** ~ Nebenschilddrüse *f*

thyroidectomise die Schilddrüse entfernen

thyroidectomy Schilddrüsenentfernung *f*, Schilddrüsenoperation *f*

thyroidomania durch Schilddrüsenerkrankung bedingte Psychose *f*

thyropathy Schilddrüsenerkrankung *f*

thyroprotein Thyreoglobulin *n*

thyrotherapy Schilddrüsenbehandlung *f*

thyrotoxicosis Thyreotoxikose *f*, Überfunktion *f* der Schilddrüse mit schwerer Vergiftung

thyrotrophin, thyrotropin Thyreotropin *n*, thyreotropes Hormon *n*

thyroxine, thyroxin Thyroxin *n*, Schilddrüsenhormon *n*, Tetrajodthyronin *n*

tic Tic *m*, Tick *m*, unwillkürliches Muskelzucken *n*, Gesichtstic *m* / ~ **convulsif** Gesichtszucken *n*, Fazialiskrampf *m* / ~ **disorders** Ticstörungen *fpl* / **chronic motor or vocal ~ disorder** chronische motorische oder vokale Ticstörung *f* / **combined vocal and multiple motor ~ disorder (de la Tourette's syndrome)** kombinierte vokale und multiple motorische Tics *mpl* (Tourette–Syndrom)/ **transient ~ disorder** vorübergehende Ticstörung *f* / **vocal ~ disorder** vokale Ticstörung *f* / ~ **douloureux** Schmerztic *m*, schmerzhafte Gesichtszuckung *f* / ~ **of an eyelid** Lidzittern *n* / **facial** ~ Gesichtstic *m*, Fazialiskrampf *m* / **laryngeal** ~ Räuspertic *m* / **mimic** ~ Gesichtstic *m*, Fazialiskrampf *m* / **organic** ~ organischer Tic *m* / **psychic** ~ psychogener Tic *m*

tickle Kitzeln *n*, Kitzelreiz *m* / kitzeln

tickling Kitzeln *n*, Kitzelreiz *m*, Kitzelgefühl *n*

tidy sauber, ordentlich, anständig

tie Verbindung *f*, Verknüpfung *f*, Bindung *f*, Nexus *m*, Paarbildung *f* / verbinden, verknüpfen, verketten / **affective** ~ Affektbindung *f* / **social** ~ soziale Bindung *f*

tilting Dreh–, Kipp–

tilting–board Wippe *f*, Kippbrett *n*

tilting–field Kippfeld *n*, Kippbrett *n*

timbre Klangfarbe *f*, Tonfarbe *f*

time Zeit *f* / **~–and–motion study** Zeit–Bewegungsstudie *f*, Zeitstudie *f* / **~–binding** Überlieferung *f* durch die Generationen / ~ **constant** Zeitkonstante *f* / **~–consuming** zeitraubend / **constant ~ delay** konstante Zeitverzögerung *f* / ~ **difference** Zeitdifferenz *f* / ~ **dimension** Zeitdimension *f* / ~ **disorientation** zeitliche Desorientiertheit *f* / ~ **error** Zeitfehler *m* / ~ **estimation** Zeitschätzung *f* / ~ **field** Zeitfeld *n* / ~ **interval** Zeitintervall *n*, Zwischenzeit *f* / **full–~ job** Ganztagsarbeit *f* / **~–keeper** Zeitnehmer *m*, Chronometer *n* / ~ **lag** Zeitverzögerung *f*, Zeitspanne *f* / **~–lapse** Zeitraffer *m* / **~–limit** Zeitbegrenzung *f*, Befristung *f*, zeitliche Begrenzung *f* / **~–limited psychotherapy** Kurztherapie *f*, zeitlich befristete Psychotherapie *f* / ~ **management** Zeitmanagement *n* / ~ **of exposure** Darbietungszeit *f*, Expositionszeit *f* / ~ **of presentation** Darbietungszeit *f*, Expositionszeit *f* / ~ **on task** effektive Arbeitszeit *f* / **~–out** Pause *f*, Auszeit *f*, Unterbrechung *f*, Time–Out *f* / ~ **perception** Zeitwahrnehmung *f* / ~ **perspective** Zeitperspektive *f* / **future ~ perspective** zukunftsgerichtete Zeitperspektive *f* / ~ **sample** Zeitstichprobe *f*, Zeitprobe *f* / ~ **sampling** Zeitprobentechnik *f*, Zeitstichprobe *f*, fraktionierte Beobachtung *f* / **~–saving** zeitsparend / ~ **schedule** Zeitplan *m* / ~ **score**

benötigte Zeit *f* / ~ **sense** Zeitsinn *m* / ~**–sense apparatus** Zeitsinnapparat *m* / ~ **series** Zeitreihe *f* / ~**–serving** Opportunismus *m* / ~**–sharing** zeitlich festgelegte Mitbenutzung *f* / ~**–signal** Zeitzeichen *n* / ~ **span** Zeitspanne *f* / ~ **study** Zeitstudie *f* / ~**–switch** Zeitschaltung *f*, Schaltuhr *f* / ~**–table** Zeittabelle *f*, Stundenplan *m* / ~**–work** Arbeit *f* im Zeitlohn / **effective** ~ nützliche Zeit *f* / **implicit** ~ Latenzzeit *f* / **interresponse** ~ Zwischenzeit *f*, Interreaktionszeit *f* / **latent** ~ Latenzzeit *f* / **psychological** ~ psychische Zeit *f*, Zeiterleben *n* / **real–**~ Realzeit *f*, „real time" / **saccadic** ~ ruckartiges Tempo *n*

timed zeitlich festgelegt, zeitlich begrenzt

timer Chronograph *m*, Zeitnehmer *m*, Zeitmessgerät *n*

timid schüchtern, verlegen, ängstlich

timidity Schüchternheit *f*, Verlegenheit *f*, Ängstlichkeit *f*

timing zeitliche Festlegung *f*

tingling Kribbeln *n*, Prickeln *n*

tinnitus Ohrgeräusch *n*, Ohrenklingen *n*, Ohrensausen *n*, Tinnitus *m* / ~ **aurium** Ohrenklingen *n*, Ohrgeräusch *n*

tinsit Situationstendenz *f*

tint Farbton *m*, Tönung *f*, Schattierung *f*

tintometer Farbenmesser *m*, Kolorimeter *n*

tintometric kolorimetrisch

tintometry Farbenmessung *f*, Kolorimetrie *f*

tiqueur Person *f* mit Gesichtszuckungen, Person *f* mit einem Tick

tire ermüden, langweilen

tiredness Müdigkeit *f*, Überdruss *m*

tissue Gewebe *n* / ~ **anoxia** Gewebeanoxie *f* / ~ **damage** Gewebsschaden *m* / ~ **donation** Gewebespende *f* / ~ **hypoxia** Gewebehypoxie *f* / ~ **impedance** Gewebewiderstand *m*, Gewebeimpedanz *f* / ~ **resistance** Gewebewiderstand *m* / ~ **respiration** Gewebebeatmung *f* / **connective** ~ Bindegewebe *n* / **epithelial** ~ Epithelium *n* / **erectile** ~ erektiles Gewebe *n*, Schwellgewebe *n* / **glandular** ~ Drüsengewebe *n* / **nervous** ~ Nervengewebe *n*

tissular zum Gewebe gehörig, Gewebs–

titillate kitzeln, erregen, reizen

titillation Kitzeln *n*, Kitzel *m*, Wohlbehagen *n*

titillomania Kratzsucht *f*, Titillomanie *f*

titubation Taumeln *n*, schwankender Gang *m* / **lingual** ~ Stottern *n*, Stammeln *n*

T cell T–Zelle *f*, T–Lymphozyt *m*

T lymphocyte T–Zelle *f*, T–Lymphozyt *m*

T maze T–förmiges Labyrinth *n*

tobacco Tabak *m* / ~ **organic mental disorder** tabakinduzierte organisch bedingte psychische Störung *f* / ~ **smoking** Rauchen *n* / ~ **withdrawal** Tabakentzug *m* / **smokeless** ~ nikotinhaltiger Ersatzstoff *m*

tobaccoism Nikotinvergiftung *f*

tocomania Wochenbettpsychose *f*

tocopherol Vitamin E *n*, Tokopherol *n*

tocophobia krankhafte Angst *f* vor der Geburt

toe Zehe *f* / ~ **reflex** Zehenreflex *m*, Babinski–Reflex *m*

toilet training Sauberkeitsgewöhnung *f*, Reinlichkeitserziehung *f*, Reinlichkeitsgewöhnung *f*

token Münze *f*, Spielgeld *n*, symbolische Anerkennung *f* / ~**–economy programme** Münz–Verstärkungsprogramm *n* / ~ **object reading** Psychometrie *f*, außersinnliche Wahrnehmung *f* über ein Objekt / ~ **payment** Münzverstärkung *f* / ~ **reinforcement** Münzverstärkung *f* / ~ **reward** Belohnung *f* mit Münzen, Eintauschverstärker *m* / ~ **system** Münzverstärkungssystem *n*

tolbutamide Tolbutamid *n*

tolerable erträglich

tolerance Toleranz *f*, Widerstandsfähigkeit *f*, Duldsamkeit *f*, Nachsicht *f*, Toleranzgrenze *f* / ~ **adaptation** Toleranzadaptation *f* / ~ **for ambiguity** Ambiguitätstoleranz *f*, Fähigkeit *f* Unsicherheit zu ertragen / ~ **to a drug** Arzneimittelgewöhnung *f*, Drogengewöhnung *f*, Immunisierung *f* / ~ **test** Belastungsprobe *f* / **immunological** ~ Immunparalyse *f*, Immuntoleranz *f*

tolerant tolerant, duldsam, widerstandsfähig

tolerate ertragen, dulden, sich gewöhnen an

toleration Toleranz *f*, Duldung *f* / ~ **of anxiety** Angsttoleranz *f*, Ertragung *f* von Angst

toluene Toluen *n*

tomo|graphy Tomographie *f* / ~ **mania** Operationssucht *f*, Tomomanie *f*

tonal Ton–, tonal

tonality Tonalität *f*, Toncharakter *m*, Farbton *m*, Tönung *f*

tonaphasia musikalische Aphasie *f*

tone Ton *m*, Klang *m*, Laut *m*, Tonus *m*, Muskeltonus *m* / ~ **brightness** Klangheftigkeit *f*, Tonhelligkeit *f* / ~ **character** Klangcharakter *m*, Toncharakter *m* / ~ **colour** Klangfarbe *f*, Tonfarbe *f*, Timbre *n* / ~ **deafness** Tontaubheit *f*, Amusie *f* / ~ **gap** Tonlücke *f* / ~ **island** Toninsel *f* / ~ **limit** Tongrenze *f*, Hörschwelle *f* / ~ **pip** Tonzeichen *n*, Zeitzeichen *n* / ~ **pulse** Tonschwingung *f* / ~ **quality** Klangfarbe *f*, Tonfarbe *f* / **vocal** ~ **recorder** Kehltonschreiber *m* / ~ **spindle** Tonnadel *f* / ~ **tint** Klangfarbe *f*, Tonfarbe *f* / ~ **variator** Tonvariator *m* / **affective** ~ Gefühlston *m* / **compound** ~ Kombinationston *m* / **differential** ~ Differenzton *m* / **emotional** ~ Gefühlston *m*, Gefühlswert *m* / **fundamental** ~ Grundton *m* / **hedonic** ~ Lustbetonung *f* / **higher** ~ **limit** obere Hörschwelle *f* / **highest audible** ~ höchster hörbarer Ton *m* / **intermediate** ~ Zwischenton *m*, Mittelton *m*, Unterton *m* / **laryngeal** ~ Kehlkopfton *m* / **lower** ~ **limit** untere Hörgrenze *f* / **lowest audible** ~ tiefster hörbarer Ton *m* / **leading** ~ 7. Ton *m* der Tonskala / **otogenic** ~ Ohrgeräusch *n* / **partial** ~ Teilton *m*, Partialton *m* / **postural** ~ Haltetonus *m* / **pure** ~ reiner Ton *m*, einfacher Ton *m* / **resting** ~ Ruhetonus *m* / **resultant** ~ Kombinationston *m* / **sharp** ~ durchdringender Ton *m* / **simple** ~ einfacher Ton *m*, Primärton *m*, reiner Ton *m* / **subjective** ~ subjektive Tonwahrnehmung *f*, Ohrgeräusch *n* / **whole** ~ Ganzton *m*

toneless klanglos, tonlos

tonelessness Tonlosigkeit *f*, Apbonie *f*

tongue Zunge *f*, menschliche Sprache *f* / ~–**bite** Zungenbiss *m*

tonic tonisch

tonicity Tonus *m*, Tonizität *f*, Spannungszustand *m*, Muskeltonus *m* / **muscular** ~ Muskeltonus *m*

tonicoclonic, tonoclonic tonisch und klonisch

tonitrophobia krankhafte Angst *f* vor Gewittern

tonograph Tonograph *m*, aufzeichnendes Tonometer *n*

tonometer Druckmesser *m*, Tonmesser *m*, Tonometer *n* / **recording** ~ aufzeichnendes Tonometer *n*

tonometry Druckmessung *f*, Tonometrie *f*

tonoscope Tonoskop *n*, Gerät *n* zur Messung der Tonhöhe

tonoscopy Tonoskopie *f*, Tonhöhenmessung *f*

tonsil Mandel *f*, Tonsille *f* / **adenoid** ~ Rachenmandel *f* / **cerebellar** ~ Kleinhirnmandel *f* / **pharyngeal** ~ Rachenmandel *f*

tonus Tonus *m*, Spannung *f*, Muskeltonus *m* / **induced** ~ induzierter Tonus *m* / **muscular** ~ Muskeltonus *m* / **myogenic** ~ Muskeltonus *m* / **neurocirculatory** ~ neurovegetativer Tonus *m* / **plastic** ~ plastischer Tonus *m*, Körperstellungstonus *m* / **postural** ~ Haltetonus *m* / **spinal** ~ Rückenmarkstonus *m*

tool Werkzeug *n*, Gerät *n*, Instrument *n* / ~ **use** Werkzeuggebrauch *m*

tooth Zahn *m*

top Spitze *f* / ~–**class sport** Hochleistungssport *m* / ~–**level manager** obere Führungskraft *f*, Top–Manager *m*, Geschäftsführer *m* / ~ **management** Unternehmensleitung *f*, Direktorium *n*, Geschäftsleitung *f*

topaesthesia, topesthesia lokalisierte Gefühlswahrnehmung *f*

topagnosis Verlust *m* der Tastlokalisation

topalgia, topoalgia umschriebener Schmerz *m*, Topalgie *f*

topectomy umschriebene Rindenexzision *f*, Topektomie *f*

topic Topik *f*, Thema *n*, Gegenstand *m*

topical örtlich, lokal, topisch, aktuell, thematisch

topoagnosia Topoagnosie *f*

topognosia, topognosis Fähigkeit *f* zur Lokalisation von Berührungsreizen, Topognosie *f*

topographic, topographical topographisch, topisch

topography Topographie *f*, Topik *f*

topological topologisch

topology Topologie *f*

toponeurosis lokalisierte Neurose *f*, örtlich begrenzte Neurose *f*, Toponeurose *f*

topoparaesthesia, topoparesthesia örtliche Parästhesie *f*

topophobia krankhafte Angst *f* vor bestimmten Orten, Topophobie *f*

topothermoaesthesiometer, topothermesthesiometer Gerät *n* zur Messung der örtlichen Wärmeempfindlichkeit

torpid empfindungslos, apathisch, stumpf, torpide

torpidity, torpidness Trägheit *f*, Stumpfheit *f*, Apathie *f*, Schlaffheit *f*, Torpor *m* / **intellectual** ~ geistige Stumpfheit *f* / **mental** ~ geistige Stumpfheit *f*

torpific betäubend, lähmend

torpor Schlaffheit *f*, Regungslosigkeit *f*, Dumpfheit *f* / Torpor *m* / **initial** ~ proaktive Hemmung *f*

torsion Drehung *f*, Torsion *f* / ~ **movement** Drehbewegung *f* / ~ **neurosis** Torsionskrampf *m* / ~ **spasm** Torsionskrampf *m*

torsional Rotations–, Drehungs–

torso Torso *n*, Rumpf *m*

torticollis Schiefhals *m*, Tortikollis *m* / **hysterical** ~ psychogener Schiefhals *m*

torture Folter *f*, Qual *f*

total total, gesamt, völlig, ganz, Gesamtsumme *f*, Gesamtheit *f* / **cumulative** ~ kumulierte Summe *f* / **grand** ~ Gesamtsumme *f* / **progressive** ~ kumulierte Summe *f*

totalisation Zusammenfassung *f*

totalise zusammenzählen, addieren

totalism Ganzheitsbewusstsein *n*

totalitarian totalitär

totalitarism Totalitarismus *m*

totality Ganzheit *f*

totem Totem *n*, Tierahn *m* / ~ **group** Totemgruppe *f*

totemic Totem–

totemism Totemismus *m*

touch Berührung *f*, Tastempfinden *n*, Tastsinn *m*, Tastgefühl *n* / berühren, tasten / ~ **corpuscle** Tastkörperchen *n*, Endkolben *m*, Meissner–Tastkörperchen *n* / ~ **pyramid** Tastpyramide *f* / ~ **receptor** Berührungsrezeptor *m* / ~ **reflex** Berührungsreflex *m* / ~ **sensation** Tastempfindung *f*, Tastgefühl *n*, Berührungsempfindung *f* / ~ **spot** Tastpunkt *m*, Berührungspunkt *m*

tough hart, fest, schwierig / **~–minded** störrisch, unbeugsam, hart

Tourette's disorder Tourette–Störung *f*, Tourette–Syndrom *n*

tourism Fremdenverkehr *m*, Tourismus *m*

town planning Städtebau *m*, Stadtplanung *f*

toxaemia, toxemia Blutvergiftung *f*, Toxämie *f*

toxaemic, toxemic Blutvergiftung betreffend, toxämisch

toxanaemia, toxanemia toxische Anämie *f*, Blutarmut *f* bei chronischen Erkrankungen

toxic, toxical toxisch, giftig

toxicity Toxizität *f* Giftigkeit *f*

toxicology Giftkunde *f*, Toxikologie *f*

toxicomania Toxikomanie *f*, krankhafte Sucht *f* Gifte einzunehmen, Giftsucht *f*

toxicomaniac Giftsüchtiger *m*

toxicophobia, toxiphobia krankhafte Angst *f* vor Giften, Furcht *f* vor Vergiftung, Toxiphobie *f*, Toxikophobie *f*

toxicosis Vergiftung *f*, Toxikose *f* / **endogenic ~** Selbstvergiftung *f*, Autointoxikation *f* / **exogenic ~** Vergiftung *f* durch äußere Einwirkung

toxin Gift *n*, Giftstoff *m*, Toxin *n*

toxoplasma Toxoplasma *n*

toxoplasmosis Toxoplasmose *f*

toy Spielzeug *n* / **~ selection** Spielzeugwahl *f* / **educational ~** pädagogisches Spielzeug *n*

trabecula cranii Schädelbalken *m*

trace Spur *f*, Skizze *f* / zeichnen, skizzieren, graphisch darstellen, nachspüren / **~ conditioning** Ausbildung *f* eines Spurenreflexes, Spurkonditionierung *f* / **~ element** Spurenelement *n* / **~ line** Aufgabenprofil *n* / **~ process** Engrammbildung *f* / **~ reflex** Spurenreflex *m* / **conditioned ~ response** konditionierter Spurenreflex *m* / **long ~ response** langer Spurenreflex *m* / **~ theory** Engrammtheorie *f* / **mnemic ~** Gedächtnisspur *f*, Engramm *n*, Neurogramm *n* / **mnemonic ~** Gedächtnisspur *f*, Engramm *n*, Neurogramm *n* / **perseverative ~** Nacherregung *f*, Perseverationsspur *f* / **short ~ response** kurzer Spurenreflex *m* / **traumatic ~** Unfallerinnerung *f*

trachea Luftröhre *f*, Trachea *f*

tracheophyma Kropf *m*

trachoma Trachom *n*, ägyptische Augenkrankheit *f*, Körnerkrankheit *f*

trachyphonia Heiserkeit *f*, Trachyphonie *f*

tracing Nachfahren *n* von Linien, Linienführen *n*, Aufzeichnung *f*

track Spur *f*, Weg *m*, Bahn *f* / aufspüren, verfolgen

tracking Spurhalten *n*, Nachfahren *n*, Tracking *n* / **visual ~** optisches Nachfahren *n*, visuelles Tracking *n*

tract Bahn *f*, Kanal *m*, Strang *m* / **~s of association** Assoziationsbahnen *fpl* / **anterior cerebellar ~** Vorderseitenstrang *m* / **anterior cerebrospinal ~** Pyramidenvorderstrangbahn *f* / **ascending ~** aufsteigende Bahn *n* / **bulbar ~** Bulbusbahn *f* / **bulbospinal ~** Olivenrückenmarksbahn *f* / **cerebellar ~** Kleinhirnbahn *f* / **cerebropontine ~** Brückenbahn *n* / **corticospinal ~** Pyramidenbahn *f* / **crossed pyramidal ~** Pyramidenseitenstrangbahn *f* / **descending ~** absteigende Bahn *f* / **digestive ~** Verdauungstrakt *m* / **direct pyramidal ~** Pyramidenvorderstrangbahn *f* / **dorsocerebellar ~** hintere Kleinhirnbahn *f* / **extrapyramidal ~** extrapyramidale Bahn *f* / **gastrointestinal ~** Magen–Darm–Trakt *m*, Gastrointestinaltrakt *m* / **intestinal ~** Darmtrakt *m* / **lateral ~** Seitenbahn *f* / **lateral cerebellospinal ~** Kleinhirnseitenstrangbahn *f* / **lateral cerebrospinal ~** Pyramidenseitenstrangbahn *f* / **lateral pyramidal ~** Pyramidenseitenstrangbahn *f* / **motor ~** motorische Bahn *f* / **olfactory ~** Riechbahn *f*, Riechstrang *m*, Tractus olfactorius *m* / **olivospinal ~** Olivenrückenmarksbahn *f* / **ophthalmic ~** Sehstrang *m* / **optic ~** Sehstrang *m*, Tractus opticus *m* / **Pontine ~** Brückenbahn *f* / **pontospinal ~** Brückenrückenmarksbahn *f* / **posterolateral ~** hintere Kleinhirnbahn *f* / **propriospinal ~** propriospinale Bahn *f* / **pyramidal ~** Pyramidenbahn *f* / **respiratory ~** Atemwege *mpl* / **rubrospinal ~** Rubrospinalbahn *f*, Tractus rubrospinalis *m* / **sensory~** sensible Nervenbahn *f* / **spinal ~** Rückenmarksstrang *m* / **spinocerebellar ~** Rückenmarkkleinhirnbahn *f* / **spinotectal ~** Haubenrückenmarksbahn *f* / **spinothalamic ~** Rückenmarkthalamusbahn *f* / **tecto–spinal ~** Haubenrückenmarksbahn *f* / **temperopontine ~** Schläfenbrückentrakt *m* / **urinary ~** Harnwege *mpl* / **vestibulospinal ~** Labyrinthrückenmarksbahn *f*

tractable lenkbar, folgsam, führbar

tractate Abhandlung *f*, Behandlung *f*

traction effect Zugeffekt *m*

tractotomy Durchtrennung *f* eines Nervenstranges, Traktotomie *f*

tractus Bahn *f*, Trakt *m* / ~ **pyramidalis** Pyramidenbahn *f*

trade Beruf *m*, Gewerbe *n*, Handel *m*, Geschäft *n*, Branche *f* / ~ **test** Berufseignungstest *m* / ~ **union** Gewerkschaft *f* / **skilled** ~ Facharbeiterberuf *m*

tradition Tradition *f*, Überlieferung *f*, Brauchtum *n*, alter Brauch *m* / **~–directed** traditionsgeleitet

traditional traditionell, herkömmlich, üblich, Traditions–

traditionalism Traditionalismus *m*, Festhalten *n* an der Tradition

traffic Verkehr *m* / **motor ~ accident** Straßenverkehrsunfall *m* / ~ **behaviour** Verkehrsverhalten *n*

train Reihe *f*, Kette *f*, Zug *m* / ausbilden, einüben, trainieren, üben / ~ **of ideas** Gedankenkette *f*, Ideenablauf *m* / ~ **nystagmus** Eisenbahnnystagmus *m* / ~ **of thought** Gedankengang *m*, Gedankenkette *f* / ~ **the trainer** Ausbildertraining *n*

trainable ausbildbar, bildungsfähig, trainierbar

trainee Auszubildender *m*, Praktikant *m*, Trainee *m*

traineeship Praktikum *n*

trainer Ausbilder *m*, Übungsleiter *m*, Trainer *m*

training Ausbildung *f*, Schulung *f*, Erziehung *f*, Übung *f*, Training *n* / ~ **analysis** Lehranalyse *f* / ~ **centre** Ausbildungsstätte *f*, Ausbildungszentrum *n* / ~ **in cleanliness** Sauberkeitsgewöhnung *f*, Reinlichkeitserziehung *f* / ~ **device** Lehrmaschine *f*, Lehrgerät *n*, Simulator *m* / ~ **group** Trainingsgruppe *f* / ~ **within industry** richtige Unterweisung *f* von Mitarbeitern / ~ **off the job** Seminartraining *n*, Schulung *f* / ~ **on the job** praktische Ausbildung *f* am Arbeitsplatz / **athletic** ~ Sporttraining *n* / **autogenic** ~ autogenes Training *n* / **cardiovascular** ~ Herz–Kreislauf–Training *n* / **civic** ~ staatsbürgerkundliche Ausbildung *f* / **inservice** ~ berufsbegleitende Weiterbildung *f* / **mental** ~ mentales Training *n* / **military** ~ militärische Ausbildung *f* / **postgraduate** ~ Postgraduiertenausbildung *f*, Doktorandenausbildung *f*, Ausbildung *f* nach dem Diplom / **professional** ~ Berufsausbildung *f* / **psychiatric** ~ Psychiatrieausbildung *f* / **psychoanalytic** ~ psychoanalytische Ausbildung *f* / **remedial** ~ Umerziehung *f*, Umschulung *f* / **psychosomatic** ~ psychosomatisches Training *n* / **vocational** ~ Berufsausbildung *f*

trait Eigenschaft *f*, Charakterzug *m*, Wesenszug *m*, Merkmal *n* / ~ **anxiety** generalisierte Angst *f* / ~ **continuity** Durchgängigkeit *f* einer Eigenschaft / ~ **difference** Charakterunterschied *m* / ~ **element** Eigenschaftselement *n* / ~ **organisation** Eigenschaftsstruktur *f* / ~ **profile** Charakterprofil *n*, Profil *n* der Eigenschaften / ~ **theory** Eigenschaftstheorie *f* / ~ **variability** Variabilität *f* der Eigenschaften / **cardinal** ~ Kardinaleigenschaft *f* / **central** ~ Zentraleigenschaft *f* / **common** ~ universelle Eigenschaft *f* / **compensatory** ~ kompensatorische Eigenschaft *f* / **constitutional** ~ konstitutionelle Eigenschaft *f* / **dominant** ~ dominantes Merkmal *n*, dominante Eigenschaft *f* / **dynamic** ~ dynamische Eigenschaft *f* / **environmental–mold** ~ umweltgeprägte Eigenschaft *f* / **ergic** ~ anlagebedingte Wurzeleigenschaft *f* / **familial** ~ Familieneigenschaft *f* / **fundamental** ~ Grundeigenschaft *f*, elementare Eigenschaft *f*, wesentliche Eigenschaft *f* / **generalized** ~ generelle Eigenschaft *f*, Durchgängigkeit *f* einer Eigenschaft / **genetic ~s** Erbanlagen *fpl* / **hereditary ~s** Erbanlagen *fpl* / **independent** ~ unabhängige Eigenschaft *f* / **metanergic** ~ umweltgeprägte Wurzeleigenschaft *f* / **native** ~ angebotener Charakterzug *m* / **objective** ~ objektives Merkmal *n* /

orthogonal ~ unabhängige Eigenschaft *f* / **personal** ~ persönliche Eigenschaft *f*, Wurzeleigenschaft *f* / **recessive** ~ rezessives Merkmal *n*, rezessive Anlage *f* / **secondary** ~ sekundäre Eigenschaft *f* / **social** ~ soziale Eigenschaft *f* / **unique** ~ singuläre Eigenschaft *f*, individuelle Eigenschaft *f*, unabhängige Eigenschaft *f* / **unitary** ~ einheitliche Eigenschaft *f* / **universal** ~ universelle Eigenschaft *f*

trance Trance *f*, Trancezustand *m* / **ecstatic** ~ Ekstase *f* / **hypnotic** ~ Hypnose *f* / **hysteric** ~ hysterischer Trancezustand *m* / **induced** ~ Hypnose *f*

tranquillisation, tranquilization Beruhigung *f*, Dämpfung *f*, Sedierung *f*

tranquillise, tranquilize beruhigen, dämpfen, sedieren

tranquilliser, tranquilizer Beruhigungsmittel *n*, Sedativum *n*, Tranquilizer *m* / **major** ~ Psycholytikum *n* / **minor** ~ Tranquilizer *m*, leichtes Beruhigungsmittel *n*

transaction Transaktion *f* / ~ **analysis** Transaktionsanalyse *f* / ~ **theory of perception** Transaktionstheorie *f* der Wahrnehmung

transactional Transaktions–

transactionalism Transaktionalismus *m*

transaminase Transaminase *f*

transceiver Sender–Empfänger *m*

transcendence Transzendenz *f*

transcendent transzendent, über alle Erfahrung hinausgehend

transcendental transzendental, über alle Erfahrung hinausgehend, übernatürlich, transzendent

transcortical transkortikal

transcription Transkription *f*

transducer Überträger *m*, Wandler *m*, Schallgeber *m* / **active** ~ aktiver Überträger *m* / **passive** ~ passiver Überträger *m*

transduction genetische Übermittlung *f*, Transduktion *f*

transect durchschneiden, quer durchtrennen

transection Durchtrennung *f*, Querschnitt *m*

transfection Transfektion *f*

transfer Übertragung *f*, Transfer *m*, unbewusste Mitübung *f* / ~ **by generalisation** Transfer *m* durch Generalisierung / ~ **of learning** Lernübertragung *f* / ~ **of principles** Übertragung *f* von Prinzipien / ~ **of response** Reaktionsgeneralisierung / ~ **student** Studienwechsler *m*, Schulwechsler *m* / ~ **surface** Übertragungsfläche *f* / ~ **of training** Übungsübertragung *f* / **applicational** ~ Transfer *m* auf die Praxis / **bilateral** ~ bilateraler Transfer *m*, beiderseitige Übertragung *f* / **interocular** ~ interokularer Transfer *m* / **negative** ~ negativer Transfer *m*, negative Übertragung *f* / **positive** ~ positiver Transfer *m*

transferase Transferase *f*

transference Übertragung *f* / ~ **neurosis** Übertragungsneurose *f* / ~ **resistance** Übertragungswiderstand *m* / ~ **of sensations** Hellsehen *n* / ~ **of thoughts** Gedankenübertragung *f*, Telepathie *f* / **countersexual** ~ Übertragung *f* auf eine gegengeschlechtliche Person / **negative** ~ negative Übertragung *f*, negative Verschiebung *f* / **positive** ~ positive Übertragung / **psychotherapeutic** ~ psychotherapeutische Übertragung *f*

transform umwandeln, umformen, umgestalten, transformieren

transformation Umgestaltung *f*, Umformung *f*, Umwandlung *f*, Transformation *f* / ~ **of instincts** Triebumwandlung *f*, Triebtransformation *f* / ~ **marker** Transformationsmarker *m* / ~ **into the opposite** Verkehrung *f* ins Gegenteil / **acoustic** ~ akustische Verarbeitung *f* / **affective** ~ Affektinversion *f* / **linear** ~ lineare Transformation *f* / **malevolent** ~ Bewusstwerden *n* der Einsicht, in einer feindlichen Welt zu leben / **perceptual** ~ Wahrnehmungstransformation *f*

transformer Transformator *m*

transformism Transformationstheorie *f*, Deszendenztheorie *f*, Evolutionstheorie *f*

transformist Anhänger *m* der Transformationstheorie / ~ **theory** Transformationstheorie *f*, Deszendenztheorie *f*

transgression Übertretung *f*, Vergehen *n*, Gesetzesverletzung *f*

transient vorübergehend, flüchtig, temporär

transition Übergang *m* / ~ **period** Übergangszeit *f* / ~ **point** Übergangspunkt *m* / ~ **training** Umschulung *f* / ~ **zone** Übergangsbereich *m*

transitional Übergangs–

transitive transitiv, Übergangs–

transitivism Transitivismus *m*

transitivity, transitiveness Transitivität *f*

transitory vorübergehend, flüchtig, transitorisch

translation Translation *f*

translocation Translokation *f*, Austausch *m* von Chromosomenstückchen

translucence, translucency Durchsichtigkeit *f*

translucent, translucid durchsichtig, transparent

transmigration Überwanderung *f*, Seelenwanderung *f* / ~ **of souls** Seelenwanderung *f*

transmissible übertragbar, vererbbar

transmission Übertragung *f*, Vererbung *f* / ~ **of excitation** Erregungsübertragung *f* / ~ **factor** Vererbungsfaktor *m* / ~ **of impulses** Reizübertragung *f* / ~ **of movement test** Transmissionstest *m*, Transmissionsaufgabe *f* / ~ **psychosis** Übertragungspsychose *f* / ~ **of stimuli** Reizübertragung *f* / ~ **theory** Übertragungstheorie *f* / ~ **unit** Übertragungseinheit *f*, Dezibel *n* / **adrenergic** ~ adrenergische Übertragung *f* / **cultural** ~ Kulturübertragung *f* / **hereditary** ~ Erbgang *m*, Vererbung *f* / **humoral** ~ humorale Übertragung *f* / **neural** ~ Erregungsfortpflanzung *f* / **neurochemical** ~ neurochemische Erregungsübertragung *f* / **neuromuscular** ~ neuromuskuläre Übertragung *f* / **social** ~ Überlieferung *f*, soziale Weitergabe *f* / **synaptic** ~ synaptische Übertragung *f*

transmit weiterleiten, fortpflanzen, fortleiten

transmitter Sender *m*, Transmitter *m*, Übertragungsubstanz *f*, Mittlersubstanz *f* / ~ **substance** Überträgersubstanz *f*, Transmittersubstanz *f*, Mittlersubstanz *f* / **inhibitory** ~ Hemmsubstanz *f*

transmutation Umwandlung *f* / ~ **of measures** Umwandlung *f* der Messwerte

transmute umwandeln, umformen, transformieren

transparency, transparence Transparenz *f*, Durchsichtigkeit *f*, Diapositiv *n*

transparent durchsichtig, transparent

transplantation, transplant Verpflanzung *f*, Umsetzung *f*, Transplantation *f* / ~ **experiment** Umsetzungsexperiment *n* / **heterologous** ~ heterologe Transplantation *f*, Xenotransplantation *f* / **neural** ~ neurale Transplantation *f*, Nerventransplantation *f*

transport Transport *m* / ~ **process** Transportprozess *m* / ~ **protein** Transportprotein *n* / **active** ~ aktiver Transport *m* / **axonal** ~ axonaler Transport *m* / **retrograde** ~ retrograder Transport *m* / **passive** ~ passiver Transport *m*

transportation accident Verkehrsunfall *m*

transpose umstellen, umsetzen, transponieren

transposition Transposition *f*, Umstellung *f*, Versetzung *f*, Transponierbarkeit *f*, Verhaltenstransposition *f* / ~ **of affect** Affektverschiebung *f* / ~ **behaviour** Transpositionsverhalten *n*

transsexual transsexuell

transsexualism Transsexualismus *m*, Transsexualität *f*, Begehren *n* nach Geschlechtsumwandlung

transudation Transsudation *f*

transvaluation Umwertung *f* / ~ **of psychic values** Umwertung *f* aller Werte

transverse quer, querverlaufend, diagonal, transversal

transvest Kleider des anderen Geschlechts anziehen

transvestism, transvestitism Transvestismus *m*, Transvestie *f* / **dual–role ~** Transvestitismus *m* unter Beibehaltung beider Geschlechtsrollen / **fetishistic ~** fetischistischer Transvestitismus *m*

transvestite Transvestit *m*

tranylcypromine Tranylcypromin *n*

trapezoid trapezförmig, trapezoid

Traube–Hering waves Traube–Hering–Wellen *fpl*

traulism Stammeln *n*, Stottern *n*

trauma Verletzung *f*, Wunde *f*, Trauma *n* / **craniocerebral ~** Schädel–Hirn–Trauma *n* / **emotional ~** emotionales Trauma *n* / **physical ~** Körperverletzung *f* / **primal ~** Urtrauma *n* / **psychic ~** psychisches Trauma *n*, psychische Schädigung *f* / **sexual ~** sexuelles Trauma *n*

traumasthenia traumatische Neurose *f*, traumatisch bedingte Nervenschwäche *f*

traumatic traumatisch, Unfall–, auf eine Verletzung zurückgehend, posttraumatisch

traumatisation Verwundung *f*, Verletzung *f*, Schädigung *f*

traumatise verwunden, verletzen, eine Schädigung erleiden

traumatism Verletzung *f*, Schädigung *f*, Trauma *n*

traumatology Traumatologie *f*, Lehre *f* von der Wundbehandlung, Unfallchirurgie *f*

traumatomania Unfallsucht *f*

traumatopathy Unfallsleiden *n*

traumatophilia Unfallsucht *f*, Unfallneigung *f*, Operationssucht *f*, Traumatophilie *f*

traumatophilic unfallsüchtig, unfallgeneigt, operationssüchtig

traumatophobia krankhafte Angst *f* vor Verletzungen, abnorme Furcht *f* vor Unfällen

travelling Reisen *n* / reisend

travesty Travestie *f*, Transvestismus *m*

trazodone Trazodon *n*

treachery Treulosigkeit *f*, Verrat *m*

treadmill ergometer Laufbandergometer *n*

treatment Behandlung *f*, Therapie *f*, systematische Veränderung *f* der Versuchsbedingungen, statistische Bearbeitung *f* der Versuchsergebnisse / **~ approach** Behandlungsansatz *m* / **~ compliance** Compliance *f* / **~ dropout** Therapieabbrecher *m* / **~ duration** Behandlungsdauer *f* / **~ effectiveness evaluation** Therapieerfolgskontrolle *f* / **~ facility** therapeutische Einrichtung *f*, Behandlungseinrichtung *f* / **~ interview** Behandlungsgespräch *n*, Beratungsgespräch *n* / **~ neurosis** Behandlungsneurose *f* / **~ of choice** Therapie *f* der Wahl / **~ of schizophrenia** Schizophreniebehandlung *f* / **~ outcome** Therapieergebnis *n* / **~ planning** Behandlungsplanung *f* / **~ programme** Behandlungsplan *m* / **~ refusal** Behandlungsverweigerung *f* / **~–resistant depression** therapieresistente Depression *f* / **~–resistant disorder** therapieresistente Störung *f* / **~ termination** Behandlungsende *n*, Therapiebeendigung *f* / **~ variable** unabhängige Variable *f* / **~ withholding** Behandlungsaussetzung *f* / **acute ~** Sofortbehandlung *f* / **causal ~** Kausalbehandlung *f* / **clinical ~** stationäre Behandlung *f* / **convulsive ~** Krampfbehandlung *f* / **cross–cultural ~** interkulturelle Behandlungssituation *f* / **dental ~** Zahnbehandlung *f* / **direct ~ effect** unmittelbarer Behandlungserfolg *m* / **eclectic ~** eklektische Behandlung *f* / **electro–convulsive ~** Schocktherapie *f* / **experimental ~** experimentelles Verfahren *n*, experimentelle Änderung *f* der Versuchsbedingungen / **fixed ~s** feste Versuchsbedingungen *fpl* / **individual ~** Einzeltherapie *f* / **institutional ~** Anstaltsbehandlung *f* / **interdisciplinary ~ approach** interdisziplinärer Behandlungsansatz *m* / **involuntary ~** Zwangsbehandlung *f* / **long–**

term ~ Dauerbehandlung *f* / **medical ~** medizinische Behandlung *f* / **mental ~** seelische Behandlung *f*, psychotherapeutische Behandlung *f* / **multimodal ~ approach** multimodaler Behandlungsansatz *m* / **outpatient ~** ambulante Behandlung *f* / **physical ~ method** physikalische Behandlungsmethode *f*, medizinisches Behandlungsverfahren *n* / **prolonged ~** Dauerbehandlung *f* / **prophylactic ~** Vorbeugungstherapie *f* / **psychotherapeutical ~** psychotherapeutische Behandlung *f* / **suggestive ~** Suggestionstherapie *f* / **symptomatic ~** symptomatische Behandlung *f*

tree Baum *m* / **~ structure** Dendrit *m* / **~ test** Baumtest *m*

tremble zittern, beben, zucken / Zittern *n*, Tremor *m*

trembling Zittern *n*, Tremor *m*

tremograph Tremograph *m*, Gerät *n* zur Aufzeichnung von Zitterbewegungen

tremolo Tremolo *n*

tremometer Tremometer *n*, Gerät *n* zur Messung von Zitterbewegungen

tremor Zittern *n*, Tremor *m* / **alcoholic ~** Alkoholtremor *m* / **coarse ~** grobschlägiger Tremor *m* / **continuous ~** Dauertremor *m* / **convulsive ~** Zitterkrampf *m*, Krampftremor *m* / **fine ~** feinschlägiger Tremor *m* / **flapping ~** grobschlägiger Tremor *m* / **hysterical ~** hysterisches Zittern *n* / **intentional ~** Intentionstremor *m* / **laryngeal ~** Stimmbandzittern *n* / **muscular ~** Muskeltremor *m*, Muskelzittern *n* / **passive ~** Ruhetremor *m* / **senile ~** seniler Tremor *m* / **volitional ~** Intentionstremor *m*

tremulation feinschlägige Zitterbewegung *f*, Tremulation *f*

tremulous zitternd, nervös

trend Neigung *f*, Tendenz *f*, Disposition *f*, Hang *m*, Strebung *f*, Streben *n*, Richtung *f*, Trend *m* / streben, sich neigen, die Tendenz haben / **~ analysis** Trendanalyse *f* / **~ of development** Entwicklungstendenz *f*, Entwicklungstrend *m* / **cognitive ~** kognitive Verhaltenstendenz *f* / **linear ~** linearer Trend *m* / **malicious ~** chronische Tendenz *f* / **neurotic ~** neurotischer Trend *m*, neurotische Tendenz *f* / **pernicious ~** chronische Tendenz *f* / **proximodistal ~** proximodistale Tendenz *f*

trepan, trephine Schädelbohrer *m*, Schädelsäge *f*, Trepan *m* / die Schädeldecke eröffnen, trepanieren

trepanation, trephination, trephinement Schädeleröffnung *f*, Trepanation *f*

trepidation Zittern *n*, Tremor *m*, nervöse Unruhe *f*, zitternde Erregung *f*

Treponema pallidum Treponema pallidum *f*, Spirochaeta pallida *f*

TRH| test TRH–Test *m* / **~ stimulation test** TRH–Test *m*, TRH–Stimulations–Test *m*

triad Triade *f*, Dreiheit *f*, Trias *f* / **anal ~** anale Trias *f*

triadic triadisch

trial Versuch *m*, Lernversuch *m*, Durchgang *m*, Erprobung *f* / **~ design** Versuchsanordnung *f* / **~ and error** Versuch *m* und Irrtum *m* / **~–and–error learning** Lernen *n* durch Versuch und Irrtum, Versuch–Irrtums–Lernen *n*, Probierverhalten *n* / **~–and–error theory** Theorie *f* des Lernens durch Versuch und Irrtum / **~ response** Antwortversuch *m*, vorläufige Reaktion *f* / **double–blind ~** Doppelblindversuch *m* / **discrete ~s** getrennte Versuche *mpl* / **massed ~s** gedrängte Übung *f* / **one–~ learning** Lernen *n* in einem Lerndurchgang / **single–blind ~** Einzelblindversuch *m* / **spaced ~s** verteilte Übung *f* / **vicarious ~–and–error behaviour** Versuchs– und Irrtumsverhalten *n*

triangle Dreieck *n* / **~ hypothesis** Dreieck–Hypothese *f* / **~ situation** Dreiecksverhältnis *n*

triazolam Triazolam *n*

tribade Tribade *f*, Lesbierin *f*, weibliche Homosexuelle *f*

tribadism, tribady Tribadie *f*, Tribadismus *m*, lesbische Liebe *f*, weibliche Homosexualität *f*

tribal Stammes–, zum Stamm gehörig

tribe Stamm *m*, Volksstamm *m*

triceptor theory Dreikomponententheorie *f*

trichaesthesia, trichesthesia, trichoaesthesia, trichoesthesia Empfindlichkeit *f* der Haare

trichinophobia Trichinenangst *f*, Trichinophobie *f*

trichoaesthesiometer, trichesthesiometer Gerät *n* zur Messung der Haarempfindlichkeit

trichoclasmania Sucht *f* sich die eigenen Haare auszureißen, Trichotillomanie *f*

trichographism Gänsehautreflex *m*, pilomotorischer Reflex *m*

trichokryptomania Sucht *f* die Haare mit den Fingernägeln abzuknipsen

trichomania Sucht *f* sich die eigenen Haare auszureißen, Trichotillomanie *f*

trichopathophobia Angst *f* vor Haarkrankheiten

trichophagia, tichphagy Haarkauen *n*, Trichophagie *f*

trichophobia krankhafte Angst *f* vor behaarten Dingen, Angst *f* vor Haaren, Trichophobie *f*

trichorrhexomania Sucht *f* die Haare mit den Fingernägeln abzuknipsen, Trichorrhexomanie *f*

trichotillomania Trichotillomanie *f*, krankhafte Sucht *f* die eigenen Haare auszureißen

trichotomous dreigeteilt, dreiteilig

trichotomy Dreiteilung *f*

trichromat normal Farbensichtiger *m*, Trichromat *m*

trichromatic farbtüchtig, normal farbensichtig, dreifarbig, trichromatisch

trichromatism Trichromasie *f*, Trichromatismus *m*, normaler Farbensinn *m* / **anomalous ~** anomale Trichromasie *f*, Farbenanomalie *f*, Farbenschwäche *f*

trichromatopsia normales Farbensehen *n*, normaler Farbensinn *m*, Trichromasie *f*, Trichromatismus *m*

trick Täuschung *f*, Illusion *f*, Selbsttäuschung *f*

tricyclic trizyklisch

tridimensional dreidimensional

trifacial Trigeminus–

trifluoperazine Trifluperazin *n*

triflupromazine Triflupromazin *n*

trigeminal Trigeminus–

trigeminus Trigeminus *m*, Nervus trigeminus *m*

trigger Auslöser *m* / auslösen / **~ action** Auslösevorgang *m*

triglyceride Triglyzerid *n*, Triglycerid *n*

trigram, trigraph Trigramm *n*, Dreierkombination *f* von Einzelbuchstaben

trihexyphenidyl Trihexyphenidyl *n*

triiodothyronine Trijodthyronin *n*

trill threshold Trillergrenze *f*

trineuric aus drei Neuronen bestehend

triolism Triolismus *m*

triplet Drilling *m*

triplopia Dreifachsehen *n*, Triplopie *f*

trireceptor theory Dreikomponententheorie *f*, Young–Helmholtzsche Dreikomponententheorie *f*

triskaidekaphobia krankhafte Angst *f* vor der Zahl dreizehn

trismus Kiefersperre *f*, Krampf *m* der Kaumuskeln, Trismus *m*

trisomic dreichromosomig

trisomy Trisomie *f*, Verdreifachung *f* eines einzelnen Chromosoms

tristimania Melancholie *f*

tristimulus values Anteile *mpl* an den drei Grundfarben

tritanomaly Blauschwäche *f*, Tritanomalie *f*

tritanopia, tritanopsia Tritanopie *f*, Blaublindheit *f*, Violettblindheit *f*

tritanopic, tritanope blaublind, violettblind, tritanop

tritone Dreiton *m*

triumph call Siegesgeschrei *n*, Triumphschrei *m*

trochlear trochlear

trochocephalus Rundkopf *m*

troilism Sex *m* zu Dritt, Ehe *f* zu Dritt

troland Troland *m*

tromomania Alkoholdelir *n*, Delirium tremens *n*

trophic Ernährungs–, trophisch

trophoneurosis Trophoneurose *f*

trophotropism Trophotropismus *m*, Raumorientierung *f* zur Nahrung hin

tropic tropisch

tropism, tropismus Tropismus *m*, Raumorientierung *f*, Taxis *f* / **positive ~** positiver Tropismus *m*

tropistic Tropismus betreffend

tropomyosin Tropomyosin *n*

tropostereoscope Tropostereoskop *n*

tropotaxis Tropotaxis *f*

trouble Störung *f*, Schwierigkeit *f*, Sorge *f*, Kummer *m* / **~–maker** Unruhestifter *m*, Störenfried *m* / **~–shooting** Störungsbeseitigung *f* / **nervous ~** nervöse Beschwerden *fpl*

truancy Schwänzen *n*, unerlaubtes Fernbleiben *n*

truant Müßiggänger *m*, Bummelant *m*, Schulschwänzer *m* / schwänzend, bummelnd die Schule schwänzen, bummeln

truculence Wildheit *f*, Grausamkeit *f*, Widerspenstigkeit *f*

truculent wild, grausam, grob, widerspenstig

true wahr, richtig, genau, wirklich

truism Binsenwahrheit *f*, Gemeinplatz *m*

truncated abgestumpft, verkürzt

trunk Stamm *m*, Strang *m* / **~ of the corpus callosum** Balkenstamm *m* / **sympathetic ~** Grenzstrang *m*

trust Vertrauen *n*, Zuversicht *f*, zuversichtliche Erwartung *f* / vertrauen

trustiness Vertrauensseligkeit *f*

trustworthiness Zuverlässigkeit *f*, Vertrauenswürdigkeit *f*

trustworthy vertrauenswürdig, zuverlässig

truth Wahrheit *f*, Wahrhaftigkeit *f*, Aufrichtigkeit *f* / **~ drug** Wahrheitsserum *n*, Wahrheitsdroge *f* / **~ serum** Wahrheitsserum *n*, Wahrheitsdroge *f*

try Versuch *m* / versuchen, probieren / **provisional ~** Versuch *m*, Ausprobieren *n*, Erproben *n*, vorläufiger Versuch *m*

trypsin Trypsin *n*

tryptamine Tryptamin *n*

tryptophan Tryptophan *n*

T scale T–Skala *f*

T score T–Wert *m*

***t* test** t–Test *m*, Student–Test

T type T–Typ *m*

tub file Karteikasten *m* / **open ~** offener Karteikasten *m*

tubal Tuben–, Eileiter–

tube Röhre *f*, Kanal *m*, Ductus *m*, Eileiter *m* / **auditory ~** Ohrtrompete *f* / **auricular ~** äußerer Gehörgang *m* / **capillary ~** Haargefäß *n*, Kapillare *f*, Kapillargefäß *n* / **cerebromedullary ~** Medullarrohr *n*, Neuralrohr *n* / **digestive ~** Verdauungskanal *m* / **Eustachian ~** Ohrtrompete *f*, Eustachi'sche Röhre *f* / **Fallopian ~** Eileiter *m* / **medullary ~** Medullarrohr *n*, Neuralrohr *n* / **neural ~** Neuralrohr *n*, Medullarrohr *n* / **pharyngo–tympanic ~** Ohrtrompete *f*

tubectomy Eileiterentfernung *f*, Tubenresektion *f*

tuber cinereum Tuber cinereum *n*

tubercle Höcker *m* / **olfactory ~** Riechwulst *m*

tuberculomania krankhafte Einbildung *f* an Tuberkulose zu leiden

tuberculophobia krankhafte Angst *f* vor Tuberkulose

tubocurarine Tubokurarin *n*

tubulin Tubulin *n*

tuition Unterricht *m*, Belehrung *f*

tuitional Unterrichts–

tumescence Schwellung *f*, Anschwellen *n*

tumescent, tumid anschwellend, angeschwollen

tumour, tumor Tumor *m*, Geschwulst *f* / **~ cell** Tumorzelle *f* / **~ of the brain** Gehirntumor *m* / **~ of the cord** Rückenmarktumor *m* / **~ of the medulla** Rückenmarktumor *m* / **benign ~** gutartiger Tumor *m* / **cerebral ~** Gehirntumor *m* / **intracranial ~** Gehirntumor *m* / **malignant ~** bösartiger Tumor *m* / **medullary ~** Rückenmarktumor *m*

tune stimmen / Melodie *f*

tuning| curve Abstimmkurve *f* / **~ fork** Stimmgabel *f*

tunnel Tunnel *m* / **~ vision** Sehfeldeinengung *f*, eingeschränktes Sehen *n*

turbid verworren, konfus, verstört, unklar

turbulence Unruhe *f*, Aufruhr *m*

turn Drehung *f*, Wendung *f*, Krise *f* / drehen, wenden / **~ of life** Wechseljahre *npl*

turner Dreher *m*, Drechsler *m* / **~'s test** Test *m* für Dreher

Turner's syndrome Turner–Syndrom *n*, Ulrich–Turner–Syndrom *n*, Morgagni–Turner–Abbright–Syndrom *n*

turning Drehung *f*, Wendung *f* / **~ backward** Rückwärtsdrehung *f*, Beugung *f* nach rückwärts / **~ round upon the subject's own self** Wendung *f* gegen die eigene Person

turnover Fluktuation *f*, Personalwechsel *m*, Schwankung *f* der Belegschaft

turricephaly Turmschädel *m*, Pyrgozephalie *f*

tutelage Leitung *f*, Unterweisung *f*, Vormundschaft *f*

tutelary Vormundschafts–, Schutz–

tutor Tutor *m*, Studienbetreuer *m*, Studienleiter *m*

tutoress Studienleiterin *f*, Tutorin *f*, Studienbetreuerin *f*

tutorial Tutor–

tutoring Studienbetreuung *f*, Tutorenunterricht *m*

tween–brain Zwischenhirn *n*

twilight Dämmerung *f* / **~ attacks** Dämmerzustand *m*, Dämmerattacken *fpl* / **~ sleep** Dämmerschlaf *m* / **~ vision** Dämmerungssehen *n*

twilight state Dämmerzustand *m* / **alcoholic ~** alkoholischer Dämmerzustand *m* / **delirant ~** deliranter Dämmerzustand *m* / **epileptic ~** epileptischer Dämmerzustand *m* / **episodic ~** episodischer Dämmerzustand *m* / **hidden ~** besonnener Dämmerzustand *m* / **hysterical ~** läppischer Dämmerzustand *m* / **infectious ~** infektiöser Dämmerzustand *m* / **juvenile ~** läppischer Dämmerzustand *m* / **masked ~** besonnener Dämmerzustand *m* / **psychogenic ~** psychogener Dämmerzustand *m* / **traumatic ~** traumatischer Dämmerzustand *m*

twin Zwilling *m* / **~ brother** Zwillingsbruder *m* / **~ helix** Doppelhelix *f* / **~ research** Zwillingsforschung *f* / **~ sister** Zwillingsschwester *f* / **binovular ~s** zweieiige Zwillinge *pl* / **conjoined ~s** siamesische Zwillinge *pl* / **dichoreal ~s** zweieiige Zwillinge *pl* / **dizygotic ~s** zweieiige Zwillinge *pl* / **enzygotic ~s** eineiige Zwillinge *pl* / **fraternal ~s** zweieiige Zwillinge *pl* / **heterozygotic ~s** heterozygote Zwillinge *pl* / **homozygotic ~s** eineiige Zwillinge *pl* / **identical ~s** eineiige Zwillinge *pl* / **monochorionic ~s** eineiige Zwillinge *pl* / **monozygotic ~** eineiige Zwillinge *pl*, monozygote Zwillinge *pl* / **monovular ~s** eineiige

Zwillinge *pl* / **siamese ~s** siamesische Zwillinge *pl* / **uniovular ~s** eineiige Zwillinge *pl*

twinge stechender Schmerz *m*

twinning Geburt *f* von Zwillingen

twitch Zuckung *f*, Kontraktion *f* / **isometric ~** isometrische Kontraktion *f*

twitching Zucken *n*, Zuckung *f* / **muscular ~** Muskelzuckung *f*

two zwei / **~-aspect theory** Leib–Seele–Theorie *f* / **~-dimensional** zweidimensional / **~-factor division** Zweifaktorenverteilung *f* / **~-factor method** Zweifaktorenmethode *f* / **~-factor theory** Zweifaktorentheorie *f* / **~-handed** beidhändig / **~-point threshold** Zweipunktschwelle *f* / **~-sided** zweiseitig / **~-tailed** zweiseitig, ungerichtet / **~-track plan** Klassenaufteilung *f* in zwei Leistungsgruppen / **~-way table** Tabelle *f*, Diagramm *n*, Streudiagramm *n* / **~-way trait** binäre Eigenschaft *f*

tympanic Trommelfell–, Paukenhöhle–tympanal

tympanism, tympanites Blähsucht *f*, Flatulenz *f*, Meteorismus *m*, Blähungen *fpl*

tympanum Trommelfell *n*, Paukenhöhle *f*

type Typ *m*, Typus *m*, Habitus *m*, Erscheinungsform *f* / **~ A personality** Persönlichkeitstyp A *m* / **~ B personality** Persönlichkeitstyp B *m* / **~ of approach** Erfassungstypus *m* / **~ of an attack** Anfallsform *f* / **~ of convulsion** Anfallsform *f*, Art *f* des Krampfanfalls / **~ I error** Typ I–Fehler *m*, Fehler *m* erster Art, Alpha–Fehler *m* / **~ II error** Typ II–Fehler *m*, Fehler *m* zweiter Art, Beta–Fehler *m* / **~ of experience** Erlebnistypus *m* / **~ fallacy** typologischer Trugschluss *m* / **~ of imagery** Vorstellungstypus *m* / **~ of personality** Persönlichkeitstypus *m* / **~ of scale** Skalentypus *m* / **~ of sequence** Sukzession *f* / **~ of succession** Sukzession *f* / **~-token ratio** Diversifikationsquotient *m* / **abdominal ~** Abdominaltypus *m* / **acoustic ~** auditiver Typus *m* / **allotropic ~** allotroper Typus *m* / **anaclitic ~** Anlehnungstypus *m* / **anaesthetic ~** anästhetischer Typus *m*, Anästhetiker *m* / **apathetic ~** apathischer Typus *m* / **apoplectic ~** apoplektischer Habitus *m*, Apoplektiker *m* / **asthenic ~** asthenischer Typ *m* / **athletic ~** athletischer Typ *m*, athletischer Körperbautyp *m* / **attitudinal ~** Einstellungstypus *m* / **audile ~** auditiver Typus *m* / **barykinetic ~** barykinetischer Typus *m* / **borderline ~** Borderline Typus *m* / **catatonic ~** katatoner Typus *m* / **cerebral ~** zerebraler Typ *m* / **cerebrotonic ~** Zerebrotoner *m*, zerebrotoner Typus *m* / **choleric ~** cholerischer Typ *m*, Choleriker *m* / **clinic ~** klinischer Typ *m* / **coarted ~** koartierter Erlebnistypus *m* / **compulsive ~** Zwangsneurotiker *m* / **constitutional ~** Konstitutionstypus *m* / **cortical ~** kortikaler Typus *m* / **depressive ~** depressiver Typ *m* / **dichotomic ~ theory** dichotome Typologie *f* / **disintegrated ~** desintegrierter Typus *m* / **disorganized ~** desorganisierter Typus *m* / **dysplastic ~** dysplastischer Typ *m*, Dysplastiker *m* / **dysthymic ~** dysthymer Typus *m*, depressiver zwangsneurotischer Typus *m* / **ectomorphic ~** ektomorpher Typus *m* / **endomorphic ~** endomorpher Typus *m* / **expansive ~** expansiver Typus *m* / **extratensive ~** extratensiver Typus *m* / **hebephrenic ~** hebephrener Typus *m* / **hippocratic ~s** hippokratische Typen *mpl* / **hyperaesthetic ~** Hyperästhetiker *m* / **hyperbolic ~** Hyperboliker *m* / **ideal ~** Idealtypus *m* / **ideational ~** Vorstellungstypus *m* / **idiotropic ~** introvertierter Typ *m* / **imaginal ~** Vorstellungstypus *m* / **impulsive ~** impulsiver Typus *m* / **intravert ~** introvertierter Typ *m* / **intraverted ~** introvertierter Typ *m* / **introversive ~** introversiver Typus *m* / **introvert ~** introvertierter Typ *m* / **introverted ~** introvertierter Typ *m* / **intuitive ~** Intuitionstypus *m*, intuitiver Typus *m* / **irrational ~** irrationaler Typ *m* / **koinotropic ~** Gesellschaftstyp *m* / **leptosome ~** leptosomer Typ *m* / **melancholic ~** melancholischer Typus *m* / **mixed ~** Mischtypus *m* / **morphological ~** Erscheinungstyp *m* / **muscular ~** muskulärer Typ *m* / **nonpurging ~** Nicht–Purging–Typus *m* / **objective ~** objektiver Typ *m* / **obsessional ~** Zwangsneurotiker *m* / **overactive ~** überaktiver Typ *m* / **paranoid ~** paranoider Typus *m* / **phlegmatic ~** Phlegmatiker *m* / **physical ~** Körperbautypus *m* / **psychological ~s** psychologische Typen *mpl* / **purging ~** Purging–Typus *m* / **pyknic ~** Pykniker *m*, pyknischer Typ *m* / **rational ~** rationaler Typ *m* / **reactive ~s** Reaktionstypen *mpl* / **residual ~** residualer Typus *m* / **restricting ~** restriktiver Typus *m* / **seclusive ~** verschlossener Typ *m* / **situational ~** situativer Typus *m* / **social ~** sozialer Typus *m* / **solitary ~** Einzelgängertyp *m* / **somatic ~** Körperbautypus *m* / **special ~** Spezialtyp *m* / **sthenic ~** muskulärer Typ *m* / **suspicious ~** misstrauischer Typ *m*, argwöhnischer Mensch *m* / **undifferentiated ~** undifferenzierter Typus *m* / **visual ~** visueller Typ *m*

typhlolexia Wortblindheit *f*, Schriftblindheit *f*, visuelle Aphasie *f*

typhomania Typhusdelirium *n*

typical typisch, charakteristisch

typicality Typisches *n*, Charakteristisches *n*

typify verkörpern, ein Beispiel sein für etwas

typing Typbestimmung *f*, Typendetermination *f*, typologische Klassifikation *f* / Maschineschreiben *n*

typological typologisch

typology Typologie *f*, Typenlehre *f* / **constitutional ~** Konstitutionstypologie *f*, Konstitutionslehre *f* / **psychodiagnostic ~** psychodiagnostische Typologie *f*, psychodiagnostische Klassifikation *f*

tyramine Tyramin *n*

tyrannize tyrannisieren

tyranny Tyrannei *f*, Despotie *f*, Willkürherrschaft *f*

tyrant Tyrann *m*, Despot *m*

tyrosine Tyrosin *n*

U

ubiquitous allgegenwärtig, ubiquitär

ubiquity Allgegenwart *f*, Ubiquität *f*

U fibres U–Fasern *fpl*

UFO psychosis Ufo–Psychose *f*

ugly hässlich, widerwärtig, niederträchtig

U hypothesis U–Hypothese *f*

ulcer Geschwür *n*, Ulkus *m*, Ulcus *m* / **duodenal ~** Zwölffingerdarmgeschwür *n* / **gastric ~** Magengeschwür *n* / **gastrointestinal ~** Magen–Darmgeschwür *n*, gastrointestinales Geschwür *n* / **peptic ~** Magen–Darmgeschwür *n*

ulna Elle *f*

ulnar zur Elle gehörig, ulnar

ulstrith spezifizierte Untergruppe *f*, Stratum *n* einer Stichprobe

ultra–audible außerhalb des Hörbereichs gelegen, Ultraschall–

ultradian ultradian

ultramodern ultramodern, hypermodern

ultrasonic außerhalb des Hörbereichs gelegen, Ultraschall–

ultrasound Ultraschall *m*

ultraviolet ultraviolett

ululation Heulen *n*, Wehklagen *n*

umbilical Nabel–

unadapted unangepasst

unadjustment Unangepasstheit *f*, fehlende Anpassung *f*

unambiguous eindeutig, unzweideutig

unambitious nicht ehrgeizig

unambivalent unzweideutig, nicht ambivalent

unanimity Einstimmigkeit *f*, Einmütigkeit *f*

unanimous einstimmig, einmütig

unassertive bescheiden, schüchtern, zurückhaltend

unassertiveness Schüchternheit *f*, Bescheidenheit *f* / **secure, discplined ~** mangelnde Selbstbehauptung *f*

unattached frei–flottierend, diffus

unavoidable unvermeidlich, unabwendbar

unaware unbewusst

unbalanced unausgeglichen, unausgewogen, im Gleichgewicht gestört, frei von systematischen Fehlern

unbearable unerträglich, untragbar

unbiased, unbiassed vorurteilsfrei, unbeeinflusst, repräsentativ, unvoreingenommen, objektiv

unbridledness Zügellosigkeit *f*

uncathected unbesetzt

uncertainty Ungewissheit *f*, Unsicherheit *f* / **~ interval** Unsicherheitsintervall *n*

unchangeable unveränderlich

unchanged unverändert, gleich

uncial Unzial– / Unzialbuchstabe *m*

uncinate hakenförmig, den Uncus gyri parahippocampalis betreffend

uncommunicative nicht mitteilsam, verschlossen

unconcernedness Sorglosigkeit *f* / **bohemian ~** Leichtlebigkeit *f*

unconditioned, unconditional unbedingt, unkonditioniert

unconditioning Wegkonditionieren *n*, Dekonditionierung *f*

unconscious unbewusst, besinnungslos / Unbewusste *n* / **absolute ~** absolutes Unbewusstes *n* / **collective ~** kollektives Unbewusstes *n* / **dynamic ~** dynamisches Unbewusstes *n* / **familial ~** familiäres

Unbewusstes *n* / **personal ~** persönliches Unbewusstes *n* / **racial ~** kollektives Unbewusstes *n*

unconsciousness Unbewusstes *n*, Unterbewusstes *n*, Bewusstlosigkeit *f*, Besinnungslosigkeit *f*

uncontrolled unkontrolliert

uncooperative nicht kooperativ

uncoordinated unkoordiniert

uncoupling Entkopplung *f*, Abkoppelung *f*

uncover aufdecken

undecided unentschieden, unschlüssig, unentschlossen, zögernd

undemonstrative zurückhaltend, unaufdringlich

underachievement Minderleistung *f* / **academic ~** schulische Minderleistung *f*, schlechtere Schulleistung als erwartet *f*

underachiever Minderleister *m*, Underachiever *m*

underage minderjährig, unmündig

underdeveloped unterentwickelt, zurückgeblieben

underdevelopment Unterentwicklung *f*, Entwicklungsretardierung *f*, Unreife *f* / **~ of an organ** Organminderwertigkeit *f*

underestimate unterschätzen / Unterschätzung *f*

underestimation Unterschätzung *f*

underfed unterernährt

underfeeding Unterernährung *f*

undergraduate Student *m*, Studentin *f* vor der Zwischen–/Abschlussprüfung / **~ education** Vordiplomausbildung *f*, Hochschulstudium *n* vor der Zwischen–/Abschlussprüfung

undergrown schwächlich, nicht ausgewachsen

underlearning unvollständiges Lernen *n*

underprivileged benachteiligt, unterprivilegiert

underproduction Unterproduktion *f*, geringe Antwortenzahl *f*

underproductive wenig produzierend, nur eine geringe Zahl Antworten produzierend

understand verstehen, begreifen, einsehen

understanding verständig, einsichtsvoll, intelligent / Verstehen *n*, Verständnis *n*, Auffassungsvermögen *n*, Auffassungsgabe *f* / **~ need** Bedürfnis *n* wahrgenommene Dinge zu verstehen

understatement Unterbewertung *f*, Untertreibung *f*

underwater effect Unterwasserwirkung *f*

underweight Untergewicht *n*

undesirable unerwünscht

undetermined unbestimmt

undeveloped unentwickelt, unreif

undifferentiated undifferenziert

undifferentiation mangelnde Differenzierung *f*, fehlende Differenzierung *f*

undisturbed ungestört, friedlich, ruhig

undo ungeschehen machen

undoing Ungeschehenmachen *n* / **~ mechanism** Verdrängungsmechanismus *m* des Ungeschehenmachens

undulant wellenförmig, oszillierend

undulation Wellenbewegung *f*

undulatory wellenförmig, Wellen–

uneasiness Unbehagen *n*, innere Unruhe *f*

uneasy unbehaglich, unruhig, ruhelos

uneducated ungebildet, unerzogen

unemployed arbeitslos, beschäftigungslos / Arbeitsloser *m*

unemployment Arbeitslosigkeit *f* / **~ neurosis** Arbeitslosigkeitsneurose *f*

unequivocal eindeutig, unzweideutig, unmissverständlich

unexcitable nicht reizbar

unfair ungerecht, parteiisch, unehrlich, unfair

unfaithful untreu, illoyal

unfeeling gefühllos, gleichgültig, kalt, unempfindlich

unfeigned echt, ehrlich, nicht geheuchelt

unfinished unvollendet, unfertig

unfit untauglich, ungeeignet, unfähig

unfitness Untauglichkeit *f*, Unfähigkeit *f*, fehlende Eignung *f* / ~ **to plead** Verhandlungsunfähigkeit *f*

unfolding technique Entfaltungstechnik *f*

ungraded ohne Klassenaufteilung, nicht abgestuft, unsortiert

ungrateful undankbar

unhealthy ungesund, krank, gesundheitsschädlich, krankhaft

uniaural einohrig, monaural

unicellular einzellig

unidextral mit einer Hand dominant

unidextrality Dominanz *f* einer Hand

unidimensional eindimensional, unidimensional

unidimensionality Eindimensionalität *f*

uniform gleichmäßig, gleichförmig, uniform, konform

uniformity Gleichförmigkeit *f*, Einheitlichkeit *f* / ~ **of nature** Einheitlichkeit *f* der Natur

unilateral einseitig, halbseitig, unilateral

unilaterality Einseitigkeit *f*

unimaginative phantasielos, einfallslos

unimanual einhändig, unimodal, eingipfelig, unimodal

unintelligence Unintelligenz *f*, Dummheit *f*

unintelligibility Unverständlichkeit *f*, Unklarheit *f*

unintelligible unverständlich, unklar

unintentional unabsichtlich, unbeabsichtigt

uniocular einäugig, mit dem einen Auge sehend, monokular

uniovular eineiig, monozygot

unipolar einpolig, unipolar

uniprocess learning theory Theorie *f* des Diskriminationslernens durch Elimination fehlerhafter Hypothesen

unique einzigartig, einmalig, einzig

uniqueness Einzigartigkeit *f*, spezifische Varianz *f* und Fehlervarianz *f*

unisexual eingeschlechtig

unisexuality Eingeschlechtigkeit *f*

unison Einklang *m*, Gleichklang *m*, Übereinstimmung *f*

unit Einheit *f* / ~ **character** Einheitsmerkmal *n* / ~ **factor** einheitlicher Faktor *m* / ~ **of measure** Maßeinheit *f* / ~ **of measurement** Maßeinheit *f* / ~ **membrane** Elementarmembran *f* / ~ **operation** Gesamtablauf *m* / ~ **plan** geschlossener Unterrichtsplan *m* / ~ **of response** Reaktionseinheit *f* / ~ **step** Einheitssprung *m* / **audio–visual** ~ audiovisuelle Einheit *f* / **developmental** ~ Entwicklungseinheit *f* / **differential** ~ unterschiedliche Einheit *f* / **elementary behavioural** ~ elementare Verhaltenseinheit *f* / **functional** ~ Funktionseinheit *f*, funktionelle Einheit *f* / **interactive** ~ Interaktionseinheit *f* / **ipsative** ~**s** ipsative Werte *mpl* / **monadic** ~ Monade *f* / **motor** ~ motorische Einheit *f* / **normative** ~**s** Standardeinheiten *fpl* / **psychiatric** ~ psychiatrische Abteilung *f* / **sensory** ~ sensorische Einheit *f*, Empfindungseinheit *f* / **spaced** ~**s** räumlich gegliederte Einheiten *fpl*

unitary einheitlich, Einheits–

unity Einheit *f*, Einheitlichkeit *f* / ~ **thema** Einheitsthema *n*, dominantes Thema *n* / **functional** ~ funktionelle Einheit *f* / **perceptual** ~ Einheit *f* der Wahrnehmung

univalent einwertig

univariate univariat, aus einer Variablen bestehend

universal universal, allgemein, Welt–

universalism Universalismus *m*

universality Universalität *f*, Allgemeingültigkeit *f*

universe Grundgesamtheit *f*, Welt *f* / ~ **of discourse** Gedankenwelt *f*, Denkbild *n*, gedanklicher Zusammenhang *m* / **statistical** ~ statistische Grundgesamtheit *f*

university Universität *f*, Hochschule *f* / ~ **education** Universitätsausbildung *f*

univitelline eineiig, monozygot

univocal eindeutig, unzweideutig

unknowable unerkennbar

unlearn verlernen

unlearned nicht gelernt, nicht erlernt, angeboren

unlearning Verlernen *n*, Umlernen *n*

unmixed ungemischt, rein, ungetrübt

unmoral amoralisch, nicht dem Sittengesetz unterworfen

unmusical unmusikalisch, unmelodisch

unnatural unnatürlich, anomal, ungewöhnlich, künstlich

unoccupied beschäftigungslos, arbeitslos

unpleasant unangenehm, unerfreulich

unpleasantness, unpleasure Unlust *f*, Unbehagen *n* / ~ **principle** Unlustprinzip *n*

unpolished ungebildet, unausgeglichen, unfein

unpretentious anspruchslos, bescheiden

unprincipled gewissenlos, charakterlos, ohne moralische Grundsätze

unproductive unproduktiv, unergiebig

unprofessional unfachmännisch

unreal unwirklich

unreality Unwirklichkeit *f*, Irrealität *f* / ~ **feeling** Gefühl *n* der Unwirklichkeit

unreasonable unvernünftig, unlogisch

unreasoning vernunftlos, vernunftwidrig

unreceptive unempfänglich

unreflective unüberlegt, gedankenlos, impulsiv

unreliable unzuverlässig, nicht reliabel

unremitting unablässig, Dauer–

unreserved freimütig, offen, uneingeschränkt

unresolved ungelöst

unresponsiveness Unansprechbarkeit *f*, mangelnde Reaktionsbereitschaft *f*

unrest innere Unruhe *f*, Bewegungsdrang *m*

unrestful unruhig, rastlos, nervös

unrestricted unbeschränkt, uneingeschränkt

unsatisfied unbefriedigt

unscrupulous gewissenlos, hemmungslos

unselected unausgewählt

unsociability Ungeselligkeit *f*, Zurückhaltung *f*, Menschenscheu *f*

unsociable ungesellig, reserviert, zurückhaltend

unsocial unsozial, asozial, ungesellig

unsocialized unsozial, asozial

unsound ungesund

unspaced massiert, unverteilt, gedrängt

unspecific unspezifisch

unspecified nicht näher bezeichnet

unstable unstet, labil, unbeständig

unstriated ungestreift, glatt

unstriped ungestreift, glatt

unstructured unstrukturiert

unsuccessful erfolglos, fruchtlos, ohne Erfolg

unsystematized unsystematisch, unzusammenhängend

unthinkable undenkbar, unvorstellbar

Unverricht's disease Unverricht–Syndrom *n*, Myoklonusepilepsie *f*, myoklonische Epilepsie *f*

unweighted ungewichtet

unwilling widerwillig, widerstrebend

unworthy unwürdig

update auf den neuesten Stand bringen, überarbeiten, revidieren

updating Überarbeitung *f*, Revision *f*

upgrading Höherbewertung *f*, Beförderung *f*

upper obere(r, s), höhere(r, s), Ober–

uprooting Entwurzelung *f* / ~ **depression** Entwurzelungsdepression *f* / ~ **neurosis** Entwurzelungsneurose *f* / ~ **reaction** Entwurzelungsreaktion *f* / ~ **psychosis** Entwurzelungspsychose *f*

upset aufregen, verwirren, aus der Fassung bringen / Verwirrung *f*, Aufregung *f*, Erregung *f* / **emotional** ~ emotionale Erregung *f*

uracil Uracil *n*

uranism Uranismus *m*, männliche Homosexualität *f*

uranist Homosexueller *m*, Invertierter *m*

uranistic homosexuell

Urban's| constant process Urbans konstantes Verfahren *n* / **~ tables** Urbans Tafeln *fpl*

urban städtisch, Stadt–

urbanization Verstädterung *f*, Urbanisierung *f*

uremia Urämie *f*

ureter Harnleiter *m*, Ureter *m*

urethra Harnröhre *f*, Urethra *f*

urethral Harnröhren–, urethral

urge Drang *m*, Impuls *m*, Trieb *m* / **~ to be active** Aktivitätsdrang *m*, Beschäftigungsdrang *m* / **~ to destroy** Zerstörungstrieb *m*, Destruktionstrieb *m* / **~–force** Antrieb *m* / **compelling ~ of overactivity** Beschäftigungszwang *m* / **creative ~** Gestaltungsdrang *m*, schöpferischer Drang *m* / **repressed ~** verdrängte Regung *f*, verdrängter Impuls *m* / **sexual ~** Geschlechtstrieb *m*

uridine Uridin *n*

urinaemia Urämie *f*

urinalysis Urinanalyse *f*, Harnuntersuchung *f*

urination Harnlassen *n*, Urinieren *n*, Wasserlassen *n*

urine Urin *m*, Harn *m*

urinology, urology Urologie *f*

urning Homosexueller *m*

urnist Homosexueller *m*

urobilinogen Urobilinogen *n*

urogenital urogenital, Urogenital–

urolagnia Urolagnie *f*, geschlechtliche Erregung *f* durch Zusehen beim Urinieren anderer, geschlechtliche Erregung *f* beim Urinieren

urophilia Urophilie *f*, pathologisches Interesse *n* am Harn

urophobia Urophobie *f*, Angst *f* vor dem Urinieren

urticaria Nesselsucht *f*, Urtikaria *f*

use Gebrauch *m*, Anwendung *f*, Brauch *m* / **~ and disuse theory** Gewöhnungs- und Entwöhnungstheorie *f* / **~–inheritance** Vererbung *f* von Gewohnheiten / **~ law** Gesetz *n* der Übung, Gesetz *n* der Gewöhnung / **harmful ~** schädlicher Gebrauch *m*

useful nützlich, brauchbar

useless nutzlos, unbrauchbar

U–shaped U–förmig

uterine uterin, Gebärmutter–, Uterus–

uteromania Nymphomanie *f*

uterus Uterus *m*, Gebärmutter *f*

U test U–Test *m*

utilisation time Nutzungszeit *f*, Hauptnutzzeit *f*

utilitarianism Utilitarismus *m*, Nützlichkeitsphilosophie *f*

utility Nützlichkeit *f*, Nutzen *m*, Brauchbarkeit *f* / **psychological ~** psychologischer Nutzen *m* / **subjectively expected ~** subjektive Nutzenerwartung *f*

utopian utopisch, visionär, erträumt / Utopist *m*, Phantast *m*, Schwärmer *m*

utricle, utriculus Utrikulus *m*, das größere Vorhofsäckchen *n* des Ohrlabyrinths

utricular sackartig, schlauchartig

utterance Äußerung *f*, Ausdruck *m*, Ausspruch *m*

U–tube U–Rohr *n*

uvea Uvea *f*

uvula Zäpfchen *n*

uvular uvulär, das Zäpfchen betreffend

uxorious unter dem Pantoffel stehend, unterwürfig

V

vacancy seelische Leere *f*, geistige Leere *f*, offene Position *f*

vacant leer, ausdruckslos, gedankenlos

vacation Urlaub *m*, Ferien *pl* / **~ benefit** Urlaubsgeld *n*

vacationing Urlaubmachen *n*, Urlaubsverhalten *n*

vaccination Impfung *f*

vaccinophobia Angst *f* vor Impfungen, Impfangst *f*

vaccinotherapy Impftherapie *f*, Vakzinetherapie *f*

vacillation Unentschlossenheit *f*, Wankelmut *m*, Unbeständigkeit *f*, Schwanken *n*

vacuity geistige Leere *f*, seelische Leere *f* / **~ of expression** Ausdruckslosigkeit *f* / **~ of mind** geistige Leere *f*, Gedankenarmut *f*

vacuum Leere *f* / **~ activity** Leerlaufverhalten *n* / **~ response** Leerantwort *f*, Leerlaufhandlung *f*

vagabondage Vagabundieren *n*, Wandertrieb *m*, Pariomanie *f*

vagal vagal

vagina Vagina *f*, Scheide *f*

vaginal vaginal, Scheiden–

vaginism, vaginismus Scheidenkrampf *m*, Vaginismus *m* / **primary ~** psychogener Vaginismus *m*, primärer Vaginismus *m* / **nonorganic ~** nichtorganischer Vaginismus *m* / **psychic ~** psychisch bedingter Scheidenkrampf *m* / **secondary ~** physiologisch bedingter Vaginismus *m*, Pseudovaginismus *m*, sekundärer Vaginismus *m*

vagomimetic parasympathikuserregend

vagotomy Vagusdurchtrennung *f*, Vagotomie *f*

vagotonia Übererregbarkeit *f* des Parasympathikus, Vagotonie *f*, Parasympathikotonie *f*

vagotonic vagoton

vagrant vagabundierend, umherwandernd, unstet / Landstreicher *m*, Person *f* ohne festen Wohnsitz

vagueness Unbestimmtheit *f*, Unklarheit *f*

vagus Vagus *m*, zehnter Hirnnerv *m* / **~ centre** Vaguszentrum *n* / **~ inhibition** Vagushemmung *f* / **~ nerve** Vagusnerv *m*, Vagus *m* / **~ neurosis** Vagusneurose *f*

vain eitel, eingebildet, großspurig

valence, valency Valenz *f*, Aufforderungscharakter *m* / **affective ~** affektive Valenz *f* / **chromatic ~** Farbvalenz *f* / **negative ~** negative Valenz *f* / **positive ~** positive Valenz *f* / **substitute ~** Ersatzvalenz *f*

valiant tapfer, heldenhaft

valid gültig / **~ negative** tatsächlich negativ / **~ positive** tatsachlich positiv

validate validieren

validation Validierung *f*, Überprüfung *f* der Validität eines Tests / **consensual ~** Validierung *f* durch Übereinstimmung / **cross ~** Kreuzvalidierung *f* / **external ~** externe Validierung *f*, kriteriumsbezogene Validierung *f* / **internal ~** interne Validierung *f*

validity Gültigkeit *f*, Validität *f* / **~ coefficient** Validitätskoeffizient *m* / **~ criterion** Validitätskriterium *n* / **a priori ~** logische Validität *f* / **common–sense ~** logische Validität *f* / **concurrent ~** Übereinstimmungsvalidität *f* / **congruent ~** Übereinstimmungsvalidität *f* / **convergent ~** Konvergenzvalidität *f* / **curricular ~** kurrikulare Validität *f*, Lehrplanvalidität *f* / **definitional ~** Konstruktvalidität *f*, konzeptionelle Validität *f*, Konzeptvaliditát *f* / **derived ~** abgeleitete Validität *f* / **ecological ~** Umweltgültigkeit *f*, Wirksamkeit *f* der Umwelt / **empirical ~** empirische Validität *f* / **external ~** äußere Validität *f*, externe Validität *f* / **factorial ~** faktorielle Validität *f* / **general ~** Allgemeingültigkeit *f* / **internal ~** innere Validität *f* / **intrinsic ~** inhaltliche Validität *f* / **logical ~** logische Validität *f* / **predictive ~** Vorhersage–Validität *f*, prädiktive Validität *f* / **rational ~** logische Validität *f* / **sampling ~** Stichprobenvalidität *f* / **statistical ~** statistische Validität *f* / **theoretical ~** Konstruktvalidität *f*

vallum Wall *m*

valuable wertvoll, teuer

valuation Bewertung *f*, Wertung *f*, Schätzung *f*

value Wert *m* / schätzen, bewerten / **~ analysis** Wertanalyse *f* / **~ of colour** Farbwert *m* / **~ judgment** Werturteil *n* / **~–orientated** wertpsychologisch orientiert / **~ system** Wertsystem *n*, Überzeugungsmatrix *f* / **absolute ~** absoluter Wert *m* / **adaptive ~** Überlebenswert *m*, arterhaltender Wert *m* / **algebraic ~** algebraischer Wert *m* / **central ~** Zentralwert *m* / **critical ~** kritischer Wert *m* / **cultural ~s** Kulturwerte *mpl* / **diagnostic ~** diagnostischer Wert *m* / **effective ~** Effektivwert *m* / **emotional ~** Gefühlswert *m* / **estimated ~** geschätzter Wert *m* / **ethnic ~s** ethnische Werte *mpl* / **expected ~** Erwartungswert *m* / **liminal ~** Schwellenwert *m*, Grenzwert *m* / **maximum ~** höchster Wert *m*, Maximalwert *m* / **mean ~** Mittelwert *m* / **median ~** Median *m*, Mittelwert *m* / **minimum ~** niedrigster Wert *m*, Minimalwert *m* / **modal ~** Modalwert *m* / **numerical ~** numerischer Wert *m* / **observed ~** beobachteter Wert *m* / **personal ~s** persönliche Werte *mpl* / **prognostic ~** prognostischer Wert *m* / **selective ~** selektiver Wert *m* / **social ~** sozialer Wert *m*, gesellschaftlicher Wert *m* / **standard ~** Standardwert *m* / **true ~** wahrer Wert *m*

valuer Schätzer *m*

vandalism Vandalismus *m*, Zerstörungswut *f*

vanishing Abbau *m* der Lernsicherung, Verminderung *f* der Lernhilfen, Schwundtechnik *f*

vanity Eitelkeit *f*, Selbstgefälligkeit *f*, Dünkel *m*

vapour, vapor Einbildung *f*, Hirngespinst *n*, Wahn *m*

variability Variabilität *f*, Veränderlichkeit *f*, Streuung *f* / **~ coefficient** Variabilitätskoeffizient *m* / **~ of individual differences** Streuung *f* individueller Unterschiede / **~ measurement** Streuungsmessung *f*, Variabilitätsmessung *f* / **absolute ~** absolute Variabilität *f* / **average ~** mittlere Variabilität *f* / **continuous ~** ständige Veränderung *f* / **impulsive ~** impulsive Veränderlichkeit *f* / **interindividual ~** Streuung *f* zwischen den Individuen / **quotidian ~** Tagesschwankung *f* / **relative ~** relative Variabilität *f*

variable veränderlich, variabel / Variable *f* / **autochthonous ~** autochthone Variable *f*, im System befindliche Variable *f* / **binary ~** binäre Variable *f*, Alternativvariable *f* / **collative ~** Vergleichsvariable *f* / **continuous ~** kontinuierliche Variable *f* / **controlled ~** kontrollierte Variable *f*, unabhängige Variable *f*, Regelgröße *f* / **dependent ~** abhängige Variable *f* / **discontinuous ~** diskrete Variable *f* / **discrete ~** diskrete Variable *f* / **distal ~** distale Variable *f* / **empirical ~** empirische Variable *f* / **experimental ~** experimentelle Variable *f* / **independent ~** unabhängige Variable *f* / **intervening ~** intervenierende Variable *f*, vermittelndeVariable *f* / **manipulated ~** Stellgröße *f* / **mediating ~** vermittelnde Variable *f* / **operational ~** operational definierte Variable *f* / **organic ~** Organvariable *f* / **or-**

ganismic ~ Organismusvariable *f* / **personal ~** Organismusvariable *f* / **statistical ~** statistische Variable *f*

variance Varianz *f*, Streuung *f*, Dispersion *f* / **~ analysis** Varianzanalyse *f* / **~ component** Varianzkomponente *f* / **~ homogeneity** Varianzhomogenität *f* / **~ of a sample** Stichprobenvarianz *f* / **between-groups ~** Varianz zwischen *f* / **relative ~** relative Varianz *f* / **true ~** wahre Varianz *f* / **within-group ~** Varianz innerhalb *f*

variant Variante *f*, Abart *f*

variate Variable *f*, Größe *f* einer Variablen

variation Variation *f*, Abweichung *f*, Änderung *f*, Unterschied *m* / **~ coefficient** Variationskoeffizient *m* / **~ of humour** Stimmungsänderung *f*, Verstimmung *f* / **concomitant ~** gleichzeitige Änderung *f* / **contingent negative ~** Erwartungswelle *f* / **continuous ~** kontinuierliche Veränderung *f* / **daily ~** Tagesschwankung *f* / **diurnal ~** Tagesschwankung *f* / **gradual ~** stufenweise Veränderung *f*, graduelle Änderung *f* / **mean ~** mittlere Abweichung *f* / **random ~** Zufallsabweichung *f* / **seasonal ~s** saisonale Schwankungen *fpl*, jahreszeitliche Schwankungen *fpl*

variational Variations–, differenziell

variator Tonvariator *m*

varied verschieden, verschiedenartig, mannigfaltig

variety Verschiedenartigkeit *f*, Verschiedenheit *f*, Abart *f*, Varietät *f*

varimax rotation Varimax–Rotation *f*, Varimax–Rotationsmethode *f*

vary ändern, variieren, abweichen, sich verändern, sich ändern

vas Gefäß *n* / **~ deferens** Samenleiter *m*

vascular gefäßbedingt, gefäßreich, vaskulär

vasectomy Samenleiterresektion *f*, Vasektomie *f*

vasiform gefäßförmig

vasocongestion Vasokongestion *f*

vasoconstriction Gefäßverengung *f*, Gefäßzusammenziehung *f*, Vasokonstriktion *f*

vasoconstrictor Vasokonstriktor *m*, gefäßverengendes Mittel *n* / **~ centre** Vasokonstriktorenzentrum *n* / **~ drug** gefäßverengendes Mittel *n*, vasokonstriktorisches Arzneimittel *n*

vasodepressor blutdrucksenkendes Mittel *n*

vasodilatation, vasodilation Gefäßerweiterung *f*, Vasodilatation *f*, Gefäßdilatation *f*

vasodilator Vasodilator *m*, gefäßerweiterndes Mittel *n* / **~ centre** Vasodilatorenzentrum *n* / **~ drug** gefäßerweiterndes Mittel *n*

vasomotor vasomotorisch, die Gefäßspannung regulierend / vasomotorischer Nerv *m*, vasomotorisch wirkendes Mittel *n*

vasoneurosis Gefäßneurose *f*, Vasoneurose *f*, Angioneurose *f*

vasoparesis Lähmung *f* vasomotorischer Nerven

vasopressin Vasopressin *n*, antidiuretisches Hormon *n*

vasoreflex Gefäßreflex *m*

vasoresection Samenleiterresektion *f*

vasospasm Gefäßkrampf *m*, Gefäßspasmus *m*

vasotonia Gefäßtonus *m*

Vater|'s corpuscles Vater–Pacini–Körperchen *npl* / **~–Pacinian corpuscles** Vater–Pacini–Körperchen *npl*

V–codes for conditions not attributable to a mental disorder that are a focus of attention or treatment V–Schlüssel *m* für Zustände, die nicht einer psychischen Störung zuzuschreiben sind, aber Anlass zur Beobachtung oder Behandlung geben

vector Vektor *m*, gerichtete Größe *f* / **~ analysis** vektorielle Analyse *f*, Vektorenanalyse *f* / **~ field** vektorielles Feld *n* / **~ psychology** Vektorenpsychologie *f* / **integral ~** Integralvektor *m*

vectorial vektoriell, Vektor–

veg Veg *n*, Skaleneinheit *f* für wahrgenommenes Gewicht

vegetable pflanzlich, vegetarisch / Pflanze *f*

vegetarian Vegetarier *m* / vegetarisch

vegetarianism vegetarische Lebensweise *f*, Vegetarismus *m*

vegetative vegetativ

vehicle Übertragungsmittel *n*, Vermittler *m*, Medium *n* / **motor ~** Kraftfahrzeug *n*

vein Vene *f*, Ader *f*

veinule Venole *f*

velleity schwacher Wunsch *m*, zögerndes Wollen *n*, Velleität *f*

vellication krampfartiges Muskelzucken *n*

velocity Geschwindigkeit *f* / **~ of flow** Strömungsgeschwindigkeit *f* / **~ of nerve conduction** Nervenleitungsgeschwindigkeit *f* / **~ of sound** Schallgeschwindigkeit *f*

venereal geschlechtlich, Geschlechts–, geschlechtskrank, venerisch

venereophobia Angst *f* vor dem Geschlechtsverkehr, Angst *f* vor Geschlechtskrankheiten, Venerophobie *f*

venery Geschlechtsgenuss *m*, Geschlechtsverkehr *m*

vengeance Rache *f*

Venn diagram Venn–Diagramm *n*, logisch–operationales Diagramm *n*

venous venös, Venen–

ventilation Ventilation *f*, Lüftung *f*, freie Erörterung *f*, Prüfung *f*

ventral ventral, Bauch–

ventricle Kammer *f*, Ventrikel *m*, Hirnkammer *f* / **~ of the brain** Hirnkammer *f*, Hirnventrikel *m* / **cerebral ~** Hirnkammer *f* / **lateral ~** Seitenventrikel *m*

ventricular Kammer–, Ventrikel–

ventriculography Röntgendarstellung *f* der Gehirnventrikel

ventriloquism Bauchredekunst *f*, Bauchreden *n*

ventriloquist Bauchredner *m*

ventrolateral ventrolateral

venule Venole *f*

verapamil Verapamil *n*

verbal wörtlich, mündlich, verbal

verbalisation Verbalisierung *f*, Ausdrucksfähigkeit *f* in Worten, Überwiegen *n* des Wortes, Wortschwall *m*

verbalism Wortausdruck *m*, Überwiegen *n* des Wortes, Wortklauberei *f*

verbalizing Ausdrücken *n* in Worten, Verbalisierung *f*

verbatim wörtlich, wortgetreu, Wort für Wort

verbiage Wortschwall *m*, Geschwätz *n*

verbigeration stereotypes Wiederholen *n* von Wörtern, Verbigeration *f*

verbomania unbeherrschbare Sprechlust *f*, Geschwätzigkeit *f*, Schwatzhaftigkeit *f*, Verbomanie *f*

verbomaniac Schwätzer *m*, Verbomaner *m*, an Redesucht Leidender *m*

verbomotor sprachmotorisch

verbose weitschweifig, wortreich

verbosity, verboseness Weitschweifigkeit *f*, Wortfülle *f*, Wortschwall *m*

vergence Drehbewegung *f* des Augapfels, Vergenz *f*

veridical wirklich, tatsächlich

verifiability Beweisbarkeit *f*, Nachprüfbarkeit *f*

verifiable beweisbar, nachprüfbar, verifizierbar

verification Nachprüfung *f*, Verifikation *f*, Verifizierung *f*

verifier Prüfmaschine *f*

verify prüfen, nachprüfen, verifizieren

verisimilar wahrscheinlich

verisimilitude Wahrscheinlichkeit *f*

verminophobia, vermiphobia krankhafte Angst *f* vor Ungeziefer, krankhafte Angst *f* vor Würmern

vermis Kleinhirnwurm *m* / **~ of the cerebellum** Kleinhirnwurm *m*

vernier Nonius *m*, beweglicher Gradteiler *m*

versatile beweglich, gewandt, vielseitig

versatility Vielseitigkeit *f*, Gewandtheit *f*

vertebra Wirbel *m*, Vertebra *f* / **~e** Wirbelsäule *f* / **~s** Wirbelsäule *f*

vertebral vertebral, Wirbel–, Wirbelsäulen–

vertebrata, vertebrates Wirbeltiere *npl*, Vertebraten *npl*

vertex Spitze *f* Gipfel *m*, Krone *f*

vertical senkrecht, vertikal

vertiginous, vertiginal schwindlig

vertigo Schwindel *m*, Vertigo *f*, Schwindelgefühl *n* / **aural ~** Ohrschwindel *m*, Menière–Schwindel *m* / **cerebellar ~** Kleinhirnschwindel *m* / **cerebral ~** Hirnschwindel *m* / **objective ~** Drehschwindel *m* / **ocular ~** Schwindel *m* infolge von Augenerkrankungen / **rotatory ~** Drehschwindel *m* / **subjective ~** Drehstuhlschwindel *m* / **true ~** Vestibularschwindel *m* / **visual ~** Sehschwindel *m*

vesical Blasen–, vesikal

vesicle Bläschen *n*, Blase *f*, Vesikel *n* / **auditory ~** Ohrbläschen *n* / **blastodermic ~** Blastula *f*, Keimblase *f* / **germinal ~** Keimbläschen *n*

vesicular bläschenförmig, vesikulär, Bläschen–

vessel Gefäß *n*, Ader *f* / **cerebral ~** Hirngefäß *n* / **coronary ~** Herzgefäß *n* / **retinal ~** Netzhautgefäß *n*

vestibular vestibulär, Vestibular–

vestibule Vorhof *m*, Vestibulum *n* / **~ of the ear** Labyrinthvorhof *m* / **~ school** Werkstrainingszentrum *n* für neue Mitarbeiter / **labyrinthine ~** Labyrinthvorhof *m*

vestibulospinal vestibulospinal

vestige Rest *m*, Überbleibsel *n*, Rudiment *n*, Spur *f*

vestigial spurenhaft, rudimentär, verkümmert

V factor Faktor *m* Sprachverständnis

viability Lebensfähigkeit *f*

viable lebensfähig

vibration Schwingung *f*, Vibration *f* / **~ cycle** Vibrationsschwingung *f* / **~ frequency** Schwingungshäufigkeit *f* / **~ rate** Schwingungshäufigkeit *f* / **~ sensation** Vibrationsempfindung *f* / **~ sense** Vibrationssinn *m* / **~ sensor** Vibrationssensor *m* / **double ~** Doppelschwingung *f* / **forced ~** Mitschwingen *n*, Resonanz *f* / **induced ~** Mitschwingung *f*, Resonanz *f* / **single ~** einfache Schwingung *f* / **sympathetic ~** Resonanz *f*, Mitschwingung *f*

vibrato Vibrato *n*

vibrator Vibrator *m*, Summer *m*

vibratory vibrierend, schwingend, Vibrations–

vibrotactile den Vibrationssinn betreffend

vicarious stellvertretend, vikariierend, Substitutions–

vice Laster *n*, Untugend *f*, Gebrechen *n*, Mangel *m* / **solitary ~** Onanie *f*, Masturbation *f*

vicious lasterhaft, unmoralisch, fehlerbehaftet

vicissitude Wechsel *m* / **~ of libido** Triebschicksal *n* / **instinctual ~s** Triebschicksale *npl*

victim Schlachtopfer *n*, Opfer *n*

victimization Viktimisierung *f*, Übervorteilung *f*, Betrug *m*, Schikanierung *f*

victimology Viktimologie *f*, Lehre *f* von der Beziehung zwischen Rechtsbrecher und Verbrechensopfer

video| display unit Bildschirm *m* / **~ game** Videospiel *n*

videotape Fernsehband *n*, Videoband *n*, Videoaufzeichnung *f* / **~ instruction** Unterricht *m* mit Videos, videounterstützter Unterricht *m* / **~ recorder** Videorekorder *m*

Vienna Circle Wiener Schule *f*, Wiener Kreis *m*

Viennese School Wiener Schule *f*

Vierordt's law Vierordt'sches Gesetz *n*

Vieth–Müller circle Vieth–Müller–Kreis *m*

view sehen, besehen, betrachten, prüfen / Sicht *f*, Anblick *m*, Standpunkt *m*, Meinung *f* / **Maxwellian ~** Maxwell'sche Sicht *f* / **retrospective ~** Rückblick *m*

viewer Viewer *m*, Programm *n* zum Ansehen bestimmer Dateiarten

viewing Seh–, Sicht–

viewmeter Rahmensucher *m*

vigil Wachen *n*, Wachsein *n*

vigilambulism rastloses Umhergehen *n* bei Schlaflosigkeit, Vigilambulismus *m*

vigilance Vigilanz *f*, Wachsamkeit *f* / **~ of consciousness** Vigilanz *f* / **~ function** Erregungsfunktion *f* / **neural ~** nervöse Anspannung *f*, gespannte Aufmerksamkeit *f*, hohe Reaktionsbereitschaft *f*

vigilant gespannt, aufmerksam

vigorous stark, kräftig, lebhaft, energisch

vigour, vigor Kraft *f*, Stärke *f*, Energie *f*

vileness Gemeinheit *f*, Niederträchtigkeit *f*

village test Dorftest *m*

villi Zotten *fpl*, Darmzotten *fpl*

Vincent| curve Vincent–Kurve *f* / **~ learning curve** Vincent–Lernkurve *f* / **~ method** Vincent–Methode *f*

vindictiveness Rachsucht *f*

violate verletzen, vergewaltigen

violation Verletzung *f*, Vergewaltigung *f*, Notzucht *f* / **~ of marital duties** Eheverfehlung *f*

violence Gewalt *f*, Gewalttätigkeit *f*

violent heftig, gewaltsam, ungestüm, erregt

violet Violett *n* / violett / **~ blindness** Violettblindheit *f*, Tritanopie *f*

viraginity Mannweibtum *n*, Viraginität *f*, Virilismus *m*

virago Mannweib *n*

virgin Jungfrau *f* / jungfräulich, rein, keusch

virginity Jungfräulichkeit *f*, Virginität *f*

virile männlich, viril

virilisation Virilisierung *f*

virilism Mannweibtum *n*, Vermännlichung *f*, Viraginität *f*

virility Männlichkeit *f*, Virilität *f* / **~ complex** Männlichkeitskomplex *m*

viripotent geschlechtsreif, heiratsfähig

virtual tatsächlich, eigentlich, virtuell

virtuality Wesen *n*, tatsächliches Sosein *n*

virtue Tugend *f*

virtuous tugendhaft, sittsam

virulence Virulenz *f*, Bösartigkeit *f*, Giftigkeit *f*, Schärfe *f*

virulent virulent, bösartig, giftig, scharf

vis a tergo Kraft *f* von hinten

viscera Eingeweide *pl*

visceral viszeral

visceroceptor, visceroreceptor Interozeptor *m*, Viszerozeptor *m*

viscerogenic viszerogen, im Körper entstanden, körperlich

viscerosensory viszerosensorisch, Organempfindung betreffend

viscerotonia Viszerotonie *f*

viscerotonic viszerotonisch

VI schedule veränderliche Zeitspannenfolge *f*

viscid klebrig

viscidity Klebrigkeit *f*

viscose Viskose *f* / viskös

viscosimeter Gerät *n* zur Messung der Zähflüssigkeit, Viskosimeter *n*, Viskositätsmesser *m*

viscosimetry Messung *f* der Viskosität, Viskosimetrie *f*

viscosity Viskosität *f*, Haften *n*

viscous zähflüssig, zäh, viskös

viscus Organ *n*, Teil *n* der Eingeweide

visibility Sichtbarkeit *f* / **~ coefficient** Sichtbarkeitskoeffizient *m*, Visibilitätskoeffizient *m* / **~ curve** Sichtbarkeitskurve *f*, Visibilitätskurve *f* / **~ meter** Gerät *n* zur Messung der Sichtbarkeit von Lichtwellen / **~ range** Bereich *m* des Sehens

visible sichtbar

visile optischer Typ *m*, Vorstellungstyp *m*

vision Sehen *n*, Sehvermögen *n*, Sehkraft *f*, Visus *m*, Gesichtshalluzination *f*, Vision *f*, Erscheinung *f* / ~ **test** Sehprüfung *f* / ~ **theory** Sehtheorie *f*, Farbtheorie *f* / **achromatic** ~ völlige Farbenblindheit *f* / **alternating** ~ alternierendes Sehen *n* / **binocular** ~ beidäugiges Sehen *n*, binokulares Sehen *n* / **central** ~ Sehen *n* im Augenmittelpunkt / **chromatic** ~ Farbensehen *n* / **coloured** ~ Farbensehen *n* / **dark** ~ Dunkelsehen *n* / **defective** ~ Sehfehler *m* / **dichromatic** ~ zweifarbiges Sehen *n*, dichromatisches Sehen *n* / **direct** ~ direktes Sehen *n* / **distant** ~ Sehweite *f* / **double** ~ Doppeltsehen *n*, Diplopie *f* / **ecstatic** ~ ekstatische Visionen *fpl* / **false** ~ Trugwahrnehmung *f* / **foveal** ~ foveales Sehen *n*, direktes Sehen *n* / **green** ~ Grünsehen *n*, Chloropsie *f* / **half** ~ Hemianopsie *f*, Halbseitenblindheit *f* / **haploscopic** ~ stereoskopisches Sehen *n* / **hysterical** ~ **disturbance** hysterische Sehstörung *f* / **indirect** ~ indirektes Sehen *n*, Randsehen *n* / **mesopic** ~ Dämmerungssehen *n* / **monochromatic** ~ einfarbiges Sehen *n* / **monocular** ~ einäugiges Sehen *n*, monokulares Sehen *n* / **near** ~ Nahsehen *n* / **normal** ~ Normalsichtigkeit *f*, Emmetropie *f* / **paracentral** ~ parazentrales Sehen *n* / **perimacular** ~ Sehen *n* mit dem Bereich um den gelben Fleck / **peripheral** ~ peripheres Sehen *n*, Randsehen *n* / **photopic** ~ Tagessehen *n* / **recurrent** ~ abwechselndes Sehen *n* von positiven und negativen Nachbildern / **scoterythrous** ~ Rotblindheit *f*, Protanopie *f* / **scotopic** ~ skotopes Sehen *n*, Dunkelsehen *n* / **stereoscopic** ~ stereoskopisches Sehen *n*

visitation right Besuchsrecht *n*

vista response perspektivische Schattierungsdeutung *f*

visual visuell

visualisation geistiges Sehen *n*, geistige Vorstellung *f* / ~ **of dimensions** Größenvorstellung *f* / ~ **of shapes** Formenvorstellung *f*

visualize sich vor Augen stellen, vorstellen, veranschaulichen

visualizer visueller Typ *m*, Vorstellungstyp *m*

visuoauditory optisch–akustisch

visuognosis optisches Erkennen *n*, visuelle Wahrnehmung *f*

visuokinaesthetic optisch–kinästhetisch

visuometer Gesichtsfeldmesser *m*, Perimeter *n*

visuomotor visuell–motorisch, visumotorisch

visuosensory Sehempfindungen betreffend, visuell–sensorisch

visuospatial optisch–räumlich

vita sexualis Geschlechtsleben *n*

vital vital, wesentlich, Lebens–

vitalism Vitalismus *m* / **creationist** ~ Vitalismus *m* mit der Annahme eines Schöpfungsglaubens

vitality Vitalität *f*, Lebenskraft *f* / **neurasthenic** ~ **deficiency** neurasthenische Leistungsschwäche *f*

vitamin Vitamin *n* / ~ **deficiency disorder** Vitaminmangelkrankheit *f*, Vitaminmangelerkrankung *f* / ~ **therapy** Vitaminbehandlung *f*, Vitamintherapie *f*

vitascope früher Tonfilmprojektor *m*

vitreous glasartig, glasig, hyalin

vivacity Lebhaftigkeit *f*, Lebendigkeit *f*, Munterkeit *f*

vivid lebhaft, lebendig

vividness Lebhaftigkeit *f*, Lebendigkeit *f*, Helligkeit *f*

vivify beleben

viviparity Lebendiggebären *n*

viviparous lebendgebährend

vivisect eine Vivisektion durchführen

vivisection Vivisektion *f*, operativer Eingriff *m* am lebenden Tier

vivisector Person *f* die eine Vivisektion durchführt

vocabulary Wortschatz *m*, Vokabular *n* / **~ burden** Umfang *m* des benutzten Wortschatzes / **~ load** Umfang *m* des benutzten Wortschatzes / **~ test** Wortschatztest *m* / **active ~** aktiver Wortschatz *m* / **passive ~** passiver Wortschatz *m* / **potential ~** passiver Wortschatz *m*

vocal vokal, Stimm–

vocalisation Stimmbildung *f*, Vokalisation *f* / **socialized ~** tierische Lautbildung *f* zur Verständigung

vocality Stimmeigenart *f*, Klangwirkung *f*

vocalize aussprechen, vokalisieren

vocation Berufung *f*, Beruf *m*, Neigung *f*

vocational beruflich, Berufs–

vocomotor sprachmotorisch, stimmmotorisch

voice Stimme *f*, Stimmhaftigkeit *f* / **~ disorder** Stimmstörung *f*, Dysphonie *f* / **~ key** Schallschlüssel *m* / **~s commenting** Begleitstimmen *fpl* / **husky ~** heisere Stimme *f* / **impaired ~** Stimmstörung *f* / **rough ~** rauhe Stimme *f* / **smooth ~** weiche Stimme *f* / **snuffling ~** näselnde Stimme *f* / **sobbing ~** schluchzende Stimme *f* / **speaking ~** Sprechstimme *f* / **whispering ~** Flüsterstimme *f*

voiceless stimmlos

volar Handflächen–, Fusssohlen–, volar, zur Hohlhand gehörend, hohlhandseitig

volition Wille *m*, Wollen *n* / **passive ~** passives Wollen *n*

volitional willensmäßig

volley Salve *f* / **~ fire** Salve *f* / **~ theory** Wellendispersionstheorie *f*

volt Volt *n*

voltage clamp Spannungsklemme *f*

voltmeter Voltmeter *n*

volume Volumen *n*, Umfang *m*, Rauminhalt *m* / **~ colour** Raumfarbe *f* / **~ of sound** Klangvolumen *n* / **~ sensor** Volumensensor *m* / **auditory ~** Hörumfang *m* / **cerebral ~** Hirnvolumen *n* / **residual ~** Residualvolumen *n* / **tonal ~** Tonumfang *m*

voluminousness Umfang *m*, Fülle *f*

voluntarism Voluntarismus *m*

voluntary willensmäßig, freiwillig, willkürlich

volunteer Freiwilliger *m* / **~ personnel** Freiwillige *pl*

voluptuous wollüstig, sinnlich, geil

vomit erbrechen, sich übergeben

vomiting Erbrechen *n*, Brechen *n*, Vomitus *m* / **~ associated with other psychological disturbances** Erbrechen *n* bei sonstigen psychischen Störungen / **~ centre** Brechzentrum *n* / **psychogenic ~** Zwangserbrechen *n* / **recurrent involuntary ~** Zwangserbrechen *n*

vomiturition Brechreiz *m*, Würgen *n*

von Frey hairs von Frey–Haare *npl*, Frey'sche Reizhaare *npl*

von Kries theory Duplizitätstheorie *f*

voodoo| death Voodoo–Tod *m*, Wodu–Tod *m* / **~ism** Zauberkult *m*, Zauberei *f*, Hexerei *f*

voting behaviour Wahlverhalten *n*

vowel Vokal *m*, Selbstlaut *m*

voyeur Voyeur *m*

voyeurism Voyeurismus *m*, Voyeurtum *n*, Schautrieb *m*

V test V–Test *m*

vulgar vulgär, allgemein üblich

vulgarity Gewöhnlichkeit *f*

vulnerability Verletzbarkeit *f*, Empfindlichkeit *f* / **concept of ~** Vulnerabilitätskonzept *n* / **primary ~** primäre Vulnerabilität *f* / **secondary ~** sekundäre Vulnerabilität *f*

vulva Vulva *f*, äußere weibliche Geschlechtsteile *mpl*

vulvismus Scheidenkrampf *m*, Vaginismus *m*

W

wage Lohn *m* / **~–cut** Lohnreduzierung *f*, Lohnminderung *f* / **~ incentive system** Lohnanreizsystem *n*, Prämiensystem *n* / **~ increase** Lohnerhöhung *f*

Wagner's corpuscle Wagner'sches Körperchen *n*, Meissner'sches Körperchen *n*, Tastkörperchen *n*

waiting Warten *n* / **~ period** Wartezeit *f*

wake wachen, erwachen, wach sein, wach bleiben, wachrufen, wach werden

wakeful wachsam, schlaflos

wakefulness Wachsein *n*, Schlaflosigkeit *f*

waking Erwachen *n*, Wachsein *n* / wachend / **~ center** Wachzentrum *n* / **~ dream** Wachtraum *m* / **~ hours** Wachstunden *fpl*

walk gehen / Gehen *n*, Gang *m* / **~ of life** soziale Schicht *f*, Stellung *f*, berufliche Laufbahn *f*

walking Gehen *n*, Spazierengehen *n* / gehend

wall, abdominal Bauchdecke *f*

walleye Auswärtsschielen *n*, Strabismus divergens *m*

walleyed auswärtsschielend

wandering Irrereden *n*, Geistesabwesenheit *f*, Träumerei *f*, Irrfahrt *f* / **~ behaviour** Umherwandern *n* / **~ effect** Phantasieeffekt *m*

want Bedürfnis *n* / **acquisitive ~** Erwerbstrieb *m*, Streben *n* nach Besitz / **altruistic ~** altruistisches Bedürfnis *n*, selbstloses Streben *n* / **maternal ~** Muttertrieb *m*

war Krieg *m* / **~ neurosis** Kriegsneurose *f*, Kampfneurose *f* / **~ psychosis** Kriegsneurose *f* / **nuclear ~** Atomkrieg *m*

warble tone Trillerton *m*

ward Krankenstation *f*, Krankenhausabteilung *f*

warfare Kriegführung *f* / **psychological ~** psychologische Kriegführung *f*

wariness Behutsamkeit *f*

warm warm / wärmen, anwärmen

warming–up Anlauf *m*, Aufwärmen *n*, Vorbereitung *f*, Anwärm–Effekt *m* / **~ decrement** Anwärm–Verlust *m* / **~ period** Anlaufzeit *f*, Eingewöhnungszeit *f*

warmth Wärme *f* / **~ sensation** Wärmeempfindung *f* / **~ spot** Wärmepunkt *m* / **paradoxical ~** paradoxe Wärmeempfindung *f*

warm–up Anlauf *m*, Aufwärmen *n*, Vorbereitung *f*, Eisbrecher *m*

warning| label Warnhinweis *m* auf Produkten / **~ sign** Warnzeichen *n*, Warnung *f*

washing Waschen *n* / **~ compulsion** Waschzwang *m* / **compulsive ~** Waschzwang *m* / **obsessional ~** Waschzwang *m*

Wassermann| reaction Wassermann–Reaktion *f* / **~ test** Wassermann–Reaktion *f*

wat Wat *n*, Einheit *f* zur Messung des Reaktionspotenzials

watch test Uhrentest *m*

water| balance Wasserhaushalt *m* / **~ deprivation** Wasserentbehrung *f*, Wasserentzug *m* / **~ fall illusion** Wasserfalleffekt *m*, Wasserfalltäuschung *f* / **~ intake** Wasseraufnahme *f* / **~ intoxication** Wasserintoxikation *f* / **~ safety** Wasserschutz *m*

Watson's psychology Behaviorismus *m*

watt Watt *n*

wave Welle *f* / ~ **amplitude** Wellenamplitude *f* / ~ **breadth** Wellenamplitude *f* / ~ **of excitation** Reizwelle *f*, Erregungswelle *f* / ~ **frequency** Wellenfrequenz *f*, Schwingungsfrequenz *f*, Frequenz *f* / **~–hollow** Wellental *n* / **~–length** Wellenlänge *f* / **~–length of equal hue** farbtongleiche Wellenlänge *f* / **~–motion** Wellenbewegung *f* / ~ **and spike** Krampfwelle *f* / **~–trough** Wellental *n* / **alpha ~** Alpha–Welle *f* / **beta ~** Beta–Welle *f* / **complementary ~** komplementäre Wellenlange *f* / **delta ~** Delta–Welle *f* / **dominant ~–length** farbtongleiche Wellenlänge *f* / **excitatory ~** Reizwelle *f*, Erregungswelle *f* / **fast ~s** schnelle Wellen *fpl* / **free progressive ~** sich frei fortpflanzende Welle *f* / **infrared ~** Infrarotstrahl *m* / **lambda ~** Lambdawelle *f* / **longitudinal ~** Längswelle *f* / **rectangular ~** rechteckige Welle *f* / **slow–~ sleep** orthodoxer Schlaf *m* / **stationary ~** stationäre Welle *f* / **theta ~** Thetawelle *f* / **transverse ~** Querwelle *f*, Transversalwelle *f* / **traveling ~** Wanderwelle *f*

wavecrest theory Wellenkammtheorie *f*

waxy wachsartig, wächsern

way Weg *m*, Art *f* / **~s of life** Lebensstil, Lebensart *f*, Lebensweise *f* / **institutional ~s** institutionelle Normen *fpl* / **one–~** einseitig, Einweg–

wayward eigensinnig, widerspenstig, unberechenbar

W compulsion starke Tendenz *f* zu Ganzantworten

we wir / **~–feeling** Wir–Gefühl *n* / **~–group** Wir–Gruppe *f* / **~/I–ratio** Wir/Ich–Verhältnis *n*

weak schwach

weakness Schwäche *f* / ~ **of character** Charakterschwäche *f* / ~ **of comprehension** Auffassungsstörung *f* / ~ **of memory** Gedächtnisschwäche *f* / ~ **of mental grasp** Auffassungsstörung *f* / ~ **of modification** Verarbeitungsschwäche *f* / ~ **sensation** Schwächegefühl *n* / **mental ~** Geistesschwäche *f*

wean entwöhnen

weaning Entwöhnung *f*, Abstillen *n* / Abbau *m* der Lernsicherung, Verminderung *f* der Lernhilfen / **psychological ~** psychologische Entwöhnung *f*

wear and tear syndrome Abnützungssyndrom *n*

web| experiment Web–Experiment *n* / ~ **page** Web–Seite *f* / Seite *f* im WWW / ~ **server** Web–Server *m* / ~ **site** Webseite *f*

Weber|'s circle Weber'scher Kreis *m* / **~–Fechner law** Weber–Fechner'sches Gesetz *n* / ~ **fraction** Weber'sche Formel *f* / **~'s law** Weber'sches Gesetz *n* / **~'s syndrome** Weber–Syndrom *n* / **~'s test** Weber–Versuch *m*

Wechsler| adult intelligence scale Wechsler–Intelligenztest *m* für Erwachsene / **~–Bellevue Scale** Wechsler–Bellevue–Test *m* / ~ **intelligence scale for children** Wechsler–Intelligenztest *m* für Kinder / ~ **memory scale** Wechsler–Gedächtnistest *m*

Wedensky| effect Wedensky–Effekt *m*, Wedensky–Hemmung *f* / ~ **inhibition** Wedensky–Hemmung *f* / ~ **phenomenon** Wedensky–Hemmung *f*

weep out ausweinen

W–effect Wirkung *f* des Wandertriebes

weigh wiegen, abwägen, sorgsam erwägen, prüfen

weighing machine Waage *f*

weight Gewicht *n*, Ladung *f* / gewichten / ~ **age** Alter *n* entsprechend der Tabelle des Durchschnittsgewichts / ~ **coefficient** Gewichtungszahl *f* / ~ **control** Gewichtskontrolle *f* / ~ **discrimination** Gewichtsunterscheidung *f* / ~ **experiment** Gewichtsexperiment *n* / ~ **perception** Gewichtswahrnehmung *f* / ~ **sensation** Gewichtsempfindung *f* / ~ **sense** Gewichtssinn *m* / **arbitrary ~** willkürliches Gewicht *n* / **beta ~** Beta–Koeffizient *m*, Standardregressionskoeffizient *m* / **effective ~** Ladung *f*, effektives Gewicht *n* / **functional ~** Ladung *f* / **ideal ~** Idealgewicht *n* / **natural ~** natürliches Gewicht *n* / **nominal ~** Nominalgewicht *n*, Gewichtungszahl *f* / **normal ~** Normalgewicht *n*

weighted gewichtet, gewogen

weighting Gewichtung *f* / **statistical ~** statistische Gewichtung *f*

weightlessness Gewichtslosigkeit *f*, Schwerelosigkeit *f*

weight training Krafttraining *n*

Weismannism Weismannismus *m*, Vererbungs– und Entwicklungstheorie *f* von Weismann

welfare Wohlfahrt *f*, Fürsorge *f*, Sozialhilfe *f* / **~ services** Wohlfahrt *f*, Fürsorgeleistungen *fpl* / **~ work** Sozialarbeit *f* / **external ~** Außenfürsorge *f* / **social ~** Sozialfürsorge *f*

well gut / **~–adjusted** angepasst / **~–balanced** ausgeglichen / **~–being** Wohlergehen *n*, Wohlbefinden *n*, Gesundheit *f* / **~–mannered** wohlerzogen / **~–thought–out** wohldurchdacht

wellness Wellness *f*, Gesundheit *f*

Wernicke's| aphasia kortikale, sensorische Aphasie *f*, Wernicke–Aphasie *f* / **~ area** Wernicke–Zentrum *n* / **~ centre** Wernicke–Zentrum *n* / **~ disease** Wernicke–Krankheit *f* / **~ encephalopathy** Wernicke–Krankheit *f* / **~ field** Wernicke–Zentrum *n* / **~ syndrome** Wernicke–Syndrom *n* / **~ zone** Wernicke–Zentrum *n*

wetness sensation Nässeempfinden *n*

wetting Bettnässen *n*, Durchnässung *f*

Wetzel grid Wetzel–Tafel *f*

Wever–Bray| effect Wever–Bray–Phänomen *n*, Mikrofoneffekt *m* des Corti–Organs / **~ phenomenon** Wever–Bray–Phänomen *n*, Mikrofoneffekt *m* des Corti–Organs

w factor W–Faktor *m*, Willensfaktor *m*

Wheatstone bridge Wheatstone–Brücke *f*

wheelchair Rollstuhl *m*

Wherry–Doolittle method Wherry–Doolittle–Verfahren *n*

whiplash Schleudertrauma *n* / **~ illusion** Peitschenriementäuschung *f* / **~ injury** Schleudertrauma *n*

whirl sensation Rotationsempfinden *n*

whisper flüstern / Geflüster *n*, Flüstern *n* / **~ test** Flüstertest *m*

whispering Flüstern *n* / flüsternd

white weiß / Weiß *n* / Weiße *m,f* / **visual ~** Sehweiß *n*, Leukopsin *n*

whiteness constancy Konstanz *f* der Farbe weiß

whole ganz, ungeteilt, vollständig, gesamt / Ganzes *n*, Ganzheit *f*, Gesamtheit *f* / **~ method of learning** Ganzheitsmethode *f* des Lernens / **~ and part learning** Lernen *n* des Ganzen und seiner einzelnen Teile / **dynamic ~** dynamisches Ganzes *n*

wholeness Ganzheit *f*, Gesamtheit *f* / **perceptual ~** Ganzheit *f* der Wahrnehmung, Wahrnehmungseinheit *f*

wholism Holismus *m*, holistische Theorie *f*, Ganzheitstheorie *f*

Whorf's hypothesis Whorf–Hypothese *f*

widow Witwe *f*

widower Witwer *m*

wild wild, unzivilisiert

Wilder's law Wilders Ausgangswertgesetz *n*

wilderness experience Wildniserleben *n*

wilful, willful eigensinnig, eigenwillig, vorsätzlich

wilfulness, willfulness Eigenwille *m*, Eigensinn *m*, Hartnäckigkeit *f*, Vorsätzlichkeit *f* / **insane ~** krankhafte Willensstärke *f*, Hyperbulie *f*

will Wille *m*, Testament *n* / **~ factor** Willensfaktor *m*, W–Faktor *m* / **~ impulsion** Willensimpuls *m* / **~ to live** Lebenswille *m* / **~ to peace** Friedenswille *m* / **~–power** Willenskraft *f* / **~ to power** Machtstreben *n* / **~ profile** Willensprofil *n* / **~–temperament test** Willens– und Temperamenttest *m* / **free ~** freier Wille *m*, Willensfreiheit *f* / **general ~** allgemeiner Wille *m* / **good ~** Vertrauen *n*, Image *n*, guter Ruf *m* / **Promethean ~** Unabhängigkeit *f* der Willensbildung / **social ~** sozialer Wille *m*

Wilson's disease Wilson–Krankheit *f*, hepatolentikuläre Degeneration *f*

windmill illusion Windmühlentäuschung *f*

window Fenster *n* / **oval ~** Vorhoffenster *n*, ovales Fenster *n* / **round ~** rundes Fenster *n* / **vestibular ~** ovales Fenster *n*, Vorhoffenster *n*

winking Blinzeln *n*, Lidschlag *m* / **~ reflex** Blinzelreflex *m*, Lidschlagreflex *m*

winter depression Winterdepression *f*

wire Draht *m* / **~–bending test** Drahtbiegeprobe *f*, Drahtbiegetest *m* / **barbed–~ disease** Gefangenenpsychose *f*, Lagerkoller *m*

wisdom Weisheit *f*, Klugheit *f*

wish Wunsch *m*, Verlangen *n*, Begehren *n* / **~ dream** Wunschtraum *m* / **~ fulfillment** Wunscherfüllung *f* / **~–fulfillment dream** Wunschtraum *m* / **~ phantasy** Wunschphantasie *f* / **instinctual ~** Triebwunsch *m* / **repressed ~** verdrängter Wunsch *m* / **unconscious ~** unbewusster Wunsch *m*

wit Verstand *m*, Geist *m*, Esprit *m*, Witz *m* / **~ work** Witzarbeit *f*

witch Hexe *f* / **~–doctor** Medizinmann *m*, Zauberer *m* / **~'s milk** Zaubermilch *f*

witchcraft Hexerei *f*, Zauber *m*, Zauberkraft *f*

withdrawal Zurückziehen *n*, Sich–Zurückziehen *n*, Coitus interruptus *m*, Entzug *m*, Retraktion *f* / **~ of affect** Affektentzug *m* / **~ of cathexis** Entziehung *f* der Besetzung / **~ delirium** Entzugsdelir *n* / **~ of the libido** Zurücknahme *f* der Libido / **~ psychosis** Entziehungspsychose *f* / **~ reflex** Fluchtreflex *m* / **~ state** Entzugssyndrom *n* / **~ state with delirium** Entzugssyndrom *n* mit Delir / **~ symptoms** Entzugssymptome *npl*, Entzugserscheinungen *fpl* / **~ syndrome** Entzugserscheinungen *fpl* / **~ treatment** Entziehungskur *f* / **autistic ~** autistische Abkapselung *f* / **social ~** soziale Isolation *f*, Kontaktarmut *f*

witness Zeugnis *n*, Zeuge *m*, Zeugin *f* / bezeugen, Zeugnis ablegen, beweisen / **~ box** Zeugenstand *m*

Witte–König paradoxical fusion effect Witte–König–Effekt *m*, Lückenphänomen *n*

Wittmaack–Ekbom syndrome Wittmaack–Ekbom Syndrom *n*, Restless–legs–Syndrom *n*

wolf child Wolfskind *n*, von Wölfen aufgezogenes Kind *n*

woman Frau *f* / **manlike ~** Mannweib *n* / **masculine ~** Mannweib *n* / **phallic ~** phallische Frau *f* / **working ~** berufstätige Frau *f*

womb Schoß *m*, Mutterleib *m*, Uterus *m* / **maternal ~** mütterlicher Schoß *m*

wonder Erstaunen *n*, Verwunderung *f*, Wunder *n* / sich wundern, sich Gedanken machen

women's lib Frauenbewegung *f*, Frauenrechtsbewegung *f*

word Wort *n* / **~ agglutination** Wortagglutination *f* / **~ association** Wortassoziation *f* / **~ association test** Assoziationsversuch *m* / **~–blind** wortblind / **~–blindness** Wortblindheit *f*, Alexie *f* / **~–building test** Wortbildungstest *m* / **~ calling** Wortnennung *f*, Wortaussprechen *n* / **~ configuration** Wortgestalt *f* / **~ count** Zählung *f* der Worthäufigkeit / **~–deaf** worttaub / **~–deafness** Worttaubheit *f*, Seelentaubheit *f*, auditorische Amnesie *f*, akustische Agnosie *f* / **~ family** Wortfamilie *f* / **~–fluency** Wortflüssigkeit *f*, Wortgewandtheit *f*, sprachliche Gewandtheit *f* / **~–formation** Wortbildung *f* / **~ frequency** Worthäufigkeit *f* / **~ hash** Wortsalat *m* / **~ magic** Wortzauber *m* / **~ meaning** Wortbedeutung *f* / **~ method** Ganzheitsmethode *f* / **~ presentation** Wortvorstellung *f* / **~ processing** Textverarbeitung *f* / **~ recognition** Worterkennen *n* / **~ salad** Wortsalat *m* / **~**

sentence Wortsatz *m* / **~–span test** Test *m* des unmittelbaren Wortgedächtnisses / **one–~ sentence** Einwortsatz *m* / **primal ~** Urwort *n* / **structural ~** Funktionswort *n* / **visual ~ centre** Lesezentrum *n*

wording Wortlaut *m*

work Arbeit *f* / **~ adjustment training** Arbeitsintegrationstraining *n* / **~ attitude** Einstellung *f* zur Arbeit / **~ cure** Beschäftigungtherapie *f* / **~ curve** Arbeitskurve *f* / **~ decrement** Leistungsabnahme *f* / **~ environment** Arbeitsumgebung *f* / **~ factor system** System *n* vorbestimmter Zeiten / **~ force** Arbeitskräfte *fpl*, Arbeiter *mpl*, Belegschaft *f* / **~ inhibition** Arbeitshemmung *f* / **~–limit procedure** zeitlich begrenztes Verfahren *n* / **~–limit test** zeitlich begrenzter Test *m* / **~ load** Arbeitsbelastung *f* / **~ method** Arbeitsmethode *f*, Arbeitsverfahren *n* / **~ of mourning** Trauerarbeit *f* / **~–related illness** Berufskrankheit *f* / **~–rest cycle** Pausenregelung *f*, Arbeits–Ruhe–Rhythmus *m* / **~ sample** Arbeitsprobe *f* / **~ sample performance test** Leistungstest *m* in Form einer Arbeitsprobe / **~ satisfaction** Arbeitszufriedenheit *f* / **~ scheduling** Arbeitseinteilung *f*, Arbeitsvorbereitung *f* / **~–shyness** Arbeitsscheu *f* / **~ simplification** Arbeitsvereinfachung *f*, Arbeitserleichterung *f* / **~ study** Arbeitsstudie *f* / **~ test** Arbeitsversuch *m*, Arbeitsprobe *f* / **~ therapy** Arbeitstherapie *f*, Beschäftigungstherapie *f* / **~ week length** Dauer *f* der Arbeitswoche / **dynamic ~** dynamische Arbeit *f* / **extramural ~** Auslandskurse *mpl*, Hochschulkurse *mpl* / **manual ~** Handarbeit *f*, manuelle Tätigkeit *f* / **mental ~** geistige Arbeit *f* / **physical ~** körperliche Arbeit *f* / **psychiatric social ~** Außenfürsorge *f* / **social ~** Sozialarbeit *f* / **static ~** statische Arbeit *f*

work|aholic Arbeitssüchtige *m,f* / **~aholism** Arbeitsbesessenheit *f*, Arbeitssucht *f*, krankhafte Arbeitswut

worker Arbeiter *m* / **~ characteristic** Arbeiter–Anforderungsprofil *n* / **agricultural ~** Landarbeiter *m* / **blue collar ~** Arbeiter *m*, gewerblicher Arbeitnehmer *m* / **foreign ~** ausländischer Arbeitnehmer *m*, Gastarbeiter *m* / **psychiatric social ~** psychiatrisch geschulter Sozialarbeiter *m* / **skilled industrial ~** Facharbeiter *m* / **social ~** Sozialarbeiter *m*, Sozialfürsorger *m* / **unskilled industrial ~** ungelernter Arbeiter *m*, Hilfsarbeiter *m* / **white collar ~** Angestellter *m*, Büroangestellter *m*

working Arbeits– / Arbeiten *n* / **~ alliance** Arbeitsbündnis *n* / **~ condition** Arbeitsbedingung *f* / **~ curve** Arbeitskurve *f* / **~ hypothesis** Arbeitshypothese *f* / **~ memory** Kurzzeitgedächtnis *n* / **~–off** Abreaktion *f* / **~–off mechanism** Mechanismus *m* der Abreaktion / **~ rhythm** Arbeitsrhythmus *m* / **~ space** Arbeitsraum *m*, Arbeitsumfeld *n* / **~ table** Arbeitstisch *m* / **~–through** Durcharbeiten *n* / **psychical ~ over** psychische Verarbeitung *f*, psychische Aufarbeitung *f* / **psychical ~ out** psychische Ausarbeitung *f*, psychische Verarbeitung *f*

workmen's compensation insurance berufsgenossenschaftliche Unfallversicherung *f*

workshop Werkstatt *f* / **sheltered ~** beschützende Werkstatt *f*, Werkstatt *f* für Behinderte

world Welt *f* / **~ of delusions** Wahnwelt *f* / **~–destruction fantasies** Weltzerstörungsideen *fpl* / **~ of ideas** Vorstellungswelt *f* / **~–reconstruction fantasies** Weltverbesserungsideen *fpl* / **~ test** Welttest *m* / **~ view** Weltanschauung *f*, Weltbild *n* / **cognitive ~** Innenwelt *f*, kognitive Welt *f* / **external ~** Außenwelt *f* / **inner ~** Innenwelt *f* / **physical ~** physikalische Welt *f*

worry Sorge *f*, Besorgnis *f* / **~ inventory** Sorgenliste *f* / **depressed ~** Kummer *m* / **excited ~** Aufregung *f*

worship Gottesdienst *m*, Kult *m*, Anbetung *f*, Verehrung *f* / **phallic ~** Phalluskult *m*

worth Wert *m* / wert

wound Wunde *f*, Verwunderung *f*

wrath Wut *f*, Zorn *m*

W response Ganzantwort *f*

wrist Handgelenk *n* / **~ reflex** Handgelenksreflex *m*

writer Autor *m* / **~'s cramp** Schreibkrampf *m*

writing Schreiben *n*, Schrift *f* / **~ accent** Schriftmerkmal *n* / **~ centre** Schreibzentrum *n* / **~ re–education** Schriftumerziehung *f* / **~ skill** Schreibfähigkeit *f* / **~ tremor** Schreibtremor *m*, Schreibzittern *n* / **ataxic ~** ungeordnete Schrift *f* / **automatic ~** Schreibautomatismus *m*, automatisches Schreiben *n* / **backhand ~** Rückwärtsschreiben *n* / **blind ~** Blind–Schreiben *n* / **creative ~** Schriftstellern *n*, Schriftstellerei *f*, kreatives Schreiben *n* / **cursive ~** Kursivschrift *f* / **developmental expressive ~ disorder** entwicklungsbedingte Schreibstörung *f* / **dextrad ~** nach rechts gerichtete Schrift *f* / **hieroglyphic ~** Hieroglyphenschrift *f* / **sinistrad ~** nach links gerichtete Schrift *f*

wry–neck Schiefhals *m*, Torticollis *m*

Wundt illusion Wundt'sche Serviettenringfigur *f*

Würzburg School Würzburger Schule *f*

XYZ

xanthic gelblich

xanthocyanopsia, xanthocyanopsy, xanthocyanopia Gelbblausichtigkeit *f*, Rotgrünblindheit *f*, Xanthozyanopie *f*

xanthoma gelbes Knötchen *n*, Xanthom *n*

xanthopsia, xanthopia Gelbsehen *n*, Xanthopsie *f*

x axis X–Achse *f*, Abszisse *f*

X chromosome X–Chromosom *n*

x coordinate Abszisse *f*, X–Achse *f*

x distance X–Abstand *m*

xenoglossophilia Drang *m* zur Benutzung unüblicher Fremdwörter, Xenoglossophilie *f*

xenoglossophobia krankhafte Angst *f* vor Fremdsprachen

xenoglossy, xenoglossia Sprechen *n* in einer sonst unbekannten fremden Sprache unter Trance, Xenoglossie *f*

xenomania übertriebene Neigung *f* zu Fremdländischem, Xenomanie *f*

xenophile Person *f* mit gesteigerter Vorliebe für Fremdländisches

xenophilia gesteigerte Vorliebe *f* für das Fremde, Xenophilie *f*

xenophobe Person *f* die unter Fremdenangst leidet

xenophobia krankhafte Angst *f* vor Fremden, Xenophobie *f*

xenotransplantation Xenotransplantation *f*

xerography Xerographie *f*, elektrostatisches Trockenkopierverfahren *n*

xerophilia, xerophily Vorliebe *f* für trockene Umgebung

xerophobia Versagen *n* des Speichelflusses vor Angst

xi Xi *n*, Gleichheitspunkt *m* auf einer subjektiven Skala

X–ray Röntgenaufnahme *f* / **~ diagnosis** Röntgendiagnose *f* / **~ equipment** Röntgengerät *n* / **~ therapy** Röntgenbestrahlung *f*, Röntgentherapie *f*

x value X–Wert *m*

XYZ grouping Eingruppierung *f* nach Fähigkeit

y array Spalte *f*

yawn gähnen

yawning Gähnen *n* / **convulsive ~** Gähnkrampf *m* / **spasmodic ~** Gähnkrampf *m*

y axis Y–Achse *f*, Ordinate *f*

Y chromosome Y–Chromosom *n*

y coordinate Y–Achse *f*, Ordinate *f*, Y–Koordinate *f*

y distance Y–Abstand *m*

year scaling Skalierung *f* nach Jahren

yell gellend schreien

yellow gelb / Gelb *n* / **~–sighted** gelbsichtig / **visual ~** Sehgelb *n*

yellowish gelblich

Yerkes–Dodson law Yerkes–Dodson–Gesetz *n*, Gesetz *n* über die Beziehung zwischen Stärke der Motivation und Diskriminationslernen

yes reaction Bestätigungsreaktion *f*

yielding unterwürfig, willfährig, ergeben

yoga Yoga *n*

yohimbine Yohimbin *n*

Young–Helmholtz theory Young–Helmholtz–Theorie *f*, Dreikomponententheorie *f*, Dreifarbentheorie *f*

youth Jugend *f*, Jugendlicher *m* / **~ centre** Jugendheim *n* / **~ custody** Jugendstrafe *f* / **~ custody centre** Jugendstrafanstalt *f* /

predelinquent ~ verwahrloste Jugend *f*, prädelinquente Jugendliche *mpl* / **wayward ~** widerspenstige Jugend *f*

y value Y–Wert *m*

z chart Z–Diagramm *n*

Z distribution Z–Verteilung *f*

zee chart Z–Diagramm *n*

Zeigarnik| effect Zeigarnik–Effekt *m* / **~ phenomenon** Zeigarnik–Effekt *m*

Zen Buddhism Zen–Buddhismus *m*, Zen–Lehre *f*

Zeno's arrow Zeno–Pfeil *m*

zenophobia krankhafte Angst *f* vor Fremden, Xenophobie *f*

zeppia weiches Überich *n*

zero Null *f* / **~ efficiency** Nulleffektivität *f* / **~ improvement** Nullverbesserung *f* / **~–order** nullter Ordnung / **~ point** Nullpunkt *m* / **~ re–set register** Registrierapparat *m* mit Rücksteflung auf null / **absolute ~** absoluter Nullpunkt *m* / **absolute ontogenetic ~** absoluter Entwicklungsbeginn *m* / **arbitrary ~** willkürlich angenommener Nullpunkt *m* / **developmental ~** Entwicklungsbeginn *m* / **non ~ sum game** Nicht–Null–Summen–Spiel *n* / **physiological ~** physiologischer Nullpunkt *m* / **true ~** absoluter Nullpunkt *m*

zest Lust *f*, Freude *f*, Genuss *m* / **~ for gambling** Spielleidenschaft *f* / **~ for life** Lebenshunger *m*

zeta Zeta *n*

zidovudine Azidothymidin *n*, AZT

Ziehen–Oppenheim disease Ziehen–Oppenheim–Krankheit *f*, Torsionsneurose *f*

zinc white Zinkweiß *n*, Deckweiß *n*, Schneeweiß *n*

zoanthropy Wahnvorstellung *f* in ein Tier verwandelt zu sein, Zooanthropie *f*

zoetrope stroboskopischer Zylinder *m*, Schnellseher *m*, Zoetrop *n*

Zöllner illusion Zöllner'sche Täuschung *f*

zomotherapy Fleischdiät *f*

zone Zone *f*, Bereich *m*, Region *f* / **~ of development** Entfaltungszone *f* / **~ of freedom** Freiheitsraum *m*, Freiheitsbereich *m* / **~ position** Bildbeigabeteil *m* / **~ primacy** Primat *m* einer Zone / **anal ~** Analbereich *m*, Analregion *f*, Analzone *f* / **erogenous ~** erogene Zone *f* / **erotogenic ~** erogene Zone *f* / **genital ~** Genitalbereich *m* / **hyperaesthetic ~** überempfindliche Zone *f* / **hysterogenic ~** hysterogene Zone *f* / **latent ~** stille Zone *f* / **motor ~ s** motorische Hirnzentren *npl* / **primary ~** erogene Urzone *f*, Primärbereich *m* / **reflexogenous ~** Reflexzone *f*, reflexogene Zone *f* / **retinal ~s** Netzhautzonen *fpl* / **sensitive ~** reizempfindliche Zone *f* / **thermoneutral ~** thermische Neutralzone *f* / **visual ~** Zone *f* des schärfsten Sehens

zonesthesia Gürtelgefühl *n*, Zonästhesie *f*

zonule Zonulafaser *f* / **ciliary ~** Zonula ciliaris *f*

zooerastia, zooerasty Sodomie *f*, Zooerastie *f*, Zoophilie *f*, Bestialität *f*

zoolagnia sexueller Drang *m* zu Tieren

zoology Zoologie *f*, Tierkunde *f*

zoomagnetism tierischer Magnetismus *m*

zoomania krankhafte Tierliebe *f*

zoomorphism tiersymbolische Götterdarstellung *f*, Tiersymbolik *f*

zoopathology Tierpathologie *f*

zoophilia, zoophily, zoophilism Tierliebe *f*, Liebe *f* zu Tieren, Zoophilie *f* / **erotic ~** Sodomie *f*

zoophilic, zoophilous Tiere liebend

zoophilist Tierliebhaber *m*, Sodomist *m*

zoophobia krankhafte Angst *f* vor Tieren, Zoophobie *f*

zoopsia Tieresehen *n*, Sehen *n* weißer Mäuse

zoopsychological tierpsychologisch

zoopsychology Tierpsychologie *f*

zoosadism Tierquälerei *f*

zooscopy Tieresehen *n*, Tierhalluzination *f*, Tierbeobachtung *f*

zoster Gürtelrose *f*, Herpes zoster *m*

z score z–Wert *m*, Standardwert *m*

z–test z–Test *m*

Zürich school Züricher Schule *f*

zygocyte, zygote Zygote *f*, befruchtete Eizelle *f*

zygotic zygotisch

LIST OF ABBREVIATIONS

ABKÜRZUNGSVERZEICHNIS

A = **adrenaline** Adrenalin *n* / = **adult** erwachsen / Erwachsener *m* / = **age** Alter *n* / = **albedo** Albedo *m* Reflektionsgrad *m* / = **American** amerikanisch / = **amplitude** Amplitude *f* / = **reaction amplitude** Erregungsamplitude *f* / = **animal content** Tierdeutung *f* / = **any number** irgendeine Zahl *f*

Å = **angstrom unit** Ångströmeinheit *f*

A_{obj} = **objects derived from the body of an animal** Tierobjekte *npl*

a = **amplitude** Amplitude *f* / = **incentive substance** Reizmittel *n*

a_1, a_2, a_3, ...a_n = **successive measurements of the same variable** Beobachtungsfolge *f* der gleichen Variablen

AA = **achievement age** Leistungsalter *n* / = **Alcoholics Anonymous** Anonyme Alkoholiker *mpl*

AAC = **antigen–antibody complex** Antigen–Antikörperkomplex *m*

AC = **alternating current** Wechselstrom *m*

Ach = **acetylcholine** Azetylcholin *n*

AChE = **acetylcholinesterase** Azetylcholinesterase *f*

ACTH = **adrenocorticotrophic hormone** adrenokortikotropes Hormon *n*, Kortikotropin *n*, Adrenokortikotropin *n*

AD = **average deviation** mittlere Abweichung *f*

Ad = **animal detail** Tierdetail *n*

ADD = **attention–deficit disorder** Störung *f* mit Aufmerksamkeitsdefizit, Aufmerksamkeitsstörung *f*

ADDH = **attention–deficit disorder with hyperactivity** Störung *f* mit Aufmerksamkeitsdefizit bei Hyperaktivität

ADH = **antidiuretic hormone** Adiuretin *n*, Vasopressin *n*

ADHD = **attention–deficit hyperactivity disorder** Aufmerksamkeits– und Hyperaktivitätsstörung

ADP = **adenosine diphosphate** Adenosindiphosphat *n*

AF = **audio–frequency** Hörfrequenz *f*

AI = **artificial insemation** künstliche Befruchtung *f* / = **artificial Intelligence** künstliche Intelligenz *f*

AIDA = **attention, interest, desire, action** Aufmerksamkeit erzielen, Interesse erregen, Verlangen wecken, Kaufentschluss herbeiführen

AIDS = **acquired immunodeficiency syndrome** erworbenes Immundefektsyndrom *n*

AL = **absolute limen** absolute Scbwelle *f* / = **adaptation level** Anpassungsniveau *n* / = **aspiration level** Anspruchsniveau *n*

ALGOL = **algorithmic language** ALGOL *n*, Programmiersprache ALGOL *f*

ALP = **anterior lobe of pituitary** Hypophysenvorderlappen *m*

alt = **alternating, alternate** abwechselnd

AMT = **anxiety management training** Angstbewältigungstraining *n*

An = **anatomy response** Anatomiedeutung *f*, Anatomieantwort *f*

Anat = **anatomy** Anatomie *f*

ANCOVA = **analysis of covariance** Kovarianzanalyse *f*

an. ex. = **anode excitation** Anodenreizung *f*

ANF = **atrial natriuretic factor** atrialer natriuretischer Faktor *m*

ANOVA = **analysis of variance** Varianzanalyse *f*

ANP = **atrial natriuretic peptide** atriales natriuretisches Peptid *n*

ANS = **autonomic nervous system** autonomes Nervensystem *n*

ant. = **anterior** vorder

AP = **action potential** Aktionspotential *n* / = **anterior pituitary** Hypophysenvorderlappen *m*

APA, A.P.A. = **American Psychiatric Association** Amerikanische Gesellschaft *f* für Psychiatrie / = **American Psychoanalytical Association** Amerikanische Gesellschaft *f* für Psychoanalyse / = **American Psychological Association** Amerikanische Gesellschaft *f* für Psychologie / = **American Psychotherapy Association** Amerikanische Gesellschaft *f* für Psychotherapie

APH = **anterior pituitary hormone** Hypophysenvorderlappenhormon *n*

App = **manner of approach** Erfassungstypus *m*

Apper = **apperceptive type** Erfassungstypus *m*

A.P.S. = **American Psychopathological Society** Amerikanische Gesellschaft *f* für Psychopathologie / = **American Psychosomatic Society** Amerikanische Gesellschaft *f* für psychosomatische Medizin

AQ = **achievement quotient** Leistungsquotient *m*

AR = **alarm reaction** Alarmreaktion *f*

Ar A = **arithmetic age** Rechenalter *n*

ARAS = **ascending reticular activating system** aufsteigendes retikuläres aktivierendes System *n*

Ar Q = **arithmetic quotient** Rechenquotient *m*

Ar R = **arithmetic ratio** Rechenquotient *m*

ARS = **arousal reaction system** System *n* der Weckreaktion

AS = **arteriosclerosis** Arteriosklerose *f*

A–S = **ascendance–submission** Überlegenheit–Unterlegenheit *f*

As = **astigmatism** Astigmatismus *m*

ASCII = **American Standard Code for Information Interchange** ASCII Zeichensatz *m*

ASL = **American Sign Language** amerikanische Zeichensprache *f*

Asn = **strength of association** Assoziationsstarke *f*

ASDC = **Association for Sleep Disorders Centers** Vereinigung *f* von Schlafzentren

ASO = **assumed similarity of opposites** angenommene Ähnlichkeit *f* zwischen Gegensätzen

AT = **achievement test** Leistungstest *m*

At = **anatomy response** Anatomiedeutung *f*

ATM = **asynchronous transfer mode** asynchrones Datenübertragungsverfahren *n*

ATP = **adenosine triphosphate** Adenosintriphosphat *n*

ATR = **Achilles tendon reflex** Achillesschnenreflex *m*

A.U. = **Angstrom unit** Ångströmeinheit *f*

A–U–D = **agree–undecided–disagree** ja–unentschieden–nein

AV = **audio–visual** audiovisuell / = **average variability** mittlere Variabilität *f*

av = **average** Durchschnitt *m* / durchschnittlich

AZT = **azidothymidine** Azidothymidin *n*

B = **behaviour** Verhalten *n* / = **response of a human being in motion** Bewegungsantwort *f* / = **body** Körper *m* / = **luminance** Leuchtdichte *f* / = **any number** irgendeine Zahl *f* / = **mean number of responses** mittlere Antwortenzahl *f*

b_{12} = regression coefficient of 1 on 2 Regressionskoeffizient *m* von 1 auf 2

B.A. = Bachelor of Arts *(Titel nach College–Graduierung)*

BAS = behavioural approach system *oder* / = behavioural activation system Annäherungssystem *n*

B.B.B. = blood–brain barrier Blut–Hirn–Schranke *f*

BC = backcross Rückkreuzung *f* / **= birth control** Geburtenkontrolle *f* / **= bone–conduction** Knochenleitung *f*

b.d. = twice daily zweimal täglich

BDNF = brain–derived neurotrophic factors *(keine deutsche Übersetzung gebräuchlich)*

beh. = behaviour Verhalten *n* / **= behaviorism** Behaviorismus *m*

BERA = brain stem evoked response audiometry Messung *f* akustisch evozierter Hirnstammpotentiale

BET = body–ego–technique Körper–Ich–Technik *f*

BIS = behavioural inhibition system Verhaltenshemm–System *n*

BM = basal metabolism Grundumsatz *m*

BMDP = biomedical computer programmes biomedizinische Computerprogramme *npl*

BMI = body mass index Körpermasseindex *m*

BMR = basal metabolic rate Grundumsatz *m*

BMT = Basic Motion Time System *n* vorbestimmter Zeiten

BO = body odour Körpergeruch *m*

B.P. = blood pressure Blutdruck *m*

BPS = British Psychological Society Britische Gesellschaft *f* für Psychologie

Bps = bits per second Bits *npl* pro Sekunde

B.Sc. = Bachelor of Science *(Titel nach College–Graduierung)*

BST = brief–stimulus therapy Behandlung *f* mit milden Schocks, Schocktherapie *f*

BT = body temperature Körpertemperatur *f* / **= brain tumour** Gehirntumor *m*

BW = birth weight Geburtsgewicht *n* / **= body weight** Körpergewicht *n*

C = centimeter Zentimeter *n* / **= class** Klasse *f*, Gruppe *f* / **= coefficient** Koeffizient *m* / **= colour response** Farbdeutung *f*, Fb–Antwort *f* / **= condition of a neuron** Zustand *m* einer Nervenzelle / **= constant** Konstante *f* / **= contingency coefficient** Kontingenzkoeffizient *m* / **= control group** Kontrollgruppe *f* / **= cortex** Rinde *f*

C' = achromatic colour response achromatische Farbantwort *f*

C. = centigrade Grad *n* Celsius

C_A = coefficient of association Assoziationsquotient *m*

C_D = drive condition Triebzustand *m*

C_{des} = colour description Farbbeschreibung *f*

C_{sum} = sum of weights for colour responses Summe *f* der Gewichtungen aller Farbantworten

C, = colour symbolism Farbsymbolik *f*

c = cervical zervikal / **= C factor** C–Faktor *m* / **= value of correction** Korrekturwert *m* / **= (as a subscript) criterion variable** (als Index) Kriteriumvariable *f* / **= shading of the inkblot with a flat surface** Schattierungsdeutung *f* ohne Perspektive

CA = chronological age Lebensalter *n*

CAD = conditioned avoidance drive konditionierter Vermeidungstrieb *m*

CAH = congenital adrenal hyperplasia adrenogenitales Syndrom *n*, Nebennierenrindenhyperplasie *f*

CAI = computer assisted instruction computerunterstützte Unterweisung *f*

cAMP = cyclic adenosine monophosphate zyklisches Adenosin–3′,5′–Phosphat *n*

CAR = conditioned avoidance reaction konditionierte Vermeidungsreaktion *f*

CAT = computer assisted testing computerunterstützte Testdurchführung *f* und –interpretation *f* / **= computerized axial tomography** Computertomographie *f*

CAVD = completion, arithmetical problems, vocabulary, directions Ergänzung *f*, Rechnen *n*, Worterklärung *f*, Aufträge *mpl* befolgen

CBF = cerebral blood flow Gehirndurchblutung *f*

CBS = chronic brain syndrome chronisches psychoorganisches Syndrom *n*

CC = coefficient of correlation Korrelationskoeffizient *m*

cc. = cubic centimeter Kubikzentimeter *m*

CCC = consonant trigram Konsonanten–Trigramm *n*, Folge *f* von 3 Konsonanten

CCK = cholecystokinin Cholezystokinin *n*

ccw = counterclockwise gegen den Uhrzeigersinn

CD = convulsive disorder krampfartige Störung *f*

cdf = cumulative distribution function kumulative Häufigkeitsfunktion *f*

CE = constant error konstanter Fehler *m*, systematischer Fehler *m*

cemf = counterelectromotive force elektromotorische Gegenkraft *f*

cent. = centigrade Grad *n* Celsius / **= central** zentral / **= centre** Zentrum *n*, Bezirk *m*

CER = conditioned emotional response konditionierte emotionale Reaktion *f*

c.e.s. = central excitatory state Erregungszustand *m* des Zentralnervensystems

CF = colour–form response Farbformantwort *f* / **= cardiac failure** Herzversagen *n*, Herzinsuffizienz *f*

CFF = critical frequency of fusion Flimmerverschmelzungsfrequenz *f* / **= critical flicker frequency** Flimmerverschmelzungsfrequenz *f*

CFS = chronic fatigue syndrome chronisches Müdigkeitssyndrom *n*

CG = control group Kontrollgruppe *f*

cg = centre of gravity Schwerpunkt *m*

CGI = Common Gateway Interface Schnittstelle *f* eines Web–Servers für externe Programme

CGM = central gray matter graue Substanz *f* des ZNS

cGMP = cyclic guanosine monophosphate zyklisches Guanosin–3′,5′–Phosphat *n*

C.G.S., cgs = centimeter–gram–second Zentimeter *n*, Gramm *n*, Sekunde *f*

Ch = pure chiaroscuro response reine Helldunkeldeutung *f*

ch = chain Kette *f* / **= child** Kind *n*

ChE = cholinesterase Cholinesterase *f*

ChF = chiaroscuro–form response Helldunkel–Formdeutung *f*

CHP = child psychiatry Kinderpsychiatrie *f*

CI = coefficient of intelligence Intelligenzkoeffizient *m*

CIA = coefficient of intellectual ability Intelligenzkoeffizient *m*, Begabungskoeffizient *m*

CJD = Creutzfeldt–Jacob disease Creutzfeld–Jakob–Krankheit *f*

CL_{alt} = comparison level for alternatives Vergleichsniveau *n* für Alternativen

cm = centimeter Zentimeter *m od. n* / **= cumulative** kumulativ

CMBD = Classification of Mental and Behavioural Diseases Klassifikation *f* der psychischen und Verhaltensstörungen

CMC = computer mediated communication Kommunikation *f* über elektronische Medien

cmps = centimeters per second Zentimeter *m od. n* pro Sekunde

Cn = colour naming Farbnennung *f*

CNS = central nervous system Zentralnervensystem *n* / **= conceptual nervous system** hypothetisch–begriffliches Nervensystem *n*

CNV = contingent negative variation negative kortikale Gleichspannungsverschiebung *f*

coef. = coefficient Koeffizient *m*

COEPS = cortically originating extrapyramidal system kortikaler Anteil *m* des extrapyramidal–motorischen Systems

COM1/COM2... = communication port 1, 2... serielle Schnittstelle *f* eines PC

cond = condition Zustand *m*, Bedingung *f*

cond ref = conditioned reflex bedingter Reflex *m*, bedingte Reaktion *f*

cond resp = conditioned response bedingte Reaktion *f*

cos = cosine Kosinus *m*

cot = cotangent Kotangens *m*, Kotangente *f*

CP = cerebral palsy Gehirnlähmung *f*

c.p. = candle power Kerzenstärke *f*

CPM = critical path method Methode *f* der Netzplantechnik

cpm = cycles per minute Schwingungen *fpl* pro Minute

cps = cycles per second Schwingungen *fpl* pro Sekunde

CPU = central processor unit zentrale Recheneinheit *f*

CR = conditioned reaction bedingte Reaktion *f*, konditionierte Reaktion *f* / **= conditioned reflex** bedingter Reflex *m* / **= conditioned response** bedingte Reaktion *f*

CRH = corticotropin releasing hormone Corticoliberin *n*

CRF = continuous reinforcement kontinuierliche Verstärkung *f*, Immerverstärkung *f*

CRT = cathode ray tube Kathodenstrahlröhre *f*

CS = cerebrospinal zerebrospinal, Gehirn und Rückenmark betreffend / **= conditioned stimulus** bedingter Reiz *m*, konditionierter Reiz *m*

Cs. = conscious bewusst / **= consciousness** Bewusstein *n*

CSF = cerebrospinal fluid Hirnflüssigkeit *f*, Gehirn– und Rückenmarksflüssigkeit *f*

CST = convulsive shock therapy Schocktherapie *f*

CT = cerebral tumour Hirntumor *m* / **= computed tomography** Computertomographie *f*

CTa = catamenia Menstruation *f*

CV = cardiovascular kardiovaskulär, Herz und Kreislauf betreffend / **= coefficient of variation** Variationskoeffizient *m* / **= controlled variable** kontrollierte Variable *f*, unabhängige Variable *f*

cva = cerebrovascular accident Apoplexie *f*

cw = clockwise im Uhrzeigersinn

D = detail response Detailantwort *f* / **= developed** entwickelt / **= deviation** Abweichung *f* / **= diameter** Durchmesser *m* / **= differential** Differential– / **= difference between D_1 and D_9** Differenz *f* zwischen dem ersten und neunten Dezil / **= difference between two scores of the same individual** Unterschied *m* zwischen zwei Ergebnissen derselben Person / **= dioptre** Dioptrie *f* / **= distance** Entfernung *f*, Distanz *f* / **= drive** Trieb *m* / **= drive stimulus** Triebreiz *m* / **= generalised drive** generalisierter Antrieb *m* / **= similarity measure between sets of scores** Ähnlichkeitsmaß *n* zwischen Gruppen von Werten *f* / **= strength of all nondominant drives** Triebstärke *f* aller nicht–dominanten Antriebe / **= strength of dominant primary drive** Stärke *f* des dominanten Primärtriebes

D. = dose Dosis *f*

D^1 = drive proper natürlicher Trieb *m*

D% = per cent of difference Unterschiedprozent *n*

d = **density** Dichte *f* / = **small detail response** Kleindetailantwort *f* / = **deviation** Abweichung *f* / = **deviation of a class from the mean of a population** Klassenabweichung *f* vom Populationsmittelwert / = **rank difference of an individual on two tests** Rangdifferenz *f* eines Probanden bei zwei Tests / = **number of j.n.d.'s lying between two stimulus aggregates** Zahl *f* der eben merklichen Schritte zwischen zwei Reizmengen / = **dioptre** Dioptrie *f* / = **distal** distal / = **dorsal** dorsal / = **drive** Trieb *m*, Antrieb *m*

d' = **strength of all the nondominant drives minus the strength of the dominant primary drive** Triebstärke *f* aller nicht–dominanten Antriebe abzüglich der Stärke des dominanten Primärtriebes

DA = **dopamine** Dopamin *n*

DAF = **delayed auditory feedback** verzögerte Gehörrückkopplung *f*

DAT = **dementia of the Alzheimer's type** Demenz *f* vom Alzheimer Typ

dB = **decibel** Dezibel *n*

DBT = **dialectic–behavioral therapy** dialektische Verhaltenstherapie *f*

DBP = **diastolic blood pressure** diastolischer Blutdruck *m*

DC = **diagnostic centre** Diagnosezentrum *n* / = **direct current** Gleichstrom *m*

DD = **differential diagnosis** Differenzialdiagnose *f*

Dd = **small detail response** Kleindetailantwort *f*

dd = **tiny–detail response** Kleinstdetailantwort *f*

D.D.A. = **Dangerous Drugs Act** Betäubungsmittelgesetz *n*

Dds = **response for which the stimulus is a minor white space** Kleinzwischenfigurdeutung *f*

DdW = **small detail — whole response** Kleindetail–Ganzantwort *f*

de = **edge detail** Randdeutung *f*, Randdetail *n*

del = **delusion** Wahn *m*

df = **degrees of freedom** Freiheitsgrade *mpl*

DHE = **dihydroergotamine** Dihydroergotamin *n*

DHEA = **dehydroepiandrosterone** Dehydroepiandrosteron *n*

DI = **increment of intensity** Intensitätsanstieg *m*, Zunahme *f* der Reizstärke

di = **inside detail** Innendetail *n*

diff = **difference** Unterschied *m*, Differenz *f*

DIMS = **disorders of initiating or maintaining sleep** Einschlaf– und Durchschlafstörungen *fpl*, EDS

dist. = **distal** distal / = **distance** Entfernung *f* / = **distribution** Verteilung *f*

DL, dl = **difference limen** Unterschiedsschwelle *f*, Differenzlimen *n*

DMT = **dimensional motion time** System *n* vorbestimmter Bewegungszeiten

DNA = **desoxyribonucleic acid** Desoxyribonukleinsäure *f* / = **did not arrive** nicht erschienen

DNS = **domain name system** System *n* zur Umwandlung von Domain–Namen in IP–Adressen

Do = **oligophrenic detail** oligophrenes Kleindetail *n*

DOB = **date of birth** Geburtsdatum *n*

DOES = **disorders of excessive somnolence** Störungen *fpl* mit exzessiver Schläfrigkeit

DOT = **Dictionary of Occupational Titles** Wörterbuch *n* der Berufsbezeichnungen

DPH = **differential–probability hypothesis** Premack–Prinzip *n*, Hypothese *f* der differentiellen Auftretenswahrscheinlichkeit

D.P.M. = **Diploma in Psychological Medicine** Diplom *n* in Psychotherapie

DQ = **deterioration quotient** Degenerationsquotient *m*, Degenerationsindex *m* / = **developmental quotient** Entwicklungsquotient *m*

DR = increment of response Reaktionszunahme *f*

dr = rare detail außergewöhnliches Detail *n*, Kleindetailantwort *f* / **= dorsal root** hintere Wurzel *f*

DRAM = dynamic random access memory dynamischer Direktzugriffsspeicher *m*

DRH = differential reinforcement of high rates differentielle Verstärkung *f* großer Häufigkeit

DRL = differential reinforcement of low rates differentielle Verstärkung *f* geringer Häufigkeit

DRNA = desoxyribose nucleic acid Desoxyribonukleinsäure *f* [DNS]

DRO = differential reinforcement of other behaviour differentielle Verstärkung *f* anderen Verhaltens

DRQ = discomfort–relief quotient Unzufriedenheits–Zufriedenheitsquotient *m*

DrS = rare white space detail Kleinzwischenfigurdeutung *f*

Ds = white space detail Zwischenfigurdeutung *f*

DSCT = dorsal spinocerebellar tract dorsaler Rückenmarkskanal *m*

DSUH = direct suggestion under hypnosis Direktsuggestion *f* unter Hypnose

DSM = Diagnostic and Statistical Manual of Mental Disorders (I, II, III, III–R, IV) Diagnostisches und Statistisches Manual Psychischer Störungen

DT = distance test Entfernungswahrnehmungstest *m*

d.t's = delirium tremens Alkoholdelir *n*, Delirium *n*

DV = dependent variable abhängige Variable *f*

D.V., d.v. = double vibration Vibrationszyklus *m*

DW = confabulated whole response konfabulatorische Ganzantwort *f*

Dws = white space detail Zwischenfigurdeutung *f*

DZ = dizygotic zweieiig, dizygotisch

DZA = set of dizygotic twins raised apart getrennt aufgewachsene zweieiige Zwillinge *pl*

E = energie Energie *f* / **= environment** Umwelt *f*, Umfeld *n* / **= probable error** wahrscheinlicher Fehler *m* / **= error variance** Fehlervarianz *f*, Fehlerstreuung *f* / **= excitatory tendency** Erregungstendenz *f* / **= experimenter** Experimentator *m*, Versuchsleiter *m* / **= experimental group** Versuchsgruppe *f*, Experimentalgruppe *f*

e = error Fehler *m*

EA, E.A. = educational age Lernalter *n*

EB = experience balance Erlebnistypus *m*

EBS = electrical brain stimulation elektrische Gehirnstimulation *f*

E/C = experiment and control Experiment *n* und Kontrolle *f*

ECC = electrocorticogram Elektrokortikogramm *n*/ **= elementary cognitive characteristics** elementare kognitive Merkmale *npl*, Bedeutungselemente *npl*

ecco = episodic communication channels in organisation ereignisbezogene Kommunikationskanäle *mpl* in einer Organisation

ECG = electrocardiogram Elektrokardiogramm *n* [EKG] / **= electrocorticogram** Elektrokortikogramm *n*

ECoG = electrocorticogram Elektrokortikogramm *n*

ECS = electroconvulsive shock Elektroschock *m* in der Krampftherapie

ECT = electroconvulsive therapy Elektrokrampftherapie *f*, Schocktherapie *f*

Ed.B. = Bachelor of Education *etwa:* Diplom–Pädagoge *m*

Ed.D. = Doctor of Education Doktor *m* der Erziehungswissenschaften

EDP = electronic data processing elektronische Datenverarbeitung *f* [EDV]

EDR = electrodermal response galvanischer Hautreflex *m*, galvanische Hautreaktion *f*, psychogalvanischer Reflex *m*

EEG, E.E.G. = electroencephalogram Elektroenzephalogramm *n*, [E.E.G.]

EFF = efficiency Leistung *f*, Effizienz *f*

eff = effects Wirkungen *fpl* / **= efferent** efferent

E group = experimental group Versuchsgruppe *f*

EGRUL = e.g. rule Beispiel–Regel–Methode *f*

E & H = environment and heridity Umwelt *f* und Vererbung *f*

Em = emmetropia Normalsichtigkeit *f*, Emmetropie *f*

emf = electromotive force elektromotorische Kraft *f*

EMG = electromyogram Elektromyogramm *n* / **= electromyography** Elektromyographie *f*

E of M = error of measurement Messfehler *m*

EOG = electrooculogram Elektrookulogramm *n*

EP = evoked potential evoziertes Potenzial *n*, Reizpotenzial *n*, Raktionspotenzial *n*

e.p.p. = end–plate potential Endplattenpotenzial *n*

EPSP = excitatory postsynaptic potential postsynaptisches Erregungspotenzial *n*

EQ, E.Q. = educational quotient Erziehungsquotient *m*, Lernquotient *m* / **= efficiency quotient** Effizienzquotient *m*, Leistungsquotient *m*

eq = equation Gleichung *f* / **= equivalent** Äquivalent *n*

ERG = electroretinogram Elektroretinogramm *n*

ERP = event–related potential ereigniskorreliertes Potenzial *n*

ESB = electrical stimulation of the brain elektrische Hirnreizung *f*

ESP = extrasensory perception außersinnliche Wahrnehmung *f*

ESR = erythrocyte sedimentation rate Blutkörperchensenkungsgeschwindigkeit *f*

EST = electroshock therapy Elektroschocktherapie *f*, Schocktherapie *f*

ETS = Educational Testing Service schulpsychologischer Testdienst *m*

Exp. = experience–type, experience balance Erlebnistyp *m*

exp = experiment Experiment *n*, Versuch *m* / **= experimental** experimentell, Versuchs–

F = face value Scheinwert *m* / **= Fahrenheit** Fahrenheit / **= female** weiblich / **= *F* factor** *F*–Faktor *m* / **= field of vision** Gesichtsfeld *n* / **= luminous flux** Lichtfluss *m* / **= form response** Formantwort *f* / **= force** Kraft *f* / **= the sum of frequencies of all classes below this class** Häufigkeitssumme *f* aller niederen Klassen / **= *F* test** *F* Test *m*

f = fluency factor Faktor *m* „Wortflüssigkeit" / **= focal** fokal, Herd– / **= frequency** Häufigkeit *f*, Frequenz *f* / **= function** Funktion *f*

F_1, F_2 = first and second filial generations erste und zweite Tochtergeneration *f*

F+ = sharp form scharfe Form *f*

F– = poor form unscharfe Form *f*

$F-_{indef.}$ = indefinite form unbestimmte Form *f*

f.a.g.r. = fractional antedating goal response teilweise antizipatorische Zielreaktion *f*

FAQ = frequently asked questions häufig gestellte Fragen *fpl*

FAS = fetal alcohol syndrome Alkoholembryopathiesyndrom *n*

FAT = file allocation table Dateizuordnungstabelle *f*

FBPsS = Fellow of the British Psychological Society Mitglied *n* der britischen Gesellschaft für Psychologie

FC = form–colour response Formfarbantwort *f*

F(C) = chiaroscuro response Helldunkeldeutung *f* / **= shading response** Schattierungsdeutung *f*

Fc = shading response Fc = Schattierungsdeutung F(Fb) *f*

fc = foot–candle Lumen *n* [Lm]

FCh = form–chiaroscuro response Form–Helldunkeldeutung *f*

FCP = final common path gemeinsame Endstrecke *f*

FFF = flicker fusion frequency Flimmerverschmelzungsfrequenz *f*

F–G = figure–ground Figur *f*–Grund *m*

FH = family history Familienanamnese *f*

FI = fixed interval gleiche Zeitspanne *f* / **= fixed interval schedule** feste Intervallverstärkung *f*

Fig. = figure Abbildung *f*

FINAPRES = finger arterial pressure Fingerarteriendruck *m*

FK = vista response perspektivische Schattierungsdeutung *f*

flybar = flying by auditory reference Fliegen *n* nach akustischen Anweisungen

FM = animal movement Tierbewegung BF *f*

FORTRAN = formula translation (spezielle Formelübersetzung *f*), FORTRAN *n*, Programmiersprache FORTRAN *f*

fpm = feet per minute Fuss *m* pro Minute

fps = feet per second Fuss *m* pro Sekunde

FR = fixed ratio in gleichem Verhältnis, in gleichem Abstand / **= fixed ratio schedule** feste Quotenverstärkung *f*

F–scale = Fascism scale Faschismus–Skala *f*

FSH = follicle stimulating hormone follikelstimulierendes Hormon *n*

ftL = foot Lambert Foot–Lambert *m*

FTP = file transfer protocol Dateitransferprotokoll *n*

FV = vista response Schattierungsdeutung *f*

FY = shading response Schattierungsdeutung *f*

FYI = for your information zu Ihrer Information

G = gain in rank Rangplatzverbesserung *f* / **= Gauss** Gauss / **= general factor** G–Faktor *m*, allgemeiner Faktor *m* / **= goal** Ziel / **= goal object** Zielobjekt *n* / **= gravity** Schwere *f*, Schwerkraft *f*, Gewicht *n*

g = general factor G–Faktor *m*, gemeinsamer Faktor *m* / **= fractional part of a goal reaction** Bruchteil *m* einer Zielreaktion / **= gramme(s), gram(s)** Gramm *n,npl* / **= mean difference** mittlere Differenz *f*

GA = guessed average vermuteter Durchschnitt *m*

GABA = gamma–amino–butyric acid Gamma–Aminobuttersäure *f*

GAF = Global Assessment of Functioning Scale Skala *f* zur globalen Erfassung des Funktionsniveaus

GAS = general adaptation syndrome allgemeines Adaptationssyndrom *n*

Ger = geriatrics Geriatrie *f* / **= german** deutsch

GFR = glomerular filtration rate glomeruläre Filtrationsrate *f*

GG = goal gradient Zielgradient *m*

GH = growth hormone Wachstumshormon *n*, Somatotropin *n*

GHIH = growth hormone inhibiting hormone Somatostatin *n*

GHRH = growth hormone releasing hormone Somatoliberin *n*, Somatotropin–releasing–Faktor *m*

GI = gastro–intestinal gastrointestinal

GIF = graphics interchange format Grafikdateiformat *n*

gir–l = German Internet Research List Deutsche Internet Forschungsliste *f*

GM = grand mal großer epileptischer Anfall *m*

G.O. = goal–orientation index Quotient *m* der Zielorientierung

GP = generator potential Generatorpotenzial *n*

gp = general paralysis Dementia paralytica *f* / **= group** Gruppe *f*

GPA = grade–point average Durchschnitt *m* der erzielten Klassennoten

GPI = general paralysis of the insane progressive Paralyse *f*

GpTh = group therapy Gruppentherapie *f*

GSR = galvanic skin response galvanische Hautreaktion *f*, psychogalvanische Reaktion *f*, galvanischer Hautreflex *m*

GTH = gonadotrophic hormone Wachstumshormon *n*

GVW = green–violet–white grün–violett–weiß

H = entropy Entropie *f* / **= harmonic mean** harmonisches Mittel *n* / **= heredity** Vererbung *f* / **= human figure** menschliche Ganzfigur *f* / **= hypermetropia** Hypermetropie *f*

h = height Höhe *f*, Größe *f* / **= hours** Stunden *fpl* / **= index of precision** Genauigkeitsindex *m*

H.C. = hypothetical construct hypothetisches Konstrukt *n*

HD = hearing distance Hörweite *f*

Hd = human detail menschliche Teilfigur *f*

H & E = heredity and environment Vererbung *f* und Umwelt *f*

HGH = human growth hormone Wachstumshormon *n*

HH = hard of hearing schwerhörig

HID = headache, insomnia, depression Kopfschmerzen *mpl*, Schlaflosigkeit *f*, Depression *f*

HIV = human immunodeficiency virus AIDS–Virus *n*

HMG = human menopausal gonadotropin Menopausengonadotropin *n*

HNC = hypothalamic neurohypophyseal complex Hypophysenzwischenhirnsystem *n*

HR = heart rate Herzfrequenz *f*

HS = hours of sleep Stunden *fpl* Schlaf

HT = hypermetropia Hypermetropie *f*

HTML = Hypertext Markup Language Befehlssprache *f* zur Umsetzung von Graphiken in Textdateien

HTML–Editor = HTML–Editor Programm *n* zur Erstellung von WWW–Seiten

HTTP = Hypertext Transfer Protocol Verfahren *n* zur Datenübertragung im WWW.

ht = height Höhe *f*, Größe *f*

Hy = hypermetropia Hypermetropie *f*

hys = hysteria Hysterie *f* / **= hysterical** hysterisch

Hz = hertz Hertz *n*

I = index Index *m*, Kennziffer *f*, Inhaltsverzeichnis *n* / **= induction** Induktion *f* / **= inhibition** Hemmung *f* / **= inhibitor** Hemmer *m* / **= luminous intensity** Lichtstärke *f*

i = imaginary quantity imaginäre Zahl *f* / **= interval** Intervall *n*

IAFI = infantile amaurotic familial idiocy infantile amaurotische familiäre Idiotie *f*

IC = immediate constituent unmittelbares Konstituent *n* / **= immune complex** Antigen–Antikörperkomplex *m*

ICD = International Classification of Diseases internationale Klassifikation *f* von Krankheiten

ICP = infantile cerebral palsy infantile Zerebralparese *f*

ICS = impulse conducting system Reizleitungssystem *n* / **= intracranial stimulation** Hirnreizung *f*

ICSH = interstitial cell–stimulating hormone Gelbkörperreifungshormon *n*

ICT = insulin coma therapy Insulinkomabehandlung *f* / **= intracranial stimulation** elektrische Hirnreizung *f*

ICW = Institute of Child Welfare Institut *n* für Kinderfürsorge

I/E = (rate of) inspiration divided by (rate of) expiration Quotient *m* von Einatmung zu Ausatmung

I.E. = introversion–extraversion Introversion *f* –Extraversion *f*

IER = Institute of Educational Research Institut *n* für Erziehungsforschung

IF = intrinsic factor intrinsic factor *m*

IFD = idealism, frustration, demoralization Idealismus *m*, Frustration *f*, Enttäuschung *f*

Ind = individual response Individualantwort *f*

ind. = individual einzeln, individuell, persönlich

inf = infant Kleinkind *n*, Säugling *m* / **= infantile** infantil, Kleinkind– / **= infected** infiziert / **= infection** Infektion *f*

inf. = inferior untergeordnet, geringer, minderwertig, untere(r,s) / **= infinity** Unendlichkeit *f*, unendliche Menge *f*

invgt. = investigation Untersuchung *f*, Forschung *f*, Erforschung *f*

IO = intraocular intraokulär

IP = Internet Protocol Internetprotokoll *n*

IPPF = International Planned Parenthood Federation Internationale Vereinigung *f* für bewusste Elternschaft

IPSA = index of problem–solving ability Index *m* der Problemlösefähigkeit

IPSP = inhibitory postsynaptic potential hemmendes postsynaptisches Potenzial *n*

IPT = information processing theory Informationstheorie *f*

IQ = intelligence quotient Intelligenzquotient *m*

IR = infra–red infrarot / **= internal resistance** innerer Widerstand *m*

I_R = reactive inhibition reaktive Hemmung *f*

IRC = Internet Relay Chat Realtime–Internet–Diskussionsforum *n*

IRI = interresponse interval Intervall *n* zwischen zwei Reaktionen

IRM = innate release mechanism angeborener Auslösemechanismus *m*

IRT = interresponse time Intervall *n* zwischen den Reaktionen, Interreaktionszeit *f*

IS = initial segment Anfangssegment *n*

ISDN = integrated services digital network digitales Telekommunikationsnetz *n* der Telekom

ISI = interstimulus interval Interstimulusintervall *n*, reizfreies Intervall *n*

IST = insulin shock therapy Insulinschocktherapie *f*

IS–TDP = intensive short–term dynamic psychotherapy intensive psychodynamische Kurztherapie *f*

I/T = intensity/duration Intensität *f* / Dauer *f*

ITA = initial teaching alphabet Unterrichtsalphabet *n* für Anfänger

IU = interval of uncertainty Unsicherheitsbereich *m*

IUD = intra–uterine device Intrauterinpessar *n*

IUPS = International Union of Psychological Science Internationale Vereinigung *f* für Psychologie

I.V. = independent variable unabhängige Variable *f* / **= intervening variable** intervenierende Variable *f*

J = joule Joule *n* / **= delay in reinforcement** Verzögerung *f* der Verstärkung

j = number of standard deviations Zahl *f* der Standardabweichungen (vom Mittelwert gemessen)

JAI = juvenile amaurotic idiocy juvenile amaurotische Idiotie *f*

jnd, JND = just noticeable difference eben merklicher Unterschied *m*, Unterschiedsschwelle *f*

jnnd = just not–noticeable difference gerade noch nicht wahrnehmbarer Unterschied *m*

JPEG = joint photographic experts group Grafikformat *n* mit hoher Bildkompression

K = diffusion response Schattierungsdeutung *f* / **= incentive** Anreiz *m* / **= motivation** Motivation *f* / **= Kelvin** Kelvin / **= kinaesthetic response** Bewegungsantwort *f*

k = coefficient of alienation Alienationskoeffizient *m* / **= diffusion response** Schattierungsdeutung *f*

k' = physical incentive physischer Anreiz *m*

kg = kilogram Kilogramm *n*

kj = knee–jerk Patellarreflex *m*, Kniesehnenreflex *m*

KPR = Kuder preference record Kuder–Interessenfragebogen *m*

KR = knowledge of result Kenntnis *f* des Erfolgs

Ku = kurtosis Kurtosis *f*, Exzess *m*

L = lambda index Lambda–Index *m* / **= Lambert** Lambert *n* / **= life** Leben *n* / **= light** Licht *n* / **= light sense** Gesichtssinn *m* / **= number of like signs** Anzahl *f* gleicher Zeichen / **= limen** Schwelle *f* / **= lumen** Lumen *n*

l = left links / **= longitudinal** Längsschnitt– / **= lower limit of a class** Klassenuntergrenze *f*

$_{s}L_{R}$ = reaction threshold Reaktionsschwelle *f*

lab = laboratory Versuchsraum *m*, Experimentierraum *m*, Laboratorium *n*, Labor *n*

LAD = language acquisition device Spracherwerbsmechanismus *m*

LAN = local area network lokales Netzwerk *n*

LBH = length, breadth, heigth Länge *f*, Breite *f*, Höhe *f*

L.C. = locus of control Ort *m* der Steuerung

LCM = lowest common multiple kleinstes, gemeinsames Vielfache *n*

LD = learning disability Lernbehinderung *f*, Lernunvermögen *n*

LDG = leaderless discussion group führerlose Diskussionsgruppe *f*, Diskussionsgruppe *f* ohne Leiter

LGB = lateral geniculate body Corpus geniculatim laterale *n*

LGD = leaderless group discussion Gruppendiskussion *f* ohne Leiter

LH = luteinising hormone luteinisierendes Hormon *n*

L–I–D = like, indifferent, dislike ja–unentschieden–nein, stimme zu–unentschieden–stimme nicht zu

lim = limit Grenze *f*

LIV = law of initial values Ausgangswertgesetz *n*

lm = lumen Lumen *n*

log = logarithm Logarithmus *m*

LP = latent period Latenzzeit *f* / **= light perception** Lichtwahrnehmung *f* / **= lumbar puncture** Lumbalpunktion *f*

LPC = least preferred coworker am wenigsten beliebter Mitarbeiter *m*

LQ = lowest quartile unterstes Quartil *n*, erstes Quartil *n*

LS = liminal sensitivity Schwellenempfindlichkeit *f*

LSD = lysergic acid diethylamide Lysergsäurediäthylamid *n*, LSD *n*

LSp = life space Lebensraum *m* / **= life span** Lebensspanne *f*

ltd. = limited begrenzt

LTM = long term memory Langzeitgedächtnis *n*

M = illumination Beleuchtung *f* / **= male** männlich / **= learning maximum** Lernmaximum *n* / **= arithmetic mean** arithmetisches Mittel *n* / **= mediator** Vermittler *m* / **= associative memory factor** assoziativer Gedächtnisfaktor *m* / **= motor neurone** Motoneuron *n* / **= movement response** Bewegungsantwort *f* / **= myopia** Kurzsichtigkeit *f*, Myopie *f*

m = meaningfulness Bedeutungshaltigkeit *f* / **= meter** Meter *m* / **= minute** Minute *f* / **= small movement response** bewegte Naturgebilde *npl* und Objekte *npl* / **= any number** jede Zahl *f*

M^1 = arbitrary origin willkürlich festgelegter Nullpunkt *m*

M_{AB} = observed frequency in cell at intersection of row A and column B beobachtete Gruppenhäufigkeit *f* am Schnittpunkt von Reihe A und Spalte B

M_G = geometric mean geometrisches Mittel *n*

MA/M.A. = mental age Intelligenzalter *n*

MAC = maximum acceptable concentration höchstzulässige Konzentration *f*

MAF = minimum audible field untere Hörschwelle *f*

MANCOVA = multivariate analysis of covariance multivariate Kovarianzanalyse *f*

MANOVA = multivariate analysis of variance multivariate Varianzanalyse *f*

MAO = monoamine oxydase Monoaminooxydase *f*

MAOI = monoamine oxydase inhibitor Monoaminooxydase–Hemmer *m*, MAO–Hemmer *m*

MAP = minimum audible pressure untere Hörschwelle *f*

MBD = minimal brain dysfunction in children frühkindliches exogenes Psychosyndrom *n*

M–C = multiple choice Mehrfachwahl–, Multiple choice

MCQ = multiple choice question Multiple–choice Frage *f*

MD = mental deficiency geistige Zurückgebliebenheit *f*

Md = median Median *m*

md = manic–depressive manisch–depressiv / **= mean deviation** mittlere Abweichung *f* / **= median** Median *m* / **= mentally deficient** geistig zurückgeblieben

MdD = median deviation Medianabweichung *f*

Mdn = median Median *m*

med = median mittlere (r, s), Median– / **= medical** ärztlich, medizinisch / **= medicine** Medizin *f* / **= medium** Medium *n*

MEG = magnetoencephalography Magnetoenzephalographie *f*

MEP = motor end–plate motorische Endplatte *f*

m.e.p.p. = miniature end–plate potential Miniatur–Endplattenpotenzial *n*

M–F = masculinity–femininity Männlichkeits–Weiblichkeits–, Maskulinität *f* — Femininität *f*

MG = maximum growth größtes Wachstum *n*, Größenwachstum *n*

mg = milligramme Milligramm *n*, Tausendstel Gramm *n*

MH = menstrual history früherer Menstruationsverlauf *m* / **= mental health** geistige Gesundheit *f*

MIME = multipurpose internet mail extension Kodierverfahren *n* für Internetdateien

MJ = marihuana Marihuana *n*, Haschisch *m*

ml = millilambert Millilambert *n*

mm. = millimeter Millimeter *m*

mμ = millimicron Millimikron *n*

Mo = mode Modalwert *m*, Modus *m*

mo = month(s) Monat *m*, Monate *mpl*

MPEG = motion picture experts group Standard *m* zur Speicherung von digitalisierten bewegten Bildern

MPS = movement producing stimulus Bewegungsreiz *m*

MPTP = methylphenyltetrahydropyridine Methylphenyltetrahydropyridin *n*

MR = mentally retarded geistig zurückgeblieben / **= metabolic rate** Grundumsatz *m*

MRI = **magnetic resonance imaging** Magnetresonanztomographie *f*, Kernspinresonanztomographie *f*

mRNA = **messenger RNA** Boten–RNA *f*

M.S. = **Master of Science** *(Titel nach College-Graduierung)*/ = **multiple sclerosis** multiple Sklerose *f* / = **muscle strength** Muskelkraft *f*

ms., msec. = **millisecond** Millisekunde *f*, tausendstel Sekunde *f*

M.Sc. = **Master of Science** *(Titel nach College-Graduierung)*

MSUD = **maple syrup urine disease** Ahornsirup–Krankheit *f*

MTM = **methods–time measurement** Methoden–Zeitmessung *f*

MU = **mental units** Einheiten *fpl* des Intelligenzwachstums

MUD = **multi–user dungeon** textbasierende Rollenspiele *npl* und Simulationen im Internet

MV = **mean variation** mittlere Abweichung *f*

mv = **millivolt** Millivolt *n*, tausendstel Volt *n*

μ = **micron** Mikron *n*, Tausendstelmillimeter *n*

μg = **microgramme** Mikrogramm *n*, Millionstel Gramm *n*

μv = **microvolt** Mikrovolt *n*, millionstel Volt *n*

mz = **monozygotic** eineiig, monozygotisch

MZA = **monozygotic twins reared apart** getrennt aufgewachsene eineiige Zwillinge *pl*

MZT = **monozygotic twins reared together** zusammen aufgewachsene eineiige Zwillinge *pl*

N = **need** Bedürfnis *n* / = **nerve** Nerv *m* / = **neurology** Neurologie *f* / = **noise** Rauschen *n* / = **number factor** Rechenfaktor *m* / = **number of instances in a total population** Zahl *f* der Fälle in einer Grundgesamtheit / = **number of reinforcements** Zahl *f* der Verstärkungen

n = **index of refraction** Brechungsindex *m* / = **need** Bedürfnis *n* / = **nerve** Nerv *m* / = **number of items in a part of a total group** Zahl *f* der Fälle in einer Teilgruppe / = **number of unreinforced elicitations of a response required to produce extinction** Zahl *f* der bis zur Auslöschung einer Reaktion erforderlichen unverstärkten Antworten / = **number of variables** Zahl *f* der Variablen

N' = **number of cases in a second group** Zahl *f* der Fälle in einer zweiten Gruppe

N I = **first nerve** erster Hirnnerv *m*, Riechnerven *mpl*, Olfaktorius *m*

N II = **second nerve** zweiter Hirnnerv *m*, Sehnerv *m*, Optikus *m*

N III = **third nerve** dritter Hirnnerv *m*, Okulomotorius *m*

N IV = **fourth nerve** vierter Hirnnerv *m*, Trochlearis *m*

N V = **fifth nerve** fünfter Hirnnerv *m*, Trigeminus *m*

N VI = **sixth nerve** sechster Hirnnerv *m*, Abduzens *m*

N VII = **seventh nerve** siebter Hirnnerv *m*, Gesichtsnerv *m*, Fazialis *m*

N VIII = **eighth nerve** achter Hirnnerv *m*, Hörnerv *m*, Nervus statoacusticus *m*

N IX = **ninth nerve** neunter Hirnnerv *m*, Zungenschlundnerv *m*, Glossopharyngeus *m*

N X = **tenth nerve** zehnter Hirnnerv *m*, Vagus *m*

N XI = **eleventh nerve** elfter Hirnnerv *m*, Beinerv *m*, Nervus accessorius *m*

N XII = **twelfth nerve** zwölfter Hirnnerv *m*, Nervus hypoglossus *m*

nAch = **need for achievement** Leistungsbedürfnis *n*, Leistungsmotiv *n*

NAD = **no appreciable disease** ohne Befund / = **nothing abnormal detected** ohne Befund

NB = **newborn** neugeboren / Neugeborenes *n*

NC = **no change** keine Veränderung *f*

NE = nerve excitability Nervenerregbarkeit *f* / **= norepinephrine** Noradrenalin *n*, Norepinephrin *n*

NGF = nerve growth factor Nervenwachstumsfaktor *m*

NM = neuromuscular neuromuskulär

NMDA = N–methyl–D–aspartate N–Methyl–D–Aspartat *n*

NMS = neuroleptic malignant syndrome malignes neuroleptisches Syndrom *n*

Nn = nerves Nerven *mpl*

NNTP = network news transfer protocol Datenübertragungsverfahren *n* für Artikel in den Newsgroups

NOS = not otherwise specified nicht näher bezeichnet

NP = near point Nahpunkt *m* / **= neuropsychiatric** neuropsychiatrisch / **= neuropsychiatry** Neuropsychiatrie *f*

NRC = normal retinal correspondence korrespondierende Netzhautpunkte *mpl*

NREM = nonrapid eye movement langsame Augenbewegung *f*

NS = nervous system Nervensystem *n* / **= neurosurgery** Neurochirurgie *f*

n.s. = nervous system Nervensystem *n*

NSFNET = National Science Foundation Network Hochgeschwindigkeitsdatennetz *n* der NSF in USA

O = observer Beobachter *m* / **= old** alt / **= organism** Organismus *m* / **= original response** Originalantwort *f* / **= oscillation** Schwankung *f* Schwingung *f*, Oszillation *f* / **= the other** der Andere *m*

OA = old age Alters– / Greisenalter *n*

OccTh = occupational therapy Arbeitstherapie *f*, Beschäftigungstherapie *f*

OCD = obsessive–compulsive disorder Zwangsstörung *f*, Zwangssyndrom *n*

OCR = optical character recognition maschinell lesbare Schreibmaschinenschrift *f*

OD = organization development Organisationsentwicklung *f*

OR = orientation response Orientierungsreflex *m*

Orig. = original response Originalantwort *f*

OT = objective test objektiver Test *m* / **= occupational therapist** Beschäftigungstherapeut *m* / **= occupational therapy** Beschäftigungstherapie *f*

P = percentile Perzentil *n* / **= percept** Wahrnehmung *f*, Wahrnehmungsinhalt *m* / **= perceptual speed** Auffassungsgeschwindigkeit *f* / **= person** Person *f* / **= personality organisation** Persönlichkeitsorganisation *f* / **= physiological drive state** physiologischer Triebzustand *m* / **= popular response** Vulgärantwort *f* / **= population** Bevölkerung *f* / **= positive** positiv / **= preference score** Vorzugswert *m*, Score *m* aller Bevorzugungen / **= probability** Wahrscheinlichkeit *f* / **= probability ratio** Wahrscheinlichkeitsquotient *m*, Wahrscheinlichkeit *f* / **= psychiatry** Psychatrie *f* / **= P technique** P–Technik *f*

p = difficulty of a test item Schwierigkeit *f* eines Testitem / **= percentage of cases** Fallprozent *n* / **= percentile** Perzentil *n* / **= probability** Wahrscheinlichkeit *f* / **= proportion of a population possessing a given characteristic** Teil *m* einer Population mit einem gegebenen Merkmal

P_1 = first parental generation erste Elterngeneration *f*

PA = paired–associate paarweise / **= psychoanalyst** Psychoanalytiker *m*

PAL = paired associate learning paarweises Assoziieren *n*

PASAR = Psychological Abstracts Search and Retrieval maschinelles Literatursuchsystem *n* das auf den „Psychological Abstracts“ basiert

P.B. = phonetically balanced phonetisch gleichgewichtig

Pb = presbyopia Alterssichtigkeit *f*

PC = personal constant persönliche Konstante *f*

pcpt = perception Wahrnehmung *f*

Pcs. = preconscious vorbewusst / Vorbewusstes *n*

PD = prisoner–dilemma game Häftlingsdilemmaspiel *n*

PE, P.E., p.e. = probable error wahrscheinlicher Fehler *m*

PEC = politicoeconomic conservatism politisch–ökonomischer Konservatismus *m*

PEG = pneumoencephalogram Pneumenzephalogramm *n* / **= pneumoencephalography** Pneumenzephalographie *f*

p.f. = phenomenal field phänomenales Feld *n*

PGP = pretty good privacy Verschlüsselungsprogramm *n* für Nachrichten und E–Mails

PGR = psychogalvanic response psychogalvanische Reaktion *f*, galvanischer Hautreflex *m*

pH = potential of hydrogen Wasserstoffionenkonzentration *f* [pH]

Ph.D. = Doctor of Philosophy Dr.phil.

PHR = point–hour ratio Durchschnitt *m* der erzielten Klassennoten

PI = proactive inhibition proaktive Hemmung *f*

PIF = prolactin inhibiting factor Prolaktin–Inhibiting–Faktor *m*

PIH = prolactin inhibiting hormone Prolaktin–Inhibiting–Hormon *n*

PIQ = performance intelligence quotient Intelligenzquotient *m* basierend auf Leistungstestwerten

PK = psychokinesis Psychokinese *f*

PKU = phenylketonuria Phenylketonurie *f*

PL = perception of light Lichtempfindung *f* / **= probability learning** Wahrscheinlichkeitslernen *n*

PM = petit mal leichter epileptischer Anfall *m*, Petit mal *m*

PMA = primary mental abilities geistige Primärfähigkeiten *fpl*, Primärfaktoren *mpl* der Intelligenz, geistige Grundfähigkeiten *fpl*

PMS = premenstrual syndrome prämenstruelles Syndrom *n*

PN = peripheral nerve peripherer Nerv *m* / **= psychiatry–neurology** Psychiatrie *f* Neurologie *f* / **= psychoneurosis** Psychoneurose *f* / **= psychoneurotic individual** Psychoneurotiker *m*

p–n = press–need Umweltsituation *f* — Bedürfnis *n*

PNAvQ = positive–negative ambivalent quotient positiv–negativer, ambivalenter Quotient *m*

PNS = parasympathetic nervous system parasympathisches Nervensystem *n* / **= peripheral nervous system** peripheres Nervensystem *n*

Po = position response Lageantwort *f*

PoP = point of presence regionaler Einwählknoten *m* eines Service–Providers

POP = post office protocol Verfahren *n* zur Übertragung von E–Mails

PPP = point–to–point protocol Punkt–zu–Punkt–Protokoll *n*

PR = percentile rank Prozentrang *m* / **= public relation** Öffentlichkeitsarbeit *f*

PRE = partial reinforcement effect Partialverstärkungseffekt *m*

PRF = prolactin releasing factor Prolaktin–Releasing–Faktor *m*

PRH = prolactin releasing hormone Prolaktin–Releasing–Hormon *n*

PsAn = psychoanalysis Psychoanalyse *f* / **= psychoanalyst** Psychoanalytiker *m* / **= psychoanalytic** psychoanalytisch

PSE = point of subjective equality Punkt *m* subjektiver Gleichheit

PSP = postsynaptic potential postsynaptisches Potenzial *n*

Psy = psychiatry Psychiatrie *f* / **= psychology** Psychologie *f*

psychiat. = **psychiatric** psychiatrisch / = **psychiatry** Psychiatrie *f*

psychoan. = **psychoanalysis** Psychoanalyse *f*

PTA = **posttraumatic anmesia** posttraumatische Amnesie *f* / = **parent–school relationship** Eltern–Schule–Beziehung *f*

PTH = **parathormone** Nebenschilddrüsenhormon *n*

PTS = **permanent threshold shift** ständige Verschiebung *f* der Hörschwelle

PTSD = **posttraumatic stress disorder** posttraumatische Stressreaktion *f*, posttraumatische Belastungsstörung *f*

PX = **past history** Anamnese *f* / = **physical examination** körperliche Untersuchung *f* / = **prognosis** Prognose *f*

Q = **luminous energy** Leuchtkraft *f* / = **quantity** Menge *f* / = **quarter** Viertel *n* / = **quartile** Quartil *n* / = **quartile deviation** Quartilabweichung *f* / = **question** Frage *f* / = **questionary, questionnaire** Fragebogen *m* / = **quotient** Quotient *m*

Q_1 = **first quartile** erstes Quartil *n*

Q_2 = **second quartile** zweites Quartil *n*, Methan *m*

Q_3 = **third quartile** drittes Quartil *n*

q = **proportion of a sample which lacks a given characteristic** Teil *m* einer Stichprobe, welcher ein bestimmtes Merkmal nicht aufweist

R = **footrule correlation** Spearmans R–Korrelation *f* / = **multiple correlation coefficient** multipler Korrelationskoeffizient *m* / = **reaction** Reaktion *f* / = **reasoning** logisches Denken *n* / = **red** rot / = **stimulus** Reiz *m* / = **response** Reaktion *f* / = **total responses** Anzahl *f* der Deutungen / = **right** rechts

r = **correlation coefficient** Korrelationskoeffizient *m* / = **product–moment correlation** Produkt–Moment–Korrelation *f*, Pearson–Maßkorrelation *f* / = **pure–stimulus act** reiner Reizvorgang *m* / = **reliability coefficient** Reliabilitätskoeffizient *m*

R_G = **goal–attaining response** Zielreaktion *f*, konsumatorische Endhandlung *f*

R_p = **response probability** Reaktionswahrscheinlichkeit *f*

R_u = **unconditioned response** unkonditionierte Reaktion *f*

$R_{1.23...n}$ = **multiple correlation coefficient** multipler Korrelationskoeffizient *m*

r_{bis} = **biserial correlation coefficient** biserialer Korrelationskoeffizient *m*

r_G = **fractional antedating goal response** fraktionelle antizipatorische Zielreaktion *f*

r, r_{tet} = **tetrachoric correlation** tetrachorische Korrelation *f*

$r_{12.34....n}$ = **partial correlation** Teilkorrelation *f*

RAS = **reticular arousal system** retikuläres aktivierendes System *n* / = **renin–angiotensin system** Renin–Angiotensin–System *n*

RB = **reactional biography** Reaktionsbeschreibung *f*

Rc = **response conditioned** bedingte Reaktion *f*, bedingter Reflex *m*, konditionierte Reaktion *f*

R & D = **research and development** Forschung *f* und Entwicklung *f*

RdA = **reading age** Lesealter *n*

RDC = **research diagnostic criteria** diagnostische Forschungskriterien *npl*

RdQ = **reading quotient** Lesequotient *m*

REM = **rapid eye movement** schnelle Augenbewegung *f* / = **rolling eye movement** Augenrollen *n*

RET = **rational–emotive therapy** rational–emotive Therapie *f*

RF = **releasing factor** Neurosekret *n*

RFC = **request for comments** Bitte *f* um Stellungnahme

R_G = **fractional antedating goal response** fraktionelle antizipatorische Zielreaktion *f*

Rh = **rhesus** Rhesusaffe *m*, Rhesusfaktor *m*

ϱ (rho) = **rho coefficient of correlation** Rangkorrelationskoeffizient *m*, Spearman–Korrelationskoeffizient *m*

RI = **retroactive inhibition** retroaktive Hemmung *f*

RIASEC = **realistic, investigative, artistic, social, enterprising and conventional** realistisch, forschend, künstlerisch, sozial, unternehmenslustig und konventionell

RL = **Reiz–Limen** Reizschwelle *f*

RM = **releasing mechanism** Auslösemechanismus *m*

RMS = **root–mean square** mittlere Quadratwurzel *f*

RNA = **ribonucleic acid** Ribonukleinsäure *f* (RNS)

Ro = **original response** ursprüngliche Reaktion *f*, zuerst erfolgte Reaktion *f*

ROC = **receiver operating characteristic** Empfänger–Verhaltenscharakteristik *f*, Leistungsfunktion *f* des Empfängers

ROT13 = **rotate 13** Kodierverfahren *n*, bei dem alle Buchatben eines Textes um 13 Zeichen verschoben werden

RP = **readiness potential** Bereitschaftspotenzial n / = **Received Pronunciation** hochsprachliche Aussprache *f*

rpm = **revolutions per minute** Umdrehungen *fpl* pro Minute

rps = **revolutions per second** Umdrehungen *fpl* pro Sekunde

RQ = **recovery quotient** Erholungsquotient *m*

RS = **reinforcing stimulus** Verstärkerreiz *m*

R/S = **response/stimulus** Reaktion *f* / Reiz *m*

RT = **rational–emotive therapy** rational–emotive Therapie *f* / = **reaction time** Reaktionszeit *f* / = **reading–test** Leseprobe *f*

R_t, r_t = **tetrachoric correlation coefficient** tetrachorischer Korrelationskoeffizient *m*

RULEG = **rule–example–method** Regel–Beispiel–Methode *f*

S = **sensation** Gefühl *n* / = **sensitive** empfindlich / = **sensory intensity** Empfindungsstärke *f* / = **space detail** Zwischenfigur–Deutung *f* / = **space factor** Faktor *m* Raumvorstellung / = **white space response, space detail** Zwischenfigur–Deutung *f* / = **standard stimulus** Standardreiz *m* / = **stimulus** Reiz *m*, Stimulus *m* / = **subject** Versuchsperson *f*

s = **sacral** Kreuzbein–, sakral / = **second** Sekunde *f* / = **see** siehe / = **sensation** Gefühl *n* / = **special ability** Sonderbegabung *f*, spezifische Fähigkeit *f* / = **standard deviation** Standardabweichung *f* / = **perseverative stimulus trace** nachwirkende Reizspur *f* / = **variable stimulus** variabler Reiz *m*

s' = **stimulus trace** Reizspur *f*

S^D = **drive stimulus** Triebreiz *m*

S_G = **goal stimulus** propriozeptiver Zielreiz *m* / = **fractional goal stimulus** fraktioneller Zielreiz *m*

SAE = **standard average European** normales Durchschnitts–Europäisch *n*

SAD = **seasonal affective disorder** saisonale depressive Störung *f*

Sb = **strabismus** Schielen *n*, Strabismus *m*

Sc = **stimulus component** Reizkomponente *f*, Reizbestandteil *m* / = **conditioned stimulus** bedingter Reiz *m*, konditionierter Reiz *m*

SCL = **skin conductance level** Hautleitfähigkeitsniveau *n*

SCR = **skin conductance response** Hautleitfähigkeitsreaktion *f*

SD = **social desirability** soziale Erwünschtheit *f* / = **standard deviation** Standardabweichung *f*

SDD = **seasonal depressive disorder** saisonale depressive Störung *f*

SDT = **signal detection theory** Signalentdeckungstheorie *f*, Signaldetektionstheorie *f*

SE = **standard error** mittlerer Fehler *m* / = **exhibitory sympathin** Noradrenalin *n*

sec = second(s) Sekunde(*n*) *f*,*fpl*

$_SE_R$ = excitatory potential oder / **= reaction potential** Reaktionspotenzial *n*, Erregungspotenzial *n*

SES = socioeconomic status sozioökonomischer Status *m*

SEU = subjectively expected utility subjektive Nutzenerwartung *f*

$_SH_R$ = habit strength Gewohnheitsstärke *f*

S.I. = inhibitory sympathin Adrenalin *n*

Σ = summation Summe *f*, Summierung *f*

σ_t = sigma Standardabweichung *f*, Millisekunde *f*

σ_M = standard error of the mean Standardfehler *m* des arithmetischen Mittels

$\sigma_{(M)}$ = standard error of measurement Standardmessfehler *m*

σ^2 = variance Streuung *f*, Varianz

SIDS = sudden infant death syndrome plötzlicher Kindstod *m*, Krippentod *m*

SIMM = single inline memory module SIMM–Modul *n*

$_SI_R$ = conditioned inhibitory potential konditionierte Hemmung *f*

sjp = small nerve junctional potential lokales Aktionspotenzial *n* der Nerv–Muskelsynapse

sk = skewness Schiefe *f*, Asymmetrie *f*

SL = serial learning Reihenlernen *n*

$_SL_R$ = reaction threshold Reaktionsschwelle *f*

SMTP = simple mail transfer protocol Datenübertragungsverfahren *n* für E–Mails über eine TCP/IP–Verbindung

SN = signal plus noise Signal *n* vor einem Rauschhintergrund

SOA = stimulus–onset asynchrony Reizbeginnasynchronie *f*

S–O–R = stimulus–organism–response Reiz *m* –Organismus *m* –Reaktion *f*

$_SO_R$ = behavioural oscillation Verhaltensschwankung *f*, Wechsel *m* des Reaktionspotenzials

SP = summation potential Summationspotenzial *n*

Sp = space Raum *m* / **= specific** spezifisch / **= spinal** spinal

SPL = skin potential level Hautpotenzialniveau *n* / **= sound pressure level** Schalldruckniveau *n*

SPR = skin potential response Hautpotenzialreaktion *f* / **= Society for Psychical Research** Gesellschaft *f* für psychologische Forschung

SQ3R = survey, question, read, recite, review Überblick verschaffen, fragen, lesen, wiedergeben, überprüfen

S–R = stimulus–response Reiz *m* –Reaktion *f*

S → R = stimulus leads to reaction Reiz *m* ruft Reaktion *f* hervor

S ↔ R = stimulus–response interaction Interaktion *f* zwischen Reiz und Reaktion

SRA = Science Research Associates Wissenschaftliche Forschungsgemeinschaft *f*

SRAM = static random access memory statischer Direktzugriffsspeicher m, statischer RAM *m*

SRL = skin resistance level Hautwiderstandsniveau *n*

SRR = skin resistance response Hautwiderstandsreaktion *f*

SRS = a stimulus leading to a response that leads to another stimulus ein Reiz *m* der zu einer Reaktion führt, die wiederum einen Reiz auslöst

SS = standard score Standardwert *m*

S–S = stimulus–stimulus Reiz *m* –Reiz *m*

$_{SS}H_R$ = summation of the habit strength Summe *f* der Gewohnheitsstärken

SSRI = serotonin selective reuptake inhibitor selektiver Serotonin–Wiederaufnahmehemmer *m*

SST = stimulus sampling theory Theorie *f* der Reizstichproben

St. = stimulus Reiz *m*

stem = space time energy material Raum *m* –Zeit *f* –Energie *f* –Material *n*

STH = somatotropic hormone Wachstumshormon *n*, somatotropes Hormon *n*

stim = stimulus Reiz *m*

STM = short term memory Kurzzeitspeicher *m*, Kurzzeitgedächtnis *n*, unmittelbares Behalten *n*

$_ST_R$ = reaction latency Reaktionslatenz *f*, Reaktionszeit *f* / **= reaction time** Reaktionszeit *f*, Latenzzeit *f*

$_St_R$ = median reaction latency mittlere Latenzzeit *f*, mittlere Reaktionszeit *f*

SU = auditory sensation unit Einheit *f* der Gehörempfindung

Su = unconditioned stimulus unkonditionierter Reiz *m*, unbedingter Reiz *m*

Succ = type of succession Sukzession *f*

$_SU_R$ = unlearned stimulus–response connections ungelernte Reiz–Reaktions–Verbindungen *fpl*, latente, nicht erlernte Reiz–Reaktions–Verbindung *f* / **= unlearned stimulus–response potentiality** ungelerntes Reiz–Reaktionspotenzial *n*

T = temperature Temperatur *f* / **= tension** Spannung *f*, Druck *m* / **= total time** Gesamtzeit *f*, Gesamtdauer *f* / **= transition point** Überschreitungspunkt *m* / **= true** wahr, echt / **= T function** T–Funktion *f*

t = any case in a series Fall *m* in einer Serie / **= time lapse** Zeitverlauf *m*, Zeitdauer *f* / **= t–test** t–Test *m*

t_{AB} = theoretical cell frequency at intersection of Ath row and B^{th} column theoretische Gitterverteilung *f* am Schnittpunkt der A^{ten} Reihe und B^{ten} Spalte

tach = tachistoscope Tachistoskop *n*

TCP/IP = transmission control protocol/ internet protocol TCP/IP

TE = time error Zeitfehler m / **= trial–and error learning** Lernen *n* durch Versuch und Irrtum, Versuch–Irrtums–Lernen *n*

Telnet = teletype network Internetprotokoll *n* für Fernverbindungen über Terminals

TENS = transcutaneous electrical nerve stimulation transkutane elektrische Nervenstimulation *f*, TENS

TF = true–false richtig–falsch

TG = training group Trainingsgruppe *f*

TH = thyroid hormone Schilddrüsenhormon *n*

th = threshold Schwelle *f*

THC = tetrahydrocannabinol Tetrahydrocannabinol *n*

Θ_1, Θ_2 = Theta Theta

TLV = threshold limit value Schwellengrenzwert *m*

TM = transcendental meditation transzendentale Meditation *f*

TO = time–out Auslösch–, Belohnungsentzugs–

TOA = type of approach Erfassungstypus *m*

TOE = type of experience Erlebnistypus *m*

TOTE = test–operate–test–exit Vergleich *m* –Veränderung *f* –Vergleich *m* –Ausführung *f*, funktionelle Regulationseinheit *f*

TPMO = time–place–mode–object Zeit *f* –Ort *m* –Weise *f* –Objekt *n*

TR = temperature range Temperaturbereich *m*

tr = trace Spur *f* / **= treatment** Behandlung *f* / **= tremor** Tremor *m*, Zittern *n*

TRH = thyrotropin releasing hormone Thyrotropin–releasing–Hormon *n*

tRNA = transfer ribonucleic acid Transfer–Ribonukleinsäure *f*

TRT = treatment Behandlung *f*, Therapie *f*

TSD = theory of signal detectability Signalentdeckungstheorie *f*, Signaldetektionstheorie *f*

TSH = thyroid–stimulating hormone Thyreotropin *n*

TTH = thyreotrophic hormone Thyreotropin *n*

TTR = type–token–ratio Diversifikationsquotient *m*

TTS = temporary threshold shift vorübergehende Schwellenabwanderung *f*

TTX = tetrododoxin Tetrododoxin *n*

TU = transmission unit Einheit *f* der Fortpflanzungswellen

TWI = training within industry richtige Unterweisung *f* von Mitarbeitern

U = unit Einheit *f* / **= number of unlike signs** Zahl *f* ungleicher Zeichen / **= upper** obere (r, s), Ober–

UCR = unconditioned reflex unbedingter Reflex *m*, unkonditionierte Reaktion *f* / **= unconditioned response** unkonditionierte Reaktion *f*, unbedingter Reflex *m*

UCS = unconditioned stimulus unkonditionierter Reiz *m*, unbedingter Reiz *m*

Ucs. = unconscious unbewusst / **= unconsciousness** Unbewusstes *n*, Unterbewusstes *n*

UCV = uncontrolled variable unkontrollierte Variable *f*

UG = universal grammar universelle Grammatik *f*

U.I. = universal index Faktorenindex *m*, Universalindex *m*

UnCS = unconditioned stimulus unkonditionierter Reiz *m*, unbedingter Reiz *m*

UNIX = Unified Conception/Multics Mehrbenutzersystem *n* für Mehrprogrammbetrieb

UnS = unconditioned stimulus unkonditionierter Reiz *m*, unbedingter Reiz *m*

UQ = upper quartile oberes Quartil *n*

UR = unconditioned response unkonditionierte Reaktion *f*, unbedingter Reflex *m*

URL = uniform resource locator Internet–Adresse *f*

US = unconditioned stimulus unkonditionierter Reiz *m*, unbedingter Reiz *m*

USENET = user network Netzwerk *n* von Diskussionsgruppen im Internet

userid = user identification Benutzername *m*, Userkennung *f*

UV = ultraviolet ultraviolett

UVr = ultraviolet rays ultraviolette Strahlen *mpl*

V = magnitude of the intensity component of a reaction potential Reiz–Intensitätsdynamik *f* / **= variable stimulus** Reizvariable *f* / **= vein** Vene *f* Ader *f* / **= verbal comprehension** Sprachverständnis *n* / **= vision** Sehen *n*, Sehkraft *f* / **= vista response** perspektivische Schattierungsdeutung *f* / **= volume** Volumen *n* / **= vulgar response** Vulgärantwort *f*

v = variable stimulus Reizvariable *f* / **= coefficient of variation** Variationskoeffizient *m* / **= volt** Volt *n* / **= volume** Volumen *n*

Va = valence Valenz *f* / **= visual acuity** Sehschärfe *f*

VC = colour vision Farbsichtigkeit *f* / **= vital capacity** Vitalkapazität *f*

VE = variable error Zufallsfehler *m*, Fehlerschwankung *f*

VF = visual field Sehfeld *n*

VI = variable interval variiertes zeitliches Intervall *n*

VIB = vocational interest blank Berufsinteressentest *m*

VR = variable ratio variiertes Verhältnis *n*

VRML = virtual reality modelling language plattformunabhängige Programmiersprache *f* zum Entwickeln dreidimensionaler Web–Seiten

v.s. = single vibration einfache Schwingung *f*

VT = variable time variable Zeit *f*

VTE = vicarious trial and error symbolisches Probierverhalten *n*

W = coefficient of concordance Konkordanzkoeffizient *m* / **= Weber fraction** Weber'sche Formel *f* / **= weight** Gewicht *n* / **= whole response** Ganzantwort *f* / **= word fluency factor** Faktor *m* „Wortflüssigkeit" / **= work in joules** Arbeit *f* ausgedrückt in Joule

w = watt Watt *n* / **= weight** Gewicht *n* / **= will factor** Willensfaktor *m* / **= with** mit / **= wrong** falsch

w_x = part of an inkblot area Teil *m* einer ganzen Kleckstafel

WAIS = wide area information system Datenbankverbund *m* im Internet

WAN = wide area network überregionales Netzwerk *n* für Langstreckenverbindungen

WFMH = World Federation for Mental Health Weltbund *m* der Psychohygiene

WHO = World Health Organisation Weltgesundheitsorganisation *f*

WL = wave length Wellenlänge *f*

wM = weighted arithmetic mean gewichtetes arithmetisches Mittel *n*

w/o = without ohne

W% = percentage of whole responses Prozentsatz *m* der Ganzantworten

WR = Wassermann reaction Wassermann Reaktion *f*

WS = whole–space response Zwischenfigurganzantwort *f*

WWW = World Wide Web Internet–Dienst *m*, Web *n*

WYSIWYG = what you see is what you get Druckbild *n* auf dem Bildschirm

X = abscissa Abszisse *f* / **= arithmetic mean** arithmetisches Mittel *n* / **= range of possible score** Bandbreite *f* eines möglichen Wertes / **= raw score of the x distribution** Rohwert *m* der X–Verteilung / **= reactance** Reaktanz *f*

x = deviation from the mean value Abweichung *f* vom Mittelwert

X_O = dependent variable abhängige Variable *f*

X_1, X_2 = predicted raw score vorhergesagter Rohwert *m*

X' = deviation from an assumed mean Abweichung *f* von einem angenommenen Mittelwert

χ^2 = chi square Chi–Quadrat *n*

XT = exotrophia Auswärtsschielen *n*

Y = dependant variable abhängige Variable *f* / **= raw score of the y distribution** Rohwert *m* der Y–Verteilung / **= year** Jahr *n*

y = value of an ordinate Ordinatenwert *m* / **= deviation from the mean ordinate value** Abweichung *f* vom mittleren Ordinatenwert

y/o = years old Jahre *npl* alt

yr = year Jahr *n*

yrs = years Jahre *npl*

ys = yellow spot gelber Fleck *m*

Z = zero Null *f* / **= standard score** Standardwert *m*